Clinical Scenarios in Surgery

DECISION MAKING AND OPERATIVE TECHNIQUE

Editors

Justin B. Dimick, MD, MPH
Assistant Professor of Surgery
Chief, Division of Minimally Invasive Surgery
Department of Surgery
University of Michigan
Ann Arbor, Michigan

Gilbert R. Upchurch Jr., MD
William H. Muller, Jr. Professor
Chief of Vascular and Endovascular Surgery
University of Virginia
Charlottesville, Virginia

Christopher J. Sonnenday, MD, MHS
Assistant Professor of Surgery
Assistant Professor of Health Management & Policy
University of Michigan
Ann Arbor, Michigan

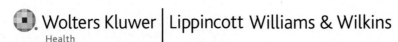
Wolters Kluwer | Lippincott Williams & Wilkins
Health

Philadelphia • Baltimore • New York • London
Buenos Aires • Hong Kong • Sydney • Tokyo

Acquisitions Editor: Brian Brown
Product Manager: Brendan Huffman
Production Manager: Bridgett Dougherty
Senior Manufacturing Manager: Benjamin Rivera
Marketing Manager: Lisa Lawrence
Design Coordinator: Joan Wendt
Production Service: SPi Global

Library of Congress Cataloging-in-Publication Data
Clinical scenarios in surgery : decision making and operative technique / [edited by]
Justin B. Dimick. — 1st ed.
      p. ; cm.
   Includes bibliographical references and index.
   ISBN 978-1-60913-972-8
 I. Dimick, Justin B.
   [DNLM: 1. Surgical Procedures, Operative—methods—Case Reports.   WO 16]
   617—dc23
                                                                      2012007290

Care has been taken to confirm the accuracy of the information presented and to describe generally accepted practices. However, the authors, editors, and publisher are not responsible for errors or omissions or for any consequences from application of the information in this book and make no warranty, expressed or implied, with respect to the currency, completeness, or accuracy of the contents of the publication. Application of the information in a particular situation remains the professional responsibility of the practitioner.

The authors, editors, and publisher have exerted every effort to ensure that drug selection and dosage set forth in this text are in accordance with current recommendations and practice at the time of publication. However, in view of ongoing research, changes in government regulations, and the constant flow of information relating to drug therapy and drug reactions, the reader is urged to check the package insert for each drug for any change in indications and dosage and for added warnings and precautions. This is particularly important when the recommended agent is a new or infrequently employed drug.

Some drugs and medical devices presented in the publication have Food and Drug Administration (FDA) clearance for limited use in restricted research settings. It is the responsibility of the health care provider to ascertain the FDA status of each drug or device planned for use in their clinical practice.

To purchase additional copies of this book, call our customer service department at (800) 638-3030 or fax orders to (301) 223-2320. International customers should call (301) 223-2300.

Visit Lippincott Williams & Wilkins on the Internet: at LWW.com. Lippincott Williams & Wilkins customer service representatives are available from 8:30 am to 6 pm, EST.

10 9 8 7 6 5 4

Contributors

Edouard Aboian, MD
Clinical Fellow in Vascular Surgery
Department of Vascular Surgery
Maimonides Medical Center
Brooklyn, New York
Lifestyle-Limiting Claudication

Daniel Albo, MD, PhD
Chief, Division of Surgical Oncology
Department of Surgery
Baylor College of Medicine
Director, GI Oncology Program
Dan L. Duncan Cancer Center
Baylor College of Medicine
Houston, Texas
Splenic Flexure Colon Cancer

Amy K. Alderman, MD, MPH
The Swan Center
Alpharetta, Georgia
Breast Reconstruction

Steven R. Allen, MD
Assistant Professor of Surgery
Department of Traumatology, Surgical Critical Care
  and Emergency Surgery
University of Pennsylvania
Philadelphia, Pennsylvania
Adrenal Insufficiency

John B. Ammori, MD
Assistant Professor
Department of Surgery
Division of General and Oncologic Surgery
Case Western Reserve University
Attending Surgeon
Department of Surgery
Division of General and Oncologic Surgery
University Hospitals Case Medical Center
Cleveland, Ohio
Gastrointestinal Stromal Tumor

Christopher D. Anderson, MD
Associate Professor of Surgery
Chief, Division of Transplant and Hepatobiliary
  Surgery
Department of Surgery
University of Mississippi Medical Center
Jackson, Mississippi
Acute Liver Failure

Stanley W. Ashley, MD
Frank Sawyer Professor of Surgery
Harvard Medical School
Chief Medical Officer
Senior Vice President for Medical Affairs
Administration
Brigham and Women's Hospital
Boston, Massachusetts
Severe Acute Pancreatitis

Samir S. Awad, MD
Associate Professor of Surgery
Chief, Section of Surgical Critical Care
Program Director Surgical Critical Care
Department of Surgery
Baylor College of Medicine
Associate Chief of Surgery
Medical Director SICU
Michael E. DeBakey VAMC
Houston, Texas
Fulminant Clostridium Difficile Colitis

Douglas C. Barnhart, MD, MSPH
Associate Professor
Division of Pediatric Surgery
University of Utah
Attending Surgeon
Pediatric Surgery
Primary Children's Medical Center
Salt Lake City, Utah
Palpable Abdominal Mass in a Toddler

William C. Beck, MD
Resident Physician, General Surgery
Department of General Surgery
Vanderbilt University
Vanderbilt University Medical Center
Nashville, Tennessee
  Cholangitis

Natasha S. Becker, MD, MPH
Fellow in Surgical Critical Care
Baylor College of Medicine
Houston, Texas
  Fulminant Clostridium Difficile Colitis

Filip Bednar, MD
House Officer
Department of Surgery
University of Michigan
Ann Arbor, Michigan
  Duodenal Injury

Jessica M. Bensenhaver, MD
Surgical Breast Oncology Fellow
Clinical Lecturer of Surgery
University of Michigan Health Systems
Ann Arbor, Michigan
  Ductal Carcinoma In Situ

Noelle L. Bertelson, MD
Laparoscopic Colorectal Surgery Fellow
Surgery
Mayo Clinic
Phoenix, Arizona
  Large Bowel Obstruction from Colon Cancer

Avi Bhavaraju, MD
Instructor in Surgery
Division of Trauma & Surgical Critical Care
Vanderbilt University
Nashville, Tennessee
  Pelvic Fracture

James H. Black, III, MD
Bertram M. Bernheim, MD
Associate Professor of Surgery
Department of Surgery
Johns Hopkins University School of Medicine
Attending Surgeon
Department of Surgery
Johns Hopkins Hospital
Baltimore, Maryland
  Acute Mesenteric Ischemia

Brendan J. Boland, MD
Department of Surgery
LAC+USC Medical Center
Los Angeles, California
  Variceal Bleeding and Portal Hypertension

Melissa Boltz, DO, MBA
Resident Physician
Department of Surgery
Penn State College of Medicine
Penn State Milton S. Hershey Medical Center
Hershey, Pennsylvania
  Incidental Adrenal Mass

Tara M. Breslin, MD
Assistant Professor of Surgery
Department of Surgery
University of Michigan
Ann Arbor, Michigan
  Ductal Carcinoma In Situ

Adam S. Brinkman, MD
Resident
Division of General Surgery
University of Wisconsin School of Medicine and
  Public Health
Madison, Wisconsin
  Malrotation and Midgut Volvulus

Malcolm V. Brock
Associate Professor of Surgery
Associate Professor of Oncology
Director of Clinical and Translational Research
  in Thoracic Surgery
The Johns Hopkins Hospital
Baltimore, Maryland
  Solitary Pulmonary Nodule

James T. Broome, MD
Assistant Professor of Surgery
Division of Surgical Oncology and Endocrine
  Surgery
Vanderbilt University
Nashville, Tennessee
  Persistent Hyperparathyroidism

Steven W. Bruch, MD, MSc
Clinical Associate Professor
Department of Surgery
University of Michigan
Pediatric Surgeon
Department of Surgery
Mott Children's Hospital
Ann Arbor, Michigan
  Tracheoesophageal Fistula

Terry L. Buchmiller, MD
Assistant Professor
Department of Surgery
Harvard Medical School
Staff Surgeon
Department of Surgery
Children's Hospital, Boston
Boston, Massachusetts
  Hepatoblastoma

Richard E. Burney, MD
Professor of Surgery
Department of Surgery
University of Michigan
Attending Surgeon
University of Michigan Hospitals
Ann Arbor, Michigan
  Perianal Abscess
  Thrombosed Hemorrhoids

Marisa Cevasco, MD, MPH
Clinical Fellow
Harvard Medical School
Resident
Department of Surgery
Brigham and Women's Hospital
Boston, Massachusetts
  Severe Acute Pancreatitis

Alfred E. Chang, MD
Professor of Surgery
Chief, Division of Surgical Oncology
Department of Surgery
University of Michigan
Ann Arbor, Michigan
  Extremity Mass (Sarcoma)

Anthony G. Charles, MD, MPH
Assistant Professor of Surgery
Director of Adult ECMO, Associate Chief of Surgical
  Critical Care
Department of Surgery
University of North Carolina
Chapel Hill, North Carolina
  Acute Renal Failure

Herbert Chen, MD
Layton Rikkers Chair in Surgical Leadership's
  Professor
Department of Surgery
University of Wisconsin
Chairman, Division of General Surgery
Surgery
University of Wisconsin Hospitals and Clinics
Madison, Wisconsin
  Medullary Thyroid Cancer

Steven Chen, MD, MBA
Associate Professor
Department of Surgery
Division of Surgical Oncology
City of Hope National Medical Center
Duarte, California
  Advanced Breast Cancer

Hueylan Chern, MD
Assistant Professor
Department of Surgery
University of California
San Francisco, California
  Crohn's Disease with Small Bowel Stricture

Albert Chi, MD
Assistant Professor of Surgery
Johns Hopkins Hospital
Division of Acute Care Surgery
Baltimore, Maryland
  Penetrating Chest Injury

Sara E. Clark, MD
Resident
Department of Surgery
University of South Florida
Tampa General Hospital
Tampa, Florida
  Small Bowel Obstruction

Robert A. Cowles, MD
Assistant Professor
Department of Surgery, Division of Pediatric Surgery
Columbia University College of Physicians and
    Surgeons
Assistant Attending Surgeon
Department of Surgery
Morgan Stanley Children's Hospital and Columbia
    University Medical Center
New York, New York
    Emesis in an Infant

Eric J. Culbertson, MD
House Officer
Department of Surgery
University of Michigan
Ann Arbor, Michigan
    Enterocutaneous Fistula

Lillian G. Dawes, MD
Professor of Surgery
Department of Surgery
University of South Florida
General Surgeon
James A. Haley Veterans Hospital
Tampa, Florida
    Small bowel obstruction

Sebastian G. De la fuente, MD
Surgical Oncology Fellow
College of Medicine
University of South Florida
H. Lee Moffitt Cancer Center & Research Institute
Tampa, Florida
    Melanoma

Ronald P. DeMatteo, MD
Professor of Surgery
Vice Chair, Department of Surgery
Head, Division of General Surgical Oncology
Leslie H. Blumgart Chair in Surgery
Memorial Sloan-Kettering Cancer Center
New York, New York
    Gastrointestinal Stromal Tumor

Charles S. Dietrich III, MD
Chief, Gynecologic Oncology Section
Department of Obstetrics and Gynecology
Tripler Army Medical Center
Honolulu, Hawaii
    Gynecologic Causes of Lower Abdominal Pain

Anastasia Dimick, MD
Laing & Dimick Dermatology
Ann Arbor, Michigan
    Nonmelanoma Skin Cancer

Justin B. Dimick, MD, MPH
Assistant Professor of Surgery
Chief, Division of Minimally Invasive Surgery
Department of Surgery
University of Michigan
Ann Arbor, Michigan
    Acute Cholecystitis
    Incarcerated/Strangulated Inguinal Hernia
    Perforated Appendicitis

Paul D. Dimusto, MD
Resident in Surgery
Department of Surgery
University of Michigan
Ann Arbor, Michigan
    Pulsatile Abdominal Mass
    Asymptomatic Carotid Stenosis

Gerard M. Doherty, MD
Chairman
Department of Surgery
Boston University
Chief of Surgery
Department of Surgery
Boston Medical Center
Boston, Massachusetts
    Papillary Thyroid Carcinoma

Bernard J. Dubray, MD
Resident Physician, Division of General Surgery
Research Fellow, Section of Abdominal
    Transplantation
Department of Surgery
Washington University in Saint Louis
Saint Louis, Missouri
    Acute Liver Failure

Gregory Ara Dumanian
Professor of Surgery
Division of Plastic Surgery
Northwestern Feinberg School of Medicine
Chief of Plastic Surgery
Division of Plastic Surgery
Northwestern Memorial Hospital
Chicago, Illinois
    Infected Ventral Hernia Mesh

Guillermo A. Escobar, MD
Assistant Professor of Surgery
Vascular Surgeon
University of Michigan
Ann Arbor, Michigan
  Ruptured Abdominal Aortic Aneurysm

David A. Etzioni, MD, MSHS
Associate Professor
Department of Surgery
Mayo Clinic College of Medicine
Rochester, Minnesota
Senior Associate Consultant
Department of Surgery
Mayo Clinic, Arizona
Phoenix, Arizona
  Large Bowel Obstruction from Colon Cancer

Heather L. Evans, MD, MS
Assistant Professor
Department of Surgery
University of Washington
Seattle, Washington
  Abdominal Compartment Syndrome

Gavin A. Falk, MD
General Surgery Resident
Department of General Surgery
Cleveland Clinic Foundation
Cleveland, Ohio
  Rectal Bleeding in a Young Child

Jonathan F. Finks, MD
Assistant Professor
Department of Surgery
University of Michigan Health System
Ann Arbor, Michigan
  Gastroesophageal Reflux Disease
  Recurrent Inguinal Hernia

Emily Finlayson, MD, MS
Assistant Professor
Department of Surgery
University of California, San Francisco
San Francisco, California
  Crohn's Disease with Small Bowel Stricture

Samuel R.G. Finlayson, MD, MPH
Kessler Director
Center for Surgery & Public Health
Harvard Medical School
One Brigham Circle
Associate Surgeon
Department of Surgery
Brigham & Women's Hospital
Boston, Massachusetts
  Acute Appendicitis

Emily M. Fontenot, MD
Surgical Resident
Department of Surgery
University of North Carolina
University of North Carolina Hospital
Chapel Hill, North Carolina
  Omphalocele

Heidi L. Frankel, MD
Assistant Professor of Surgery
Departments of Surgery and Surgical Critical Care
University of Maryland Medical Cetner
Baltimore, Maryland
  Adrenal Insufficiency

Timothy L. Frankel, MD
Surgical Oncology Fellow
Department of Surgery
Memorial Sloan-Kettering Cancer Center
New York, New York
  Extremity Mass (Sarcoma)
  Obstructive Jaundice

Michael G. Franz, MD
Vice President Global Clinical and Medical Affairs
LifeCell Corporation
Branchburg, New Jersey
  Enterocutaneous Fistula

Danielle Fritze, MD
House Officer
Department of Surgery
University of Michigan
Ann Arbor, Michigan
  Acute Cholecystitis
  Bleeding Gastric Ulcer

Samir K. Gadepalli, MD
Pediatric Surgery Fellow
Department of Pediatric Surgery
University of Michigan
CS Mott Children's Hospital
Ann Arbor, Michigan
Gastroschisis

Wolfgang B. Gaertner, MS, MD
Surgical Chief Resident
Department of Surgery
University of Minnesota
University of Minnesota Medical Center
Minneapolis, Minnesota
Appendiceal Carcinoid Tumor

Paul G. Gauger, MD
William J. Fry Professor of Surgery
Department of Surgery
University of Michigan
Ann Arbor, Michigan
Adrenal Cancer

James D. Geiger, MD
Professor of Surgery
Section of Pediatric Surgery
CS Mott Children's Hospital
University of Michigan
Executive Director
Medical Innovation Center
University of Michigan
Ann Arbor, Michigan
Intussusception
Gastroschisis

Philip P. Goodney, MD, MS
Assistant Professor
Center for Health Policy Research
The Dartmouth Institute
Hanover, New Hampshire
Assistant Professor
Department of Surgery, Section of Vascular Surgery
Dartmouth Hitchcock Medical Center
Lebanon, New Hampshire
Lifestyle-Limiting Claudication

Sarah E. Greer, MD, MPH
Clinical Fellow
Department of Surgery
Hospital of the University of Pennsylvania
Philadelphia, Pennsylvania
Acute Appendicitis

Tyler Grenda, MD
Resident in General Surgery
Department of Surgery
University of Michigan Health System
Ann Arbor, Michigan
Achalasia

Erica R. Gross, MD
Research Fellow
Pediatric Surgery
College of Physicians and Surgeons, Columbia
    University
Pediatric ECMO Fellow
Pediatric Surgery
Morgan Stanley Children's Hospital, New York
New York, New York
Emesis in an Infant

Travis E. Grotz, MD
Resident
General Surgery
Mayo Clinic
Rochester, Minneapolis
Palpable Breast Mass

Oliver L. Gunter, MD
Assistant Professor of Surgery
Biomedical Research Education & Training
Vanderbilt University Medical Center
Nashville, Tennessee
Pelvic Fracture

Jeffrey S. Guy, MD, MSc, MMHC
Associate Professor
Department of Surgery
Vanderbilt University
Director-Regional Burn Center, Director-Acute
    Operative Services
Department of Surgery
Vanderbilt University Medical Center
Nashville, Tennessee
Burns

Adil H. Haider, MD, MPH
Associate Professor of Surgery
Anesthesiology and Health Policy and Management
Director
Center for Surgical Trials and Outcomes Research
    (CSTOR)
Johns Hopkins Hospital
Division of Acute Care Surgery
Baltimore, Maryland
Penetrating Chest Injury

Ihab Halaweish
House Officer II
Department of Surgery
University of Michigan
Ann Arbor, Michigan
Neuroblastoma

A.L. Halverson
Associate Professor of Surgery
Northwestern University
Feinberg School of Medicine
Department of Surgery
Chicago, Illinois
Anal Carcinoma

Allen Hamdan, MD
Associate Professor of Surgery
Department of Surgery
Harvard Medical School
Attending Surgeon
Division of Vascular and Endovascular Surgery
Beth Israel Deaconess Medical Center
Boston, Massachusetts
Diabetic Foot Infection

James Harris Jr., MD
Surgical Resident
Department of Surgery
Johns Hopkins Hospital
Baltimore, Maryland
Solitary Pulmonary Nodule

Elliott R. Haut, MD
Associate Professor of Surgery
Anesthesiology/Critical Care Medicine (ACCM) and
    Emergency Medicine
Division of Acute Care Surgery, Department of
    Surgery
The Johns Hopkins University School of Medicine
Director
Trauma/Acute Care Surgery Fellowship
The Johns Hopkins Hospital
Baltimore, Maryland
Nutritional Support in the Critically Ill Surgery Patient

A.V. Hayman
General Surgical Resident
Northwestern Memorial Hospital
Chicago, Illinois
Anal Carcinoma

David W. Healy, MD, MRCP, FRCA
Assistant Professor
Anesthesiology
University of Michigan
Director, Head & Neck Anesthesia
Department of Anesthesiology Health Systems
University of Michigan Hospital and Health Systems
Ann Arbor, Michigan
Airway Emergency

Mark R. Hemmila, MD
Associate Professor of Surgery
Acute Care Surgery
University of Michigan
Ann Arbor, Michigan
Duodenal Injury
Perforated Appendicitis

Samantha Hendren, MD, MPH
Assistant Professor
Department of Surgery
University of Michigan
Colorectal Surgeon
Department of General Surgery
Ann Arbor VA Healthcare System
Ann Arbor, Michigan
Medically Refractory Ulcerative Colitis

Peter K. Henke, MD
Professor of Surgery
Surgery
University of Michigan
Ann Arbor, Michigan
Acute Limb Ischemia

Richard Herman, MD
Instructor of Surgery
University of Michigan Hospital and Health Systems
Department of Pediatric Surgery
Ann Arbor, Michigan
Necrotizing Enterocolitis

Michael G. House, MD
Assistant Professor
Department of Surgery
Indiana University School of Medicine
Indianapolis, Indiana
Symptomatic Pancreatic Pseudocyst

Gina M.S. Howell, MD
Surgery Resident
Department of Surgery
University of Pittsburgh
Pittsburgh Hospital
University of Pittsburgh Medical Center
Pittsburgh, Pennsylvania
Stab Wound to the Neck

Thomas S. Huber, MD, PhD
Professor and Chief
Division of Vascular Surgery and Endovascular
    Surgery
University of Florida College of Medicine
Gainesville, Florida
Need for Hemodialysis Access

David T. Hughes, MD
Assistant Professor
Department of Surgery
Albert Einstein College of Medicine
Attending Surgeon
Department of Surgery
Montefiore Medical Center
Bronx, New York
Adrenal Cancer

Alicia Hulbert
Clinical Fellow
Department of Oncology
School of Medicine
Baltimore, Maryland
Solitary Pulmonary Nodule

Justin Hurie, MD
Assistant Professor
Department of Vascular and Endovascular Surgery
Wake Forest University
Attending Surgeon
Department of Vascular and Endovascular Surgery
North Carolina Baptist Hospital
Winston-Salem, North Carolina
Deep Venous Thrombosis

Neil Hyman, MD
Samuel B. and Michelle D. Labow Professor of
    Surgery
Codirector, Digestive Disease Center
Department of Surgery
University of Vermont College of Medicine
Burlington, Vermont
Anastomotic Leak After Colectomy

Angela M. Ingraham, MD, MS
General Surgery Resident
Department of Surgery
University of Cincinnati
Cincinnati, Ohio
Postoperative Dehiscence

Kamal M.F. Itani, MD
Professor of Surgery
Department of Surgery
Boston University
Boston, Massachusetts
Chief of Surgery
Department of Surgery
VA Boston Health Care System
Worcester, Massachusetts
Ventral Incisional Hernias

Alexis D. Jacob, MD
Vascular Surgery Fellow
Division of Vascular Surgery and Endovascular
    Surgery
University of Florida College of Medicine
Gainesville, Florida
Need for Hemodialysis Access

Lisa K. Jacobs, MD
Assistant Professor of Surgery
Director of Clinical Breast Cancer Research
Departments of Surgery and Oncology
Johns Hopkins University
Baltimore, Maryland
Suspicious Mammographic Abnormality

James W. Jakub, MD
Assistant Professor of Surgery
General Surgery
Mayo Clinic
Rochester, Minnesota
Palpable Breast Mass

Jennifer E. Joh, MD
The Hoffberger Breast Center at Mercy
Baltimore, Maryland
Breast Cancer During Pregnancy

Jussuf T. Kaifi, MD, PhD
Assistant Professor of Surgery and Medicine
Department of Surgery
Penn State College of Medicine
Assistant Professor of Surgery and Medicine
Department of Surgery
Penn State Hershey Medical Center
Hershey, Pennsylvania
  Gastric Cancer

Jeffrey Kalish, MD
Laszlo N. Tauber Assistant Professor
Department of Surgery
Boston University School of Medicine
Director of Endovascular Surgery
Department of Surgery
Boston Medical Center
Boston, Massachusetts
  Diabetic Foot Infection

Lillian S. Kao, MD, MS
Associate Professor
Department of Surgery
University of Texas Health Science Center at Houston
Houston, Texas
Vice-Chief
Department of Surgery
LBJ General Hospital
Houston, Texas
  Necrotizing Soft Tissue Infections

Muneera R. Kapadia, MD
Clinical Assistant Professor
Department of Surgery
University of Iowa Hospitals and Clinics
Iowa City, Iowa
  Ischemic Colitis

Srinivas Kavuturu, MD, FRCS
Assistant Professor of Surgery
Department of Surgery
Michigan State University, College of Human
  Medicine
Attending Physician
Department of Surgery
Sparrow Hospital
Lansing, Michigan
  Gastric Cancer

Sajid A. Khan, MD
Surgical Oncology Fellow
Department of Surgery
The University of Chicago Medical Center
Chicago, Illinois
  Refractory Pain from Chronic Pancreatitis

Hyaehwan Kim, MD
Surgery Resident
Brookdale University Hospital and Medical Center
Newyork
  Rectal Cancer

Andrew S. Klein, MD, MBA
Professor
Department of Surgery
Director
Comprehensive Transplant Center
Cedars Sinai Medical Center
Los Angeles, California
  Variceal Bleeding and Portal Hypertension

Carla Kohoyda-Inglis, MPA
Program Director
International Center for Automotive Medicine
Ann Arbor, Michigan
  Blunt Abdominal Trauma from Motor Vehicle Crash

Geoffrey W. Krampitz, MD
General Surgery Resident
Department of Surgery
Stanford Hospital and Clinics
Stanford, California
  Gastrinoma

Andrew Kroeker, MD
Resident Surgeon
Department of Otolaryngology
University of Michigan
Ann Arbor, Michigan
  Melanoma of the Head and Neck

Hari R. Kumar, MD
Chief Resident
Department of Surgery
Indiana University School of Medicine
Indianapolis, Indiana
  Cortisol-secreting Adrenal Tumor

Adriana Laser, MD
Resident in Surgery
University of Maryland
Baltimore, Maryland
  Ruptured Abdominal Aortic Aneurysm

Christine L. Lau, MD
Associate Professor
Surgery, Thoracic & Cardiovascular
University of Virginia Health System
Charlottesville, Virginia
  Esophageal Perforation

Constance W. Lee, MD
Surgical Resident
Department of Surgery
University of Florida College of Medicine
Gainesville, Florida
  Perforated Duodenal Ulcer

Marie Catherine Lee, MD
Assistant Professor of Sciences
Division of Oncologic Science
University of South Florida
Assistant Member
Women's Oncology—Breast Division
Moffitt Cancer Center
Tampa, Florida
  Breast Cancer During Pregnancy

Jules Lin, MD
Assistant Professor
Section of Thoracic Surgery
University of Michigan Medical School
Assistant Professor
Section of Thoracic Surgery
University of Michigan Health System
Ann Arbor, Michigan
  Achalasia

Peter H. Lin, MD
Professor of Surgery
Chief of Division of Vascular Surgery and
  Endovascular Therapy
Michael E. DeBakey Department of Surgery
Baylor College of Medicine
Houston, Texas
  Symptomatic Carotid Stenosis

Pamela A. Lipsett, MD, MHPE
Warfield M Firor Professor of Surgery
Program Director
General Surgery and Surgical Critical Care
Co-Director of the Surgical Intensive Care Units
Johns Hopkins Hospital
Baltimore, Maryland
  Septic Shock

Ann C. Lowry, MD
Clinical Professor of Surgery
Division of Colon and Rectal Surgery
University of Minnesota
St. Paul, Minnesota
  Ischemic Colitis

Dennis P. Lund, MD
Surgeon-in-Chief, Phoenix Children's Hospital
Executive Vice President, Phoenix Children's Medical
  Group
Professor, Department of Child Health
Academic Division Chief, Pediatric Surgery,
  Department of Child Health
University of Arizona College of Medicine—Phoenix
Phoenix, Arizona
  Malrotation and Midgut Volvulus

Paul M. Maggio, MD, MBA
Assistant Professor of Surgery
Department of Surgery
Stanford University
Associate Director of Trauma
Department of Surgery
Stanford University Hospital
Stanford, California
  Symptomatic Cholelithiasis in Pregnancy

Ali F. Mallat, MD, MS
Assistant Professor of Surgery
Department of General Surgery
University Of Michigan
General Surgery Service Chief
Department of Surgery
Ann Arbor VA Medical Center
Ann Arbor, Michigan
  Cholecystoduodenal fistula

Sean T. Martin, MD
Associate Staff Surgeon
Colorectal Surgery
Cleveland Clinic
Cleveland, Ohio
  Complicated Diverticulitis

Jeffrey B. Matthews, MD
Dallas B. Phemister Professor of Surgery
Chairman, Department of Surgery
Surgery-In-Chief
Department of Surgery
The University of Chicago
Chicago, Illinois
   Refractory Pain from Chronic Pancreatitis

Haggi Mazeh, MD
Clinical Instructor
Surgery
University of Wisconsin
Madison, Wisconsin
   Palpable Thyroid Nodule

Timothy W. McCardle, MD
Assistant Member
Pathology
Moffitt Cancer Center
Tampa, Florida
   Melanoma

Erin McKean, MD
Assistant Professor
Department of Otolaryngology—Head and Neck
   Surgery
University of Michigan Medical School
Assistant Professor
Department of Otolaryngology—Head and Neck
   Surgery
University of Michigan Health System
Ann Arbor, Michigan
   Melanoma of the Head and Neck
   Head and Neck Cancer

Sean E. McLean, MD
Assistant Professor of Surgery
Department of Surgery
University of North Carolina at Chapel Hill
Staff Surgeon
Department of Surgery
UNC Hospitals
Chapel Hill, North Carolina
   Omphalocele

Michelle K. McNutt, MD
Assistant Professor of Surgery
Surgery
University of Texas Medical School at Houston
Houston, Texas
   Necrotizing Soft Tissue Infections

Genevieve Melton-Meaux, MD, MA
Assistant Professor
Department of Surgery, Institute for Health
   Informatics
University of Minnesota
Staff Surgeon
University of Minnesota Medical Center
Minneapolis, Minnesota
   Appendiceal Carcinoid Tumor

April E. Mendoza, MD
Trauma Research Fellow
Department of Surgery
University of North Carolina
Department of Surgery
UNC Memorial Hospital
Chapel Hill, North Carolina
   Acute Renal Failure

Evangelos Messaris, MD, PhD
Assistant Professor
Division of Colon and Rectal Surgery
Pennsylvania State University
Faculty
Division of Colon and Rectal Surgery
Milton S. Hershey Medical Center
Hershey, Pennsylvania
   Symptomatic Primary Inguinal Hernia

Stacey A. Milan, MD
Assistant Professor of Surgery
General Surgery
Jefferson Medical College
Assistant Professor of Surgery
General Surgery
Thomas Jefferson University Hospital
Philadelphia, Pennsylvania
   Pancreatic Neuroendocrine Tumors

Barbra S. Miller, MD
Assistant Professor
Surgery
University of Michigan
Ann Arbor, Michigan
   Primary Hyperaldosteronism

Judiann Miskulin, MD
Assistant Professor of Surgery
Endocrine Surgery
Department of Surgery
Indiana University Health
Indianapolis, Indiana
   Cortisol-secreting Adrenal Tumor

Derek Moore, MD, MPH
Assistant Professor of Surgery
Department of Surgery, Division of Liver, Kidney and
    Pancreas Transplantation
Vanderbilt University Medical Center
Nashville, Tennessee
    End-Stage Renal Disease (Renal Transplantation)

Arden M. Morris, MD
Associate Professor
Department of Surgery
Chief, Division of Colorectal
Surgery
University of Michigan
Ann Arbor, Michigan
    Colonic Vovulus

Monica Morrow, MD
Professor of Surgery
Weill Medical College of Cornell University
New York, New York
Chief, Breast Service
Department of Surgery
Anne Burnett Windfohr Chair of Clinical Oncology
Memorial Sloan-Kettering Cancer Center
New York, New York
    Inflammatory Breast Cancer

John Morton, MD, MPH
Associate Professor of Surgery
Director of Bariatric Surgery
Department of Surgery
Stanford University
Stanford, California
    Morbid Obesity

Michael Mulholland, MD, PhD
Professor and Chair
Department of Surgery
University of Michigan
Surgeon in Chief
University of Michigan Hospital
Ann Arbor, Michigan
    Bleeding Gastric Ulcer

Alykhan S. Nagji, MD
Resident
Department of Surgery
University of Virginia Hospital System
Charlottesville, Virginia
    Esophageal Perforation

Lena M. Napolitano, MD
Professor
Department of Surgery
University of Michigan
Division Chief, Acute Care Surgery
Director, Trauma & Surgical Critical Care
Department of Surgery
University of Michigan
Ann Arbor, Michigan
    Acute Respiratory Distress Syndrome (ARDS)

Avery B. Nathens, MD, MPH, PhD
Professor
Department of Surgery
University of Toronto
Division Head in General Surgery
Director of Trauma
General Surgery & Trauma
St. Michael's Hospital
Toronto, Ontario
    Postoperative Dehiscence

Erika Newman, MD
Assistant Professor in Pediatric Surgery
Edith Briskin Emerging Scholar
CS Mott Children's Hospital
Department of Surgery
A. Alfred Taubman Medical Research Institute
The University of Michigan Medical School
Ann Arbor, Michigan
    Neuroblastoma

Lisa A. Newman, MD, MPH
Professor of Surgery
Director, Breast Care Center
Department of Surgery
Ann Arbor, Michigan
    Lobular Carcinoma In Situ

Jeffrey A. Norton, MD
Professor of Surgery
Chief, Division of General Surgery
Stanford University Medical Center
Stanford, California
    Gastrinoma

Babak J. Orandi, MD, MSc
General Surgery Resident
Department of Surgery
Johns Hopkins University
Johns Hopkins Hospital
Baltimore, Maryland
    Acute Mesenteric Ischemia

Mark B. Orringer, MD
Professor of Surgery
Section of Thoracic Surgery
University of Michigan
Ann Arbor, Michigan
Esophageal Cancer

Paul Park, MD, MA
Chief Resident
Department of Surgery
Section of General Surgery
University of Michigan Medical School
University of Michigan Hospital
Ann Arbor, Michigan
Cholecystoduodenal fistula

Pauline K. Park, MD
Associate Professor
Department of Surgery
University of Michigan
Co-Director Surgical Intensive Care Unit
Department of Surgery
University of Michigan Health System
Ann Arbor, Michigan
Acute Respiratory Distress Syndrome (ARDS)

Timothy M. Pawlik, MD, MPH
Associate Professor
Department of Surgery
Johns Hopkins University
Johns Hopkins Hospital
Baltimore, Maryland
Metastatic Colorectal Cancer

Shawn J. Pelletier, MD
Associate Professor
Surgical Director of Liver Transplantation
Department of Surgery
University of Michigan Health System
Ann Arbor, Michigan
Incidental Liver Mass

Peter D. Peng, MD, MS
Surgical Oncology Fellow
Department of Surgery
Johns Hopkins Hospital
Baltimore, Maryland
Metastatic Colorectal Cancer

Catherine E. Pesce, MD
Department of Medical Oncology
The Sidney Kimmel Comprehensive Cancer Center
   at Johns Hopkins
Baltimore, Maryland
Suspicious Mammographic Abnormality

Rebecca Plevin, MD
Department of Surgery
University of Washington Medical Center
Seattle, Washington
Abdominal Compartment Syndrome

Benjamin K. Poulose, MD, MPH
Assistant Professor
Department of Surgery
Vanderbilt University School of Medicine
Associate Director, Endoscopy Suite
Department of Surgery
Vanderbilt University Medical Center
Nashville, Tennessee
Cholangitis

Sandhya Pruthi, MD
Associate Professor of Medicine
General Internal Medicine
Mayo Clinic
Rochester, Minnesota
Palpable Breast Mass

Krishnan Raghavendran, MD
Associate Professor
Surgery
University of Michigan Hospital and Health
   Systems
Ann Arbor, Michigan
Ventilator-Associated Pneumonia
Acute Respiratory Distress Syndrome (ARDS)

Matthew W. Ralls, MD
Surgical House Officer
Department of Surgery
University of Michigan
Ann Arbor, Michigan
Incarcerated/Strangulated Inguinal Hernia

John E. Rectenwald, MD
Associate Professor of Surgery & Radiology
Program Director, Vascular Surgery
Section of Vascular Surgery
University of Michigan Health System
Ann Arbor, Michigan
  Asymptomatic Carotid Stenosis

John W. Rectenwald, MD
Associate Professor of Surgery
Surgery
University of Michigan
Ann Arbor, Michigan
  Acute Limb Ischemia

Scott E. Regenbogen, MD, MPH
Assistant Professor
Department of Surgery
University of Michigan
Ann Arbor, Michigan
Staff Surgeon
Department of Surgery
University of Michigan Health System
Ann Arbor, Michigan
  Lower Gastrointestinal Bleeding

Amy L. Rezak, MD
Assistant Professor
Department of Surgery
University of North Carolina at Chapel Hill School of
  Medicine
Trauma, Critical Care Surgeon
Department of Surgery
UNC Health Care
Chapel Hill, North Carolina
  Severe Acute Pancreatitis

William P. Robinson III, MD
Assistant Professor of Surgery
Division of Vascular and Endovascular Surgery
University of Massachusetts Medical School
Division of Vascular and Endovascular Surgery
UMass Memorial Medical Center
Worcester, Massachusetts
  Tissue Loss Due to Arterial Insufficiency

Michael J. Rosen, MD
Associate Professor of Surgery
Chief Division of GI and General Surgery
Department of Surgery
Case Western Reserve University
Cleveland, Ohio
  Complex Abdominal Wall Reconstruction

Michael S. Sabel, MD
Associate Professor
Surgery
University of Michigan
Ann Arbor, Michigan
  *Melanoma Presenting with Regional Lymph Node
  Involvement*
  Merkel Cell Carcinoma

Vivian M. Sanchez, MD
Assistant Professor of Surgery
Department of Surgery
Boston University
Boston, Massachusetts
Minimally Invasive and Bariatric Surgery
Department of Surgery
VA Boston Health Care System
West Roxbury, Massachusetts
  Ventral Incisional Hernias

George A. Sarosi Jr., MD
Associate Professor of Surgery
Department of Surgery
University of Florida College of Medicine
Staff Surgeon
Surgical Service
North Florida/South Georgia VA Medical Center
Gainesville, Florida
  Perforated Duodenal Ulcer

Brian D. Saunders, MD
Assistant Professor
Departments of Surgery and Medicine
Penn State College of Medicine
Assistant Professor
Departments of Surgery and Medicine
Penn State Milton S. Hershey Medical Center
Hershey, Pennsylvania
  Incidental Adrenal Mass

C. Max Schmidt, MD, PhD, MBA
Associate Professor
Surgery
Indiana University School of Medicine
Indianapolis, Indiana
Incidental Pancreatic Cyst

Maureen K. Sheehan, MD
Assistant Professor
Division of Vascular Surgery
University of Texas Health Science Center at
San Antonio
San Antonio, Texas
Chronic Mesenteric Ischemia

Terry Shih, MD
House Officer
Department of Surgery
University of Michigan
University of Michigan Health System
Ann Arbor, Michigan
Perforated Appendicitis

Andrew Shuman, MD
Chief Resident
Department of Otolaryngology—Head and Neck
Surgery
University of Michigan Hospitals
Ann Arbor, Michigan
Melanoma of the Head and Neck

Sabina Siddiqui, MD
Pediatric Surgical Critical Care Fellow
Department of Pediatric Surgery
University of Michigan, Ann Arbor
Fellow
Department of Pediatric Surgery
C.S. Mott's Children's Hospital
Ann Arbor, Michigan
Intussusception

Matthew J. Sideman, MD
Associate Professor
Department of Surgery
University of Texas Health Science Center
at San Antonio
San Antonio, Texas
Chronic Mesenteric Ischemia

Rebecca S. Sippel, MD
Assistant Professor
Department of Surgery
University of Wisconsin
Chief of Endocrine Surgery
Department of Surgery
University of Wisconsin Hospitals and Clinics
Madison, Wisconsin
Palpable Thyroid Nodule

Alexis D. Smith, MD
General Surgery Resident
Department of General Surgery
University of Maryland School of Medicine
Baltimore, Maryland
Pheochromocytoma

Vance L. Smith, MD, MBA
Attending Surgeon/Surgical Intensivist
Department of Surgery
Division of Trauma Surgery
Eden Medical Center—Sutterhealth
Castro Valley, California
Symptomatic Cholelithiasis in Pregnancy

Oliver S. Soldes, MD
Staff Pediatric Surgeon
Department of Pediatric Surgery
Cleveland Clinic Foundation
Cleveland, Ohio
Rectal Bleeding in a Young Child

Vernon K. Sondak, MD
Professor
Surgery and Oncologic Sciences
University of South Florida
Department Chair
Cutaneous Oncology
H. Lee Moffitt Cancer Center & Research Institute
Tampa, Florida
Melanoma

Christopher J. Sonnenday, MD, MHS
Assistant Professor of Surgery
Assistant Professor of Health Management & Policy
University of Michigan
Ann Arbor, Michigan
Bile Duct Injury
Liver Mass in Chronic Liver Disease
Obstructive Jaundice

Julie Ann Sosa, MD, MA
Associate Professor of Surgery and Medicine
    (Oncology)
Dept of Surgery, Divisions of Endocrine Surgery and
    Surgical Oncology
Yale University School of Medicine
New Haven, Connecticut
    Primary Hyperparathyroidism

Matthew Spector, MD
Chief Resident
Department of Otolaryngology
University of Michigan
Ann Arbor, Michigan
    Head and Neck Cancer

Jason L. Sperry, MD, MPH
Assistant Professor of Surgery and Critical Care
    Medicine
University of Pittsburgh Medical Center
Pittsburgh, Pennsylvania
    Stab Wound to the Neck

Kevin F. Staveley-O'Carroll, MD, PhD
Professor of Surgery, Medicine, Microbiology
    and Immunology
Department of Surgery
Penn State College of Medicine
Penn State Hershey Medical Center
Hershey, Pennsylvania
    Gastric Cancer

John F. Sweeney, MD
W. Dean Warren Distinguished Professor of Surgery
Department of Surgery
Emory University School of Medicine
Atlanta, Georgia
    Splenectomy for Hematologic Disease

Kevin E. Taubman, MD
Assistant Professor
Department of Surgery
University of Oklahoma College of Medicine
Tulsa, Oklahoma
    Chronic Mesenteric Ischemia

Daniel H. Teitelbaum, MD
Professor
Department of Surgery, Section of Pediatric Surgery
University of Michigan
Ann Arbor, Michigan
    Necrotizing Enterocolitis

Pierre Theodore
Associate Professor
Van Auken Chair in Thoracic Surgery
UCSF Medical Center
San Francisco, California
    Spontaneous Pneumothorax

Thadeus Trus
Associate Professor of Surgery
Department of Surgery
Dartmouth Medical School
Lebanon, New Hampshire
    Paraesophageal Hernia

Douglas J. Turner, MD
Associate Professor
Department of Surgery
University of Maryland School of Medicine
Chief, General Surgery
Baltimore VA Medical Center
Baltimore, Maryland
    Pheochromocytoma

Gilbert R. Upchurch Jr., MD
William H. Muller, Jr. Professor
Chief of Vascular and Endovascular Surgery
University of Virginia
Charlottesville, Virginia
    Pulsatile Abdominal Mass
    Ruptured Abdominal Aortic Aneurysm
    Asymptomatic Carotid Stenosis

Kyle J. Van Arendonk, MD
Halsted Resident
Department of Surgery
Johns Hopkins Hospital
Baltimore, Maryland
    Nutritional Support in the Critically Ill Surgery Patient

Chandu Vemuri, MD
Vascular Surgery Fellow
Department of Surgery
Washington University in St. Louis
St. Louis, Missouri
    Retroperitoneal Sarcoma

Jon D. Vogel, MD
Staff Colorectal Surgeon
Cleveland Clinic
Cleaveland, Ohio
    Complicated Diverticulitis

Wendy L. Wahl, MD
Professor of Surgery
Department of Surgery
University of Michigan Health System
Ann Arbor, Michigan
Bleeding Duodenal Ulcer

Thomas W. Wakefield, MD
S. Martin Lindenauer Professor of Surgery
Department of Vascular Surgery
University of Michigan
Head, Section of Vascular Surgery
Department of Vascular Surgery
University of Michigan Health Systems
Ann Arbor, Michigan
Deep Venous Thrombosis

Jennifer F. Waljee, MD, MS
House Officer
Department of Surgery
University of Michigan
University of Michigan Medical Center
Ann Arbor, Michigan
Breast Reconstruction

Stewart C. Wang, MD, PhD
Endowed Professor of Surgery
Director, International Center for Automotive
    Medicine
University of Michigan
Ann Arbor, Michigan
Blunt Abdominal Trauma from Motor Vehicle Crash

Joshua A. Waters, MD
Resident
Department of Surgery
Indiana University School of Medicine
Indianapolis, Indiana
Incidental Pancreatic Cyst

Sarah M. Weakley, MD
Michael E. DeBakey Department of Surgery
Baylor College of Medicine
Houston, Texas
Symptomatic Carotid Stenosis

Walter P. Weber, MD
Assistant Professor
Department of Surgery
University of Basel
Attending Surgeon
Department of Surgery
University Hospital of Basel
Basel, Switzerland
Inflammatory Breast Cancer

Martin R. Weiser, MD
Associate Member
Surgery
Memorial Sloan-Kettering Cancer Center
New York, New York
Associate Professor
Surgery
Cornell Weill Medical School/New York Presbyterian
    Hospital
New York, New York
Rectal Cancer

Bradford P. Whitcomb, MD
Associate Residency Program Director
Department of Obstetrics and Gynecology
Tripler Army Medical Center
Honolulu, Hawaii
Gynecologic Causes of Lower Abdominal Pain

Elizabeth C. Wick, MD
Assistant Professor
Department of Surgery
Johns Hopkins University
Staff Surgeon
Department of Surgery
Johns Hopkins Medical Institutions
Baltimore, Maryland
Appendiceal Carcinoid Tumor

Sandra L. Wong, MD, MS
Assistant Professor
Department of Surgery
University of Michigan
Ann Arbor, Michigan
Staff Physician
Department of Surgery
University of Michigan Hospital and Health Systems
Ann Arbor, Michigan
Retroperitoneal Sarcoma

Derek T. Woodrum, MD
Assistant Professor
Department of Anesthesiology
University of Michigan Medical School
Faculty Anesthesiologist
Department of Anesthesiology
University of Michigan Medical Center
Ann Arbor, Michigan
  Airway Emergency

Leslie S. Wu, MD
Attending surgeon
Department of Surgery
Maine Medical Center
Portland, Maine
  Primary Hyperparathyroidism

Charles J. Yeo, MD
Samuel D. Gross Professor and Chairman
Department of Surgery
Thomas Jefferson University
Chief
Department of Surgery
Thomas Jefferson University Hospital
Philadelphia, Pennsylvania
  Pancreatic Neuroendocrine Tumors

Barbara Zarebczan, MD
General Surgery Resident
Surgery
University of Wisconsin
Madison, Wisconsin
  Medullary Thyroid Cancer

Foreword

In preparing a generation of surgical residents to enter practice, there are some pointers that I may offer. There are also some rules that I have picked up while writing and editing chapters for surgical textbooks. Most of us are not born surgeons. If you are the exception—accomplished, articulate, and confident; if surgical principles come effortlessly, you may stop reading now. Still, you might want to take a look. Here are three thoughts:

1. Start reading right away.

For most surgeons, the most difficult reading assignment is the first assignment. The problem lies not in realizing the high stakes of a board exam; the trouble comes with the commitment that board preparation requires. The form of most contemporary texts is part of the problem. A glance shows the chapters to be long, devoid of illustrations, a textual sensory deprivation. *Clinical Scenarios in Surgery* is so inviting with its crisp writing, generous illustrations, and telegenic presentation that it begs to be read. Get started.

2. Grab hold of the present and look to the future.

Modern surgery is forward looking, seeking to improve the care of current patients and to prevent disease in potential future patients. Given the pace of modern biomedical research, no lone individual can be expected to find, read, synthesize, and apply all new knowledge relevant to any clinical problem. All surgeons need an occasional guide through the surgical literature. In the midst of this information overload, the experienced, energetic editors of *Clinical Scenarios in Surgery* strike just the right balance. Keep going.

3. Keep reading, even just a little bit, every day.

Reading is a skill, sharpened with practice, perfected by *continuous* practice. Operative surgery reinforces this notion. The physical skills, sense of prioritized organization, personal confidence, and intuition of the accomplished surgeon result from attention to the craft. That is the reason it is called the practice of surgery. Like the scalpel, a book becomes much friendlier with frequent use. Enjoy the journey.

Michael W. Mulholland, M.D., Ph.D.

Preface

Despite remarkable technical advances and rapid scientific progress, it has never been more challenging to become a safe and proficient surgeon.

Young surgeons are challenged by both the pace of new information and the subspecialization occurring in every surgical discipline. Traditional surgical textbooks, which have grown to keep pace with these changes, are becoming encyclopedic reference books, which we turn to only when we need a comprehensive overview. With the vast amount of information available, it is often difficult to sort out the basic principles of safe surgery for a given clinical scenario. The mismatch between existing education materials and the need for a solid understanding of general surgical principles becomes most apparent when young surgeons sit down to prepare to take their written and oral board exams.

Young surgeons also learn differently than those in the past. Modern surgical trainees do not sit down and read for hours at a time. They are multitaskers who demand efficiency and immediate relevance in their learning materials. Most medical schools have responded to these changes by transitioning to curricula based on case-based learning. Clinical narratives are extremely effective learning tools because they use patient stories to teach essential surgical principles. Most existing surgical textbooks have not kept pace with these broader changes in medical education.

We wrote this book to fill these gaps. We have created a case-based text that communicates core principles of general surgery and its specialties. We believe the patient stories in these clinical scenarios will provide context to facilitate learning the principles of safe surgical care. Students, residents, and other young surgeons should find the chapters short enough to read between cases or after a long day in the hospital. We hope this book will be particularly useful for senior surgical residents and recent graduates as they prepare for the American Board of Surgery oral examination.

Justin B. Dimick
Gilbert R. Upchurch, Jr.
Christopher J. Sonnenday

Contents

xxxii Contents

Chapter 99
Melanoma Presenting with Regional Lymph Node Involvement 505
Michael S. Sabel

Chapter 100
Merkel Cell Carcinoma 508
Michael S. Sabel

Chapter 101
Nonmelanoma Skin Cancer 511
Anastasia Dimick

Chapter 102
Necrotizing Soft Tissue Infections 514
Michelle K. Mcnutt
Lillian S. Kao

Chapter 103
Extremity Mass (Sarcoma) 518
Timothy L. Frankel
Alfred E. Chang

Chapter 104
Retroperitoneal Sarcoma 524
Chandu Vemuri
Sandra L. Wong

Trauma
Chapter 105
Penetrating Chest Injury 529
Albert Chi
Adil H. Haider

Chapter 106
Stab Wound to the Neck 535
Gina M.S. Howell
Jason L. Sperry

Chapter 107
Burns 540
Jeffrey S. Guy

Chapter 108
Blunt Abdominal Trauma from Motor Vehicle Crash 546
Carla Kohoyda-Inglis
Stewart C. Wang

Chapter 109
Duodenal Injury 550
Filip Bednar
Mark R. Hemmila

Chapter 110
Pelvic Fracture 555
Avi Bhavaraju
Oliver L. Gunter

Critical Care
Chapter 111
Airway Emergency 560
Derek T. Woodrum
David W. Healy

Chapter 112
Acute Renal Failure 566
April E. Mendoza
Anthony G. Charles

Chapter 113
Adrenal Insufficiency 571
Steven R. Allen
Heidi L. Frankel

Chapter 114
Acute Respiratory Distress Syndrome (ARDS) 574
Pauline K. Park
Krishnan Raghavendran
Lena M. Napolitano

Chapter 115
Ventilator-associated Pneumonia 581
Krishnan Raghavendran

Chapter 116
Septic Shock 584
Pamela A. Lipsett

Chapter 117
Abdominal Compartment Syndrome 589
Rebecca Plevin
Heather L. Evans

Chapter 118
Nutritional Support in the Critically Ill Surgery Patient 594
Kyle J. Van Arendonk
Elliott R. Haut

Transplant

Head and Neck

1 Symptomatic Primary Inguinal Hernia

EVANGELOS MESSARIS

Presentation

A 55-year-old male patient with a history of hypertension and diabetes presents with right groin discomfort. He reports having right groin discomfort for the last 3 months. He also noticed a bulge in his right groin several months ago. He has no fever, chills, nausea, vomiting or dysuria. His vitals are normal. On exam it is noted that he has a mass in the right groin that extends into his scrotum. The mass is reducible, but it immediately recurs after reduction.

Differential Diagnosis

Groin discomfort usually is associated with an inguinal or femoral hernia or a process involving the spermatic cord or round ligament structures. Although, inguinal hernias are common, there are other medical conditions that can have similar presentation. Femoral hernias, enlarged inguinal nodes, hydroceles, testicular torsion, epididymitis, varicocele, spermatocele, epididymal cyst, and testicular tumors are less frequent but should be included in the differential diagnosis of a patient presenting with a symptomatic groin mass or groin discomfort.

Workup

The patient undergoes more extensive physical exam of his abdomen, in the standing and supine position, demonstrating a reducible inguinal mass at the level of the external ring of the inguinal canal with minimal overlying tenderness, suggestive of a right inguinal hernia.

The diagnosis of an inguinal hernia is based on physical examination. Reported sensitivity and specificity of physical examination for the diagnosis of inguinal hernia are 75% and 96%, respectively. In males, the index finger of the examiner should invaginate the scrotum in an attempt to find the external opening of the inguinal canal. The patient should then be asked to cough or perform a Valsalva maneuver. The examiner should then feel the hernia sac with all its contents at the tip of his index finger. Similarly, in female patients the examiner can feel for the hernia sac by palpating the inguinal area just laterally of the pubic tubercle. It should be noted that the exam is performed above the inguinal ligament, because if the protruding mass is below the inguinal ligament, then it is a femoral hernia. This distinction is not often easy, especially in obese patients. In all cases both sides should be examined (not only the symptomatic side) to rule out bilateral inguinal hernias. No laboratory studies can help with the diagnosis of an inguinal hernia.

Rarely the use of imaging studies is helpful in moving from the differential diagnosis to a single working diagnosis. Imaging studies are mostly used in obese patients where physical exam has limitations **(Figure 1)**. An ultrasound can demonstrate or rule out enlarged inguinal nodes, hydroceles, testicular torsion, varicocele, spermatocele, epididymal cyst, and testicular tumors. Furthermore, an experienced ultrasonographer can demonstrate an inguinal hernia sac and identify its contents. Computed tomography is mostly used on cases of very large inguinal hernias, to depict the contents of the sac and to identify aberrant anatomy in the inguinal canal **(Figure 2)**.

Diagnosis and Treatment

Ascertaining whether patients have symptoms from their hernia is important for decision making. For truly asymptomatic hernias, a watchful waiting strategy can be followed. Younger patients are almost always symptomatic because they are invariably active. However, older patients who are not physically active may not be bothered by their hernia and repair can be deferred indefinitely.

Inguinal hernias can present with many different symptoms. A reducible hernia will often present with groin discomfort that is exacerbated with activity. Patients with incarceration or strangulation will present with more severe pain and, potentially overlying skin erythema. The treatment of all symptomatic inguinal hernias is surgical repair. The goals of the repair are to relieve the symptoms and prevent any future incarceration or strangulation of the hernia. The timing for symptomatic hernia repairs depends on whether the hernia is reducible, incarcerated, or

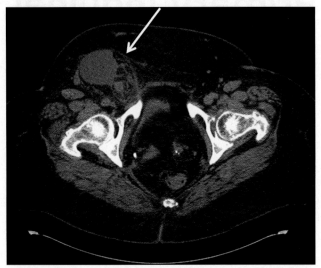

FIGURE 1 • Axial cut of a CT demonstrating a moderate-size right inguinal hernia with omentum in the hernia sac in an obese patient where physical exam findings would be limited.

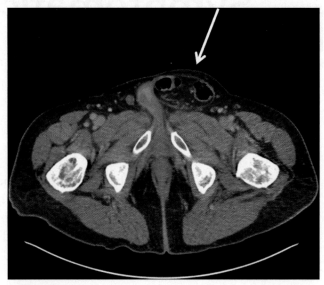

FIGURE 2 • Axial cut of a CT, demonstrating a left inguinal hernia with sigmoid colon in the hernia sac.

strangulated. Reducible hernias can be repaired in an elective outpatient fashion, incarcerated hernias warrant urgent repair within 12 hours of presentation, and strangulated hernias need to go to the operating room emergently, since the viability of an organ in the hernia sac is compromised.

Surgical Approach

The surgical approach for a symptomatic inguinal hernia could be open or laparoscopic, with local, spinal, or general anesthesia. In the open procedures the repair can be suture based (Bassini, McVay, Shouldice) or using mesh (e.g., Lichtenstein). Mesh is also used in all the laparoscopic cases that can be further divided in total extraperitoneal (TEP) and transabdominal preperitoneal (TAPP), depending on whether the peritoneal cavity is used for access to the inguinal region or not. Although many suggest using open repair for unilateral primary hernias and laparoscopic repair for bilateral and recurrent inguinal hernias, surgeon's experience should guide the choice of repair. Laparoscopic inguinal hernia repair has a steep learning curve, and most experts suggest 100 to 250 cases are necessary to develop proficiency. For surgeons who are not proficient at laparoscopic herniography, open mesh repair is the best choice, even for recurrences and bilateral repairs.

Regardless of the technique employed, the main goal of surgical therapy is a tension-free repair of the defect to decrease the recurrence rate. All elective and the majority of the emergent repairs, except those where bowel is compromised and a bowel resection is performed, achieve this goal by placing mesh over the defect, or in the case of the laparoscopic approach, behind the defect. In contaminated cases, a suture-based technique (Bassini, McVay, or Shouldice) or biologic mesh can be used. However, these patients will have a higher recurrence rate.

Preoperative Care

All patients are placed in a supine position on the operating table. Patients should have thigh-length sequential compression devices and in our practice we give 5,000 units of unfractionated heparin subcutaneously if they are older than 40 years. Administration of a first-generation cephalosporin intravenously within 1 hour prior to incision is recommended, especially in cases where mesh is going to be used. Skin preparation should be done with chlorhexidine and should include the scrotum, in case manipulation is needed for the hernia sac reduction or to facilitate the return of the testicle into its proper location.

Local anesthesia can be given either as a nerve block of the ilioinguinal and iliohypogastric nerves or as direct infiltration into the incision site, always in combination with some conscious sedation. Alternatively, spinal or general anesthesia can be used.

All patients should void prior to the procedure, otherwise intraoperative bladder decompression with a bladder catheter is advised.

Open Inguinal Hernia Repair

Lichtenstein open, tension-free hernioplasty is considered the "gold standard" for open hernia repair **(Table 1)**. The skin incision is placed over the inguinal

TABLE 1. Key Steps to Open Lichtenstein Tension-free Hernioplasty

1. The skin incision is placed over the inguinal canal for exposure of the pubic tubercle.
2. The cord structures are dissected from the cremasteric muscle and transversalis fascia fibers and retracted off the inguinal canal floor.
3. The cord is explored for an indirect hernia sac or cord lipoma.
4. Polypropylene mesh is secured inferiorly to the shelving edge of the inguinal ligament and superiorly to the rectus sheath and internal oblique muscle.
5. The internal ring is reconstructed by suturing the two leaves of the mesh together.
6. The spermatic cord is returned to its original position and the aponeurosis of the external oblique is reapproximated.
7. Check that testicles are still in the proper anatomical position in the scrotum.

Potential Pitfalls

- The pubic tubercle must be completely covered with mesh; if not there is higher risk for recurrence.
- Avoid entrapment of ilioinguinal, iliohypogastric, or genitofemoral nerves.
- Mesh fixation should be tension free.
- Confirm that spermatic vessels are intact and that testicles are in proper position at the end of the procedure.

TABLE 2. Key Steps to Laparoscopic Totally Extraperitoneal Repair of Inguinal Hernia

1. Enter rectus sheath through dissection from a infraumbilical skin incision.
2. A bluntly dissecting balloon is placed in the space between the rectus muscle anteriorly and the posterior fascia, and directed down to the pubis.
3. Two 5-mm trocars are placed in the lower midline between the rectus muscles.
4. Proper identification of critical anatomical landmarks is essential (the inferior epigastric vessels superiorly, Cooper's ligament medially, and the ileopubic tract laterally).
5. Hernia sac is reduced and separated off the cord structures.
6. A preformed or custom-made polyester mesh is positioned from a medial to lateral direction under the cord structures paying particular attention to cover the internal ring both laterally and superiorly, while its medial aspect is tucked below the Cooper's ligament.
7. Mesh fixation is not needed.

Potential Pitfalls

- Blunt dissection in the wrong plane or previous surgery in the pelvic or inguinal region may provide poor visualization of the landmark structures.
- Injury to the inferior epigastric vessels should be avoided.
- Incomplete hernia sac reduction and dissection off the cord structures may lead to incomplete repair and early recurrence.
- Nerve injuries are more common in laparoscopic repairs.

canal and angled only slightly cephalad as it progresses laterally. The major anatomical landmark is exposure over the pubic tubercl, medially. The incision is carried down to the abdominal wall fascia that consists of the external oblique aponeurosis to expose the external inguinal ring. The aponeurosis is incised in the direction of its fibers. The cord structures are dissected from the cremasteric muscle and transversalis fascia fibers and retracted off the inguinal canal floor. The cord is explored for an indirect hernia sac or cord lipoma. All hernia sacs and cord lipomas are transected at the level of the internal ring. An appropriate size polypropylene mesh is secured to the shelving edge of the inguinal ligament from the pubic tubercle to past the insertion of the arch of the internal oblique to Poupart's ligament using running or interrupted 2-0 Prolene suture. Similarly, the upper edge of the mesh is sutured to the rectus sheath and internal oblique muscle. The internal ring is reconstructed by suturing the two leaves of the mesh together lateral to the cord. The spermatic cord is returned to its original position and the aponeurosis of the external oblique is reapproximated using 2-0 absorbable suture in a running fashion, avoiding injuries of the ilioinguinal nerve.

Laparoscopic Inguinal Hernia Repair

The TEP repair of inguinal hernias was developed out of concern for possible complications related to intra-abdominal access required for transabdominal approach **(Table 2)**. In detail, the skin incision is made at the inferior aspect of the umbilicus and the anterior rectus sheath is incised lateral to the midline. Blunt dissection is used to sweep the rectus muscle laterally from the midline to expose the posterior rectus sheath fascia. A dissecting balloon is placed in the space between the rectus muscle anteriorly and the posterior fascia, and directed down to the pubis. Under direct visualization, the dissector is inflated. The balloon is then replaced by a standard blunt port and the previously created extraperitoneal space is insufflated with CO_2 to reach 12 mm Hg. Two 5-mm trocars are placed in the lower midline. After identification of the inferior epigastric vessels superiorly, Cooper's ligament medially, and the ileopubic tract laterally, the hernia sac is reduced, paying particular attention to completely detach the sac off the cord structures. A preformed or custom-made polyester mesh can be used for the repair. The mesh is positioned from a medial to lateral direction under the cord structures paying particular attention to cover the internal ring both laterally and superiorly, while its medial aspect is tucked below the Cooper's ligament. When the mesh is correctly positioned, it can be fixated using tacks, staples, fibrin glue, or just be left in place without any fixation.

Special Intraoperative Considerations

In all inguinal hernia repair cases, all types and all approaches, the major key point for a successful operation is knowing the anatomy of the inguinal canal **(Tables 1 and 2)**.

For open repairs, attention should be paid to the dissection and preservation of the ilioinguinal and iliohypogastric nerve. Nerve entrapment can cause significant neuralgia in the postoperative period. If during the procedure a nerve is injured, then complete transection of the nerve is advised.

During laparoscopic repairs, the dissection in the groin area will cause some lacerations to the peritoneum and the peritoneal cavity contents maybe encountered. Each defect of the peritoneum should be closed using an endo-loop ligature (2-0 vicryl), and if the peritoneal cavity is insufflated with CO_2, then it can be decompressed using a Veress needle.

Intraoperative complications include femoral vessel or inferior epigastric vessel injuries, bladder or testicular injuries, and vas deferens injury or nerve injury.

Postoperative Management

For elective cases or cases with omental incarceration, the patient usually can be discharged within 3 to 4 hours postoperatively. The patient should void without any problems and have adequate pain control before being discharged. Urinary retention is frequent after inguinal surgery and it is associated with the use of narcotics, the type of surgery, and the amount of intravenous fluids administered to the patients.

For urgent or emergent cases if no bowel was affected usually 24 hours of observation are adequate before discharge. In cases where bowel was found strangulated and bowel resection was done, the patients are usually followed in the hospital for 2 to 3 days.

Follow-up in all cases usually is scheduled 3 to 4 weeks postoperatively to check the wound healing (rule out any wound infections—rare <1%, or seromas or hematomas). Routine examination should rule out early recurrence and any neuralgia from nerve injury or entrapment. Most patients are able to return to work within 2 weeks from surgery, and even earlier if performed laparoscopically. No heavy weight lifting is advisable up to 3 months from the operation.

Case Conclusion

The patient underwent a successful laparoscopic right inguinal repair with mesh and was discharged 4 hours postoperatively. He returned to the office in 3 weeks with well-healed port sites and was pain free. During his routine postoperative appointment, the patient reported feeling a bulge in the right groin that was similar to the hernia that he had before. Exam did not reveal a recurrence and an ultrasound demonstrated a seroma at the repair site. No intervention was performed and the patient was seen 3 months postoperatively and the seroma was completely resolved.

TAKE HOME POINTS

- Inguinal hernias are common, comprising three-fourths of all abdominal wall defects. Lifetime risk for developing an inguinal hernia is 15% for males and 5% for females.
- All symptomatic inguinal hernias need to be surgically repaired to relieve symptoms and prevent any future incarceration or strangulation of the hernia.
- There are several described procedures for inguinal hernia repair and they can be open or laparoscopic.
- Regardless of the technique employed, the main goal of surgical therapy is a tension-free repair of the defect to decrease the recurrence rate.
- Seromas, neuralgia, and recurrence are some of the most frequent postoperative complications.

SUGGESTED READINGS

Amato B, Moja L, Panico S, et al. Shouldice technique versus other open techniques for inguinal hernia repair. Cochrane Database Syst Rev. 2009;(4):CD001543.

Langeveld HR, van't Riet M, Weidema WF, et al. Total extraperitoneal inguinal hernia repair compared with Lichtenstein (the LEVEL-Trial): a randomized controlled trial. Ann Surg. 2010;251(5):819–824.

Messaris E, Nicastri G, Dudrick SJ. Total extraperitoneal laparoscopic inguinal hernia repair without mesh fixation: prospective study with 1-year follow-up results. Arch Surg. 2010;145(4):334–338.

Neumayer L, Giobbie-Hurder A, Jonasson O, et al.; Veterans Affairs Cooperative Studies Program 456 Investigators. Open mesh versus laparoscopic mesh repair of inguinal hernia. N Engl J Med. 2004;350(18):1819–1827.

Nordin P, Zetterström H, Gunnarsson U, et al. Local, regional, or general anaesthesia in groin hernia repair: multicentre randomised trial. Lancet. 2003;362(9387):853–858.

2 Recurrent Inguinal Hernia

JONATHAN F. FINKS

Presentation

A 50-year-old obese man with a large pannus is referred for evaluation of a recurrent right inguinal bulge occurring 5 years following open mesh repair of a right inguinal hernia. He has noticed the bulge for the last several months. Although reducible, the patient has noted increasing discomfort associated with the bulge over the last few weeks. He denies any obstructive symptoms and has had no symptoms on the left side. Physical exam demonstrates some fullness in the right groin, but the exam is limited by the patient's body habitus.

Differential Diagnosis

The leading diagnosis based on these symptoms is a recurrent right inguinal hernia. Other considerations would include lymphadenopathy; soft tissue mass, such as a lipoma or a sarcoma; and hematoma related to trauma.

Workup

To evaluate for recurrent hernia, the best imaging study is a CT of the abdomen and pelvis, with at least oral contrast. Two sets of images should be obtained: the first using a standard technique and the second with the patient performing a Valsalva maneuver. This test will allow for better identification of hernia contents in the inguinal canal.

Diagnosis and Treatment

In this case, cross-sectional imaging demonstrated a recurrent right inguinal hernia containing nonobstructed loops of small bowel. The left inguinal canal was normal in appearance. Given the symptomatic nature of this hernia, repair is warranted. There are several options for surgical management. An anterior approach would be very difficult and unlikely to produce durable results, given the patient's body habitus and the presence of previously placed mesh. A preperitoneal approach is preferred in this case because the repair would be done in an unviolated tissue plane. Furthermore, this technique results in coverage of the direct, indirect, and femoral spaces. This could be done using an open preperitoneal technique but would be difficult given the patient's obesity and large pannus. Similarly, a total extraperitoneal (TEPP) approach would also be hindered by a thick abdominal wall and limited working space due to adipose tissue in the preperitoneal space. In this case, I believe the best technique would be a transabdominal preperitoneal (TAPP) approach. The transabdominal route allows access to the preperitoneal space, while avoiding the thick lower abdominal wall pannus. The TAPP repair is also useful in cases of large scrotal hernias, as these can be more easily reduced from the peritoneal cavity than from the preperitoneal space. The transabdominal approach also allows for assessment of bowel viability in cases of strangulated hernias. Finally, conversion to TAPP repair may also be required during an attempted TEPP repair if, for example, the peritoneum is violated while attempting to develop the preperitoneal space with a balloon dissector. This latter scenario often occurs in patients with lower abdominal incisions (e.g., Pfannenstiel).

Surgical Approach

In essence, the TAPP procedure for inguinal hernia repair involves entry into the preperitoneal space by incision of the lower abdominal wall peritoneum from inside the peritoneal cavity **(Table 1)**. Once in the preperitoneal space, the hernia sac is dissected free from the cord structures and reduced from within the deep inguinal ring (indirect hernia), Hesselbach's triangle (direct hernia), and/or the femoral space (femoral hernia). Once the hernia contents have been reduced, the peritoneum is dissected well off of the cord structures to make room for placement of the mesh. Mesh is then placed such that it adequately covers the direct, indirect, and femoral spaces. The peritoneum is then secured up to the abdominal wall to cover the mesh.

The procedure is performed under general anesthesia with the patient supine, both arms tucked to the side, in slight Trendelenburg position. A Foley catheter is inserted to decompress the bladder. Access to the peritoneum is obtained using a closed (Veress) or an open (Hasson) technique, and pneumoperitoneum is established. The surgeon stands on the side opposite the hernia, with the assistant on the ipsilateral side **(Figure 1)**. An 11-mm trocar is placed above the umbilicus in the midline for placement of the laparoscope and later insertion of the mesh into the peritoneal cavity. Many surgeons prefer to work through ports on both sides of the midline so as to effect proper triangulation **(Figure 1)**. However, in the obese individual, the surgeons' working ports (both 5-mm ports) should both be on the side contralateral to the hernia, usually on either side of the midclavicular line and below the level of the umbilicus. In some cases, an additional 5-mm assistant's port may be placed on the ipsilateral side, at the midclavicular line above the level of the umbilicus. In the case of bilateral inguinal hernia repair, the working trocars are generally placed at or above the level of the umbilicus. A 10-mm 30° laparoscope is employed, although some surgeons prefer a 0° laparoscope in nonobese patients.

The procedure begins with an inspection of the lower abdominal wall on both sides. **Figure 2** shows the anatomy and landmarks in the right lower abdomen. The median umbilical ligaments and epigastric vessels should be identified on either side of the bladder. Any obvious hernia defects should be identified, although some of these may not be apparent until the peritoneum is taken down. Indirect hernias are located lateral to the inferior epigastric vessels. Direct hernias occur through Hesselbach's triangle, bordered laterally by the inferior epigastric vessels, medially by lateral edge of the rectus muscle, and inferiorly by the inguinal ligament. Femoral hernias occur through the femoral space, bordered laterally by the femoral vein, posteriorly by Cooper's ligament, and anteriorly by the inguinal ligament.

The preperitoneal space is then developed beginning with an incision in the peritoneum using electrocautery. The incision begins vertically along the ipsilateral median umbilical ligament down to its root. The incision is carried transversely above the level of the hernia defects, across to the anterior superior iliac spine **(Figure 3)**. In cases of a bilateral inguinal hernia,

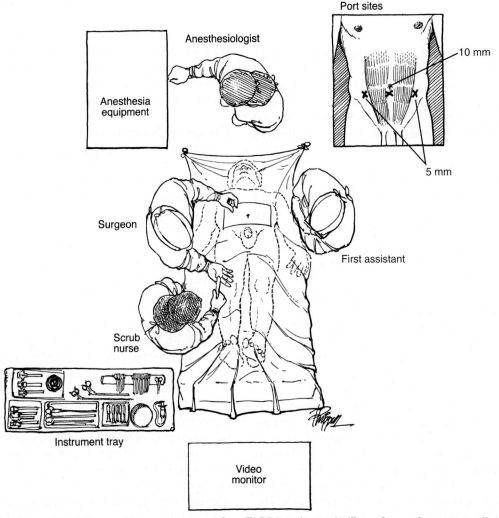

FIGURE 1 • Operating room setup and trocar placement for a TAPP hernia repair. (From Soper, Swanstrom, Eubanks. Mastery of Endoscopic and Laparoscopic Surgery. 3rd ed. Lippincott Williams and Wilkins, 2009, Figure 53-13.)

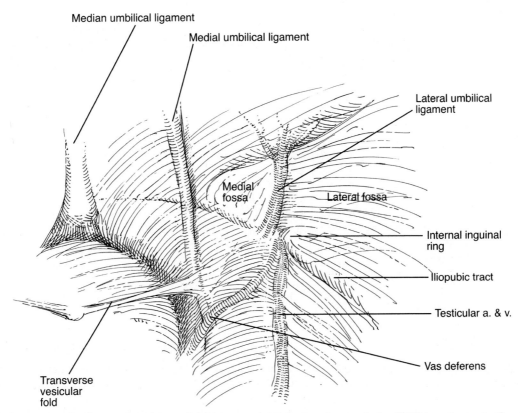

Median umbilical ligament

Medial umbilical ligament

Lateral umbilical ligament

Medial fossa

Lateral fossa

Internal inguinal ring

Iliopubic tract

Testicular a. & v.

Vas deferens

Transverse vesicular fold

FIGURE 2 • Laparoscopic view and anatomy of right lower abdominal wall seen during TAPP hernia repair. (From Soper, Swanstrom, Eubanks. Mastery of Endoscopic and Laparoscopic Surgery. 3rd ed. Lippincott Williams and Wilkins, 2009, Figure 53-14.)

a mirror incision is made on the opposite side. Separate dissections and pieces of mesh are used to repair bilateral hernias. Blunt and sharp dissection with electrocautery is then used to develop the preperitoneal space, staying close to the peritoneum. This dissection begins lateral to the cord structures, in Bogros' space, advances medially toward the retropubic space, and extends proximally to expose the femoral vessels, psoas muscle, and retroperitoneum **(Figure 3)**. Medially, the bladder is carefully dissected off of the anterior abdominal wall, exposing the symphysis pubis and Cooper's ligament. Care must be taken not to injure *corona mortis*, which refers to the venous connection between the inferior epigastric and obturator veins. This structure courses inferiorly along the lateral aspect of Cooper's ligament and, because of its location on the pubic bone, can be difficult to control if lacerated or avulsed.

An assessment for femoral and direct hernia defects occurs during the medial dissection. Careful attention is paid to identify the critical structures: inferior epigastric vessels, Cooper's ligament, and the femoral vein. Direct and femoral hernias may contain only preperitoneal fat or they may contain a hernia sac. It is not uncommon for direct hernias to contain the urinary bladder. The hernia contents are reduced with gentle

blunt dissection. With a direct hernia, there is usually a clear transition between the transversalis fascia and the hernia sac. These structures can often be separated by applying cephalad and posterior retraction of the sac and anterior and caudad retraction of the transversalis fascia. In the setting of a large direct defect, large seromas may develop. To help minimize the risk for seroma formation, the transversalis fascia may be reduced from within Hesselbach's triangle and tacked to Cooper's ligament. When reducing femoral hernias, care must be taken to carefully delineate between hernia contents and the fat and lymphatic tissue intimately associated with the femoral vein. Injudicious dissection can lead to injury to the femoral vein. The medial dissection may also reveal an obturator hernia, located posterior to Cooper's ligament through the obturator foramen. These are also reduced by blunt dissection and may require an additional medially placed mesh to cover the defect.

An indirect hernia is identified during the lateral dissection. The hernia sac is bluntly dissected away from the underlying spermatic cord structures, namely the vas deferens and the testicular vessels. The sac must be dissected free from the cord structures prior to reduction of the sac from within the deep inguinal

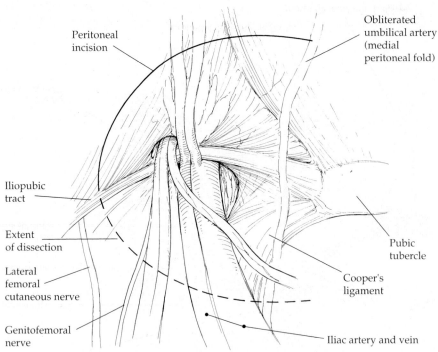

Peritoneal
incision

Obliterated
umbilical artery
(medial
peritoneal fold)

Iliopubic
tract

Extent
of dissection

Lateral
femoral
cutaneous nerve

Genitofemoral
nerve

Pubic
tubercle

Cooper's
ligament

Iliac artery and vein

FIGURE 3 • Peritoneal incision (*solid line*) and extent of dissection (*dashed line*) in a left-sided TAPP hernia repair. (From Soper, Swanstrom, Eubanks. Mastery of Endoscopic and Laparoscopic Surgery. 3rd ed. Lippincott Williams and Wilkins, 2009, Figure 53-1.)

ring to avoid inadvertent laceration or transection of the vas deferens or testicular vessels. The hernia sac is then reduced by application of cephalad and posterior retraction on the hernia sac, with anterior and caudad retraction of the transversalis fascia. We do not employ cautery during this dissection, especially in the space lateral to the cord structures, to avoid injury to the genital branch of the genitofemoral nerve, which courses anterior to the psoas muscle in the pelvis and passes through the inguinal canal along with the cord in the lateral bundle of the cremasteric fascia.

Care must be taken to ensure that the hernia sac remains free from the cord structures during this entire process, particularly in the setting of a large scrotal sac. If the peritoneal sac is very large and cannot be easily reduced, it may be transected, with the distal aspect allowed to retract into the scrotum. The proximal aspect of the sac must then be secured during reperitonealization following the mesh repair to prevent bowel adhesions to the mesh. Transection of the sac is safe but may lead to development of a hydrocele in some cases. Preperitoneal fat within the deep inguinal ring (cord lipomas) should be completely reduced from that space in order to prevent the patient's sensation of a persistent bulge following hernia repair.

Once the hernia sac has been reduced, the peritoneum is dissected off of the cord structures in a cephalad direction. Adequate parietalization of the cord is essential, as it prevents peritoneum from slipping underneath the bottom edge of the mesh, which leads to lateral recurrences. Similarly, herniated preperitoneal fat must also be dissected well off of the cord so that it cannot slip beneath the mesh. This dissection continues cephalad to the level of the anterior superior iliac spine and laterally to the iliac wing, allowing for exposure of the psoas muscle. Medially, this continues to the transition to the urinary bladder, which is then itself dissected off of Cooper's ligament and the pubis in order to clear a space for placement of the mesh. Gentle medial retraction on the bladder allows for better delineation between prevesicular fat and fat associated with the femoral vein and helps reduce the risk of inadvertent injury to the vein.

Once hemostasis has been ensured, the next step involves placement of a large piece of nonabsorbable mesh. We employ an anatomically contoured, lightweight, woven polypropylene mesh that is 10 cm in height by 16 cm in width. The mesh must be large enough to cover the direct, indirect, and femoral spaces (myopectineal orifice) and the posterior aspect of Cooper's ligament. In the case of bilateral hernias, two pieces of mesh are used. The mesh is rolled and inserted into the abdomen through the 10-mm port. It is inserted into the preperitoneal space and unrolled such that the inferior aspect is draped over the cord structures and psoas muscle laterally and Cooper's ligament and pubic symphysis medially. The superior aspect of mesh then covers the anterior abdominal wall above the level of the iliopubic tract, including the inferior epigastric vessels and the rectus muscle medially. We tack the mesh medially to Cooper's ligament with a single 5-mm spiral tack to prevent the mesh from sliding and will tack to the rectus muscle in cases of a large direct hernia to prevent the mesh from herniating through the defect. We avoid any tack placement laterally to prevent injury to the ilioinguinal and iliohypogastric nerves.

Once the mesh has been placed, the peritoneum is closed. This is facilitated by reducing the pneumoperitoneum pressure as low as possible, while still permitting adequate visualization. The entire peritoneum must be secured and the mesh covered to prevent bowel adhesions to the mesh or incarceration of a bowel loop within the preperitoneal space. This can be accomplished using spiral tacks, suture, or a combination of these.

Special Intraoperative Considerations

In general, it is easy to get disoriented during laparoscopic inguinal hernia repairs, whether done as a TEPP or a TAPP procedure, and this can lead to disastrous consequences. In the setting of a large indirect hernia sac, particularly in an obese patient, it can be difficult to identify the cord structures and this can lead to

dissection in the deeper "triangle of doom" with inadvertent injury to the femoral artery or vein. It is worthwhile to periodically identify known landmarks, such as Cooper's ligament and the symphysis pubis as well as the inferior epigastric vessels. Such periodic reorienting is often very helpful in keeping the dissection in the proper plane. In the event of a femoral vein injury, conversion to open will most likely be required. First, however, the surgeon should increase the pneumoperitoneum pressure to 25 mm of mercury or higher as necessary to help tamponade the bleeding. Direct pressure with a Raytec opened completely and inserted through the 10-mm trocar will allow for direct compression of the vessel. These two maneuvers should provide adequate hemostasis and time for a deliberate conversion to open with all members of the surgical team prepared and ready.

TAKE HOME POINTS

- The TAPP approach should be considered for patients with an indication for a preperitoneal repair (e.g. bilateral or recurrent inguinal or femoral hernia) in whom a TEPP approach is not feasible (e.g. due to obesity, previous pfannenstiel incision, or inadvertent peritoneal entry during access in an attempted TEPP repair).
- The right and left preperitoneal spaces should be dissected separately and 2 pieces of mesh used in cases of bilateral hernias to reduce the risk of recurrent hernia.
- Initial dissection in the preperitoneal space should remain close to the peritoneum to avoid inadvertent injury to the femoral vessels.
- Adequate closure of the peritoneum after hernia repair is essential to prevent adhesions between bowel and mesh and to prevent internal herniation of bowel loops within the preperitoneal space.

TABLE 1. Key Technical Steps and Potential Pitfalls

Key Technical Steps

1. Incision of the peritoneum and development of the preperitoneal space.
2. Reduction of direct and/or femoral hernias medially.
3. Dissection of an indirect hernia sac off of the cord structures and subsequent reduction of the sac and the cord lipoma from within the deep inguinal ring.
4. Extensive peritoneal dissection with parietalization of the cord.
5. Placement of nonabsorbable mesh to cover the entire myopectineal orifice.
6. Closure of the peritoneum.

Potential Pitfalls

- Injury to femoral vessels from dissection in the "triangle of doom" deep to the cord structures.
- Injury to genital branch of the genitofemoral nerve from injudicious use of cautery in the "triangle of pain" lateral to the cord structures.
- Traction injury to the cord structures during reduction of an indirect hernia if the sac is not adequately dissected off of the cord prior to reduction of the sac.
- Early recurrence if the peritoneum is not adequately dissected prior to mesh placement.

SUGGESTED READINGS

Felix E. Causes of recurrence after laparoscopic hernioplasty. A multicenter study. Surg Endosc. 1998;12(3):226–231.

Lovisetto F. Laparoscopic transabdominal preperitoneal (TAPP) hernia repair: surgical phases and complications. Surg Endosc. 2007;21(4):646–652.

McCormack K. Laparoscopic techniques versus open techniques for inguinal hernia repair. Cochrane Database Syst Rev. 2003;(1):CD001785.

Rebuffat C. Laparoscopic repair of strangulated hernias. Surg Endosc. 2006;20(1):131–134.

Rosenberger RJ. The cutaneous nerves encountered during laparoscopic repair of inguinal hernia: new anatomical findings for the surgeon. Surg Endosc. 2000;14(8):731–735.

3 Incarcerated/Strangulated Inguinal Hernia

MATTHEW W. RALLS and JUSTIN B. DIMICK

Presentation

A 61-year-old man presents to the emergency department with obstipation and left groin mass for 3 days. His past medical history was notable for chronic obstructive pulmonary disease, type II diabetes, obesity, hyperlipidemia, and schizophrenia. His surgical history was significant for two prior inguinal hernia repairs on the left side. Due to his schizophrenia, he resides in an assisted living facility and comes in with a caregiver today. He describes an increase in abdominal pain and distention over the 3-day period. His oral intake has decreased, and he reports minimal urine output over the past 2 days. Physical exam is notable for a well-healed scar in the right lower quadrant at McBurney's point and a large, 12- × 12-cm bulge in the left inguinal region. The mass is tender to palpation, erythematous, and nonreducible. Although the bulge has intermittently been present, both the patient and caregiver state that the size and tenderness are new in the past 2 days. Laboratory values were notable for a WBC of 8.7 and hematocrit of 42.4.

Differential Diagnosis

In a patient with an intermittent groin bulge that is now fixed, tender, and erythematous, complications of a groin hernia should be first consideration in the differential diagnosis. However, there are several other possible etiologies to consider. Subcutaneous pathology, such as lipoma, groin abscess, or inguinal adenopathy, can present as a groin mass. Testicular pathology comprising torsion and epididymitis should also be considered, especially when the mass involves the scrotum. Vascular etiologies, such as aneurysmal or pseudoaneurysmal disease, should be considered in patients with a history of vascular disease and/or previous interventions at or near the femoral vessels.

Once the surgeon suspects groin hernia, it is important to discern inguinal from femoral hernia. To some degree, this can be ascertained on physical exam. For a femoral hernia, the bulge is below (and lateral) to the medial end of the inguinal ligament. In contrast, in an inguinal hernia, the bulge would be above the inguinal ligament (Figure 1). However, this distinction can be difficult to assess if the bulge is large, tender, and inflamed.

Most importantly, early identification of complications of groin hernia, such as incarceration or strangulation, is essential. Such complications change the time course of intervention. Incarcerated hernias cannot be reduced and therefore may progress to strangulation if they have not already. Strangulated hernia is by definition a hernia in which the blood supply of the herniated viscus is compromised. For a reducible groin hernia, repair can be delayed and scheduled electively. But suspected incarceration and strangulation are surgical emergencies.

Workup

History and physical examination in patients with suspected incarcerated and/or inguinal hernia are often diagnostic. The decision to operate can often be made without further evaluation (Figure 2). Laboratory values such as complete blood count, comprehensive metabolic panel, and lactate level can provide information about the patient's hydration status and whether there is systemic inflammatory response, which are important in assessing the likelihood of strangulation. However, these tests have a high sensitivity and low specificity, that is, most patients with incarceration and strangulation will have normal or near-normal laboratory values. To avoid a high false-negative rate (i.e., missing the diagnosis when it is present), surgeons should err on the side of exploring patients when incarceration/strangulation are suspected. If there is substantial uncertainty regarding the diagnosis, imaging studies can be obtained. If the patient is obstructed at the site of incarceration, plain films of the abdomen will show signs of distended loops of bowel and air fluid levels if the patient is obstructed (Figure 3). However, computed tomography (CT) imaging is the standard in emergency evaluation (Figure 4) if the clinical diagnosis is in question after history, physical, and plain abdominal radiographs.

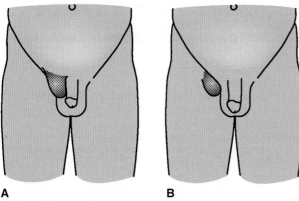

FIGURE 1 • Landmarks in discerning inguinal (**A**) versus femoral (**B**) hernia. (From Mulholland MW, et al. Greenfield's Surgery: Scientific Principles & Practice. 4th ed. Philadelphia, PA: Lippincott Williams & Wilkins, 2006, with permission.)

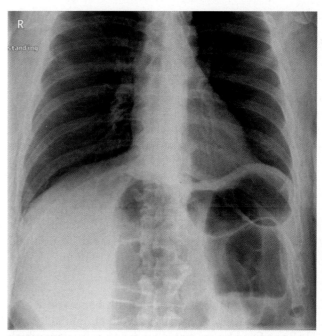

FIGURE 3 • Plain film of patient described in this clinical scenario. Distended loops of large bowel are concerning for a distal large bowel obstruction.

Discussion

Inguinal hernia repair is one of the most commonly performed surgical procedures worldwide. Over 800,000 inguinal hernia repairs are performed in the United States each year. Despite being a very common operation, the relevant anatomy is complex and often difficult for students and surgical trainees to fully understand. An intimate knowledge of this anatomy, however, is important, especially for addressing incarcerated or recurrent inguinal hernias. In these settings, the distortion of the tissues makes operative repair extremely challenging. In 1804, Astley Cooper stated, "No disease of the human body, belonging to the province of the surgeon, requires in its treatment a greater combination of accurate anatomic knowledge, with surgical skill, than hernia in all its varieties."

Over the past two centuries, there have been many advances in groin hernia repair. The most frequently used technique in contemporary surgical practice is the tension-free mesh repair, or Lichtenstein repair. The laparoscopic totally extraperitoneal (TEP) is emerging as the most frequent minimally invasive approach and

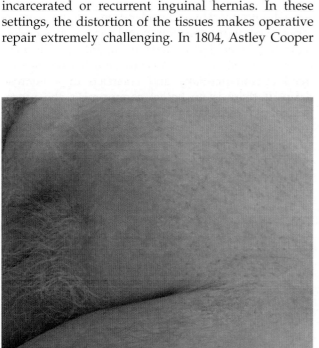

FIGURE 2 • Erythema and swelling over left groin concerning for incarcerated hernia. This exam finding, coupled with appropriate presentation, is sufficient cause for exploration.

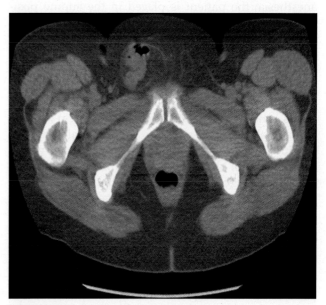

FIGURE 4 • CT showing left inguinal hernia.

allows for quicker recovery, less pain, and similar or lower recurrence rates in experienced hands. Primary tissue repairs, such as the Bassini and McVay, are rarely used. However, in certain settings, such as contaminated fields with infection or bowel resection, a working knowledge of primary tissue repairs is essential.

Symptomatic inguinal hernias that are reducible should be repaired on an elective basis. As discussed above, incarcerated hernias should be addressed more expeditiously. Surgery within 6 hours may prevent loss of bowel. Emergent repair differs little from elective repair. Either open or laparoscopic techniques are acceptable, although it is the preference of the author to utilize the open procedure if there is concern for strangulation. This is due to the tissue distortion and friability associated with acute inflammation.

Diagnosis and Treatment

The patient in our case presents with a scenario worrisome for incarcerated or strangulated inguinal hernia. He has a fixed bulge that is tender to palpation, which is typical of incarceration. He also presents with erythema in the overlying skin, which suggests possible strangulation. The patient also presents with radiographic evidence of large bowel obstruction (**Figure 3** is his abdominal radiograph) with resultant obstipation and abdominal pain, with associated nausea and vomiting. Given the bowel obstruction in this patient, and the possible risk of strangulation, we will perform an open repair, beginning with an inguinal exploration.

Surgical Approach for Open Mesh Repair of Incarcerated Inguinal Hernia Repair (Table 1)

Open repair can often be done under general, spinal, or local anesthetic with sedation. Regardless of the anesthesia, the patient is placed in the supine position. Reverse Trendelenburg position is advocated by some to aid in reduction of the hernia. The patient is prepped and draped in the standard sterile fashion. Local anesthetic is injected in the subcutaneous space above and parallel to the inguinal ligament. The patient can be further anesthetized with varying forms of nerve block if necessary. A 6- to 8-cm incision is made above and parallel to the inguinal ligament. The incision is deepened through the soft tissue with a combination of blunt dissection and Bovie electrocautery to the level of the external oblique aponeurosis. The muscle is then cut along the line of the external oblique fibers from the level of the internal ring and through the external ring.

At this point, groin exploration is warranted in the case of suspected incarceration/strangulation. If the viability of the bowel is in question, a resection can be performed via the inguinal incision. If that is not feasible, it may be necessary to perform laparotomy (see

TABLE 1. Key Technical Steps in Open Inguinal Hernia Repair with Mesh

1. Verify laterality.
2. Prophylax with antibiotics.
3. Groin incision.
4. Expose and incise the external oblique in the direction of the fibers to the external ring.
5. Identify and protect the ilioinguinal nerve.
6. Mobilize flaps of external oblique.
7. Attempt reduction of hernia contents to better establish anatomical landmarks.
8. Encircle the spermatic cord (round ligament if female) at the external ring with a Penrose drain.
9. Identify the hernia sac on the anteromedial surface of cord and dissect it free from the surrounding structures.
10. In the case of an indirect hernia, open the sac, reduce the contents, and highly ligate with suture ligature.
11. If direct hernia, free sac from surrounding attachments and reduce into the abdomen.
12. Assess the floor of the canal and prepare the mesh.
13. Begin medially at the pubic tubercle and secure the mesh in place to the shelving edge inferiorly and the conjoined tendon superiorly.
14. Avoid narrowing the internal ring or incorporating nervous tissue into the repair.
15. Ensure hemostasis.
16. Close the external oblique aponeurosis and Scarpa's fascia in layers.
17. Approximate the skin edges and apply a dressing.

special intraoperative considerations). Great care is taken to not injure the ilioinguinal nerve that is underlying this layer. Tissue flaps are mobilized. Through blunt finger dissection, the cord (and hernia sac) are freed circumferentially and encircled in a Penrose drain. If there is no bowel compromise, the procedure moves forward as with an uncomplicated hernia repair.

The dissection is now turned to identification and separation of the hernia sac from the cord structures with division of the cremasteric fibers. Classically the sac will be anterior and medial with respect to the cord. The internal ring is inspected for evidence of indirect hernia. If found, the sac is dissected free and ligated under direct vision. Care is taken to avoid injury to the contents of the hernia. If a direct hernia is encountered, the hernia is reduced. The inguinal floor should be inspected for weakness.

Attention is then turned to repairing the ring and floor with mesh. A polypropylene mesh (precut or 6-in^2) is typically used. The medial point is secured to the lateral aspect of the pubic tubercle, suturing to the periosteum and not the bone itself. The prosthesis is positioned over the inguinal floor and secured to the lateral edge of the rectus sheath (i.e., the conjoint tendon or area). The cord structures are placed through a

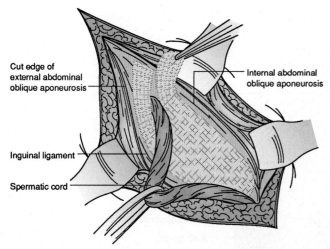

Cut edge of
external abdominal
oblique aponeurosis

Internal abdominal
oblique aponeurosis

Inguinal ligament

Spermatic cord

FIGURE 5 • Mesh placement during standard open (Lichtenstein) hernia repair. (From Mulholland MW, et al. Greenfield's Surgery: Scientific Principles & Practice. 4th ed. Philadelphia, PA: Lippincott Williams & Wilkins, 2006, with permission.)

TABLE 2. Key Technical Steps in TEP Inguinal Hernia Repair with Mesh

1. Verify laterality.
2. Prophylax with antibiotics.
3. Infraumbilical incision for the 10–12-mm trocar.
4. Identify the anterior rectus sheath on the contralateral side of the midline. Identify and retract the medial border of the rectus.
5. Insert a finger over the posterior rectus sheath and develop a plane.
6. Insert the balloon-tipped trocar into this space aimed toward the symphysis pubis, and the preperitoneal space is insufflated under direct visualization.
7. Place additional trocars in the midline 5 and 12 cm above the symphysis.
8. Clear the areolar tissue from the ipsilateral pubic tubercle with care to not injure the communicating branch between the inferior epigastric and the obturator vessels (the corona mortis).
9. Free the lateral attachments of the peritoneum from the anterior abdominal wall.
10. Skeletonize the cord structures.
11. If direct: Reduce the sac and preperitoneal from the internal ring by gentle traction.
12. If indirect: mobilize the sac from the cord structures, and reduce into the peritoneum.
13. Place precut lateralized mesh in proper orientation to completely cover direct, indirect, and femoral spaces.
14. Place tacking suture on the medial aspect of the mesh in Cooper's ligament.
15. Ensure peritoneal edge is free from entrapment under the newly placed mesh, and desufflate under direct visualization.

slit in the lateral portion of the mesh, and the two tails are secured to each other to create a new internal ring. The inferior leaflet of the mesh is secured to the shelving edge of the inguinal ligament **(Figure 5)**. The external oblique aponeurosis and Scarpa's fascia are closed in layers. The skin is approximated.

Surgical Approach to Laparoscopic Repair of Incarcerated Inguinal Hernia (Table 2)

The author's preference is to approach recurrent hernias laparoscopically, even when presenting with incarceration. If the incarcerated bowel is viable, and can be reduced laparoscopically, the laparoscopic repair allows for repair of the hernia through tissue planes that are undisturbed by prior surgery. We begin by placing the laparoscope intra-abdominally to reduce and evaluate the viability of any incarcerated bowel. Once this step is complete, and we are convinced the bowel is viable, we withdraw the ports and convert to a TEP laparoscopic repair.

General anesthesia is used so the preperitoneal space can be insufflated. The patient is placed in the supine position and then prepped and draped in standard sterile fashion. The umbilical port from the prior exploration is used to place the initial port. Blunt dissection is used to identify the anterior rectus sheath on the contralateral side of the midline. The medial border of the rectus abdominus is identified and retracted laterally. Gentle insertion of a finger over the posterior rectus sheath past the arcuate line is done to develop a plane in the preperitoneal space. The balloon-tipped trocar is then inserted into this space and aimed toward the symphysis pubis, and the preperitoneal

space is insufflated under direct visualization. Two 5-mm working ports are placed in the lower midline. The complex anatomy must be well understood by the surgeon **(Figure 6)**. Blunt graspers are used to free the cord and hernia sac from the surrounding areolar tissue.

Two pitfalls of this portion of the operation are to dissect in the triangle of doom and the triangle of pain. The triangle of doom is bordered by the vas deferens medially, spermatic vessels laterally, and external iliac vessels inferiorly. The contents of this space comprise the external iliac artery and vein and the deep circumflex iliac vein. Damage to these vessels can obviously cause major bleeding and should be avoided. The triangle of pain is defined as spermatic vessel medially, the iliopubic tract laterally, and inferiorly the inferior edge of skin incision. This triangle contains the lateral femoral cutaneous nerve and anterior femoral cutaneous nerve of thigh. Manipulation, dissection, and tacking should be avoided as nerve damage or entrapment can cause neuralgia.

The hernia sac should be gently freed from the cord structures and the peritoneum retracted superiorly and medially. A precut lateralized mesh is put through

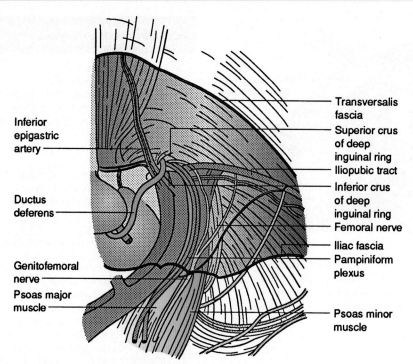

FIGURE 6 • Deep inguinal region from an intra-abdominal point of view demonstrating crucial landmarks and vital structures. (From Mulholland MW, et al. Greenfield's Surgery: Scientific Principles & Practice. 4th ed. Philadelphia, PA: Lippincott Williams & Wilkins, 2006, with permission.)

the infraumbilical port. When in proper position and orientation, the mesh should completely cover direct, indirect, and femoral spaces. Place tacking suture on the medial aspect of the mesh in Cooper's ligament. Ensure the peritoneal edge is free from entrapment under the newly placed mesh and desufflate under direct visualization. The procedure is finished with closure of the 10-mm port and skin approximation.

Special Intraoperative Considerations

As with many urgent or emergent general surgery situations, intraoperative decision making is essential to optimize outcomes. Incarceration or strangulation increases the odds of gross spillage of bowel contents. In the case of bowel resection or other contamination, the surgeon will need to utilize biologic mesh or primary tissue repair. For a straightforward primary inguinal hernia with contamination, a Bassini repair would be a good choice. For this procedure, the lateral edge of the rectus sheath (i.e., conjoined tendon) is approximated to the inguinal ligament. A relaxing incision is made if there is any tension. For a femoral hernia with contamination, a Bassini repair will not be adequate because the femoral canal has not been addressed. In this case, a McVay (Cooper's ligament) repair is appropriate. With a McVay repair, the lateral edge of the rectus sheath (i.e., conjoined tendon) is approximated to Cooper's ligament. To perform these primary tissue repairs, the surgeon must be able to

correctly identify these anatomical structures. In recurrent hernias or where acute inflammation obscures the anatomy, an alternative is to perform a Lichtenstein repair with biologic mesh. However, using biologic mesh will likely result in recurrent hernia as it is incorporated and weakens.

In certain circumstances, a laparotomy may be necessary. If there is any question of bowel compromise during inguinal exploration that cannot be managed through the inguinal incision, a laparotomy should be performed to further inspect the bowel and perform resection. In some cases, intra-abdominal adhesions may be too dense to adequately reduce the hernia through an inguinal incision. When forced to make a laparotomy, a lower midline laparotomy below the umbilicus is usually adequate. With this approach, the operator can choose to enter the peritoneal cavity or stay preperitoneal. Once a laparotomy is performed, it is also possible to perform an open preperitoneal repair, which is useful in recurrent hernias with anterior scarring and distortion of the relevant anatomy.

Postoperative Management

Postoperative care for patients undergoing surgery for incarcerated inguinal hernias is mostly supportive, including correcting lab aberrations, providing intravenous hydration, optimizing pain control, and awaiting the return of bowel function. The period of observation should be dictated by the severity of presenting illness as well as postoperative clinical progression. It is important to avoid the reduction of necrotic bowel into the peritoneal cavity. If this is the case, the patient will likely have continued or worsening bowel obstruction with overall deterioration of the clinical picture. If left untreated, abdominal sepsis will ensue.

Case Conclusion

The patient was taken emergently to the Operating room (OR) for open repair. Portions of the small bowel as well as the sigmoid colon were found to be in a large direct hernia sac. A lower midline laparotomy was made due to the difficulty in reduction of the sac and questionable bowel viability. Once fully reduced, it was apparent that all bowel was viable. Because of the distorted anterior anatomy from previous hernia repair, an open preperitoneal repair with prosthetic mesh was performed through the lower midline incision. An open preperitoneal approach is an excellent option for multiply recurrent hernias where a laparotomy is necessary. We perform our open preperitoneal repair using the same technique described for a laparoscopic approach **(Table 2)**. The patient was monitored in the intensive care unit for the initial resuscitation. His postoperative course was otherwise uncomplicated.

TAKE HOME POINTS

- Suspected incarceration or strangulation mandates immediate surgical intervention.
- The gold standard approach to suspected incarceration or strangulation is groin exploration to assess bowel viability and repair hernia.
- If the hernia cannot be managed through a groin incision, due to questionable bowel viability, intra-abdominal adhesions, or an inability to safely reduce the hernia contents, a lower midline laparotomy should be made.
- When bowel resection is necessary due to strangulation, prosthetic mesh should not be used. Instead, a primary tissue repair (e.g., Bassini or McVay) can be performed.
- Laparoscopic or open preperitoneal approaches can be used for multiply recurrent hernias, but it is essential to ensure viability of hernia contents before proceeding with these techniques.

SUGGESTED READINGS

Eklund AS, Montgomery AK, Rasmussen IC, et al. Low recurrence rate after laparoscopic (TEP) and open (Lichtenstein) inguinal hernia repair: a randomized, multicenter trial with 5-year follow-up. Ann Surg. 2009;249:33–38.

Ferzli G, Shapiro K, Chaudry G, et al. Laparoscopic extraperitoneal approach to acutely incarcerated inguinal hernia. Surg Endosc. 2004;18:228–231.

Kouhia ST, Huttunen R, Silvasti SO, et al. Lichtenstein hernioplasty versus totally extraperitoneal laparoscopic hernioplasty in treatment of recurrent inguinal hernia—a prospective randomized trial. Ann Surg. 2009;249:384–387.

Sevonius D, Gunnarsson U, Nordin P, et al. Repeated groin hernia recurrences. Ann Surg. 2009;249:516–518.

4 Ventral Incisional Hernias

VIVIAN M. SANCHEZ and KAMAL M.F. ITANI

Presentation

A 74-year-old male smoker with diabetes, obesity, and hypertension presents to the outpatient clinic with complaints of intermittent periumbilical abdominal pain of 3 months' duration. The pain is not associated with eating, does not radiate, and is occasionally associated with nausea and emesis. On examination, his vital signs are stable and his body mass index (BMI) is 41. He has a long midline scar with a 5- × 6-cm ventral incisional hernia (VIH) in the periumbilical area (Figure 1). There are no overlying skin changes. The hernia is partially reducible and tender only to deep palpation. He does have loss of abdominal domain. His past surgical history is notable for perforated diverticulitis 5 years prior, requiring emergency colectomy with diverting sigmoid colostomy. His colostomy was reversed 2 years ago and was complicated by a wound infection that healed by secondary intention. The patient is a retired police officer who used to be quite active but has recently been experiencing increased shortness of breath when climbing stairs.

Differential Diagnosis

In patients presenting with a reducible abdominal bulge, it is not difficult to diagnose a VIH, especially with a history of prior abdominal surgery. However, it is important to distinguish ventral hernias from rectus diastasis (i.e., separation of the right and left recti abdominis muscle from the midline), which is a relatively common problem in postpartum women and obese men. Rectus diastasis presents as a symmetric, midline bulge extending from the umbilicus to the xiphoid process. With rectus diastasis, the fascia is intact and therefore there is no need for surgical repair. It is also important to distinguish a reducible or chronically incarcerated ventral hernia from an acutely incarcerated hernia that would require urgent surgery. Patients with acute incarceration may present with bowel obstruction, an acutely tender bulge, or even erythema of the abdominal wall, particularly if they have progressed to strangulation and compromised bowel.

Workup

The patient undergoes workup of his abdominal pain with laboratory studies, flat and upright films of the abdomen, and right upper-quadrant ultrasound. All studies are normal. A CT scan of the abdomen is obtained to further evaluate the pain. The CT reveals a large 5- × 6-cm ventral hernia along the midline (Figure 2). It contains the transverse colon without adjacent stranding or fluid and without a transition point; there are no gallstones or other abnormalities of the biliary system or pancreas.

Diagnosis and Treatment

The patient has a 5- × 6-cm VIH at his prior laparotomy incision. The hernia is reducible and nontender to palpation. Other causes of periumbilical pain such as biliary colic, pancreatitis, and small bowel obstruction are ruled out. Laboratory tests including liver function tests, amylase, and white blood cell counts are normal. Plain abdominal films and RUQ ultrasound were normal. A CT scan did not demonstrate any evidence of a bowel obstruction or other intra-abdominal pathology. It did demonstrate the hernia defect.

The patient is diagnosed with a symptomatic VIH after other etiologies of his symptoms were ruled out. A laparoscopic VIH repair with mesh is planned. The risks and benefits of the procedures were explained. He was further evaluated by medicine for his shortness of breath, history of diabetes, hypertension and smoking, and the possibility of cardiac symptoms. A cardiac stress test was performed which revealed a fixed myocardial defect, no reversible ischemia, and an ejection fraction of 50%. He was started on beta blockers and categorized as a low/intermediate risk for myocardial event after surgery.

Discussion

VIHs are iatrogenic, occurring after laparotomy with an incidence of 2% to 11%. Most (90%) occur within 3 years of laparotomy but can continue to occur over the lifetime of the patient. Followed by small bowel obstruction, VIH is the most common cause of reoperation postlaparotomy. Strangulation or incarceration is the reason for repair in approximately 17% of patients,

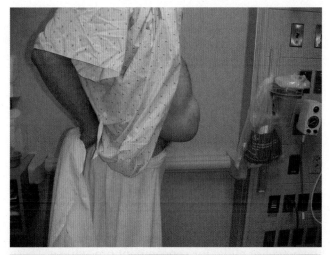

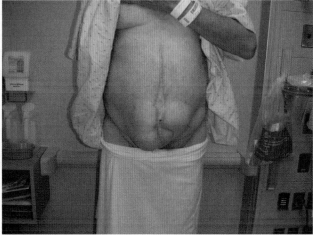

FIGURE 1 • Patient with a previous midline laparotomy an a perumbilical 5-×6-cm ventral incisional hernia.

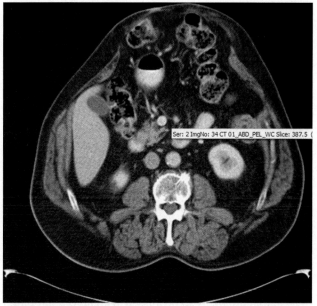

FIGURE 2 • CT scan revealing a large 5- × 6-cm ventral hernia along the midline.

whereas gradual enlargement leading to loss of domain, pain, and other structural abnormalities accounts for the majority of hernia repairs. In the absence of prohibitive medical comorbidities, the presence of a ventral hernia after laparotomy is in itself an indication for VIH repair. More specific indications for repair include the following: (1) bothersome symptoms; (2) bulges affecting the patient's quality of life; (3) hernias with a narrow neck, which are at higher risk for strangulation.

Causes of VIH are multifactorial but most commonly include technical factors during abdominal wall closure, surgical site infections, connective tissue disorders, immunosuppressants, diabetes, obesity or other causes of increased intra-abdominal pressure after surgery, malnourishment, low oxygen tension such as chronic obstructive pulmonary disease (COPD), and smoking. An association with abdominal aortic aneurysms has been described.

This diabetic patient who is also a smoker had an emergency laparotomy in a contaminated field and was therefore at higher risk for developing a VIH.

The utilization of mesh has significantly reduced the recurrence rates of VIH. In a prospective randomized trial of VIH < 6 cm, the recurrence rate was 24% and 43% (at 3 years) and 32% and 63% (at 10 years) for primary repair and repair with mesh, respectively. All current data support the utilization of mesh in VIH repair.

Choice of mesh depends on the surgeon's preference, technique, and contamination. Polypropylene (PP) and extended polytetrafluoroethylene (ePTFE) meshes are the most commonly used types of meshes. PP meshes should not come in contact with bowel, as they can lead to fistulization. Newer generations of PP meshes contain an adhesive barrier or PTFE on the side exposed to bowel to prevent this dreaded complication. Biologic meshes are useful in cases where there is contamination or when the prosthetic material cannot be covered by skin. Although biologic meshes have performed well in short-term follow-up, long-term results are still unavailable.

Open VIH mesh placement techniques include inlay (bridging the defect with mesh), onlay (covering the defect with mesh and fascia overlap), and underlay repair (placing the mesh in a retrorectus position, above the posterior rectus fascia or intraperitoneally with fascia overlap). The underlay technique is the most widely advocated open technique because of lower recurrence rates. The inlay technique carries the highest rates of recurrence. By definition, a laparoscopic VIH repair involves an underlay intraperitoneal mesh placement.

Surgical Repair of Ventral Incisional Hernias

Open Versus Laparoscopic Approach

Recent studies suggest that laparoscopic repair is the favored approach in experienced hands, with some exceptions. Laparoscopic VIH repair has been shown to be associated with less overall complications than open repair, although the complications of laparoscopic repair tend to be more severe. The risks of postoperative surgical site infections and other wound complications are definitely lower with the laparoscopic repair which also results in a shorter hospital stay, and lower costs. The disadvantage of open repair comes from raising large flaps and/or extensive devitalization of soft tissues. Most importantly, there is a trend toward lower recurrence rates with the laparoscopic approach. The laparoscopic approach provides the ability to better visualize and inspect the abdominal wall and detect clinically silent defects that are likely to be missed with an open repair.

In addition, the laparoscopic approach allows for a large intraperitoneal working space that enables repair of multiple and large hernias alike without the need for an extended incision.

Caution must be exercised when considering a laparoscopic VIH repair in patients with severe COPD or low cardiac reserve as these patients are at risk for CO_2 retention and preload reduction/afterload increase, respectively.

The open approach can be beneficial in patients in whom severe adhesions are anticipated or those who have a large loss of domain, making the laparoscopic approach difficult secondary to a lack of working space. In addition, open repair is advocated in patients with incarcerated/strangulated hernias to avoid damage to the bowel or allow for concomitant procedures. These historical contraindications to laparoscopic surgery have become relative contraindications for experienced laparoscopic surgeons **(Table 1)**.

TABLE 1. Key Steps to Laparoscopic Ventral Hernia Repair

1. Enter the abdomen under direct visualization, via an open Hasson technique, or using an optical trocar (after abdomen insufflated with CO_2). If using a Veress needle, perform a saline insufflation test.
2. Place ports lateral enough to allow for at least 4-cm overlap of mesh to fascia.
3. Perform sharp adhesiolysis to free viscera from the abdominal wall. Electrocautery is avoided, if possible, given potential for delayed bowel injury through propagation of electrical current and undetected burns.
4. At least 4 cm of healthy fascia circumferentially around the hernia defect must be exposed.
5. The hernia sac is usually left in place.
6. A spinal needle is used to identify the boundaries of the defect and the defect is measured with low insufflation pressure.
7. There is a growing trend to approximate the fascial edges prior to placement of the mesh in order to medialize the recti the muscles and improve abdominal wall function postoperatively.
8. Select a mesh with minimal adhesions to bowel. In case of prior infection, consider avoiding the utilization of ePTFE.
9. Size the mesh, adding 4 to 5 cm to each side. For example, if a defect is 4 × 10 cm, the mesh should be at least 12 × 18 cm.
10. Place 0 or 1 prolene or PDS sutures in each quadrant of the mesh with knots facing away from the bowel. Mark one surface of the mesh with permanent marker to ensure proper orientation towards the abdominal wall.
11. Roll the mesh tightly around a grasper. Avoid injuring the sutures with the grasper. Insert via a 12-mm port. If unable to insert given the large size of the mesh, remove port and place mesh through skin incision.
12. Roll out the mesh in correct orientation with sutures facing toward the abdominal wall.
13. Make four small 1-mm incisions on the abdominal wall corresponding to sutures placed on the mesh. Pierce the fascia with a suture passer in two different sites via the same skin incision, grasping each end of the suture. Ensure the tip of the suture passer is visualized to minimize potential for bowel injury.
14. After all four transfacial sutures are placed, hold up the mesh to ensure all defects are covered appropriately. The mesh should lie flat, without any tension.
15. If appropriate position, tie each suture.
16. Use a 5-mm circular tacker to secure the mesh at 1- to 2-cm intervals around the periphery, approximately 1 cm from the edge of the mesh. Make a ledge with your hand to cradle the tip prior to deployment.
17. Place more transabdominal sutures every 5 to 6 cm all the way around the mesh.
18. Inspect for intraperitoneal injuries and proper hemostasis.
19. Close any port >10 mm.

Potential Pitfalls

- Hernias close to the bladder require preoperative placement of a Foley catheter. Intraoperatively, the bladder is dissected free and the space of Retzius which is entered by creating a peritoneal flap. The mesh is tacked to Cooper's ligament bilaterally. The Foley is then insufflated with saline to ensure there are no injuries to the bladder.
- Delayed or missed enterotomies occur after laparoscopic VIH repair approximately 1% to 3% of the cases. Every effort should be made to check the bowel prior to closure. Utilization of cautery can lead to burns that may present in a delayed manner and should be minimized or avoided.
- Lack of space to work in patients with large meshes and loss of domain.
- If ports are not placed laterally enough, it becomes difficult to work once the mesh is placed.

Special Intraoperative Considerations

Intraoperative findings that would change management include an intraoperative enterotomy. If diagnosed, the enterotomy needs to be repaired (either open or laparoscopically) and contamination addressed. The amount of spillage and location of injured bowel (small bowel or colon) determines whether mesh will be utilized. In general, if significant bowel spillage is encountered, one could consider utilizing a biologic mesh (open or laparoscopic). Some surgeons have advocated aborting the procedure after repair of the bowel injury, administering antibiotics for few days in the hospital, and then returning within the same hospitalization once the contamination is clear to place a nonbiologic mesh.

Postoperative Management

Many small VIH repairs are performed as outpatient procedures. However, those patients who require extensive adhesiolysis should be observed overnight. Pain control is the most common postoperative issue after laparoscopic VIH repair. Transabdominal sutures can lead to significant pain. Intraoperative utilization of Marcaine and postoperative administration of Toradol should be considered. Seromas are observed very commonly after laparoscopic repair and the vast majority are self-limited and will resolve over time (1 to 3 months). Aspiration of a seroma should be avoided unless the seroma is symptomatic. Aspiration can lead to infection by inoculating the seroma with bacteria. Utilization of abdominal wall binders is advocated to decrease seroma formation but remains unproven. Other possible complications include ileus (2% to 3%), as well as hematoma, trocar site infections, and pulmonary complications.

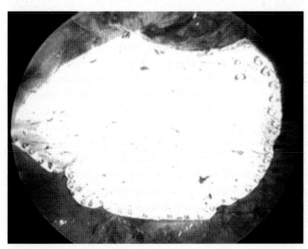

FIGURE 3 • Completed laparoscopic repair.

Case Conclusion

The patient underwent a laparoscopic repair. The adhesions to the anterior abdominal wall were challenging and were carefully taken down. Intraoperative measurement of the defect revealed a 4- × 5-cm defect necessitating a 12- × 15-cm PP composite mesh with an antiadhesion barrier. A total of 12 transabdominal sutures were placed at approximately 6-cm intervals in addition to the tacks at 1-cm interval circumferentially **(Figure 3)**.

The patient was discharged home on the second postoperative day. On follow-up, he was found to have a seroma that was observed and ended up disappearing after 2 months of follow-up. At 2 years, the patient is doing well with no recurrence.

TAKE HOME POINTS

- Incisional hernia is a common complication following laparotomy.
- Repair is usually performed for pain/discomfort and gradual loss of domain more frequently than for incarceration or strangulation.
- The laparoscopic repair is safe, allows the surgeon to visualize most defects, and is associated with lesser wound complications, shorter hospitalizations, and equivalent to lower recurrence rates compared to open repairs.
- At least 4- to 5-cm mesh to fascia overlap is needed to ensure the defect is appropriately covered.
- Avoidance of an enterotomy is critical.

SUGGESTED READINGS

Carlson MA, Frantzides CT, Laguna LE, et al. Minimally invasive ventral herniorrhaphy: an analysis of 6,266 published cases. Hernia. 2008;12:9–22.

Flum DR, Horvath K, Koepsell T. Have outcomes of incisional hernia repair improved with time? A population-based analysis. Ann Surg. 2003;237(1):129–135.

Itani KMF, Hawn MT, eds. Advances in abdominal wall hernia repair. Surg Clin North Am. 2008;88:xvii–xix.

Itani KMF, Hur K, Neumayer L, et al. Comparison of laparoscopic and open repair with mesh for the treatment of ventral incisional hernia: a randomized trial. Arch Surg. 2010;145:322–328.

Luijendijk RW, Hop WCJ, van den Tol MP, et al. A comparison of suture repair with mesh repair for incisional hernia. N Engl J Med. 2000;343(6):392–398.

5 Complex Abdominal Wall Reconstruction

MICHAEL J. ROSEN

Presentation

The patient is a 56-year-old obese (BMI 41 kg/m²) male with a past medical history of hypertension and non–insulin-dependent diabetes. Three years prior to this presentation, he underwent an elective sigmoid colectomy for multiply recurrent sigmoid diverticulitis. He developed a postoperative wound infection and his wound healed by secondary intention. Within 1 year, he noted a bulge along his incision that was becoming increasing uncomfortable. He was noted to have an incisional hernia and underwent elective repair. He was repaired in an open fashion with a 10- × 15-in piece of Composix mesh (Polypropylene and PTFE). He initially did well and was discharged on postoperative day 3. However, on his 2-week postoperative visit, he was noted to have erythema of the wound and purulent drainage. He was explored in the operating room, the wound was opened, the fascia appeared intact, and cultures revealed MRSA. He was placed on a negative pressure wound therapy for approximately 6 months and presents to you with a chronic draining sinus. An abdominal computerized tomography scan reveals fluid around the mesh. The patient reports generalized malaise, denies fevers, and has no erythema on exam. His laboratory evaluation is unremarkable.

Differential Diagnosis

This case presentation considers the workup of a patient with a chronic draining sinus after an open ventral hernia repair with prosthetic mesh. The differential diagnosis of a draining sinus after an open ventral hernia repair depends on the time of presentation. In the early postoperative period, multiple factors can lead to wound issues. Superficial surgical site infections are common and often are a result of skin flora contamination. Deep space infections involving the mesh in the early postoperative period are more concerning. While these are most often associated with prosthetic contamination with skin flora, potential bowel injury and missed enterotomy must be considered. Culture results revealing gram-negative or anaerobic bacteria should raise concern for the surgeon. Patients presenting with chronic draining sinuses many months after open ventral hernia repair often represent some form of an infected foreign body. Occasionally, these can be the result of a suture sinus abscess, and removal of the suture can be curative. Unfortunately, most often this involves contamination of the graft, signaling lack of incorporation, and will not resolve without surgical intervention. If patients present with a draining sinus long after their initial surgery, the possibility of mesh erosion into the viscera should be entertained. Careful evaluation for a fistula is imperative to guide preoperative planning.

Discussion

Abdominal wall reconstruction represents a broad spectrum of disease. Patients can range from those with a small umbilical hernia (<2 cm) up to some of the most challenging reconstructive problems such as patients with massive hernias and an enterocutaneous fistula. The reconstructive surgeon dealing with the full spectrum of these problems must have multiple reconstructive techniques at hand. It is impossible for one procedure or one form of prosthetic to address all of the unique problems these patients can display. This chapter focuses on the complex spectrum of these scenarios. It is important to mention that there is no single definition of a "complex" ventral hernia. In fact, multiple factors can make a ventral hernia complex, and often recognizing these issues preoperatively can avoid potential postoperative morbidity. In general, ventral hernias become complex based on certain patient, defect, and surgical technique characteristics. Patient comorbidities linked to postoperative complications include obesity, smoking, COPD, immunosuppression, malnutrition, and diabetes. Optimization of each of these parameters preoperatively is important for ultimate success of the repair. Complex defect characteristics include the presence of contamination or infection (i.e., infected prosthetic material, enterocutaneous fistulas, or concomitant elective bowel surgery), large defects with substantial tissue loss, massive hernias with loss of abdominal domain (more viscera outside the abdominal cavity than within it), and multiply recurrent hernias with fixed noncompliant abdominal walls. Finally, at times the reconstructive techniques chosen by the surgeon can complicate the repair. For instance, a commonly performed procedure, component separation, typically involves elevation of large subcutaneous flaps that can be associated with wound morbidity of up to 40% in some series. In this chapter, I will address a common clinical scenario of a complex abdominal wall problem: infected prosthetic mesh.

Workup

The initial workup of any patient presenting with problem after surgery is to obtain all operative reports and determine exactly what was done before. It is important to identify what mesh was placed, and in what compartment in the abdominal wall. The management of an onlay mesh can be significantly different than an intraperitoneally placed mesh. Likewise, the composition of the mesh material can have implications in management. For example, macroporous mesh (polypropylene and polyester mesh) can often be salvaged with partial mesh excision. However, microporous mesh (ePTFE, Goretex) can almost never be salvaged and requires complete mesh excision. I obtain an abdominal computerized tomography scan for all patients with complex abdominal wall problems. This imaging test gives important information with regard to whether there is uncontrolled infection (i.e., undrained fluid collections), the size of the mesh, the layer of the abdominal wall where the mesh was placed, whether bowel is involved, and the extent of remaining uninvolved abdominal wall that can be used for eventual reconstruction.

It is never an emergency to remove an infected piece of prosthetic material from the abdominal wall. If there is extensive soft tissue inflammation/erythema, a course of antibiotics is warranted. If there are undrained fluid collections causing systemic inflammatory response, these should be drained surgically or by interventional radiology. Although it is not likely that this will cure the infection, these measures will reduce soft tissue inflammation and preserve these important structures for eventual abdominal wall reconstruction. Appropriate treatment of any skin breakdown is also important. Optimization of nutrition prior to formal abdominal wall reconstruction is paramount. In patients with a chronic nidus of infection it is often impossible to normalize their metabolic profile, but maximizing nutrition is important for a successful result. If a fistula is present, I rarely keep patients NPO unless they are high output and cannot control the effluent with an ostomy appliance.

Diagnosis and Treatment

In this patient, the timing of the early wound infection followed by a chronic draining sinus and the presence of MRSA suggests a deep surgical site infection involving the prosthetic. Given the fact that it is a PTFE-based mesh, complete surgical excision of the graft is warranted. In these situations, it is important to have clear goals between the surgeon and the patient as to what must be accomplished and what would be the ideal situation if possible. After 6 months of conservative therapy, it is not necessary to continue with any other nonoperative measures and the patient should be optimized for resection of the mesh as previously mentioned. The most important principle in managing infection of a prosthetic device regardless of its location, is complete resection of all foreign material whenever possible. Fortunately, in cases of infected microporous mesh, the graft is often not well incorporated and can be easily removed.

When planning the operation, the surgeon will be faced with several potential scenarios. Occasionally, the peritoneal cavity is not violated during resection of the mesh. In this case, I often will leave the wound open, allow it to heal by secondary intention, and perform my formal reconstruction 6 months to 1 year later in a clean field. Alternatively, if the peritoneal cavity is violated, the surgeon must stabilize the abdominal wall. Rapidly absorbable synthetic mesh (Vicryl or Dexon) are reasonable alternatives; however, they often result in very large defects to repair in the future. Single-staged reconstruction with biologic mesh is another alternative. There are multiple products available and it is beyond the scope of this chapter to evaluate these differences, but certain reconstructive principles remain constant. These materials do not function as an interposition graft to prevent hernias. They should be used with advanced reconstructive techniques such as a Rives-Stoppa or component separation to function as a reinforcement of a primary facial repair. When used accordingly they have reported successful reconstructions in up to 80% of contaminated single-staged repairs.

Surgical Approach

As described above, the principles of the operation are to perform complete excision of all prosthetic material. This often requires a full midline laparotomy to expose the entire abdominal wall to ensure complete mesh removal and definitive abdominal wall reconstruction if necessary. Key technical points of the reconstruction are described in **Table 1**.

Component Separation

Begin by performing a complete laparotomy and removing all prosthetic material, and address any

TABLE 1. Key Technical Steps and Potential Pitfalls to Component Separation

1. Remove all prosthetic material, and address any bowel issues as necessary.
2. Perform complete adhesiolysis of the entire anterior abdominal wall to the paracolic gutters to allow muscular components to slide to the midline during reconstruction.
3. Elevate lipocutaneous flaps 2 cm lateral to the linea semilunaris, edge of the rectus muscle.
4. Incise the external oblique fascia and separate the external and internal oblique muscles in their avascular plane.
5. Continue the dissection 3–4 cm above the costal margin, and inferiorly to the inguinal ligament.
6. Release the posterior rectus sheath, 2 cm lateral to the linea semilunaris.
7. Place an appropriately sized biologic graft as an underlay, redistributing tension across the graft to help medialize the rectus complex.
8. Drains placed over the mesh.
9. Midline fascia reapproximated with interrupted figure-of-eight sutures.
10. Remove excess devascularized skin, and close over multiple drains.

Potential Pitfalls

- Not dissecting the adhesions free from the undersurface of the abdominal wall, which prevents the muscular blocks from medializing after release.
- Inadvertent injury to the linea semilunaris, which results in full thickness defect in the lateral abdominal wall and a troublesome hernia to repair.
- Skin flap necrosis from excessive undermining and division of the medial row (periumbilical) perforators.

bowel issues as necessary. Perform a complete adhesiolysis of the entire anterior abdominal wall to the paracolic gutters. This will allow muscular components to mobilize toward the midline during reconstruction. Elevate lipocutaneous flaps 2 cm lateral to the linea semilunaris to the lateral edge of the rectus muscle. Take care to avoid the periumbilical perforators during this mobilization by leaving an "island" of subcutaneous tissue in the middle of the flap. This maneuver will prevent problems with abdominal wall ischemia (Table 1).

Incise the external oblique fascia just lateral to the rectus sheath and separate the external and internal oblique muscles in their avascular plane. Continue the dissection 3 to 4 cm above the costal margin, and inferiorly to the inguinal ligament. Release the posterior rectus sheath, 2 cm lateral to the linea semilunaris. Place an appropriately sized biologic graft as an underlay, redistributing tension across the graft to help medialize the rectus complex. Place closed suction drains over the mesh. Reapproximate the midline fascia with interrupted figure-of-eight sutures.

Remove excess devascularized skin, and close in several layers.

Special Intraoperative Considerations

In certain cases of infected and contaminated abdominal wall reconstruction, the field will be grossly contaminated. It is imperative that appropriate bioburden reduction techniques are employed, including debridement of all devitalized tissue, and copious pulse lavage irrigation of the wound. If the wound cannot be grossly decontaminated, then reconstructive efforts should be postponed. The patients can be placed on dressings for several days and formal reconstruction performed after the wound has been decontaminated.

Postoperative Management

These reconstructive procedures performed in the setting of infection and contaminations are fraught with postoperative wound complications. Recognizing and managing these appropriately is important to eventual success of the operation. In cases of MRSA prosthetic infections, I feel there is often a biofilm present in the wound that cannot be eradicated. Therefore, I place these patients on suppressive antibiotic therapy for at least 6 months after removal of the graft (Bactrim SS QD). I also feel it is important to keep the drains in place in cases of biologic mesh utilization. Despite the term "mesh," these are actually grafts that are often not perforated and therefore are prone to fluid buildup around the graft. This fluid will prevent incorporation and often contains collagenases that will degrade the graft. Therefore, I leave the drains in place for at least 2 weeks in most cases. These reconstructive procedures are also major surgical endeavors and epidurals can help pain management, and most patients should be observed in an intensive care unit setting for the immediate postoperative period.

TAKE HOME POINTS

- Set realistic expectations for the patients and the surgeons about what can actually be accomplished in one setting in these difficult problems.
- Remove all infected prosthetic material whenever possible.
- Single-staged reconstruction of infected and contaminated fields is reasonable in most patients, although it does not always have to be performed. Know when you are in a difficult situation and know when to bail out.
- Optimize patients preoperatively with adequate nutrition, infection control, and preservation of soft tissues.
- Do not wait forever to remove infected synthetic mesh. If the wound is not healed by 3 to 6 months, the prosthetic is almost always infected.

Enterocutaneous Fistula

6

ERIC J. CULBERTSON and MICHAEL G. FRANZ

Presentation

A 61-year-old man with a history of morbid obesity, hypertension, and hiatal hernia repair underwent ventral incisional hernia repair with synthetic mesh 2 years ago. That operation was complicated by infected mesh that was explanted 4 weeks ago. The patient presents now with a nonhealing abdominal wound that for the past few days is draining increasing amounts of foul-smelling fluid. He complains of pain at the wound site and skin irritation from the drainage, but denies fevers, chills, nausea or vomiting, and has a normal appetite and bowel movements. The patient is afebrile and vital signs are normal. He weighs 140 kg (BMI, 38.6). Mucous membranes are noted to be dry. Focused examination reveals a 12 × 12 cm open, granulating wound in the midabdomen with two sinus tracts from which is expressed a thin, foul-smelling, light brown fluid **(Figure 1)**. There is significant abdominal wall laxity at the wound site.

Differential Diagnosis

Postoperative abdominal wound drainage most often signifies the presence of infection, seroma, hematoma, or enterocutaneous fistula. Foul-smelling, purulent discharge in this patient most likely indicates a deep-space wound infection, including possible retained infected mesh, or a gastrointestinal fistula with drainage of bowel contents. The majority of enterocutaneous fistulas develop postoperatively (75% to 85%), following surgery for inflammatory bowel disease (IBD), cancer, or bowel obstruction (i.e., lysis of adhesions). Presentation is usually during the first 5 to 7 postoperative days. Enterocutaneous fistulas may also occur spontaneously (15% to 25%) as a result of radiation, malignancy, or a number of inflammatory conditions including IBD and diverticular disease. Other factors that contribute to fistula development or delay fistula healing include the presence of distal bowel obstruction, foreign body inflammation, infection, irradiated bowel, local malignancy, or antiproliferative drugs **(Table 1)**.

Workup

History and physical examination can be diagnostic. Food or feculent drainage from the wound is diagnostic, as is visible intestinal mucosa. Serum laboratory studies are important to evaluate for signs of infection, electrolyte disturbances, and malnutrition.

The patient in our scenario has normal white blood cell and platelet counts and hemoglobin. Potassium and chloride are somewhat low at 3.4 and 95 mmol/L, respectively; the remainder of the electrolytes are normal, but BUN and creatinine are elevated at 32 and 1.5 mg/dL, respectively. Liver function tests are within normal limits but the albumin is low at 3.0 g/dL. The electrolyte and renal tests indicate that the patient is suffering the effects of fluid loss and dehydration and will need resuscitation. A low albumin suggests that the patient also may be malnourished despite his obesity.

A CT scan of the abdomen and pelvis is conducted to assess for intra-abdominal abscess or other source of deep-space infection. The CT scan will also evaluate for abscess or retained infected mesh and assess the source and anatomy of a possible fistula. The patient in our scenario has no evidence of abscess, infected mesh, inflammation, or wound infection on CT scan. However, there is a loop of bowel that is in close approximation to the skin surface, which may indicate the presence of an enterocutaneous fistula is identified **(Figure 2A)**. A fistulogram, in which the external opening of the fistula tract is cannulated and injected with water-soluble contrast and evaluated by immediate and delayed radiographs, is subsequently performed. This is important to identify the source and location of the fistula and any possible intra-abdominal leakage, as well as to rule out the presence of a distal bowel obstruction, which may keep the fistula open and prevent future closure. In our patient, a fistulogram of the two wound tracts identifies an opening corresponding to an efferent limb of distal small bowel with contrast flowing easily past the ileocecal valve and filling the colon with no evidence of distal obstruction or intra-abdominal leakage **(Figure 2B)**. The other external opening is identified as the afferent bowel limb, which also fills easily without leakage (image not shown).

Diagnosis and Treatment

Based on the imaging studies, the patient in this scenario has an enterocutaneous fistula involving the distal small bowel with two openings corresponding

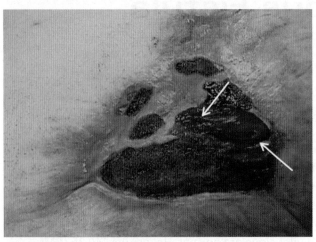

FIGURE 1 • Nonhealing surgical wound with two visible mucosal openings (*white arrows*).

TABLE 1. Factors Associated with Nonhealing Fistulas

FRIENDS Mnemonic:
- **F**oreign body
- **R**adiation
- **I**nflammation/infection
- **E**pithelialization
- **N**eoplasm
- **D**istal obstruction
- **S**teroids or other antiproliferative drugs

to the afferent and efferent bowel limbs, without evidence of distal bowel obstruction or intra-abdominal leakage. Fistula formation is a dreaded surgical complication with mortality of 5% to 20%. Treatment initially beings with replacing fluid and electrolyte losses and controlling infection. Depending on the fistula location and the degree of fistula output, patients may present with profound fluid and electrolyte losses. In the patient in our scenario, lab results suggest that the

patient is dehydrated and hypokalemic and hypochloremic from enteric fluid loss. Resuscitation is begun with intravenous normal saline supplemented with potassium chloride. Although this patient does not show signs of sepsis and no clear infection is seen on CT imaging, patients with fistulas often present with overt infection and sepsis and prompt administration of broad-spectrum antibiotic therapy along with resuscitation is warranted in these cases. Abscesses should be drained either percutaneously or surgically, and in some cases surgical bowel diversion may be necessary. Skin and soft tissue surrounding the injury must also be aggressively protected in anticipation of surgical correction, if necessary.

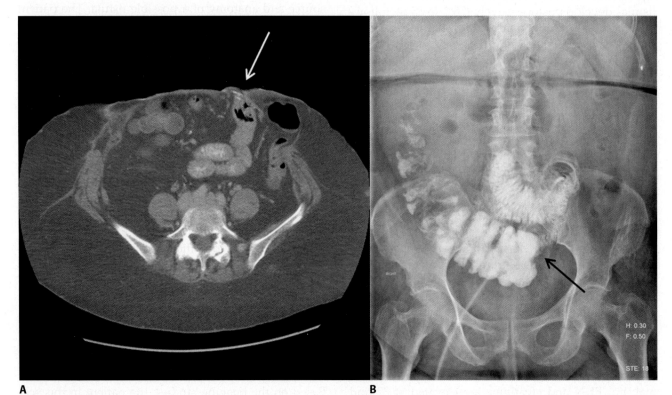

A   **B**

FIGURE 2 • **A:** CT scan demonstrating a loop of small intestine in close approximation to the skin surface constistent with a possible enterocutaneous fistula (*white arrow*). **B:** Fistulogram with contrast flowing past the ileocecal valve (*black arrow*) and filling the colon.

Once the patient is stabilized, and ongoing support established, attention can be turned to managing the fistula output and improving the patient's nutritional status. Patients should be made NPO and parenteral nutrition given to minimize fistula output, restore ongoing fluid and electrolyte losses, and maintain caloric and protein goals to optimize the patient's nutrition and wound-healing capability. Electrolytes and blood sugar should be followed closely and the parenteral nutrition adjusted accordingly. Proton pump inhibitors are given to reduce gastric secretions. Underlying disorders such as IBD should be controlled. Fistula output should be measured or estimated and recorded on a daily basis. The output is classified as either low (<500 mL/d) or high (>500 mL/d). High-output, gastric, duodenal, and ileal fistulas are associated with a lower rate of spontaneous closure, whereas low-output, esophageal, pancreatobiliary, jejunal, and colonic fistulas are more likely to close with conservative management alone. If fistula output remains low after an initial period of NPO status and parenteral nutrition, oral feedings may be attempted, especially for more distal fistulas, and should be adjusted to ensure minimal fistula output. In some cases enteral feedings alone may be possible, although most often parenteral nutrition is required in order to maintain optimal wound healing and readiness for potential surgery. In cases of persistent high fistula output in which it is difficult to maintain adequate fluid intake and electrolyte balance, subcutaneous somatostatin or an analog may be trialed. Somatostatin inhibits gastrointestinal tract secretions and increases intestinal water and electrolyte absorption, and may reduce high fistula output. Our patient is initially made NPO and started on parenteral nutrition. Fistula output remains well below 500 mL/d, and small amounts of supplemental oral liquids and soft foods are permitted for comfort.

Adequate wound care is important but can often be challenging and requires considerable patient education and outpatient management. Assistance of a specialized wound or enterostomal care team can often be helpful but is not always available. Skin barriers (powders, creams, foam, etc.) should be used to protect the skin from irritation. Low-output fistulas may be managed with frequent dressing changes, whereas high-output fistulas usually require an ostomy pouch or a similar device. Another management technique often employed with success is negative pressure wound therapy, which may improve nonsurgical fistula closure rates and manage or close fistulas in patients with contraindications to surgery.

For the patient in our scenario, we chose negative pressure therapy for initial management. A sponge is placed over the entire wound up to the skin edges. Holes are created through the sponge for each fistula opening and rubber catheters passed through. One catheter is advanced into the afferent bowel limb, and the other into the efferent limb. The sponge and catheters are then sealed with clear adhesive sheets and continuous suction applied. In this manner, the skin is protected, fistula output is well controlled and can be accurately recorded, and wound healing is promoted **(Figure 3)**. In the case of a more proximal fistula, tube feedings can be given through a catheter in the efferent bowel limb.

In general, a conservative management approach should be taken for the initial 4 to 6 weeks to assess the possibility of spontaneous fistula closure, which occurs in as many as one-third of cases. After this time, fistulas are unlikely to heal on their own. Patients with small, superficial fistulas or those who are deemed not to be surgical candidates may be considered for fibrin glue treatment of the fistula site for potential closure. Surgical repair is delayed until at least 4 to 6 months, and sometimes up to a year from the time of the most recent abdominal operation to allow for bowel adhesions to soften and to optimize the patient's infectious, nutritional, and wound status.

Surgical Approach

After careful consideration of the timing and patient optimization, surgical repair with the goal of restoring intestinal continuity may be considered **(Table 2)**. Extensive discussion should be had with the patient regarding risks and expected outcomes. Although definitive repair at the initial operation is usually

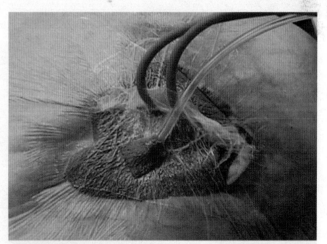

FIGURE 3 • Negative pressure wound therapy device in place on the fistula wound. The two red rubber catheters are placed in the afferent and efferent bowel limbs to control the effluent. The clear tubing applies a vacuum to the black sponge dressing to stabilize the abdominal wall and to promote wound healing. A nonadherent, nonocclusive dressing is placed deep into the wound to protect against further bowel injury. Compulsive wound examinations and adjustments to negative pressure therapy are required for safety and effectiveness.

TABLE 2. Key Technical Steps and Potential Pitfalls to Enterocutaneous Fistula Repair

Key Technical Steps

1. Wait up to 1 year to allow inflammation and intense fibroplasia to resolve.
2. Incision through uninjured abdominal wall.
3. Meticulous dissection and lysis of adhesions to achieve full bowel exposure and eliminate distal obstructions.
4. Remove all foreign body synthetic material to reduce chronic inflammation.
5. Identification and excision of the fistula tract and any involved or pathologic intestine.
6. Careful inspection to insure bowel viability, repair of any bowel injuries, and drainage of any abscesses.
7. If appropriate, primary bowel anastomosis to restore intestinal continuity.
8. Thorough abdominal irrigation.
9. Abdominal wall closure.

Potential Pitfalls

- Enterotomy or other iatrogenic injury.
- Significant bowel resection with <100-cm small intestine remaining, leading to short gut syndrome.
- Presence of significant peritoneal infection or gross spillage during lysis of adhesions and fistulectomy necessitating enterostomy placement.
- Fascial defect requiring use of mesh and/or musculofascial advancement techniques for adequate abdominal closure.

the goal, in many cases a temporary diverting enterostomy is needed to allow for adequate bowel and wound healing, and in some cases the fistula cannot be safely repaired necessitating permanent fistula or enterostomy. Consider marking potential stoma sites prior to surgery. Preoperatively, bowel preparation should be considered and appropriate antibiotic and deep venous thrombosis (DVT) prophylaxis should be given.

It is often advantageous to approach the peritoneum and intra-abdominal organs through a new incision, typically midline above or below previous scars, to minimize the risk of bowel injury due to adhesions to the abdominal wall at prior surgical sites. Meticulous dissection and lysis of adhesions is carried out to expose the peritoneal cavity. Selective adhesiolysis from the ligament of Treitz to the rectum is considered with the goal of preparing bowel for reconstruction and eliminating distal obstructions, and weighed against the risk of further intestinal injury due to injudicious dissection. Any sites of abscess should be drained and thoroughly irrigated. The fistula site is carefully isolated and separated from the abdominal wall **(Figure 4A)**. The fistula tract is excised and segmental resection of any involved bowel is performed using clamps or a stapler with preservation of as much

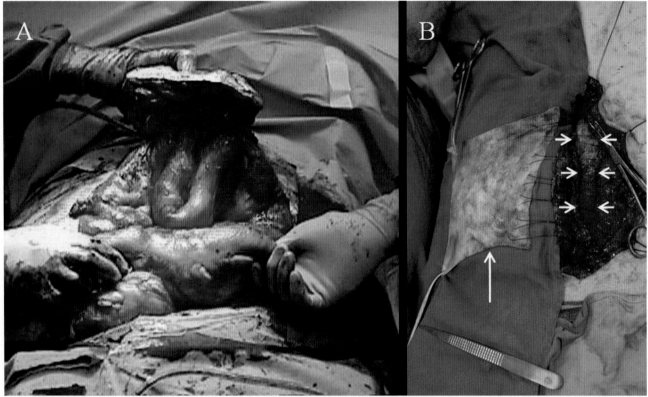

FIGURE 4 • Intraoperative view of an enterocutaneous fistula repair. **A:** After extensive lysis of adhesions, the fistula with involved bowel and abdominal wound are identified and separated from normal intestine and abdominal wall prior to excision. **B:** Human cadaveric dermis (*single white arrow*) is sutured into place with minimized bridging of a remaining fascial defect (*white arrow heads*) after fistula repair.

unaffected bowel as possible. Simple closure of the fistula site alone is associated with a high rate of recurrence. The entire bowel should be inspected along its length and any diseased (such as from IBD, diverticular disease, ischemia, etc.) segments resected. Every effort should be made to preserve at least 100 cm of small intestine to avoid short gut syndrome. If conditions are appropriate and contamination is minimal, bowel continuity can be restored with either a stapled or two-layer hand-sewn primary anastomosis under physiologic tension. Given the extensive adhesions that are often present in these cases, unplanned enterostomy may occur. These should be carefully repaired using absorbable suture and reinspected before abdominal closure to ensure bowel viability and adequate repair. After the fistula has been excised, bowel reanastomosed, other injuries repaired, and bowel reinspected, the abdomen is thoroughly irrigated. The abdominal wall is then closed beginning with the fascia using permanent or slowly absorbing suture. In cases of active wound or peritoneal infection or gross contamination, the skin should be left open and allowed to heal by secondary intention or a delayed-primary closure may be considered.

Special Intraoperative Considerations

If significant intra-abdominal infection is present, gross contamination occurs during the operation, underlying disease processes such as IBD or malignancy are inadequately controlled, or the patient has significant comorbidities, placement of a proximal diverting enterostomy may be necessary to allow distal anastomoses to adequately heal. Placement of a decompressive gastrostomy and feeding jejunostomy should be considered based on patient status and the magnitude of the operation. All patients with fistulas have associated fascial defects (hernias). If the fascial defects are small enough to be closed with minimal tension, the fascia is repaired primarily. Many hernias will require use of mesh, typically an absorbable synthetic mesh or a biologic mesh such as a dermal allograft or xenograft due to the greater risk of recurrent fistulization or mesh infection with permanent synthetic material **(Figure 4B)**. In some cases, musculofascial advancement flaps, such as a components separation procedure, may also be necessary to allow adequate abdominal wall closure. Local cutaneous flaps or skin grafts may be needed to cover areas of extensive skin loss.

Postoperative Management

Ensuring adequate postoperative nutrition is essential for anastomotic and laparotomy wound healing. Parenteral nutrition, if used preoperatively, is continued until the patient is taking an adequate oral diet. Postoperative ileus may require several days to resolve and recovery is assisted with nasogastric tube decompression. Resumption and advancement of an oral diet may be slow, particularly in patients who have not eaten for weeks or months. Antibiotic coverage should be discontinued within 24 hours postoperatively unless there is suspected or documented infection to minimize the risk of antibiotic resistance. Any underlying conditions associated with the fistula formation, such as IBD, should be medically controlled. While in the hospital, the patient's wound should be assessed regularly for signs of infection or fistula recurrence. If an open wound or ostomy is present, the patient should be educated in proper wound and/or stomal care prior to discharge or provided with home nurse visitation. Close outpatient follow-up with regular clinic visits until the wound is well healed is warranted. If a diverting enterostomy was placed at the time of repair, consideration for restoring bowel continuity will depend greatly on individual patient factors but should be delayed for at least 6 to 12 weeks, and longer if possible, to allow the wound to heal, assure that fistulization does not recur, treat inciting disease processes (IBD, malignancy, etc.), and allow adhesions to soften.

Case Conclusion

Our patient is deemed an appropriate surgical candidate following 6 months of negative pressure wound management and parenteral nutrition with oral supplementation. The abdomen was entered through a fresh incision superior to the previous incisions and wound site, extensive adhesiolysis was performed, the bowel was mobilized, and the fistula tract and the involved abdominal wall were excised **(Figure 4A)**. No abscesses or peritoneal contamination were identified and primary anastomosis of the remaining healthy bowel ends after removal of pathologic segments was performed without complication. A residual fascial defect was repaired using human cadaveric dermis **(Figure 4B)**. Parenteral nutrition was continued in the initial postoperative period. The patient was started on a clear liquid diet on postoperative day 6, advanced to soft foods the following day, and parenteral nutrition was discontinued. At the time of most recent follow-up, 1 year after fistula repair, the incision has healed well without signs of fistula recurrence or significant abdominal wall laxity.

TAKE HOME POINTS

- Identify and treat sepsis, dehydration, electrolyte imbalances, and malnutrition, which are frequently seen in these patients.
- Radiologic evaluation with CT imaging and fistulogram aids in identifying potential sources of infection, intestinal obstruction, and delineating the fistula anatomy.
- Parenteral nutrition and NPO status are implemented initially. If the fistula is located distally and output is low, oral feedings may be considered.
- Wound care is rigorous and focused on controlling fistula output, protecting the surrounding skin and soft tissues and promoting wound healing.
- Up to one-third of fistulas will close with nonoperative management. Fistulas that do not close within 4 to 6 weeks are unlikely to do so.
- Fistula repair is delayed for at least 4 to 6 months and up to a year to allow bowel adhesions to soften, treat any underlying disease, and optimize the patient's infectious, nutritional, and wound status.
- Postoperatively, nutritional status should be maintained, and the patient should be followed closely for signs of infection or refistulization until wounds are fully healed.

SUGGESTED READINGS

Berry SM, Fischer JE. Classification and pathophysiology of enterocutaneous fistulas. Surg Clin North Am. 1996;76: 1009–1018.

Draus JM Jr, Huss SA, Harty NJ, et al. Enterocutaneous fistula: are treatments improving? Surgery. 2006;140: 570–576; discussion 576–578.

Evenson AR, Fischer JE. Current management of enterocutaneous fistula. J Gastrointest Surg. 2006;10:455–464.

Gunn LA, Follmar KE, Wong MS, et al. Management of enterocutaneous fistulas using negative-pressure dressings. Ann Plast Surg. 2006;57:621–625.

Martinez JL, Luque-de-Leon E, Mier J, et al. Systematic management of postoperative enterocutaneous fistulas: factors related to outcomes. World J Surg. 2008;32: 436–443; discussion 444.

Schecter WP, Hirshberg A, Chang DS, et al. Enteric fistulas: principles of management. J Am Coll Surg. 2009; 209:484–491.

Torres AJ, Landa JI, Moreno-Azcoita M, et al. Somatostatin in the management of gastrointestinal fistulas. A multicenter trial. Arch Surg. 1992;127:97–99; discussion 100.

Visschers RG, Olde Damink SW, Winkens B, et al. Treatment strategies in 135 consecutive patients with enterocutaneous fistulas. World J Surg. 2008;32:445–453.

Wainstein DE, Fernandez E, Gonzalez D, et al. Treatment of high-output enterocutaneous fistulas with a vacuum-compaction device. A ten-year experience. World J Surg. 2008;32:430–435.

7 Infected Ventral Hernia Mesh

GREGORY ARA DUMANIAN

Presentation

A 55-year-old diabetic smoker with a BMI of 27 kg/m² is referred 4 months after a ventral hernia repair with mesh because he has persistent drainage along the midline of his incision. His surgery was uneventful apart from a serosal tear that was identified and repaired immediately. One month postoperatively, he developed a seroma that was drained in the office, and since that time he has noted drainage and a small opening along the middle of the incision, requiring the use of dressing changes twice daily (**Figure 1**). He is otherwise healthy.

Differential Diagnosis

The differential diagnosis for this patient includes a mesh infection, persistent noninfected seroma, and an enterocutaneous fistula. A distinction should be made between acute and chronic mesh infections. Acute mesh infections are processes with high levels of inflammation, pyogenic bacteria that can invade local tissue, and tissue necrosis. They occur early after a ventral hernia repair and are associated with a stormy postoperative course, reexploration, and prolonged use of antibiotics. The hallmark of chronic mesh infection (colonization) is nonincorporation of the mesh by the soft tissues and fluid collections, but often without the high levels of inflammation in surrounding tissues. Chronic mesh infections are characterized by a more indolent course (>3 months) and associated with persistent fluid collections, drainage, fistula formation, and ultimately mesh extrusion. Both acute and chronic mesh infections will often require mesh excision and reconstruction, but there are subtle differences in the procedure selected for each condition.

Workup

Workup begins with a thorough physical exam, obtaining cultures of the draining fluid, and assessing the patient's wound characteristics for the quality of the surrounding skin (erythema, extent of tissue loss) as well as the quality of the drainage (color, odor, consistency). The wound should be gently probed to determine if the mesh is exposed. Mesh colonization is easy to diagnose when the mesh can be visualized or palpated. If the mesh cannot be felt, a CT scan is warranted and may reveal a fluid collection in close proximity to the mesh, although this alone is not diagnostic of mesh colonization. Oral contrast will locate a fistula if present. Fluid around a colonized foreign body does not necessarily enhance, and therefore IV contrast is not always necessary. Secondary signs of infection including pain, erythema, and a leukocytosis can help distinguish between mesh colonization and persistent noninfected seromas. Sampling of the fluid under radiographic guidance can be helpful in differentiating a sterile seroma from an infection. However, low-grade mesh colonization in patients on suppressive antibiotics may not grow any bacteria.

In our case, polypropylene mesh could be palpated at the base of the wound, which tracks into a large cavity. The surrounding tissues are inflamed and woody over an area of approximately 5 × 8 cm. The drainage is yellow-green tinted, approximately 20 mL per day. His WBC is 13,000 per μL, and blood glucose is 300 mmol/L. The patient is otherwise in good health. A CT scan reveals a fluid collection anterior to the abdominal wall overlying the permanent mesh (**Figure 2**). There are no fistulae visualized. The fluid is drained under radiographic guidance and the culture shows *Staphylococcus aureus*.

Diagnosis and Treatment

The most likely diagnosis for the patient in this scenario is chronic mesh colonization. Patients with chronically infected abdominal wall mesh are best thought of as wound problems. The wounds will resolve when the foreign material is removed. While antibiotics alone on occasion can solve a mesh problem, the biofilms present often cannot be penetrated and the bacteria remain present in a dormant state. Before this patient is taken to surgery, the surgeon must (i) anticipate the abdominal wall integrity after mesh removal, which depends on the type of mesh in place and the timing since the last surgery, and

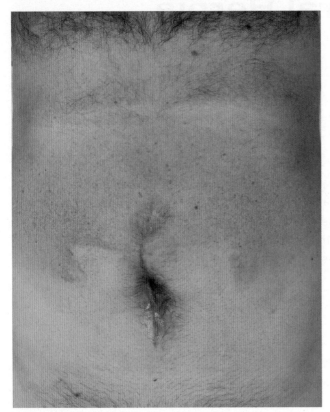

FIGURE 1 • A 55-year-old diabetic smoker, 4 months after ventral hernia repair with polypropylene mesh. The midline draining wound has been present for 3 months.

(ii) assess the patient's overall health status and evaluate the quality of the local tissues.

Abdominal Wall Integrity

The surgeon must anticipate whether or not the mesh can be excised without putting the patient at risk for

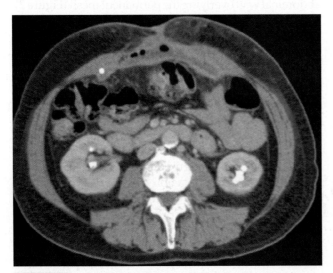

FIGURE 2 • A CT scan reveals a fluid collection anterior to the abdominal wall overlying the permanent mesh.

an evisceration. If the mesh can be excised and scar/granulation tissue is present to hold the bowel within the abdominal cavity, then a wound closure and delayed reconstruction with a plan for hernia repair in the future is the optimal treatment. If removal of the mesh is only possible with a full laparotomy and bowel mobilization, then a one-stage mesh excision and abdominal wall reconstruction is performed. The timing since the last surgery and the type of mesh present will lead the surgeon to one of these two pathways. Within 2 weeks of the initial implantation of the mesh, removal will often necessitate a procedure to prevent evisceration, such as placement of a temporary polyglactin mesh or a bioprosthetic mesh. Both of these materials are not prone to colonization by bacteria like prosthetic mesh. After 3 weeks from implantation, bowel adhesions are typically strong enough to avoid evisceration despite removal of the mesh.

The type of mesh present also dictates what the expected strength of the scar tissue between bowel loops will be after removal of the material. Polytetrafluoroethylene (PTFE) meshes can be removed even 3 weeks after implantation without evisceration, because a fibrous rind develops posterior to the mesh. This rind represents granulated viscera and omentum and has enough structural integrity to prevent a postoperative evisceration after the mesh removal. PTFE meshes are used to decrease the chance of problematic visceral adhesions. Unfortunately, the sheet-like nature of the mesh and the relative lack of tissue ingrowth facilitate the spread of bacteria along the surface of the material when contaminated. While it is theoretically possible to rearrange the soft tissues to provide coverage and help clear infection, this can only be done with early exposures before the development of a bacterial biofilm. In general, all PTFE mesh exposures will require explantation of the mesh and wound closure. The resulting hernia that develops 3 to 6 months later can be treated with a prosthetic mesh in a clean field. Polypropylene or polyester meshes act quite differently than do PTFE meshes, and this is related to the tissue ingrowth that occurs with these materials. If the amount of mesh exposed is small and the majority of mesh appears incorporated, *local excision of visible mesh may be performed, but only by an experienced abdominal wall surgeon* with great care to avoid a bowel injury. Wound contracture of the soft tissues can then occur with local wound care. Larger pieces of exposed polypropylene or polyester mesh must be removed in their entirety. Unlike PTFE meshes, the adhesions between the polypropylene or polyester mesh and the viscera are such that they cannot be stripped out of their location without a formal laparotomy. An associated procedure to prevent evisceration and restore the abdominal wall then becomes a necessity. It is difficult to predict whether composite meshes (comprising both PTFE as adhesion barriers and polypropylene to aid incorporation) will leave behind enough of a rind to contain the abdominal contents. In these situations, both the surgeon and the patient must be ready for the longer mesh dissection and full abdominal wall reconstruction.

Health Status and Quality of Local Tissues

It is imperative for the surgeon to attempt to optimize this patient's nutritional parameters, ensuring tight blood glucose control (history of diabetes), encouraging weight loss (BMI of $27 \text{kg}/\text{m}^2$) and tobacco cessation. Improving these parameters will reduce but not eliminate his risk of wound-healing problems. In general, the inflamed and stiff tissues of a patient with a mesh infection will not hold sutures well and tend not to heal *per primam*. For these patients, a radical *en bloc* excision of the wound and mesh can be performed **(Figures 3–5)**, and the abdominal wall reconstruction performed with noninflamed mobilized lateral tissues (i.e., component separation).

In our case, the patient is informed of the diagnosis and the need for explant of the mesh with single-stage reconstruction using the component separation technique. The possibility of bowel resection, blood transfusion, wound-healing problems, prolonged

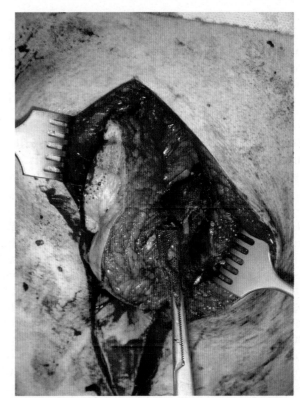

FIGURE 4 • Great care is taken to dissect the polypropylene mesh free from underlying bowel.

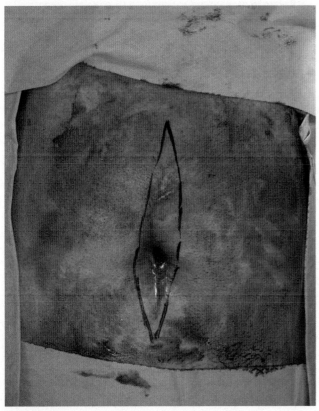

FIGURE 3 • An elliptical incision is marked to encompass the draining wound and surrounding inflamed tissues.

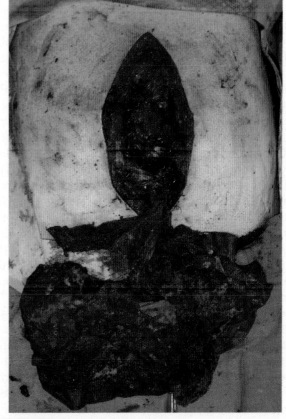

FIGURE 5 • Removal of the polypropylene mesh in its entirety.

hospital stay, and risk of recurrence are explained. An initial incision and drainage in the office is performed to better drain the fluid collection and to temporize the wound until the major procedure is performed. Surgery is scheduled after he has stopped smoking, controlled his blood sugars, and has been cleared by his medical doctor.

Surgical Approach for Mesh Removal and Abdominal Wall Reconstruction

This patient's polypropylene mesh is colonized and must be removed. As discussed above, colonization of a large portion of this type of mesh requires *en bloc* removal with entry into the abdomen and dissection of bowel under direct vision. In the operating room, an elliptical incision is made through the soft tissues to encompass the inflamed soft tissues and mesh **(Figures 3–5)**. A dissecting finger is introduced between the mesh and the medial aspect of the rectus muscles, and Bovie electrocautery is used to divide the tissue and to excise *en bloc* the central inflamed mesh and soft tissues located between the rectus muscles. The omentum and bowel are typically stuck to the undersurface of the mesh. With this inflamed central tissue now elevated out of the abdomen, the viscera are now dissected off the undersurface of the mesh with improved visualization to complete the *en bloc* resection. Pinpoint fistulas may require a bowel excision and resection **(Table 1)**.

The component separation technique is chosen for abdominal wall reconstruction for this patient because it will allow for resection of the chronically inflamed tissue in the midline in exchange for healthy well-vascularized lateral tissue. The components separation technique **(Figures 6–8)** involves dividing the external oblique muscle and fascia from their insertion into the anterior rectus fascia from above the rib cage to near the symphysis pubis to create bilateral myofascial rectus abdominis flaps. Skin vascularity is important in these contaminated wounds. The releases along the semilunar lines can be performed through 6-cm transverse incisions located just inferior to the ribs. This preserves the periumbilical perforators that supply the skin blood flow to the abdominal wall. There is a 20-25% recurrence rate when using the component separation technique in this setting without any supporting mesh. As an alternative to component separation, bioprosthetic mesh alone can be used to restore abdominal wall integrity as a nonvascularized "patch." However, there must be adequate soft tissue coverage for closure over the bioprosthetic. Unless component separation is performed, the tissue used for closure is the undermined medial skin, which is more prone to breakdown. In addition, the long-term integrity of these bioprosthetic meshes is still under great debate.

TABLE 1. Key Technical Steps

1. An elliptical incision is marked in the skin to include the wound bed and surrounding inflamed tissues.
2. Careful dissection is performed to gain entry into the abdomen, assuming the bowel may be adherent to the undersurface of the mesh.
3. The mesh and the overlying scarred tissue are dissected free from the intestines and removed *en bloc*.
4. Releases of the external oblique muscle and fascia are performed through bilateral transverse 6-cm incisions located at the inferior border of the rib cage **(Figure 6A)**. This maintains skin blood flow in the midline by avoiding division of the periumbilical perforators. Tissues over the semilunar line are elevated by blunt dissection.
5. The external oblique muscle and fascia are then divided under direct vision from above the rib cage to the level of the inguinal ligament **(Figures 6B and C)**.
6. The inferior aspect of the release is completed under a small tunnel that joins the lower aspect of the midline laparotomy incision with the lateral dissection.
7. The external oblique is then bluntly dissected off of the internal oblique, allowing the muscles to slide relative to each other.
8. The medial aspect of the rectus muscles sewn together with 0-polypropylene suture, and the incision is closed with vicryl suture and staples over drains.

Potential Pitfalls

- Failure to appreciate the overall health of the patient and optimize his health preoperatively.
- Failure to recognize the risk of evisceration after removal of the colonized polypropylene mesh.
- Failure to prepare the patient for a laparotomy, potential bowel resection, extended hospital stay, and risk of recurrence.

Chronic Seromas with Mesh Present

Chronic fluid collections that do not appear to be infected can occur in association with abdominal wall mesh. Despite a thorough workup, on occasion it cannot be decided preoperatively whether or not there is mesh colonization. For these patients, intraoperative assessment of mesh incorporation must be made. A completely incorporated mesh without a hernia is probably a chronic seroma that can be treated with excision of the bursal cavity and reclosure without the risks of an intra-abdominal procedure. Mesh with areas of wrinkled or nonincorporation associated with a chronic seroma may be better treated with total mesh excision and abdominal wall reconstruction.

Postoperative Management

After a full laparotomy, mesh excision, and reconstruction, a typical hospital stay is 6 to 7 days. An ileus is expected and usually resolves after 4 days, at which point oral food intake can begin. Binders are useful to help compress the skin down to the abdominal wall, but do not prevent hernia recurrences. Drains between the skin and abdominal wall are left in routinely until

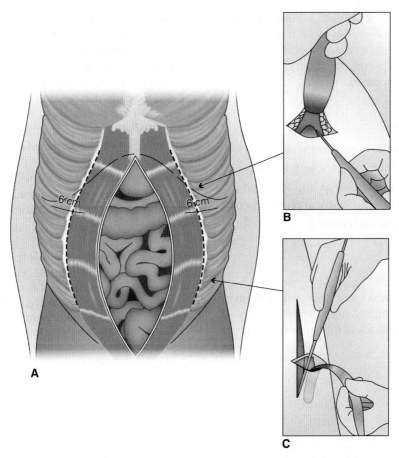

FIGURE 6 • Releases of the external oblique muscle and fascia are performed through bilateral transverse 6-cm incisions located at the inferior border of the rib cage (Figure 6A). The external oblique muscle and fascia are then divided under direct vision from above the rib cage to the level of the inguinal ligament (Figure 6B and C).

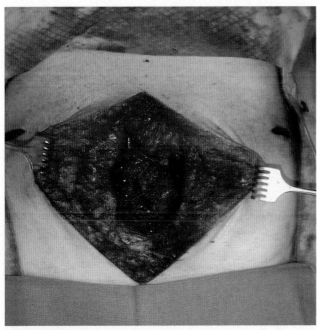

FIGURE 7 • The medial aspect of the rectus muscles are debrided of any nonviable tissue.

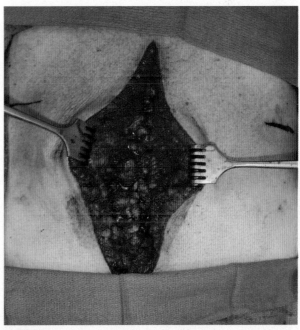

FIGURE 8 • The rectus muscles are brought together easily without tension using 0-polypropylene interrupted sutures.

drainage is < 30 mL over 24 hours. Long-term antibiotics are not necessary when the mesh has been completely removed and *en bloc* excisions of inflamed tissue performed. Routine follow-up for wound healing and hernia formation is performed.

Case Conclusion

The patient tolerates the procedure well. He remains in the hospital for 6 days, and is discharged home without antibiotics and tolerating a general diet. He shows no signs of hernia recurrence at 18 months postoperatively.

TAKE HOME POINTS

- Before treatment, knowledge of the previous surgeries is mandatory. The timing since the last surgery and type of mesh in place will influence the surgery sequence.

- Mesh exposures and infections should be treated with mesh removal. Some of these patients will require simultaneous abdominal wall reconstruction, depending on the integrity of the abdominal wall after removal of the mesh.
- PTFE-based meshes can often be removed and the skin closed primarily over drains. Abdominal wall reconstruction is performed at a later time, when the patient is well nourished and the tissues are soft and pliable.
- Infected polypropylene and polyester meshes often will require a one-stage excision and reconstruction given the loss of abdominal wall integrity after mesh removal.

SUGGESTED READINGS

Ko JH, Wang EC, Salvay DM, et al. Abdominal wall reconstruction: lessons learned from 200 "components separation" procedures. Arch Surg. 2009;144(11):1047–1055.

Szczerba SR, Sukkar SM, Dumanian GA. Definitive surgical treatment of infected or exposed mesh. Ann Surg. 2003;237:437–441.

8 Postoperative Dehiscence

ANGELA M. INGRAHAM and AVERY B. NATHENS

Presentation

A 59-year-old male with a history of type 2 diabetes mellitus, hypertension, and a 30-pack-year smoking history underwent a left colectomy for an obstructing colon cancer. He tolerated the procedure well except for some hypotension in the operating room due to bleeding. On postoperative day 5, he was febrile to 38.7°C, was found to have a white count of 12.3, and was noted to have some erythema of the inferior aspect of the wound for which he was started on cefazolin. On postoperative day 6, he was getting out of bed when he noticed the abrupt onset of copious serosanguineous drainage from the wound.

Fascial dehiscence is the postoperative separation of the reapposed musculoaponeurotic layers of the abdomen. Failure of acute surgical wounds occurs when the load being placed across the wound exceeds the resistive capacity of the suture line and temporary matrix. Surgical wound strength increases rapidly from the first week until the fourth to sixth week postoperatively. At that time, the wound strength is between 50% and 80% of unwounded tissue. Wound strength following this initial postoperative period increases at a slower rate and never achieves the strength of unwounded tissue.

The incidence of postoperative fascial dehiscence varies depending on the study but has been reported to be between 1% and 5%. Despite the advances in antimicrobial prophylaxis, anesthesia, and suture materials, the incidence of this complication has not significantly decreased over time.

Fascial dehiscence is typically recognized within several days of the index procedure. Postoperative fascial dehiscence has been reported between postoperative days 1 and 21 with the average occurrence being on postoperative day 7. Patients often report that "something has given way" or experiencing a "ripping sensation." In 23% to 84% of cases, serosanguineous fluid drains from the wound prior to a dehiscence. Rarely, and most commonly in late fascial dehiscence (>7 to 10 days), the fascia separates while the superficial wound layers remain intact.

Differential Diagnosis

Postoperative fascial dehiscence is easily diagnosed if evisceration is present. On the other end of the spectrum, when evisceration is not the presenting sign, there may be a delay in the recognition of a fascial dehiscence, as the superficial layers of the wound remain intact while there remains a defect in the abdominal wall. Other issues regarding the wound, such as seroma or infection, may make the identification of a postoperative fascial dehiscence more challenging.

Workup

A thorough examination of the wound, potentially including probing a draining wound, is performed. The role of advanced imaging in the diagnosis of fascial dehiscence is limited. However, a CT scan may be useful if the dehiscence is identified late in the postoperative course, a subfascial fluid collection is suspected, and operative management is not planned. The incidence of intra-abdominal infection with fascial dehiscence has been reported to be as high as 44% in some series.

When evaluating a patient for postoperative fascial dehiscence, the risk factors predisposing to the complication should also be considered. Risk factors for fascial dehiscence fall into two broad categories, those related to the patient's comorbidities and those indicative of surgeon technique and decision making.

Patient characteristics identified as predictors of postoperative fascial dehiscence include age >65, wound infection, pulmonary disease, hemodynamic instability, presence of an ostomy within the incision, hypoproteinemia, sepsis, obesity, uremia, use of hyperalimentation, malignancy, ascites, steroid use, and hypertension. In a case control study, patients with five risk factors were reported to have an incidence of 30%, while those with eight or more comorbidities all had postoperative dehiscence.

Although patient factors are important in dehiscence, there are important technical factors to consider. The most common cause of postoperative fascial dehiscence is the suture tearing through fascia. "Bites" of tissue should reapproximate the fascia without impeding perfusion of the healing tissue. Excessive suture tension impedes blood flow causing muscle/fascial necrosis. Failure of the suture to hold occurs in the area just adjacent to the wound edge. In this area, the native tissue integrity is reduced due to proteases, which have been activated during the tissue repair process. Other causes of postoperative fascial dehiscence include a broken suture, a slipped knot, a loose stitch, and excessive travel between stitches. Lastly, whether continuous versus interrupted, closure techniques to decrease the risk of postoperative fascial dehiscence continue to be debated in the literature. A meta-analysis of 23 randomized, controlled studies found that interrupted closure is associated with a significantly decreased risk of dehiscence (Odds ratio: 0.58, $P = 0.014$). However, a second meta-analysis of 15 randomized studies with at least 1 year of follow-up found no difference in the risk of fascial dehiscence using continuous versus interrupted suture. Furthermore, a multicenter randomized trial comparing three parallel groups (interrupted Vicryl, continuous polydioxanone, and continuous Monoplus) found no significant difference in the incidence of fascial dehiscence.

Finally, characteristics of the incision have also been proposed as risk factors for fascial dehiscence, although this remains controversial. Retrospective data have suggested that upper abdominal incisions are at higher risk for dehiscence than those in the lower abdomen. Retrospective data have also found a higher incidence of fascial dehiscence in midline as compared to transverse incisions due to abdominal wall contractions approximating the edges of transverse incisions while separating those of midline incisions.

Diagnosis and Treatment

As fascial dehiscence can be complicated to treat, attention should be directed toward preventing fascial dehiscences and making a prompt diagnosis when appropriate. Surgical techniques that can minimize the incidence of fascial dehiscence include appropriate antibiotic coverage, improved operative technique (minimizing dead space, appropriate use of electrocautery currents in making incisions), controlling intraoperative risk factors (minimizing operative time, avoiding hypothermia), and proper closure technique (appropriate choice of suture material, utilization of drains). Proper suture placement improves bursting strength of abdominal incisions.

Decreased tissue strength along the border of the acute wound has prompted investigations into the identification of an ideal suture length to wound length (SL-to-WL) ratio for primary closure of midline celiotomies. An SL-to-WL ratio of 4:1 reduces the occurrence of fascial dehiscence and incisional hernia formation. This is the basis for the surgical dogma of 1-cm "bites" with progress between bites of 1 cm. The ideal SL-to-WL ratio allows the wound to be approximated with an appropriate amount of tension along the suture line. Increased tension causes the wound to

fail at the suture–native tissue interface. Studies have found no difference in acute fascial wound dehiscence with mass abdominal wall closures versus layered closures. Randomized trials comparing one-layer (peritoneum not reapproximated) and two-layer closures (peritoneum reapproximated) have found no difference in the rate of fascial dehiscence of paramedian and midline incisions.

Surgical Approach

Management of dehiscence follows several surgical principles with customization of the treatment based upon the patient's condition and the available resources. The management of fascial dehiscence must take into account the most probable cause of the complication. Primary closure is acceptable if the cause of the dehiscence was technical in nature and occurred in an otherwise healthy patient. In more complicated patients, options for closure include component release, temporary packing with an overlying plastic silo or packs, use of mesh or bioprosthesis, and skin closure only.

In less complicated cases of fascial dehiscence (i.e., without evisceration), the operative management of fascial dehiscence is dependent upon when the dehiscence occurs in the postoperative course. Dehiscence in the early postoperative period when adhesions are at a minimum potentially warrants immediate operative repair. However, if a dehiscence has occurred later in the postoperative course when new adhesions are more likely to be encountered, the risks of inadvertent enterotomies and fistulas may outweigh the development of a hernia that can be repaired at a later date. When early repair of the dehiscence is pursued, intestinal decompression via a nasogastric tube is often utilized to facilitate closure. The patient is placed under general anesthesia with adequate use of muscle relaxants to minimize abdominal wall tension. The abdomen should be explored to identify any injury related to the dehiscence. Wide debridement of compromised fascia and subcutaneous tissues is carried out. Fascial edges should be debrided back to healthy/bleeding tissue. Debridement should not be compromised due to a concern of having inadequate tissue for closure. If adequate healthy tissue is present and primary closure can be accomplished without tension, the fascia can be primarily repaired. Closure technique (use of internal and external retention sutures and running versus interrupted stitches) is primarily surgeon dependent.

When there is inadequate tissue for primary repair, a mesh closure can be considered. Since most wounds are contaminated, biologic mesh is usually used after acute wound failure. This is especially true for patients with perforation, gross spillage, or intra-abdominal abscess. However, if the fascia cannot be closed primarily, the placement of an absorbable mesh (e.g., polyglycolic acid—Vicryl or Dexon) or a bioprosthesis

(Surgisis or Alloderm) is recommended. Although the use of biologic mesh may result in hernia formation, using prosthetic mesh could result in chronic mesh infection, a dreaded complication. Similar to the use of mesh in elective general surgical cases, when using mesh to treat a fascial dehiscence, an attempt should be made to place omentum between the bowel and the mesh to minimize the development of fistula.

Special Intraoperative Considerations

The intraoperative management of fascial dehiscence is heavily directed by individual patient factors. Due to excessive tension on the wound, primary closure may not be feasible in patients with significant intra-abdominal edema. Closing an abdominal wall under excess tension predisposes the patient to a repeated dehiscence, respiratory compromise, and even compartment syndrome. Therefore, in patients with anasarca or visceral edema, a temporary wound closure, such as the abdominal wound vac, should be considered.

Postoperative Management

Patients whose index surgery was complicated by fascial dehiscence will often require intensive care and will have prolonged hospital stays. It is important to note that the same comorbidities that placed the patient at risk for fascial dehiscence predispose them to developing other postsurgical complications.

After closure of a fascial dehiscence, particular attention should be paid to modifying risk factors to prevent repeat dehiscence. Patients should be educated regarding their postoperative surgical and wound care. They should be instructed to avoid straining and heavy lifting for a minimum of 6 weeks. An abdominal binder is often prescribed to reduce tension of the wound. Finally, the patient's nutritional status should be optimized to promote healing **(Table 1)**.

TABLE 1. Key Technical Steps and Potential Pitfalls

Key Technical Steps
1. Debride nonviable fascia.
2. Maintain a suture length to wound length ratio of 4:1.
3. One-centimeter "bites" with 1-cm travel between bites
4. Reinforce wound with biologic mesh if necessary to achieve tension-free closure.
5. Consider temporary abdominal closure for patients at risk for abdominal compartment syndrome.

Potential Pitfalls
- Inadequate wound debridement due to a concern of not being able to primarily close the wound.
- Excessive tension on the wound as this promotes fascial necrosis.

Case Conclusion

The patient's wound was opened at the bedside. Examination of the wound revealed an approximately 10-cm area where the fascia had dehisced and the suture had torn through the fascia. The patient was taken back to the operating room emergently. No visceral injuries from the fascial dehiscence were identified. After debridement of some of the fascial edges, the musculoaponeurotic layer was reapproximated without tension using interrupted, figure of eight stitches with 0-Prolene suture, paying special attention to suture placement. The superficial wound was packed with moist gauze.

TAKE HOME POINTS
- The incidence of postoperative fascial dehiscence has not decreased significantly despite advances in surgical care.
- Both patient- and surgeon-dependent factors contribute to postoperative fascial dehiscence.
- Emphasis on appropriate surgical technique will decrease the modifiable risk of fascial dehiscence.

SUGGESTED READINGS

Carlson MA. Acute wound failure. Surg Clin North Am. 1997;77(3):607–636.

Cliby WA. Abdominal incision wound breakdown. Clin Obstet Gynecol. 2002;45(2):507–517.

Diener MK, Voss S, Jensen K, et al. Elective midline laparotomy closure: the INLINE systematic review and meta-analysis. Ann Surg. 2010;251(5):843–856.

Dubay DA, Franz MG. Acute wound healing: the biology of acute wound failure. Surg Clin North Am. 2003;83(3):463–481.

Graham DJ, Stevenson JT, McHenry CR. The association of intra-abdominal infection and abdominal wound dehiscence. Am Surg. 64(7):660–665.

Gupta H, Srivastava A, Menon GR, et al. Comparison of interrupted versus continuous closure in abdominal wound repair: a meta-analysis of 23 trials. Asian J Surg. 2008;31(3):104–114.

Seiler CM, Bruckner T, Diener MK, et al. Interrupted or continuous slowly absorbable sutures for closure of primary elective midline abdominal incisions: a multicenter randomized trial. Ann Surg. 2009;249(4):576–582.

van 't Riet M, Steyerberg EW, Nellensteyn J, et al. Meta-analysis of techniques for closure of midline abdominal incisions. Br J Surg. 2002;89(11):1350–1356.

Webster C, Neumayer L, Smout R, et al. Prognostic models of abdominal wound dehiscence after laparotomy. J Surg Res. 2003;109(2):130–137.

9 Splenectomy for Hematologic Disease

JOHN F. SWEENEY

Presentation

A 44-year-old female presented to her primary care doctor several months ago complaining of a recent onset of easy bruising and gum bleeding. A CBC demonstrated a platelet count <10 × 10⁹/L. She was diagnosed with immune thrombocytopenic purpura (ITP) and admitted to the hospital for treatment. She was started on high-dose intravenous immunoglobulin and high-dose corticosteroids with an excellent response in her platelet count. She was discharged home on a gradual prednisone taper. As her prednisone doses were weaned below 20 mg per day, the patient experienced a recurrence in her thrombocytopenia with associated recurrence of easy bruising.

Differential Diagnosis

Excluding trauma, benign hematologic diseases are the most common indication for splenectomy **(Table 1)**. ITP is the most common indication for splenectomy and constitutes >70% of patients undergoing splenectomy for benign disease. ITP is a disorder characterized by antiplatelet antibodies to platelet membrane glycoprotein. This results in opsonization of platelets and their premature removal from the circulation by the spleen. Adult patients typically present with petechiae, purpura, and bruising tendency. Mucosal bleeding, including epistaxis and hematuria, tend to be more frequent when the platelet count decreases to <20 × 10⁹/L. The incidence of severe bleeding (e.g., intracranial hemorrhage) increases with platelet counts below 10 × 10⁹/L.

Additional benign hematologic conditions that are indications for splenectomy include patients with congenital hemolytic anemia, metabolism abnormalities, hemoglobinopathies, and erythrocyte structure abnormalities (e.g., hereditary spherocytosis and elliptocytosis). Splenectomy may be indicated as a diagnostic tool or for palliation in patients with malignant hematologic disease. Surgical staging is utilized most often in Hodgkin's disease, resulting in a change in diagnosis and subsequent impact on therapy and prognosis in up to 30% to 40% of patients. Splenectomy can also provide relief to patients with symptomatic splenomegaly, which may or may not be accompanied by hypersplenism. Patients with malignant hematologic diseases are more likely to have massively enlarged spleens (>1,000 g), resulting in significant discomfort and pain as well as early satiety. When splenomegaly is accompanied by cytopenias (hypersplenism), the cytopenia often improved or sometimes cured by removal of the spleen.

Workup

Although the presumptive diagnosis is ITP, the patient undergoes a bone marrow aspirate that demonstrates normal marrow cellularity with specific mention of adequate megakaryocytes. Review of the peripheral blood smear does not demonstrate platelet clumping.

Discussion

First-line therapy for ITP includes oral corticosteroids and IV immunoglobulin. The majority of patients will initially respond to medical management of ITP, but recurrent thrombocytopenia is common. The indication and timing of splenectomy is often individualized according to response to treatment and patient and physician preferences. Splenectomy is indicated for ITP in patients with episodes of severe bleeding related to thrombocytopenia, patients who fail to respond to 4 to 6 weeks of medical therapy, patients who require toxic doses of immunosuppressive medications to achieve remission, or patients who relapse following an initial response to steroids. Patients with ITP are ideal candidates for a minimally invasive approach because they are frequently young, otherwise healthy patients with normal to only slightly enlarged spleens.

Technique for Laparoscopic Splenectomy

Removal of the spleen laparoscopically is facilitated by the fact that the anatomic landmarks are relatively consistent, the operation is extirpative and does not require reconstruction, and in most cases the spleen does not need to be preserved for pathology so it can be morcellated in the abdominal cavity prior to

TABLE 1. Hematologic Indications for Splenectomy

Diagnosis	Incidence
Benign	
Immune thrombocytopenic purpura (ITP)	21%–68%
Thrombocytopenic thrombotic purpura (TTP)	2%–6%
Hereditary spherocytosis	4%–13%
Autoimmune hemolytic anemia	3%–10%
Evan's syndrome	1%
Hemoglobinopathies	1%
Sickle cell anemia	
Beta-Thalassemia	
Hemoglobin S/C disease	
Malignant	
Lymphoma	10%–55%
Hodgkin's disease	
Non-Hodgkin's lymphoma	
Leukemia	7%–10%
Chronic lymphocytic leukemia	
Chronic myelogenous leukemia	
Hairy cell leukemia	3%–6%
Other	
Myeloproliferative disorders (myelofibrosis)	
Idiopathic hypersplenism	
Sarcoidosis	
Splenomegaly with portal hypertension	
Splenic tumor/cyst	

TABLE 2. Key Steps for Laparoscopic Splenectomy

1. Patient positioned in modified right lateral decubitus position.
2. Abdominal access via open Hasson technique with 12-mm trocar ~ 3–4 cm below the left costal margin in the midclavicular line.
3. Two 5-mm trocars are placed along the costal margin between xiphoid process and Hasson trocar.
4. Divide the splenocolic ligament and mobilize of the splenic flexure caudad.
5. Additional 12-mm trocar is placed in the left anterior axillary line below the costal margin.
6. The short gastric vessels are divided in their entirety up to the level of the superior pole of the spleen.
7. Mobilize inferior pole of the spleen by dividing splenorenal ligament.
8. Mobilize the superior pole of the spleen to isolate the splenic hilum.
9. The splenic hilar vessels are divided with an endoscopic stapler.
10. Spleen is placed in endobag, which is exteriorized through the Hasson trocar site so the spleen can be morcellated.
11. Upon completion, the abdomen is then reinspected laparoscopically to ensure hemostasis.
12. All ports are withdrawn under direct vision. The lateral 12-mm port is closed with absorbable suture using an endoclose device, and the Hasson Trocar site is close in layers with absorbable sutures.

Potential Pitfalls
- Injury to the splenic artery or vein results in significant and rapid blood loss, mandating conversion to HALS or open splenectomy.
- Injury to the short gastric vessels results in significant and rapid blood loss; if not controlled quickly, mandates conversion to HALS or open splenectomy.
- Injury to the tail of the pancreas leads to pancreatic leak, with resulting pancreatitis, pancreatic abscess, or pancreatic fistula.

removal **(Table 2)**. Laparoscopic splenectomy (LS) has been shown in several retrospective studies to have equivalent or superior short- and long-term outcomes when compared to open splenectomy.

Preoperative Preparation

The patient's preoperative preparation includes administration of polyvalent pneumococcal vaccine at least 2 weeks before surgery. The evening before surgery, patients commence a clear liquid diet and take a mild laxative several hours before bedtime to decompress the colon and facilitate laparoscopic visualization of the left upper quadrant and spleen. Several units of packed red blood cells are crossmatched, and in patients with idiopathic thrombocytopenic purpura, platelets are crossmatched for administration after the splenic artery has been ligated intraoperatively if there is failure of clot formation.

Immediately preoperatively, pneumatic compression boots are applied and a preoperative antibiotic (1 gs cephazolin) is given. Patients who have been receiving corticosteroids within 6 months of surgery are given stress doses of intravenous corticosteroids. Before transport to the operating room, a beanbag-stabilizing device is placed on the operating table to enable subsequent patient positioning and stabilization. After endotracheal induction of general anesthesia, a Foley catheter and an orogastric tube are placed.

The patient is positioned in the incomplete right lateral decubitus position at an angle of 45°. This allows the patient's position to be changed from nearly supine to nearly lateral by tilting the operating table. In this way, a combined supine and lateral approach can be realized. It is important to position the patient with the iliac crest immediately over the table's kidney rest and mid–break point. The kidney rest is elevated and the table flexed, allowing more distance between the iliac crest and the left lower costal margin in the midaxillary line. The beanbag-stabilizing device is activated, and the patient's hip is secured to the table with loosely applied tape. Legs are padded with pillows, and an axillary roll is placed. The left arm is hung over the chest on a sling. The arm must be far enough cephalad to clear the operative field and allow obstruction-free use of the laparoscopic instruments. All pressure points are adequately padded.

The skin is prepared and draped so that either laparoscopy or open surgery can be performed. The table is tilted 30° to the left to place the patient in the near-supine position. Before incisions are made, the area is anesthetized with long-lasting local anesthetic.

Laparoscopic Splenectomy

We prefer to obtain intra-abdominal access via an open technique with placement of a 12-mm Hasson trocar approximately 3 to 4 cm below the costal margin in the left midclavicular line **(Figure 1A)**. The abdomen is then insufflated to a pressure of 15 mm Hg with carbon dioxide and a 10-mm, 30° laparoscope is introduced into the abdomen. Two 5-mm trocars are then placed in the upper midline or to the left of the midline along the costal margin. The first 5-mm trocar is placed 3 to 4 cm below the xiphoid process and the second trocar is placed in between the subxiphoid 5-mm trocar and the Hasson trocar. The abdomen is inspected with special attention paid to the greater omentum and splenocolic regions that are common locations for

● 5 mm   ● 12 mm

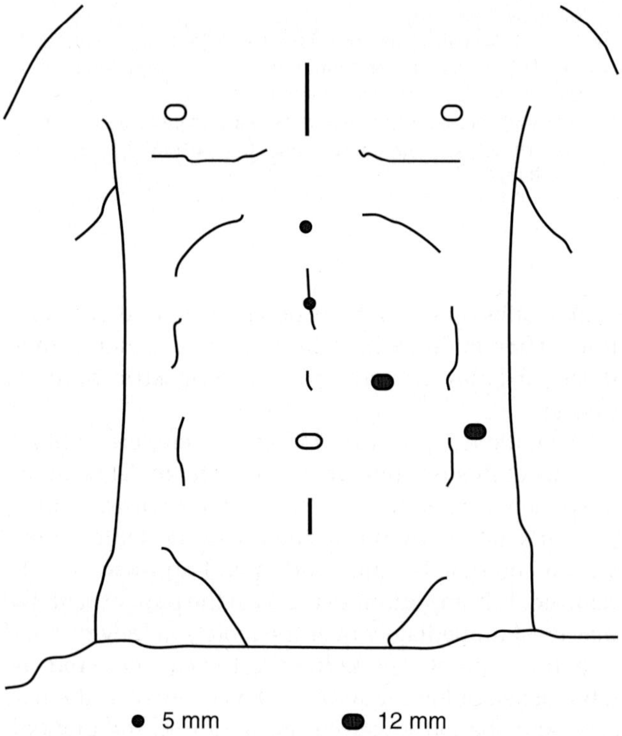

A

FIGURE 1A • Laparoscopic Splenectomy Port Placement.

accessory splenic tissue. Accessory spleens are found in 10% to 15% of patients with hematologic disease and have been associated disease recurrence in patients with ITP when they are not removed.

Following division of the splenocolic ligament and mobilization of the splenic flexure, an additional 12-mm trocar is placed in the left anterior axillary line, below the costal margin. The patient is then placed in steep reverse Trendelenburg position and the table rolled to the patient's right giving a true left lateral decubitus position. Ultrasonic shears are used to divide the gastrosplenic ligament and short gastric blood vessels, allowing the stomach to fall to the patient's right and providing excellent exposure to the splenic hilum. The splenic artery can then be easily identified and ligated with hemoclips if desired at this point of the case. Attention is then turned toward mobilization of the lower pole of the spleen. The splenophrenic and the splenorenal ligaments are divided using ultrasonic shears. If a lower pole vessel is encountered at this point, it is divided using an endoscopic stapling device with a vascular cartridge. This approach allows for visualization of the splenic hilum and the tail of the pancreas by retracting the spleen toward the abdominal wall. The superior splenophrenic attachments to the upper pole of the spleen are left intact to prevent torsion of the spleen during division of the hilum. The endoscopic stapling device with a vascular cartridge is then used to divide the well-exposed splenic hilum. Several fires of the stapler may be necessary. Following division of the remaining upper pole attachments, the spleen is placed into a specimen retrieval bag. The mouth of the bag is brought through the 12-mm Hasson trocar site, and the spleen is then morcellated with sponge forceps and removed in pieces. Special care must be taken to avoid ripping the endoscopic bag during this process in order to prevent spillage of splenic tissue in the abdomen. The left upper quadrant is irrigated and inspected for hemostasis. A second search for accessory splenic tissue is undertaken before the 12-mm fascial openings are securely closed with absorbable suture and the skin incisions are closed. The orogastric tube is removed in the operating room, and the patient is taken to the recovery room.

Hand-assisted Laparoscopic Splenectomy

The LS can be converted to hand-assisted laparoscopic splenectomy (HALS) if difficult anatomy, dense adhesions due to a previous upper abdominal surgery or excessive splenomegaly, is encountered. Preoperatively, the decision to proceed with HALS is made for patients with very large spleens or if the spleen must be removed intact for pathologic examination. When HALS is indicated preoperatively, we still place all trocars as described for a LS and proceed with division of the gastrosplenic ligament and short gastric blood vessels **(Table 3)**. This provides excellent exposure to the splenic hilum and allows for early ligation of the splenic artery, which we feel is an essential step in patients with significant splenomegaly. We then create an incision connecting the

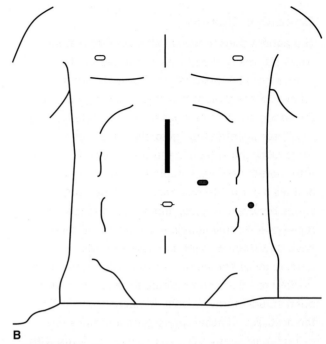

B

FIGURE 1B • Hand-assisted Laparoscopic Splenectomy (HALS) Port Placement.

TABLE 3. Key Steps for Hand-assisted Laparoscopic Splenectomy

1. Patient is positioned in modified right lateral decubitus position.
2. Abdominal access via open Hasson technique with 12-mm trocar ~ 3–4 cm below the left costal margin in the midclavicular line.
3. Two 5-mm trocars are placed in the paramedian position ~ 7–8 cm apart with the first being just below xiphoid process.
4. Divide the splenocolic ligament and mobilize of the splenic flexure caudad.
5. Additional 12-mm trocar is placed in the left anterior axillary line below the costal margin.
6. The short gastric vessels are divided in their entirety up to the level of the superior pole of the spleen.
7. Connect the 5-mm skin incisions and open the subcutaneous tissue and fascia.
8. Place hand port. Utilize left hand to protect and retract the spleen and the right hand to use dissecting instruments.
9. Mobilize inferior pole of the spleen by dividing splenorenal ligament.
10. Mobilize the superior pole of the spleen to isolate the splenic hilum.
11. The splenic hilar vessels are divided with an endoscopic stapler.
12. Spleen placed in large endobag or sterile x-ray cassette cover and exteriorized through the hand-port site, so the spleen can be morcellated or removed in its entirety.
13. Close hand-port site with heavy monofilament suture. Upon completion, the abdomen is then reinspected laparoscopically to ensure hemostasis. All ports are withdrawn under direct vision. The lateral 12-mm port is closed with absorbable suture using an endoclose device and the Hasson Trocar site is close in layers with absorbable sutures.

Potential Pitfalls

- Injury to the splenic artery or vein results in significant and rapid blood loss, mandating conversion to HALS or open splenectomy.
- Injury to the short gastric vessels results in significant and rapid blood loss; if not controlled quickly, mandates conversion to HALS or open splenectomy.
- Injury to the tail of the pancreas leads to pancreatic leak, with resulting pancreatitis, pancreatic abscess, or pancreatic fistula.
- Hand-port site at increased risk for development of Incisional hernia over time.

two 5-mm trocars about 7 cm in size in the left paramedian position **(Figure 1B)**. The left hand is then placed into the abdomen, which is then reinsufflated. There are several commercially available hand-port devices that can be used for HALS. The spleen is then mobilized as described for a total LS with the left hand providing gentle traction while at the same time preventing injury to the splenic capsule by the ultrasonic shears or a laparoscopic grasper. After the splenic hilum is divided and the spleen completely mobilized, it is placed in a specimen retrieval bag. A sterile radiograph cassette bag can be placed in the abdomen through the hand incision to retrieve those spleens that do not fit in the large specimen retrieval bags. The fascia is closed with appropriate strength suture and the abdomen then reinsuflated and inspected for hemostasis as described above.

Postoperative Care

Postoperatively, the patient is allowed clear liquids orally and ambulates the night of surgery. The Foley catheter is removed the following morning. Pain is controlled with intermittent parenteral narcotics until the patient is able to take oral pain medication. Diet is advanced on postoperative day 1, and the patient is discharged when oral intake is tolerated and pain is controlled with oral analgesics usually on postoperative day 2.

Case Conclusion

The patient does very well after LS. Her platelet count returns to the normal range before discharge from the hospital. At 6- and 12-month follow-up, the patient has no clinical evidence of thrombocytopenia and has normal platelet counts.

LS has become the "gold standard" for removal of the spleen in the setting of ITP. Although the increase in platelet number that defines a complete response to splenectomy varies between studies, numerous retrospective reviews and prospective nonrandomized trials have determined that the response rates (80% to 89%) and long-term remission rates (50% to 70%) to LS are comparable to those following open splenectomy, despite initial concern about the accuracy of accessory spleen identification using laparoscopy. LS also provides patients with improved short-term morbidity. Reductions in postoperative morbidity characteristic of minimally invasive procedures such as reduced length of hospital stay and reduced postoperative ileus have been consistently demonstrated in patients with ITP who undergo LS.

TAKE HOME POINTS

- Immune thrombocytopenic purpura (ITP) is the most common indication for splenectomy excluding trauma.
- Splenectomy is indicated for treatment of ITP in patients with episodes of severe bleeding related to thrombocytopenia, patients who fail to respond to 4 to 6 weeks of medical therapy, patients who require toxic doses of immunosuppressive medications to achieve remission, or patients who relapse following an initial response to steroids.
- Laparoscopic splenectomy (LS) is the optimal approach for removal of the spleen in the setting of ITP. It is associated with a shorter hospital stay, decreased postoperative pain, and earlier return to regular activities.
- Accessory spleens are found in 10% to 15% of patients and if not removed at the time of splenectomy will lead to recurrence of ITP.
- LS for ITP is associated with short-term response rates of 80% to 89% and complete long-term remission rates of 50% to 70% that are compatible with outcomes for open splenectomy.

SUGGESTED READINGS

Bresler L, Guerci A, Brunaud L, et al. Laparoscopic splenectomy for idiopathic thrombocytopenic purpura: outcome and long-term results. World J Surg. 2002;26:111–114.

Brunt LM, Langer JC, Quasebarth MA, et al. Comparative analysis of laparoscopic versus open splenectomy. Am J Surg. 1996;172:596–599;discussion 599–601.

Friedman RL, Fallas MJ, Carroll BJ, et al. Laparoscopic splenectomy for ITP. The gold standard. Surg Endosc. 1996;10:991–995.

Mikhael J, Northridge K, Lindquist K, et al. Short-term and long-term failure of laparoscopic splenectomy in adult immune thrombocytopenic purpura patients: a systematic review. Am J Hematol. 2009;84(11):743–748.

Rescorla FJ, Engum SA, West KW, et al. Laparoscopic splenectomy has become the gold standard in children. Am Surg. 2002;68:297–301;discussion 301–302.

Targarona EM, Espert JJ, Cerdan G, et al. Effect of spleen size on splenectomy outcome. A comparison of open and laparoscopic surgery. Surg Endosc. 1999;13:559–562.

10 Acute Appendicitis

SARAH E. GREER and SAMUEL R.G. FINLAYSON

Presentation

A 24-year-old woman presents to the emergency department with abdominal pain, nausea, vomiting, and anorexia that began the previous evening. She describes her abdominal pain as initially periumbilical, but now localized to the right lower quadrant (RLQ). Her temperature is 37.9. Her vital signs are otherwise normal. On abdominal exam, her abdomen is soft and nondistended, but tender to palpation over McBurney's point. She has no signs of peritonitis.

Differential Diagnosis

In the United States, acute appendicitis is the most common time-sensitive surgical problem. The signs and symptoms of acute appendicitis are believed to develop as a result of obstruction of the appendiceal lumen. This obstruction leads to bacterial proliferation, which can result in appendiceal necrosis and perforation.

While the classic symptoms of abdominal pain migrating to the RLQ, nausea, and anorexia occur in a majority of patients with acute appendicitis, symptoms may be less specific, requiring clinicians to consider a broad differential diagnosis, including gastrointestinal, urologic, and gynecologic pathology. Alternative gastrointestinal diagnoses that must be considered include gastroenteritis, colitis, ileitis, diverticulitis, and inflammatory bowel disease. Infectious causes, such as mesenteric adenitis, urinary tract infection, and pyelonephritis, should also be considered. In women, it is important to include Mittleschmirz, salpingitis, tuboovarian abscess, ovarian torsion, and ruptured ovarian cyst in the differential diagnosis.

Workup

A full history and physical exam must be performed to help establish the diagnosis. In addition to eliciting a history of symptoms and their temporal evolution, the surgeon should ask the patient about any family history of inflammatory bowel disease and a complete menstrual and pregnancy history in women.

On physical exam, pain over McBurney's point (one-third the distance from the anterior superior iliac spine to the umbilicus) is a classic presenting sign of acute appendicitis. Additional physical exam findings may suggest appendicitis as a diagnosis. *Rovsing's sign* is pain in the RLQ when pressure is applied in the left lower quadrant (LLQ); an obturator sign is pain with passive rotation of the flexed right hip; and a psoas sign describes pain on extension of the right hip, the latter commonly present in patients with a retrocecal appendix that lies in contact with the iliopsoas muscle. A pelvic exam in women of childbearing age must not be omitted, as it may reveal gynecologic conditions to which the patient's symptoms can be attributed.

Laboratory tests that should be obtained include a complete blood count, which will typically reveal a low-grade leukocytosis. Other laboratory tests that should be ordered include a coagulation profile, type and screen (if an operation is anticipated), and a urinalysis to exclude urinary pathology. A pregnancy test should also be performed in women of childbearing age.

In the patient above, pelvic exam reveals no adnexal mass or cervical motion tenderness. Laboratory evaluation reveals a leukocytosis of 16,000. The patient is otherwise healthy, with no history of previous abdominal surgery and no pertinent family history.

Diagnostic Imaging

In young males with symptoms and signs consistent with acute appendicitis, imaging studies to confirm the diagnosis are generally unnecessary prior to proceeding to surgery. In many cases, however, when the diagnosis is not clear after thorough history taking and physical examination, imaging may be helpful in making the decision whether or not to proceed with surgery. Many clinicians are more liberal in the use of imaging in young female patients, both because of the presence of gynecologic conditions in the differential diagnosis and because of the risk of infertility associated with ruptured appendicitis that might result from a delay in diagnosis.

The two most common imaging modalities used in the diagnosis of appendicitis are ultrasound and computed tomography (CT). CT has demonstrated significantly higher sensitivity for the diagnosis of appendicitis, 94% versus 83% to 88%. However, because CT scans expose patients to ionizing radiation, this modality should be used judiciously, especially in children.

Although CT scans are an expensive technology, a focused contrast CT scan limited to the appendix may actually be cost saving. A study by Rao et al. found that routine appendix-focused CT in patients with suspected appendicitis prevented unnecessary appendectomies as well as unnecessary hospitalization for observation, with a net reduction in use of hospital resources and cost per patient.

In the patient in this case, a CT scan was performed that demonstrates a dilated, thickened appendix with surrounding inflammatory changes, consistent with acute appendicitis (Figure 1).

Diagnosis and Treatment

Although a few studies in the surgical literature support nonoperative management of nonperforated acute appendicitis, surgical appendectomy represents the standard of care in the United States. Management of the 15% to 30% of patients who present with perforated appendicitis is controversial. Perforated appendicitis with abscess can be treated initially with antibiotics and image-guided percutaneous drainage, with interval appendectomy 6 to 12 weeks later to prevent recurrence. This approach has been advocated to decrease complication and reoperation rates associated with immediate appendectomy for perforated appendicitis. However, others have argued that an immediate operative approach to perforated appendicitis may improve long-term outcomes and consume fewer healthcare resources.

Surgical Approach

The technique for open appendectomy was described by McBurney in 1894 and has been used with little modification throughout the 20th century. In 1983, Semm introduced the option of laparoscopic appendectomy. Since then, there has been much debate regarding the superiority of one approach versus the

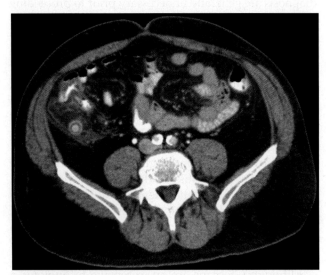

FIGURE 1 • CT radiograph showing appendiceal dilation, wall thickening, and periappendiceal fat stranding consistent with acute appendicitis.

other. Advantages of laparoscopic appendectomy include the ability to perform diagnostic laparoscopy if the appendix is found to be normal. Laparoscopic appendectomy is also associated with less postoperative pain, faster recovery, and lower wound infection rates. In contrast, open appendectomy has been found to be less costly and less time-consuming.

Open Appendectomy

Following administration of preoperative antibiotics and induction of general anesthesia, with the patient in a supine position, an incision is made in an oblique or transverse direction overlying McBurney's point. The subcutaneous fat and Scarpa's fascia are divided to expose the external oblique aponeurosis. The aponeurosis is sharply opened along the direction of its fibers. The fibers of the internal oblique muscle and transverses abdominus are then bluntly separated. The underlying peritoneum is then elevated into the wound and sharply opened along the length of the incision (Table 1).

Upon entering the abdominal cavity, presence of purulent fluid or foul smell should be noted. If the appendix is not immediately visualized, exploration with the index finger may reveal an inflammatory mass. Alternately, the teniae coli of the right colon can be followed proximally to the base of the appendix, which is then delivered into the wound with gentle traction, taking care not to avulse the appendix.

The mesoappendix including the appendiceal artery is divided between clamps and ligated. The base of the appendix once free of the mesentery is doubly ligated close to the cecum and sharply divided. The stump mucosa is often cauterized to prevent the development of a mucocele, and then the stump is invaginated into the cecum with a purse-string suture or Z-stitch.

After copious irrigation and ensuring hemostasis, the wound is closed in layers with absorbable suture. The skin may be closed primarily with a subcuticular suture, or may be left open for a delayed primary closure in the setting of significant contamination.

Laparoscopic Appendectomy

Similar to an open approach, the patient receives preoperative antibiotics and general anesthesia and is positioned supine on the operating table. Gastric decompression should be accomplished with an orogastric tube, and a urinary catheter should be placed to decompress the bladder. Once the abdomen has been sterilely prepped and draped, a three-port-site approach is used: one at the umbilicus and the other two according to surgeon preference. The abdomen is systematically explored to confirm the diagnosis and rule out other pathology (Table 2).

The appendix is then mobilized to expose its base. A window in the mesoappendix is created near the base of the appendix using blunt dissection, and then an endoscopic stapler may be used to divide the

---

TABLE 1. Key Steps of Open Appendectomy

Open Appendectomy

1. Incise the skin and subcutaneous tissues in a transverse (Rocke-Davis) or oblique (McBurney) orientation over McBurney's point.
2. Divide the external oblique aponeurosis, internal oblique muscle, and transversus abdominus muscle in the direction of their fibers.
3. Elevate and sharply divide the peritoneum.
4. Digitally explore the abdomen and deliver the appendix into the wound.
5. Divide the mesoappendix.
6. Ligate and divide the appendix at its base.
7. Invaginate the appendiceal stump using a purse-string suture or Z-stitch.
8. Irrigate the abdomen with sterile saline.
9. Close the abdominal wall layers.

appendix. If the tissue at the base of the appendix is not deemed viable, a small portion of the cecum may be removed with the appendix to ensure that the staple line traverses tissue that will heal well. The mesoappendix and appendiceal artery are then divided with cautery and clips, or with a stapler using a vascular load. A specimen bag is typically used to remove the appendix through the largest port site.

The RLQ is then copiously irrigated and hemostasis assured. Provided no other pathology is noted, the ports are removed under direct vision to ensure the absence of abdominal wall bleeding. The fascia is reapproximated with absorbable suture at port sites larger than 5mm. The skin is then closed with a subcuticular suture.

Special Intraoperative Considerations

When the appendix is found to be normal, the abdominal cavity must be searched diligently for an alternative explanation for the patient's symptoms. In female

TABLE 2. Key Steps of Laparoscopic Appendectomy

Laparoscopic Appendectomy

1. Incise the skin adjacent to the umbilicus and create pneumoperitoneum using Hassan or Veress needle technique.
2. Place an 11-mm trocar at the umbilical incision.
3. Inspect the abdominal cavity laparoscopically to confirm the diagnosis.
4. Place two additional trocars (5mm) in positions that facilitate access to the RLQ.
5. Dissect open a "window" in the mesoappendix adjacent to the base of the appendix.
6. Divide the base of the appendix.
7. Divide the mesoappendix.
8. Remove the appendix through the 11-mm trocar incision.
9. Irrigate the abdomen with sterile saline.
10. Close the trocar incisions.

patients, the ovaries and uterus should be inspected carefully for pathologic findings, such as tubo-ovarian abscess, ovarian torsion, tumor, or cyst. The small bowel should be systematically inspected for sources of inflammation, such as Crohn's disease or Meckel's diverticulitis. The gallbladder should also be inspected for signs of cholecystitis.

Traditionally, a normal appendix is removed when it is discovered during open appendectomy, mainly to prevent future surgeons from assuming that the appendix is absent on the basis of a RLQ scar. This traditional approach has been called into question since the advent of laparoscopic appendectomy.

Appropriate management of the normal appendix requires judgment when Crohn's disease is found as the cause of the patient's illness. If the base of the appendix and cecum appear to be uninvolved in the inflammatory process, appendectomy is likely safe. The major benefit of appendectomy in the setting of Crohn's disease is that subsequent episodes of RLQ pain will not be confused with appendicitis.

Appendiceal tumors are rare, but given the prevalence of appendectomy, most surgeons will occasionally encounter them. Carcinoid tumors comprise the majority of appendiceal tumors. If a carcinoid tumor is suspected at the time of surgery, the appendix should be sent to the pathology laboratory for a frozen section histologic diagnosis. For carcinoids <2cm, simple appendectomy is sufficient. For larger carcinoids, right hemicolectomy with ileocolic lymphadenectomy is recommended. If the histology shows adenocarcinoma of the appendix, a right hemicolectomy is also warranted.

Postoperative Management

For patients with acute appendicitis in the absence of perforation, abscess, or gangrene, a single dose of prophylactic antibiotics is sufficient. Antimicrobial therapy for established intra-abdominal infection should be continued until after the resolution of all clinical signs of infection, including resolution of leukocytosis and fever.

SUGGESTED READINGS

Addiss DG, Shaffer N, Fowler BS, et al. The epidemiology of appendicitis and appendectomy in the United States. Am J Epidemiol. 1990;132:910–925.

Chung RS, Rowland DY, Li P, et al. A meta-analysis of randomized controlled trials of laparosopic versus conventional appendectomy. Am J Surg. 1999;177:250–256.

Rao PM, Rhea JT, Novelline RA, et al. Effect of computed tomography of the appendix on treatment of patients and use of hospital resources. N Engl J Med. 1998;338:141–146.

Silen W, ed. Cope's Early Diagnosis of the Acute Abdomen. 19th ed. New York, NY: Oxford University Press, 1996.

Simillis C, Symeonides P, Shorthouse AJ, et al. A meta-analysis comparing conservative treatment versus acute appendectomy for complicated appendicitis. Surgery. 2010;147:818–829.

11 Perforated Appendicitis

TERRY SHIH, MARK R. HEMMILA, and JUSTIN B. DIMICK

Presentation

A 25-year-old man with no previous medical or surgical history presents to the emergency room with 5 days of abdominal pain. His pain was initially periumbilical, but has since migrated to his right lower quadrant (RLQ), and finally became diffuse. For the past 3 days, he has had nausea, vomiting, and fevers. He presents now as he could no longer tolerate oral intake. His vital signs include a fever of 39.2°C, tachycardia, with a heart rate in the 110s, and a normal blood pressure. On physical examination, his abdomen is nondistended and he has tenderness to palpation in the RLQ with focal rebound tenderness and voluntary guarding.

Differential Diagnosis

RLQ pain with fevers, nausea, and vomiting with localized tenderness is the classic presentation of acute appendicitis. In a young, otherwise healthy male, there is a limited list of other potential diagnoses, such as gastroenteritis or the initial presentation of Crohn's disease. In a female patient, gynecologic pathologies must be considered, including ovarian torsion, ectopic pregnancy, ruptured ovarian cyst, or pelvic inflammatory disease.

This patient has a delayed presentation (5 days) with a high fever, which raises suspicion for perforated appendicitis, as perforation typically occurs 24 to 36 hours following onset of symptoms. Patients with perforation often also present with more substantial systemic inflammatory response, including higher fevers and tachycardia. Patients may have more substantial abdominal pain and tenderness as the underlying inflammatory process may be more significant (e.g., phlegmon or abscess). Because of the different presentation, the differential diagnosis is different for early acute appendicitis and should include right-sided diverticulitis, perforated right-sided colon cancer, cecal perforation due to a distal obstruction (cancer or diverticular stricture), and typhlitis in immunosuppressed patients.

Workup

Patients with suspected appendicitis, either early or late in their course, should undergo laboratory tests, including a complete blood count (CBC) and basic metabolic panel (i.e., electrolytes, BUN, and creatinine). In our patient, the CBC and basic metabolic panel reveal a leukocytosis with a white blood cell count of 18,000 with an elevated creatinine 1.8 mg/dL. All other laboratory tests are within normal limits.

In young healthy males who present with signs and symptoms of classic appendicitis, routine further imaging with computed tomography (CT) scan may not be necessary before proceeding to surgery. However, female patients should be evaluated with further imaging such as a CT scan or transabdominal and transvaginal ultrasound, as pathology of RLQ structures may mimic the presentation of appendicitis.

This case demonstrates several key differences from early appendicitis. The patient has had pain for 5 days with high fevers and tachycardia, increasing the chance of perforation, abscess, or phlegmon. Contrary to early appendicitis, where CT scan is used selectively, cross-sectional imaging is always warranted when perforation is suspected. In our patient, a CT scan of the abdomen and pelvis reveals a dilated appendix to 1.2 cm with extraluminal air and fat stranding surrounding the appendix. There is a periappendiceal fluid collection that measures 4 × 5 cm with rim enhancement **(Figure 1)**.

Discussion

Once the diagnosis of perforated appendicitis is established, treatment depends on the extent of the inflammatory process. Patients with evidence of early perforated appendicitis without a large abscess may benefit from appendectomy at the time of presentation. However, if the patient has evidence of a large amount of inflammation (i.e., periappendiceal phlegmon or abscess), immediate surgical intervention may do more harm than good. In this setting, appendectomy is associated with a significantly higher rate of complications and concomitant bowel resection (e.g., ileocecectomy or right colectomy) than an operation performed for nonperforated appendicitis.

Patients with phlegmon but no definitive abscess **(Figure 2)** will often improve with intravenous antibiotics alone. Patients with evidence of abscess (e.g., contained collections of air and fluid on CT scan) **(Figures 1 and 3A–C)** potentially benefit from radiology-guided

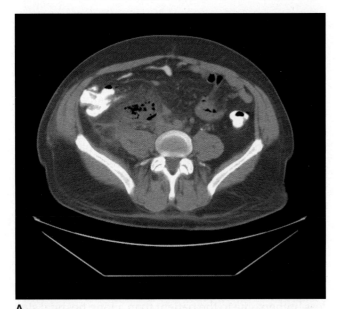

FIGURE 1A • Right lower quadrant abscess.

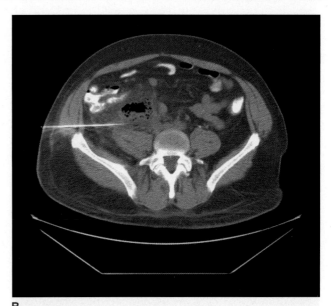

FIGURE 1B • Drain placement for abscess 1.

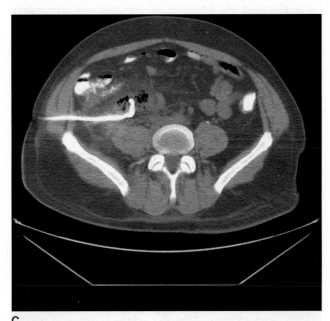

FIGURE 1C • Drain placement 2.

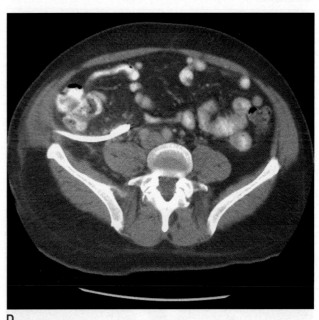

FIGURE 1D • Drain placement with resolution of abscess.

percutaneous drainage, in addition to intravenous antibiotics. **Figures 2A–D** demonstrate CT-guided percutaneous aspiration with placement of a drain. Resolution of symptoms and leukocytosis will determine the duration of IV antibiotics. Typically, antibiotics may be transitioned to an oral regimen for the patient to complete a 1- or 2-week course as an outpatient.

Once the inflammation in the area has decreased after 6 to 8 weeks, the patient may proceed with interval appendectomy. Although recent studies suggest routine interval appendectomy may not be warranted in an asymptomatic patient, it is still our practice to perform subsequent appendectomy to eliminate the risk of recurrent appendicitis. Patients who are of appropriate age (>50 years) or have suspicious findings on imaging should undergo colonoscopy to rule out malignancy.

Surgical Approach

The decision to operate in a patient with perforated appendicitis should be made after a careful assessment of the degree of inflammation. Most patients will be

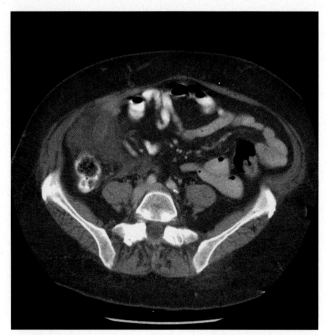

FIGURE 2 • Phlegmon without definite abscess.

managed nonoperatively with intravenous antibiotics with (abscess) or without (phlegmon) percutaneous drainage. Operation in patients with advanced degrees of inflammation could result in a much larger operation (e.g., ileocecetomy) because the base of the appendix may be involved in the process, making it unsafe to remove the appendix in isolation.

There are two specific clinical scenarios where surgery should be considered with perforated appendicitis. First, prompt exploratory laparotomy should be pursued in patients who present with diffuse peritonitis due to free perforation of appendicitis. Often the precise diagnosis will be unknown at the time of exploration. However, if a patient with perforated appendicitis becomes clinically worse (e.g., develops diffuse peritonitis and/or worsening systemic inflammatory response) despite conservative management, emergent laparotomy should be undertaken. Exploratory laparotomy, ileocecetomy, and irrigation are usually necessary in this scenario. Second, appendectomy can be pursued in patients with early perforation (e.g., insignificant inflammation but small amounts of extra-appendiceal fluid and air on CT scan). This latter scenario is somewhat controversial and clinical practice varies across surgeons. In our practice, we believe that a laparoscopic appendectomy and irrigation in early perforated appendicitis will be less bothersome to the patient than a long hospital stay for intravenous antibiotics and bowel rest.

As with early acute appendicitis, appendectomy can be performed via an open or laparoscopic approach. Studies comparing these approaches have shown a decrease in the incidence of wound infection but an increase in the incidence of intra-abdominal abscess with the laparoscopic approach. Patients who undergo laparoscopic appendectomy also experience less postoperative pain, have shortened hospital stays, and return to normal activity earlier. However, the advantages in this regard are very small.

There are several clinical scenarios where laparoscopy may be favored over an open approach.

A

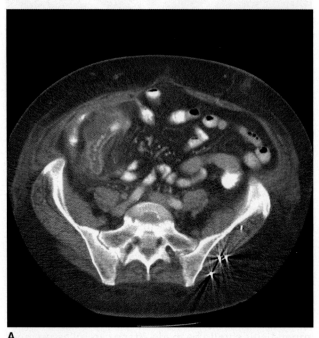

FIGURE 3A • Small perforation on lateral wall of appendix.

B

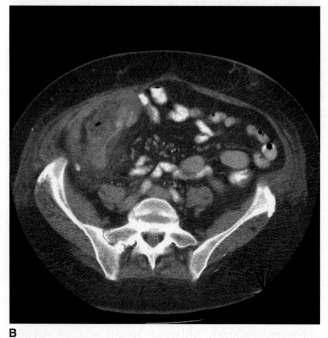

FIGURE 3B • Perforation with small pocket of air.

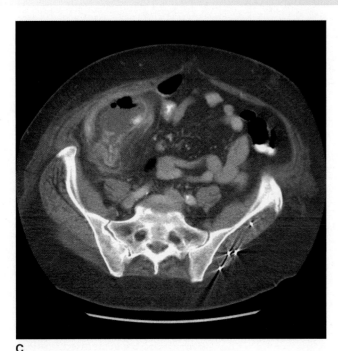

C

FIGURE 3C • Periappendiceal abscess.

Laparoscopy may be favored in women or in men with an unclear diagnosis because it allows more thorough abdominal exploration. In patients with obesity, an open approach may be difficult due to the depth of the incision, potentially requiring a large incision to navigate successfully into the peritoneal cavity. Laparoscopy allows for easier access to the peritoneal cavity in such cases.

Laparoscopic Appendectomy

The procedure is performed in the supine position with the left arm tucked under general anesthesia. An orogastric tube and Foley catheter is placed. The entire abdomen is prepped and draped. A 12-mm infraumbilical incision can be made either curvilinearly or vertically in the midline. Access to the abdomen is made either with Veress needle or open Hasson technique. The abdomen is insufflated with CO_2 to 15 mm Hg. A 5-mm 30° laparoscope is then inserted and diagnostic laparoscopy is performed.

Thorough exploration is crucial in patients with perforation. The degree of inflammation should be assessed carefully. In case of abscess or phlegmon or if it looks like a "bomb went off" in the RLQ, the procedure can be aborted and the patient treated conservatively with antibiotics and percutaneous drainage, if indicated.

If the decision is made to proceed, two additional 5-mm ports are placed, one in the midline above the pubic symphysis and another in the upper midline. Transillumination of the abdominal wall is recommended to allow avoidance of abdominal wall blood vessels during the additional port placement process.

Port placement may vary with position of the appendix and the patient's body habitus. For example, in young, thin patients, ports should be placed further away from the appendix to ensure adequate working room. Placement of the patient in Trendelenburg position with right side up will improve exposure of the cecum and appendix. Attention is turned to the RLQ, and the appendix may be identified by following the teniae of the cecum toward its base. Terminal ileum and all loops of small bowel are swept away from the pelvis. Adhesions may often be encountered, especially in the case of previous perforated appendicitis (i.e., interval appendectomy). These adhesions can often be divided using blunt dissection, but may require sharp dissection or cautery. Once free of adhesions, the appendix is retracted anteriorly and a window in the mesentery at the base of the appendix is created using a Maryland dissector. Prior to dividing the appendix, carefully assess the degree of inflammation at its base. If the base is inflamed, a cuff of uninvolved cecum should be included. If this is not possible, ileocecectomy should be considered. The mesoappendix is divided with an Endo-GIA with a 2.5-mm (vascular) staple load and the appendix is then divided at its base with 3.5-mm staples (bowel load). The appendix is retrieved with an Endocatch bag and removed through the infraumbilical incision. The appendiceal and mesoappendiceal staple lines are thoroughly inspected to assure hemostasis. If the appendix is perforated, the RLQ should be thoroughly irrigated. The 5-mm ports are removed under camera visualization followed by desufflation of the abdomen. The infraumbilical port is then removed and the fascia is closed with absorbable sutures. Skin is closed with either monofilament suture or Indermil glue **(Table 1)**.

Open Appendectomy

The patient is placed in supine position under general anesthesia. The entire abdomen is prepped and draped. A transverse skin incision is made at McBurney's point, two-thirds the distance from the umbilicus to the anterior superior iliac spine. The incision is carried down to the external oblique aponeurosis using Bovie electrocautery. The aponeurosis is opened sharply parallel to the direction of its fibers to expose the internal oblique muscle. The muscle fibers are bluntly separated at right angles. The peritoneum is identified, elevated, and incised sharply, avoiding abdominal viscera.

The appendix is then identified and delivered into the incision. The appendix can often be found by locating the cecum and grasping the teniae with Babcock forceps and following the teniae down to their convergence at the base of the cecum. The mesoappendix is then divided between clamps and ligated with silk sutures. A silk purse-string suture is placed at the base of the appendix.

TABLE 1. Key Technical Steps and Potential Pitfalls in Laparoscopic Appendectomy

Key Technical Steps

1. Infraumbilical 12-mm incision and abdominal access via Veress needle or open Hasson technique.
2. Insert two 5-mm ports in low midline above pubic symphysis and left lower quadrant.
3. Divide adhesions in RLQ to expose appendix.
4. Create mesenteric window at base of appendix with Maryland dissector.
5. Divide mesoappendix and appendix with endoscopic GIA stapler.
6. Retrieve appendix with Endocatch device.
7. Remove ports, close fascia at infraumbilical incision, and close skin.

Potential Pitfalls

- Injury to inferior epigastric vessels or abdominal viscera with port placement.
- Dense adhesions require conversion to open appendectomy.
- Injury to cecum, small bowel, or iliac vessels during dissection.
- Division of the appendix with inflammation at the base, resulting in staple line leak.

TABLE 2. Key Technical Steps and Potential Pitfalls in Open Appendectomy

Key Technical Steps

1. Skin incision at McBurney's point or point of maximal tenderness.
2. Open external oblique aponeurosis and bluntly separate internal oblique and transverse abdominis muscles.
3. Incise peritoneum.
4. Identify appendix and deliver into operative field.
5. Divide mesoappendix.
6. Place purse-string suture around base of appendix.
7. Clamp crush base of appendix and ligate and divide appendix at its base.
8. Invaginate appendiceal stump into base of cecum.
9. Close peritoneum, fascia, and skin in individual layers.

Potential Pitfalls

- Damage to cecum.
- Retrocecal appendix may be difficult to expose.
- Inability to inspect other abdominal structures with limited incision.

A straight clamp is used to crush the appendix at its base and then moved distally and applied again. The appendix is then ligated with absorbable suture and divided sharply proximal to the clamp. Electrocautery is used to obliterate the mucosa of the appendiceal stump. The appendiceal stump is then invaginated into the cecum with the purse-string silk suture.

The surgical field is then irrigated and the peritoneum, fascia, and skin are closed in layers. In cases with gross contamination, leaving the wound open or a loose closure may be a better option **(Table 2)**.

Special Intraoperative Considerations

If extensive inflammation is encountered involving the base of the appendix or cecum, it may be necessary to perform a larger resection such as an ileocecectomy or right colectomy. The resection should extend to healthy noninflamed bowel both proximally and distally. This may be performed laparoscopically, depending on the surgeon's experience. The anastomosis may be either stapled or hand-sewn based on surgeon preference.

Postoperative Management

In the setting of acute perforation, the patient often has an ileus. Broad spectrum intravenous antibiotics are administered and the patient is kept NPO. The patient's diet may be advanced as tolerated once symptoms improve. Antibiotics can be transitioned to an oral regimen and the patient may be discharged home with close follow-up.

After allowing inflammation to subside (6 to 8 weeks), an interval appendectomy may be performed. Pain is usually controlled with oral narcotics or NSAIDs. Interval appendectomy may be performed as an outpatient procedure. The patient should be educated to monitor for signs of postoperative infection: fevers, chills, fatigue, nausea, vomiting, or diarrhea from possible pelvic abscess.

Case Conclusion

The patient undergoes ultrasound-guided percutaneous drain placement upon admission. He is made NPO, given fluid hydration, and treated with IV piperacillin/tazobactam for broad-spectrum coverage of enteric flora. This is transitioned to oral amoxicillin/clavulanic acid when his leukocytosis resolves after 3 days and he is able to tolerate an oral diet. He is discharged home to complete a 2-week course of antibiotics and seen in clinic in 2 weeks. His drain is discontinued in clinic as its output is <30 mL per day. He is seen 8 weeks after initial presentation, at which time a CT scan reveals no residual abscess. He is taken to the operating room for an interval laparoscopic appendectomy and discharged home on the same day of his procedure. He is seen in clinic 2 weeks after surgery and noted to be doing well.

TAKE HOME POINTS

- Patients with RLQ pain with delayed presentation, high fevers, or marked leukocytosis should receive CT scan as they may have perforated rather than early appendicitis.
- Perforated appendicitis with intra-abdominal abscess should initially be managed conservatively with percutaneous drain placement and intravenous antibiotics.
- There is no significant difference in patient outcomes between laparoscopic and open appendectomy in perforated appendicitis.
- Interval appendectomy may no longer be routinely indicated for carefully selected patients.

SUGGESTED READINGS

Brown CV, Abrishami M, Muller M, et al. Appendiceal abscess: immediate operation or percutaneous drainage? Am Surg. 2003;69:829.

Hemmila MR, Birkmeyer NJ, Arbabi S, et al. Introduction to propensity scores: a case study on the comparative effectiveness of laparoscopic vs open appendectomy. Arch Surg. 2010;145:939–945.

Kaminski A, Liu IL, Applebaum H, et al. Routine interval appendectomy is not justified after initial nonoperative treatment of acute appendicitis. Arch Surg. 2005;140(9):897.

Oliak D, Yamini D, Udani VM, et al. Initial nonoperative management for periappendiceal abscess. Dis Colon Rectum. 2001;44:936.

Sauerland S, Lefering R, Neugebauer EA. Laparoscopic versus open surgery for suspected appendicitis. Cochrane Database Syst Rev. 2004;4:CD001546.

Simillis C, Symeonides P, Shorthouse AJ, et al. A meta-analysis comparing conservative treatment versus acute appendectomy for complicated appendicitis (abscess or phlegmon). Surgery. 2010;147(6):818.

12 Gynecologic Causes of Lower Abdominal Pain

CHARLES S. DIETRICH III and BRADFORD P. WHITCOMB

Presentation

A 35-year-old female with no significant prior history presents to the emergency department with acute-onset severe right lower-quadrant pain that started earlier that day and has been progressively worsening. Her vital signs are significant for a low-grade temperature, mild tachycardia, and a normal blood pressure. On abdominal examination, tenderness to deep palpation is noted in the right pelvic region, and rebound tenderness is elicited. Her pelvic examination is remarkable for exquisite right-adnexal tenderness that further precludes adequate examination.

Differential Diagnosis

Acute pelvic pain can be caused by a number of possible diagnoses that include not only gynecologic causes but also gastrointestinal, urologic, and musculoskeletal etiologies. The most common gynecologic causes for lower-abdominal pain include complications of pregnancy (ectopic pregnancy or spontaneous abortion), hemorrhagic or ruptured ovarian cysts, pelvic inflammatory disease (PID), ovarian torsion, dysmenorrhea, degenerating uterine leiomyomas, endometriosis, and pelvic adhesive disease. Nongynecologic causes that should be considered include appendicitis, diverticulitis, acute cystitis, and urinary calculi **(Table 1)**.

Workup

The patient undergoes ultrasound evaluation of the pelvis revealing an 8-cm solid/cystic right ovarian mass resting anterior to the uterus **(Figure 1)**. Doppler studies reveal no internal ovarian flow. A small amount of pelvic fluid surrounds the ovary and fills the pelvic cul-de-sac. The endometrial lining is approximately 8 mm in maximal diameter. The uterus and left adnexa are normal in shape and size. Serum laboratory assessment is notable for a white blood count of $12.2 \times 10^3/\mu L$, a hemoglobin of 12 g/dL, and a normal platelet count. Quantitative β-hCG is <5 mIU/mL. Serum chemistries, liver function tests, and urinalysis are unremarkable. Tumor markers including a CA125, AFP, LDH, and inhibin levels are collected but are pending. CT imaging is ordered for further evaluation confirming the right

complex ovarian mass **(Figure 2)**. Further findings include a normal caliber appendix, no suspicious pelvic or paraaortic lymphadenopathy, and no evidence of metastatic disease.

Discussion

Female patients presenting with acute pelvic pain should be initially evaluated with a thorough history and physical exam. An accurate menstrual history should be collected including age of menarche, start date of the last menstrual period, duration of menstrual flow, quantification of flow, and time interval between menses. Any intermenstrual bleeding should also be documented. Other important aspects of the history include a sexual history, contraceptive techniques, and a history of prior pregnancies, sexually transmitted diseases, abnormal cervical cytology, or other gynecologic problems. Abdominal examination should be performed to assess for signs of a surgical abdomen. Pelvic examination should include direct visualization of the cervix, assessment for cervical motion tenderness, and bimanual examination to determine uterine size and the presence of pelvic masses as well as regions of tenderness. Rectovaginal examination is also useful to help localize any masses that may be found.

All women of reproductive age presenting with acute pain should have pregnancy testing. If qualitative testing is positive, further clarification with a quantitative β-hCG is warranted. Other important laboratory assessments include a complete blood count, basic chemistries, liver function tests, and urinalysis.

The best initial imaging modality for assessing pelvic pain is ultrasound. Ultrasound can accurately identify ovarian pathology, and morphology indexing to stratify the risk for malignancy can be

The views expressed in this manuscript are those of the authors and do not reflect the official policy or position of the Department of the Army, Department of Defense, or the United States Government.

TABLE 1. Common Causes for Acute Pelvic Pain

Gynecologic	Urologic/ Gastrointestinal
Spontaneous abortion	Urinary tract infections
Ectopic pregnancy	Nephroureterolithiasis
Pelvic inflammatory disease	Interstitial cystitis
Endometritis	Gastrointestinal
Salpingitis	Appendicitis
Tubo-ovarian abscess	Diverticulitis
Degenerating uterine leiomyomas	Inflammatory bowel disease
Endometriosis	Irritable bowel syndrome
Dysmenorrhea	Gastroenteritis
Mittelschmerz	
Ruptured ovarian cysts	
Hemorrhagic ovarian cysts	
Ovarian torsion	
Pelvic adhesive disease	

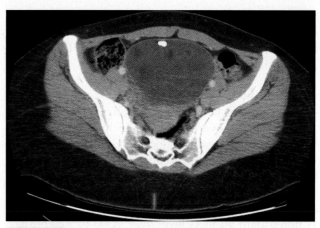

FIGURE 2 • CT image of the complex right ovarian mass. The calcific density within the mass is suggestive of a teratoma.

performed if an ovarian mass is noted. Ultrasound is invaluable in assessing early pregnancy complications as well. Doppler studies are often used to establish the presence of ovarian blood flow and to further assess the risk for a malignant process. CT imaging may also be useful to exclude other diagnoses such as appendicitis.

Diagnosis and Treatment

The findings in this case are most consistent with acute ovarian torsion. Ovarian torsion is the fifth most common emergency room presentation for acute pain in females (following ectopic pregnancy, hemorrhagic ovarian cyst, PID, and appendicitis). While it can occur in all age groups, the majority of females

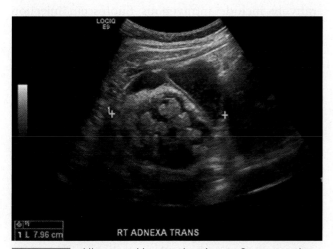

FIGURE 1 • Ultrasound image showing an 8-cm complex solid/cystic right ovarian mass.

affected are under 50 years. In most cases involving adnexal torsion, an ovarian or tubal tumor is present. The risk for torsion increases linearly with ovarian size. In one series, 83% of affected patients had an ovarian tumor ≥5 cm. Conversely, very large tumors become less likely to undergo torsion, as mobility decreases. Normal-sized ovaries can also undergo torsion, but this presentation is more prevalent in children and early adolescents. Histologically, any ovarian tumor can twist; however, dermoid tumors are more commonly seen secondary to their prevalence and greater tissue density when compared to other diagnoses. Fortunately, malignancy is rarely encountered in cases of ovarian torsion, occurring in <2% of adult patients.

When an ovarian torsion occurs, the ovary's vascular pedicle becomes compromised. Initially, venous flow is more affected than arterial flow, causing ovarian engorgement. As the torsion becomes more complete, ischemia results, which eventually leads to necrosis and peritonitis. Pain is the most common presenting complaint and is often associated with nausea. The pain can come in waves, especially with activity, if an intermittent torsion is present. Fevers occasionally are noted and are usually low grade. Mild leukocytosis is often the only laboratory abnormality, although mild anemia can also occur from secondary hemorrhage. Unfortunately, the clinical presentation is often nonspecific, making diagnosis challenging in many cases. Ultrasound is highly sensitive for identifying ovarian masses, and the presence of an adnexal mass should raise the suspicion for torsion if acute pain is present. Doppler studies are usually reported when a tumor is identified; however, diminished or absent flow can be found in normal adnexa. Conversely, the presence of flow does not exclude an intermittent torsion. Maintaining a high index of suspicion with early operative intervention confirms the diagnosis and maximizes the chance for ovarian conservation.

Further Discussion

Other diagnoses to consider for acute gynecologic pain that can mimic ovarian torsion include ectopic pregnancy, PID, and hemorrhagic ovarian cysts. Pain associated with an ectopic pregnancy can be similar to a torsion presentation. The key difference, however, is an elevated hCG level. Ultrasound, again, is critical to the diagnosis. When no intrauterine gestational sac is noted with an hCG level over 1,500 to 2,000 mIU/mL, then an ectopic pregnancy should be strongly considered. If the hCG level rests below this discriminatory zone, then serial hCG levels can be helpful to differentiate between a normal and abnormal early gestation as the levels usually rise at least 66% over 48 hours. While an adnexal mass can be found with an ectopic pregnancy, it is usually smaller than those associated with torsion and often is paraovarian in location. Historically, surgical removal was the standard approach to treatment. With accurate hCG assays and improving ultrasound technology, earlier diagnosis has made medical management with methotrexate more prevalent.

Acute PID can also have a similar presentation to torsion, although the onset of pain tends to be more insidious. Severe cases of PID are often associated with a tubo-ovarian abscess, which on ultrasound can be quite sizable and associated with diminished Doppler flow. Fevers and leukocytosis tend to be more prominent in PID. A mucopurulent cervical discharge and cervical motion tenderness are also typically seen. Most acute cases are associated with gonorrhea or chlamydia, although many presentations are polymicrobial. Antibiotics, in most cases, quickly lead to resolution. Occasionally, surgical or percutaneous drainage of a tubo-ovarian abscess is required.

Hemorrhagic or ruptured ovarian cysts also present similarly to ovarian torsion. Pain often has an acute onset, and an adnexal mass is obviously noted on ultrasound. Fevers and leukocytosis are typically absent, while anemia may be more pronounced if active bleeding is ongoing. On ultrasound, pelvic fluid may also be more prominent. Management is usually conservative with ultrasound abnormalities often resolving within 6 weeks, although cases involving hemodynamic instability require urgent surgical intervention.

Surgical Approach

Surgical management of ovarian pathology in the acute setting can be accomplished by several routes including laparoscopy, minilaparotomy, and laparotomy. The decision on the approach should be based on operator experience, available resources, ovarian size and mobility, the risk for a malignant process, and patient comorbidities. Relatively large ovarian masses can be removed laparoscopically if they are predominantly cystic and can be decompressed once placed inside an endobag. If there is concern for a malignant process, care should be taken not to rupture the tumor, as this upstages the malignancy and usually necessitates postoperative chemotherapy. Predominantly solid tumors cannot be adequately decompressed, and are more amenable to removal via open laparotomy. When performing a laparotomy, most benign pelvic pathology can be addressed via a Pfannenstiel incision. If further lateral exposure is needed, conversion to a Cherney incision can be accomplished by detaching the rectus muscles from their tendonous insertions on the pubic symphysis. If malignancy is suspected, or if distorted fixed anatomy is anticipated, then a midline vertical approach is indicated. Maximal pelvic exposure is achieved by developing the space of Retzius and ensuring the fascial incision extends completely to the pubic symphysis.

When faced with twisted adnexa, the primary intraoperative decision to make revolves around ovarian salvage. Historically, salpingo-oophorectomy was the procedure of choice as it was thought that reduction of the torsion would release clots or inflammatory cells into the ovarian vein. Recent reports, however, have confirmed the efficacy of conservative, ovarian-sparing approaches. Conservation is significantly more common in children, adolescents, and women early in their reproductive years. Timing is critical, as the risk for ovarian necrosis significantly increases after 24 hours of torsion. Following conservation, the ovary will often remain dark or dusky, but subsequent ovarian function is usually noted. Adjuncts to assess ovarian perfusion intraoperatively include intravenous fluorescein injection and ovarian bivalving. The primary risk associated with ovarian conservation is necrosis in cases where irreversible ischemic injury has occurred, leading to peritonitis and systemic infection. Fortunately this risk is low, but necessitates close surveillance immediately following surgery. Oophoropexy is sometimes performed following ovarian conservation, especially in cases of recurrent torsion, and in children or adolescents.

Ovarian cystectomy is a relatively simple surgical procedure allowing for ovarian conservation in reproductive-aged individuals. It should be reserved for benign pathology or for an interval procedure where the diagnosis is uncertain. Initially, either a linear or elliptical incision over the top antimesenteric portion of the ovarian mass is created in the serosa with either a scalpel or Bovie cautery. Blunt and sharp dissection with Metzenbaum scissors or endoshears is then used to identify the underlying tumor and to separate it from the surrounding stroma. The ease of dissection is highly variable, depending on tumor histology and other cofactors such as infection or prior surgeries. Bleeding is usually minimal until the base of the tumor is reached where the ovarian vessels enter the ovarian hilum. Care should be taken to avoid tumor rupture; however, this is not an uncommon event, especially with thin-walled tumors. Once the tumor is removed, bleeding is controlled with suture ligation and cautery. The ovarian serosa can either be left open, or reapproximated with fine suture **(Table 2)**.

Salpingo-oophorectomy is also a relatively straightforward procedure. It is indicated for malignant pathology, nonviable ovarian tissue following torsion, definitive management of recurrent benign pathology, and in postmenopausal patients. The first step is to develop the pararectal space to allow for identification of important retroperitoneal structures **(Figure 3)**. The infundibulopelvic ligament is located on the pelvic sidewall and the peritoneum 1 cm lateral to this structure is incised in a parallel fashion from the round ligament toward the line of Toldt. The external iliac artery and vein can then be identified. Careful blunt dissection of the loose areolar tissue medial to these vessels will open up the pararectal space, which can be further developed inferiorly until the sacrum is reached. The ureter should then be directly visualized as it courses along the medial peritoneal reflection. By following the iliac vessels cephalad and gently lifting anteriorly on the infundibulopelvic ligament, it is usually easy to locate the ureter as it crosses over the external iliac artery and vein near the bifurcation of the common

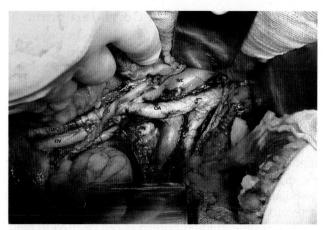

FIGURE 3 • Retroperitoneal pelvic anatomy. IVC, inferior vena cava; CIA, common iliac artery; U, Ureter; EIA, external iliac artery; EIV, external iliac vein.

iliac vessels. Once the ureter has been positively identified, a window is then made between the ureter and ovarian vessels. The ovarian vessels can then be safely transected with suture ligation or laparoscopic vessel sealant devices. Once the ovarian vessels are ligated and divided, the ovary and fallopian tube should be placed on anterior traction and the remainder of the sidewall peritoneum skeletonized toward the utero-ovarian ligament. Finally, the fallopian tube and utero-ovarian ligament are transected close to the uterus, freeing the remaining ovarian attachments in the process **(Table 3)**.

TABLE 2. Key Technical Steps for Ovarian Cystectomy

1. Expose and stabilize the ovarian mass.
2. Create a superficial incision in the ovarian serosa over the anterior surface of the mass.
3. Use blunt and sharp dissection to identify the mass, and to separate it from its serosal and stromal attachments.
4. Hemostasis within the remaining ovarian cavity is achieved with either ligation using fine absorbable suture or with cautery.
5. The ovarian serosa can either be left open or reapproximated with absorbable suture.

Potential Pitfalls

- Avoid tumor rupture if possible.
- If rupture occurs, ensure that all portions of the cyst wall are removed.
- Most significant bleeding occurs at the base of the tumor where ovarian vessels enter the ovarian hilum. If hemostasis cannot be achieved with conservative approaches, oophorectomy may be indicated.

TABLE 3. Key Technical Steps for Salpingo-Oopherectomy

1. Expose the pelvic sidewall and identify the infundibulopelvic and round ligaments.
2. Incise the peritoneum approximately 1 cm lateral to the infundibulopelvic ligament and develop the pararectal space.
3. Identify important retroperitoneal structures including the ureter, external and internal iliac arteries, and the external iliac vein.
4. Create a window through the peritoneum isolating the ovarian vessels from the ureter.
5. Ligate and divide the ovarian vessels.
6. Place the ovary and fallopian tube on anterior traction while transecting the inferior peritoneal attachments toward the utero-ovarian ligament.
7. Ligate the fallopian tube and utero-ovarian ligaments close to the uterine cornua.

Potential Pitfalls

- Failure to properly develop the pararectal space and identify the ureter can lead to ureteral injury.
- Adherent pathology may necessitate radical dissection with ureterolysis to the bladder insertion.
- Avoid tumor rupture if possible.
- If tumor size or adhesions prohibit adequate visualization, controlled tumor decompression may be needed.

Special Intraoperative Considerations

While ovarian cystectomy and salpingo-oophorectomy are relatively straightforward procedures, several dilemmas may arise intraoperatively regarding management of adnexal masses. The first issue that is commonly encountered is management of an incidental adnexal mass found during surgical evaluation for a separate indication. Key issues surrounding this problem include consent parameters, the impact intervention might have on reproductive potential, the risk for malignant pathology, and the potential morbidity associated with nonintervention (future tumor rupture, hemorrhage, or torsion). While there is no definitive answer, several guiding principles can be used to help make decisions. Simple ovarian cysts in reproductive-aged females <5 cm in diameter are usually functional in nature and will resolve on their own. Solid tumors, masses ≥10 cm, or those associated with excrescences are more likely to be malignant, and removal should be considered. Finally, any mass found intraoperatively in a postmenopausal patient should be considered for removal. Intraoperative consultation with a gynecologist is recommended if possible. If the indications are unclear or resources unavailable for management, it is always appropriate to refer the patient postoperatively for treatment counseling. While this approach may result in a second operation, it allows for better planning and gives the patient time to deal with potential impacts on fertility, hormonal status, or a malignant diagnosis.

Another potential challenge that may arise when dealing with pelvic pathology is distorted or fixed masses. In this case, rushing into the surgery without a well-thought-out approach can lead to unintended injuries and hemorrhage. In this event, the operative team should be alerted of the situation, and blood products should be readily available. Experienced assistance should be called. The first step should be to optimize exposure. If a large tumor is present that limits pelvic sidewall exposure, controlled tumor decompression or partial debulking may be necessary to improve visualization. Development of avascular pelvic spaces will improve visualization of important retroperitoneal structures. Vascular control should be obtained as early in the surgical process as is feasible. Ureteral stenting can help with identification of the ureters; however, the risk for injury is not decreased, and ureterolysis is often required to ensure ureteral integrity. During this process, care should be taken as the tunnel of Wertheim is entered since the uterine artery crosses over the ureter near this point. Bowel adhesions usually can be freed from the pelvis; however, on occasion, en bloc resection with dense intestinal adhesions is necessary.

Postoperative Management

Postoperative care for a patient who has recently undergone laparoscopic or open ovarian cystectomy or oophorectomy is relatively straightforward and is similar to any patient having abdominal surgery. Postoperative complications such as bleeding, venous thromboembolism, or infection occur at rates comparable to other similarly classed procedures. Pelvic rest is often recommended during the convalescent period. In general, most patients recover quickly and are able to resume normal activities in 4 to 6 weeks after open procedures or sooner after laparoscopic procedures.

Questions that often arise in the postoperative setting in patients who have had a unilateral salpingo-oophorectomy include the impact on future fertility in reproductive-aged women as well as the possibility for earlier menopause. In most cases, fertility is minimally impacted as long as the contralateral ovary and fallopian tube are normal. However, fertility rates are challenging to generalize as the disease process requiring surgery in the first place can impact reproductive potential. There are a number of studies that suggest patients who have had unilateral oophorectomy reach menopause slightly earlier than those who did not; however, in many of these studies, the patients also had concurrent hysterectomy.

Case Conclusion

The patient was taken to the operating room for a diagnostic laparoscopy, where a right-ovarian torsion was noted. Following reduction, no vascular flow was identified and necrotic tissue was evident. Conversion to an open laparotomy was necessary as the tumor was predominantly solid. A right salpingo-oophorectomy was performed without complications (**Figure 4**). The patient's final pathology was consistent with a mature cystic teratoma with significant regions of necrosis. Her postoperative course was uneventful and she was released from the hospital 2 days later.

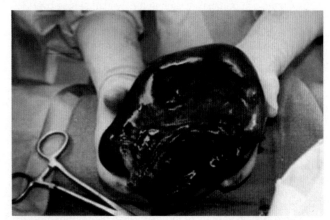

FIGURE 4 • A necrotic right ovarian mass following salpingo-oophorectomy. Final pathology was consistent with a mature teratoma.

TAKE HOME POINTS

- Leading diagnoses for acute pelvic pain in females include ectopic pregnancy, hemorrhagic ovarian cyst, pelvic inflammatory disease, appendicitis, and adnexal torsion.
- All women of reproductive potential with pelvic pain should have hCG testing as part of their initial evaluation.
- Ultrasound is the best initial modality for imaging pelvic pathology.
- Adnexal torsion can be difficult to diagnose. Therefore, any patient presenting with acute pain in the presence of an ovarian mass should raise suspicion. Early surgical intervention confirms the diagnosis and increases the chance for ovarian conservation.
- Reducing adnexal torsion does not increase the risk for clot embolization and will help determine if ovarian salvage is possible.

- Optimal pelvic exposure and development of the avascular pelvic spaces minimize the risk for adjacent structural injury during salpingo-oophorectomy.

SUGGESTED READINGS

Baggish MS, Karram MM, eds. Atlas of Pelvic Anatomy and Gynecologic Surgery. 3rd ed. Philadelphia, PA: Saunders Elsevier, 2010.

Cass DL. Ovarian torsion. Semin Pediatr Surg. 2005;14:86–92.

Dietrich CS, Martin RF. Obstetrics and gynecology for the general surgeon. Surg Clin North Am. 2008;88(2).

Dolgin SE, Lublin M, Shlasko E. Maximizing ovarian salvage when treating idiopathic adnexal torsion. J Pediatr Surg. 2000;35:624.

13 Paraesophageal Hernia

THADEUS TRUS

Presentation

A 66-year-old man presents to the clinic for evaluation of a large hiatal hernia discovered on chest x-ray. He has a significant history of gastroesophageal reflux disease (GERD) characterized by substernal burning and regurgitation, which is controlled by a proton pump inhibitor taken daily. More recently, he is experiencing mild postprandial chest discomfort and early satiety and has lost 20 lb. He also notes occasional dysphagia and vomiting. On exam, he is well appearing. Heart sounds are normal and his lungs are clear. Occasional bowel sounds are heard on auscultation of the chest. On examination, his abdomen is soft without tenderness or palpable masses, and he has no palpable lymphadenopathy. Upon laboratory investigations, he is noted to have a hemoglobin level of 10.5. Recent colonoscopy was negative.

Differential Diagnosis

The patient's nonspecific symptoms can be associated with a variety of conditions such as GERD, biliary disease such as cholelithiasis and colic, cardiac disease, esophageal pathology including esophagitis and hiatal hernia, and malignancy. His heartburn and spontaneous regurgitation may reflect a hiatal hernia. Additionally, his symptom progression and current dysphagia and vomiting can be indicative of a paraesophageal hernia or intrathoracic stomach.

Workup

All patients, particularly older patients, with atypical chest pain should be evaluated for underlying coronary artery disease as the cause of their symptoms. Once this is excluded, along with other potential pathology, suspected paraesophageal hernias should be evaluated with a barium swallow. This study provides a "snap shot" of the esophagogastric anatomy and allows for classification of the type of hiatal hernia. Any organoaxial rotation of the stomach can be seen as well. It is less sensitive for the evaluation of mucosal pathology and esophageal motility. Endoscopy (EGD) should be performed on all patients to assess for esophagitis, Barrett's esophagus, peptic stricture, Cameron's ulcers, and malignancy. Of note, Cameron's ulcers are the most common source of anemia in these patients but are not always found on endoscopy; they are transient in nature and can be difficult to visualize in the distorted gastric anatomy associated with large paraesophageal hernias. Peptic strictures, if found, should be biopsied and dilated as needed preoperatively. Although esophageal manometry can be done, it is often difficult to pass the probe effectively in the setting of a paraesophageal hernia or an intrathoracic

stomach. Manometry is not critical to the preoperative workup.

The patient in this scenario undergoes further workup of his hiatal hernia. A barium swallow demonstrates a large paraesophageal hernia: The gastroesophageal junction (GEJ) remains at the level of the diaphragm with gastric antrum herniating into the chest (Figure 1). An EGD is then performed, which confirms a large hiatal hernia with a paraesophageal component. A Cameron's ulcer is found near the hiatal hernia (Figure 2A,B). The surveyed mucosa is otherwise normal.

Type I — sliding (90%)
II — paraesophageal
III — mixed
IV — hiatal + organ (spleen/colon)

Discussion

The patient in this scenario has a Type II hiatal hernia. There are four types of hiatal hernias. Type I or the sliding hiatal hernia is the most common, accounting for 90% to 95% of hiatal hernias. It is characterized by migration of the GEJ through the hiatus. Type II hernias are true paraesophageal hernias where the GEJ remains in its normal anatomic position below the diaphragm; the gastric fundus herniates above the GEJ though the hiatus. Type III or mixed-type hiatal hernias are characterized by herniation of both the GEJ and gastric fundus above the diaphragm. These tend to be large hernias with more than 50% of the stomach located in the mediastinum. Finally, Type IV hiatal hernias occur when a Type II or III hernia exists and other organs (e.g., spleen and/or colon) migrate into the thorax as well.

Paraesophageal hernias are more common in elderly patients aged 60 to 70 years. It remains unclear as to why certain individuals develop paraesophageal hernias. It is theorized that hernia formation is likely related to the progression of a hiatal hernia in

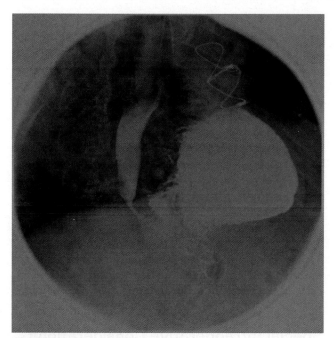

FIGURE 1 • Barium contrast study showing a large paraesophageal hernia.

conjunction with increased intra-abdominal pressure, as is seen in obesity and COPD.

Diagnosis and Treatment

Symptomatic patients with paraesophageal hernias warrant surgical repair. Rarely, patients present with acute obstruction secondary to gastric volvulus. These patients should be decompressed with a nasogastric tube. If necessary, endoscopy can be utilized for decompression. This will often provide relief of the patient's

symptoms and allows for preoperative resuscitation. These patients should be definitively repaired within a few days of presentation. Controversy exists regarding the surgical management of asymptomatic paraesophageal hernias. Historically, studies suggest that up to 30% of asymptomatic patients with paraesophageal hernias will develop potentially devastating complications such as strangulation and perforation. However, recent data suggests that the incidence of developing such complications is much lower than the previously reported. Because of this there is some support for the observation of asymptomatic patients aged 65 years or older. For the most part however, most patients with paraesophageal hernias are at a minimum, mildly symptomatic with occasional bloating, heartburn, or episodic dysphagia. Given the likelihood of symptom progression over time in this elderly population, we advocate early elective repair.

Surgical Approach

Various approaches to paraesophageal hernia repair have been described, including open transabdominal, transthoracic (thoracotomy), or laparoscopic transabdominal. Recently, the laparoscopic approach has become the preferred method of repair. Yet controversy exists in the literature regarding the long term efficacy of laparoscopic paraesophageal hernia repair versus open repair. Advocates of an open approach argue that there is a lower recurrence rate with a repair performed via laparotomy or thoracotomy. Laparoscopic advocates contend that not all recurrences warrant surgical intervention as many are asymptomatic. Furthermore, the use of biomesh as part of the paraesophageal hernia repair has been shown to decrease recurrence rates at least in the short term. Because of the less invasive approach, we advocate laparoscopic repair of

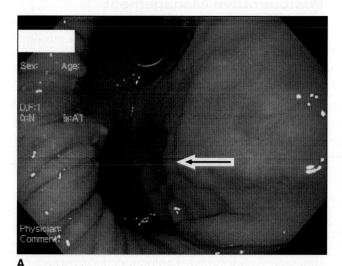

A

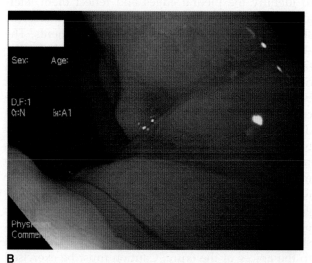

B

FIGURE 2 • Upper endoscopy demonstrating a large paraesophageal hernia with Cameron's ulcer (*arrow*) and otherwise normal mucosa.

paraesophageal hernias. In this elderly patient population, the proven benefits related to perioperative recovery far outweigh the potential for a recurrence of unclear clinical significance.

Regardless of the surgical approach, there are four fundamental steps to paraesophageal hernia repair:

1. Complete reduction of the stomach and GEJ into the abdominal cavity without tension
2. Complete reduction and excision of the hernia sac
3. Crural closure
4. Fixation of the stomach in the abdomen with fundoplication or gastropexy

Laparoscopic paraesophageal hernia repair is performed with the patient positioned split-legged or in lithotomy with the surgeon standing between the patient's legs. Access to the abdominal cavity can be gained with an open or closed technique. The camera port should be placed approximately 15 to 17 mm inferior to the xiphoid process and to the left of midline, through the rectus muscle. Five-millimeter ports are placed under direct vision along the left and right costal margin, each approximately 10 cm away from the xiphoid process. These serve as the surgeon's operating ports. A lateral 5-mm port is placed further along the right costal margin for the atraumatic liver grasper; this is used to elevate the left liver lobe facilitating exposure of the hiatus. Another 5-mm port is placed in the right upper quadrant for the assistant. The hernia is first reduced with gentle traction. Excessive traction can lead to injury to the stomach and should be avoided. Dissection of the hernia sac begins along the inner border of the crura—we prefer starting this dissection along the left crus, continuing over the crural arch to the right crus. This plane between the hernia sac and the crura is developed bluntly and dissection proceeds into the mediastinum. Care must be taken to identify the pleural edges and reflect them laterally. Once reduced intra-abdominally, any excess sac should be removed from its gastric attachments. The short gastric vessels are then divided which further facilitates exposure of the base of the crura. There is often a large posterior esophageal fat pad which must be reduced to allow for complete visualization of the crural base. This allows for placement of a Penrose drain around the esophagus and vagus nerves for traction. Esophageal lengthening is achieved with circumferential dissection of the esophagus within the mediastinum. The crural defect is then closed posterior to the esophagus using multiple, nonabsorbable pledgeted sutures. A partial or full fundoplication over a 60-French bougie is then fashioned. Any large defect is should be reinforced with a U-shaped biomesh sutured to the apices of the crura. Caution must be exercised in large, long-standing paraesophageal hernias, as the vena cava can be pulled quite close to the right crus.

Potential pitfalls of the operation include pneumothorax, injury to the vagus, serosal injury to the stomach, and esophageal injury. If a pneumothorax is recognized, one can usually continue the operation with the patient on positive-pressure ventilation without difficulty. These more often occur on the left, where it can be difficult to identify pleural edge from hernia sac. At the conclusion of the case, the pneumothorax can be evacuated with a red-rubber catheter placed through the hiatal closure and put to water-seal. Injury to the anterior vagus nerve can occur during reduction of the hernia sac. One must be sure to identify the nerve that is often lifted off of the esophagus, making it more susceptible to injury. Excessive traction on the stomach during reduction can result in serosal tears. These should be primarily repaired at the time of injury. Finally, although esophageal perforations are rare, inadvertent myotomies during dissection of the hernia sac are not infrequent.

Special Intraoperative Considerations

Gastric perforation may occur in the patient with acute gastric volvulus. This can usually be avoided with early decompression and surgical intervention. These perforations usually occur on the anterior surface of the fundus and can be repaired primarily laparoscopically.

Short esophagus can be a challenge, limiting esophageal mobilization to allow for 3 to 4 cm of tension-free, intra-abdominal esophagus. Esophageal length can usually be achieved by high mediastinal dissection. Rarely, a Collis gastroplasty is warranted.

Management of the critically ill patient can be difficult. If the patient cannot tolerate extensive surgery, the surgeon should attempt separation of the sac from the esophagus and stomach, crural closure, and gastropexy (G-tube or suture pexy).

Postoperative Management

Postoperative CXR is not routinely performed unless clinically indicated. Small pneumothoraces are often seen and not treated. Routine nasogastric decompression is not warranted. Patients are left NPO the day of surgery and antiemetics are given prophylactically to prevent retching. Patients are started on a clear liquid diet without carbonated beverages on postoperative day 1 and advanced to a mechanical soft diet as tolerated. Patients are usually discharged home on postoperative day 1 or day 2, depending on oral intake and mobility.

Unexplained tachycardia or shortness of breath mandates immediate UGI study with gastrograffin followed by barium to evaluate for a leak. If a leak is found, immediate exploration with primary repair and drainage is warranted. Exploratory laparoscopy can also be liberally used to rule out postoperative bleeding or leak.

Case Conclusion

The patient undergoes a laparoscopic paraesophageal hernia repair with Toupet fundoplication. He does well postoperatively and is discharged to home on postoperative day 2.

TAKE HOME POINTS

- Paraesophageal hernias are common in the elderly.
- Symptoms may be vague and nonspecific.
- Most paraesophageal hernias should be repaired electively.
- Paraesophageal hernias can be safely repaired through a laparoscopic approach.
- Principles of repair include complete reduction of the hernia sac, crural closure, and fundoplication/gastropexy.

SUGGESTED READINGS

Edye MB, Canin-Endres J, Gattorno F, et al. Durability of laparoscopic repair of paraesophageal hernia. Ann Surg. 1998;228(4):528–535.

Lal DR, Pellegrini CA, Oeslschlager BK. Laparoscopic repair of paraesophageal hernia. Surg Clin N Am. 2005;85:105–118.

Oelschlager BK, Pellegrini CA. Paraesophageal hernias: open, laparoscopic, or thoracic repair? Chest Surg Clin N Am. 2001;11(3):589–603.

Skinner DB, Belsey RH. Surgical management of esophageal reflux and hiatus hernia. Long term results with 1030 patients. J Thorac Cardiovasc Surg. 1967;53(1):33–54.

14 Gastroesophageal Reflux Disease

JONATHAN F. FINKS

Presentation

A 55-year-old otherwise healthy, mildly obese (body mass index 33) woman is referred for evaluation of refractory heartburn and regurgitation. Her symptoms have been present for approximately 10 years. She initially attempted lifestyle changes, including cessation of smoking and caffeine use, as well as weight loss, but did not have significant relief. Her symptoms have improved with use of twice daily proton pump inhibitors (PPIs), but she continues to have breakthrough symptoms, especially after eating and when lying down.

Differential Diagnosis

The leading diagnosis based on these symptoms is gastroesophageal reflux disease (GERD). An important consideration is whether or not there is an accompanying hiatal hernia, as this can influence the choice of treatment. The differential diagnosis also includes achalasia. Patients with achalasia most often present with dysphagia, but they will occasionally present with complaints of regurgitation and heartburn. In the case of achalasia, heartburn occurs several hours after eating and usually results from fermentation of undigested food within the esophagus. Certain "alarm" symptoms, including dysphagia, odynophagia, weight loss, anemia, and gastrointestinal bleeding, should prompt a search for esophagogastric malignancy.

Workup

For patients with classic symptoms (heartburn and regurgitation), a good therapeutic response to a trial of PPI therapy is diagnostic of GERD. Further workup is indicated, however, in patients over 50, those with frequent breakthrough symptoms or whose symptoms have persisted for over 5 years, and those with alarm symptoms as mentioned above.

For patients with dysphagia, a *barium swallow* is a good first study, as it allows for assessment of esophageal strictures (benign and malignant) and diverticula. Furthermore, the barium swallow provides a detailed view of the anatomic relationships of the stomach, esophagus, and diaphragm, allowing for identification of hiatal hernias (**Figure 1**). A barium swallow is also a good confirmatory study for patients with manometric evidence of achalasia.

Upper endoscopy offers direct visualization of esophageal mucosa, allowing for identification of esophagitis, Barrett's esophagus, and esophagogastric malignancies. It is especially useful for patients with atypical, or extraesophageal, symptoms, such as cough, sore throat, and hoarseness, and is indicated in any patient for whom antireflux surgery is considered. The presence of esophagitis on upper endoscopy, in association with typical reflux symptoms (heartburn and regurgitation), is generally considered adequate evidence of reflux disease to justify antireflux surgery.

Ambulatory esophageal pH testing is indicated for patients with atypical symptoms and those with nonerosive disease for whom antireflux surgery is being considered. Generally, this study should be performed with the patient off of any antacid medicine (e.g., PPIs). A more recent alternative is the combined pH and impedance monitor, which allows for detection of both acid and nonacid reflux. This study is particularly useful for patients with persistent symptoms despite the use of maximum medical therapy as well as those with atypical symptoms.

Esophageal manometry offers a functional assessment of the lower esophageal sphincter as well as the motility in the body of the esophagus. It is indicated for patients with dysphagia, where malignancy and hiatal hernia have been ruled out by other studies. Most surgeons also consider esophageal manometry essential before antireflux surgery in order to rule out a significant motility disorder, such as achalasia or scleroderma.

Diagnosis and Treatment

The patient from our clinical scenario had classic symptoms of reflux and demonstrated improvement with the use of PPIs. However, because of her age and the duration of symptoms, she underwent an upper endoscopy that demonstrated a small hiatal hernia but no evidence of esophagitis. Ambulatory pH testing demonstrated that the fraction of time with a pH <4 was 8% (upper limit of normal is <4%), and manometry was normal. All of these findings are consistent with GERD.

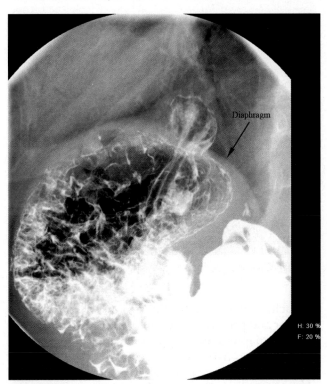

FIGURE 1 • Barium swallow demonstrating a sliding hiatal hernia.

In patients with refractory symptoms, as the one in the clinical scenario, or in those who do not tolerate PPIs, antireflux surgery is warranted. Although there are a number of endoluminal devices to treat GERD, some of which fire full-thickness plicators to recreate a competent antireflux valve at the gastroesophageal junction, the long-term efficacy of these devices does not appear promising in early clinical trials. Therefore, we focus instead on surgical approaches, specifically laparoscopic Nissen fundoplication.

Surgical Approach

Antireflux surgery involves restoration of the normal anatomic position of the stomach and gastroesophageal junction and recreation of the antireflux valve. There are several key elements to successful antireflux surgery. First, any hiatal hernia must be completely reduced. This process involves an extensive mediastianal dissection to ensure adequate esophageal mobilization. Second, any defect in the diaphragmatic crura must be adequately closed. Third, the fundus should be completely mobilized by division of the short gastric vessels in order to prevent twisting of the wrap, which could lead to dysphagia. Finally, a 2-cm long "floppy" fundoplication is performed around the distal esophagus over a large dilator, also for prevention of dysphagia.

The procedure is performed under general anesthesia with the patient in the split-leg position. Access to the periotoneum is obtained using a closed (Veress) or open (Hasson) technique and pneumoperitoneum is established. We employ a five-port approach with a camera port placed 15 cm below the top of the xiphoid process. The surgeon stands between the patient's legs using two upper-quadrant ports. The assistant stands to the patient's left, using a port in the left upper quadrant and operating the laparoscope. A final port is placed in the subxiphoid position for the liver retractor. Once the ports are placed, the patient is put into the reverse Trendelenberg position and a Nathanson retractor is used to elevate the left lateral segment of the liver.

First, the stomach is manually reduced into the abdomen in the event of a hiatal hernia. Then the gastrohepatic ligament is incised with the ultrasonic dissector, beginning in the avascular portion and extending toward the diaphragm in order to expose the right crus **(Table 1)**. We recommend preserving the hepatic branch of the vagus nerve, both to reduce risk for subsequent gallstone formation and also to avoid injury to the accessory left hepatic artery, which can be present in up to 12% of patients **(Figure 2)**. Next, the phrenoesophageal ligament anterior to the esophagus is opened, with care taken to avoid injury to the underlying esophagus and anterior vagus nerve. Blunt dissection is then used to develop a plane between the right crus and the esophagus. This dissection is continued until the decussation of the left and right crura is visualized. Some retroesophageal dissection may be done from the right side during this portion of the

---

TABLE 1. Key Technical Steps and Potential Pitfalls

Key Technical Steps

1. Incision of the gastrohepatic ligament through the avascular space to expose the right crus.
2. Blunt dissection to develop a plane between the esophagus and the crus until the crural decussation is visualized.
3. Complete mobilization of the fundus.
4. Extensive mediastinal dissection to deliver at least 2.5–3 cm of distal esophagus into the abdomen.
5. Closure of the crural defect with nonabsorbable pledgeted sutures.
6. Creation of a 2-cm long 360° posterior fundoplication using nonabsorbable suture.

Potential Pitfalls

- Injury to accessory or replaced left hepatic artery running with the hepatic branch of the vagus nerve in the gastrohepatic ligament.
- Injury to anterior and posterior vagus nerves. The posterior nerve often falls away from the esophagus and is most susceptible to injury.
- Injury to the proximal short gastric vessels. These are fragile and difficult to control if avulsed or torn.
- Esophageal injury from inadvertent contact with energy source, such as the ultrasonic dissector, during mediastinal dissection.

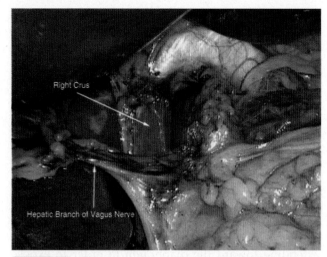

FIGURE 2 • Exposure of the right crus of the diaphragm.

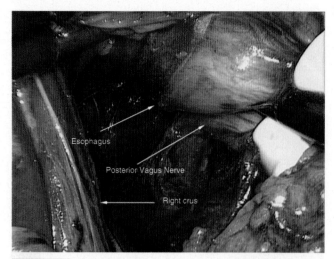

FIGURE 4 • Mediastinal dissection.

procedure. Care should be taken to prevent injury to the posterior vagus nerve and to keep the nerve up with the esophagus during the dissection.

Attention then turns to mobilization of the fundus **(Figure 3)**. The short gastric vessels are divided with the ultrasonic dissector, beginning at the level of the inferior pole of the spleen and extending toward the left crus. The posterior attachments of the stomach should also be divided to ensure full mobilization of the fundus. At this point, the retroesophageal dissection is completed from the left side and a penrose drain is placed around the esophagus, with the ends anchored anteriorly using an endoscopic loop. The penrose drain facilitates retraction of the esophagus.

What follows is an extensive mediastinal mobilization, using both blunt and ultrasonic dissection to free the esophagus from its mediastinal attachments **(Figure 4)**. This dissection continues until at least 2.5 to 3 cm of distal esophagus remains within the abdomen without having to apply traction to the

stomach. Care should be taken to avoid injury to the anterior and posterior vagus nerves during this dissection. The diaphragmatic crura are then reapproximated using nonabsorbable suture secured with felt pledgets to prevent the suture from tearing through the muscle of the diaphragm. The closure should be snug, but not tight, around the esophagus. Calibration with a 56- to 60-French dilator may be helpful during the closure.

The fundus of the stomach is brought behind the esophagus and a 360° fundoplication is then performed over a large dilator (56 to 60 French) **(Figure 5)**. The fundoplication is secured at the right anterolateral aspect of the esophagus with three nonabsorbable sutures. The sutures are placed 1 cm apart, with the most superior suture placed 2 cm above the gastroesophageal junction. Each suture incorporates a full-thickness bite of stomach on either side of the esophagus, as well as a partial thickness bite of esophagus, in order to prevent slippage of the fundus behind the wrap.

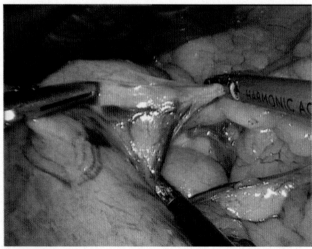

FIGURE 3 • Mobilization of the fundus.

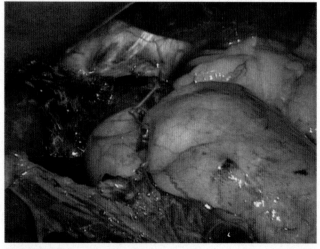

FIGURE 5 • Fundoplication.

Special Intraoperative Considerations

During the mediastinal dissection, especially in the setting of a hiatal hernia, the pleura can be adherent to the hernia sac and is then susceptible to injury. A pleural tear can result in capnothorax with resultant hypercarbia, acidosis, hypoxia, and reduced lung volumes on the affected side. There are typically no lasting consequences, as the gas will absorb rapidly once the pneumoperitoneum has been released. If untreated, however, capnothorax may require conversion to an open procedure. In the event of a pleural tear, there are several steps that will diminish the impact on the patient. First, the tear is enlarged to prevent a tension capnothorax. Next, a 14-French red rubber catheter is inserted into the abdomen. One end of the catheter is then inserted into the pleural space and the other end is left in the abdomen. This will help equalize the pressure between the two cavities. At the end of the procedure, the abdominal end of the catheter is pulled out through the left subcostal port while the pneumoperitoneum is released. The end of the catheter is placed into a water seal while deep Valsalva breaths are administered. This will allow for evacuation of any remaining gas from the affected pleural space. The red rubber catheter is then removed. A postoperative chest x-ray is useful to confirm lung reexpansion.

Postoperative Management

The Foley catheter is typically removed at the end of the procedure. Patients are placed on a scheduled antiemetic, such as ondansetron, for 24 to 48 hours, and may have PRN orders for additional antiemetics, in order to prevent nausea and retching, which can result in disruption of the wrap or early recurrent hiatal hernia. On the first postoperative night or the following day, patients are started on a clear liquid diet and then advanced to a full liquid diet. They are typically discharged on the first or second postoperative day and may advance to a mechanical soft diet within the first week after surgery.

Side effects of antireflux surgery include dysphagia and bloating. Mild dysphagia is not uncommon in the first week or two following the procedure. Because of this problem, patients are advised to avoid tough or dry meat, raw vegetables, and bread for at least 4 to 6 weeks following surgery. In the case of severe dysphagia or dysphagia persisting beyond 6 to 8 weeks,

patients should undergo barium swallow to rule out a recurrent hiatal hernia or slipped fundoplication (fundus slipped behind the wrap). If neither of these findings is present, patients should undergo endoscopic dilation. The cause of bloating after antireflux surgery is not clear, but may relate to vagal stretch during the dissection or simply to competence of the wrap which does not permit belching as freely as before surgery. This side effect often resolves after several weeks and can be minimized by avoiding carbonated beverages and eating smaller meals five to six times per day.

TAKE HOME POINTS

- Careful patient selection is essential to success with antireflux surgery. Those selected for surgery should have objective evidence for reflux and symptoms that are attributable to GERD.
- All patients selected for surgery should undergo upper endoscopy and esophageal manometry. Ambulatory 24-hour pH testing should be reserved for patients with nonerosive disease and those with atypical symptoms (e.g., cough, hoarseness).
- Dysphagia is a common complaint following antireflux surgery. The risk for dysphagia can be reduced by full mobilization of the fundus and creation of a "floppy" fundoplication over a 56- to 60-French dilator.
- Recurrent hiatal hernia is the most common cause for failure of antireflux surgery. Adequate crural closure and a thorough mediastinal mobilization of the esophagus, allowing for a minimum of 2.5 to 3 cm of intra-abdominal esophageal length, will help reduce the risk for this complication.

SUGGESTED READINGS

Campos GM, Peters JH, DeMeester TR, et al. Multivariate analysis of factors predicting outcome after laparoscopic Nissen fundoplication. J Gastrointest Surg. 1999;3(3):292–300.

Hunter JG, Trus TL, Branum GD, et al. A physiologic approach to laparoscopic fundoplication for gastroesophageal reflux disease. Ann Surg. 1996;223(6):673–685.

Jobe BA, Kahrilas PJ, Vernon AH, et al. Endoscopic appraisal of the gastroesophageal valve after antireflux surgery. Am J Gastroenterol. 2004;99(2):233–243.

Malhi-Chowla N, Gorecki P, Bammer T, et al. Dilation after fundoplication: timing, frequency, indications and outcome. Gastrointest Endosc. 2002;55(2):219–223.

15 Gastric Cancer

SRINIVAS KAVUTURU, JUSSUF T. KAIFI, and KEVIN F. STAVELEY-O'CARROLL

Presentation

A 52-year-old male presents with history of epigastric discomfort and dysphagia for 6 months. He describes two previous episodes of black tarry stools and a 30-lb weight loss over the past 3 months. His past medical history is significant for hypertension, hypercholesterolemia, and benign prostatic hypertrophy. He had an open appendectomy as a child. He drinks about eight beers a day and has a 30-pack-year history of smoking cigarettes. He has family history of heart disease and hypertension. His medications include tamsulosin, metoprolol, omeprazole, and Lipitor. He is not allergic to any known medications.

Differential Diagnosis

Based on his age and clinical presentation (e.g., dysphagia, weight loss, and melena), esophageal/gastric cancer should be considered as the first differential but the following alternative diagnoses could also be taken into account. Benign diseases to consider include esophagitis, gastritis, peptic ulcer disease, or esophageal varices. Malignant diseases to consider include gastric or esophageal carcinoma, MALT (mucosa-associated lymphoid tissue) lymphoma of the stomach, primary gastric lymphoma (non-MALT type), and gastrointestinal (GI) stromal tumor.

Workup

Workup includes a thorough history and physical examination, laboratory testing, diagnostic imaging, and invasive tests (e.g., endoscopy). In case it turns out to be a malignancy, the diagnostic workup should have two goals: (1) determine the extent of disease, that is, clinical staging and (2) risk stratification for any proposed surgery.

Personal history of previous gastric surgery and family history of upper GI cancers (e.g., Lynch syndrome II, BRCA2 mutation, and familial polyposis coli) are strongly suggestive of malignancy.

Most patients with malignancy have normal physical exams. Positive findings on physical examination are most often associated with locally advanced or metastatic disease. These findings may include palpable abdominal mass from a large primary tumor, liver or ovarian metastases (Krunkenberg's tumor), palpable left supraclavicular node (Virchow's node), periumbilical nodule (Sister Mary Joseph node), pelvic deposits (rectal Blummer's shelf), jaundice, or ascites. Paraneoplastic syndromes associated with gastric cancer include acanthosis nigricans, thrombophlebitis, circinate erythemas, dermatomyositis, pemphigoid, and seborrheic keratosis.

When malignancy is suspected, flexible endoscopy is the diagnostic modality of choice. The diagnostic accuracy of upper GI endoscopy for gastric cancer approaches 98%. In a study of 100 randomly selected patients, endoscopy was more sensitive (92% vs. 54%) and specific (100% vs. 91%) than double-contrast barium studies. Barium studies also cannot distinguish benign from malignant ulcers.

Preoperative staging evaluates local extent of the tumor, resectability, lymph node involvement, and presence of metastasis. Imaging modalities include computerized tomography (CT) scan, upper endoscopy, endoscopic ultrasound (EUS), positron emission tomography (PET), magnetic resonance imaging (MRI) and laparoscopic exploration. CT scan of the abdomen is valuable in determining hepatic metastasis (≥ 1 cm), bulky lymphadenopathy, visceral metastasis, ascites, and extragastric extension to surgically unresectable structures. CT scan also helps in planning the extent of surgery if en bloc resection of nearby organs is necessary. However, its value is limited in detecting peritoneal disease and hepatic metastasis less than 1 cm in size. CT scan of the chest should be included for tumors at the gastroesophageal (GE) junction to evaluate the extent of disease in the mediastinum. EUS can assess the depth of the tumor (T stage) and local nodal status (N stage) with overall accuracy of up to 80%. Although limited by technical challenges, EUS-guided fine needle aspiration (FNA) biopsy of the regional lymph nodes, aspiration of small volume ascites, and accessible distant metastatic sites (e.g., mediastinal lymph nodes, liver) improve the accuracy of lymph nodal staging and could prove distant metastasis avoiding noncurative laparotomy. PET-CT improves preoperative staging of gastric adenocarcinoma and can alter treatment options in up to 20% of patients. PET combined with CT is more accurate for preoperative staging than either modality alone and can facilitate the selection of patients for a curative resection by confirming a nodal status identified by CT. PET-CT is also the most sensitive noninvasive imaging modality for the diagnosis of hepatic metastases from gastric cancer.

Performing diagnostic laparoscopy prior to definitive surgery has several advantages. Laparoscopy detects small metastases (<0.5 cm) of the peritoneum and liver in up to 40% patients who are eligible for potentially curative resection based on CT scan. Laparoscopy also helps in staging by cytopathologic analysis of peritoneal fluid for free intraperitoneal gastric cancer cells, placement of feeding jejunostomy in obstructing GE junction mass, and in palliation by avoiding nontherapeutic laparotomy in advanced gastric cancer. Currently, staging laparoscopy is recommended in select patients with high probability of having distant metastatic disease in the abdomen, based on the tumor location (GE junction and whole-body tumors), and in patients who are medically fit but have unresectable disease by noninvasive staging investigations. The role of laparoscopic intraoperative ultrasonography to stage the gastric cancer is still to be defined by systematic studies.

Preoperative risk stratification for surgery includes nutritional, cardiovascular, pulmonary, central nervous system and functional assessment, clinically and by appropriate investigations and to optimize the medical comorbidities.

The patient described in the scenario above had an unremarkable clinical examination. He had no relevant family history. He had an upper GI endoscopy that revealed a Siewert type III GE junction tumor (i.e., tumor lying within 2 to 5 cm distal to the GE junction). Upper endoscopy revealed an irregular mass below the GE junction. Biopsies from the mass were consistent with moderately differentiated adenocarcinoma. A multiphase CT scan of his chest, abdomen, and pelvis with contrast revealed thickening of stomach wall at the GE junction and a few perigastric lymph nodes less than 1 cm in size. There was no evidence of invasion/encasement of any major vascular structures, distant metastasis, or peritoneal seeding. PET-CT showed an FDG (flurodeoxyglucose) avid lesion in the proximal stomach corresponding to the lesion seen on the CT scan. The subcentimeter lymph nodes seen on the CT scan were also FDG avid on the PET-CT, indicating metastatic spread. EUS showed the lesion to be invading muscularis propria (T2) and EUS-guided FNA of the perigastric lymph nodes were positive for adenocarcinoma (N1).

Diagnosis and Treatment

The diagnosis of gastric cancer is established by histopathologic assessment of biopsies or cytology from gastric washes/brushing. Two most commonly used pathologic classifications of gastric cancer based on microscopic configuration are that of Lauren and World Health Organization (WHO) systems. The Lauren classification divides gastric cancer into two major histologic types: intestinal and diffuse. The intestinal form is often seen arising in a setting of chronic atrophic gastritis (e.g., *Helicobacter pylori* and autoimmune gastritis), whereas the diffuse form is less related to environmental influences and may arise as single cell mutations within normal gastric glands. The WHO classification has five subtypes: adenocarcinoma (intestinal and diffuse), papillary, tubular, mucinous, and signet-ring cell. Staging of gastric cancer is currently based on the American Joint Committee on Cancer recommendation of the TNM staging (seventh edition, 2010) with the addition of the term "R status" denoting the status of resection margins after surgery (R0, negative margins; R1, microscopic residual disease; R2, gross residual disease).

Surgical resection is the mainstay of treatment of gastric cancer. However, a multidisciplinary team approach with combined modality therapy (surgery, chemotherapy, and radiation) is most effective especially in patients who have locoregional disease. Clinically, gastric cancer can be classified into early, locoregionally advanced (but resectable), nonresectable, and metastatic.

For patients with early gastric cancer (Tis, T1 tumors limited to mucosa), gastrectomy with D1/D2 lymphadenectomy remains the treatment of choice. Endoscopic mucosal resection (EMR) is being performed on select patients but is not yet the standard of care.

For patients with locoregionally advanced resectable gastric cancer, recent evidence supports neoadjuvant therapy prior to surgery. In a recent randomized trial, preoperative chemotherapy has been shown to improve survival, improve local failure rates, and increase the proportion of patients with R0 resection rates (MAGIC trial).

For patients with locally advanced but initially nonresectable disease, neoadjuvant chemotherapy or chemoradiotherapy has also been tried in with an intention to convert it into a potentially resectable disease with a curative intent, but the approach has not yet been standardized. Patients with metastatic disease need palliative therapy, depending on their symptoms and functional status.

Postoperatively, after gastric resection, current NCCN guidelines recommend adjuvant chemoradiation with 5FU following R0 resection of T3, T4, or node-positive cancers.

Surgical Approach

The extent of gastric resection is a crucial part of surgical plan. Since gastric carcinoma has the propensity to spread via submucosal and subserosal lymphatics, a resection margin of at least 5 cm is advocated. Curative resection with microscopically negative margins (R0 resection) involves resection of the tumor with lymphatics and lymph nodes and any adjacent organ involved by direct extension of the tumor (e.g., tail of pancreas, spleen). Hence, selection of appropriate surgical procedure is determined by location of the tumor, lymph nodal status, and extragastric extension into the adjacent organs.

A total gastrectomy with esophagojejunostomy is appropriate for proximal (upper third) gastric tumors. GE junction tumors predominantly involving cardia (Siewert type III—tumor lying within 2 to 5 cm distal to the "Z" line) should be treated by an extended total gastrectomy with a segment of esophagus for a safe margin. On the other hand, GE junction tumors with predominant involvement of the esophagus (Siewert type I— tumor lying within 1 to 5 cm proximal to the "Z" line) should be treated by transhiatal/transthoracic esophagectomy with proximal gastrectomy and gastric pull-up with cervical/thoracic esophagogastrostomy. The necessary extent of resection for Siewert type II (tumor lying within 1 cm proximal or 2 cm distal to the "Z" line) has been controversial and intraoperative assessment of the tumor by an experienced surgeon and frozen section of the resected margins help decide the course—either a total gastrectomy or a transhiatal esophagectomy. For tumors in the distal stomach (lower two-thirds), a subtotal gastrectomy with Bilroth II or Roux-en-Y reconstruction is appropriate (Tables 1 and 2).

The extent of lymphadenectomy for gastric cancer remains controversial. Western as well as Asian studies could not show any survival benefit with D2 dissections (lymph nodes along the named arteries of the stomach) over D1 (immediate perigastric lymph nodes). Moreover, few studies demonstrated increased morbidity and mortality with extended lymph nodal dissections. Current AJCC guidelines state that pathologic examination of at least 15 lymph nodes is required for adequate staging (Tables 3 and 4).

It is our preference and practice to perform gastrectomy with D2 lymphadenectomy after neoadjuvant chemotherapy. Depending on the extent of tumor, a splenectomy and/or a distal pancreatectomy is performed to achieve negative margins (R0 resection). This strategy maximizes the chances of R0 resection and provides adequate number of lymph nodes for accurate staging of the disease.

The patient in our case scenario had a moderately differentiated adenocarcinoma of the stomach (Siewert type III) with T3, N1, M0—stage IIB, that is, locally

TABLE 2. Total Gastrectomy—Potential Intraoperative Pitfalls

1. Accessory/replaced left hepatic artery arising from the left gastric artery (15%–20%)
2. Injury to the spleen
3. Positive tumor margins of esophagus and stomach
4. Ischemic-looking duodenal stump

TABLE 3. American Joint Committee on Cancer (AJCC) TNM Staging Classification for Staging of the Stomach (7th ed., 2010)

Primary Tumor (T)

TX	Primary tumor cannot be assessed
T0	No evidence of primary tumor
Tis	Carcinoma in situ: intraepithelial tumor without invasion of the lamina propria
T1a	Tumor invades lamina propria or muscularis mucosae
T1b	Tumor invades submucosa
T2	Tumor invades muscularis propria
T3	Tumor penetrates subserosal connective tissue without invasion of visceral peritoneum or adjacent structures
T4a	Tumor invades serosa (visceral peritoneum)
T4b	Tumor invades adjacent structures

Regional Lymph Nodes (N)

NX	Regional lymph node (s) cannot be assessed
N0	No regional lymph node metastasis
N1	Metastasis in 1–2 regional lymph nodes
N2	Metastasis in 3–6 regional lymph nodes
N3	Metastasis in 7 or more regional lymph nodes
N3a	Metastasis in 7–15 regional lymph nodes
N3b	Metastasis in 16 or more regional lymph nodes

Distant Metastasis (M)

M0	No distant metastasis
M1	Distant metastasis

Histologic Grade (G)

GX	Grade cannot be assessed
G1	Well differentiated
G2	Moderately differentiated
G3	Poorly differentiated
G4	Undifferentiated

Used with the permission of the American Joint Committee on Cancer (AJCC), Chicago, Illinois. The original source for this material is the *AJCC Cancer Staging Manual*, 7th ed. (2010) published by Springer Science and Business Media LLC, www.springer.com.

TABLE 1. Total Gastrectomy—Key Technical Steps

1. Midline laparotomy and full exploration
2. Mobilize GE junction and esophagus, taking a margin of diaphragmatic crura.
3. Separate the omentum and lesser sac lining en bloc from the transverse colon.
4. Divide the short gastric vessels and skeletonize the celiac, splenic, and common hepatic arteries, taking their lymph nodes.
5. Ligate left and right gastric and gastroepiploic arteries at their bases.
6. Divide esophagus, stomach, and jejunum.
7. Reconstruction with esophagojejunostomy and jejunojejunostomy

TABLE 4. American Joint Committee on Cancer (AJCC) TNM Staging Classification for Staging of the Stomach (7th ed., 2010, Table 2)

Stage	T	N	G
Stage 0	Tis	N0	M0
Stage IA	T1	N0	M0
Stage IB	T2	N0	M0
	T1	N1	M0
Stage IIA	T3	N0	M0
	T2	N1	M0
	T1	N2	M0
Stage IIB	T4a	N0	M0
	T3	N1	M0
	T2	N2	M0
	T1	N3	M0
Stage IIIA	T4a	N1	M0
	T3	N2	M0
	T2	N3	M0
Stage IIIB	T4b	N0	M0
	T4b	N1	M0
	T4a	N2	M0
	T3	N3	M0
Stage IIIC	T4b	N2	M0
	T4b	N3	M0
	T4a	N3	M0
Stage IV	Any T	Any N	M1

Used with the permission of the American Joint Committee on Cancer (AJCC), Chicago, Illinois. The original source for this material is the *AJCC Cancer Staging Manual.* 7th ed. (2010) published by Springer Science and Business Media LLC, www.springer.com.

advanced but was resectable. Hence, as a part of multimodality treatment, he underwent neoadjuvant chemotherapy with Etoposide, Cisplatin, and 5-FU. He then underwent a total gastrectomy with Roux-en-Y esophagojejunostomy.

Operative procedure The patient is placed in a supine position with consideration given to the possibility of right thoracic or cervical approach in case of GE junction tumors needing esophagectomy. The skin from the chin to the pubic symphysis is prepared and draped. We prefer a midline incision extending from the xiphoid process to just below the umbilicus for most patients undergoing a total gastrectomy. A fixed retractor (e.g., Thomson) is used for adequate exposure of the GE junction. Careful methodical exploration of the abdomen is performed to exclude metastasis, assess extent of resection, resectability, and local extension to other viscera. The gastrohepatic omentum is divided closer to the liver, closely watching for accessory left hepatic artery, which should be preserved in most cases. Dissection in the region of the esophagus and the fundus of the stomach starts by taking a ring of diaphragmatic crura, dividing the phrenic vein en route and taking the pericardial lymph node packet en bloc with the specimen (**Figure 1**). The omentum and the lesser sac with the lining are

separated en bloc from the transverse colon. The short gastric vessels along the greater curvature of the stomach are divided close to the spleen (**Figure 2**), dissection facilitated by a vessel-sealing device. The celiac, splenic, and common hepatic arteries are skeletonized and the nodal tissue swept up the left gastric artery. The left and right gastric arteries and the gastroepiploic vessels are ligated at their bases and the lymph nodes are taken with the specimen. Duodenum is then divided with a GIA stapler 2 to 3 cm distal to the pyloric vein (**Figure 3**). GE junction is mobilized and esophagus is divided with a transverse anastomosis (TA) stapler. The specimen is sent to pathology and a frozen section obtained from the proximal and distal margins of the specimen to check for adequacy of resection. Reconstruction after a standard D2 total gastrectomy is by a Roux-en-Y esophagojejunostomy (**Figure 4**). We prefer to perform this with an end-to-end anastomosis (EEA) stapling device. Alternately a hand-sewn anastomosis or anastomosis to a jejunal pouch could also be performed. A jejunostomy feeding tube is placed routinely. We use two closed suction drains to drain the duodenal stump and the esophagojejunal anastomosis.

There are several potential pitfalls during a routine gastrectomy. The gastrohepatic ligament might contain an accessory left hepatic artery (15% to 20%) and sometimes it represents the only arterial flow to the left lobe of the liver. Proximal ligation of left gastric artery in such case may result in hepatic ischemia. Injury to the spleen or its vessels may sometimes need splenectomy to control hemorrhage. Positive esophageal resection margin may require re-resection of the distal esophageal margin. When a transhiatal esophagetomy

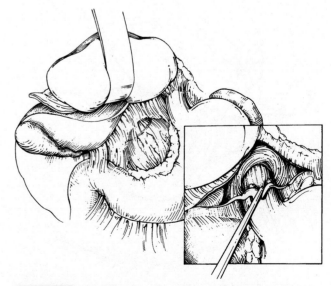

FIGURE 1 • Mobilization of esophageal hiatus is completed by detaching the peritoneal reflection from the diaphragm. (From Fischer et al. Mastery of Surgery. 5th ed. Philadelphia, PA: Lippincott Williams & Wilkins, 2007, with permission.)

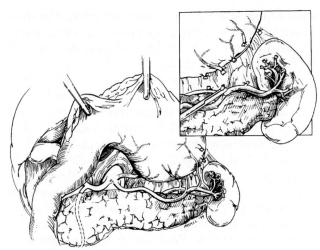

FIGURE 2 • Division of the short gastric vessels close to the spleen. (From Fischer et al. Mastery of Surgery. 5th ed. Philadelphia, PA: Lippincott Williams & Wilkins, 2007, with permission.)

is attempted for a GE junction tumor, a positive gastric resection may sometimes need a total esophagogastrectomy with colon/jejunum interposition. Stapled duodenal stump often does not need further reinforcement with additional sutures; however, when it looks ischemic, we recommend oversewing it with Lembert sutures to prevent duodenal stump leak, which is a disastrous postoperative complication.

Special Intraoperative Considerations

GE junction tumors extending into the body of the stomach, where a 5 cm margin could not be achieved, will require total gastrectomy with esophagectomy.

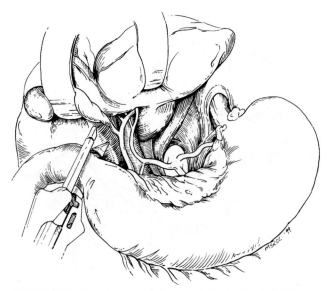

FIGURE 3 • The duodenum being divided with the GIA stapler. (From Fischer et al. Mastery of Surgery. 5th ed. Philadelphia, PA: Lippincott Williams & Wilkins, 2007, with permission.)

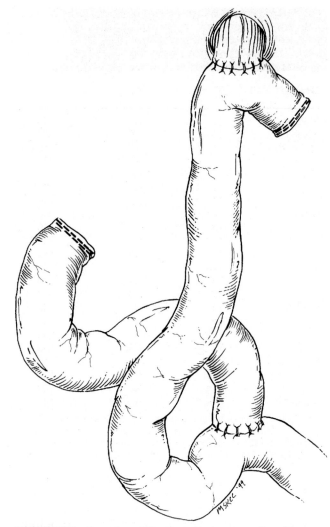

FIGURE 4 • Completed Roux-en-Y reconstruction. (From Fischer et al. Mastery of Surgery. 5th ed. Philadelphia, PA: Lippincott Williams & Wilkins, 2007, with permission.)

We prefer colon interposition in this situation. The left colonic segment based on the ascending branch of the left colic vessels is used. When the colon is absent or has extensive diverticulosis, jejunal conduit can be used.

Postoperative Management

We place a nasogastric tube (threaded beyond the gastrojejunal anastomosis intraoperatively), which is maintained on low intermittent suction. Postoperative pain control and early ambulation is the key to faster recovery. Jejunostomy feeding is started on post-op day 2. Drains are removed on the fourth postoperative day if the bilirubin and amylase in the drain fluid is less than three times the serum values. Oral feeding is started once it is established that the patient does not have an intra-abdominal leak from esophagojejunostomy. A contrast swallow study can effectively rule out a leak in this situation if it is suspected. A dietitian can help the patient adapt to the changed eating habit of small frequent meals.

Multivitamin, B_{12}, and iron supplementation will be needed for life in case of total gastrectomy. If the patient does not experience complications, they are discharged home around sixth to seventh postoperative day.

TAKE HOME POINTS

- Upper GI endoscopy is diagnostic and EUS provides the tumor and lymph node stage.
- PET-CT is emerging as a vital diagnostic tool in diagnosing regional as well as distant metastasis.
- Most Siewert type II GE junction tumors are staged and treated like an esophageal cancer.
- Neoadjuvant chemotherapy has shown to improve survival rate in locally advanced tumors and is being recommended by many surgeons and oncologists.
- Total gastrectomy with Roun-en-y esophagojejunostomy remains the operation of choice for locally advanced resectable proximal (upper one-third) gastric carcinoma.
- Current NCCN guidelines state that at least 15 lymph nodes should be retrieved for adequate staging, mostly achieved through a D2 lymph nodal dissection.
- Postoperative chemotherapy and radiation is advised for locally advanced cancers.

SUGGESTED READINGS

Ajani JA, Komaki R, Putnam JB, et al. A three-step strategy of induction chemotherapy then chemoradiation followed by surgery in patients with potentially resectable carcinoma of the esophagus or gastroesophageal junction. Cancer. 2001;92(2):279–286.

Avella D, Garcia L, Staveley-O' Carroll K, et al. Esophageal extension encountered during transhiatal resection of gastric or gastroesophageal tumors: attaining a negative margin. J Gastrointest Surg. 2009;13(2):368–373.

Bonenkamp JJ, Hermans J, Sasako M, et al. Extended lymph-node dissection for gastric cancer. N Engl J Med. 1999;340(12):908–914.

Bozzetti F, Bonfanti G, Bufalino R, et al. Adequacy of margins of resection in gastrectomy for cancer. Ann Surg. 1982;196(6):685–690.

Cascinu S, Scartozzi M, Labianca R, et al. High curative resection rate with weekly cisplatin, 5-fluorouracil, epidoxorubicin, 6S-leucovorin, glutathione, and filgastrim in patients with locally advanced, unresectable gastric cancer: a report from the Italian Group for the Study of Digestive Tract Cancer (GISCAD). Br J Cancer. 2004;90(8):1521–1525.

Chen J, Cheong JH, Yun MJ, et al. Improvement in preoperative staging of gastric adenocarcinoma with positron emission tomography. Cancer. 2005;103(11):2383–2390.

Chua YJ, Cunningham D. The UK NCRI MAGIC trial of perioperative chemotherapy in resectable gastric cancer: implications for clinical practice. Ann Surg Oncol. 2007;14(10):2687–2690.

Cunningham D, Allum WH, Stenning SP, et al. Perioperative chemotherapy versus surgery alone for resectable gastro-esophageal cancer. N Engl J Med. 2006;355(1):11–20.

Cuschieri A, Fayers P, Fielding J, et al. Postoperative morbidity and mortality after D1 and D2 resections for gastric cancer: preliminary results of the MRC randomized controlled surgical trial. The Surgical Cooperative Group. Lancet. 1996;347(9007):995–999.

Dooley CP, Larson AW, Stace NH, et al. Double-contrast barium meal and upper gastrointestinal endoscopy. A comparative study. Ann Intern Med. 1984;101(4):538–545.

Ganpathi IS, So JB, Ho KY. Endoscopic ultrasonography for gastric cancer: does it influence treatment? Surg Endosc. 2006;20(4):559–562.

Gotoda T, Iwasaki M, Kusano C, et al. Endoscopic resection of early gastric cancer treated by guideline and expanded National Cancer Centre criteria. Br J Surg. 2010;97(6):868–871.

Kinkel K, Lu Y, Both M, et al. Detection of hepatic metastases from cancers of the gastrointestinal tract by using noninvasive imaging methods (US, CT, MR imaging, PET): a meta-analysis. Radiology. 2002;224(3):748–756.

Lee YT, Ng EK, Hung LC, et al. Accuracy of endoscopic ultrasonography in diagnosing ascites and predicting peritoneal metastases in gastric cancer patients. Gut. 2005;54(11):1541–1545.

Power DG, Schattner MA, Gerdes H, et al. Endoscopic ultrasound can improve the selection for laparoscopy in patients with localized gastric cancer. J Am Coll Surg. 2009;208(2):173–178.

Saikawa Y, Kubota T, Kumagai K, et al. Phase II study of chemoradiotherapy with S-1 and low-dose cisplatin for inoperable advanced gastric cancer. Int J Radiat Oncol Biol Phys. 2008;71(1):173–179.

Sarela AI, Lefkowitz R, Brennan MF, et al. Selection of patients with gastric adenocarcinoma for laparoscopic staging. Am J Surg. 2006;191(1):134–138.

Smith JW, Moreira J, Abood G, et al. The influence of (18) flourodeoxyglucose positron emission tomography on the management of gastroesophageal junction carcinoma. Am J Surg. 2009;197(3):308–312.

Yang SH, Zhang YC, Yang KH, et al. An evidence-based medicine review of lymphadenectomy extent for gastric cancer. Am J Surg. 2009;197(2):246–251.

16 Bleeding Gastric Ulcer

DANIELLE FRITZE and MICHAEL MULHOLLAND

Presentation

A 58-year-old man presents to the emergency room following several episodes of coffee ground emesis. While awaiting evaluation, he suddenly vomits a large volume of bright red blood. As he is urgently transported to a resuscitation bay, his wife explains that he is generally healthy except for the stomach ulcer he had the previous year. He completed a course of two antibiotics for the ulcer and continues to take omeprazole daily. He has never had an operation and takes no other medications. On exam, the patient is distressed but alert, oriented, and no longer vomiting. Initial vital signs reveal tachycardia with a pulse of 115 and blood pressure of 100/70. He has mild discomfort with deep palpation in the epigastrium, and the remainder of his exam is unremarkable.

Differential Diagnosis

For patients presenting with upper gastrointestinal (GI) bleeding, the source may be located in any portion of the GI tract, from the oropharynx through the ligament of Trietz **(Figure 1)**. Peptic ulcers are the most common cause of upper GI hemorrhage requiring hospitalization, implicated in nearly half of all cases. Mallory-Weiss tears, esophageal varices, and erosive disease each account for an additional 10%. While neoplasms such as adenocarcinoma or gastrointestinal stromal tumor (GIST) are less common sources, their accurate identification is particularly important for treatment planning. Rare causes of GI hemorrhage include Dieulafoy's lesions, gastric varices, and hemobilia.

Although the differential diagnosis for upper GI bleeding is broad, individual patient risk factors may point to a particular source. For example, patients with portal hypertension are at particular risk of variceal bleeding. In anyone who has had an aortic aneurysm repair, aortoenteric fistula must be immediately considered as a potentially lethal source of GI hemorrhage. This patient's ulcer history makes a recurrent gastric ulcer the most probable source of hematemesis.

Workup

Immediate management of upper GI bleeding is dictated by the patient's clinical condition. If the airway may be compromised by bleeding or diminished mental status, the patient should be intubated. Adequate intravenous access should be established promptly, with administration of crystalloid or blood products as appropriate for the patient's vital signs and rate of blood loss. Patients taking warfarin or antiplatelet agents are likely to require reversal of their coagulopathy. Nasogastric (NG) tube placement can be diagnostic

of an upper GI bleed if bright red blood is aspirated. NG tube placement also allows for evacuation of gastric contents and a rough estimation of the rate of bleeding.

History and physical exam are rarely diagnostic for a bleeding ulcer but may provide information useful in its management. Most patients with gastric ulcers report symptoms of gnawing or burning epigastric pain with a waxing and waning course. Classically, discomfort from gastric ulcers is exacerbated by oral intake. Slow, chronic blood loss may cause melena and lead to symptoms of anemia. Identification of risk factors for ulcer development such as nonsteroidal anti-inflammatory drug (NSAID) use, smoking, or multiple endocrine neoplasia type I syndrome (MEN I) lends insight into the underlying etiology of the ulcer. Knowledge of any anticoagulant or antiplatelet agents taken by the patient allows for appropriate management of the associated coagulopathy. Physical exam is often unremarkable in ulcer patients, but some will exhibit epigastric tenderness. Peritoneal signs raise concern for perforation that infrequently accompanies hemorrhage. In the acutely bleeding patient, the main utility of physical exam is to identify signs of shock and estimate the degree of blood loss.

In parallel with the initial resuscitation, diagnostic studies are undertaken. Serum hematocrit, coagulation profile, and blood type and screen are obtained; hematocrit is followed serially. Peritoneal signs should prompt an upright chest x-ray to evaluate for pneumoperitoneum. In the absence of peritonitis, no imaging studies are necessary. Esophagogastroduodenoscopy (EGD) is the most effective means of locating the source of upper GI bleeding, with successful identification of the responsible lesion in 95% of patients. In rare cases where the source of bleeding is not located on initial endoscopy, repeat EGD, angiography, or technetium-99m–labeled red blood cell scan may be successful.

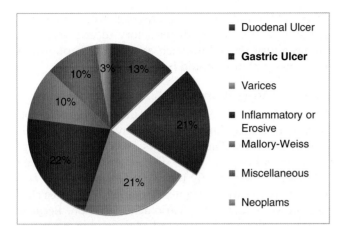

- ■ Duodenal Ulcer
- ■ **Gastric Ulcer**
- ■ Varices
- ■ Inflammatory or Erosive
- ■ Mallory-Weiss
- ■ Miscellaneous
- ■ Neoplams

FIGURE 1 • Sources of upper gastrointestinal bleeding.

Diagnosis and Treatment

Once a gastric ulcer is identified, endoscopic therapy is guided by the risk of recurrent hemorrhage and the patient's clinical stability. Although bleeding frequently resolves spontaneously, specific stigmata of hemorrhage predict continued or recurrent bleeding and the need for intervention **(Table 1)**. Ulcers with evidence of active bleeding or a visible vessel within the lesion (Forrest grade 1a, 1b, and 2a) are at highest risk. Ulcers with an adherent clot and underlying oozing are also prone to recurrent bleeding. Endoscopic intervention is indicated for each of these high-risk lesions. Options include the application of clips, thermal coagulation, or injection of a vasoconstricting or sclerosing agent. When feasible, biopsy of the ulcer is important to identify any associated malignancy. Antral biopsies are used to establish a histologic diagnosis of *Helicobacter pylori*. For patients with a bleeding ulcer, endoscopic interventions carry a 90% success rate in achieving initial hemostasis. If a patient rebleeds after endoscopic intervention, a second endoscopic attempt at hemostasis is made and has been demonstrated in a randomized trial to be safer than proceeding to surgery. However, for bleeding that cannot be controlled endoscopically (after two attempts), or for patients with hemorrhagic shock, surgery may be lifesaving.

Following initial hemostasis, the etiology of the ulcer must be identified and addressed. *H. pylori* and NSAIDs are the two most important factors contributing to the development of gastric ulcers **(Table 2)**. Each is implicated in over 50% of cases, with additive effects. Tobacco use is also contributory. Four percent of gastric ulcers harbor an underlying malignancy, most commonly gastric adenocarcinoma. In rare cases, Zollinger-Ellison syndrome, either sporadic or associated with MEN I, may be at fault. Ulcer location may also offer insight into etiology. Prepyloric and duodenal ulcers are typically related to acid hypersecretion, whereas NSAID-induced ulcers may be located anywhere in the stomach **(Table 3)**.

Medical therapy directed at ulcer etiology is an important adjunct to endoscopic and surgical interventions. Acid suppression with a proton pump inhibitor (PPI) decreases the risk of rebleeding after endoscopic hemostasis, aids in ulcer healing and prevents ulcer recurrence. NSAIDs should be withheld if medically possible. If NSAIDs are to be continued, concurrent acid suppression or use of misoprostol is imperative. Smoking cessation is strongly encouraged. For patients with *H. pylori*, eradication of the bacteria results in lower ulcer recurrence rates than acid suppression therapy alone. In over 90% of colonized patients, this can be accomplished with a single course of "triple therapy"—two antibiotics active against *H. pylori* and a PPI. Confirmed clearance of *H. pylori*, in combination with a maintenance PPI, is associated with <2% risk of recurrent bleeding in the first year. Endoscopy should be performed after 6 weeks to document ulcer healing. Almost uniformly, recurrence is related to *H. pylori* reinfection or NSAID use.

Surgical Approach

While surgery remains the primary means of managing anatomic complications of ulcer disease, the development of effective pharmacotherapy for acid suppression and *H. pylori* clearance has reduced the role of surgery in addressing the underlying etiology. When treating anatomic complications, the operation should be carefully tailored to the patient's clinical scenario. The appropriate surgical procedure for a bleeding gastric ulcer is also dependent upon the patient's condition **(Figure 2)**. For unstable patients, midline laparotomy is followed by anterior gastrotomy. Once the lesion is identified, the ulcer is oversewn, biopsied

TABLE 1. Forrest Classification of Peptic Ulcers

Grade	Stigmata		30-day Risk of Rebleeding After Endoscopic Therapy (%)
1a	Actively bleeding	Pulsatile	20
1b	Ulcer	Nonpulsatile	<10
2a	Nonbleeding ulcer	Visible vessel	15
2b		Adherent clot	<5
2c		Hematin-covered base	7
3	Nonbleeding ulcer	Clean base	3

TABLE 2. Etiology of Gastric Ulcer

NSAIDS
H. pylori
Zollinger-Ellison
Neoplasm

TABLE 3. Modified Johnson Classification of Gastric Ulcers

Type	Location	Etiology
I	Lesser curve	Varies, not related to acid hypersecretion
II	Two ulcers, stomach body and duodenum	Acid hypersecretion
III	Prepyloric	Acid hypersecretion
IV	GE junction	Varies, not related to acid hypersecretion
V	Any location	NSAIDs

(if possible) and the gastrotomy repaired. For stable patients with a history of refractory ulcer disease, an antisecretory procedure such as truncal vagotomy or distal gastrectomy should be considered.

Truncal Vagotomy

In patients with bleeding gastric ulcers, truncal vagotomy is indicated for those who have failed previous medical therapy. These patients usually have a long-standing history of ulcer disease and have proven refractory to (or serially noncompliant with) PPIs and *H. pylori* eradication. Vagotomy markedly reduces cholinergic stimulation of gastric acid secretion. Because vagotomy also results in pyloric denervation, a concurrent procedure such as pyloroplasty or antrectomy is thus necessary to ensure gastric drainage.

To perform a truncal vagotomy, the left hepatic lobe is retracted cephalad and laterally with division of the triangular ligament as needed to expose the hiatus. The overlying peritoneum is incised and the esophagus dissected circumferentially for several centimeters about the gastroesophageal (GE) junction. Anteriorly, the vagal trunk is found closely applied to the esophageal wall. In contrast, the posterior vagus may reside

Algorithm for Management of Bleeding Gastric Ulcer

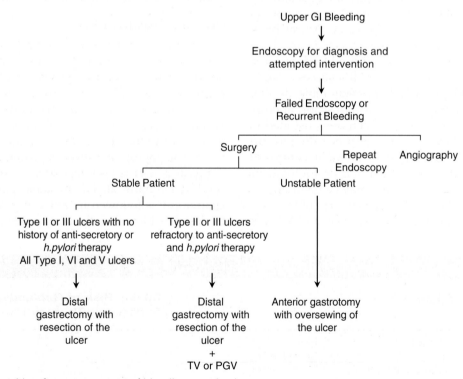

FIGURE 2 • Algorithm for management of bleeding gastric ulcer.

1 cm or more posterolateral to the esophagus. Palpation may aid in initial identification of the nerves. Once both trunks are located, proximal and distal clips are placed to allow for resection of a 2-cm intervening segment of nerve. These specimens are sent to pathology for histologic confirmation. There may be several divisions of each vagal trunk, so the area of the GE junction is carefully inspected to determine that all vagal fibers have been divided. Prior to closure, cruroplasty may be required to prevent development of a hiatal hernia.

Distal Gastrectomy

If a patient with bleeding gastric ulcer is stable, there are a few scenarios in which a distal gastrectomy can be considered. As with truncal vagotomy, patients are usually only considered candidates for distal gastrectomy if they have a history of failed medical management, especially patients with large antral ulcers that cannot be easily oversewn or patients with ulcers suspicious for cancer. Risks of operative death and complications are much higher for distal gastrectomy than simple oversewing or vagotomy, so this procedure should only be undertaken when clear indications exist.

To perform distal gastrectomy, a vertical incision in the supraumbilical midline affords adequate exposure in most cases. Following exploration of the abdomen, a Kocher maneuver is performed to mobilize the duodenum. Mobilization of the distal stomach begins with division of the gastrocolic ligament. Entry into the lesser sac permits examination of the posterior gastric wall. The omentum is then divided along the greater curvature, from the duodenum halfway to the GE junction. The right gastroepiploic vessels are ligated and divided near the gastroduodenal artery (GDA). The gastrohepatic ligament is then incised. The right gastric artery is identified, ligated, and divided near the superior border of the duodenum. Branches of the left gastric artery are divided along the lesser curve in preparation for resection and anastomosis. An area of healthy proximal duodenum is chosen and transected with a stapling device. The proximal extent of the resection is determined by the location of the ulcer and the condition of the gastric wall. The stomach is also divided with a stapling device and all staple lines are oversewn. Continuity of the GI tract can be reestablished via either Billroth I or II reconstruction, depending upon the length and health of the duodenal stump.

Special Intraoperative Considerations

Type IV gastric ulcers can be particularly challenging to manage due to their proximity to the GE junction. In most cases, the ulcer can be resected as part of the distal gastrectomy with an extension along the lesser curve. Traditional Billroth I or II reconstruction is avoided as

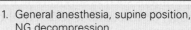

TABLE 4. Key Technical Steps in Distal Gastrectomy and Truncal Vagotomy

1. General anesthesia, supine position, NG decompression.
2. Supraumbilical vertical midline incision.

Distal gastrectomy

3. Kocher maneuver.
4. Divide the gastrocolic ligament to enter the lesser sac.
5. Examine the stomach and identify the region of the ulcer to determine the appropriate extent of resection.
6. Divide the greater omentum along the greater curve from duodenum halfway to the GE junction.
7. Ligate and divide the right gastroepiploic vessels near the GDA.
8. Incise the gastrohepatic ligament.
9. Ligate and divide the right gastric artery proximally.
10. Divide the duodenum and stomach with a stapling device.
11. Oversew both staple lines, leaving a portion of the gastrotomy closure available for reconstruction.
12. Reestablish GI tract continuity via either Billroth I or II reconstruction.

Truncal vagotomy

13. Retract the left hepatic lobe laterally, with division of the triangular ligament as needed to expose the esophageal hiatus.
14. Incise the peritoneum and dissect the esophagus circumferentially.
15. Identify and dissect the anterior and posterior trunks of the vagus nerves.
16. Place proximal and distal clips ~2 cm apart on each trunk and then resect the intervening nerve segments.
17. Inspect the esophagus to ensure that all portions of the vagus nerves have been divided.
18. As needed, perform a cruroplasty to prevent hiatal hernia.
19. Confirm NG tube placement and then close the abdomen.

Potential Pitfalls

- Failure to identify an associated neoplasm.
- Injury to the porta or inferior vena cava with Kocher maneuver and duodenal dissection.
- Injury to the middle colic vessels with division of the gastrocolic ligament.
- Billroth I reconstruction under tension or with inflamed duodenum.
- Failure to divide all vagal branches.

it is likely to result in narrowing of the GE junction. Instead, roux-en-Y gastrojejunostomy permits construction of a wide anastomosis, incorporating the distal GE junction and the entirety of the gastrotomy. In rare circumstances, the ulcer may be oversewn and left *in situ*. A concurrent antisecretory procedure with *H. pylori* eradication, PPI, and cessation of NSAIDs results in satisfactory ulcer healing in most patients.

Postoperative Management

Following surgery for a bleeding gastric ulcer, patients remain on bowel rest with NG decompression. These measures may be discontinued as gastric emptying resumes. Patients should be observed for potential postoperative complications such as surgical site infection (SSI), hemorrhage, or anastomotic leak. For those with a Billroth II reconstruction, duodenal stump leak is a particularly morbid complication.

With initiation of oral intake, patients who undergo gastrectomy should also be monitored for postgastrectomy dumping syndrome. This is characterized by postprandial GI and vasomotor symptoms, such as nausea, abdominal pain, dizziness, and even syncope. In most patients, these symptoms are temporary, and easily managed with frequent small meals. In a small minority of patients, however, dumping symptoms can become debilitating. Octreotide may be helpful in this circumstance. At discharge, all patients are counseled to avoid tobacco and NSAIDs as well as to continue PPI therapy. Those colonized with *H. pylori* receive triple therapy and eradication is confirmed at follow-up.

Case Conclusion

The patient's immediate management included placement of two large-bore ivs, crystalloid resuscitation, and a pantoprazole infusion. His initial hematocrit was 28%, with normal coagulation studies. Endoscopy performed while the patient was still in the emergency room revealed a 2-cm gastric ulcer in the prepyloric region (type III) with a nonbleeding visible vessel. Clips were applied and biopsies performed endoscopically. He was then admitted to the hospital for observation. The following day, he had another episode of hematemesis. Endoscopy was again attempted, but unsuccessful in controlling the bleeding. He required two units of packed red blood cells but remained hemodynamically stable. He was taken to the operating room emergently for surgical intervention. Given the history of recurrent type III gastric ulcer following *H. pylori* eradication and long-term acid suppression, an antisecretory procedure was deemed appropriate. Truncal vagotomy was performed in conjunction with distal gastrectomy. The patient tolerated the procedure well, and recovered without recurrent bleeding or serious complication. Final surgical pathology confirmed a benign gastric ulcer.

TAKE HOME POINTS

- Although decreasing in incidence, peptic ulcer remains the most common cause of upper GI bleeding, with significant associated mortality.
- *H. pylori* infection and NSAID use are the most frequent inciting factors in bleeding gastric ulcers.
- Endoscopy is the first-line diagnostic intervention and is therapeutically effective in a majority of patients.
- Surgery is indicated in patients with massive bleeding, failure of endoscopic therapy, recurrent hemorrhage, or neoplasm.
- Anterior gastrotomy, ulcer oversewing, and biopsy is the procedure of choice for patients without a history of refractory ulcer disease.
- Truncal vagotomy is indicated only for patients with ulcers refractory to adequate PPI therapy and *H. pylori* eradication.
- Distal gastrectomy with inclusion of the ulcer in the specimen is the procedure of choice in stable patients with refractory ulcer disease who have large antral ulcers.
- Acid suppression and clearance of *H. pylori* decrease the risk of recurrent bleeding gastric ulcer.

SUGGESTED READINGS

Enestvedt BK, Gralnek IM, Mattek N, et al. An evaluation of endoscopic indications and findings related to nonvariceal upper-GI hemorrhage in a large multicenter consortium. Gastrointest Endosc. 2008;67(3):422–429.

Gisbert JP, Khorrami S, Carballo F, et al. H. pylori eradication therapy vs. antisecretory non-eradication therapy (with or without long-term maintenance antisecretory therapy) for the prevention of recurrent bleeding from peptic ulcer. Cochrane Database Syst Rev. 2004(2):CD004062.

Gralnek IM, Barkun AN, Bardou M. Management of acute bleeding from a peptic ulcer. N Engl J Med. 2008;359(9):928–937.

17 Bleeding Duodenal Ulcer

WENDY L. WAHL

Presentation

A 57-year-old man with multiple medical problems presents to the emergency department feeling light-headed with hematemesis and melena. His medical history includes end-stage renal disease and bladder cancer, for which he recently underwent cystectomy with an ileal conduit. He is hypotensive, and placement of a nasogastric tube yielded bright red blood clots. He is currently on hemodialysis three times each week and has no prior history of ulcers. He does not take nonsteroidals or aspirin on a regular basis. Large-bore intravenous access is established and his blood pressure improves with fluid resuscitation. His abdomen is mildly distended but nontender on palpation. He has a healing midline abdominal incision with a pink ileal conduit with minimal dark-appearing urine. Digital rectal examination reveals dark, tarry stool, which is guaiac positive.

Differential Diagnosis

His recent major surgery, and the attendant lack of oral intake, place him at risk for stress gastritis or peptic ulcer disease. His history of renal failure may also make him more likely to have arterial–venous malformations or bleeding from gastritis from platelet dysfunction. He could also have esophageal disease such as a Mallory-Weiss tear from vomiting and, less likely, variceal hemorrhage since he provides no history of cirrhosis. But with his history of hemodialysis and renal failure, he does have a higher risk of hepatitis. Less likely in this scenario, given the acute onset, would be upper gastrointestinal tract neoplasms such as esophageal, gastric, or duodenal tumors.

Workup

At this point, if a nasogastric tube were not in place, one should be placed for gastric lavage and evacuation of the stomach. Given his history of hematemesis, an esophagogastroduodenoscopy (EGD) would be the next diagnostic and potentially therapeutic procedure of choice. If there is any concern over perforation in addition to bleeding, an abdominal radiograph should be performed prior to EGD. Laboratory tests that should be drawn to establish baseline values would be a complete CBC with platelets, PT with INR, PTT, type and screen, a comprehensive metabolic panel to assess for electrolyte abnormalities. An arterial blood gas should be drawn to evaluate for metabolic acidosis due to underresuscitation.

Diagnosis and Treatment

In severely ill patients, endotracheal intubation should be considered prior to EGD, especially in patients who are in shock or unable to protect their airway. This patient is awake and alert and has normal vital signs after fluid resuscitation. An EGD is performed, which reveals a large clot and active bleeding in the first portion of the posterior duodenum **(see Figure 1)**.

This patient is at high risk for rebleeding (active bleeding during endoscopy—90% chance of recurrence, visible vessel—50% chance of rebleeding, adherent clot—25% to 30% chance of recurrence). Despite this risk, attempts at endoscopic control of the bleeding should be made. Recent experience suggests that removing the clot in order to treat the underlying ulcer can reduce the risk of rebleeding. Studies show that epinephrine injection alone is inferior to combined therapies with epinephrine injection and thermal coagulation or placement of a hemoclip.

Administration of proton pump inhibitors (PPIs) has been shown to reduce the risk of rebleeding. Most of these studies used intravenous omeprazole, although other PPIs can serve as reasonable alternatives. No studies have shown that high-dose infusions are more effective than routine intravenous doses of PPIs. In addition to PPIs, any potentially precipitating medications such as aspirin or nonsteroidal anti-inflammatory agents should be discontinued. The patient should also be evaluated with gastric biopsies for the presence of *Helicobacter pylori* as a precipitating factor for ulcer formation.

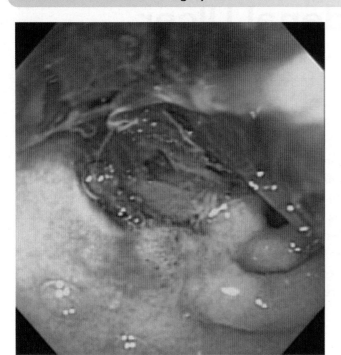

FIGURE 1 • Endoscopic view of bleeding duodenal ulcer.

Presentation Continued

The patient stabilizes after a total of four units of PRBCs. Three days after his initial EGD he develops recurrent hematemesis with an associated drop in his blood pressure. Blood transfusion and fluids are started.

Discussion

Based on a controlled trial that assessed efficacy of endoscopic therapy compared to surgery for recurrent bleeding, patients who had a second therapeutic endoscopy had fewer complications than those who underwent operative intervention, although mortality was equivalent. Given that this patient has had a recent midline incision and has not failed a second endoscopic attempt, a repeat EGD is indicated. In our case, at his second EGD, the endoscopist is able to slow the bleeding down with epinephrine injections but cannot reliably use cautery or other methods for hemostasis.

Although endoscopy is the best initial diagnostic and therapeutic procedure, failure to achieve hemostasis leaves surgery and transcatheter arterial intervention (TAI) as possible therapeutic modalities. At this point, indications for surgery for active rebleeding from a duodenal ulcer include hemodynamic instability or shock despite blood transfusion, rebleeding after two attempts at endoscopic therapy, or continued slow bleeding requiring blood transfusion exceeding more than three units per day. In our case, after discussion with the family and patient, they do not wish to pursue surgery at this time and opt for TAI. Active bleeding is identified **(Figure 2A)**, and successful coil embolization of the gastroduodenal artery (GDA) is performed and the bleeding has stopped **(Figure 2B)**. On the day of discharge, the patient has recurrent, large-volume hematemesis with hemodynamic instability. At this point, the patient has failed two endoscopic therapies and angiographic embolization. Surgical intervention is warranted. Depending on institutional resources, this

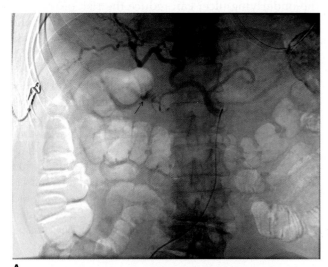

A

FIGURE 2A • Active bleeding during angiography.

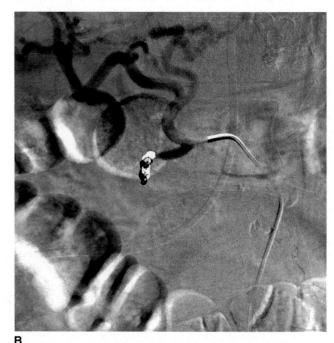

B

FIGURE 2B • Cessation of bleeding after embolization coils.

may have been the selected therapeutic option after the second failed endoscopy.

Surgical Approach

Much of the literature surrounding choices for operative management for complicated peptic ulcer disease heralds from the era that predated the use of H₂-blockers and PPI therapy. Controversy exists as to whether a definitive ulcer operation is now required, particularly for perforated peptic ulcers. The priority for patients undergoing operation for a bleeding duodenal ulcer is to control the bleeding. If the exact site of the bleeding is not known, a longitudinal pyloroduodenotomy allows for inspection of the duodenal bulb and the gastric antrum. Otherwise, the proximal duodenum can be incised directly over the ulcer site. Suture of the bleeding vessel in the base of the ulcer can be performed with sutures placed superiorly and inferiorly to the ulcer crater **(Figure 3)**. If bleeding continues, the GDA can be ligated superiorly to the duodenum. While placing the sutures, the surgeon must be aware that the common bile duct courses posteriorly, and if the location cannot be determined, a Fogarty or similar biliary catheter should be inserted into the duct to avoid injury. After achieving hemostasis, attempts to approximate the ulcer crater should be made. The longitudinal pyloroduodenotomy should then be closed transversely to avoid narrowing of the pylorus and duodenum (Heineke-Mikulicz pyloroplasty).

After control of hemorrhage from the GDA, an acid-reduction procedure is generally recommended for patients with a history of refractory peptic ulcer disease (i.e., a history of long-standing PPI use or noncompliance). The type of procedure is dependent on patient stability and surgeon experience. The most expeditious procedure is a truncal vagotomy; however, if the patient has stabilized and the surgeon is experienced, a parietal cell vagotomy (highly selective vagotomy) is a reasonable alternative. Maneuvers for truncal vagotomy include retracting the left lobe of the liver for exposure. The serosa overlying the esophagus

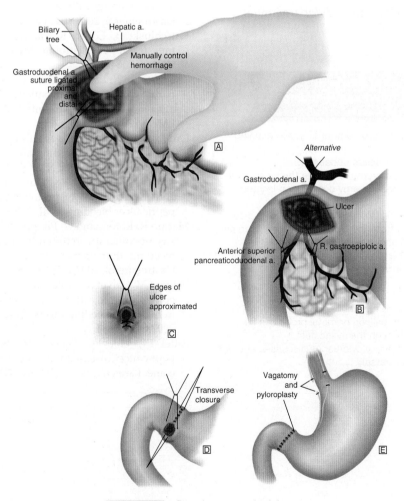

FIGURE 3 • Duodenotomy incision.

is opened and using a combination of blunt and sharp dissection, the esophagus is encircled with a Penrose drain. By retracting the esophagus caudally and palpating, the firm "violin string" of the vagus nerve is felt. The anterior vagus is easier to find and larger. If the posterior vagus is not felt, it may not be included in the Penrose drain contents, and the search should continue. After identification, the nerves should be clipped proximally and distally and a small segment excised.

Case Conclusion

The patient undergoes exploratory laparotomy, pyloroduodenotomy, and oversewing of a posterior duodenal bulb ulcer **(Table 1)**. Given his hemodynamic instability, and the fact that he has not previously been treated with PPIs, an acid reduction procedure is not performed. He recovers well from surgery without further bleeding. Gastric biopsies from his EGD return *H. pylori* positive. He is sent home on PPIs and *H. pylori* treatment.

TABLE 1. Key Technical Steps to Maneuvers in Oversewing a Bleeding Duodenal Ulcer

1. Midline laparotomy with placement of a self-retaining retractor.
2. Kocher maneuver to mobilize duodenum.
3. Create a pyloroduodenotomy to expose the ulcer in the duodenal bulb (or duodenotomy over ulcer if located elsewhere).
4. Place sutures superior, inferior, and medial to the ulcer.
5. Refractory bleeding from the GDA can be addressed by ligation of the GDA above the duodenum.
6. Close the incision transversely to avoid narrowing the pylorus or duodenum.

Potential Pitfalls

- Oversewing the distal common bile duct. To avoid this complication, a Fogarty balloon or metal probe can be passed from above through the cystic duct.
- Narrowing the duodenum or pylorus. As discussed above, close the incision transversely.

TAKE HOME POINTS

- Ensure adequate intravenous access and an adequate airway prior to any procedure.
- EGD is the most important assessment tool since it can be both diagnostic and therapeutic.
- Treat patients with a PPI and evaluate for *H. pylori* infection.
- EGD is a reasonable approach for patients who rebleed and are not profoundly unstable.
- Angiographic embolization is an option for patients who fail endoscopic therapy or have contraindications to surgery, but this option must be readily available.
- The operative approach should focus on cessation of bleeding followed by an acid reduction procedure, if appropriate.

SELECTED READINGS

Bleau BL, Gostout CJ, Sherman KE, et al. Recurrent bleeding from peptic ulcer associated with adherent clot: a randomized study comparing endoscopic treatment with medical therapy. Gastrointest Endosc. 2002;56:1–6.

Elmunzer BJ, Young SD, Inadomi JM, et al. Systematic review of the predictors of recurrent hemorrhage after endoscopic hemostatic therapy for bleeding peptic ulcers. Am J Gastroenterol. 2008;103:2625–2632.

Katschinski B, Logan R, Davies J, et al. Prognostic factors in upper gastrointestinal bleeding. Dig Dis Sci. 1994;39:706–712.

Lau JY, Sung JJ, Lam YH, et al. Endoscopic retreatment compared with surgery in patients with recurrent bleeding after initial endoscopic control of bleeding ulcers. N Engl J Med. 1999;340:751–756.

Lau JY, Sung JJ, Lee KK, et al. Effect of intravenous omeprazole on recurrent bleeding after endoscopic treatment of bleeding peptic ulcers. N Engl J Med. 2000;343:310–316.

Leontiadis GI, Sharma VK, Howden CW. Systematic review and meta-analysis of proton pump inhibitor therapy in peptic ulcer bleeding. BMJ. 2005;330:568.

Marmo R, Rotondano G, Piscopo R, et al. Dual therapy versus monotherapy in the endoscopic treatment of high-risk bleeding ulcers: a meta-analysis of controlled trials. Am J Gastroenterol. 2007;102:279–289.

Vergara M, Calvet X, Gisbert JP. Epinephrine injection versus epinephrine injection and a second endoscopic method in high risk bleeding ulcers. Cochrane Database Syst Rev. 2007;CD005584.

Zittel TT, Jehle EC, Becker HD. Surgical management of peptic ulcer disease today–Indication, technique and outcome. Langenbecks Arch Surg. 2000;385:84–96.

18 Perforated Duodenal Ulcer

CONSTANCE W. LEE and GEORGE A. SAROSI Jr.

Presentation

A 70-year-old man presents to the emergency department (ED) with a 1-hour history of generalized abdominal pain that began abruptly and now radiates to both shoulders. The patient has a prior history of peptic ulcer disease but is not currently on acid-suppression therapy. He is also on low-dose aspirin for peripheral vascular disease. He has never had an abdominal surgery. He has no known drug allergies. He does not smoke tobacco or drink alcohol.

On physical examination, his temperature is 36.5°C, heart rate is 100, blood pressure is 125/70, and his abdomen is diffusely tender to palpation.

Differential Diagnosis

The differential diagnosis for this patient includes the following: perforated hollow viscus secondary to peptic ulcer disease (PUD), carcinoma, gastrinoma, mesenteric ischemia, small bowel obstruction, Crohn's disease, and Boerhaave's syndrome; pancreatitis, appendicitis, diverticulitis, ruptured abdominal aortic aneurysm, ruptured ectopic pregnancy, pneumonia, pulmonary infarction, and renal or biliary colic.

Peptic ulcers are most frequently found in the stomach and duodenum. They are most often associated with *Helicobacter pylori* infection or the use of nonsteroidal anti-inflammatory drugs (NSAIDs), including aspirin. Risk factors for the development of NSAID-related ulcers include advanced age, history of prior ulcer, serious systemic illness, concomitant use of anticoagulants or corticosteroids, and high NSAID doses. Less common causes of PUD include gastrinoma, systemic mastocytosis, carcinoma, sarcoidosis, Crohn's disease, and carcinoid syndrome.

Ulcer complications include perforation, obstruction, and bleeding. In a review of 88 patients with a perforated peptic ulcer, the most common location of perforation was the duodenal bulb (62%), followed by the pyloric region (20%), and then the gastric body (18%). Ulcer perforation is associated with prior history of ulcer disease and use of NSAIDs. In the setting of NSAID therapy, the risk factors associated with ulcer perforation include a history of prior ulcer, age >60 years, and the concomitant use of steroids, anticoagulants, selective serotonin reuptake inhibitors, or alendronate.

The classic clinical presentation of a perforated peptic ulcer has been described as a three-stage process:

1. Early (onset to 2 hours): The abdominal pain begins abruptly, with the patient often being able to remember the exact time the pain started. The pain may first localize to the epigastrum but quickly becomes generalized. The pain may radiate to the shoulders if the diaphragm is irritated. On examination, the patient may be tachycardic, have a low body temperature, and the abdomen is tender to palpation.
2. Intermediate (2 to 12 hours): The patient may report an improvement in pain. However, on physical exam the patient often displays increased pain with movement, and the abdominal wall is rigid. In addition, there may be significant pain with palpation of the hypogastrum and right lower quadrant secondary to drainage of enteric contents from the perforation.
3. Late (after 12 hours): The patient may complain of increased pain and fevers, signs of hypovolemia, and abdominal distension. Although the patient may vomit during any stage, it is most common at this stage.

Workup

It is important to quickly diagnose a perforated peptic ulcer because the prognosis is good if treatment is provided within the first 6 hours, whereas delayed treatment beyond 12 hours is associated with decreased survival and increased morbidity.

Imaging Studies

An upright chest x-ray or an abdominal x-ray may reveal the presence of intraperitoneal free air. A computed tomography (CT) scan may also be used to identify intraperitoneal free air or free fluid. However, approximately 10% to 20% of patients with a perforated duodenal ulcer will not have direct findings of perforation. If free air is present, no other test is required to confirm the diagnosis. An upper GI study or an abdominal CT scan with water-soluble contrast may demonstrate the leak if free air is not present and a confirmatory test is required for diagnosis.

Laboratory Studies

Laboratory studies are not necessary for the diagnosis of a perforated duodenal ulcer. However, they contribute to the complete evaluation and appropriate management of the patient. A basic metabolic panel will guide fluid and electrolyte resuscitation. A complete blood count may demonstrate leukocytosis with a left shift in a patient with a perforated ulcer. A serum gastrin level may assist in the diagnosis of gastrinoma, though the result of the test will likely not return in time to influence the operative strategy. Given that *H. pylori* infection is present in 70% to 90% of duodenal ulcers and 30% to 60% of gastric ulcers, patients with peptic ulcer disease should be tested. Noninvasive testing for *H. pylori* infection includes urea breath testing, stool antigen testing, and serology. Ideally, *H. pylori* infection is identified preoperatively, as it can influence operative strategy. A monoclonal stool antigen test is available that has 94% sensitivity, 97% specificity, and may be performed in about an hour. There is also a rapid stool antigen test for the diagnosis of *H. pylori* that can be done in 5 minutes. However, its sensitivity and specificity have been shown to be 76% and 98%, respectively.

In our scenario, the patient's presenting signs and symptoms, combined with his risk factors place the diagnosis of a perforated peptic ulcer high on the list of differential diagnoses. An upright chest x-ray demonstrates free intraperitoneal air. A stool antigen test is positive for *H. pylori* infection. The ED physician consults general surgery, starts fluid resuscitation, initiates nasogastric decompression, places a Foley catheter, and administers omeprazole, ampicillin, metronidazole, ceftriaxone, and fluconazole.

Diagnosis and Treatment

The medical/nonoperative management of a perforated peptic ulcer includes fluid resuscitation, nasogastric decompression, acid suppression, and empiric antibiotic therapy for coverage of enteric gram-negative rods, oral flora, anaerobes, and fungus. In the setting of a perforated duodenal ulcer without peritonitis, the application of a nonoperative management strategy has been proposed, especially for patients at high risk for operative complications. However, delaying the surgical repair of a perforated peptic ulcer more than 12 hours after presentation has been associated with increased morbidity and mortality. Furthermore, a randomized trial of nonoperative treatment for perforated peptic ulcers by Crofts et al. demonstrated that patients over 70 years of age were less likely to improve with conservative management. Operative management is the preferred treatment strategy in most patients, especially the elderly.

In our clinical scenario, you evaluate the patient 2 hours after the start of the symptoms, at which time the patient notes an improvement in generalized pain.

However, on examination the heart rate is 110, the blood pressure is 90/50, and the abdomen is rigid, with the patient more sensitive to changes in position. You decide to proceed to the operating room for management of this problem. On exploration of our patient you identify a 1 cm anterior duodenal perforation.

Surgical Approach

Elective operations for peptic ulcer disease have become uncommon with the successful medical management of acid and *H. pylori* infection. However, surgical management is almost always indicated for a perforated ulcer, especially when the patient is hemodynamically unstable, has signs of peritonitis, or has evidence of free contrast extravasation on imaging. Although operative treatment is the appropriate plan, the patient should receive fluid resuscitation and antibiotic treatment while preparing the operating room. It should be noted that emergency surgery for peptic ulcer perforation has up to 30% risk of mortality. The presence of comorbid disease has been shown to increase mortality. Furthermore, in patients requiring emergency surgery, variables identified as being independently associated with mortality include age, American Society of Anesthesiologists (ASA) class, shock on admission, hypoalbuminemia on admission, preoperative metabolic acidosis, and an elevated serum creatinine.

Surgical Procedure(s) for the Management of Perforated Duodenal Ulcers

1. *Omental patch repair* (**Table 1**): The safest technique for the management of a perforated duodenal ulcer, especially in the setting of delayed repair (>24 hours after presentation), hemodynamic instability, or significant intra-abdominal contamination is a patch repair with an omental pedicle. This technique combined with the appropriate medical therapy is likely sufficient in the case of a patient with a history of *H. pylori* infection or NSAID use.

The repair may be performed laparoscopically or open. The perforation is repaired by taking a seromuscular bite from one side of the perforation, taking a bite of omentum, followed by another seromuscular bite from the other side of the perforation, and then tying to fix the omental pedicle in place. Typically, three to four sutures are required to secure the patch. Follow the repair by irrigation of the peritoneal cavity with large volumes of warm saline.

Pitfalls

- The optimal repair of duodenal ulcer perforations >2 cm can be challenging, and the omental patch repair may be associated with increased risk of failure. Performing a definitive repair has been suggested, as have less standard repairs, including tube duodenostomy.

TABLE 1. Omental Patch Key Points

Laparoscopic or open approach

Fix omental pedicle in place.

No need to suture the perforation closed.

Irrigate peritoneal cavity.

TABLE 2. Truncal Vagotomy and Pyloroplasty Key Points

Isolate the distal esophagus.

Identify, dissect, and transect the vagal trunks—send nerve biopsy to pathology.

Dissect the distal 6 cm of the esophagus to ensure complete division of vagal fibers.

Mobilize the duodenum.

Make an incision from the antrum onto the proximal duodenum.

Place stay sutures at either end of the incision to facilitate transverse closure.

- On exploration, the omentum, liver, or gallbladder may have already "patched" the perforation, in which case the surgeon must decide whether to remove the natural patch and surgically repair the defect, or to simply irrigate the peritoneal cavity.
- If the ulcer perforation is located at the distal end of the pyloric channel, the duodenum may need to be mobilized to provide adequate exposure of the defect.

2. A definitive ulcer procedure may be performed if the patient is hemodynamically stable, has minimal intra-abdominal contamination, and either (1) has a history of PUD with unknown *H. pylori* status or (2) is unable to stop NSAID therapy.

   a. *Truncal vagotomy and pyloroplasty (drainage) (V&D)* **(Table 2)**: A truncal vagotomy reduces basal acid secretion by 80% and stimulated acid secretion by 50%. It reduces acid secretion by preventing direct cholinergic stimulation for acid secretion and by decreasing the response of parietal cells to histamine and gastrin. Unfortunately, a truncal vagotomy also damages the stomach's receptive relaxation and antral grinding, in addition to the pyloric sphincter's coordination required for gastric emptying. To compensate for these changes, a pyloroplasty is performed to facilitate stomach drainage. The benefit of V&D is that it is safe and may be done relatively quickly. The drawbacks of the procedure are that 10% of patients later report diarrhea or dumping syndrome, and 10% have a recurrent ulcer.

   Procedure: Access the esophageal hiatus by dividing the left triangular ligament and retracting the left lateral lobe of the liver. Open the peritoneum overlying the esophagus by dividing the lesser omentum and the esophagophrenic ligament. Use blunt dissection between the esophagus and the adjacent crux to allow two fingers behind the esophagus. Careful dissection is critical to avoid iatrogenic esophageal perforation. Downward traction on the gastroesophageal junction facilitates identification of the vagus nerve. Identify the anterior and posterior vagal trunks, dissect them from the esophagus, and then transect them **(Figure 2)**. Mark the transected vagal margins with hemoclips and send biopsies of both nerves to pathology to confirm that the transected structures were nerves. Note that the criminal nerve of Grassi coming off the posterior vagus trunk can be missed if the vagotomy is performed lower on the esophagus; to avoid this, complete circumferential dissection of the distal 6 cm of the esophagus ensures division of these nerve fibers.

   A Heinecke-Mikulicz pyloroplasty is performed by mobilizing the second part of the duodenum using a Kocher maneuver. Then a 5 cm incision is made from the antrum, over the pyloric sphincter, and onto the proximal duodenum. Place seromuscular tacking sutures to the cephalad and caudad ends of the incision to facilitate the transverse closure of the wound **(Figure 1)**. The incision is closed in one or two layers. If closed in two, start with an inner layer of full-thickness interrupted absorbable sutures, followed by a seromuscular layer of Lembert sutures. Alternatively, a stapled closure may be performed using a TA-55 stapler containing 4.8 mm staples. Note that if the duodenum is severely scarred or inflamed, then a gastrojejunostomy may be used in place of a pyloroplasty.

Pitfalls

- Failure to perform careful esophageal dissection and injuring/perforating the esophagus
- Forgetting to perform biopsies of the vagal nerves for confirmation of the appropriate resection of nerve tissue
- Causing splenic injury when applying traction on the stomach
- Causing a postoperative hiatal hernia from not repairing defects at the esophageal hiatus at the time of vagotomy

   b. Vagotomy and antrectomy **(Table 3)**: The combination of the vagotomy and antrectomy eliminates basal acid secretion and decreases stimulated acid secretion by 80%. The benefits

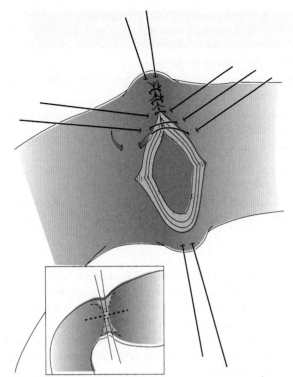

FIGURE 1 • Pyloroplasty. (Figure 46.2 in Mulholland MW. Gastroduodenal ulceration. In: Mulholland MW, Lillemoe KD, Doherty GM, et al., eds. Greenfield's Surgery: Scientific Principles and Practice. 4th ed. Baltimore, MD: Lippincott Williams & Wilkins, 2006:722–735).

of a vagotomy with antrectomy are that the procedure may be applied to a variety of situations, and that the ulcer recurrence rate is very low. The disadvantages are that the operative mortality is higher than with V&D or highly selective vagotomy (HSV), and that there may be complications associated with the subsequent Billroth I or Billroth II reconstructions. In the modern era, the antrectomy should be reserved for healthy/stable patients with refractory ulcer disease and/or anatomic indications (e.g., large antral gastric ulcers, pyloric scarring).

TABLE 3. Antrectomy

Antrectomy

Free the greater curvature of the stomach.

Dissect the first part of the duodenum from the pancreas.

Divide the stomach.

Ligate the right gastric artery at the level of the pylorus.

Divide the duodenum just distal to the pylorus—send duodenal stump margin for pathology.

Complete with either a Billroth I or Billroth II anastomosis.

Procedure: The vagotomy proceeds as described above.

The antrectomy is begun by separating the distal half of the greater curvature by dissecting the greater omentum from the proximal half of the transverse colon, carefully isolating and ligating the branches from the gastroepiploic arcade. Then the posterior wall of the first part of the duodenum is dissected from the pancreas. The gastrohepatic ligament is divided proximally along the lesser curvature and the left gastric vessels along the lesser curvature are ligated and divided. The stomach is divided with the goal to remove all the antral mucosa. The upper margin of the antrum may be approximated by identifying the halfway point on the lesser curvature between the gastroesophageal junction and the pylorus. The stomach is divided with a GIA-style linear stapler using 4.8 mm staples. Next, the right gastric artery is identified above the pylorus, ligated, and divided. To facilitate manipulation of the duodenum, dissect approximately 1.5 cm of the posterior duodenum off of the pancreas. Divide the duodenum just distal to the pylorus with a GIA-style linear stapler. Send a frozen section biopsy of the margin of duodenal stump to confirm the presence of duodenal Brunner's glands to avoid retained antrum. Following the antrectomy, either a Billroth I gastroduodenal anastomosis or a Billroth II gastrojejunostomy is constructed. A Billroth I requires at least 1 cm of healthy duodenum and in the case of significant scarring it is difficult to perform. A Billroth II is the default reconstruction and can almost always be performed. For a Billroth I reconstruction, the staple line of the transected duodenum is excised and an end-to-end gastroduodenal anastomosis is performed in two layers. The inner layer consists of full-thickness continuous sutures. The outer layer consists of interrupted seromuscular Lembert sutures. A crown stitch is placed at the "angle of sorrow" of the gastroduodenal anastomosis. If a Billroth II is to be constructed, then the duodenal stump is closed in two layers. The Billroth II gastrojejunostomy is begun by choosing a loop of proximal jejunum and bringing it antecolic or retrocolic to the stomach. If a retrocolic approach is chosen, care must be taken to close the mesenteric defect to reduce the risk of a future internal hernia. The jejunum is aligned along the gastric pouch and a two-layered gastrojejunostomy is performed. A crown stitch is placed at the "angle of sorrow" at the medial margin of the gastrojejunal anastomosis. Any exposed staples from the antrectomy should be oversewn.

TABLE 4. Parietal Cell Vagotomy Key Points

Divide the lesser omentum from the lesser curvature.

Encircle the trunks with Penrose drain and apply tension to facilitate exposure of branches.

Dissect and ligate neurovascular branches of the vagal trunks proximal to the crow's foot of the nerve of Latarjet.

Skeletonize the distal 6 cm of the esophagus to ensure complete division of criminal nerve of Grassi.

Pitfalls

- Incomplete removal of the antrum increases the risk of developing a marginal ulcer.
- For the Billroth II reconstruction, it is important to properly close the duodenal stump to prevent future leaks that could be complicated by fistula formation or pancreatitis.
- Splenic injury may occur secondary to downward traction on the greater curvature of the stomach.

c. Parietal cell/proximal vagotomy **(Table 4) (Figure 2)**: The goal of the parietal cell vagotomy is to eliminate vagal stimulation of the acid-secreting portion of the stomach, while retaining motor innervation to the antrum and pylorus. The receptive relaxation of the stomach is still affected by this procedure, and liquid emptying from the stomach is accelerated, but solid emptying is normal. This procedure reduces the basal acid secretion by 75% and the stimulated acid secretion by 50%. The HSV has low mortality (risk < 0.5%) and morbidity but has a high ulcer recurrence rate especially with inexperienced surgeons.

Procedure: The initial exploration is as described for truncal vagotomy. The anterior nerve of Latarjet, which is the termination of the left vagus nerve, is identified and encircled. Then the lesser sac is examined for adhesions to the pancreas and then entered by dividing the gastrocolic ligament, while preserving the gastroepiploic arcade. Next, the lesser omentum is divided from the lesser curvature between the incisura angularis and the cardia, by dividing all of the blood vessels and nerves that enter the lesser curvature. The dissection begins just proximal to the crow's foot of the nerve of Latarjet and proceeds proximally along the lesser curvature to the left side of the gastroesophageal junction. The neurovascular branches should be ligated with 3-0 or 4-0 silk sutures and divided. Then the stomach is reflected upward and the posterior denervation is conducted in a similar manner. Then the nerve fibers and blood vessels on the lower 5 to 7 cm of the esophagus must be dissected and ligated.

Pitfalls

- Recurrent ulcers may be the consequence of an inadequate proximal vagotomy.

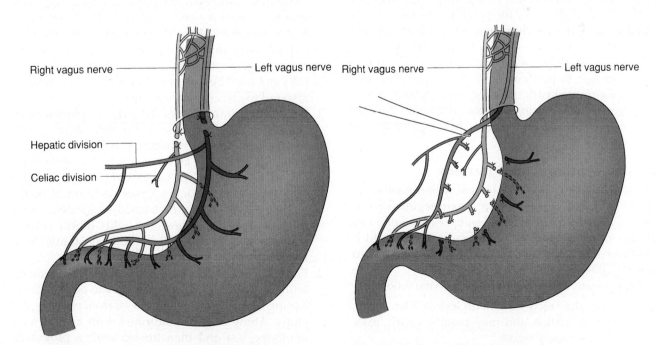

FIGURE 2 • Truncal and proximal vagotomy. (Figure 46.1 in Mulholland MW. Gastroduodenal ulceration. In: Mulholland MW, Lillemoe KD, Doherty GM, et al., eds. Greenfield's Surgery: Scientific Principles and Practice. 4th ed. Baltimore, MD: Lippincott Williams & Wilkins, 2006:722–735).

- Careful dissection around the lesser curvature of the stomach is important to decrease the risk of injury to the lesser curve.

Special Intraoperative Considerations

Laparoscopic repair: Omental patch repair of ulcers <1.0 cm may be performed by either an open or laparoscopic approach. A randomized controlled trial of 121 patients with perforated peptic ulcers reported that the laparoscopic group had significantly lower analgesic requirements, postoperative hospital length of stay, and returned to work significantly earlier than the open group. There were no significant differences between the two groups in mortality, incidence of reoperation, or postoperative intra-abdominal fluid collections.

Giant perforated ulcers: There is no standard management for giant perforated ulcers (>2 to 3 cm). Recommendations for repair have included omental patch, controlled tube duodenostomy, jejunal pedicled graft, jejunal serosal patch, free omental plug, partial gastrectomy, and pyloric exclusion. The choice of repair will be influenced by the patient's status, the size of the perforation, the degree of intraperitoneal contamination, and the surgeon's experience.

Posterior perforation: Spontaneous posterior perforation of a duodenal ulcer is rare. A definitive ulcer operation is typically undertaken, though there is no standard treatment.

Perforated gastric cancer: Though perforation is a rare complication (<1%) of gastric cancer, a biopsy and frozen section should be taken during surgery for all gastric perforations. Options for the surgical repair of a perforated gastric cancer include omental patch, emergency gastrectomy, and a two-stage radical gastrectomy.

Perforation at the gastroesophageal junction: The operative approach to perforation of an ulcer located next to the esophagogastric junction may include a subtotal gastrectomy to include the ulcer with a Roux-en-Y esophagogastrojejunostomy or a vagotomy with antrectomy.

Postoperative Management

H. pylori infection should be treated with triple therapy for 10 to 14 days; a common treatment regimen is clarithromycin, amoxicillin, and omeprazole. Following treatment conclusion, *H. pylori* eradication should be confirmed. Patients should receive counseling regarding NSAID use.

Postoperative complications include the following:

1. An early ulcer recurrence with leak is often treated with reexploration and may require gastric resection to adequately repair.
2. An uncontained leak after omental patch may require reexploration and gastric resection with a Billroth II.
3. Subphrenic and subhepatic abscesses are associated with a surgery delay >12 hours.
4. A patient should be evaluated for duodenal obstruction if gastric emptying is not normal by the eighth postoperative day.
5. Wound infection
6. Pneumonia
7. Pancreatitis

In patients following a definitive ulcer surgery there are also the following risks:

1. Diarrhea following truncal vagotomy occurs in 5% to 10% of patients. It typically occurs 1 to 2 hours following a meal. This problem usually resolves without intervention. Persistent symptoms may be improved by cholestyramine and/or loperamide. If medical therapy does not improve symptoms, a surgical option includes placement of a reversed jejunal interposition placed 100 cm distal to the ligament of Treitz.
2. Dumping syndrome occurs in 5% to 10% of patients following distal gastrectomy, pyloroplasty, or pyloromyotomy. It is classified as either early dumping, occurring within 30 to 60 minutes of eating; or late dumping, occurring 2 to 3 hours following a meal. Symptoms of early dumping include fatigue, facial flushing, lightheadedness, diaphoresis, palpitations, cramping abdominal pain, nausea, vomiting, and diarrhea. Symptoms of late dumping are typically limited to vasomotor symptoms. Treatment of these symptoms with dietary manipulation is often successful. Octreotide may be useful in severe cases. Octreotide, administered prior to meals, has been shown to improve both gastrointestinal and vasomotor symptoms. Remedial surgery is an option for patients with dumping symptoms resistant to medical management; however, this approach is typically not used because most patients do eventually respond to conservative therapy.
3. Following elimination of the pyloric sphincter bile can reflux into the stomach. Alkaline reflux gastritis develops in 2% of patients. It is characterized by epigastric pain and nausea that is provoked by meals. Medical therapy with cholestyramine may improve symptoms. Cases resistant to medical management may be treated surgically with a Billroth II gastrojejunostomy with Braun enteroenterostomy, Roux-en-Y gastrojejunostomy, or a Henley loop.
4. Early satiety with epigastric fullness and emesis with meals may develop secondary to gastric stasis, having a small gastric remnant, or from postsurgical atony. Atony may be confirmed with a solid food emptying test and then treated with a prokinetic agent, or if that fails, gastric pacing or completion gastrectomy. Symptoms of a small gastric remnant typically improve with small frequent meals.

5. Following Billroth II construction, the limb may become obstructed and cause afferent and efferent loop syndromes. Afferent loop syndrome is characterized by postprandial epigastric pain and non-bilious vomiting that is relieved following bilious vomiting. Efferent loop syndrome is characterized by epigastric pain, distention, and bilious vomiting. Both syndromes are treated with a surgical approach.

TAKE HOME POINTS

- Early diagnosis and operation are associated with improved outcome.
- It is important to identify prior NSAID use.
- It is important to identify *H. pylori* infection.
- Surgical goals are to control the perforation and lavage the abdominal cavity.
- Although rarely required, definitive ulcer operation may be required in select patients.
- Gastric perforation should prompt consideration of underlying gastric cancer.

SUGGESTED READINGS

Adachi Y, Mori M, Maehara Y, et al. Surgical results of perforated gastric carcinoma: an analysis of 155 Japanese patients. Am J Gastroenterol. 1997;92:516–518.

Ashley SE, Evoy D, Daly JM. Stomach. In: Schwartz S, ed. Principles of Surgery. New York: McGraw-Hill, 1999:1181.

Bank S, Marks IN, Louw JH. Histamine- and insulin-stimulated gastric acid secretion after selective and truncal vagotomy. Gut. 1967;8:36–41.

Cellan-Jones CJ. A rapid method of treatment in perforated duodenal ulcer. BMJ. 1929;1:1076–1077.

Crofts TJ, Park KG, Steele RJ, et al. A randomized trial of nonoperative treatment for perforated peptic ulcer. N Engl J Med. 1989;320:970–973.

Dempsey DT. Stomach. In: Brunicardi FC, Andersen DK, Billiar TR, et al., eds. Schwartz's Principles of Surgery. 9th ed. Columbus: McGraw-Hill, 2010:889–948, Chapter 26.

Donovan AJ, Berne TV, Donovan JA. Perforated duodenal ulcer: an alternative therapeutic plan. Arch Surg. 1998;133:1166–1671.

Gabriel SE, Jaakkimainen L, Bombardier C. Risk for serious gastrointestinal complications related to use of nonsteroidal anti-inflammatory drugs. A meta-analysis. Ann Intern Med. 1991;115:787–796.

Gisbert JP, de la Morena F, Abraira V. Accuracy of monoclonal stool antigen test for the diagnosis of H. pylori infection: a systematic review and meta-analysis. Am J Gastroenterol. 2006;101:1921–1930.

Grabowski MD, Dempsey DT. Concepts in surgery of the stomach and duodenum. In: Scott-Conner C, ed. Chassin's Operative Strategy in General Surgery: An Explosive Atlas. New York: Springer Science Business Media, 2002.

Graham DY, Malaty HM. Alendronate and naproxen are synergistic for development of gastric ulcers. Arch Intern Med. 2001;161:107–110.

Grassi R, Romano S, Pinto A, et al. Gastro-duodenal perforations: conventional plain film, US and CT findings in 166 consecutive patients. Eur J Radiol. 2004;50:30–36.

Gunshefski L, Flancbaum L, Brolin RE, et al. Changing patterns in perforated peptic ulcer disease. Am Surg. 1990;56:270–274.

Gupta S, Kaushik R, Sharma R, et al. The management of large perforations of duodenal ulcers. BMC Surg. 2005;5:15.

Jordan PH Jr, Thornby J. Perforated pyloroduodenal ulcers. Long-term results with omental patch closure and parietal cell vagotomy. Ann Surg. 1995;221:479–486; discussion 486–488.

Lal P, Vindal A, Hadke NS. Controlled tube duodenostomy in the management of giant duodenal ulcer perforation: a new technique for a surgically challenging condition. Am J Surg. 2009;198:319–323.

Lanas A, Serrano P, Bajador E, et al. Evidence of aspirin use in both upper and lower gastrointestinal perforation. Gastroenterology. 1997;112:683–689.

Lanza FL. A guideline for the treatment and prevention of NSAID-induced ulcers. Members of the Ad Hoc Committee on Practice Parameters of the American College of Gastroenterology. Am J Gastroenterol. 1998;93:2037–2046.

Lee SC, Fung CP, Chen HY, et al. Candida peritonitis due to peptic ulcer perforation: incidence rate, risk factors, prognosis and susceptibility to fluconazole and amphotericin B. Diagn Microbiol Infect Dis. 2002;44:23–27.

Leodolter A, Wolle K, Peitz U, et al. Evaluation of a near-patient fecal antigen test for the assessment of Helicobacter pylori status. Diagn Microbiol Infect Dis. 2004;48:145–147.

Lew E. Peptic ulcer disease. In: Greenberger RBN, Burakoff R, eds. Current Diagnosis and Treatment: Gastroenterology, Hepatology, and Endoscopy. Columbus, OH: McGraw-Hill, 2009:175–183.

Li-Ling J, Irving M. Therapeutic value of octreotide for patients with severe dumping syndrome–a review of randomised controlled trials. Postgrad Med J. 2001;77:441–442.

McColl KE. Clinical practice. Helicobacter pylori infection. N Engl J Med. 2010;362:1597–1604.

Moller MH, Shah K, Bendix J, et al. Risk factors in patients surgically treated for peptic ulcer perforation. Scand J Gastroenterol. 2009;44:145–152, 2 p following 152.

Mort JR, Aparasu RR, Baer RK. Interaction between selective serotonin reuptake inhibitors and nonsteroidal antiinflammatory drugs: review of the literature. Pharmacotherapy. 2006;26:1307–1313.

Roviello F, Rossi S, Marrelli D, et al. Perforated gastric carcinoma: a report of 10 cases and review of the literature. World J Surg Oncol. 2006;4:19.

Sarosi GA Jr. Dumping Syndrome. In: Johnson LR, ed. Encyclopedia of Gastroenterology. Academic Press, San Diego, CA, 2003:634–636.

Shan YS, Hsu HP, Hsieh YH, et al. Significance of intraoperative peritoneal culture of fungus in perforated peptic ulcer. Br J Surg. 2003;90:1215–1219.

Sharma SS, Mamtani MR, Sharma MS, et al. A prospective cohort study of postoperative complications in the management of perforated peptic ulcer. BMC Surg. 2006;6:8.

Silen W. Cope's Aarly Diagnosis of the Acute Abdomen. 19th ed. New York: Oxford University Press, 1996:xiv, 315 p., 24 p. of plates.

Siu WT, Leong HT, Law BK, et al. Laparoscopic repair for perforated peptic ulcer: a randomized controlled trial. Ann Surg. 2002;235:313–319.

Svanes C, Lie RT, Svanes K, et al; Adverse effects of delayed treatment for perforated peptic ulcer. Ann Surg. 1994;220:168–175.

Wolfe MM, Lichtenstein DR, Singh G. Gastrointestinal toxicity of nonsteroidal antiinflammatory drugs. N Engl J Med. 1999;340:1888–1899.

Wong CH, Chow PK, Ong HS, et al. Posterior perforation of peptic ulcers: presentation and outcome of an uncommon surgical emergency. Surgery. 2004;135:321–325.

Yamada TA, Alpers DH, Kaplowitz N, et al. Textbook of Gastroenterology. 4th ed. Philadelphia, PA: Lippincott Williams & Wilkins, 2003.

19 Small Bowel Obstruction

SARA E. CLARK and LILLIAN G. DAWES

2/2; adhesions
incarcerated hernias
neoplasms
Crohn's / IBD

Presentation

A 78-year-old man with a history of hypertension, diabetes, and coronary artery disease presents with a 2-day history of diffuse abdominal pain, nausea, and several episodes of emesis. He has not been able to tolerate any oral intake. His bowel movements have been normal up until the previous day when he had a liquid bowel movement. He has not had any flatus for at least 2 days. On physical exam, his abdomen is distended and tympanitic, and he has diffuse abdominal tenderness without guarding. He has a midline abdominal scar and a right subcostal scar. He has had multiple abdominal surgeries including an open aortic aneurysm repair, a cholecystectomy, and a right hemicolectomy for colon cancer.

Differential Diagnosis

The constellation of abdominal pain, nausea, vomiting, and decreased flatus/bowel movements is nonspecific but may represent a small bowel obstruction. A mechanical small bowel obstruction results when there is blockage of the lumen of the small bowel. Neurogenic causes of bowel dilatation such as a paralytic ileus can cause distention due to a lack of bowel motility. In this patient with a history of multiple abdominal surgeries, a mechanical bowel obstruction is a concern.

Adhesions from prior surgery are the most common cause of a mechanical small bowel obstruction, accounting for up to two-thirds of all bowel obstructions. Incarcerated hernias and neoplasms are the next most common cause. Crohn's disease or inflammatory bowel disease can cause a mechanical obstruction in diseased segments of bowel. Less common causes of a small bowel obstruction include volvulus, bezoar, gallstone ileus, or intussusception **(Table 1)**.

Small bowel neoplasms can progressively occlude the lumen or serve as a leading point for intussusception. Symptoms may be intermittent as the onset is slow, and patients usually have chronic anemia. Extrinsic neoplasms may entrap loops or cause external compression. Comprehensive physical exam looking for a hernia is a must—patients with incarcerated hernias can present with small bowel obstruction and bowel compromise. Internal hernias, which may not be apparent on physical examination, can occur through the obturator foramen, acquired adhesive defects or lateral to surgical defects (e.g., parastomal hernias). Volvulus results from rotation of bowel loops from a fixed point due to congenital anomalies or acquired adhesions. Patients with volvulus will usually have acute onset of symptoms and strangulation often occurs rapidly. Malrotation of the intestine is a cause of volvulus in children but is very rare in adults.

Other rare causes of obstruction include foreign bodies (bezoar, ingested), gallstone ileus (passage of large stone through cholecystenteric fistula), and inflammatory bowel disease (secondary to inflammation and fibrosis of small bowel wall).

Workup

The patient undergoes further evaluation with laboratory workup significant for a mild leukocytosis, hypokalemia and hypochloremia. He has no evidence of acidosis on his initial labs and his creatinine is normal. His acute abdominal series shows air-fluid levels and dilated loops of small bowel with no evidence of free air. He undergoes computed tomography (CT) scan of the abdomen and pelvis showing large fluid filled stomach, dilated loops of small bowel with possible transition point in the pelvis. His distal ileum and colon are decompressed **(Figure 1)**.

When presented with this clinical scenario, several things need to be considered.

1. Is this a mechanical small bowel obstruction or is this an ileus?
2. If a mechanical bowel obstruction, is the blockage partial or complete?
3. Is this a simple or strangulating obstruction?

Workup for small bowel obstruction to help answer these questions should include a combination of radiographic and laboratory investigations. Initially an acute abdominal series should be performed to look for free air, dilated small bowel or stomach, air-fluid levels in small bowel, and presence or absence of air/fluid in colon. A CT scan is often performed as a second evaluation to look at integrity of small bowel, and assess for the presence or absence of signs of bowel ischemia including pneumatosis, complete obstruction with a transition point, presence of small bowel volvulus, intussusception, hernias, or neoplasm.

TABLE 1. Causes of Small Bowel Obstruction	
Causes	**Incidence (%)**
Adhesions	60–74
External hernia	8–15
Neoplasms	8–10
Intrinsic (Primary small bowel—20%)	
Extrinsic (Metastatic—80%)	
Inflammatory bowel disease	5
Miscellaneous	10
Intussusception	
Volvulus gallstone ileus	
Infections/abscess, bezoar	

TABLE 2. Causes of Ileus
Causes
Postoperative
Metabolic and or electrolyte imbalance
Hypokalemia
Hyponatremia
Hypomagnesemia
Uremia
Drugs
Inflammation
Sepsis

Laboratory evaluation may reveal leukocytosis, anemia if there is a bleeding mass or elevated hematocrit if the patient is volume contracted. Electrolyte abnormalities may be present because of gastric losses and creatinine may be elevated if the patient is dehydrated. If there is significant bowel compromise, the lactic acid may be elevated.

An ileus can at times mimic a small bowel obstruction. Conditions that may cause an ileus are listed in **Table 2**. An ileus tends to affect the entire gastrointestinal tract and there should not be a transition point on CT scan. With an ileus, the large bowel is usually dilated as well as the small bowel.

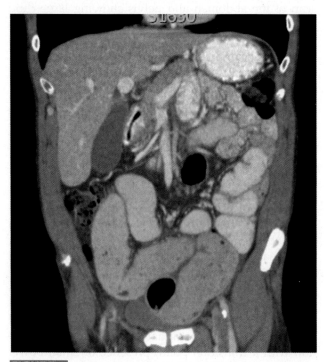

FIGURE 1 • Dilated small bowel is evident as is a collapsed colon. A transition point was found to be in the pelvis.

Diagnosis and Treatment

In the patient from our scenario, a nasogastric tube (NGT) is placed and 1 L of bilious material is immediately drained. He has partial resolution of his abdominal pain following placement. Conservative treatment is elected and he is placed on intravenous fluids and kept NPO.

Typically, if the patient is thought to have a partial small bowel obstruction secondary to adhesions, a trial of conservative (nonsurgical) management is pursued initially. This includes NGT decompression, bowel rest, intravenous fluid resuscitation, and correction of electrolyte abnormalities. If the patient fails to improve clinically over 48 hours, it is likely that the patient requires an operation.   *2d trial — surgery*

The challenge with treating a small bowel obstruction is deciding when to operate. Sixty-five to eighty-five percent of partial small bowel obstructions will resolve with conservative management. The old dictum of "never let the sun rise nor set on a bowel obstruction" is still true for complete small bowel obstruction, large bowel obstruction, or when there is concern of strangulation or bowel compromise. Delay in surgical therapy in these cases can lead to irreversible bowel ischemia. However, proceeding with immediate operation in patients with a partial small bowel obstruction may lead to an unnecessary intervention.

Indications for immediate operation include peritonitis, sepsis, hemodynamic instability, acidosis, or radiographic evidence of small bowel compromise, such as pneumatosis, perforation, signs of bowel ischemia, internal hernia, or volvulus. Physical findings suggesting the need for early operation are fever, tachycardia, and pain out of proportion to physical findings. CT scanning provides additional useful information. Although the presence of a transition point on CT scan has failed to reliably predict the need for operation, there are some findings that should alert the surgeon that earlier surgery is warranted. Bowel compromise is associated with intraperitoneal fluid and decreased

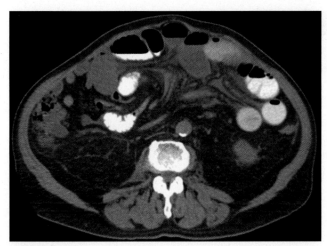

FIGURE 2 • In the center of this CT scan image, there are mesenteric vessels that move in a circular pattern to the left. This is known as a "swirl sign" and is concerning for a potential volvulus. At operation, a loop of bowel twisted around an internal hernia was found. Untwisting of the mesentery restored blood flow and relieved the obstruction.

enhancement of the bowel wall. Pneumatosis and portal venous air can also be seen with bowel ischemia. The presence of a "whirl sign" is concerning for a volvulus or internal hernia **(Figure 2)**.

One special case worth mentioning is postbariatric surgery patients presenting with bowel obstruction. Because of the mesenteric defects from the gastrojejunostomy (often antecolic) and the jejunojejunostomy, bariatric surgery patients are at very high risk for internal hernias. If a large amount of small bowel is involved, these patients can have catastrophic midgut volvulus, even leading to short gut syndrome. In these patients, the surgeon should look carefully for evidence of internal hernia or volvulus (e.g., mesenteric "swirl"

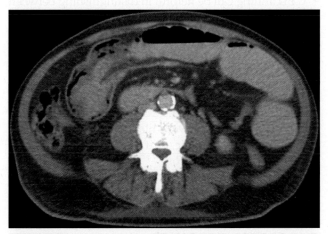

FIGURE 3 • Small bowel intussusception is demonstrated here with a mass as the lead point. A spindle cell tumor was found at operation causing the intussusception and bowel obstruction.

sign on CT scan) and promptly explore patients with any suggestion of an internal hernia.

Small bowel obstruction due to intussusception in adults is often due to a tumor of the small bowel that serves as a lead point. The hallmark of intussusception on CT scan is the presence of a "target sign." A target sign on CT scan may at times be seen with normal peristalsis. However, when evidence of intussusceptions on CT scan is associated with a bowel obstruction or a mass **(Figure 3)**, operative intervention and small bowel resection with removal of the abnormal segment are indicated.

Surgical Approach

The usual approach to patients with bowel obstruction is through a midline incision **(Table 3)**. Entering the abdomen away from a prior incision may be beneficial if possible (e.g., entering the midline just above or below a prior laparotomy site). The abdomen is entered carefully with sharp dissection in order to avoid bowel injury. The bowel is freed from the anterior abdominal wall and is carefully inspected. All adhesions that could possibly cause obstruction are taken down and the small bowel is inspected in its entirety. It is important to try and identify the point of obstruction, or "transition point" where the bowel goes from dilated to decompressed. It is much more satisfying when the causative adhesions are lysed. However, oftentimes the transition point will not be obvious. For very dense adhesions, dissection with a scalpel is often useful. Any areas of enterotomy can be repaired if the bowel is viable. If it is not viable or the damage is extensive, a small bowel resection must be performed. In order to determine viability you must assess the vascular supply of the small bowel. This can be done by standard clinical judgment (i.e., color and appearance), Doppler ultrasound of mesentery, and, in rare cases, fluorescein dye evaluation.

The less common causes of small bowel obstruction are usually apparent on inspection of the small bowel. When the small bowel is inspected, any volvulus will be reduced. Intussusception can be reduced by gentle traction, and any masses/neoplasms can be resected. With all circumstances, bowel viability must be assessed. Hernias can be approached through an incision over the hernia (umbilical, inguinal) with low threshold for conversion to open laparotomy if there is concern for bowel strangulation to assess intra-abdominal bowel. For hernias where incarcerated and strangulated bowel is suspected, one should not attempt reduction of the hernia until operative intervention to allow inspection of the involved loop of bowel.

During the operation, it is essential to be aware of any enterotomies and spillage from small bowel. Missed enterotomies and spillage can lead to postoperative intra-abdominal abscess, sepsis, and other morbidities.

TABLE 3. Key Technical Steps and Potential Pitfalls

Key Technical Steps

1. Run the entire small bowel; multiple points of obstruction can be present.
2. Assess the bowel blood supply. If there is uncertainty consider a "second look" operation.
3. Carefully inspect for potential enterotomy. Missed enterotomy will lead to intestinal fistula, a devastating postoperative complication. The best treatment of a bowel fistula is prevention.
4. Preserve as much bowel as possible. With an intact duodenum and colon, 200 cm or more of residual small bowel is usually sufficient to prevent symptoms of short gut syndrome. If a lot of small bowel needs to be resected, the remaining length should be measured to aid in postoperative management should there be symptoms of short bowel.

Potential Pitfalls

- Missed enterotomy.
- Missed intraluminal lesion.
- Lack of recognition of compromised bowel.
- Recurrent bowel obstruction in the future.

Special Intraoperative Considerations

During exploration for small bowel resection, it is important to be aware of findings of Crohn's disease. Findings of Crohn's disease at laparotomy include fibrotic strictures, usually short and multiple with "skip" areas of normal interposed bowel. There is often "creeping fat" onto the small bowel. Strictures from Crohn's disease can cause obstruction and abdominal pain and often are managed with strictureplasty rather than resection to avoid excessive loss of small bowel and the development of short bowel syndrome.

If an obstructing stone is found in the ileum just proximal to the ileocecal valve, a "gallstone ileus" is likely the cause. Inspection of the gallbladder is warranted to investigate the possibility of a cholecystoenteric fistula. Often this is diagnosed preoperatively due to the presence of air in the bile ducts without any history of iatrogenic or surgical intervention. Inspection of the entire small bowel for multiple stones should be performed as there can be more than one stone present. Relieving the obstruction by performing an enterotomy with removal of the stone is all that is usually required for treatment. Repair of the cholecystoenteric fistula is usually not necessary but can be considered in a low-risk patient.

Postoperative Management

Postoperatively, the NGT should be continued until there is return of bowel function with flatus. Care should be taken to maintain the patient's volume status and all electrolyte abnormalities should be aggressively corrected. If the patient has been in a fasted state for a long period of time, consideration should be given to starting parenteral nutrition. Patients with chronic obstructive problems may have prolonged ileus following lysis of adhesions. Nutritional status is important to prevent complications including wound infection and dehiscence.

Case Conclusion

Two days after admission, our patient still has output from his NGT of 600 mL per shift and he has not passed any flatus. He is taken to surgery where he is found to have dense adhesions with a transition point in the ileum. The adhesions are taken down and postoperatively he has an uneventful course.

TAKE HOME POINTS

- Complete bowel obstructions or when bowel ischemia is suspected requires early surgical intervention
- Partial bowel obstructions can be initially conservatively managed with NGT decompression, intravenous fluids, and close observation.
- CT scanning can be helpful in distinguishing between ileus and obstruction (i.e., determining the presence of a "transition point" and identifying complications that require immediate operative intervention, e.g., internal hernia, volvulus, or ischemic bowel).
- Careful inspection for potential enterotomy will help avoid the serious complication of postoperative small bowel fistula.
- Evaluation of the bowel's blood supply is important. Resect if ischemic, or if in doubt, consider a "second look" operation.
- Preserve as much small bowel as possible and if significant amount of small bowel needs to be resected, measure the amount of remaining small bowel.

SUGGESTED READINGS

Colon MJ, Telem DA, Wong D, et al. The relevance of transition zones on computed tomography in the management of small bowel obstruction. Surgery. 2010;147(3):373–377.

Diaz JJ Jr, Bokhari F, Mowery NT, et al. Guidelines for management of small bowel obstruction. J Trauma. 2008;64(6):1651–1664.

Kendrick ML. Partial small bowel obstruction: clinical issues and recent technical advances. Abdom Imaging. 2009; 34:329–334.

O'Day BJ, Ridgway PF, Keenan N, et al. Detected peritoneal fluid in small bowel obstruction is associated with the need for surgical intervention. Can J Surg. 2009;52(3):201–206.

Olasky J, Moazzez A, Barrera K, et al. In the era of routine use of CT scan for acute abdominal pain, should all adults with small bowel intussusceptions undergo surgery? Am Surg. 2009;75(10):958–961.

Zielinski MD, Eiken PW, Bannon MP, et al. Small bowel obstruction-who needs an operation? A multivariate prediction model. World J Surg. 2010;34(5):910–929.

20 Morbid Obesity

JOHN MORTON

Presentation

A 42-year-old woman with history of a BMI of 55, type II diabetes, depression, hypertension, hyperlipidemia, and gastroesophageal reflux disease (GERD) presents for surgical consultation. She has previously attempted weight loss on multiple occasions with initial success but subsequent weight regain. The patient has previous history of two cesarean sections and right knee arthroscopy for a torn meniscus. Her medications include NPH Insulin, Prozac, Hydrochlorothazide, Aciphex, and Zocor.

Differential Diagnosis

This patient suffers from the disease of obesity and qualifies as stage IV obese. While consideration of secondary causes of obesity must be considered, primary obesity is the overwhelming diagnosis. Rarely, secondary causes of obesity may be genetic (Prader-Willi), endocrine (hypothyroidism), or iatrogenic (steroids or pituitary resection). For this patient, the diagnosis and staging is complete.

Workup

All patients considering surgical weight loss must have a comprehensive history and physical examination with a special consideration to determining full burden of obesity and obesity-related diseases. A comprehensive cataloguing of obesity comorbidity is necessary to report their subsequent remission or improvement, a requirement for bariatric surgery center of excellence. Often, the obese patient will have undiagnosed or untreated medical concerns. By default, the bariatric surgeon assumes many primary care responsibilities for the obese patient.

The physical examination in the obese may be challenging but is nonetheless important. Anthropometric measurements such as neck or waist circumference may indicate sleep apnea or metabolic syndrome. The abdominal exam may display a hernia potentially affecting operative decision making. The stigmata of venous stasis disease are an important finding given that it may raise the risk of postoperative deep venous thrombosis (DVT).

In addition to the history and physical examination, the preoperative evaluation of the bariatric surgery patient should include upper endoscopy and psychological and nutritional consultation. Upper endoscopy or upper gastrointestinal (GI) series helps determine severity of GERD or masses in a stomach that may not be accessible postoperatively. Both nutritional and psychological counseling are critical tools

for patients who must change their ingrained eating behaviors. Psychological contraindications to bariatric surgery include schizophrenia, developmental delay, active substance abuse, recent major depression with hospitalization or suicidal attempts, and severe bipolar disease. The psychological evaluation can also provide coping and stress management skills.

Serologic evaluation should incorporate complete blood count, liver function tests, biochemical cardiac risk factors, prothrombin time/partial thromboplastic time, glucose parameters, and nutritional markers. Often, obese patients may be calorically replete but nutritionally depleted.

Additionally, cardiac evaluation of obese patients is paramount. Frequently, these patients may have occult cardiac disease that may be misdiagnosed as asthma. Initial assessment should include a comprehensive history, EKG and, in certain patients, a stress echo. While rare, patients reporting a history of taking fenfluramine/phentermine, should have a cardiac echo to rule out valvular disorders. Further cardiac risk stratification can be gained through a biochemical cardiac risk factor assessment.

In the patient in this scenario, on history and exam, she has diabetes for 4 years, prior DVT, and has severe venous stasis disease. Her serologic testing demonstrates an elevated hemoglobin A1C of 9.8 and triglycerides of 250 mg/dL.

Diagnosis and Treatment

This patient has stage IV obesity and has repeatedly demonstrated failure of medical management. Her psychological evaluation does not reveal any contraindications. Based on her history, this patient will require more aggressive prevention of venous thromboembolism given her high risk as demonstrated by previous history of DVT and venous stasis disease.

Given her diagnosis of stage IV obesity (BMI > 50), this patient is at higher risk for any operative approach. A method for reducing risk is preoperative weight loss. Preoperative weight loss is a method for "down-staging," acting in the same manner as preoperative chemoradiation therapy does for cancer. The objective for preoperative weight loss should not be a number or time period but an approach that ensures education and understanding of the tools needed postoperatively. Even a modest amount of weight loss will ensure a smaller liver and shorter OR times.

All major surgical options for weight loss are presented to the patient including gastric banding, gastric sleeve, and gastric bypass. As part of any preoperative discussion, risks and benefits are elaborated. Given this patient's weight and comorbidities, the recommendation of gastric bypass is made for this patient and she agrees. For this particular patient, gastric bypass will afford her the most consistent and profound weight loss and comorbidity improvement for her GERD and diabetes.

Surgical Approach

A laparoscopic gastric bypass is scheduled **(Table 1)**. The laparoscopic approach is superior to the open approach with considerably lower complications particularly wound-related complications. She lost 5% of her excess weight and her hemoglobin A1C improved to 8 mg/dL by doubling her Metformin. She also had a temporary IVC filter placed in preparation for her surgery.

At the time of surgery, care is taken to appropriately position the patient to facilitate intubation and prevent nerve compression and skin breakdown. In order to prevent postoperative nausea and vomiting, several strategies are employed including IV hydration, a small steroid dose, and Zofran®. An orogastric tube is placed to prevent any gastric distension or aspiration.

During the surgical timeout, prophylactic subcutaneous 5,000 units of subcutaneous heparin, sequential compression devices, and 2 g of Cefoxitin® are confirmed as being administered. Availability of special equipment such as gastroscope and longer instruments is also confirmed during the surgical timeout.

Surgery is begun by placing an index trocar at 18 cm below the xiphoid in the midline after the Veress needle has been introduced to provide pneumoperitoneum. After remaining trocars are placed, laparoscopic exploration of the abdomen is conducted. The greater omentum is elevated and the ligament of Treitz is identified. The jejunum is divided into a biliopancreatic and Roux limbs at 20 cm distal to ligament of Treitz. Next, the jejunojejunostomy is performed after a 75- to 150-cm Roux limb is run, potential internal hernia sites are closed, and the liver retractor is placed. The gastric pouch at 15 to 30 mL in size is constructed based on the lesser curve and begun horizontally at the second vascular arcade and finished vertically up to the angle of His. Finally, the gastrojejunostomy is constructed either

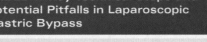

TABLE 1. Key Technical Steps and Potential Pitfalls in Laparoscopic Gastric Bypass

Key Technical Steps

1. Pneumoperitoneum, trocar placement and exploration.
2. Identify ligament of Treitz and divide jejunum.
3. Split mesentery and run a 75-to 150-cm Roux limb.
4. Construct jejunojejunostomy and close potential internal hernia sites.
5. Place liver retractor and construct lesser-curve–based gastric pouch.
6. Perform gastrojejunostomy.

Potential Pitfalls

- Bleeding from the staple line, liver or spleen.
- Pronounced fulcrum effect from thickened abdominal wall and redundant omentum.
- Tension at the gastrojejunostomy anastomosis.

through circular-stapled, linear-stapled, or hand-sewn techniques with a surgical drain placement. Potential pitfalls that can occur include bleeding, inability for the Roux limb to reach the gastric pouch without tension, and unexpected anatomy such as malrotation, enlarged liver, excessive omentum, and thick abdominal wall.

Special Intraoperative Considerations

Though rare, unexpected findings during a laparoscopic gastric bypass may influence the operative course. For example, previous surgery may yield tenacious adhesions requiring lysis, malrotation of the ligament of Treitz necessitates a mirror image approach to the technique, hernia findings will require a change in port placement, or cirrhosis that may require biopsy or even aborting the case if varices or ascites is noted. The above image demonstrates a gastrointestinal stromal tumor (GIST) that may not have been revealed with preoperative assessment **(Figure 1)**. In this circumstance, the tumor may be resected in its entirety and the gastric bypass be completed.

Postoperative Management

Postoperatively, the patient develops shortness of breath (SOB), increased heart rate, and per nurse, the Jackson-Pratt drain now has a cloudy discharge.

Bariatric surgery has increasingly become exceeding safe with a 30-day mortality of 0.2%. While rare, the two leading causes of mortality following bariatric surgery include pulmonary embolus (PE) and anastomotic leak. In this particular circumstance, this patient had an IVC filter filtered placed preoperatively reducing risk of PE, but the risk of anastomotic leak remains. Intraoperatively, a leak may be identified by endoscopic surveillance of the anastomosis while postoperatively, an upper GI study (as in the above image) or amylase levels from the drain might help identify

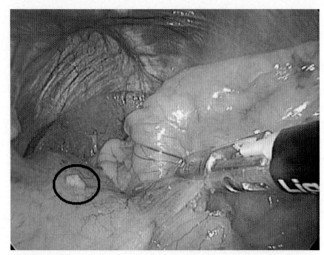

FIGURE 1 • GIST tumor (*circled*) on anterior aspect of stomach. (From Morton, Obesity Surgery. 2005.)

the leak **(Figure 2)**. Treatment includes NPO status, IV antibiotics, drainage and/or reoperation if a patient is unstable.

While early complications like PE, leaks, or bleeding can occur, late complications like bowel obstruction from internal hernias or anastomotic concerns like ulcers or strictures are also possible. Other complications may be psychological such as substance abuse or depression. Tracking of complications is a

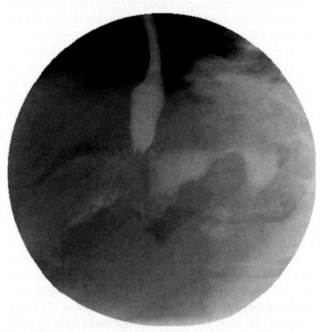

FIGURE 2 • Upper GI contrast study demonstrating a leak from the gastrojejunal anastomosis. (From Morton, Obesity Surgery. 2007.)

requirement for all bariatric surgery centers of excellence. Another component of outcomes reporting includes demonstration of the effective weight loss and comorbidity remission that accompanies bariatric surgery.

TAKE HOME POINTS

- All bariatric surgery patients require a thorough preoperative evaluation due to the high burden of disease of the obese.
- All patients should have a full description of major bariatric procedures including indications, risks, and benefits.
- The laparoscopic approach has substantial benefit for the bariatric patient.
- Serious complications following gastric bypass include PE, anastomotic leak, and bleeding.
- Obesity is a chronic disease and long-term surveillance is required for all postoperative patients.

SUGGESTED READINGS

Birkmeyer NJ, Dimick JB, Share D, et al. Hospital complication rates with bariatric surgery in Michigan. JAMA. 2010;304(4):435–342.

Buchwald H, Avidor Y, Braunwald E, et al. Bariatric surgery: a systematic review and meta-analysis. JAMA. 2004;292(14):1724–1737.

Flum DR, Belle SH, King WC, et al. Perioperative safety in the longitudinal assessment of bariatric surgery. Longitudinal Assessment of Bariatric Surgery (LABS) consortium. N Engl J Med. 2009;361(5):445–454.

Hernandez-Boussard T, Ahmed SM, Morton JM. Obesity disparities in preventive care: findings from the National Ambulatory Medical Care Survey, 2005–2007. Obesity. 2011.

Lee JK, Van Dam J, Morton JM. Endoscopy is accurate, safe, and effective in the assessment and management of complications following gastric bypass surgery. Am J Gastroenterol. 2009;104(3):575–582.

Raman R, Raman B, Raman P, et al. Abnormal findings on routine upper GI series following laparoscopic Roux-en-Y gastric bypass. Obes Surg. 2007;17(3):311–316.

Sanchez BR, Morton JM, et al. Incidental finding of gastrointestinal stromal tumors (GISTs) during laparoscopic gastric bypass. Obes Surg. 2005;15:1384–1388.

Schuster R, Hagedorn JC, Morton JM. Retrievable inferior vena cava filters may be safely applied in gastric bypass surgery. Surg Endosc. 2007;21(12):2277–2279.

Solomon H, Liu GY, Alami R, et al. Benefits to patients choosing preoperative weight loss in gastric bypass surgery: new results of a randomized trial. J Am Coll Surg. 2009;208(2):241–245.

Santry HP, Gillen DL, Lauderdale DS. Trends in bariatric surgical procedures. JAMA. 2005;294(15):1909–1917.

Williams DB, Morton JM. Gastric bypass reduces biochemical cardiac risk factors. Surg Obes Relat Dis. 2007;3(1):8–13.

Woodard GA, Downey J, Hernandez-Boussard T, et al. Impaired alcohol metabolism after gastric bypass surgery: a case-crossover trial. J Am Coll Surg. 2011;212(2):209–214.

21 Gastrointestinal Stromal Tumor

JOHN B. AMMORI and RONALD P. DEMATTEO

Presentation

A 68-year-old, otherwise healthy man presents with early satiety and vague upper abdominal pain, which became progressively worse over the past several months. His symptoms are unrelieved by proton pump inhibitors and have worsened in the past 2 weeks prompting him to see his primary physician. His past medical history is significant for hypertension and hyperlipidemia controlled with medications. His surgical history is unremarkable. Review of systems is negative for any other symptoms. Vital signs are normal. Physical examination reveals an upper abdominal mass, no associated jaundice, and no generalized lymphadenopathy. Contrast-enhanced CT scan of the abdomen and pelvis demonstrates a large, heterogeneous, partially necrotic left upper-quadrant mass inseparable from the gastric fundus (**Figure 1**). There is no radiographic evidence of metastatic disease.

Differential Diagnosis

The differential diagnosis of a gastric mass includes gastric adenocarcinoma, gastrointestinal stromal tumor (GIST), leiomyosarcoma, leiomyoma, gastric lymphoma, and neuroendocrine tumor. Given the large size of the mass, its exophytic nature, and lack of intra-abdominal metastatic disease in this case, gastric adenocarcinoma and neuroendocrine tumor are unlikely to be the diagnosis. Gastric lymphoma is an unlikely diagnosis since there was no lymphadenopathy on clinical and radiologic examination. Leiomyomas are homogenous and usually well marginated, making this diagnosis unlikely in this case. The most likely diagnoses in a patient presenting with a large, necrotic exophytic gastric mass are GIST and leiomyosarcoma.

Workup

Esophagogastroduodenoscopy (EGD) demonstrates a submucosal mass in the gastric body. Biopsy of the mucosa overlying the mass revealed no pathologic abnormality. Endoscopic ultrasound (EUS) showed a large heterogeneous mass contiguous with the gastric wall without perigastric lymphadenopathy. Fine needle aspiration (FNA) biopsy showed spindle cells; immunohistochemistry was not performed.

As in this case, endoscopic biopsies are often unable to make diagnosis because the mass is submucosal. If the tumor has eroded into the gastric mucosa and caused bleeding, biopsy may yield a diagnosis. EUS is not mandatory in the workup of these tumors, but it can be useful in assessing the extent of disease is some cases. In a patient with a resectable tumor who is fit

for surgery, FNA is not necessary. Biopsy of GIST may lead to complications, such as hemorrhage or tumor rupture, which may lead to tumor dissemination. FNA, or core needle biopsy, is useful for patients with the following indications: (1) metastatic or unresectable disease; (2) when neoadjuvant therapy is considered; or (3) if lymphoma is strongly suspected. Good quality cross-sectional imaging of the abdomen and pelvis is crucial to evaluate local and distant extent of disease. The typical imaging finding is a large, hypervascular, exophytic, heterogeneous mass, often with central necrosis. The liver and peritoneum are the most common metastasic sites and must be carefully evaluated.

Diagnosis and Treatment

Approximately 3,000 GISTs are diagnosed each year in the United States. The stomach is the most common primary site of GIST. Sixty percent of tumors arise from the stomach, while 30% arise in the small intestine. Less common sites include the duodenum and rectum, accounting for approximately 5% each.

The clinical presentation of GIST depends on both its size and location. Nearly 30% of GISTs are asymptomatic and discovered incidentally. Symptoms generally result from mass effect of these extraluminal masses. They are usually nonspecific symptoms such as nausea, emesis, early satiety, abdominal distension, or pain. The median size of GIST in symptomatic patients is approximately 9 cm compared with nearly 3 cm in asymptomatic patients. Patients may also present with microcytic anemia due to subclinical gastrointestinal

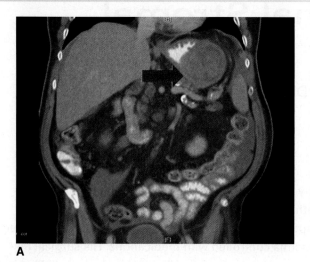
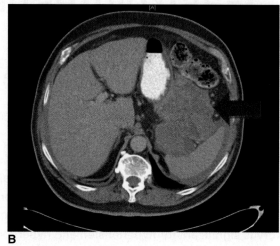

A   **B**

FIGURE 1 • CT scan demonstrating a large, heterogeneous, partially necrotic left upper-quadrant mass inseparable from the gastric fundus. Also note reactive perisplenic fluid.

bleeding into the gastrointestinal tract lumen. Some patients with GIST manifest significant bleeding due to erosion into the gastrointestinal tract or intraperitoneal tumor rupture.

GISTs have three histologic patterns: spindle cell type (70%), epitheloid cell type (20%), and mixed (10%). The definitive diagnosis of GIST is made by immunohistochemical expression of the KIT receptor tyrosine kinase (CD117 antigen). Approximately 95% of GISTs are positive for KIT expression. Approximately 80% of KIT-negative GISTs have a mutation in the platelet-derived growth factor receptor alpha (PDGFRA). The most frequent site of KIT mutation is exon 11 (70%), followed by exon 9 (10%), and exons 13 and 17 (rare). GISTs with an exon 9 mutation have a poorer clinical course compared to those with an exon 11 mutation.

Surgery is the mainstay of treatment for resectable GIST. The goal is a margin negative resection. Segmental resection of the organ from which the tumor originates is adequate. For example, if it is anatomically feasible, segmental gastric resection is appropriate as opposed to formal gastrectomy. When the tumor is adherent to contiguous organs, en bloc resection to attain negative surgical margins should be performed. There is no role for routine lymphadenectomy since metastases to lymph nodes are extremely rare. However, if regional lymph nodes are suspicious for metastatic disease, lymphadenectomy should be performed.

Imatinib is the mainstay of adjuvant therapy for GIST. Imatinib is a targeted tyrosine kinase inhibitor that competitively inhibits KIT. Approximately 60% of patients have a partial response and 25% have disease stability. Tumors with KIT exon 11 mutations are more sensitive to imatinib therapy than tumors with KIT exon 9 mutations, with approximately 75% achieving

a partial response compared to 45%, respectively. Imatinib is first-line therapy for metastatic GIST. The role of adjuvant imatinib following complete resection has been studied in a randomized, phase III, double-blind, placebo-controlled multicenter trial. One-year recurrence-free survival was significantly improved in patients treated with adjuvant imatinib for 1 year after resection (98% vs. 83%, $P < 0.001$). The rate of recurrence increased 6 months following the completion of imatinib therapy. Trials are currently underway assessing longer courses of adjuvant therapy. Neoadjuvant imatinib should be considered in clinical situations in which downsizing of the tumor would assist in achieving negative resection margins, such as large tumors that may require adjacent organ resection. Preoperative therapy may also be beneficial for tumors in surgically difficult locations such as the gastroesophageal junction, duodenum, and rectum. The tumor is reassessed with cross-sectional imaging and surgery is often performed after 6 months of treatment.

CT scan can be used to assess response to imatinib. Tumors do not decrease substantially in size, but instead the tumor appearance changes from hypervascular to hypoattenuating, homogeneous, and cystic **(Figure 2)**. Primary resistance to imatinib therapy is seen in 15% of tumors. Secondary resistance to imatinib often occurs after approximately 18 months of therapy, often due to additional mutations in the KIT gene. CT scan will demonstrate a new solid enhancing focus within a responding mass **(Figure 2)**. Patients who develop resistance to imatinib may respond to second-line sunitinib therapy.

Liver and peritoneum are the most likely sites of metastatic disease. The three major factors predicting metastases following resection are primary site, size, and mitotic rate **(Table 1)**. Standard treatment for

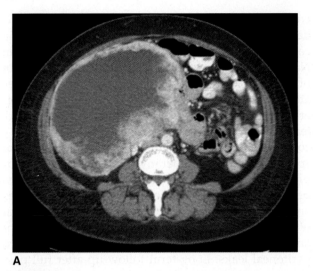
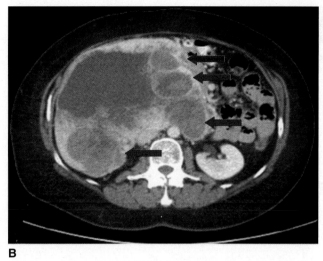

A   **B**

FIGURE 2 • CT imaging of imatinib response and secondary resistance. **A:** Characteristic hypoattenuating, homogeneous, and cystic appearance of tumor indicating response to imatinib. **B:** New solid enhancing foci (*arrows*) within a responding mass indicating secondary resistance to imatinib.

metastatic disease is imatinib. There are three main indications for cytoreductive surgery in metastatic or recurrent GIST. These are (1) emergencies such as hemorrhage, bowel perforation, or obstruction; (2) resectable disease that is stable or responsive to imatinib; and (3) focal progression defined as the development of secondary drug resistance to imatinib in one or a few sites, while other sites of disease remain stable. In the latter case, one may consider resecting only the drug resistant tumors if complete resection is not possible. Cytoreductive surgery is generally not indicated for debulking unresectable progressive disease or diffuse progression defined as multiple sites of progressive disease.

Surgical Approach

Complete surgical resection with negative microscopic margins is the treatment of choice for resectable tumors without evidence of metastasis. Segmental resection of the stomach or small intestine is appropriate. Formal gastrectomy for wider clearance of uninvolved tissue is unnecessary. Since lymph node metastases are rare, lymphadenectomy is unnecessary unless there is clinical suspicion of lymph node involvement. GISTs are often exophytic from the stomach or small bowel and can typically be lifted away from adjacent organs. Tumors with pedunculated or limited attachment can often be resected with a gastric wedge. Tumors with broad-based attachment that cannot be resected with a wedge generally require partial gastrectomy, typically with a Billroth II gastrojejunal reconstruction. Large lesions near the gastroesophageal junction may require total gastrectomy with roux-en-y esophagojejunostomy. Some tumors can densely adhere to surrounding organs requiring en bloc resection in order to achieve complete resection. In general, one may

TABLE 1. Risk Factors for Recurrence of GIST Based on Mitotic Rate, Tumor Size, and Site of Origin

Tumor Parameters		Risk for Progressive Disease, Based on Site of Origin			
Mitotic Rate	**Size**	**Stomach**	**Jejunum/Ileum**	**Duodenum**	**Rectum**
≤5/50 HPFs	≤2 cm	0%	0%	0%	0%
	>2, ≤5 cm	1.9%	4.3%	8.3%	8.5%
	>5, ≤10 cm	3.6%	24%	Insufficient data	Insufficient data
	>10 cm	10%	52%	34%	57%
> 5/50 HPFs	≤2 cm	0%	50%	Insufficient data	54%
	>2, ≤5 cm	16%	73%	50%	52%
	>5, ≤10 cm	55%	85%	Insufficient data	Insufficient data
	>10 cm	86%	90%	86%	71%

HPFs, high power fields.
Adapted from Miettinen M, Lasota J. Gastrointestinal stromal tumors: pathology and prognosis at different sites. Semin Diagnostic Pathol. 2006;23:70.

approach surgical resection of GIST by either an open or a laparoscopic approach depending on technical concerns as well as surgeon preference and experience.

The key technical steps for resection of a gastric GIST are as follows **(Table 2)**. The abdomen is explored, paying particular attention to the peritoneal surfaces and liver. The lesser sac is entered through the gastrocolic ligament. The tumor is identified. A partial gastrectomy is performed with 1-cm gross margins. This can usually be done with GIA stapling devices. Care should be taken to avoid narrowing the gastric lumen. If the tumor is located near the pylorus, incisura, or gastroesophageal junction, and a formal gastrectomy should be performed, as discussed above.

The patient in the case presented in this chapter underwent tumor resection using an open approach due to the large tumor size and the anticipated need for a complex resection. At laparotomy, initial exploration revealed no evidence of peritoneal or liver metastases. A large tumor arising from the greater curvature of the stomach was identified. It was densely adherent to the pancreatic tail and splenic hilum. A complete resection was achieved with an en bloc resection including wedge partial gastrectomy, splenectomy, and distal pancreatectomy.

Meticulous and careful intraoperative handling of GISTs is critical. These tumors are usually fragile with extensive necrosis or hemorrhage. If the pseudocapsule is torn, bleeding and tumor rupture may occur, increasing the risk of peritoneal recurrence.

Special Intraoperative Considerations

Metastatic disease may be discovered at exploration. If there is limited and resectable metastases, resection of all disease should be performed. This may require liver resection and resection of limited peritoneal disease.

Postoperative Management

As with all abdominal surgery, pain control, early ambulation and aggressive pulmonary toilet are crucial for postoperative recovery. Prophylaxis for deep venous thrombosis is achieved with sequential compression devices and/or subcutaneous heparin. Nasogastric tube decompression is at the discretion of the surgeon. Diet is advanced as the patient tolerates. Surgery-specific complications include postoperative surgical site infections, bleeding, and gastric leak. Surgical site infections are the most common complication, ranging from wound cellulitis to organ space infections. Postoperative bleeding is a rare complication that may occur early in the postoperative period. Gastric or enteric leak is rare and usually presents approximately 1 week postoperatively. These can often be controlled with percutaneous drainage and antibiotics, but reoperation is necessary for free intraperitoneal leaks. Long-term follow-up after full postoperative recovery includes history and physical as well as CT scan every 3 to 6 months for 3 to 5 years and annually thereafter. Patients with low-risk tumors can be managed with less frequent follow-up.

The patient in the case presented in this chapter recovered well without surgical complication. He is taking adjuvant imatinib and is without recurrence 9 months following surgery.

TAKE HOME POINTS

- GIST is the most common mesenchymal tumor of the gastrointestinal tract.
- Characterized by expression of the KIT receptor tyrosine kinase
- May present with nonspecific symptoms or with gastrointestinal hemorrhage
- Tumors are exophytic, and often necrotic and hemorrhagic. Endoscopy shows a submucosal mass, occasionally with an overlying ulcer.
- Surgery with negative margins is the mainstay of treatment for nonmetastatic GIST.
- Patients at high risk for recurrence should receive adjuvant imatinib for at least 1 year.
- Imatinib is the treatment of choice for metastatic GIST. Treatment should be continued until secondary resistance develops.
- Surgery plays a role in selected patients with resectable metastatic disease that is stable or responsive to imatinib and in selected patients with focal progression.

SUGGESTED READINGS

Dematteo RP, Ballman KV, Antonescu CR, et al. Adjuvant imatinib mesylate after resection of localised, primary gastrointestinal stromal tumour: a randomised, double-blind, placebo-controlled trial. Lancet. 2009;373:1097–1104.

Demetri GD, von Mehren M, Antonescu CR, et al. NCCN Task Force report: update on the management of patients with gastrointestinal stromal tumors. J Natl Compr Canc Netw. 2010;8(suppl 2):S1–S41; quiz S2–S4.

Gold JS, Gonen M, Gutierrez A, et al. Development and validation of a prognostic nomogram for recurrence-free survival after complete surgical resection of localised primary gastrointestinal stromal tumour: a retrospective analysis. Lancet Oncol. 2009;10:1045–1052.

Miettinen M, Lasota J. Gastrointestinal stromal tumors: pathology and prognosis at different sites. Semin Diagn Pathol. 2006;23:70–83.

van der Zwan SM, DeMatteo RP. Gastrointestinal stromal tumor: 5 years later. Cancer. 2005;104:1781–1788.

Zalinski S, Palavecino M, Abdalla EK. Hepatic resection for gastrointestinal stromal tumor liver metastases. Hematol Oncol Clin North Am. 2009;23:115–127, ix.

22 Symptomatic Cholelithiasis in Pregnancy

VANCE L. SMITH and PAUL M. MAGGIO

Presentation

A 32-year-old woman, 28 weeks pregnant with her second child, with no significant past medical history presents to the emergency department with a 2-day history of right upper-quadrant (RUQ) abdominal pain and nausea. Her obstetrician-gynecologist, who had evaluated her earlier in the day, thought it was unlikely that her symptoms were related to her pregnancy. In the emergency department, she is afebrile and her vital signs are remarkable for mild tachycardia of 102. Her pain is episodic, lasting approximately 90 minutes after eating. On abdominal exam, the fundal height measures 29 weeks, consistent with her pregnancy. She has focal tenderness in the RUQ and reports that the pain radiates through to her back on the same side. She is anorexic but has been able to keep liquids down.

Differential Diagnosis

Symptomatic cholelithiasis is a common cause of RUQ abdominal pain and is second only to appendicitis as a cause of abdominal emergencies during pregnancy. Although gallstones have been reported in up to 10% of patients during pregnancy, the incidence of gallstone-related diseases causing complications during pregnancy is <1%. Contributing factors include hormonal changes associated with increased bile stone formation and altered gallbladder contractility.

Diagnosing symptomatic cholelithiasis during pregnancy can be a challenge for any physician particularly when compounded by efforts to limit radiologic exposure. The presenting signs and symptoms of symptomatic cholelithiasis may be nonspecific and difficult to distinguish from those associated with pregnancy itself, and the changing position of intra-abdominal contents during pregnancy may complicate the examination of the gravid abdomen. For example, the appendix is typically located at McBurney's point early in pregnancy but is later displaced laterally and upward into the RUQ by the enlarging uterus **(Figure 1)**. As a consequence, appendicitis may present as RUQ pain in the pregnant patient, especially in patients late in their pregnancy. Less common causes of RUQ pain during pregnancy include peptic ulcer disease, pancreatitis, pyelonephritis, HELLP syndrome (syndrome of hemolysis, elevated liver enzymes, and low platelets), acute fatty liver, and hepatitis.

Workup

Laboratory evaluation including a complete blood count and liver function tests was obtained. The white blood cell count was mildly elevated at $13 \times 10^3/\mu L$. Liver and pancreatic enzymes were normal (total bilirubin 1.0 mg/dL, indirect bilirubin 0.5 mg/dL, alkaline phosphatase 90 U/L, lipase 35 U/L). A RUQ abdominal ultrasound was performed **(Figure 2)** and demonstrated a normal gallbladder wall with multiple hyperechoic shadowing consistent with gallstones. The common bile duct measured 0.7 cm.

Diagnosis and Treatment

The imaging modality of choice in diagnosing symptomatic cholelithiasis is ultrasonography. Transabdominal ultrasound is sensitive (>95% for gallstones), inexpensive, and safe without exposing the patient to radiation. For the diagnosis of acute cholecystitis, it yields a sensitivity of 88% and a specificity of 80%.

When choledocholithiasis is suspected (e.g., bilirubin or alkaline phosphatase is elevated), endoscopic retrograde cholangiopancreatography can be safely performed with minimal radiation exposure as long as proper shielding is used. Magnetic resonance cholangiopancreatography (MRCP) is an alternative, but it is only diagnostic and its safety in regard to the fetus has not been well established.

The timing of surgical intervention for symptomatic cholelithiasis in the pregnant patient remains controversial. Historical recommendations were to delay surgical intervention until the second trimester. In the intervening time, these patients were managed with intravenous fluids, bowel rest, narcotics, broad-spectrum antibiotics, and a fat-restricted diet. More recent evidence suggests that an operation can be performed safely during any trimester of pregnancy.

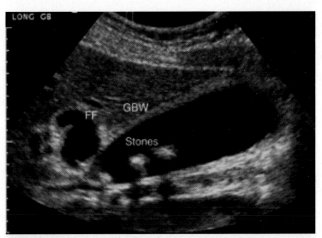

FIGURE 2 • RUQ abdominal ultrasound revealing cholelithiasis.

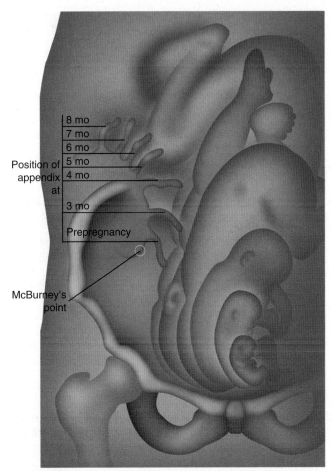

FIGURE 1 • As the uterus grows, there is upward displacement of the appendix in counterclockwise fashion.

In fact, some surgeons have argued that delaying surgery may have devastating consequences for the fetus. When managed nonoperatively, symptomatic cholelithiasis has a high recurrence rate and its associated complications, such as gallstone pancreatitis, can lead to spontaneous abortion and preterm labor. Recurrence rates for symptomatic patients have been reported to be as high as 92% in the first trimester, 64% in the second trimester, and 44% in the third trimester.

Once the decision to perform an operative intervention has been made, laparoscopic cholecystectomy is the preferred approach. It carries the same benefits of laparoscopy performed in the nonpregnant patient. Specifically, laparoscopic surgery results in a decreased requirement for narcotics, a lower rate of wound complications, shorter hospital stays, and a decreased risk of venous thromboembolism secondary to early ambulation. An obstetric consultation should be obtained for all cases involving a viable

fetus (>24 weeks gestation) and will typically include preoperative and postoperative monitoring of fetal heart rate and uterine activity.

Surgical Approach for Laparoscopic Cholecystectomy

The patient is placed supine on the operating table. For the gravid patient, she can lie in the left lateral recumbent position to decrease compression of the vena cava. Access to the abdomen is obtained via an open Hasson, Veress needle, or optical trocar, depending on surgeon preference and level of experience. While there is no evidence that any of the above options is superior to others, many surgeons would opt to enter via an open Hasson technique. This allows direct visualization of the abdominal wall and intra-abdominal viscera prior to trocar insertion. Port location should be adjusted for fundal height, which should be measured before and after induction of general anesthesia. More recent advances such as single-port laparoscopy should be reserved for high-volume centers with surgeons experienced in this technique, and only in pregnant patients whose fundal height permits entry at the umbilicus.

Pneumoperitoneum can usually be achieved by CO_2 insufflation of 10 to 15 mm Hg, although it is important to remember that some pregnant patients may demonstrate restrictive lung physiology due to elevation of their diaphragm. These patients are prone to arterial desaturation and may be better managed with insufflation pressures <12 mm Hg. In all cases, adequate visualization of the gallbladder and biliary anatomy must be maintained.

Once all ports are placed, the fundus of the gallbladder is retracted toward the abdominal wall

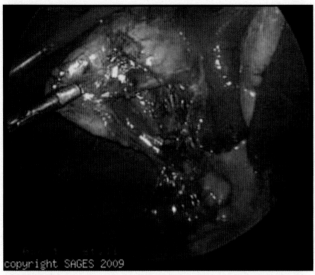

copyright SAGES 2009

FIGURE 3 • Critical view during laparoscopic cholecystectomy. Note the clear delineation of the junction of the cystic duct with the gallbladder as well as the clear space between the gallbladder and liver, devoid of any other structure other than the cystic artery.

TABLE 1. Key Technical Steps and Potential Pitfalls to Laparoscopic Cholecystectomy in the Pregnant Patient

Key Technical Steps

1. Appropriate port placement based on fundal height of uterus preferably through an open Hasson technique.
2. Position the patient in the supine position, and a left lateral recumbent position for third-trimester patients.
3. Insufflate abdomen to 10–15 mm Hg, 12 mm Hg in patients with restrictive lung physiology.
4. Adequately retract gallbladder toward abdominal wall.
5. Dissect peritoneum from the gallbladder neck to the common bile duct in order to gain the critical view of safety.
6. Identify the cystic artery as it courses from the right hepatic artery to the gallbladder.
7. Divide and ligate both the cystic duct and the cystic artery.
8. Use electrocautery or Harmonic scalpel to dissect the gallbladder from the liver fossa.
9. Remove ports under direct visualization and close port sites.

Potential Pitfalls

- Improper port placement.
- Failure to achieve the critical view.
- Failure to recognize replaced right hepatic artery.

and superiorly over the liver, and the peritoneum is dissected from the gallbladder neck. Dissection should be carried out from the gallbladder neck to the common bile duct in order to gain the critical view of safety **(Figure 3)**. The critical view is achieved by clearing all fat and fibrous tissue in Calot's triangle, after which the cystic structures can be clearly identified, occluded, and divided. This helps to avoid bile duct injuries and failure to successfully create this view is an indication for conversion to an open cholecystectomy.

The cystic duct and artery are then clipped and divided, and the gall bladder is removed from its fossa using electrocautery or the Harmonic scalpel. If there is spillage of bile from the gallbladder, the abdomen should be irrigated and the fluid aspirated. The ports are withdrawn under direct visualization and the abdomen desufflated. Each incision is closed **(Table 1)**.

Surgical Approach for Open Cholecystectomy

For patients in whom laparoscopic cholecystectomy cannot be performed safely, an open cholecystectomy is indicated. This is accomplished through a right subcostal incision. After retractors are placed and the bowel and gravid uterus packed away from the surgical field, the gallbladder is grasped and dissection is performed via a top-down approach. The cystic duct and artery are identified, ligated,

and divided. Once adequate hemostasis is obtained, the viscera are returned to their normal anatomic position and the incision is closed in two layers **(Table 2)**.

Postoperative Management

After undergoing laparoscopic cholecystectomy, patients are usually admitted overnight for observation. Fetal monitoring is required in cases that involve a viable fetus to evaluate fetal heart rate and uterine activity. An oral diet can be started on the day of surgery and oral pain medications shortly thereafter. Patients undergoing an open cholecystectomy typically require a 3- to 5-day hospital stay to achieve adequate pain control and sufficient oral intake.

TABLE 2. Key Technical Steps to Open Cholecystectomy in the Pregnant Patient

Key Technical Steps

1. Make a right subcostal incision.
2. Pack visceral and uterus from the operative field.
3. Grasp gallbladder and dissect via a top-down approach.
4. Identify the cystic duct and artery just beyond gallbladder neck.
5. Ligate and divide the cystic duct and cystic artery.
6. Use electrocautery to dissect the gallbladder from the liver fossa.
7. Close the abdomen in two layers.

Case Conclusion

Once diagnosed with symptomatic choleli-thiasis, the patient is admitted to the Obstetrics Antepartum unit for preoperative pain control and fetal monitoring. That afternoon she undergoes a laparoscopic cholecystectomy and is admitted postoperatively for 24 hours of fetal monitoring. After an uneventful stay, she is discharged on postoperative day 1. Her follow-up visit reveals no further pain, and her pregnancy progressed uneventfully to term.

TAKE HOME POINTS

- The presenting signs and symptoms of symptomatic cholelithiasis may be nonspecific and difficult to distinguish from those associated with pregnancy.
- The changing position of intra-abdominal contents during pregnancy complicates the examination of the gravid abdomen.
- Asymptomatic cholelithiasis, even found during pregnancy, is not an indication for cholecystectomy.
- For symptomatic cholelithiasis, a cholecystectomy can be safely performed in all trimesters of pregnancy.

- Nonoperative management of symptomatic cholelithiasis exposes the patient to a high rate of recurrence and associated complications.
- Laparoscopic cholecystectomy is preferred to an open procedure and carries the same benefits as in the nonpregnant patient.
- An obstetric consultation should be obtained for all cases involving a viable fetus (>24 weeks gestation) and will typically include preoperative and postoperative fetal monitoring.

SUGGESTED READINGS

Basso L, McCollum PT, Darling MR, et al. A study of cholelithiasis during pregnancy and its relationship with age, parity, menarche, breast-feeding, dysmenorrhea, oral contraception and a maternal history of cholelithiasis. Surg Gynecol Obstet. 1992;175:41–46.

Date RS, Kaushal M, Ramesh A. A review of the management of gallstone disease and its complications in pregnancy. Am J Surg. 2008;196:599–608.

Ko CW. Risk factors for gallstone-related hospitalization during pregnancy and the postpartum. Am J Gastroenterol. 2006;101:2263–2268.

Oto A, Ernst RD, Ghulmiyyah LM, et al. MR imaging in the triage of pregnant patients with acute abdominal and pelvic pain. Abdom Imaging. 2009;34:243–250.

Shea JA, Berlin JA, Escarce JJ, et al. Revised estimates of diagnostic test sensitivity and specificity in suspected biliary tract disease. Arch Intern Med. 1994;154:2573–2581.

23 Acute Cholecystitis

DANIELLE FRITZE and JUSTIN B. DIMICK

Presentation

A 70-year-old woman with multiple chronic medical conditions presents to the emergency room with 36 hours of right upper-quadrant (RUQ) pain and subjective fever. She describes numerous prior episodes of postprandial RUQ abdominal pain that resolves after several hours. While her pain is occasionally accompanied by nausea and vomiting, she denies jaundice, alcoholic stools, or dark urine. On exam, she is febrile to 38.5°C with otherwise normal vital signs. Her abdomen is soft with a well-healed vertical midline incision. She has marked tenderness to palpation in the right subcostal region and a positive Murphy's sign.

Differential Diagnosis

While this patient's symptoms of fever, RUQ pain, and vomiting represent the classic manifestations of acute cholecystitis, the clinical presentation is not always straightforward. Frequently, acute cholecystitis must be distinguished from other complications of cholelithiasis. Biliary colic results from temporary impaction of a gallstone in the gallbladder neck. It is characterized by postprandial abdominal pain, nausea, and vomiting that resolve over several hours. Signs of systemic inflammation, such as fever and elevated white blood cell count, are usually absent. Gallstones in the common bile duct (CBD), that is, choledocholithiasis, may cause RUQ pain with spontaneous passage of a stone or could progress to ascending cholangitis or biliary pancreatitis. Acalculous biliary disease is also a diagnostic consideration. Sphincter of Oddi dysfunction or biliary dyskinesia with low gallbladder ejection fraction often mimics the symptoms of biliary colic. Acute acalculous cholecystitis may be the end result of gallbladder hypoperfusion but usually is limited to critically ill patients. Nonbiliary abdominal pain due to gastroenteritis, acute hepatitis, ulcer disease, or bowel obstruction must also be excluded.

Workup

The diagnosis of acute cholecystitis is strongly suggested by this patient's history and is supported by characteristic findings on her physical exam. Constant, burning, RUQ pain is the most common presenting symptom in patients with cholecystitis. The pain occurs following ingestion of a high-fat meal and may awaken the patient from sleep. Many patients have known gallstones and nearly half report prior episodes of biliary colic. Approximately 5% to 10% of patients with biliary colic will go on to develop acute cholecystitis or another complication of gallstones each year. Physical exam reveals fever and right subcostal or epigastric tenderness, possibly with localized guarding.

Occasionally, a tender mass is palpable just inferior to the right costal margin. Inspiratory arrest with deep palpation in the RUQ, known as Murphy's sign, is a classic finding in acute cholecystitis.

Further evaluation of RUQ pain includes laboratory tests and imaging. This patient had an elevated white blood count of 13,000, bilirubin of 1 mg/dL, and normal liver and pancreatic enzymes. Leukocytosis with a predominance of neutrophils is common and helps to distinguish acute cholecystitis from biliary colic. Serum transaminases, bilirubin, and pancreatic enzymes are within the normal range or mildly elevated. Elevated liver enzymes or bilirubin should raise suspicion for choledocholithiasis but may also result from extrinsic compression of the common hepatic duct by a stone impacted in the neck of the gallbladder (Mirizzi syndrome). Elevated amylase and lipase indicate pancreatitis, potentially related to choledocholithiasis.

While acute cholecystitis may be diagnosed by several imaging modalities, abdominal ultrasound (US) is considered first line in the evaluation of RUQ pain. This patient's US was consistent with acute cholecystitis, demonstrating gallstones with gallbladder wall thickening, pericholecystic fluid, and a normal caliber CBD (Figure 1). Some patients experience a sonographic Murphy's sign, that is, pain caused by the US probe pressing directly on an inflamed gallbladder. Although CBD stones are not consistently identified by US, dilation of the CBD (>8 mm) suggests biliary obstruction. However, bile duct dilation on US is a specific but not very sensitive indicator of obstruction. Often, patients with elevated bilirubin or alkaline phosphatase levels will have normal size bile ducts on US.

While characteristic US findings are sufficient to diagnose acute cholecystitis in a patient with a concordant history and exam, other imaging modalities may be helpful in cases of diagnostic uncertainty. hepatobiliary iminodiacetic acid (HIDA) scan is considered the gold standard for diagnosis of acute cholecystitis

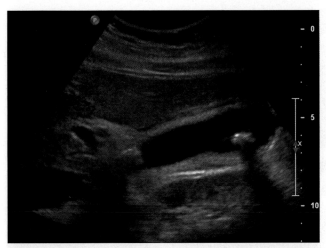

FIGURE 1 • US with classic findings of cholecystitis: cholelithiasis, thickened gallbladder wall and pericholecystic fluid.

in this setting, with sensitivity and specificity >95%. It is particularly useful in distinguishing cholecystitis from biliary colic and other nonbiliary processes but may have false-positive results in the setting of chronic cholecystitis. Nonvisualization of the gallbladder at 60 minutes is diagnostic for cholecystitis **(Figure 2)**. Gallbladder contraction may be stimulated by morphine or cholecystokinin to further increase HIDA's accuracy in diagnosing cholecystitis. Measurement of the gallbladder ejection fraction by HIDA also allows for identification of biliary dyskinesia.

In patients for whom there is a suspicion of choledocholithiasis, visualization of the biliary tree with Magnetic resonance cholangiopancreatography (MRCP) may help with the diagnosis **(Figure 3)**. Therapeutic sphincterotomy and stone extraction may be accomplished by ERCP in those patients with signs or symptoms of persistent biliary obstruction. While CT scan should not routinely be used to evaluate suspected cholecystitis given its low sensitivity and specificity, abdominal CT may suggest the diagnosis by revealing cholelithiasis, an enhancing and thickened gallbladder wall, pericholecystic fluid, and surrounding inflammatory fat stranding **(Figure 4)**.

Diagnosis and Treatment

The initial management of acute cholecystitis includes NPO status with systemic broad-spectrum antibiotics and resuscitation as dictated by the patient's condition. Ideally, cholecystectomy is performed upon diagnosis, within 48 hours of the onset of symptoms. Surgery is performed during the same hospitalization if possible, despite how long the patient has had symptoms. Although some advocate delaying operation if the patient has had symptoms >72 hours, we do not follow this practice. Despite the myth that cholecystectomy is easier after a "cooling off" period, evidence indicates

that interval cholecystectomy, performed more than 6 weeks after recovery from acute cholecystitis, does not result in fewer operative complications and is associated with a longer length of hospital stay. During this time, the acute process progresses to chronic fibrotic scarring, which can make dissection even more difficult. Thus, we believe early urgent cholecystectomy is the treatment of choice if at all feasible.

Cholecystectomy may be accomplished via either a laparoscopic or an open approach. Laparoscopic cholecystectomy is associated with decreased length of hospital stay, less patient discomfort, and shorter recovery time. Patients with a hostile abdomen, known aberrant anatomy, significant inflammation, or who are unlikely to tolerate pneumoperitoneum are best served with open cholecystectomy.

In patients whose comorbidities or clinical condition pose a prohibitive operative risk, drainage of the gallbladder may be accomplished via percutaneous or laparoscopic cholecystostomy. Decompensated cardiac failure, unstable angina, and severe or poorly controlled chronic lung disease are among the conditions that may render surgery unnecessarily high risk. Critically ill patients who develop acute cholecystitis in the setting of multiorgan failure or septic shock are particularly well served with cholecystostomy tube. A cholecystostomy tube may remain in place indefinitely, especially for patients with a limited life expectancy, or serve as a bridge to cholecystectomy when and if the patient's condition improves. Any trial of tube removal must be preceded by contrast injection to confirm a patent cystic duct. Up to 50% of patients will develop recurrent cholecystitis following tube removal; thus, most patients benefit from cholecystectomy if they are a fit operative candidate. Performing cholecystectomy after a tube placement poses a unique technical challenge given the chronic nature of the inflammation and fibrosis around the triangle of Calot. In this setting, the risk of conversion to an open procedure, or the necessity to perform a partial cholecystectomy, is quite high and should be considered prior to taking the patient to the operating room.

Although this particular patient has multiple comorbidities, these do not constitute a prohibitive operative risk, so the choice is made to proceed with cholecystectomy. An attempt at laparoscopy is planned with anticipated conversion to an open operation should adhesions from her prior colectomy inhibit reasonable progress or obscure relevant anatomy. In order to avoid disrupting the mesh from her ventral hernia repair, alternate port placement will be used.

Surgical Approach

Laparoscopic cholecystectomy is performed under general anesthesia with the patient in supine position **(Table 1)**. Access to the abdomen is generally obtained

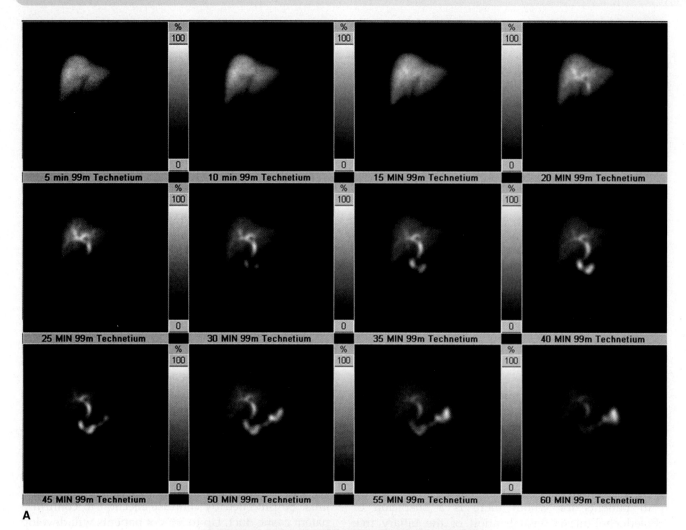

A

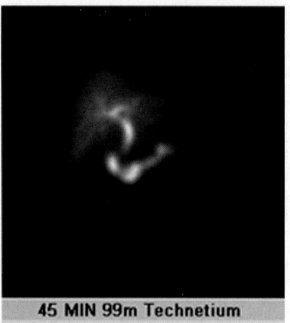

B

FIGURE 2 • HIDA scan consistent with acute cholecystitis. At 45 minutes after injection of contrast, there is opacification of the intra- and extrahepatic biliary tree and duodenum. The gallbladder is not visualized.

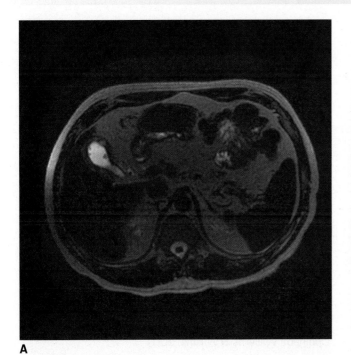

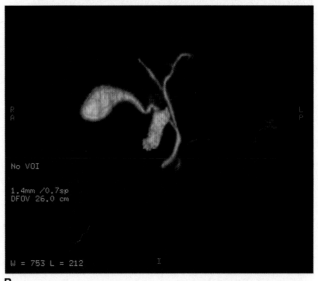

A

B

FIGURE 3 • MRCP demonstrating a thickened gallbladder wall and gallstones within the cystic duct, but no biliary dilation or choledocholithiasis. The filling defects within the gallbladder likely represent small polyps. Reformatted images delineate the patient's biliary anatomy.

inferior to the umbilicus via open Hassan or closed Veress needle technique. Pneumoperitoneum is established and a 30-degree laparoscope inserted. Two additional operating ports are inserted in the RUQ and one in the subxiphoid epigastrium. Reverse Trendelenburg and tilting the operating table to the patient's left facilitate displacement of the small bowel and omentum out of the operative field. The fundus of

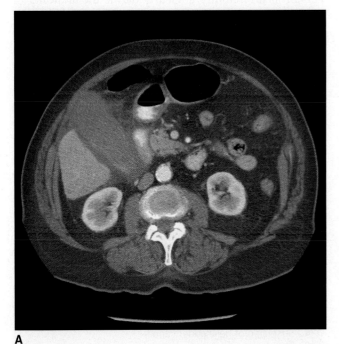

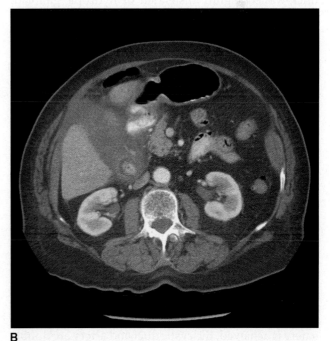

A

B

FIGURE 4 • CT scan consistent with acute cholecystitis demonstrating a dilated, thick-walled gallbladder with surrounding inflammatory stranding. A large gallstone is lodged in the gallbladder neck.

TABLE 1. Key Technical Steps and Potential Pitfalls in Laparoscopic Cholecystectomy

Key Technical Steps

1. Access the peritoneum.
2. Place ports: umbilical, subxiphoid, medial, and lateral right subcostal.
3. Retract the gallbladder fundus cranially and the infundibulum laterally to open the triangle of Calot.
4. Incise and divide the peritoneu.m overlying the gallbladder and the triangle of Calot.
5. Establish the critical view of safety: completely dissect the triangle of Calot until the cystic duct and the cystic artery are the only structures remaining.
6. Clip and divide the cystic duct and artery only after the critical view of safety has been definitively achieved.
7. Elevate of the gallbladder off of the liver bed with electrocautery.
8. Place the gallbladder in a specimen bag and then remove from the abdomen.
9. Assure hemostasis, release the pneumoperitoneum, and close all port sites.

Potential Pitfalls

- Complicated abdominal entry with damage to abdominal viscera or great vessels.
- Aberrant biliary or vascular anatomy.
- Inability to define the relevant anatomy.
- Injury to portal structures, liver, or duodenum.
- Choledocholithiasis.
- Perforation of the gallbladder.

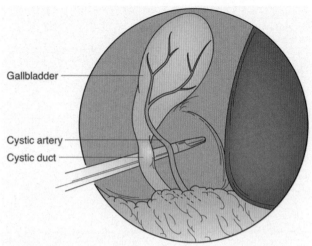

FIGURE 5 • The critical view of safety. The triangle of Calot has been neatly cleared of all tissue except the cystic artery and cystic duct. These two remaining structures are seen directly entering the gallbladder and may be safely divided. (From Mulholland, M., Greenfield's Surgery, 5th ed. Lippincott Williams & Wilkins, 2011)

the gallbladder is grasped and retracted cephalad over the edge of the liver via the lateral subcostal port. A thick-walled, tightly distended or hydropic gallbladder may be extremely difficult to grasp. Needle aspiration of gallbladder contents facilitates grasping the gallbladder for retraction. The remainder of the operation is conducted through the subxiphoid and medial right subcostal ports. Any adhesions to the gallbladder are taken down to reveal the triangle of Calot. The infundibulum is retracted laterally to open the triangle, separating the cystic duct from the common hepatic duct. The overlying peritoneum is incised and the triangle of Calot is cleared of soft tissue. Dissection continues until the cystic duct and artery are the only remaining structures in the triangle and can be seen directly entering the gallbladder. This constitutes the "critical view of safety" (Figure 5). Opening the peritoneal reflections over the gallbladder and elevating the distal gallbladder off of the liver with electrocautery may facilitate this portion of the operation. This technique is particularly helpful in the setting of acute cholecystitis with dense inflammation of the gallbladder and surrounding structures. Once the critical view of safety is achieved, the cystic duct and artery are doubly clipped and divided. The gallbladder is dissected off of the liver with electrocautery, placed into a specimen

bag, and removed from the abdomen. After hemostasis is assured, pneumoperitoneum is released, all port sites are closed, and the patient is allowed to emerge from anesthesia.

Special Intraoperative Considerations

Approximately 10% of attempts at laparoscopic cholecystectomy for acute cholecystitis result in conversion to an open operation. The primary indication for conversion is an inability to clearly define the anatomy of the biliary tract. Failure to establish the critical view of safety mandates conversion. Other indications include significant inflammation, failure to make satisfactory progress, any suspicion of injury to ductal or vascular structures, and concern for gallbladder cancer (Table 2).

Intraoperative cholangiography (IOC) may be used routinely in cholecystectomy or reserved for select circumstances (Table 3). Direct imaging of the biliary tree may demonstrate choledocholithiasis in patients suspected of having common duct stones due to biliary dilatation, elevated liver enzymes, or pancreatitis (Figure 6). Stones may be removed via CBD exploration

TABLE 2. Indications for Conversion to Open

1. Inability to define relevant biliary and vascular anatomy
2. Suspected injury to the biliary tree, vasculature, or bowel
3. Uncontrolled hemorrhage
4. Suspicion of gallbladder cancer
5. Failure to make satisfactory progress
6. Patient intolerance of pneumoperitoneum

TABLE 3. Indications for Intraoperative Cholangiogram

1. Inability to define relevant biliary anatomy
2. Suspicion of biliary injury
3. Suspicion of choledocholithiasis:
    Dilated CBD
    Elevated liver or pancreatic enzymes
    CBD stones identified on preoperative imaging
4. Routine use

or ERCP, either during the operation or postoperatively. Additionally, IOC may aid in delineating biliary anatomy or identification of biliary injury.

Patients with severe inflammation pose a particular challenge. Needle decompression of a tense gallbladder allows for more effective retraction. IOC may be necessary to define ductal anatomy. Occasionally, it is not possible to definitively attain the critical view of safety due to unclear anatomy or inflammation, which would render further dissection unsafe. Frequently in these circumstances, the operation may be safely completed with conversion to open. In select cases, however, the patient may be better served with a partial cholecystectomy. The gallbladder is elevated off of the liver bed starting proximally with the fundus. It is then transected at the level of the gallbladder neck or infundibulum without complete dissection of the triangle of Calot. Remaining stones can then be removed through the gallbladder lumen. The distal gallbladder can then be oversewn with absorbable suture. Drains should be left in place, given the risk of a bile leak from

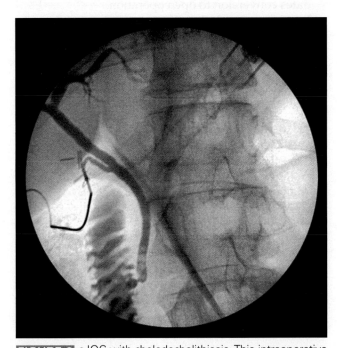

FIGURE 6 • IOC with choledocholithiasis. This intraoperative cholangiogram revealed stones stacked within the CBD.

the oversewn gallbladder. If partial cholecystectomy is performed, care must be taken to remove almost all of the gallbladder and any remaining stones. Otherwise, the patient could develop recurrent cholecystitis. If this approach is also ill-advised due to severe inflammation and/or anatomical distortion, a cholecystostomy tube may be placed laparoscopically.

Prior abdominal operations are not an absolute contraindication to an attempt at laparoscopic cholecystectomy, but may necessitate deviation from standard port placement. The initial access to the abdomen should be obtained in a location remote from prior operations where possible to minimize the risk of visceral injury. The left subcostal region is often an excellent location. In cases where this is not practical, an open approach to placement of the first port allows direct visualization of any adhesion to the abdominal wall. Alternate port placement may also be considered in patients with indwelling mesh from a prior herniorrhaphy. The camera port and the right subcostal ports may often be placed lateral and superior to the anticipated margins of the mesh. Placing a port directly through indwelling synthetic mesh is technically possible but carries a risk of contamination of the prosthetic and subsequent infection, and may compromise the integrity of the hernia repair. While laparoscopic cholecystectomy is technically possible in many patients with prior abdominal surgery, primary open cholecystectomy must also be considered. The ultimate choice of surgical approach must be tailored to the individual.

Postoperative Management

Most patients with acute cholecystitis are able to return home the day after laparoscopic cholecystectomy. Regular diet may be resumed immediately after surgery, and oral pain medications usually provide ample analgesia. Antibiotics are not indicated beyond the immediate perioperative period. Some patients experience diarrhea associated with altered bile salt storage after cholecystectomy, but this is typically mild and temporary.

Persistent abdominal pain, fever, or hyperbilirubinemia should prompt evaluation for retained CBD stone, biliary leak, or biliary injury. US should be the initial imaging study as it noninvasively demonstrates biliary dilation and fluid collections. Similar information may be derived from abdominal CT. Biliary dilation should be further evaluated with ERCP to identify a retained CBD stone or biliary injury causing obstruction. During the same procedure, interventions such as stent placement, stone extraction, or sphincterotomy may be accomplished **(Figure 7)**. Postoperative fluid collections may represent hematoma, biloma, or abscess. Percutaneous CT- or US-guided drain placement allows for adequate drainage of the collection as well as identification

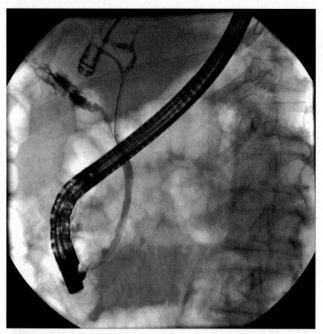

FIGURE 7 • ERCP with bile leak. Postoperative ERCP demonstrating a cystic duct stump leak. A wire is seen within the common hepatic duct, which traverses the CBD and terminates in the duodenum. A stent is placed across this wire to encourage bile flow into the duodenum rather than through the leak.

of its source. Return of bilious fluid should prompt ERCP to pinpoint the leak. During ERCP, an endobiliary stent may then be placed to encourage bile flow through the biliary tree into the duodenum rather than into the peritoneum.

Case Conclusion

The patient underwent laparoscopic cholecystectomy for acute cholecystitis. Despite residual adhesions from the patient's right hemicolectomy, the critical view is achieved and the operation completed laparoscopically. The patient recovers without incident and is discharged on postoperative day 1. On postoperative day 4, she returns to the ER with fever, increasing abdominal pain, leukocytosis, and hyperbilirubinemia. She is

admitted to the hospital and treated with antibiotics. US demonstrates a fluid collection in the gallbladder fossa. A percutaneous drain is placed with return of bilious fluid. ERCP identifies a cystic duct stump leak, and a biliary stent is inserted endoscopically **(Figure 7)**. The patient's condition improves and she returns home 2 days later. The volume of drain output decreases over the course of several weeks, and the drain is subsequently removed. The patient suffers no further complications and no recurrence of her biliary symptoms.

TAKE HOME POINTS

- Acute cholecystitis presents with RUQ pain, fever, and leukocytosis.
- RUQ ultrasound is the first-line diagnostic test.
- Acute cholecystitis must be distinguished from other biliary pathology such as biliary colic, choledocholithiasis, cholangitis, or biliary pancreatitis.
- Urgent laparoscopic cholecystectomy is the treatment of choice for most patients, even those presenting after 72 hours.
- During laparoscopic cholecystectomy, no structures should be divided until the critical view of safety is established.
- Inability to achieve the critical view of safety mandates conversion to open operation.
- Intraoperative cholangiogram may be useful in defining the patient's biliary anatomy and identifying choledocholithiasis or biliary injury.
- Persistent postoperative pain, fever, or hyperbilirubinemia are concerning for retained CBD stone or biliary leak.

SUGGESTED READINGS

Csikesz N, Ricciardi R, Tseng JF, et al. Current status of surgical management of acute cholecystitis in the United States. World J Surg. 2008;32(10):2230–2236.

Gurusamy KS, Samraj K. Early versus delayed laparoscopic cholecystectomy for acute cholecystitis. Cochrane Database Syst Rev. 2006;(4):CD005440.

Strasberg SM. Clinical practice. Acute calculous cholecystitis. N Engl J Med. 2008;358(26):2804–2811.

Bile Duct Injury

CHRISTOPHER J. SONNENDAY

Presentation

A 38-year-old woman presents to the emergency room with right upper-quadrant pain, nausea, emesis, and subjective fever. She underwent a laparoscopic cholecystectomy 4 days ago for acute cholecystitis. Past medical history is notable for obesity and two uncomplicated pregnancies.

On physical exam, the patient appears uncomfortable and diaphoretic. She is alert and oriented. Vital signs are notable for a temperature of 38.7°C, pulse of 110 beats per minute, blood pressure of 130/80, respiratory rate of 18, and an oxygen saturation of 99%. Her sclerae are anicteric. The abdomen is mildly distended with diffuse tenderness to light palpation, and more focal tenderness in the right upper quadrant. Her laparoscopic port site incisions are dry and intact without erythema or induration.

Differential Diagnosis

Abdominal pain following laparoscopic cholecystectomy, particularly pain significant enough to require an emergency room evaluation, should immediately prompt evaluation for technical complications of the procedure. Postoperative pain following laparoscopic cholecystectomy, now often accomplished as an outpatient operation, is generally moderate and should improve each subsequent postoperative day. It is unusual for otherwise healthy patients to require narcotic analgesics after the first 3 to 5 postoperative days. Patients who do not follow this expected course should be evaluated thoroughly, as early recognition and treatment of postcholecystectomy complications are paramount to limiting the impact of these events on the patient.

Complications common to any laparoscopic procedure should always be considered when evaluating the patient with abdominal pain following laparoscopic cholecystectomy. Inadvertent injury to bowel from trocar placement or instrument passing may present with peritonitis and postoperative sepsis. Evidence of urinary tract or surgical site infection should be queried. Constipation or ileus may also be seen in some patients, but lack of return of bowel function should lead to consideration of a more serious underlying complication.

The major complications specific to laparoscopic cholecystectomy include postoperative hemorrhage, a retained common bile duct stone, and bile duct injury. Bleeding complications following cholecystectomy are rare and often present in the first 24 to 48 hours postoperatively. Common etiologies include hemorrhage from the cystic artery stump or liver parenchyma along the gallbladder fossa. A retained common bile duct stone may present days to weeks following cholecystectomy and is typically associated with signs and symptoms of obstructive jaundice, cholangitis, and/or pancreatitis. Bile duct injury represents the most feared technical complication of cholecystectomy and can present in protean ways dependent on whether the primary injury results in a biliary leak or obstruction. Maintaining a high index of suspicion for bile duct injury in patients with unexpected problems following cholecystectomy is essential to making an early and definitive diagnosis. Sending a patient with unusual postoperative pain home from the clinic or emergency room without proper assessment can have catastrophic consequences if underlying intra-abdominal sepsis or biliary obstruction is left to go unaddressed.

Workup

Evaluation of the postcholecystectomy patient with suspected complications should proceed in a methodical manner. Initial maneuvers include administration of appropriate analgesia and fluid resuscitation as indicated. Laboratory evaluation should include a complete blood count, metabolic panel, liver profile, amylase, lipase, coagulation profile, and urinalysis. The initial laboratory results can be helpful in guiding the selection of appropriate imaging procedures and other interventions. Laboratory evaluation may initially be underwhelming, though a leukocytosis may be present. The total bilirubin may be normal or only slightly elevated (2 to 4 mg/dL) in the case of a complete biliary transection with free leak. Reabsorption of bile from the peritoneum may elevate the bilirubin slightly. Marked elevation of the transaminases is not typical and should raise concern of an associated vascular injury when present. Biliary injuries are typically not associated with abnormalities of the serum amylase and lipase. When associated with an obstructive pattern to the liver profile, biochemical evidence of pancreatitis may indicate a retained common bile duct stone rather than a bile duct injury.

Initial diagnostic imaging may include ultrasound, to assess for perihepatic fluid collections and biliary ductal dilatation, or computed tomography (CT) in select patients. If identified, significant perihepatic collections may be percutaneously drained. If bilious, a biliary leak is diagnosed, and the evaluation should proceed with direct cholangiography either by endoscopic retrograde cholangiography (ERC) or percutaneous transhepatic cholangiography (PTC). If the fluid visualized on ultrasound or CT is not easily drained, or if the question of a biliary injury is still open, a hepatobiliary iminodiacetic acid (HIDA) nuclear medicine scan may be performed. HIDA scans can detect extravasation of biliary drainage and may also demonstrate failure of bile excreted from the liver to enter the duodenum. Further anatomic detail is not available from HIDA scans, but the test may be sufficient to confirm a suspicion of biliary injury before proceeding to more invasive means of cholangiography. CT angiography, with dual arterial and portal venous phases, can be used to define associated vascular injury. Magnetic resonance cholangiopancreatography (MRCP) is an attractive noninvasive imaging option if the diagnosis of a biliary injury is still in doubt. MR cholangiography can define an interrupted or strictured bile duct, and contrast agents (e.g., Eovist) with biliary excretion can be used to document biliary leaks on delayed images.

ERC is the best initial invasive study in a patient with a suspected or confirmed biliary injury following cholecystectomy. In injuries in which the continuity of the extrahepatic biliary tree is preserved, ERC may be both diagnostic and therapeutic. Endoscopic sphincterotomy and placement of an endobiliary stent is often sufficient to treat biliary leaks from the cystic duct stump or small accessory ducts. Incomplete transections may be bridged by endobiliary stents, with the need for subsequent operative intervention determined over time. In cases of common bile duct ligation, or in instances where a segment of the extrahepatic duct is excised with the gallbladder leaving an open proximal and distal extrahepatic bile duct, ERC may not be adequate to provide anatomic detail of the proximal biliary tree, nor able to facilitate crossing the injury. In these cases, PTC with placement of transhepatic biliary drains is typically necessary, and PTC should be performed in all patients with suspected bile duct injury in whom ERC was either not technically feasible or not definitive.

PTC in a patient with a recent ductal ligation or leak, and thus a decompressed biliary system, is difficult and often requires sophisticated interventional radiology resources and expertise. It is often necessary to place additional percutaneous drains to control bile leakage and drain infected bilomas until the biliary drainage is adequately diverted. These patients truly require multidisciplinary management to ensure that procedures are coordinated with the goals of improving the patient's condition, defining the relevant anatomy, and facilitating eventual definitive repair. For this reason, the hepatobiliary surgeon needs to be involved in all decisions about placement of drains and transhepatic catheters, and the timing of these procedures.

Direct cholangiography allows classification of the type of biliary injury **(Figure 1)** according to the Bismuth-Strasberg classification. Type A injuries occur due to leakage from the cystic duct stump or accessory

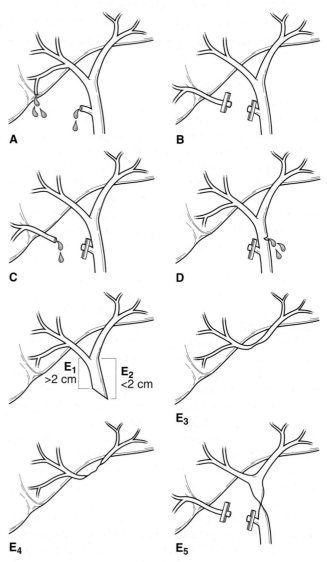

FIGURE 1 • The Bismuth-Strasberg classification of biliary injuries following laparoscopic cholecystectomy. (Reproduced from Winslow ER, Fialkowski EA, Linehan DC, et al. "Sideways": results of repair of biliary injuries using a policy of side-to-side hepaticojejunostomy. Ann Surg. 2009;249(3):426–434, with permission.)

ducts draining directly into the gallbladder (ducts of Luschka) and present as a biliary leak and/or subhepatic biloma. Type B injuries are defined as ligation and division of an anomalous segmental hepatic duct, typically the duct draining segment 6 (± segment 7). This injury is often facilitated by the associated anomaly where the cystic duct drains into the right posterior duct. The proximal and distal ends of the anomalous segmental duct are clipped and divided during control of the cystic duct. Type B injuries are often asymptomatic or may present late with abdominal pain or cholangitis involving the occluded liver segment. Normally, the liver behind a type B injury will atrophy over time, often indolently. Type C injuries occur in the same anatomic setting as type B injuries, though the proximal ductal segment is not ligated and leaks freely into the peritoneal cavity. The difficulty in type C injuries lies in their diagnosis, as ERC typically misses the leaking segment as it is not opacified via the main biliary tree. Cholangiograms should be carefully inspected to make sure all liver segments are visualized; when the posterior segment is not seen, PTC may be diagnostic and allow control of the leak.

In type D injuries, a lateral injury to the extrahepatic bile duct occurs, either sharply or by thermal injury. The biliary tree remains in continuity, and the injury may manifest with a leak initially or a stricture in a delayed presentation. These injuries may be diagnosed accurately by ERC, which can also provide definitive treatment via endobiliary stenting.

Type E injuries are defined by complete disruption of biliary–enteric continuity due to transection, excision, and/or ligation of the extrahepatic biliary tree. Injuries that include a free biliary leak will prevent early with bile peritonitis and sepsis. Injuries with occlusion of the proximal hepatic drainage may present in a delayed fashion with jaundice and/or cholangitis, although still typically within 2 weeks of cholecystectomy as all biliary drainage is occluded. Type E injuries are further described according to the Bismuth classification (E1 to E5, as depicted in **Figure 1**), with important implications about the complexity of definitive repair. The majority of type E injuries will require PTC to definitively reveal the anatomic details of the injury and to establish stable biliary drainage.

In the present case, CT demonstrates the patient to have a large right upper-quadrant fluid collection. The collection is percutaneously drained, revealing frank bilious output that grows gram-negative organisms in culture. Antibiotics are initiated. ERC reveals an obstructed bile duct at the level of the cystic duct. PTC is performed demonstrating a complete transection of the hepatic duct within 2 to 3 mm of the bifurcation (type E3 injury, **Figure 2, panel A**). A transhepatic biliary drain is left in place, providing external biliary drainage **(Figure 2, panel B,C)**.

Diagnosis and Treatment

The management of bile duct injuries should be catered to the condition of the patient, timing of the injury, and anatomic details according to the Bismuth-Strasberg classification. Principles that apply in all cases include control of sepsis, drainage of all bile collections, and establishment of secure biliary drainage. Ongoing

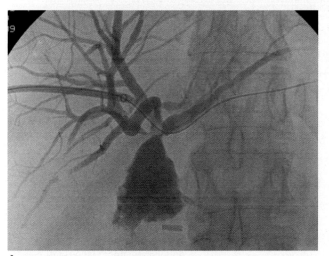
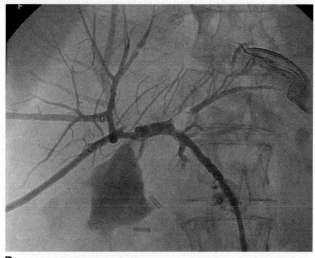

A   **B**

FIGURE 2 • Type E3 biliary injury managed with U tube percutaneous biliary drainage and delayed Roux-en-Y hepaticojejunostomy. PTC on postoperative day 5 following laparoscopic cholecystectomy reveals type E3 injury with biliary leak (**panel A**). A wire was able to be passed from percutaneous access to the right hepatic across the hepatic duct bifurcation and retrieved from percutaneous access to the left hepatic duct, allowing placement of a U tube for external biliary drainage (**panel B**).

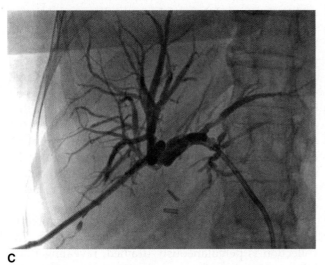

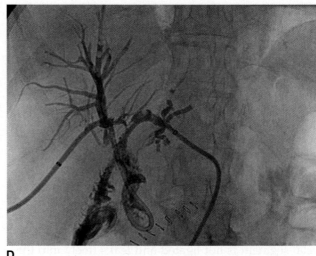

C   D

FIGURE 2 • *(Continued)* The patient recovered over the ensuing 12 weeks, during which time the biliary leak resolved with stable U tube drainage (**panel C**). At the time of hepaticojejunostomy, the U tube was exchanged for individual bilateral biliary catheters placed across the anastomosis. The catheters were removed 3 weeks after repair when cholangiogram revealed a well-healed patent hepaticojejunostomy (**panel D**).

reassessment of the patient's clinical condition, with reimaging as clinically indicated to detect undrained bilomas, will get even the frailest patients through what can be tenuous early stages of their injury, allowing definitive repair to be performed in an elective fashion on a healthy patient. Timing of definitive repair for those patients that require biliary reconstruction is an individualized decision that requires careful surgical judgment.

Specific treatment strategies for bile duct injuries can be determined according the Bismuth-Strasberg classification, as summarized in **Table 1**. The decision making about the urgency of intervention and the need for surgical reconstruction varies based upon the timing of the patient's presentation, and the patient's clinical condition. Injuries recognized at the time of cholecystectomy, or within the immediate postoperative period (48 to 72 hours), can be considered for early repair.

TABLE 1. The Bismuth-Strasberg Classification of Biliary Injuries Following Laparoscopic Cholecystectomy

Bismuth-Strasberg Classification	Description	Extrahepatic Bile Duct in Continuity?	Treatment
Type A	Bile leak from cystic duct or accessory hepatic duct (duct of Luschka)	Yes	Endoscopic sphincterotomy and endobiliary stent placement
Type B	Ligation of posterior segment hepatic duct	Partially (posterior segment[s] excluded)	Hepaticojejunostomy in symptomatic patients
Type C	Bile leak from injured posterior hepatic duct	Partially (posterior segment[s] excluded)	Percutaneous transhepatic biliary drainage, followed by hepaticojejunostomy
Type D	Lateral injury with incomplete transection of the extrahepatic bile duct	Yes	Endoscopic sphincterotomy and endobiliary stent placement; hepaticojejunostomy if refractory stricture develops
Type E	Circumferential injury (ligation and/or transection) to hepatic duct(s)	No	Percutaneous transhepatic biliary drainage, followed by hepaticojejunostomy

In the case of injuries recognized intraoperatively at the time of cholecystectomy, immediate repair should only be performed when adequate surgical experience and expertise are available and the extent of the injury is completely understood. The inability to perform good quality cholangiography, or the lack of surgical experience with biliary–enteric anastomoses, are examples of contraindications to immediate repair. Other relative contraindications to early repair include an associated vascular injury, hemodynamic instability, excessive blood loss, or a thermal injury to the duct with extensive devitalized tissue.

In the case of patients who present in the first 48 to 72 hours after cholecystectomy, early repair may be considered if the patient is clinically well without signs of sepsis or hepatic dysfunction, and the anatomic details of the injury are well understood with cholangiography. Relative contraindications to early repair include associated vascular injury, thermal injury with extensive devitalized tissue, and Class E3 or greater injuries where achieving a quality repair to healthy tissue can be difficult in the acute setting.

In patients presenting beyond 72 hours from cholecystectomy, and/or with signs of intra-abdominal sepsis, the initial priorities should be appropriate resuscitation, broad-spectrum antibiotics, cross-sectional imaging, and percutaneous drainage of all significant fluid collections. Direct cholangiography via ERC or PTC is the next step, with an attempt to obtain definitive internal or external biliary drainage. Once biliary drainage is established, the pressure of time is removed and the patient should be allowed to recover from the cholecystectomy and any associated sepsis. Most hepatobiliary surgeons will wait 6 to 8 weeks or more before proceeding with biliary reconstruction. This delay allows for the resolution of any associated peritonitis, provides time for collateralized biliary blood flow to be established, and allows the patient to rehabilitate physically.

Surgical Approach

The preferred method for repairing most injuries is a Roux-en-Y hepaticojejunostomy **(Table 2)**, and the key principles include creation of a tension-free anastomosis to healthy hepatic ducts that drain all biliary segments. Direct end-to-end repair of the extrahepatic bile duct is often unsatisfactory when a significant section of the duct has been devitalized or removed, and is associated with a high rate of additional complications especially stricture.

Care should be taken to choose a part of the proximal jejunum that reaches easily to the right upper quadrant. The small bowel should be divided at an appropriate place with a GIA stapler, and the mesentery divided to allow the Roux limb maximum mobility. Division of the first vascular arcade of the small bowel mesentery

TABLE 2. Key Technical Steps and Potential Pitfalls in Roux-en-Y Hepaticojejunostomy Procedure

Key Technical Steps

1. Right subcostal incision, meticulous lysis of adhesions.
2. Careful portal dissection—mobilizing duodenum, omentum, hepatic flexure away from porta.
3. "Anterior-only" dissection of the hepatic duct.
4. Lowering of the portal plate to allow exposure of the anterior aspect of the hepatic duct bifurcation.
5. Starting along the long extrahepatic portion of the left hepatic duct may facilitate exposure of hepatic duct bifurcation.
6. Creation of tension free Roux-en-Y limb, brought up to right upper quadrant via defect in transverse mesocolon to the right of the middle colic vessels.
7. Broad biliary–enteric anastomosis using absorbable monofilament suture.
8. Closed suction drainage.

Potential Pitfalls

- Electing to perform repair too early, when peritonitis and adhesions from time of injury have not improved.
- Creation of the biliary–enteric anastomosis at the site of injury, to devitalized biliary tissue.
- Circumferential dissection of the hepatic duct, interrupting important collateral blood supply.
- Tension on the biliary–enteric anastomosis, caused by either failure to adequately mobilize the jejunum or placing the Roux limb in an antecolic position.

can usually be done safely, though the end of the Roux limb should always be inspected for sufficient perfusion. A retrocolic Roux-en-Y hepaticojejunostomy, brought to the right upper quadrant through a defect made in the mesocolon to the right of the middle colic vessels and above the duodenum, provides the most direct route to the porta and can avoid any undue tension created by draping the Roux limb over the colon. In patients with previous abdominal surgery, time should be taken to meticulously lyse any adhesions that tether the small bowel mesentery. In cases where patients have a foreshortened mesentery, due to previous surgery, radiation, or other conditions, a medial visceral rotation of the right colon will expose the root of the small bowel mesentery that can be mobilized up to the level of the duodenum and neck of the pancreas.

A few important principles apply to the dissection of the porta in the setting of a biliary injury. The mechanism of bile duct injury in these cases often arises from unintentional dissection of a long segment of the bile duct, which can strip the duct of its blood supply that runs through the periductal adventitial tissue. In early repair cases, it is therefore important to identify a portion of the duct that has not been completely dissected, and carefully expose or shorten the hepatic duct in a location that is amenable to construction of the biliary anastomosis. In E1 or E2 injuries, it may be possible therefore to stay below the true hepatic duct bifurcation, but care should be taken not to sew to a traumatized end of the hepatic duct. Opening the duct on its anterior surface, with a ductotomy extended toward the long extrahepatic portion of the left hepatic duct can expose healthy tissue and avoid further dissection behind the duct which can further compromise ductal blood supply. In later repair cases, avoiding dissection behind the hepatic duct is really essential, as this allows preservation of any collateralized blood supply that has been created at the site of the injury. This principle of "anterior-only" dissection also avoids creating additional vascular injury, as the right hepatic artery is often directly behind the hepatic duct at this level and can be obscured or difficult to identify in a chronically inflamed or scarred field.

All biliary anastomoses should be performed under loupe magnification, using fine monofilament absorbable suture, typically in an interrupted fashion. Placement of subhepatic drains to monitor for biliary leak is typically performed. After completion of the biliary anastomosis, the Roux limb can be further anchored to relieve tension by taking seromuscular bites of the jejunum and tacking it to the former gallbladder fossa, portal plate, or umbilical fissure.

Special Intraoperative Considerations

For E3 injuries or higher, the hepatic duct bifurcation needs to be exposed by lowering the portal plate. This involves incising into the liver parenchyma to get above the hepatic duct bifurcation, beginning above the long extrahepatic course of the left hepatic duct. This can often be done with a blunt technique and judicious use of electrocautery but can be facilitated in difficult cases by the use of an ultrasonic or hydrojet dissector. Bleeding may be encountered during this technique, but can be stopped by packing gauze or other hemostatic material into the hepatotomy for a period of time. Returning to this area after completing other tasks, such as creating the enteroenterostomy of the Roux limb, allows performance of the biliary anastomosis in a dry and controlled field.

Controversy exists over the need for transhepatic biliary catheters to serve as a stent across a fresh biliary–enteric anastomosis. In the case of early repairs, many surgeons will go to the operating room without transhepatic catheters. Intraoperative placement of retrograde transhepatic biliary catheters is difficult and potentially adds additional trauma to the liver. Therefore in these cases, routine postoperative stenting is not possible or advised. In the case of delayed repairs, a transhepatic biliary catheter is typically in place at the time of repair, and may be passed across the new biliary–enteric anastomosis. These tubes typically can be capped off ("internalized") in the immediate postoperative period if no evidence of anastomotic leak, used for postoperative cholangiography to interrogate the new anastomosis, and removed 3 to 6 weeks after repair.

Associated vascular injury is not uncommon in bile duct injury and may be associated with both acute liver injury and delayed biliary stricture due to ischemia. Significant vascular injury associated with a measurable rise in liver enzymes and systemic inflammatory response is a relative contraindication to early repair of bile duct injury, as the patient may not be optimized for a complex operation. Delayed repair also allows for collateral blood flow to involved biliary segments to mature over time. Fortunately, segmental hepatic vascular injuries do not typically require reconstruction due to the redundant blood flow to the liver. Exceptions to this general rule would include ligation or severe stenotic injury to the main portal vein or proper hepatic artery.

Postoperative Management

The postoperative period in patients undergoing a biliary–enteric anastomosis is typical of other major upper abdominal operations. Appropriate analgesia, early mobilization, and sequential advancement in diet should occur in all patients. Wounds should be monitored for signs of infection, especially in patients with indwelling percutaneous biliary drains, which predispose to surgical site infection. Patients should be monitored for biliary leak or other signs of intra-abdominal infection. In cases where a closed suction drain is left at the time of operation, the output should be monitored for bilious fluid. Typically the drain(s) can be removed in 3 to 4 days once the patient has resumed a diet if the output is nonbilious. In the case of a low-volume biliary leak, observation with continued external drainage may be the only necessary intervention, as such leaks will resolve. In the case of a more significant leak, or a leak associated with signs of sepsis, percutaneous biliary drainage may be necessary if not already in place. Reoperation is typically not necessary for management of a biliary leak.

In the intermediate and long term, biliary stricture is the most significant potential postoperative event. As many as 15% of patients undergoing biliary reconstruction may develop an anastomotic stricture, with the vast majority able to be managed by percutaneous transhepatic dilatation and stenting without the need for operative revision. As most biliary strictures may present indolently, a liver profile should be followed for signs of cholestasis. Often an isolated rise in the alkaline phosphatase is the initial sign of a biliary stricture. A liver profile should be checked every 3 to 6 months for the first 2 years, and then annually thereafter. The majority of anastomotic strictures will present in the first 2 years postoperatively, though rarely may present even in a markedly delayed fashion.

Case Conclusion

With percutaneous biliary drainage and antibiotics, the patient improves and is sent home. After an 8-week delay, biliary reconstruction is performed with a Roux-en-Y hepaticojejunostomy. The biliary catheter is passed across the new biliary enteric anastomosis and removed after a follow-up cholangiogram at 3 weeks postoperatively reveals a widely patent anastomosis **(Figure 2, panel D)**. At 3-year follow-up, the patient is clinically well with a normal liver profile.

TAKE HOME POINTS

- Patients who present following cholecystectomy with unusual pain or signs of infection should be considered to have a bile duct injury until proven otherwise.
- Initial diagnostic imaging of a patient with a suspected bile duct injury should include ultrasound and/or CT to assess for perihepatic fluid collections.
- Initial management of bile duct injury should include control of sepsis, drainage of all bilomas, and establishment of secure internal or external biliary drainage.
- Patients who present beyond 48 to 72 hours from the time of their injury, and/or who show signs of intra-abdominal sepsis, are best managed with a delayed operative repair.
- A broad, tension-free anastomosis using absorbable suture is the preferred method for reestablishing biliary–enteric continuity.
- Biliary stricture is the primary significant long-term complication of hepaticojejunostomy; serial liver profile monitoring may detect an indolent stricture before clinically apparent.

SUGGESTED READINGS

Couinaud C. Exposure of the left hepatic duct through the hilum or in the umbilical of the liver: anatomic limitations. Surgery. 1989;105(1):21–27.

Melton GB, et al. Major bile duct injuries associated with laparoscopic cholecystectomy: effect of surgical repair on quality of life. Ann Surg. 2002;235(6):888–895.

Sicklick JK, et al. Surgical management of bile duct injuries sustained during laparoscopic cholecystectomy: perioperative results in 200 patients. Ann Surg. 2005;241(5):786–792; discussion 793–795.

Winslow ER, et al. "Sideways": results of repair of biliary injuries using a policy of side-to-side hepatico-jejunostomy. Ann Surg. 2009;249(3):426–434.

25 Cholangitis

WILLIAM C. BECK and BENJAMIN K. POULOSE

Presentation

A 68-year-old man with a history of adult-onset diabetes, obesity, and tobacco use presents to the emergency department. He is febrile on arrival with a temperature of 102.7, a blood pressure of 95/50, and a heart rate of 106. His primary complaint is of right upper-quadrant pain of 24-hour duration. He notes that he has had similar pain on occasion before but always had complete resolution of pain within a couple of hours. He reports his urine has been very dark for the last 12 hours. On exam, he has tenderness of his right upper quadrant with voluntary guarding. The sclerae are mildly icteric. No jaundice is present.

Differential Diagnosis

The typical presentation of cholangitis involves the combination of right upper-quadrant pain, fever, and jaundice, commonly known as Charcot's triad. Only 50% to 70% of patients, however, present with all three elements. The addition of mental status changes and hypotension comprise Reynold's pentad, which is indicative of systemic sepsis. Although biliary colic may be elicited, patients with cholangitis usually also manifest with fever and jaundice. In a patient presenting with a history of gallstones or right upper-quadrant pain, the presence of jaundice, hypotension, or altered mental status should alert the provider to the diagnosis of cholangitis. Peritonitis is uncommon and should prompt the examiner to look for other causes of abdominal pain such as diverticulitis, perforated ulcer, or pancreatitis. Careful consideration should be given to acute cholecystitis in the differential diagnosis, as the immediate treatment would differ considerably. A previous history of biliary interventions should prompt providers to consider the diagnosis of acute cholangitis. Those patients with prior biliary operations, endoscopically or radiologically placed biliary stents, and history of chronic biliary conditions (i.e., primary sclerosing cholangitis) are at increased risk of developing cholangitis.

Workup

An abdominal ultrasound (US) is the preferred initial imaging study. In the above patient, it reveals cholelithiasis with mild intra- and extrahepatic biliary duct dilation. Computed tomography (CT) scan and magnetic resonance cholangiopancreatography (MRCP) are not needed for the diagnosis of cholangitis but may prove helpful to identify the underlying etiology of the biliary obstruction that predisposed the patient to cholangitis, such as benign or malignant biliary strictures, or periampullary mass. In the case of malignant causes of biliary obstruction, pain is usually less of a component of presentation and the onset is more insidious. In general, a single, good-quality noninvasive study (US, CT, or MRCP) can suffice to establish biliary ductal dilation and provide clues to the etiology of biliary obstruction. A high suspicion for common bile duct stones is present with clinical ascending cholangitis without other obvious etiology, or total bilirubin >4 mg/dL. Other strong predictors of common bile duct stones include a dilated common bile duct (>6 mm) on US with gallbladder *in situ* and bilirubin between 1.8 and 4 mg/dL.

Many patients do not present with Charcot's triad, and in 2006 an international consensus meeting was held in Tokyo, Japan, with the goal of developing guidelines useful in establishing the diagnosis of acute cholangitis. The consensus was reached that Charcot's triad was sufficient to diagnose acute cholangitis. Additionally, the Tokyo guidelines suggest that if two of the three elements of Charcot's triad are present, along with (1) laboratory evidence of inflammatory response, (2) abnormal liver function tests, and (3) abnormal imaging studies demonstrating biliary dilatation, inflammatory findings, or the presence of an etiology such as a biliary stricture, calculus, stent,

Presentation Continued

This patient undergoes further evaluation of his abdominal pain, fevers, and jaundice with a complete blood count (CBC), comprehensive metabolic panel (CMP), amylase, lipase, coagulation profile, and two sets of blood cultures. He has a leukocytosis of 13,300/mL with a left shift, a bilirubin of 4.4 mg/dL, and alkaline phosphatase of 500 IU/L. Both the AST and the ALT are elevated at 210 and 334 IU/L, respectively.

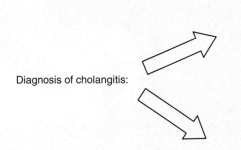

Charcot's triad: (1) Fever
(2) Jaundice
(3) Right upper quadrant pain

Diagnosis of cholangitis:

Tokyo Criteria

(1) Presence of 2/3 elements of Charcot's triad +
(2) Laboratory evidence of inflammation: +

i. Elevated WBC
ii. Elevated CRP
iii. Increased ESR

(3) Abnormal LFT's +
(4) Abnormal imaging studies

i. Biliary dilatation
ii. Inflammation
iii. Etiology

1. Stones
2. Stents
3. Mass

FIGURE 1 • Diagnosis of cholangitis may be made using either the traditional Charcot's triad, or Tokyo criteria.

or mass that the diagnosis of cholangitis can be made **(Figure 1)**.

Blood test results can vary in patients with acute cholangitis, and must be taken in the context of the history and physical exam of the individual patient. The white blood cell count is elevated above 10,000/mL in 60% to 80% of patients that present with acute cholangitis and is the most often noted abnormal result. The absence of an elevated total bilirubin should question the diagnosis of cholangitis. Liver tests (AST, ALT, GGT) are usually elevated, but no specific pattern has been demonstrated. Alkaline phosphatase is also usually elevated and is typically more elevated in biliary obstruction due to malignant etiologies as compared to choledocholithiasis.

Diagnosis and Treatment

In this patient presenting with two elements of Charcot's triad (fever, abdominal pain, and jaundice), biliary disease should be at the top of the differential diagnosis. In the setting of altered mental status and relative hypotension in a normally hypertensive man, the provider should strongly suspect cholangitis as the diagnosis. Many patients have a history of prior calculous biliary disease or biliary operation. In Western countries, choledocholithiasis is the most common etiology, followed by benign and malignant biliary strictures. Other etiologies include autoimmune cholangitis, parasitic infections, prior biliary operations, indwelling stents, and chronic pancreatitis.

When cholangitis is suspected, the patient should be admitted to the hospital for intravenous fluid resuscitation, initiation of appropriate antibiotics, hemodynamic monitoring, and prompt biliary decompression if indicated. Blood cultures should be sent prior to the initiation of antibiotics to allow for the tailoring of antibiotic therapy after the causative organism is identified. Timely initiation of empiric intravenous antibiotic therapy is crucial to successful treatment. Therapy should target gram-negative bacteria and anaerobes. A fluoroquinolone with added metronidazole or extended-spectrum beta lactam (piperacillin–tazobactam) can provide adequate empiric coverage. Occasionally, coagulopathy is present, which needs to be corrected prior to undergoing any intervention. If the patient responds well to antibiotic therapy, and there is no hemodynamic instability, further imaging (CT or MRCP) may be performed to better elucidate the underlying cause of the cholangitis. However, if the patient appears septic, urgent biliary decompression is required either by endoscopic, percutaneous, or surgical means.

Those patients who respond well to initial resuscitation and antibiotic therapy without biliary drainage are deemed as having mild cholangitis. Continued clinical improvement in these patients may delay the urgency of biliary decompression as the etiology for biliary obstruction is sought. Patients who do not respond to resuscitation and antibiotics alone will need urgent biliary decompression.

Surgical Approach

Urgent endoscopic decompression of the biliary tree has been established as the treatment of choice for the management of acute cholangitis. Endoscopic retrograde cholangiography (ERC) is successful in over 90% of patients in decompressing the biliary tree. The timing of endoscopic biliary decompression should be individualized and often occurs within 24 to 48 hours of initial admission. The urgency of intervention should be dictated by the patient's clinical response to resuscitation and antibiotic therapy. An initially good response followed by clinical deterioration prompts urgent biliary decompression. More urgent or emergent decompression is required in patients who remain hypotensive despite aggressive resuscitation and antibiotic therapy. When ERC expertise is not readily available and urgent biliary decompression is needed, percutaneous or surgical biliary decompression should be employed.

ERC can be performed under moderate or deep sedation and is associated with decreased rates of postoperative mechanical ventilation and death as opposed to traditional open bile duct exploration. ERC is typically performed with the patient in the prone or semiprone position. The duodenoscope is advanced through the oropharynx, esophagus, and stomach to the second portion of the duodenum. The ampulla is visualized and engaged with a cannula or sphincterotome. Wire access to the biliary tree is achieved and the cannula advanced into the bile duct. Before a large volume of contrast in instilled into the biliary tree, bile is aspirated to assist with decompression and to obtain biliary cultures. The act of biliary cannulation alone will often result in rapid biliary decompression in patients with acute suppurative cholangitis **(Figure 2)**. Radiopaque contrast is then injected into the bile duct and cholangiography performed to ascertain the etiology of biliary obstruction. Should a common bile duct calculus be discovered, a judgment is made regarding appropriateness of biliary sphincterotomy prior to stent placement. If the calculus is relatively small and there is little associated ampullary edema, biliary sphincterotomy can usually be safely performed to help facilitate ductal clearance either with a biliary extraction balloon or a Dormia basket. A temporary transampullary biliary stent is then placed to ensure continued biliary drainage **(Figure 3)**. If during cholangiography a large, challenging stone or complex stricture is encountered, the main priority should be biliary decompression with stenting to quickly improve the patient's clinical condition. This is done at the expense of repeated diagnostic and therapeutic procedures to help define the precise etiology of biliary obstruction and definitively treat the patient. However, these additional procedures can often be performed on

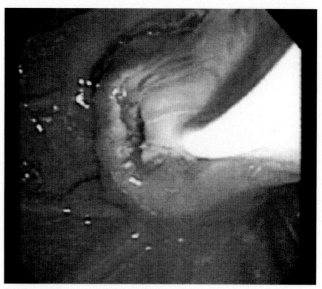

FIGURE 2 • Suppurative cholangitis.

an elective basis. In experienced hands, ERC can be performed with minimal risk. Post-ERC pancreatitis is the most frequently encountered complication, followed by hemorrhage, cholangitis, and perforation. In patients with severe sepsis and hypotension who do not have suppurative cholangitis at the time of ERC, serious consideration should be given to an alternate diagnosis.

If ERC is not available, other options for biliary decompression include percutaneous transhepatic drainage and surgical decompression. If the intrahepatic ducts are dilated, thus providing a transhepatic target for biliary access, a percutaneous route to biliary drainage is favored as it is less invasive than surgical

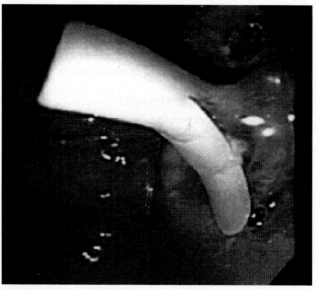

FIGURE 3 • Transampullary stent placement.

decompression and provides adequate drainage. In addition, a percutaneously placed biliary drain drainage can usually be converted to an internal endoscopically placed stent once acute issues have resolved via a rendezvous technique.

Surgical decompression of the biliary tree is largely of historical interest given the high success of ERC and percutaneous techniques, avoiding the additional physiologic insult of a major operation. However, there are scenarios where surgical decompression may be the preferred method of decompression. These atypical scenarios arise in patients with altered upper gastrointestinal anatomy (e.g., post Roux-en-Y gastric bypass) and where endoscopic or percutaneous radiologic expertise is not readily available. If a patent cystic duct can be demonstrated with an *in situ* gallbladder, an open or laparoscopic cholecystostomy tube may be an efficient, life-saving intervention until further expertise can be obtained. If common bile duct access is necessary, an open approach is usually employed for common bile duct exploration and t-tube placement **(Table 1)**. Surgeons with advanced laparoscopic skills and experience may consider a laparoscopic approach. If a laparotomy is performed, an upper midline or right subcostal incision is utilized to approach the biliary tree. A self-retaining retractor is used to retract the liver cephalad and colon caudally. If a gallbladder is present, it is mobilized in a dome-down fashion until the cystic duct is identified. Calot's triangle is defined and the cystic artery is ligated and divided. The anterior surface of the cystic duct is dissected toward the common bile duct, which usually is readily identified. Care is then taken to dissect the anterior surface of the bile duct only to avoid the flanking blood supply coursing at the 3 and the 9 o'clock positions. The caliber of the bile duct and associated inflammation are assessed to help further guide surgical intervention. The cholecystectomy is completed. The intended area of choledochotomy should be 1 to 2 cm distal to the insertion of the cystic duct toward the ampulla. Two separate mural sutures, using a fine 4-0 or 5-0 suture, are placed on either side of the anterior portion of the bile duct and a longitudinal choledochotomy made with a no. 15 blade scalpel. At this point, a decision is made to proceed with common bile duct exploration or to insert a t-tube for decompression in the unstable patient. If common bile duct stones are suspected, simple irrigation of the ductal lumen with a small bore red rubber catheter is usually adequate to mobilize most calculi out through the choledochotomy. The red rubber catheter can be advanced both proximally and distally to clear the bile duct. A balloon-tipped catheter ("biliary Fogarty") may also be used. Rigid instrumentation and extraction forceps should be avoided especially with inflamed tissues increasing the chance of ductal injury. Choledochoscopy is a very useful adjunct to ensure ductal clearance. A 3-mm or a 5-mm choledochoscope can be used with continuous saline irrigation to adequately and efficiently visualize the ductal lumen. Difficult stones can be retrieved with wire baskets placed through the scope. It is essential that the surgeon be familiar with the equipment intended for choledochoscopy prior to the procedure. In addition, biliary endoscopy can be challenging even for experienced surgical endoscopists; familiarity with endoscopic techniques in general greatly facilitates this procedure, especially when through-the-scope therapeutics are employed. Once the duct is cleared, a t-tube is usually placed in the setting of acute cholangitis. For adequate drainage, a 14 F or 16 F guttered t-tube should be placed within the bile duct. The choledochotomy is closed using absorbable sutures over the t-tube, which is brought through the abdominal wall. Some redundancy of the tubing should be left within the abdomen to avoid tension, but a long and tortuous course should be avoided to help facilitate possible future percutaneous techniques. If time and resources permit, a completion t-tube cholangiogram can be performed to confirm bile duct clearance and integrity of the ductal closure. A closed-suction drain is placed in the area of the choledochotomy and the abdomen closed in the standard fashion.

TABLE 1. Key Technical Steps and Potential Pitfalls of Open Biliary Decompression

Key Technical Steps

1. Upper midline or right subcostal laparotomy.
2. Self-retaining retractor used to lift liver cephalad, and retract colon caudally.
3. If present, gallbladder is dissected using "dome-down" technique until Calot's triangle is identified. The cystic artery is ligated and divided.
4. Cystic artery is followed antegrade to the common bile duct, which is dissected anteriorly.
5. The cholecystectomy is completed.
6. A longitudinal choledochotomy is made 1–2 cm distal to the confluence of the cystic duct and the common bile duct.
7. The common bile duct is cleared with irrigation or a Fogarty catheter.
8. The choledochotomy is closed using absorbable suture over a t-tube and a closed suction drain is left in the area of the choledochotomy.

Potential Pitfalls

- Dissection on the common bile duct laterally, thereby compromising the blood supply.
- Rigid instrumentation of the CBD, causing injury.
- Failure to correctly identify the CBD prior to making choledochotomy.

Special Intraoperative Considerations

The surgical approach to the common bile duct should be avoided in patients with smaller ducts (<5 mm) where identification and manipulation would be technically difficult, especially in an inflamed field. In these situations, cholecystostomy tube placement may be an ideal method of biliary decompression, should endoscopy not be feasible. Should the surgeon encounter severely inflamed tissues around the main portal triad, every effort to minimize dissection and safely enter the common bile duct need to be employed. Keen judgment should be used to avoid injury to the portal vein, hepatic artery, or duodenum in the inflamed field. Identification of the common bile duct can be facilitated by using a small needle (22 to 25 g) to aspirate bile from the duct before an incision is made within it. This technique is especially helpful in patients who have had prior cholecystectomy. Laparoscopy has limited use in the acute decompression of the common bile duct except among surgeons and surgical teams who have considerable expertise with these techniques.

Postoperative Management

Following biliary decompression, patients are observed in the hospital for resolution of their symptoms. Antibiotics may be tailored following the results of cultures and continued for 5 to 7 days. A CBC and CMP may be sent to follow improving white blood cell counts and liver profile. Definitive therapy is dictated by the underlying cause of biliary obstruction. In most patients who undergo ERC for choledocholithiasis, elective cholecystectomy can be performed at a later date with ductal clearance usually achieved via ERC.

For those patients in whom a t-tube was placed, the tube is initially left to gravity drainage in the acute setting. After discharge, a contrast study is obtained via the tube to confirm clearance of the bile duct and patency of the biliary tree. With this study, usually performed 2 to 3 weeks after insertion, decision can then be made to "internalize" biliary drainage (i.e., cap the t-tube). Another study is repeated at 4 to 6 weeks and the tube is removed should this study demonstrate normal patency and drainage of the biliary system.

Case Conclusion

In the patient presented, a high suspicion of common bile duct stones exists based on documented cholelithiasis, extrahepatic biliary ductal dilation, clinical ascending cholangitis, and a total bilirubin level greater than 4mg/dL. The patient underwent successful ERC with biliary sphincterotomy and extraction of common bile duct stones. Once discharged, an elective laparoscopic cholecystectomy was performed.

TAKE HOME POINTS

- Prompt diagnosis, antibiotic administration, and fluid resuscitation are of utmost importance in the patient with acute cholangitis.
- The most common cause of acute cholangitis in Western countries is choledocholithiasis, followed by malignancy.
- Urgent biliary decompression is the essential treatment in acute cholangitis not responsive to resuscitation and antibiotics.
- Endoscopic biliary decompression is associated with lower morbidity and mortality than with conventional surgical bile duct exploration.
- Percutaneous or surgical decompression should be employed when endoscopic intervention is not feasible.

SUGGESTED READINGS

ASGE Standards of Practice Committee, Maple JT, Ben-Manachem T, et al. The role of endoscopy in the evaluation of suspected choledocholithiasis. Gastrointest Endosc. 2010;71:1–9.

Boey JH, Way LW. Acute cholangitis. Ann Surg. 1980;191:264–270.

Lai EC, Mok FP, Tan ES, et al. Endoscopic biliary drainage for severe acute cholangitis. N Engl J Med. 1992;326:1582–1586.

Mayumi T, Takada T, Kawarda Y, et al. Results of the Tokyo Consensus Meeting Tokyo Guidelines. J Hepatobiliary Pancreat Surg. 2007;14:114–121.

Thompson JE, Tompkins RK, Longmire WP. Factors in management of acute cholangitis. Ann Surg. 1982;195:137–145.

26 Severe Acute Pancreatitis

MARISA CEVASCO, STANLEY W. ASHLEY, and AMY L. REZAK

Presentation

A 39-year-old male with a history of alcohol abuse presents to the emergency department complaining of epigastric abdominal pain for the past 36 hours. He describes the pain as constant and radiating to his back. He also complains of nausea and has vomited several times. He had a normal bowel movement one day prior to presentation and denies melena. The patient is currently unemployed and recently divorced from his wife. He admits to drinking a case of beer each day for the past week. He denies smoking and illicit drug use. His family history is significant for hypertriglyceridemia.

Physical exam reveals abdominal distension and diffuse tenderness to palpation, worse over the epigastrium, but no guarding or rigidity. He is not jaundiced and has no Grey-Turner or Cullen signs. His vital signs are notable for a temperature of 101°F, sinus tachycardia, and hypotension with a blood pressure of 90/60 mm Hg. He has palpable distal pulses and no pretibial edema.

Differential Diagnosis

Epigastric abdominal pain radiating to the back, in a patient with a history of heavy alcohol consumption and a family history of hypertriglyceridemia, suggests acute pancreatitis. However, in a patient who is tachycardic, hypotensive, and vomiting, the differential diagnosis would also include perforated gastroduodenal ulcer disease and esophageal rupture (Boerhaave's syndrome). Cholecystitis and cholangitis are other important considerations, as these patients may present with fever, tachycardia, hypotension, and abdominal pain.

Presentation Continued

The patient has been hospitalized in the past for acute pancreatitis. He has no history of gallstone disease. Laboratory tests were notable for lipase of 18,200 U/L, amylase of 7,800 U/L, and mildly elevated transaminases (AST of 124 IU/L and ALT of 79 IU/L). Alkaline phosphatase, total bilirubin, and creatinine were within normal limits. Serum glucose was elevated at 230 mg/dL and lactate dehydrogenase (LDH) was 411 IU/L. He had a hematocrit of 48% and an elevated white blood cell (WBC) count of 16,400 cells/cm³. Triglycerides were 1,100 mg/dL. His respiratory rate was 16 and an arterial blood gas was notable for a pH of 7.31 and a P_aO_2 of 72 mm Hg. A Ranson score of 3 was calculated upon admission (Table 1).

A contrast-enhanced computerized tomographic (CT) scan of the abdomen and pelvis reveals stranding, inflammation, and edema within the peripancreatic area and extending inferiorly along the paracolic gutters to the pelvis (Figure 1). The low attenuation area in the tail of the pancreas is consistent with necrosis and represents approximately 30% of the pancreatic parenchyma (Figure 2). Bowel wall thickening was also seen at the hepatic flexure of the transverse colon. There was no free air or evidence of biliary disease, and no occlusion or thrombosis of the peripancreatic vasculature.

Workup

This patient presents with severe acute necrotizing pancreatitis. The most common etiology of acute pancreatitis is obstructive biliary tract disease, responsible for up to 40% of cases. Excessive alcohol use is the second most common cause of pancreatitis, responsible for approximately 35% of cases. Other causes include hypertriglyceridemia, endoscopic retrograde pancreatography (ERCP), anatomic abnormalities (e.g., pancreatic divisum), and abdominal trauma.

Nearly 20% to 30% of patients with acute pancreatitis have pancreatic necrosis; therefore, it is vital to determine the severity of pancreatitis. The Ranson score, based on the presence of 11 clinical signs (five measured at the time of admission and six measured

TABLE 1. Ranson Criteria

On Admission	After 48 Hours
Age > 55 years	Calcium < 8.0 mg/dL
WBC count > 16,000 cells/mm³	Hematocrit decreased > 10%
Blood glucose > 200 g/dL	Hypoxemia (P_aO_2 < 60 mm Hg)
AST > 250 IU/L	BUN increased by > 5 mg/dL
LDH > 350 IU/L	Base deficit > 4 mEq/L
	Sequestration of fluids > 6 L

Ranson score of:
1–2: 1% mortality
3–4: 15% mortality
5–6: 40% mortality

48 hours after admission), indicates the risk of systemic complications and the likelihood of pancreatic necrosis **(Table 1)**. The presence of three or more Ranson criteria (or if the patient is in shock, renal insufficiency, or pulmonary insufficiency) indicates severe pancreatitis and a greater likelihood of necrosis. Severe pancreatitis is associated with multiple organ dysfunction syndrome (MODS) and mortality rates that typically exceed 15%. In contrast, patients with mild disease generally recover completely with conservative management.

Contrast-enhanced abdominal CT is the gold standard for noninvasive diagnosis of pancreatic necrosis. CT is >90% accurate in diagnosing necrosis if more than 30% of the gland is affected. There are several CT-based classification schemes that predict disease severity and mortality. However, several recent

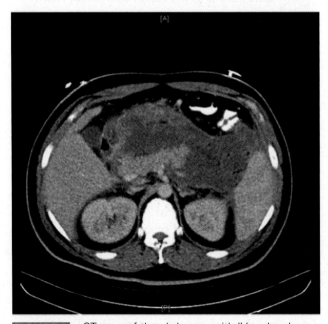

FIGURE 1 • CT scan of the abdomen with IV and oral contrast reveals stranding, inflammation, and edema within the peripancreatic area.

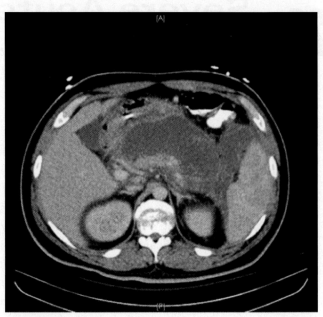

FIGURE 2 • CT scan of the abdomen with IV and oral contrast reveals low attenuation of the tail of the pancreas. This is consistent with necrosis and represents approximately 30% of the pancreatic parenchyma.

studies revealed that the associated radiation exposure was significant and that, after CT imaging, changes in clinical management were infrequent. Subsequently, it is recommended that the use of CT be restricted to patients with severe pancreatitis.

Diagnosis and Treatment

Initial treatment of the patient with severe pancreatitis includes monitoring, fluid resuscitation, and pain control with patient-administered or epidural analgesia (PCA). A Foley catheter to measure urine output should be considered. Oxygenation should be monitored closely and early intubation should be considered in the patient whose respiratory function is deteriorating. Caloric support should be initiated early in the hospital course, and enteral feeding via a nasojejunal tube is preferred if the patient's ileus is not too severe.

In patients who are appropriately resuscitated, infectious complications are considered to be the main cause of mortality in severe pancreatitis. Multiple trials have examined the value of prophylactic antibiotics and this remains controversial; selection for resistant organisms and *Candida* species may be associated with even worse outcomes.

For patients with MODS and signs of sepsis, CT-guided (FNA) of the necrotic areas should be performed to determine the presence of bacterial contamination. Although these developments may be the result of infection, MODS and the systemic inflammatory response syndrome can result from pancreatic necrosis alone. Infected pancreatic necrosis is an indication for intervention with either surgical or radiologic drainage. In extremely ill patients, a percutaneous drain placed at the time of the FNA can help stabilize the patient prior to surgery, and may be used to temporize or even definitively treat infected necrosis. If possible, waiting at least 4 weeks prior to necrosectomy will allow demarcation of necrosis, thereby minimizing resection of viable pancreas and the accompanying morbidity. Sterile necrotizing pancreatitis, on the other hand, has not been shown to benefit from drainage or debridement and may be managed nonoperatively. In patients who develop abdominal compartment syndrome, surgical decompression may improve respiratory, cardiovascular, and renal parameters, but it is unclear if this is associated with an improvement in mortality.

Presentation Continued

The patient was admitted to the intensive care unit. His pain was controlled with a PCA, and his electrolytes were closely monitored. A postpyloric feeding tube was placed under endoscopic guidance. Although he initially stabilized, on the eighth hospital day, the patient became tachycardic and hypotensive. His WBC count continued to rise, and his creatinine became elevated. An intra-abdominal pressure was measured at 15 mm Hg. He became increasingly dyspneic and required intubation. CT-guided FNA revealed gram-negative rods, and a percutaneous drain was placed. Despite this, the patient continued to deteriorate and the decision was made to proceed with surgical debridement.

Surgical Approach

The approach to pancreatic debridement is determined by the interval to operation. Over time, the pancreatic necrosis becomes increasingly organized, permitting a more focused and even minimally invasive approach. In patients undergoing operation prior to a month after onset, open pancreatic necrosectomy is often required.

Open pancreatic necrosectomy **(Table 2)**. Preoperative imaging should be used to guide placement of the incision. A vertical midline or Chevron incision may be employed. The greater omentum is usually separated from the middle of the transverse colon for a distance sufficient to expose the pancreas. When the collection extends into the mesocolon and the small bowel

TABLE 2. Key Technical Steps and Potential Pitfalls in Open Pancreatic Necrosectomy

Key Technical Steps
1. Midline vertical or Chevron incision and full exploration.
2. Access to the lesser sac obtained through the gastrocolic ligament or mesocolon.
3. Drainage of purulent material.
4. Debridement of necrotic tissue.
5. Placement of feeding jejunostomy.
6. JP drains placed into the lesser sac for postoperative irrigation and drainage.

Potential Pitfalls
- Generalized venous bleeding requiring intra-abdominal packing.
- Recurrent necrosis after initial operative debridement requiring return to the operating room.
- Enzymatic damage to the bowel or vasculature resulting in hemorrhage.
- Bowel wall edema caused by generous resuscitation resulting in an open abdomen.

mesentery, a direct approach from below the transverse colon may be more appropriate. Once the pancreas is exposed, the capsule is opened and all purulent material and necrotic tissue is removed from the pancreatic bed, being careful to preserve viable pancreatic tissue. Sharp dissection is usually avoided; it is typically sufficient to remove tissue that comes easily with a ring forceps or irrigation. The transverse colon should be inspected for viability; if the colon is compromised, an extended right hemicolectomy should be performed. Care should be taken to minimize intra-operative hemorrhage. Depending on the organization of the necrosis, the anticipated need for further debridement, and the degree of hemorrhage, it may be appropriate to pack the pancreatic bed and plan reoperation. In cases where the laparotomy incision will be closed, Jackson-Pratt (JP) drains should be placed to maximize postoperative drainage of debris. Closed continuous lavage of the retroperitoneum may be appropriate in patients where ongoing necrosis is anticipated.

Laparoscopic pancreatic necrosectomy. For critically ill, hemodynamically unstable patients or if the necrosis is not yet organized, laparoscopic intervention is contraindicated. However, some case series suggest that laparoscopic necrosectomy is appropriate in patients who have undergone prior percutaneous drainage and/or have limited areas of necrosis that will benefit from a single-stage procedure. Full laparoscopic procedures with carbon dioxide pneumoperitoneum and modified laparoscopic procedures aided by a hand port have been described. Postoperative drainage is recommended with both techniques. Other minimally invasive techniques, such as endoscopic transgastric or transduodenal necrosectomy or retroperitoneal percutaneous necrosectomy, may be alternatives to surgical intervention, but a full description of these techniques and their indication is beyond the scope of this text.

Special Intraoperative Considerations

Pancreatic necrosectomy may be combined with cholecystectomy if exposure is simple and mobilization is thought to be safe. However, in the patient with severe pancreatitis, even if secondary to gallstones, cholecystectomy should be deferred to a later date if the gallbladder is not easily accessible.

A subcostal incision can be performed if focal areas of necrosis are in the tail or in the head of the gland. Formal mobilization of the gastrocolic gutters is typically not performed but all areas of necrosis, identified by preoperative CT, need to be addressed. Postoperative closed irrigation with JP drains placed into the lesser sac through separate small incisions should be considered in patients with ongoing necrosis.

Postoperative Management

Postoperative complications are common and significant. They include organ failure, retroperitoneal and intra-abdominal hemorrhage, endocrine dysfunction, and secondary fungal infections. Fistulae from the pancreatic duct and gastrointestinal tract, pseudocyst formation, pancreatic abscess, and vascular complications (e.g., mesenteric or splenic venous thrombosis and arterial pseudoaneuryms) are also late complications of acute pancreatitis. Follow-up with repeat imaging is required to identify and manage these sequelae of pancreatic necrosectomy.

Case Conclusion

The patient underwent pancreatic necrosectomy via a vertical midline incision. His abdomen was left open and he returned to the operating room for two additional irrigation and debridement procedures. He tolerated these procedures well. During the second take-back, he underwent placement of a feeding jejunostomy, and his abdomen was closed. Postoperatively, he remained hemodynamically stable and was successfully weaned from the ventilator. Follow-up imaging was notable for the development of a pancreatic pseudocyst, which was managed via endoscopic cystogastrostomy. He was ultimately discharged from the hospital to a subacute care facility, on tube feeds, and starting to tolerate a small amount of oral intake.

TAKE HOME POINTS

- Postpyloric enteral feeding is the preferred method of nutritional support.
- Patients with acute necrotizing pancreatitis and a question of infection should undergo CT-guided FNA of necrotic regions of the pancreas to differentiate between sterile and infected pancreatic necrosis.
- Infected pancreatic necrosis in patients is an indication for intervention, including radiologic drainage and/or surgery.
- Surgical intervention should favor an organ-preserving approach. Resection procedures such as partial or total pancreatectomy that remove vital pancreatic tissue are associated with postoperative exocrine and endocrine insufficiency and high mortality rates.
- Cholecystectomy should be performed when safe to avoid recurrence of gallstone-associated pancreatitis.

SUGGESTED READINGS

Ashley SW, Perez A, Pierce EA, et al. Necrotizing pancreatitis: a contemporary analysis of 99 consecutive cases. Ann Surg. 2001;234:572–580.

Baron TH, Morgan DE. Acute necrotizing pancreatitis. N Engl J Med. 1999;340:1412–1417.

Clancy TE, Benoit EP, Ashley SW. Current management of acute pancreatitis. J Gastrointest Surg. 2005;9:440–452.

Connor S, Alexakis N, Raraty GT, et al. Early and late complications after pancreatic necrosectomy. Surgery. 2005;137:499–505.

Dellinger EP, Tellado JM, Soto NE, et al. Early antibiotic treatment for severe acute necrotizing pancreatitis: a randomized, double blind, placebo-controlled study. Ann Surg. 2007;245:674–683.

27 Incidental Liver Mass

SHAWN J. PELLETIER

Presentation

A 38-year-old woman with a history of a thyroid nodule and use of an ethinyl estradiol and etonogestrel vaginal ring presents with epigastric pain and early satiety. She states her pain has been present for months but now has increased in severity and limits her quality of life. On physical exam, she is noted to have epigastric fullness and mild epigastric tenderness. An ultrasound of her liver demonstrates an incidental 15-cm mass in the left lateral segment of her liver.

Differential Diagnosis

The potential differential diagnoses are listed in **Table 1.** Most incidental liver masses identified in an otherwise healthy individual are benign, but the possibility of a malignant etiology needs to be investigated. While most metastatic liver masses come from a colorectal origin, neuroendocrine tumors and other cancers are possible. In addition, primary liver cancers should be considered including hepatocellular carcinoma (HCC), cholangiocarcinoma, and gallbladder cancer.

The most likely etiology of the tumor described in this patient setting is one of several benign tumors. Cavernous hemangiomas are benign vascular lesions of unclear etiology. They are the most common benign liver tumor and can be found in all age groups. Hemangiomas >4 cm in diameter have been termed "giant hemangiomas." Eleven to fourteen percent of cases may be symptomatic. Regardless of size, the risk of rupture and hemorrhage is minimal. In rare cases, large cavernous hemangiomas may lead to high cardiac output heart failure or Kasabach-Merritt syndrome.

Focal nodular hyperplasia (FNH) is the second most common benign lesion. In general, FNH is viewed as hyperplastic and not neoplastic. Recent studies demonstrate that these evolve from portal tract injury that leads to oxidative stress and activation of hepatic stellate cells forming a central scar. FNHs are typically found in women between the ages of 30 and 50 years. There is some association with the use of oral contraceptives, but it is felt that the use of oral contraceptives has a low likelihood to lead to progression.

Hepatocellular adenomas are typically found in women between 30 and 50 years and can enlarge particularly with the use of oral contraceptives or during pregnancy. Hepatic adenomas tend to have more heterogeneous imaging characteristics. In general, the management of adenomas is more aggressive than most other benign lesions because rupture and hemorrhage have been reported to occur between 11% and 29% of cases and the risk is greatest if the tumor is more than

5 cm in diameter. Malignant transformation into HCC has also been reported to occur in up to 5% to 10% of lesions. Liver adenomatosis can occur and has been previously defined as having more than 3 to 10 adenomas.

Workup

The algorithm for the evaluation of a patient with a liver mass is depicted in **Figure 1.** Laboratory evaluation includes a complete blood count, coagulation studies, hepatitis screen, liver function tests, and tumor markers (CEA, AFP, CA-19-9).

Incidental solid and cystic lesions within the liver are being detected more commonly due to increased utilization of modern imaging. In otherwise healthy individuals, most incidental masses are benign. Radiologic characteristics and clinical features can often define the etiology of the liver mass, thus reducing the need for percutaneous biopsy. However, after adequate imaging has been performed, 10% of lesions that remain indeterminate may be malignant. Obtaining an accurate diagnosis is critical because management ranges from observation to surgical resection.

The patient undergoes further evaluation of this liver mass with a multiphasic liver MRI, which reveals a 15-cm mass arising from the left lateral segment of the liver, displacing the spleen and the stomach. In addition, four lesions, all <2 cm in size, are noted in the right lobe of her liver **(Figure 2).** These lesions have peripheral nodular enhancement during the arterial phase of the MRI and progressive centripetal enhancement during the venous phase. All lesions are consistent with cavernous hemangiomas.

Diagnosis and Treatment

Once adequate imaging is obtained, if a diagnosis of FNH is made, the patient can be observed. If an FNH liver mass is symptomatic and no other cause for the symptoms can be identified, resection may be considered. For most hepatic adenomas, consideration should be given to the risk of resection compared to

TABLE 1. Differential Diagnosis of Incidental Liver Mass

Primary Liver Malignancies
  HCC
  Cholangiocarcinoma
  Gallbladder cancer
Metastatic Liver Malignancies
  Colorectal cancer
  Neuroendocrine tumors
  Others
Benign Liver Lesions
  Hepatic cyst (simple or complex)
  Hemangioma
  Adenoma
  Focal nodular hyperplasia
  Biliary hamartoma
  Intrahepatic abscess
  Focal fat sparing

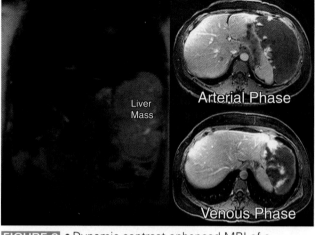

FIGURE 2 • Dynamic contrast-enhanced MRI of a 38-year-old woman with a liver mass.

serial imaging. Adenomas with a diameter >5 cm have an increased risk of hemorrhage or malignant transformation. Therefore, resection is preferred if it can be performed safely.

If the diagnosis is uncertain after adequate imaging, consideration can be given to obtaining a percutaneous core liver biopsy. Biopsy should be performed only when the results will change management. In other words, if the lesion is symptomatic or has radiologic findings concerning for malignancy, proceeding with resection without biopsy is reasonable. In general, biopsies can be obtained safely in most clinical settings and have an approximate 1% risk of either bleeding or peritoneal seeding if the tumor is malignant. Also, because the histologic architecture is necessary for the diagnosis of many of these lesions, obtaining a fine needle aspiration is often unhelpful. If the diagnosis remains indeterminate after biopsy, resection should be performed.

- • History and Physical Exam
  – Abdominal pain / weight loss
  ----- Jaundice / Scleral icterus
  – Liver disease / cirrhosis / alcohol use
  – Palpable Mass / HSM
  – Hepatitis / blood transfusion / tattoos
  – Portal hypertension
  – OCP / hormone use / cancer history

- • Laboratory tests
  – CBC / platelets / coags / hepatitis screen / albumin
  – LFTs / ammonia
  – Tumor markers (CEA, AFP, CA 19-9)
- • Abdominal imaging studies
  – US / CT or MRI
  – Nuclear medicine / angiogram / PET
- • Liver biopsy (if needed)
  » Occult primary evaluation (if malignancy)
  » EGD / colonoscopy
  » Mammogram / Gyn exam / pap smear
- • Diagnosis

FIGURE 1 • Algorithm for evaluation of a liver mass.

Some authors have suggested that a laparoscopic approach to liver tumors is associated with an easier recovery and therefore may expand the indications for surgical resection. However, even with a laparoscopic approach, the risk of complications remains and many of these lesions have a low risk for developing malignant degeneration or bleeding. In addition, an operation performed for pain from a liver tumor may be associated with postoperative pain as well and patient selection for this indication is critical.

Overall, significant advances have been made with liver surgery so that mortality rates are often reported to be <2% and even as low as 0.2% in some populations. This is partly due to improvements in anesthesia and critical care as well as an increased understanding of intrahepatic anatomy. Preoperative and intraoperative imaging, including intraoperative liver ultrasound, allows for better preoperative planning and performing segmental resections. Performing portal vein embolization of the affected side may allow for hypertrophy of the future surgical remnant in highly selective cases. In addition, the development of "bloodless" liver surgery has improved outcomes using techniques such as intermittent inflow occlusion (Pringle maneuver), isohemodilution, total vascular isolation, maintenance of low central venous pressures, and improved dissection instruments (hydrojet dissection, ultrasonic dissection, saline-cooled coagulation, bipolar cautery, surgical stapling techniques, among others), argon beam coagulation, and fibrin sealants.

Surgical Approach

Laparoscopic Resection

To perform laparoscopic liver resection safely, the surgeon must have extensive experience with both open liver surgery and advanced laparoscopic techniques.

In general, experience can be accumulated by starting with peripheral lesions within the left lateral segment or on the inferior aspect of the liver. As skills develop, resection of lesions within segments five and six can be attempted. Resection of tumors within segments seven and eight are more difficult but can be performed safely with appropriate experience. Ultimately, more than 75% of all patients with liver tumors can be approached with a laparoscopic technique, even including trisegmentectomy. As with any laparoscopic procedure, a surgeon should not hesitate to convert to an open procedure if there is inadequate exposure, hemorrhage, or concern for obtaining an adequate surgical margin.

While laparoscopic liver resections can be performed using a straight laparoscopic or hybrid approach, the hand-assisted approach offers many advantages. This allows for palpation and direct examination of the liver and abdominal cavity, adequate retraction of the relatively large liver, an improved ability to obtain a negative margin, and the ability to manually control hemorrhage. The patient is placed in the supine position and adequately secured to the table to allow for steep reverse Trendelenburg and rotation of the operative table. The hand-assist device is almost always placed in the midline near the umbilicus. For lesions in the superior aspect of the liver, the hand-assist device may be placed slightly higher on the abdomen. Positioning of the trochars depends on the location of the tumor for resection but attention should be paid to placing 12-mm trochars strategically so that laparoscopic staplers can be utilized. After the liver and the abdomen are visually inspected and palpated, ligamentous attachments are divided. An intraoperative liver ultrasound is performed, using either a T probe through the hand port or a laparoscopic ultrasound probe. Attention is first turned to a formal evaluation of the liver with particular attention paid to identifying lesions within the liver that were not identified on preoperative imaging. The known lesion is then evaluated and the vascular and biliary anatomy are noted. Margins for resection can be marked on the capsule of the liver using cautery. For lesions that are very close to major vascular or biliary structures and the lesion is known to be benign, consideration can be given to enucleating the tumor near these areas. If the tumor is concerning for malignancy, a margin should be obtained. Intermittent inflow occlusion can be utilized by placing a Penrose drain around the porta hepatis. The liver parenchyma is then divided using any of a number of different techniques, such as using ultrasonic dissection until major vascular structures are encountered. Small- to medium-sized vascular structures can be clipped and divided. Larger vascular structures and the portal plate are usually divided using an endovascular stapler. The tumor can then be removed via the

hand port. Hemostasis on the cut edge of the liver can be obtained using the argon beam coagulation or standard cautery. The cut edge of the liver is also carefully inspected for potential bile leaks that can be oversewn. The use of a sealant agent can be considered to minimize postoperative biliary leaks. Placement of a drain near the cut edge of the liver may be considered for observation and potential treatment of a postoperative biliary leak **(Table 2)**.

Open Resection

In general, the technique used for open resection is similar to that of a laparoscopic resection. Placement of an epidural for postoperative pain management should be considered preoperatively. With the patient in the supine position, a right subcostal incision with upper midline extension is made. This allows adequate exposure to the left and right lobes of the liver as well as exposure to the suprahepatic vena cava and the lower abdomen if a Roux-en-Y hepaticojejunostomy needs to be constructed. Prior to placing a fixed retractor, the round and falciform ligament should be divided and any adhesions of the liver to the anterior abdominal wall should be mobilized to avoid tearing of the hepatic capsule leading to bleeding. As described in the laparoscopic approach, the abdomen and the liver are inspected, the lobe of the liver to be resected is mobilized, and an intraoperative liver ultrasound is performed. The liver resection itself is performed using similar techniques to divide the liver parenchyma. Inspection of the cut edge of the liver is also carefully performed to help avoid postoperative bile leaks. The abdomen is closed in the standard fashion, and a drain

TABLE 2. Key Steps to Laparoscopic Liver Resection

1. Placement of trochar or hand-assisted device and induction of pneumoperitoneum.
2. Laparoscopic evaluation of abdomen and liver.
3. Placement of additional trochars.
4. Mobilization of liver as necessary.
5. Intraoperative liver ultrasound.
6. Resection of liver mass/segment(s)/lobe.
7. Insure adequate hemostasis.
8. Evaluate adequate perfusion of the liver remnant and look for potential bile leaks.
9. Placement of drain as indicated.
10. Close abdomen.

Potential Pitfalls
- Central lesions and large bulky tumors.
  - Compromise laparoscopic working space.
  - Can be difficult to resect laparoscopically.
- Control of potential hemorrhage.
- Risk of air embolism related to pneumoperitoneum.
- Skills in open and lap liver surgery are required.

TABLE 3. Key Steps to an Open Liver Resection

1. Subcostal incision.
2. Evaluation of abdomen and liver.
3. Mobilization of liver as necessary.
4. Intraoperative liver ultrasound.
5. Resection of liver mass/segment(s)/lobe.
6. Insure adequate hemostasis.
7. Evaluate adequate perfusion of the liver remnant and look for potential bile leaks.
8. Placement of drain as indicated.
9. Close abdomen.

Potential Pitfalls

- Central lesions and large bulky tumors.
  ○ Can be difficult to resect.
- Control of potential hemorrhage.
- Risk of air embolism if large inadvertent venotomy occurs.

may be placed to diagnose and treat potential postoperative bile leaks **(Table 3).**

Special Intraoperative Considerations

Several unexpected findings or complications may be encountered. The liver mass may ultimately be identified as a metastasis from another primary source. In this setting, biopsies to obtain an accurate diagnosis should be obtained and intraoperative staging should be performed. If appropriate, proceeding with resection of the liver tumor along with the primary tumor can be considered. This may be encountered in the setting of a colorectal malignancy or a neuroendocrine tumor. Additional hepatic lesions may also be identified that were not identified on preoperative imaging. If possible, consideration can be given to resection of these lesions as well. If there is concern for leaving an inadequate remnant, these lesions may also be treated using radiofrequency or microwave ablation.

During resection, preparation should always be made for unexpected hemorrhage. This includes preoperative communication with the anesthesia team to insure that adequate vascular access is present. Depending on the location of bleeding, control can often be obtained with manual compression or packing. A Pringle maneuver can also be used. In cases of extreme bleeding, total vascular isolation of the liver can be obtained by performing a Pringle maneuver as well as clamping the vena cava in a supra- and infrahepatic position.

Postoperative Management

While most patients undergoing liver resection do not require treatment in an ICU, a low threshold for ICU care should be maintained if there is any concern for bleeding, hepatic insufficiency, need for observation of renal function, or other concerns based on the patient's comorbidities. The patient's volume status, hepatic, and renal function should be closely monitored and managed in the postoperative period.

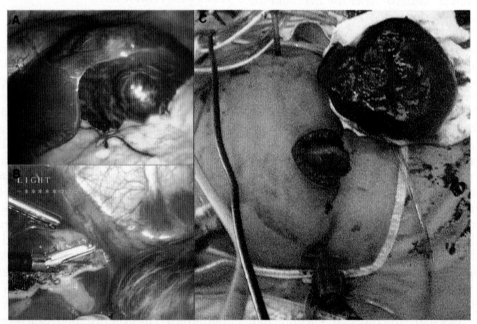

FIGURE 3 • Laparoscopic resection of a liver mass using a hand-assisted technique. **A:** Laparoscopic image of a 15-cm left lateral segment hepatic hemangioma. **B:** Transection of the liver parenchyma using an ultrasonic dissector. **C:** 15-cm hemangioma removed from a 7-cm laparoscopic hand port incision.

Pain can be controlled with either patient-controlled analgesia using intravenous opioids or an epidural. While an ileus may occur, this is usually limited if the majority of the surgical procedure occurred in the right upper abdomen; therefore, a postoperative nasogastric tube is usually unnecessary, and oral intake can be advanced relatively quickly. If bile is not present within the closed suction drain, the drain can be removed within several days postoperatively. If bile is present within the drain and is at a relatively low volume, the drain should be left in place and can be removed as an outpatient once the bile leak has resolved. If a high-volume leak is present, placement of an endobiliary stent to decompress the biliary tree may be necessary.

Case Conclusion

The patient undergoes successful laparoscopic resection of the largest left lobe liver mass using a hand-assisted technique **(Figure 3)** and is discharged from the hospital without complications on postoperative day 4. The final pathology returns confirming a giant cavernous hemangioma. Two years later, she remains pain free.

TAKE HOME POINTS

- Modern imaging has led to increased detection of incidental liver masses.
- In otherwise healthy individuals, most incidental masses are benign.
  - 10% of indeterminant lesions may be malignant.
- Better definition of radiologic characteristics and clinical features has led to
  - Accurate radiologic diagnosis
  - Reduced need for biopsy
- Management ranges from observation to surgical resection.

SUGGESTED READINGS

Buell JF, Cherqui D, Geller DA, et al. The international position on laparoscopic liver surgery: the Louisville statement, 2008. Ann Surg. 2009;250:825–830.

Clavien PA, Petrowsky H, DeOliveira ML, et al. Strategies for safer liver surgery and partial liver transplantation. N Engl J Med. 2007;356:1545–1559.

Jarnagin WR, Gonen M, Fong Y, et al. Improvement in perioperative outcome after hepatic resection: analysis of 1,803 consecutive cases over the past decade. Ann Surg. 2002;236:397–406; discussion 406–407.

Koffron AJ, Auffenberg G, Kung R, et al. Evaluation of 300 minimally invasive liver resections at a single institution: less is more. Ann Surg. 2007;246:385–392; discussion 392–394.

Yoon SS, Charny CK, Fong Y, et al. Diagnosis, management, and outcomes of 115 patients with hepatic hemangioma. J Am Coll Surg. 2003;197:392–402.

28 Liver Mass in Chronic Liver Disease

CHRISTOPHER J. SONNENDAY

Presentation

A 59-year-old man with cirrhosis secondary to chronic hepatitis C infection undergoes an annual screening liver ultrasound. A 2.5-cm solid, well-circumscribed mass in the posterior aspect of the right hepatic lobe is identified. The liver is noted to be nodular in appearance.

Differential Diagnosis

While the differential diagnosis of a liver mass is broad and includes infectious lesions as well as both benign and malignant lesions, a new mass detected in a patient with chronic liver disease should be presumed to be a primary hepatic malignancy until proven otherwise. Hepatocellular cancer (HCC) is the leading cause of death in clinically compensated cirrhotics, and individuals with cirrhosis secondary to viral hepatitis have a 10% to 20% 5-year cumulative risk of developing HCC. For this reason, HCC screening has been shown to have a profound impact on HCC-related mortality among cirrhotics. The American Association for the Study of Liver Disease currently recommends serial hepatic ultrasound and serum alpha-fetoprotein (AFP) every 6 to 12 months in at-risk populations (e.g., any patient with cirrhosis).

While the evaluation of a liver mass in a patient with cirrhosis is aimed at diagnosing HCC, other etiologies may be considered. Regenerative nodules may appear mass-like and may represent an early stage in the development of hepatocellular neoplasms. Similarly, adenomas may be diagnosed in patients with chronic liver disease. These lesions are at high risk for malignant transformation, especially in this population, and imaging characteristics alone may be insufficient to distinguish hepatic adenomas from well-differentiated HCC. Thus, surgical resection or ablative therapies should be considered in adenomas. Other benign lesions that typically do not require surgical resection include focal nodular hyperplasia (FNH) and hemangioma.

Patients with chronic liver disease and cirrhosis are also at increased risk for developing intrahepatic cholangiocarcinoma, the other major primary hepatic malignancy. While classically described in patients with cholestatic liver disease (e.g., primary sclerosing cholangitis), patients with cirrhosis are also more prone to developing cholangiocarcinoma and mixed tumors that include both HCC and cholangiocarcinoma cell types.

Workup

Any mass lesion suspected on screening ultrasound should be further investigated with contrast-enhanced cross-sectional imaging, either computed tomography (CT) or magnetic resonance imaging (MRI). MRI appears to be slightly more sensitive and specific than CT, and particular imaging characteristics—arterial phase enhancement with early washout of contrast on the delayed phases of the scan—are considered diagnostic for HCC (Figure 1). Contrast-enhanced MRI may provide definitive diagnosis of FNH and hemangioma as well. Image-guided percutaneous biopsy is reserved for cases in which the diagnosis is in doubt following adequate imaging or in cases where it is thought to change management based on clinical suspicion.

Once the diagnosis of HCC is established by imaging or biopsy, the choice of appropriate therapy is made based upon tumor burden, severity of underlying liver disease, and patient performance status. Staging evaluation should include measurement of serum AFP and chest CT. Bone scan may be appropriate when clinically indicated by symptoms or suspicion on cross-sectional imaging.

Evaluation of underlying liver function and synthetic reserve is critical to providing safe treatment for HCC. While multiple clinical classification systems exist to predict severity of liver disease, the Child-Turcotte-Pugh (CTP) classification may be the simplest and most helpful (Table 1). Consensus exists that CTP class C patients should not undergo hepatic resection due to excessive perioperative mortality, and CTP class B patients should only be considered for minor hepatic resections (resection of two or fewer Couinaud segments) when they have excellent performance status. The evaluation of CTP class A patients for hepatic resection is more difficult, as these patients can vary

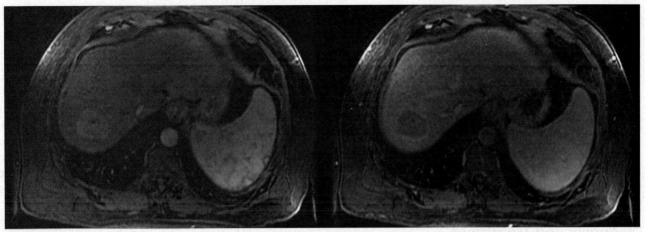

FIGURE 1 • MRI of hepatocellular carcinoma, demonstrating characteristic enhancement on arterial phase imaging (**left panel**) with washout of contrast on delayed-phase imaging (**right panel**).

substantially in their risk of perioperative mortality and postoperative liver failure.

CTP class A patients with overt evidence of portal hypertension are generally considered suboptimal candidates for hepatic resection. Clinical signs of portal hypertension, such as a history of variceal hemorrhage, esophageal or gastric varices on upper endoscopy, visible upper abdominal varices on cross-sectional imaging, or grossly apparent ascites are all contraindications to resection. Thrombocytopenia is another critical clinical indicator of surgical risk with hepatic resection, reflecting the hypersplenism of advanced cirrhosis and portal hypertension. A platelet count under 100,000 is considered a contraindication to major hepatectomy.

A number of quantitative liver function tests have been investigated to assess hepatic reserve prior to hepatic resection, including indocyanine green (ICG) clearance, galactose elimination capacity, and technetium-99m galactosyl human serum albumin scan, among others. The ICG clearance study is the most

commonly used internationally, though it is not commonly used or available in the United States. Many surgeons use volumetric assessment as a proxy for hepatic reserve. This technique relies on the use of manual or automated serial measurement of cross-sectional liver volumes produced from a thin-section helical CT scan. The volume of the liver segments to be preserved following resection is then divided by the total estimated liver volume, which produces a percentage of future liver remnant (FLR) volume. In patients with normal liver parenchyma and function, an FLR of 25% to 30% is considered adequate, if two contiguous Couinaud segments are preserved. In patients with cirrhosis, an FLR of 40% to 50% is desired.

Presentation Continued

In the present case, contrast-enhanced MRI reveals arterial phase enhancement with delayed phase contrast washout of a 2.5-cm solitary lesion in

TABLE 1. The CTP Classification of Liver Disease Severity

Clinical Criteria	Points		
	1	2	3
Albumin (g/dL)	>3.5	2.8–3.5	<2.8
Bilirubin (mg/dL)	<2.0	2.0–3.0	>3.0
International normalized ratio	<1.7	1.7–2.3	>2.3
Ascites	None	Moderate (or suppressed by diuretics, not requiring regular paracentesis)	Severe (tense ascites, refractory to medication, or requiring regular paracentesis)
Encephalopathy	None	Grade I–II (or controlled with medication)	Grade III–IV (or refractory to medication)

CTP class A	**5–6 points**
CTP class B	**7–9 points**
CTP class C	**10–15 points**

segment 6 of the right hepatic lobe. Chest CT shows no evidence of metastasis. The patient is active and independent in his activities of daily living and works full-time. He has no history of ascites or hepatic encephalopathy. Upper endoscopy shows no esophageal varices. Laboratory evaluation reveals an albumin of 4.1 g/dL, total bilirubin of 1.1 mg/dL, and a platelet count of 148,000. CT volumetry suggests that resection of the posterior sector (segments 6 and 7) would leave an FLR of 65%.

Diagnosis and Treatment

Treatment options for HCC are diverse and require careful consideration of both tumor stage and liver disease severity. Resection offers the best likelihood of survival in select patients with resectable disease, superior to nonsurgical therapies with 30% to 70% 5-year survival. In patients with CTP class B or C liver disease, liver transplantation may be the more appropriate choice of therapy. Posttransplant survival has been shown to be excellent (65% to 80% 5-year survival) when patients are selected for transplant according to strict selection criteria, known as the Milan criteria (solitary tumor under 5 cm, or 3 or fewer tumors each under 3 cm). Obviously donor organ availability and the significant medical risks and costs associated with liver transplantation limit its expansion to all patients with HCC.

Among patients with more extensive tumor burden, and/or decompensated liver disease, ablative therapies may be considered. Radiofrequency ablation may offer prolonged survival and local tumor control, particularly in small solitary lesions (<3 to 4 cm). Transarterial chemoembolization has been shown to extend survival in patients with unresectable disease, though the procedure may also precipitate hepatic decompensation and is best applied to CTP class A or select CTP class B patients. In patients with metastatic or recurrent disease, systemic chemotherapy with the multikinase inhibitor sorafenib may provide additional months of survival in patients not eligible for other therapies.

In cirrhotic patients without an adequate predicted FLR who are otherwise good candidates for surgical therapy, portal vein embolization (PVE) may be considered as a way to augment the size of the remnant liver. PVE takes advantage of the contralateral hypertrophy and ipsilateral atrophy that takes place in response to selective portal vein occlusion. Repeat imaging is typically performed 3 to 6 weeks following embolization, with repeat liver volume estimates. Failure to respond to PVE portends a poor outcome following resection and should be considered a contraindication to proceeding with surgical therapy. Most centers will aim to operate on patients with an appropriate response at 21 to 30 days following PVE, capitalizing on the peak hypertrophic response at this time period.

Surgical Approach

While hepatic resection can be accomplished safely by both open and minimally invasive techniques, cirrhotic patients present particular challenges in terms of transection of the fibrotic hepatic parenchyma and risk of blood loss. Therefore, only experienced laparoscopic liver surgeons should take on minimally invasive hepatic resections in cirrhotic patients. Laparoscopic liver surgery is discussed elsewhere in this text; this section describes open hepatic resection (**Table 2**).

Perioperative management of the hepatic resection patient can have a profound influence on outcomes, with maintenance of a low central venous pressure as a central tenet in intraoperative management. Establishment of large-bore venous access is essential, and arterial line placement for systemic blood pressure monitoring is also advised. Central venous access, which has been advocated both for large-volume resuscitation and for CVP monitoring, can be helpful in the most complex cases but is probably not necessary in limited resection cases. Use of large-bore peripheral intravenous catheters (14 or 16 gauge) and conservative volume resuscitation can achieve similar goals.

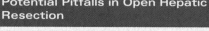

TABLE 2. Key Technical Steps and Potential Pitfalls in Open Hepatic Resection

Key Technical Steps

1. Right subcostal incision with midline extension.
2. Thorough laparotomy to assess for metastatic disease.
3. Limited mobilization of the liver to allow exposure for ultrasound.
4. Intraoperative ultrasound (IOUS):
   a. Define segments by portal and hepatic venous anatomy.
   b. Scan liver for all visible lesions.
   c. Plan resection, with marking of capsule along line of transection.
5. Portal dissection—encircle porta with tape to allow Pringle maneuver.
6. Extrahepatic ligation of segmental portal structures when indicated.
7. Parenchymal transection.
8. Obtain meticulous hemostasis and observe for biliary leaks.
9. Completion IOUS to document adequate inflow and outflow to liver remnant.

Potential Pitfalls

- Failure to leave an adequate liver remnant (≥40%–50% total liver volume in cirrhotic).
- Missing additional lesions due to inadequate IOUS.
- Excessive blood loss due to failure to control inflow and outflow vascular pedicles.
- Compromise of the surgical margin due to failure to reassess margin by IOUS during parenchymal transection.

Incision choice is critical to exposure and efficiency. Left-sided hepatic lesions can be approached from an upper midline incision, but typically a right subcostal incision is preferred. A right subcostal incision with midline extension is a very versatile incision, allowing exposure to the suprahepatic vena cava, making a bilateral subcostal or Chevron incision necessary only for cases with difficult exposure due to body habitus or large tumors. The abdomen should be carefully explored to assess for metastatic disease. Limited mobilization of the liver is performed to allow access for intraoperative ultrasound (IOUS).

Careful IOUS should follow a consistent three-step sequence, beginning with definition of the Couinaud segments based on the portal and hepatic venous anatomy. Attention is paid to important anatomic variants such as early or late division of the right portal pedicle or large accessory hepatic veins. The second phase of the IOUS exam should be a methodical scan through the entire liver parenchyma, with identification and measurement of all lesions. The final step in an IOUS exam is planning of intended resection with note taken of the important critical vasculature to be included or avoided in a segmental resection.

The dissection phase of the operation begins with isolation of the portal structures by opening the pars flaccida (gastrohepatic ligament) and passing a finger through the foramen of Winslow such that the porta can be encircled with a tape. This maneuver facilitates quick access to the porta when necessary, and can facilitate episodic inflow occlusion (Pringle maneuver). The amount of portal dissection necessary is then determined by the extent of hepatectomy planned. A peripheral nonanatomic or segmental resection will not require much additional portal dissection. A formal or extended lobectomy may be approached with a formal portal dissection and pedicle control prior to parenchymal transection.

Parenchymal transection may be performed by multiple techniques, with use of surgical energy devices, clips, or ligatures to control small vessels. Stapling devices may be used to control larger pedicles, including the hepatic veins. The role of inflow occlusion (Pringle maneuver) during parenchymal transection may be utilized to limit excessive blood loss when appropriate. While some surgeons use this technique routinely, others try to limit any potential ischemic injury to the liver remnant, preferring selective pedicle isolation and ligation. When inflow occlusion is utilized, it appears that intermittent periods of clamping followed by periods of reperfusion can limit the ischemic injury to the liver remnant.

Once the parenchymal transection is completed, achieving final hemostasis is critical. Significant bleeding vessels should be controlled with nonabsorbable fine sutures or clips. The argon beam coagulator is effective for small vessels and raw surfaces. Application of additional hemostatic agents such as fibrin- and thrombin-based agents can also be helpful. Care should be taken to identify occult biliary leaks from the parenchymal surface, which should be controlled with fine sutures when identified. Leaving a surgical drain after hepatectomy is a controversial practice and appears to be only partially successful in allowing diagnosis and adequate drainage of a postoperative biliary leak. Selective use of drains for cases with concomitant biliary reconstruction and/or difficult perihilar dissection is probably a reasonable strategy.

Special Intraoperative Considerations

IOUS should be used throughout the hepatectomy operation, not just at the stage of planning the resection. Surgeons should use IOUS to reassess margin status throughout the parenchymal transection. Furthermore, IOUS can be used to identify large vascular pedicles that will need to be controlled in the parenchymal division. Finally, a completion IOUS with Doppler exam can assess the preserved inflow and outflow to the liver remnant, especially in larger segmental resections.

While obtaining a clear surgical margin has obvious oncologic applications, preservation of hepatic parenchyma is of particular concern in patients with cirrhosis. Thus, resection should be planned by IOUS to include an adequate but not excessive margin, with preservation of inflow and outflow to adjacent segments. In the case of hepatic surgery, it appears that the size of the margin is not oncologically relevant, as long as it proves to be histologically negative.

Improved outcomes with hepatic resection have allowed the cautious expansion of advanced hepatobiliary techniques to allow resection of more locally advanced tumors, including those with vascular involvement. Total vascular isolation of the liver may allow resection and reconstruction of tumors involving the vena cava, hepatic veins, or portal structures. However, given the increased risk of postoperative hepatic dysfunction in patients with cirrhosis, these techniques are not advisable in these patients.

Postoperative Management

Perioperative monitoring should include observation for evidence of hemorrhage, particularly in thrombocytopenic or coagulopathic patients. While surgical site infections in hepatectomy patients are relatively rare when compared to patients undergoing gastrointestinal operations, biliary leaks from the cut surface of the liver may predispose to biloma and abscess formation. Typically low-volume leaks can be controlled with adequate percutaneous drainage and observation, but larger, more central leaks may benefit from endoscopic sphincterotomy and endobiliary stent placement to divert bile flow away from the site of leak.

Obviously in the cirrhotic patient, monitoring for signs of hepatic dysfunction is the most important postoperative strategy. Mild hepatic dysfunction can present with progressive jaundice or ascites. If the patient remains otherwise clinically well and free of infection, these clinical problems will often resolve over the first 1 to 2 postoperative weeks. More ominous signs of liver failure include progressive coagulopathy, lactic acidosis, renal dysfunction, vasodilatation, and encephalopathy. Evaluation of a patient with progressive liver dysfunction should include liver duplex to establish patent hepatic vascular inflow and outflow. Renal replacement therapy should be considered in more severe cases to address volume overload and more hepatic injury from congestion. Supportive care is the only intervention in most cases, although salvage liver transplantation may be considered in patients who are otherwise appropriate candidates who have surgical pathology revealing tumors within Milan criteria and without vascular invasion.

Case Conclusion

The patient undergoes an open segment 6/7 resection with IOUS. The liver is stiff and cirrhotic, making division of the hepatic parenchyma challenging. Estimated blood loss is 800 mL. Postoperatively, the patient develops mild ascites and lower extremity edema, and his bilirubin rises to 2.1 mg/dL by postoperative day 5.

Over the ensuing week, the ascites resolves with gentle diuresis, and the bilirubin is corrected. Final pathology from the resection specimen reveals a 2.3-cm moderately differentiated HCC with negative margins and no vascular invasion.

At 18 months postoperatively, the patient remains free of disease with stable liver function.

TAKE HOME POINTS

- A liver mass identified in a patient with cirrhosis should be considered malignant until proven otherwise.
- Contrast-enhanced MRI is the preferred confirmatory diagnostic study for investigation of a liver mass in a cirrhotic patient.
- Arterial phase enhancement with delayed phase washout is diagnostic for HCC.
- Evaluation of a cirrhotic patient for hepatic resection includes careful assessment of both tumor burden and severity of underlying liver disease.
- CTP class B and C patients, and patient with obvious portal hypertension, are not appropriate candidates for hepatic resection.

SUGGESTED READINGS

Azoulay D, Castaing D, Smail A, et al. Resection of non-resectable liver metastases from colorectal cancer after percutaneous portal vein embolization. Ann Surg. 2000; 231:480–486.

Bruix J, Sherman M. Management of hepatocellular carcinoma. Hepatology. 2005;42:1208–1236.

Fattovich G, Stroffolini T, Zagni I, et al. Hepatocellular carcinoma in cirrhosis: incidence and risk factors. Gastroenterology. 2004;127:S35–S50.

Marrero JA, Hussain HK, Nghiem HV, et al. Improving the prediction of hepatocellular carcinoma in cirrhotic patients with an arterially-enhancing liver mass. Liver Transpl. 2005;11:281–289.

29 Metastatic Colorectal Cancer

PETER D. PENG and TIMOTHY M. PAWLIK

Presentation

A 62-year-old man is referred to your office 2 years after a right hemicolectomy for T3N1M0 colon cancer detected on screening colonoscopy. Following surgery, the patient received adjuvant chemotherapy with 5-fluorouracil, leucovorin, and oxaliplatin (FOLFOX). Now, 2 years later, he presents with an elevated carcinoembryonic antigen (CEA) of 80 ng/mL and a CT scan demonstrating four new masses in his right hemiliver.

Differential Diagnosis

The differential diagnosis of a liver mass includes both benign (cyst, hemangioma, focal nodular hyperplasia, hepatic adenoma) and malignant (metastatic disease, primary hepatocellular carcinoma, intrahepatic cholangiocarcinoma, gallbladder cancer) disease processes. However, in a patient with a history of colon cancer and a rising CEA, metastatic colon cancer is the most likely diagnosis. Approximately one-half of patients with a history of colon cancer will either present with synchronous hepatic metastasis or develop them during the course of their disease. In general, about 15% to 25% of patients will present with synchronous disease, while 20% to 25% will develop metachronous colorectal liver metastasis. In about 30% to 50% of patients with colorectal liver metastasis, the liver will be the only site of metastatic disease, and these patients will be candidates for local surgical therapy.

Workup

Patients being considered for resection of colorectal liver metastasis should have preoperative cross-sectional imaging. A helical triphasic CT scan is the most commonly employed imaging modality. On CT imaging, metastases from colorectal cancer are visualized best on the venous phase and appear as hypointense, low-attenuating masses within the liver if the scan is obtained when the contrast is in the portal circulation (Figure 1). With multidetector helical CT, the sensitivity of identifying liver metastasis is about 80% to 90%. MRI is another imaging modality that can be utilized. On contrast-enhanced MRI with agents such as gadolinium, colorectal liver metastases are best seen on the T2-weighted images and give MRI an 80% to 90% sensitivity in detecting colorectal liver metastasis. Chest imaging should be considered before resection of colorectal liver metastasis to rule out pulmonary metastasis. The use of positron emission tomography (PET), either alone or in combination with CT (PET/CT), may also be useful and should, in general, be obtained prior to surgery to assess the extent of metastatic disease.

Some studies have reported that PET may change clinical management in up to 20% of patients with colorectal liver metastasis being considered for surgical resection. Identification of extrahepatic metastases is a relative contraindication to hepatic metastectomy, especially when it is non-pulmonary in location and multi-focal in nature.

Resectable lesions should not be routinely biopsied. In most cases, biopsy is unnecessary to make the diagnosis in the appropriate clinical context, associated with elevation of serum CEA and pathognomonic radiologic features on cross-sectional imaging/PET (Figure 2). Although the risk is small, biopsy can result in tumor dissemination and therefore should be reserved only for those situations when there is diagnostic uncertainty or when the biopsy will provide needed data to allow for the administration of chemotherapy or other nonresectional treatment options. Finally, depending on the situation and timing of the last colonoscopy, a repeat colonoscopy should be considered in the patient with a history of colon cancer.

Diagnosis and Treatment

Surgical therapy for liver metastasis remains the only therapy that promises a potential cure. Long-term survival after surgery for colorectal liver metastasis has been demonstrated in numerous studies, with the overall 5-year survival reported to range from 35% to 58%. In addition to resection, ablative techniques, such as radiofrequency or microwave ablation, can also be utilized to destroy the tumor via the application of heat. In general, tumor ablation should not be viewed as a replacement for resection, but more as a supplement or an extension of localized therapy for those patients with extensive disease or those patients who otherwise are not resection candidates. Ablation should not be used for lesions near the hilum due to the risk of bile duct injury and stricture.

In the past, tumor number ≥4, bilobar disease, metastasis within 1 cm of the planned transection margin, or extrahepatic disease were all considered

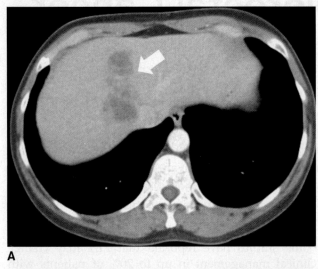

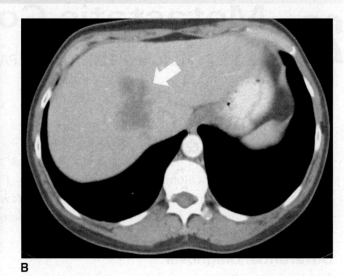

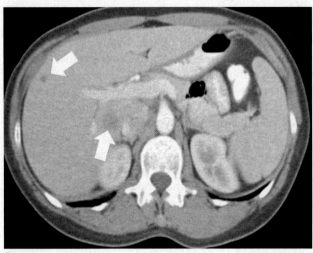

FIGURE 1 • Select CT axial images of colorectal liver metastases (arrows), venous phase. Note that the metastases are hypointense and low attenuating. The larger mass at the dome of the liver abuts the right and the middle hepatic vein.

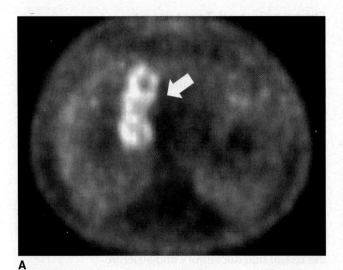

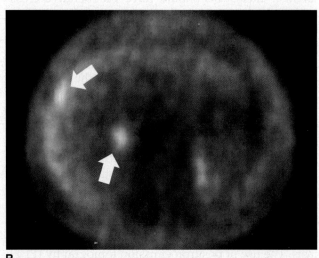

FIGURE 2 • PET scan demonstrating multiple FDG-avid lesions (arrows) in the liver that correlate with the metastases identified on cross-sectional CT imaging.

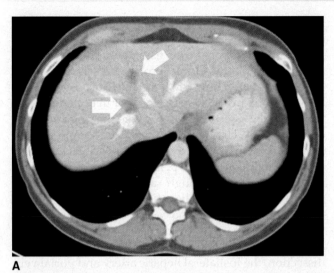 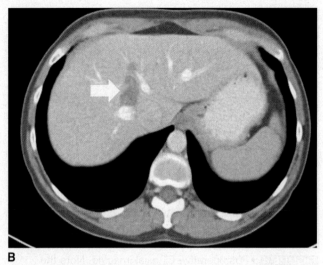

FIGURE 3 • Repeat CT axial imaging following treatment with neoadjuvant treatment with four cycles of FOLFOX plus bevacizumab chemotherapy. Note the cytoreduction in the size of the liver metastases (arrows).

strong relative contraindications to liver-directed surgery. However, with improvements in operative technique and systemic chemotherapy, more recent data have demonstrated that these clinicopathologic factors should not be considered absolute contraindications to surgery. Rather, decisions regarding resectability have shifted in focus away from criteria based on the metastatic disease (tumor size, number, margin width, etc.). Decisions regarding resectability now are more based on whether all the metastatic disease can be removed (R0 resection) while preserving enough volume of liver after the resection to avoid liver insufficiency/failure. In general, following liver resection at least two contiguous hepatic segments with adequate inflow, outflow, and biliary drainage need to be preserved with a functional liver remnant (FLR) volume of at least 20%.

Given this new therapeutic approach, there has been a shift to try to expand the pool of patients who might be candidates for surgical therapy. Over the past two decades, chemotherapeutic and biologic agents have been found that have significant increased activity against colon cancer. The improved efficacy of chemotherapy agents has not only increased patient survival in the noncurative setting, but has also allowed a subset of previously unresectable patients to undergo potentially curative liver surgery after tumor downsizing. The use of chemotherapy in the preoperative setting for patients with resectable colorectal liver metastasis is more controversial. The rationale for using neoadjuvant chemotherapy is supported, in part, by the better prognosis obtained with preoperative chemotherapy and surgery among patients with multifocal colorectal liver metastasis compared with immediate surgery alone. The decision to give chemotherapy before or

after surgery needs, however, to be individualized and be based on the specific clinical situation **(Figure 3)**.

In a small subset of patients with extensive disease, portal vein embolization (PVE) or a two-stage hepatectomy may be warranted. Some patients with extensive intrahepatic disease will require an extended hepatectomy (right hepatectomy plus segment 4) to extirpate all disease. To avoid operating on patients with low-volume FLR, PVE can be considered to induce hypertrophy. In PVE, the portal vein to the tumor-bearing side of the liver is embolized inducing contralateral liver hypertrophy. The selective use of PVE may enable the performance of an extended hepatectomy in a subset of patients who otherwise would not be considered candidates for surgery. In those patients with multiple metastases with a bilobar distribution, a sequential—or two-stage—hepatectomy may be more appropriate. For example, the left hemiliver can be cleared of disease during the first operation. A right portal vein ligation can be performed intraoperatively or a right PVE can be performed postoperatively. The remnant left liver is then allowed to hypertrophy and a right or an extended right hepatectomy is performed as the second stage **(Figure 4)**.

In general, the goals of surgical therapy are to extirpate all disease (R0) with the use of either resection alone or, if necessary, in combination with ablation. While not supported with robust level one data, adjuvant chemotherapy is usually employed given that the majority of patients with hepatic colorectal metastasis will experience a recurrence after surgery.

Surgical Approach

Liver resection can be performed using both a traditional open or a laparoscopic approach **(see Table 1)**.

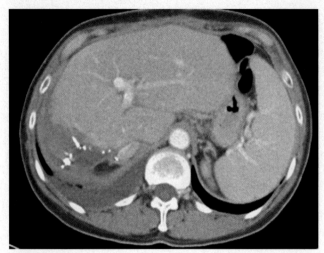

FIGURE 4 • Postoperative CT axial imaging. Note the hypertrophy of the remnant left hemiliver, especially segments 2 and 3.

While there are increasing data emerging about the use of laparoscopic liver resection to treat malignancies, most major liver resections are still performed using an open technique. For an open approach, either a midline or a right subcostal incision can be used. Upon entering the abdomen, the ligamentum teres and falciform ligament are taken down and a full evaluation of the liver is performed visually, by palpation, and with intraoperative ultrasound (IOUS). IOUS is an important tool for accurately staging liver tumors, assessing the true extent of disease, and making intraoperative decisions. IOUS is usually performed using a midfrequency (5.0 and 7.5 MHz) transducer probe, with the 7.5-MHz probe able to penetrate 6 to 8 cm. IOUS needs to always be performed in a systematic manner in both the transverse and the sagittal planes to avoid missing any small occult lesions. The hepatic vasculature should also be examined with IOUS to identify possible anatomic variants and to aid in the planning of the resection.

Inflow control through an intermittent Pringle maneuver of the porta hepatis can be utilized to help decrease blood loss. In the case of a formal hemihepatectomy, the hepatic inflow pedicle is often dissected out at the level of the hilum. With an extrahepatic pedicle dissection, the ipsilateral hepatic artery and portal vein are divided outside the substance of the liver after lowering the hilar plate. Following division of the hepatic artery and the portal vein, the liver usually demarcates along the principal plane of the liver. Depending on the location of the lesion (i.e., for those lesions not near the hilum), an intrahepatic technique can alternatively be utilized to obtain pedicle control. The intrahepatic technique has the potential advantages of being faster and more unlikely to cause injury to the biliary or vascular structures to the contralateral liver.

The extent of liver mobilization is dictated by the extent and type of procedure to be performed. The coronary ligament at the top of the liver is taken down

TABLE 1. Key Technical Steps and Potential Pitfalls to Open Major Hepatectomy

Key Technical Steps

1. Midline or subcostal incision.
2. Exploration to rule out extrahepatic disease.
3. Exposure with self-retaining retractor (Thompson, Bookwalter, "Upper-Hand," etc.).
4. Liver mobilization (taking down ligamentous attachment of the liver, exposing retrohepatic cava for right hepatectomy, etc.).
5. Intraoperative ultrasound.
6. Inflow control (Pringle maneuver).
7. Extra- or intrahepatic control of ipsilateral hepatic pedicle with division of the hepatic artery and the portal vein.
8. Extrahepatic division of the right hepatic vein when performing right hepatectomy; in general, when performing a left hepatectomy, the left hepatic vein is divided within the substance of the liver during the parenchymal transection (depending on location of lesion in left hemiliver).
9. Parenchymal transection in setting of low CVP.
10. Hemostasis. Larger bleeding structures are controlled surgically with sutures, while smaller parenchymal bleeding is controlled topically.
11. Examination for bile leak; oversew any possible small bile leaks.
12. Placement of closed suction drain in select situations (e.g., diaphragm or bile duct resection/reconstruction performed in conjunction with liver resection, etc.). Drains not placed for routine major liver resections.
13. Close abdomen.

Potential Pitfalls

- Failure to mobilize the liver adequately prior to initiation of hepatic transection.
- Failure to identify all hepatic disease due to inadequate IOUS.
- Injury/stricturing of bile duct in remnant liver due to inappropriate division of bile duct in hilum.
- Injury/stricturing of bile duct in remnant liver due to inappropriate ablation of lesion too close to hilum.
- Bleeding from middle hepatic vein during division along parenchymal plane.
- Failure to obtain negative surgical margin due to poor planning of parenchymal transection plane.

with cautery to expose the suprahepatic vena cava and hepatic veins. In the case of a right hemihepatectomy, the right hemiliver is mobilized by taking down the right triangular ligament, exposing the bare area of the liver along the right diaphragm. The right hemiliver is further mobilized by taking down the retroperitoneal attachments along the inferior aspect of the right liver and the attachments along the right adrenal gland. With the right liver rotated medially and superiorly, the retrohepatic vena cava is exposed and several small venous branches traveling directly from the cava to the liver are ligated and divided. The hepatocaval ligament (Makuuchi's ligament) is dissected free and divided, often with an endovascular stapler. The right hepatic vein is circumferentially dissected free and can be divided between clamps or with an endovascular stapling device.

For a left hemihepatectomy, the left hemiliver is mobilized by taking down the left triangular ligament. The ligamentum venosum is dissected free and divided to better expose the left hepatic vein. For a left hepatectomy, the left hepatic vein is often not dissected out at this point, but instead is divided later within the substance of the liver during the hepatic parenchymal transection. The specifics of the dissection are, however, dictated by the size and location of the lesion relative to the hepatic vein.

A number of techniques can be utilized for parenchymal transection. Some of these techniques include, but are not limited to, crush-clamp, bipolar or monopolar cautery, radiofrequency ablation (Habib device), harmonic scalpel, as well as ultrasonic aspirator or hydrojet devices. While different surgeons advocate different transection techniques, no technique has clearly been shown to be superior to another. As such, the most important factor in choosing a method of liver transection should be the surgeon's comfort and familiarity with the technique so as to ensure minimal blood loss and an R0 surgical margin. In general, major liver surgery should be performed in the setting of a low central venous pressure (CVP) (<5 mm Hg) before and during parenchymal transection. A low CVP helps ensure less back-bleeding from the cava/hepatic veins and, therefore, less blood loss. Larger bleeding structures are controlled surgically with sutures. Hemostasis of the transected liver margin may also require topical hemostatic agents such as methylcellulose, collagen sponges, thrombin sealants, and argon beam coagulation. The liver margin should then be carefully inspected for bile leakage, which can be oversewn.

Intraoperative pathologic confirmation of an R0 margin is critical after removal of the specimen. While attaining an R0-negative margin is important, the width of the negative margin has not been demonstrated to correlate with recurrence rates.

Routine placement of closed suction drains is unnecessary following major liver resections. Placement of close suction drain should, however, be placed in select situations (e.g., diaphragm or bile duct resection/reconstruction performed in conjunction with liver resection, etc.).

Special Intraoperative Considerations

The surgeon needs to be aware of aberrant arterial anatomy. Hepatic artery variants should be identified prior to the initiation of hepatic resection. The lesser omentum should be examined to identify a replaced/accessory left hepatic artery that would normally course through the middle of the lesser omentum as it travels into the base of the umbilical fissure. In contrast, a replaced/accessory right hepatic artery originating from the superior mesenteric artery usually courses posterior and lateral to the common bile duct.

Not infrequently, IOUS may identify disease not recognized on preoperative imaging. New findings may necessitate a change in the operative plan, including either a revision in the type of planned hepatic resection or the addition of ablation. When unsuspected extrahepatic disease is encountered, in general, hepatic resection is not warranted. Patients with unsuspected peritoneal disease or gross hilar adenopathy probably do not derive long-term survival benefit from hepatic resection. Rather, this subset of patients is probably best treated with systemic chemotherapy and should only be considered for liver-directed surgery after restaging and careful multidisciplinary consideration.

Postoperative Management

Following major hepatic resection, most patients are monitored in the intensive or intermediate care unit overnight. During this time, standard crystalloid resuscitation and postoperative care is instituted. Electrolytes, liver function tests, hemoglobin, and prothrombin (PT) are checked after the operation and then daily. Hypophosphatemia is common after a major hepatic resection; phosphate levels should therefore be checked and repeated as necessary. Following an extended hepatic resection (removal of 70% to 80%), liver insufficiency/failure can sometimes occur. In these circumstances, the PT may be elevated and is treated with fresh frozen plasma when the PT is longer than 17 seconds. In most circumstances, a regular diet can be started on postoperative day 2 or 3, with an anticipated discharge on day 4 or 5.

Although uncommon, bile leaks can be a potential complication of liver resection. Usually, patients have a fever and an elevated bilirubin level in the setting of a normal alkaline phosphatase. A CT scan should be obtained and can easily identify a biloma.

Intra-abdominal collections can usually be adequately drained using percutaneous techniques. Most bilomas will subsequently resolve following drainage with expectant management.

Case Conclusion

The patient received four cycles of FOLFOX plus bevacizumab with a measureable decrease in the size of the intrahepatic metastases. The patient underwent an extended right hemihepatectomy with complete extirpation of all intrahepatic disease. Postoperatively, the patient received adjuvant chemotherapy and remains disease free.

TAKE HOME POINTS

- Resection of solitary colorectal hepatic metastasis is associated with approximately 50% 5-year survival.
- Resectability is now defined as the ability to achieve an R0 resection while preserving two or more contiguous segments with vascular inflow, outflow, biliary drainage, as well as an adequate liver volume (~20%).
- Chemotherapy for colorectal liver metastasis can result in response rates >50%; chemotherapy should often be integrated into the overall therapeutic plan (i.e., neoadjuvant, conversion, or adjuvant depending on the situation).
- Resection resulting in R0-negative margins is the most important operative goal.

SUGGESTED READINGS

Abdalla EK, Adam R, et al. Improving resectability of hepatic colorectal metastases: expert consensus statement. Ann Surg Oncol. 2006;13(10):1271–1280.

Charnsangavej C, Clary B, et al. Selection of patients for resection of hepatic colorectal metastases: expert consensus statement. Ann Surg Oncol. 2006;13(10):1261–1268.

Nordlinger B, Sorbye H, et al. Perioperative chemotherapy with FOLFOX4 and surgery versus surgery alone for resectable liver metastases from colorectal cancer (EORTC Intergroup trial 40983): a randomised controlled trial. Lancet. 2008;371(9617):1007–1016.

Pawlik TM, Choti MA. Surgical therapy for colorectal metastases to the liver. J Gastrointest Surg. 2007;11(8):1057–1077.

Pawlik TM, Schulick RD, et al. Expanding criteria for resectability of colorectal liver metastases. Oncologist. 2008;13(1):51–64.

Poston GJ, Figueras J, et al. Urgent need for a new staging system in advanced colorectal cancer. J Clin Oncol. 2008;26(29):4828–4833.

30 Obstructive Jaundice

TIMOTHY L. FRANKEL and CHRISTOPHER J. SONNENDAY

Presentation

A 58-year-old man with a 50-pack-year smoking history presents to his primary care doctor after family members noted that his eyes were turning yellow. He notes that over the past 2 weeks, he has developed pruritus and clay-colored stools. He describes darkening of his urine and a 15-lb weight loss over the past 2 months. Vital signs are within normal limits. On examination, he appears jaundiced with scleral icterus. He has no abdominal pain and no palpable masses. He has no prior medical problems and is a construction worker.

Differential Diagnosis

Jaundice can be caused by either altered metabolism of bilirubin (i.e., overproduction of bilirubin, impaired uptake of bilirubin by the liver, or decreased conjugation of bilirubin) or ineffective excretion of bile into the gastrointestinal tract. Serum bilirubin can be fractionated into direct and indirect values, which correspond to conjugated and unconjugated bilirubin, respectively. Causes of unconjugated hyperbilirubinemia include increased production from hemolysis, congenital diseases (such as Crigler-Najjar and Gilbert's syndrome), and intrinsic liver failure such as cirrhosis or hepatitis. Conjugated or direct bilirubin elevation results from obstruction of biliary outflow from benign causes (such as chronic pancreatitis or choledocholithiasis) or malignancy including cholangiocarcinoma or periampullary tumors. Painless jaundice in a middle-aged or elderly person without overt liver disease should be assumed to be a malignancy until proven otherwise.

Workup

Initial evaluation of the jaundiced patient should include a detailed history and physical exam, with attention paid to risk factors for, or evidence of, underlying chronic liver disease, pancreatitis, or gallstone disease. Progressive jaundice, particularly of a malignant cause, may be associated with weight loss and malnutrition. The patient's overall health status and fitness for diagnostic and therapeutic procedures should be assessed. On physical exam, assessment should be done for lymphadenopathy, ascites, abdominal masses, and organomegaly that may indicate more advanced malignant disease and/or hepatic insufficiency.

Laboratory evaluation should include a complete blood count, which may provide signs of infection, anemia, and/or thrombocytopenia, as well as a comprehensive metabolic panel and a PT/INR. In addition to assessment of the liver profile for confirmation of hyperbilirubinemia and an obstructive pattern, attention should be paid to electrolyte deficiencies, evidence of dehydration, and any hypoalbuminemia. Patients with obstructive jaundice, particularly when long-standing, will have a relative vitamin K deficiency from poor absorption and therefore may have an elevated INR and bleeding risk.

The least invasive initial imaging test is an abdominal ultrasound, which allows for the assessment of liver contour and morphology that may indicate occult liver disease, assessment for biliary ductal dilatation, identification of gallbladder pathology and documentation of gallstones, and may allow assessment for periampullary masses depending on image quality. Cross-sectional imaging, typically with a high-resolution thin-slice CT scan, is the most appropriate test to assess the patient with obstructive jaundice who appears to have a distal biliary obstruction. MRI with magnetic resonance cholangiopancreatography is another reasonable alternative and may augment CT findings in some cases, particularly when complex biliary pathology is present.

Patients with a documented distal biliary obstruction, particularly when a malignant cause is suggested by imaging, should undergo an evaluation by a surgeon with expertise in diseases of the liver and pancreas. Decisions about the need for more invasive procedures aimed at palliating jaundice or providing a tissue diagnosis should be made in the context of the patient's operative candidacy and resectability. Malnourished or debilitated patients, and patients with marked hyperbilirubinemia (total bilirubin > 12 mg/dL), would benefit from biliary decompression and optimization of nutritional and functional status prior to consideration of surgical therapy. Patients with clearly resectable disease and good overall health status, who have a periampullary mass with obstructive jaundice and no evidence of metastases, may appropriately be taken to the operating room for resection without a tissue diagnosis in many cases. Preoperative biliary decompression has been associated with an increased risk of postoperative infection and therefore should be avoided if not indicated.

When biliary decompression is warranted, or in cases where the etiology of biliary obstruction is not clear by noninvasive means, direct cholangiography is necessary. The most common initial technique is endoscopic retrograde cholangiography (ERC), with percutaneous transhepatic cholangiography (PTC) reserved for patients in whom endobiliary access is either not possible (e.g., following gastric bypass) or unsuccessful. ERC allows placement of an endobiliary stent across the distal biliary obstruction which typically leads to prompt resolution of jaundice, and biliary strictures may be brushed or biopsied intraluminally to achieve a tissue diagnosis. In the case of ampullary or duodenal masses associated with distal biliary obstruction, the tumors may be biopsied directly at the time of endoscopy. Biliary decompression and tissue sampling from biliary strictures may also be accomplished by PTC.

When a tissue diagnosis is needed and cannot be established by endobiliary means, endoscopic ultrasound (EUS), with fine needle aspiration of any identified periampullary mass, is the preferred modality. EUS allows assessment of the pancreatic parenchyma for endosonographic evidence of chronic pancreatitis and careful inspection for small or subtle pancreatic masses, and may allow evaluation of the relationship of periampullary tumors to the mesenteric and hepatic vessels, which can add to the information gathered from contrast-enhanced cross-sectional imaging regarding resectability.

In cases where a malignant diagnosis is established, staging for metastatic disease should include a CT scan of the chest. Positron emission tomography scan should be reserved for patients with extrapancreatic CT findings that may be suggestive of metastases, especially when not amenable to percutaneous biopsy. A serum CA 19-9 level may assist in providing additional prognostic information, and may be followed to assess response to treatment, but its absolute value is not helpful in determining a malignant diagnosis or establishing the presence or absence of metastatic disease. The serum CA 19-9 should ideally be drawn after the patient's jaundice is palliated, as it may be falsely elevated in cases of biliary obstruction or cholangitis.

Presentation Continued

In the patient presented in this scenario, a more thorough history fails to identify any risk factors for viral hepatitis. Initial laboratory values are remarkable for an elevated bilirubin to 12 mg/dL with fractionation revealing primarily direct hyperbilirubinemia. Abdominal ultrasound identifies both intrahepatic and extrahepatic biliary ductal dilation and fails to find stones in either the gallbladder or the common bile duct (CBD). A CT scan is obtained which reveals a mass in the head of the pancreas causing dilation of both the CBD and the pancreatic duct **(Figure 1)**. ERC confirms a malignant-appearing distal CBD stricture **(Figure 2)**, and an endobiliary stent is placed, with resolution of the patient's jaundice over the ensuing week. EUS confirms a 3-cm pancreatic head mass, and fine needle aspiration biopsy is consistent with adenocarcinoma.

Diagnosis and Treatment

The diagnostic evaluation in this case confirms the presence of a pancreatic adenocarcinoma. As curative treatment for pancreatic adenocarcinoma must include definitive surgical resection, the initial decision making in regard to treatment must include assessment of the patient's appropriateness for surgery. Metastatic disease should be ruled out as mentioned above. In addition to assessing the patient's overall health status and comorbid disease, resectability must be definitively assessed by an experienced surgeon. If not already obtained, a dedicated pancreatic protocol CT with distinct arterial and mesenteric venous phases should be obtained. Involvement or abutment of the superior mesenteric artery (SMA) and vein, hepatic

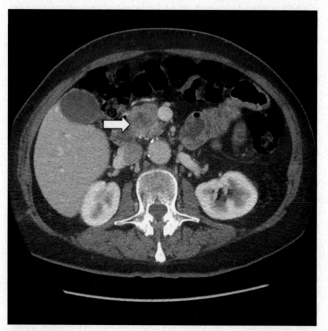

FIGURE 1 • Pancreatic protocol CT of patient with obstructive jaundice. Hypodense mass (*arrow*) is noted in the head of the pancreas, with abutment of the adjacent SMV.

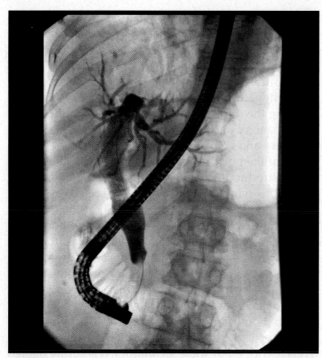

FIGURE 2 • ERC of patient with a malignant-appearing distal bile duct stricture in a patient with a mass in the head of the pancreas.

artery, and portal vein (PV) should be assessed. Direct arterial involvement is most often considered a contraindication to surgical resection, and the degree of mesenteric venous involvement and options for venous reconstruction must be considered carefully as well. In patients considered "borderline" resectable due to either long segment venous involvement or questionable arterial involvement, neoadjuvant chemoradiation may be given in order to improve the likelihood of a margin-negative resection. Unresectable patients, or patients with obvious metastatic disease, should be referred for palliative systemic chemotherapy or appropriate clinical trials.

Surgical resection, while necessary for cure of pancreatic cancer, should not be considered sufficient. A multidisciplinary approach to pancreatic malignancy, combining surgical therapy with systemic chemotherapy and radiation therapy, has been shown to provide the optimal patient outcomes for this complicated disease. Decision making regarding offering neoadjuvant chemoradiation for pancreatic cancer is best made in a collaborative manner, considering patient performance status, comorbidity, and tumor resectability. Given the high recurrence rate of pancreatic cancer even for patients with optimal pathology, all patients with appropriate performance status should be considered for adjuvant chemotherapy ± radiation. Ideally, adjuvant therapy should be started within 6 to 10 weeks of the date of surgical resection.

Surgical Approach

With advances in cross-sectional imaging, the likelihood of finding occult metastatic or locally unresectable disease at the time of surgical exploration has decreased significantly. While CT is quite sensitive in determining local tumor extent and visceral metastatic disease, it often misses small volume peritoneal disease. Thus, some surgeons advocate beginning any planned operative intervention with a laparoscopic exploration with or without peritoneal washings. Once obvious peritoneal metastases have been excluded, open operative intervention should proceed. If the laparoscopic exploration is not performed initially, an upper midline incision should be made, which is large enough to allow visualization of omental and mesenteric surfaces and palpation and inspection of the liver. Any lesions suspicious for metastatic disease should be biopsied and sent for frozen section analysis prior to proceeding with resection of the primary tumor.

The pancreaticoduodenectomy dissection begins with mobilization of the hepatic flexure, exposing the duodenum and proximal pancreas. This allows reflection of the hepatic flexure and transverse colon inferiorly. Care should be taken not to avulse the middle colic vein or its distal branches when reflecting the transverse mesocolon off the pancreatic head; there is often a small crossing branch that connects the middle colic vein with the gastroepiploic venous drainage which can be inadvertently injured at this stage of the operation. Next, a complete Kocher maneuver is performed separating the duodenum and posterior aspect of the pancreatic head from retroperitoneum, which exposes the anterior surface of the inferior vena cava. This dissection should be carried medially until the origin of the SMA is encountered. A helpful landmark in identifying the origin of the SMA is the left renal vein, which crosses immediately inferior to the SMA origin as it crosses anterior to the aorta. Tumor involvement that obliterates the plane between the SMA and the uncinate process of the pancreas is most often considered a contraindication to surgical resection and should prompt aborting the resection and consideration of operative palliation.

Continuation of the Kocher maneuver along the third portion of the duodenum until one encounters the root of the small bowel mesentery crossing the duodenum allows access to the lateral aspect of the superior mesenteric vein (SMV). With the transverse mesocolon retracted inferiorly and ventrally, the course of the middle colic vein should indicate the location of the SMV as it approaches the inferior border of the pancreas. Careful dissection of the mesenteric adventitial tissue at this level will expose the anterior and lateral aspects of the SMV. If tumor infiltration or other aberrant anatomy makes exposure of the SMV difficult, the lesser sac should be opened broadly by taking the omentum off the transverse mesocolon. Filmy attachments between the posterior wall of the stomach and the retroperitoneum are divided, exposing the anterior aspect of the pancreas. Dissection along the inferior border of the pancreas from the proximal pancreatic body toward the head should bring the anterior aspect of the SMV into view. Again the course of the middle colic and gastroepiploic veins can provide clues to the location of the SMV, particularly in obese patients in whom the SMV may be obscured by mesenteric fat.

Once the SMV is identified, dissection should proceed meticulously toward the inferior border of the pancreas (Figure 3). The drainage of the middle colic and gastroepiploic veins should be identified; in some patients, they will merge as a common trunk. Ideally, the middle colic vein should be preserved if not involved with tumor. The gastroepiploic should be divided, which opens the space between the SMV and inferior border of the pancreas nicely and will allow rotation of the distal stomach and duodenum completely off the pancreatic neck. With gentle retraction on the inferior edge of the pancreas with a vein retractor or similar instrument, the space between the anterior aspect of the SMV and the posterior aspect of the pancreatic neck should be developed, typically by pushing the anterior aspect of the vein gently dorsally. As one proceeds cephalad, the confluence with the splenic vein and the drainage of the inferior mesenteric vein can often be identified. Once this plane is developed, attention is turned to the superior border of the

pancreas and the portal dissection. If SMV invasion is encountered at this level, plans for venous reconstruction should be made or the operation aborted and referral to an appropriate institution made.

With the duodenum gently retracted inferiorly, the peritoneum over the portal structures is divided, allowing the duodenum to roll off the superior border of the pancreas at the pancreatic head. The right gastric artery and vein are often encountered at the medial aspect of the porta and should be ligated and divided. The gastroduodenal artery (GDA) is identified as it enters the pancreatic head and dissected free from surrounding tissues back to its origin at the common hepatic artery. Safe division of the GDA without compromise of hepatic arterial blood flow is facilitated by two maneuvers: (1) dissection of the GDA origin completely with exposure of a short distance of the proper hepatic artery proximally and the common hepatic artery distally and (2) test occlusion of the GDA with confirmation of a retained pulse in the hepatic artery distally near the liver hilum. Once the GDA is definitively identified by these techniques, it is suture ligated and divided. Division of the GDA exposes the anterior aspect of the PV immediately posteriorly, as it passes behind the superior border of the pancreas (Figure 3). Immediately laterally to this space is the distal CBD. The CBD is encircled and elevated with a vessel loop, further exposing the anterior PV. Care should be taken

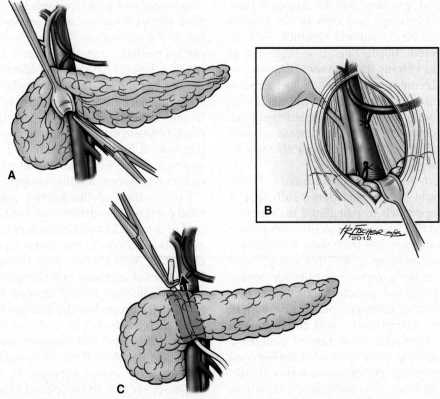

FIGURE 3 • Illustration of the critical landmarks allowing safe dissection of the SMV at the inferior border of the pancreas (A), and the PV at the superior border of the pancreas after division of the GDA (B). Panel C demonstrates passing an umbilical tape behind the neck of the pancreas after the inferior and superior dissection planes are connected.

at this point to inspect carefully for a replaced right hepatic artery that typically traverses laterally and posteriorly to the CBD. When present, a replaced right hepatic artery can be often dissected completely off the posterior aspect of the pancreatic head, freeing it down to its origin at the proximal SMA.

Cholecystectomy is then performed. The CBD is divided above the level of the pancreatic head, with a margin sent for frozen section analysis. A Bulldog or similar atraumatic small clamp may be used to control the proximal CBD and prevent bile spillage. The distal CBD is then reflected inferiorly, further rolling the head and neck of the pancreas off the anterior aspect of the PV. The plane between the anterior aspect of the PV and posterior aspect of the pancreatic neck is developed bluntly until the previous area of the inferior pancreatic dissection is encountered, thus completing the retropancreatic tunnel. An umbilical tape or Penrose drain is passed through this tunnel, allowing elevation of pancreatic neck off the PV–SMV confluence.

Depending on surgeon preference and the condition of the proximal duodenum, either proximal duodenal transection with pylorus preservation or distal gastrectomy may be performed next. Contraindications to pylorus preservation include direct tumor involvement of the proximal duodenum or gastric outlet, clinical evidence of gastric outlet obstruction, extensive primary duodenal tumors, and treatment with preoperative radiation therapy. When preserving the pylorus, the duodenum should be divided no closer than 2 to 4 cm from the pylorus. This prevents the subsequent duodenojejunostomy from being immediately adjacent to the pylorus, which may contribute to pyloric edema and delayed gastric emptying.

Once the foregut is divided, the pancreatic neck is transected. The superior and inferior pancreatic vascular arcades are controlled with figure of eight sutures at the inferior and superior border of the pancreas, placed proximally and distally to the line of transection. The pancreatic neck is divided sharply with a fresh scalpel, and a pancreatic neck margin sent for frozen section. When the margin returns positive, the proximal pancreatic body may need to be mobilized off the splenic vein to allow resection of additional pancreatic parenchyma. The cut pancreatic margin often bleeds initially; small arterial vessels should be controlled with sutures with other hemostasis obtained by pressure, avoiding the temptation to excessively cauterize the cut pancreatic surface.

The proximal jejunum is then divided and the mesentery of the distal duodenum taken with clamp and ties or a surgical energy device. Encroaching on the SMV or SMA with the mesenteric transection is avoided by staying immediately adjacent to the small bowel wall when dividing the mesentery. The proximal jejunum is then passed through the defect at the ligament of Treitz toward the right upper quadrant. The remainder of the

resection phase includes division of the uncinate process attachments to the retroperitoneum. This portion of the case has the most potential for blood loss or mesenteric vessel compromise, and therefore it should be accomplished methodically. Freeing of the SMV and its initial branches from the specimen allows the SMV to be elevated off the uncinate process and SMA. Finding the plane immediately adjacent to the SMA adventitia is actually the safest plane and provides the most definitive retroperitoneal margin. Typically there are two pancreaticoduodenal branches (superior and inferior) off the SMA entering the uncinate process that should be ligated with fine suture. Once the specimen is freed completely, the uncinate process margin should be marked and the specimen sent to pathology. The right upper quadrant is irrigated and inspected for hemostasis.

Reconstruction begins with closure of the defect at the ligament of Treitz, which is best accomplished with a continuous nonabsorbable suture. The proximal jejunum is then brought through a defect in the bare area of the transverse mesocolon just to the right of the middle colic vessels. A number of techniques exist for the pancreaticojejunostomy including a two-layer duct-to-mucosa anastomosis, invagination of the pancreatic remnant end to side into the jejunum, or end-to-end intussusception technique. No method of pancreaticojejunostomy has been definitively shown to be superior in terms of preventing pancreatic fistula, and each method may have its place depending on the size and texture of the pancreatic remnant and the caliber of the pancreatic duct. The biliary reconstruction is accomplished next, typically 10 to 20 cm distal to the pancreaticojejunostomy. Circumferential bile duct to mucosal stitches are placed using a monofilament suture. The mesenteric defect in the transverse mesocolon is then closed around the jejunum using interrupted absorbable sutures.

Gastrojejunostomy or duodenojejunostomy is the final stage of the pancreaticoduodenectomy reconstruction. This is best accomplished in an antecolic position, approximately 50 cm distal to the biliary anastomosis. Closed suction drains are typically placed adjacent to the pancreatic anastomosis, though some centers have debated the necessity of drainage in all patients. Surgeons who favor use of perioperative drains typically value the practice of testing the drain effluent for amylase in the postoperative period, allowing the diagnosis of pancreatic fistula early before infectious or other complications occur. Opponents of routine drain usage argue that most pancreatic fistula likely resolve without intervention, and monitoring of drain output and amylase content can extend length of stay unnecessarily in some patients **(Table 1)**.

Special Intraoperative Considerations

Improvements in surgical technique and patient selection have allowed the gradual expansion of pancreaticoduodenectomy to patients previously considered

TABLE 1. Key Technical Steps and Potential Pitfalls in Pancreaticoduodenectomy Procedure

Key Technical Steps

1. Midline laparotomy and inspection to rule out occult metastatic disease.
2. Mobilize hepatic flexure and perform complete Kocher maneuver.
3. Identify the origin and course of the SMA.
4. Identification of the SMV at the inferior border of the pancreas and development of plane posterior to pancreatic neck.
5. Portal dissection with definitive identification and safe division of the GDA.
6. Division of the pancreatic neck with immediate evaluation of distal margin.
7. Safe division of the small bowel mesentery along the proximal jejunum and distal duodenum.
8. Division of the uncinate process attachments to the retroperitoneum in the plane adjacent to the SMA adventitia.
9. Tension-free, precise anastomoses of the pancreas and bile duct to the proximal jejunum.
10. Antecolic gastrojejunostomy (or duodenojejunostomy if pylorus preserving).
11. Closed suction drainage.

Potential Pitfalls

- Failure to recognize tumor involvement of the SMA following completion of a complete Kocher maneuver.
- Failure to safely expose the SMV at the root of the mesentery.
- Compromise of hepatic arterial blood flow by inaccurate identification of the GDA origin and/or hepatic artery anatomic variants.
- Failure to safely develop the tunnel between the posterior aspect of the pancreatic neck and the anterior aspect of the PV—SMV confluence.
- Failure to identify the proper plane of dissection between the uncinate process of the pancreas and the adventitial margin of the SMA.

unresectable, specifically those patients with locally advanced tumors and mesenteric vascular involvement. Resection and reconstruction of the SMV, hepatic artery, and SMA have all been described during pancreaticoduodenectomy, typically in the context of comprehensive treatment strategies that include neoadjuvant chemoradiation. In experienced hands, vascular reconstruction can be performed safely and may improve the ability to obtain a margin-negative outcome. However, the ability of pancreaticoduodenectomy with vascular resection and reconstruction to produce improved overall survival has not been definitively proven. Therefore, the addition of vascular resection to pancreaticoduodenectomy should only be performed by surgeons experienced in these procedures and ideally in the context of a multidisciplinary neoadjuvant treatment protocol. SMV resection and reconstruction is the most well-studied

and proven adjunct to pancreaticoduodenectomy, with major pancreatic centers demonstrating perioperative and oncologic outcomes in SMV resection patients equivalent to patients without vascular involvement. Reconstruction options for the SMV can include primary repair, patch venoplasty, segmental resection and primary anastomosis, and resection with interposition vein graft. Synthetic conduits for SMV reconstruction have also been utilized, though are typically avoided due to concerns about diminished long-term patency and increased infection risk.

In recent years, some surgeons and institutions have begun to gather experience with minimally invasive approaches to pancreaticoduodenectomy. Both completely laparoscopic and robotic approaches have been developed, with good perioperative outcomes in limited series. Purported advantages of minimally invasive pancreaticoduodenectomy include decreased postoperative pain, decreased wound complications, and faster return to normal activities. At this point, there are no data to suggest that minimally invasive techniques diminish the rate of the most common and problematic complications of pancreaticoduodenectomy, including pancreatic fistula and delayed gastric emptying.

Postoperative Management

Patients are ideally monitored on a dedicated surgical unit following pancreaticoduodenectomy. Intensive care unit stay may be indicated in patients with significant comorbidities or a complicated intraoperative course, depending on institutional resources. As with all major operative procedures, early mobilization facilitated by appropriate postoperative analgesic strategies is paramount to avoiding pulmonary and thromboembolic complications. Unfractionated or low molecular weight subcutaneous heparin should be administered preoperatively and continued in the postoperative period.

Nasogastric decompression is typically utilized during the first 24 to 48 hours postoperatively, though some centers have debated the necessity of this historic standard. Oral intake is typically advanced sequentially and gradually, with patients encouraged to eat small frequent portions until gastric function improves. Up to 20% of patients will experience delayed gastric emptying, manifest by persistent postoperative nausea, emesis, and gastric distention. Most patients will gradually improve with observation and antiemetics, though nasogastric decompression may be necessary in patients with persistent emesis. Supplemental nutrition, given parenterally or ideally via a nasojejunal tube placed fluoroscopically, may be necessary in patients unable to resume oral intake within the first postoperative week. Prospective clinical trials of prophylactic postoperative medications such as metoclopramide or the motilin agonist erythromycin have failed to demonstrate a profound impact on the incidence of delayed gastric emptying, and no clear advantage to pylorus preservation or distal gastrectomy during pancreaticoduodenectomy has been shown in randomized clinical trials.

Pancreatic fistula, defined as high-output amylase-rich drain fluid after postoperative day 5, occurs in approximately 8% to 20% of patients, and may be associated with the texture of the pancreas found at the time of resection. In patients without associated infectious complications, management includes adequate drainage and observation. Enteral nutrition may be maintained in patients without septic complications and low-output fistulae (typically defined as <200 mL per 24-hour period). Low-output fistulae will typically resolve spontaneously, and can often be managed as an outpatient following hospital discharge, with drain removal once fistula output is consistently <30 mL per 24-hour period. In patients with high-volume fistulae, and/or associated infectious complications, bowel rest with subcutaneous octreotide administration should be initiated. Parenteral nutrition is often necessary in these patients. Pancreatic fistula can be associated with other postoperative complications including ileus and delayed gastric emptying, wound infection or dehiscence, or bleeding complications. Pseudoaneurysm formation at the GDA stump can occur as a complication of a known or occult pancreatic fistula; management for this potentially life-threatening complication includes appropriate resuscitation and angiographic intervention with occlusion or exclusion of the GDA pseudoaneurysm. All but rare catastrophic complicated pancreatic fistulae can and should be managed nonoperatively. Revision pancreaticojejunostomy is likely a futile procedure, and completion pancreatectomy can be a near-impossible procedure in a reoperative and contaminated field. In patients without adequate percutaneous drainage and uncontrolled sepsis, surgical intervention for washout and placement of additional peripancreatic drains may be appropriate.

Case Conclusion

The patient underwent successful pancreaticoduodenectomy with negative margins. The postoperative course was complicated by a pancreatic fistula, diagnosed by low-volume amylase-rich drain output. The patient was sent home postoperative day 7, on a low-fat diet with the surgical drains in place. Drain output was minimal by the third postoperative week, and drains were removed. The patient completed adjuvant chemotherapy and at 18 months postoperatively has no evidence of recurrent disease.

TAKE HOME POINTS

- Painless obstructive jaundice should be considered indicative of a malignancy until proven otherwise.
- Obstructive jaundice with intrahepatic and extrahepatic biliary ductal dilatation, consistent with a distal biliary obstruction, should first be evaluated with a pancreatic protocol CT when possible.
- In a patient with a pancreatic head mass, decisions about the need for biliary decompression and/or biopsy should be made by an experienced hepatopancreaticobiliary surgeon while considering resectability and the overall treatment plan.
- Surgical resection is necessary, but not sufficient, as curative therapy for pancreatic adenocarcinoma. Definitive treatment for pancreatic cancer should include multidisciplinary oncologic care including surgery, systemic chemotherapy, and radiation therapy.
- Venous resection and reconstruction can be performed safely with appropriate oncologic outcomes in appropriately selected patients by experienced surgeons.
- All operations for pancreatic cancer should begin with a thorough exploration to assess for metastatic disease and to determine resectability.
- Postoperative complications, including delayed gastric emptying and pancreatic fistula, can be safely managed when recognized early and treated comprehensively.

SUGGESTED READINGS

Abrams RA, Lowy AM, O'Reilly EM, et al. Combined modality treatment of resectable and borderline resectable pancreas cancer: expert consensus statement. Ann Surg Oncol. 2009;16:1751–1756.

Bassi C, Dervenis C, Butturini G. Postoperative pancreatic fistula: an international study group (ISGPF) definition. Surgery. 2005;138(1):8–13.

Evans DB, Farnell MB, Lillemoe KD, et al. Surgical treatment of resectable and borderline resectable pancreas cancer: expert consensus statement. Ann Surg Oncol. 2009;16(7):1736–1744.

Simeone DM. Complications of pancreatic surgery. In: Doherty GM, ed. Complications in Surgery. 1st ed. Philadelphia, PA: Lippincott, Williams & Wilkins, 2006:463–476.

van der Gaag NA, Rauws EA, van Eijck CH, et al. Preoperative biliary drainage for cancer of the head of the pancreas. N Engl J Med. 2010;362:129–137.

31 Incidental Pancreatic Cyst

JOSHUA A. WATERS and C. MAX SCHMIDT

Presentation

A 57-year-old, previously healthy woman is referred to the surgical clinic with a newly diagnosed 2-cm cystic lesion within the body/tail of the pancreas. The cyst lesion was identified incidentally on a computed tomography (CT) scan performed during a workup for hematuria. The patient is without any significant gastrointestinal complaint, has no history of pancreatitis, and denies weight loss or diarrhea. Her physical examination is unremarkable. The patient is physically active and works full-time as an elementary school teacher.

Differential Diagnosis

The differential diagnosis of pancreatic cystic lesions can be subdivided into inflammatory and neoplastic. Pancreatic pseudocysts are inflammatory and generally arise as sequelae of acute pancreatitis. The majority of incidentally discovered asymptomatic pancreatic cystic lesions fall into the neoplastic category. This group can then be further divided into cystic lesions with or without malignant potential. Serous cystic neoplasms (SCNs), lymphoepithelial pancreatic cysts, and simple pancreatic cysts are regarded as benign entities, whereas intraductal papillary mucinous neoplasms (IPMNs), mucinous cystic neoplasms (MCNs), solid pseudopapillary neoplasms, and cystic neuroendocrine tumors (pNETs) represent cystic neoplasms with varying degrees of malignant potential. The most common neoplastic cystic lesions encountered in practice will be IPMN, MCN, and SCN.

Workup

Although a pancreatic cystic lesion may be detected as an "incidental finding" as in this case, a complete history and physical examination will often reveal subtle but characteristic symptoms and signs. In taking a history, patient demographics, specifically gender and age, should be considered in the diagnosis and treatment of pancreatic cystic lesions. Symptoms and signs caused by a pancreatic cystic lesion are important to characterize because they may increase the likelihood of the lesion being malignant. Alternative causes of symptoms/signs must be ruled out since these should not impact this risk assessment. Symptoms/signs are typically abdominal/back pain, pancreatitis, steatorrhea, unintentional weight loss, and new-onset diabetes. These findings may be due to mass-effect, inflammation, ductal obstruction, or pancreatic (exocrine or endocrine) failure. Persistent or recurrent upper abdominal pain with/without radiation to the back may represent pain of pancreaticobiliary origin. In IPMN, this is potentially caused by intermittent pancreatic ductal obstruction with mucus that is most common when the main pancreatic duct is involved. Such pain may also occur in MCN and SCN possibly due to the effects of inflammation or local pressure on the pancreatic parenchyma and ductal system. Sequelae of pancreatic exocrine failure may occur, characterized by steatorrhea and unintentional weight loss that may result in malnutrition. In protracted untreated cases, the cachexia that results may be significant enough to be confused with cancer cachexia. Exocrine failure occurs most commonly in patients with main duct IPMNs but may occur in side-branch IPMNs, MCNs, or SCNs. Often, exocrine failure presents with more subtle findings such as bloating or foul-smelling flatulence. These symptoms will resolve with administration of oral pancreatic enzyme supplementation. Pancreatic endocrine failure manifested by glucose intolerance or diabetes may indeed occur and should be suspected particularly if there is no other obvious explanation (e.g., high body mass index or positive family history of diabetes).

Finally, a social and family history is important to delineate further risks of pancreatic cancer (e.g., tobacco, obesity, family) to arrive at a cumulative risk assessment for the patient. Some of pancreatic cystic lesions can be seen a part of familial syndromes (e.g., SCN and von Hippel-Lindau syndrome; IPMN and familial pancreatic cancer).

Physical exam findings aside from abdominal tenderness are uncommon. A palpable abdominal mass, enlarged supraclavicular lymph nodes, cachexia, or jaundice may occur, but are uncommon except in cases of advanced pancreatic malignancy.

The primary *diagnostic modalities* for identification and characterization of pancreatic cysts are cross-sectional imaging and endoscopy. Thin-slice helical CT with dual-phase intravenous contrast administration or magnetic resonance cholangiopancreatography (MRCP) with gadolinium and secretin injection are both useful in the characterization of pancreatic cystic lesions. MRCP is

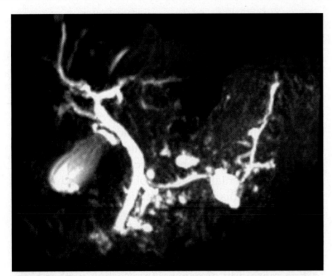

FIGURE 1 • This MRCP ductogram demonstrates multifocal side-branch IPMN with the largest lesion situated within the body/tail junction of the pancreas. Additional small dilated branch ducts may be seen within the pancreatic head and throughout.

more sensitive at detecting small lesions in part because it produces a detailed pancreatic ductogram **(Figure 1)**. The presence of ductal connectivity suggests an IPMN. Multifocality in the absence of a history of pancreatitis such as in this case is virtually diagnostic of IPMN. The presence of a central stellate scar is classic for microcystic SCN but is unreliable for macrocystic serous lesions. Cystic dilation of the main pancreatic duct is typical of main duct–involved IPMN but may also be present in other cystic lesions (MCN, pNET) and is associated with high rates of malignant transformation. Intracystic mural nodules are characteristic of IPMNs and MCNs and also serve as predictors of malignancy. Mucus or dependent debris may resemble mural nodularity in static imaging, so suspected mural nodules on CT or MRI–MRCP should be confirmed by a dynamic test such as endoscopic ultrasound (EUS).

EUS is more invasive than cross-sectional imaging, but allows for dynamic visualization. If there are contraindications to MRI–MRCP, EUS should be strongly considered. In addition, EUS allows fine needle aspiration (FNA) of cyst fluid, intracystic mural nodules, and adjacent masses. Endoscopic retrograde cholangiopancreatography (ERCP) is uncommonly used due to its higher risk profile, but ERCP in combination with pancreatic ductoscopy with directed biopsies may be indicated in patients with main pancreatic duct dilation to establish a diagnosis of neoplasia versus pancreatitis and to assist in operative planning in patients with diffusely dilated main pancreatic duct and suspected main duct–involved IPMNs.

Cyst fluid *cytopathology*, second only to surgical pathology, remains the "gold standard" and most accurate and specific predictor of malignancy. Unfortunately, it is not as sensitive, and this is most often due to low cellularity. Cyst fluid may also be assessed for *biochemical* (carcinoembryonic antigen [CEA], amylase) and *molecular (DNA) analyses*. Pancreatic cyst fluid CEA >192 ng/mL predicts a mucinous lesion (MCN or IPMN) but has no value in determination of malignant character. Elevated pancreatic cyst fluid amylase suggests ductal connectivity (IPMN or pseudocyst), but in ductal obstruction (e.g., mucin plug), it may be consistent with serum levels even in the presence of ductal connectivity. Molecular analyses may detect KRAS mutations that predict a mucinous lesion (compliments CEA). Quantity of DNA and number of DNA mutations may predict malignant potential.

Finally, *serum* studies may be useful in the workup of the incidental pancreatic cyst. Serial elevations of serum hemoglobin A1C (or fasting glucose) or cancer antigen 19-9 may predict malignant progression. Alkaline phosphatase elevation, particularly in pancreatic head cysts, may indicate early biliary obstruction, which correlates with malignancy in pancreatic head cystic lesions. Finally, elevated pancreatic inflammation markers, serum amylase and lipase, even in the absence of clinical pancreatitis, may indicate a pancreatic cyst with greater malignant potential.

Presentation Continued

Upon further clinical interview and exam, this patient recalls that she has experienced intermittent but prolonged epigastric pain radiating to her back over the past several months that she has attributed to dyspepsia. An MRI–MRCP demonstrates a 2-cm multiloculated cyst located in the body/tail junction of the pancreas with a 5-mm mural nodule, a ductal connection, and a main pancreatic duct that is 4 mm in close proximity to the cyst. Also identified on the MRCP is a 5-mm cyst within the head of the pancreas. EUS–FNA was performed on the 2-cm pancreatic body/tail cyst with the biopsy needle directed at the 5-mm mural nodule **(Figure 2)**. Cyst fluid analysis reveals a CEA level of 429 ng/mL and an amylase of 2,000 IU. Cyst fluid cytopathology is negative for high-grade atypia but demonstrates mucinous epithelium and abundant extracellular mucin. DNA analysis of the pancreatic cyst fluid reveals high DNA quantity and a high clonality KRAS mutation, the combination reported as a pancreatic cyst with aggressive behavior. Serum amylase and lipase on random check are elevated.

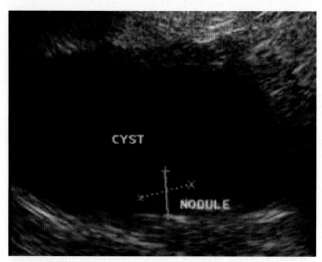

FIGURE 2 • EUS demonstrating a discreet unilocular cyst within the pancreatic gland with a mural nodule.

Diagnosis and Treatment

In a patient with side-branch IPMN without attributable symptoms, concerning radiographic features, or suspicious cytopathologic findings, surveillance in lieu of surgery is an acceptable approach. Surveillance may be less acceptable, however, in young patients due to the anticipated length of surveillance. This is due both to the cumulative risk of malignant transformation over time as well as cost to the individual and society of prolonged surveillance.

In this patient, based upon imaging features (main pancreatic duct connection and cyst multifocality), pancreatic cyst fluid markers (CEA > 192 ng/μL and cyst fluid amylase > serum amylase), and cytopathology (mucinous epithelium), the diagnosis of the tail of pancreas cystic lesion is likely to be a side-branch IPMN. Mucin contamination may occur due to the transgastric route utilized for the EUS–FNA leading to the possibility of false positive results, but there are enough data in this case for the diagnosis to stand without a definitive cytopathologic diagnosis.

Upon arriving at IPMN as the most likely diagnosis for this pancreatic cyst, the remainder of the management of this lesion hinges on the formation of an oncologic risk assessment. IPMNs represent a wide spectrum of potential to progress to invasive carcinoma. Consequently, accurate assessment of this risk allows for optimal prevention of pancreatic cancer development. Various predictors of this potential have been derived from numerous retrospective clinical studies focusing on clinical factors associated with the presence of, or eventual progression to, carcinoma within these cysts. The most basic distinction when developing an oncologic risk assessment relies on the presence or absence of main pancreatic duct involvement. Main duct–involved IPMNs have been reliably associated with elevated rates of invasive cancer, up to 50% to 60%, whereas side-branch IPMNs represent a risk of harboring invasive cancer of 10% to 20%. An additional radiographic/ endoscopic finding that has been associated with an increased rate of invasive cancer is the presence of a mural nodule within the cystic lesion. The presence of a mural nodule within a branch-type IPMN has been validated as an independent predictor of invasive carcinoma. Finally, concerning cyst cytology (i.e., high-grade atypia) is useful as a predictor only when positive, as it is not a sensitive test. The surgical treatment of IPMN involves segmental resection of the affected pancreatic segment. This is often complicated by the fact that IPMN presents as multifocal lesions affecting more than one region of the pancreatic gland (as demonstrated in this case by the synchronous 5-mm cyst within the head of the pancreas). Additionally, the substantial postoperative morbidity of pancreatic resection further highlights the importance of oncologic risk stratification and preoperative characterization of IPMN.

In the described patient scenario, the presence of symptoms, possible early main pancreatic duct involvement (4-mm MPD diameter), and the presence of a mural nodule all elevate the risk of malignancy. The combination of these findings in the setting of a relatively young and fit patient would typically not be acceptable from an oncologic risk standpoint and would warrant consideration for resection of the pancreatic segment containing the most concerning lesion—in this case the 2-cm tail cyst containing a mural nodule.

Surgical Approach

In this case, the risk of malignancy significantly outweighs the risk of surgical resection. Thus, the patient is offered segmental resection targeted to the tail of the pancreas. The additional cyst in the head of the pancreas is almost certainly a side-branch IPMN. Despite this and the patient's young age, total pancreatectomy is not recommended in this setting. The pancreatic head cyst has no concerning radiographic, cytopathologic, or molecular features. Thus, we would recommend surveillance to avoid the inevitable complications of pancreatic endocrine and exocrine failure associated with total pancreatectomy.

A minimally invasive distal pancreatectomy is one approach particularly well suited for cystic lesions of the distal pancreas. Although randomized clinical trials are not available to compare outcomes of minimally invasive to open distal pancreatectomy, case control studies suggest minimally invasive distal pancreatectomy is associated with decreased blood loss, decreased hospital length of stay, and a quicker recovery compared to open distal pancreatectomy. Preoperatively, the patient may be prepared with splenic vaccinations in case the spleen is sacrificed. The spleen may be salvaged in the setting of premalignant lesions of the distal pancreas, while it should be taken en bloc with the pancreatic resection in the setting of cancer. Spleen preservation may take one of two forms, either vessel-preserving or vessel-ligating (Warshaw) techniques.

The operation is commenced by performing a vertical incision above (laparoscopic) or below (robotic) the umbilicus. The laparoscopic video camera is introduced into the peritoneum using an open, needle localization or trocar visualization technique. Resection for IPMN, as in operations for known cancer, requires a thorough laparoscopic exploration to rule out metastatic disease to liver and visceral surfaces. Four additional 10 to 12-mm trocars are placed under direct laparoscopic vision, two in the left and two in the right hemiabdomen. The lesser sac is entered with a laparoscopic energy device through the greater gastrocolic omentum preserving the gastroepiploic vasculature. The posterior wall of the stomach is then retracted cephalad to expose the dorsal aspect of the pancreas in the retroperitoneum. Often a segmental portion of the splenic artery is visualized as it courses anteriorly from the celiac trunk and makes a tortuous course along the superior border of the pancreas. If these landmarks are not readily appreciated (e.g., fatty pancreas/peripancreatic retroperitoneum), laparoscopic ultrasound may help with localization. A plane is established along the inferior border of the pancreas using a laparoscopic energy device. Care must be taken to identify and preserve the splenic vein as the plane inferior to the pancreas is developed. The splenic vein is dissected free from the overlying pancreas using a laparoscopic energy device to seal and transect splenic vein branches to the pancreas. A vessel loop is placed around the splenic vein to retract the vein posteriorly to facilitate dissection. With the splenic vein retracted posteriorly, the proximal splenic artery underneath the neck of the pancreas is often visualized where it branches from the celiac trunk. A vessel loop may likewise be placed around the splenic artery to facilitate its dissection from the pancreas. Laparoscopic energy devices are less reliable on arterial branches, so the surgeon should have a low threshold for suture ligation.

Spleen preservation is preferred except in cases where there is a high index of suspicion preoperatively or intraoperatively for invasive cancer. In addition to spleen preservation, splenic artery and vein preservation are also desirable as case control studies suggest superior outcomes compared to splenic vessel sacrifice. Splenic vessel preservation when unsuccessful fails most often as dissection of the splenic vessels approaches the splenic hilum. Deliberate and meticulous dissection in this area is important, as upstream pancreatic tail anatomy can be quite variable particularly if the cystic lesion is located in this area. Foreshortening and disfigurement of the pancreas from inflammation may also complicate this dissection. Optimal preoperative imaging to understand the relationship between the upstream pancreas and the splenic vasculature is critical. These images should be consulted liberally intraoperatively. Laparoscopic ultrasound may also be used but is likely to be less helpful in the splenic hilum. Once the pancreatic tail is separated from the splenic vasculature, the pancreatic neck is transected. In thin pancreata, a stapling device, with or without buttress material, may be employed successfully. In thick or firm pancreata, transaction should be performed with laparoscopic energy device followed by oversewing (absorbable suture) of the pancreatic neck and pancreatic duct (if visualized). A closed suction drain although often used has no proven benefit. If a closed suction drain is placed, optimally the drain is removed early postoperatively, but if the output is >50 mL/d, drain amylase should be tested to guide timing of removal.

Special Intraoperative Considerations

One of the most challenging aspects in the operative management of IPMN comes as a result of its commonly multifocal and multicentric character. Even when prepared with the most robust preoperative imaging, the surgeon is often greeted with difficult intraoperative decisions. During resection for suspected IPMN, intraoperative frozen section of the proximal margin should be obtained routinely. Even in patients with a radiographically normal-appearing pancreatic ductal system at the site of transection, involvement with mucinous papillary epithelium may be noted. When the intraoperative margin is negative, no further action is necessary. When the main duct is involved with IPMN at the margin, re-resection should be undertaken. The management of low-grade main duct IPMN at the resection margin when further resection would require total pancreatectomy (particularly in cases of normal sized main pancreatic duct) is more controversial and should be considered on a case-by-case basis, weighing such things as the fitness and projected life expectancy of the patient. In side-branch IPMN, a commonly multifocal condition, it is important to remove the most threatening lesion(s), but try to preserve the remainder of the gland. Low-grade side-branch IPMN at the margin need not be re-resected unless this involves the lesion targeted preoperatively for removal. High-grade or invasive IPMN at the margin regardless of duct localization (branch vs. main) mandates re-resection to negative margins in fit candidates, even to the extent of total pancreatectomy. In the case presented, the operative goal is targeted resection of the highest-risk side-branch lesion. Due to the multifocal nature of this IPMN, we anticipate side-branch IPMN will be left in the remnant pancreatic head. As always, the risks of additional resection should be weighed against the resulting morbidity including pancreatic exocrine/endocrine failure (Table 1).

TABLE 1. Key Technical Steps to
Laparoscopic Distal Pancreatectomy

Key Technical Steps

1. Place one supraumbilical camera port and four additional working ports, two in each hemiabdomen.
2. Explore the liver and peritoneal surfaces for evidence of metastases.
3. Enter lesser sac through gastrocolic ligament; retract posterior stomach cephalad.
4. Establish plane inferior to pancreas; identify and preserve splenic vessels.
5. Dissect the pancreas free from splenic vessels out to the splenic hilum.
6. Transect pancreatic parenchyma with a buttressed linear cutting stapler or energy device with oversewing of main pancreatic duct and parenchyma if indicated.
7. Retrieve specimen with Silastic bag, morsellation of the spleen (if necessary), and enlargement of supraumbilical incision to accommodate removal.

Potential Pitfalls

- Relationship of the cystic lesion to the splenic vessels may dictate a different approach. A cystic lesion in the splenic hilum may preclude splenic preservation. If the cystic lesion is remote from the hilum but intimately associated with the splenic vessels, the splenic vessels should be resected en bloc with the distal pancreas. The spleen may yet be preserved on the short gastrics.
- A thick and/or firm pancreatic gland may "crack" if a stapled transection is attempted. In these cases, division with an energy device with identification and oversewing of the main pancreatic duct and stump is optimal.
- A calcific plaque in the splenic artery makes stapled transection ineffective. Suture ligation is optimal to combat this finding.

Postoperative Management

The most common serious morbidity associated with resection of the distal pancreas is related to leak of exocrine pancreatic secretions from the cut end of the pancreatic gland. Although the clinical impact of pancreatic fistulae (PF) varies, the overall rate of PF in distal pancreatectomy is between 15% and 25%. The subset of patients undergoing distal pancreatectomy in the setting of pancreatic cyst is at particularly high risk for fistula as they often have a soft pancreatic gland texture and a small pancreatic duct. Traditionally, intra-operatively placed closed suction drains are left at the cut edge of pancreas. Contemporary practice suggests that this may offer limited benefit or even detriment. PF may present late, in some cases after removal of operatively placed drains, or even after discharge, consequently the patient and clinician should be vigilant for clinical signs including fever, tachycardia, delayed return of bowel function, or worsening abdominal pain.

The long-term surveillance for IPMN varies based on the status of the remnant gland and the pathology of the primary lesion. Patients with unifocal low-grade IPMNs with a radiographically negative or positive remnant should undergo annual surveillance with history/physical, cross-sectional imaging (MRI–MRCP, CT) and serum studies. Patients with a positive low-grade main duct margin, patients with high-grade dysplasia on pathology, and patients who develop a new lesion in a previously negative remnant are at higher risk for malignancy and should undergo at least semiannual surveillance with the studies listed above. Surveillance in these high-risk groups should also include EUS–FNA with cytopathology and molecular analyses on an annual or biannual basis to monitor the remnant gland for recurrence or progression of existing unresected IPMN.

Case Conclusion

The patient ultimately elects to undergo robotic distal pancreatectomy given the relative risk of malignancy. The operation is completed robotically with splenic vessel and spleen preservation, and the patient is discharged from the hospital on postoperative day 3. Permanent pathology reveals an isolated branch-type IPMN with high-grade dysplasia **(Figure 3)**. In light of the high-grade dysplasia, this patient is placed in a high-risk surveillance protocol to monitor the remnant pancreas, which includes a small unresected cystic lesion in the pancreatic head.

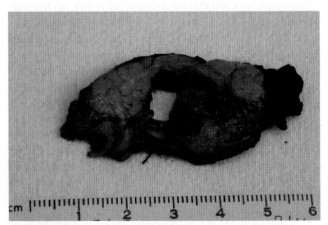

FIGURE 3 • Pathologic cross section of a distal pancreatectomy specimen, which demonstrates a cystic lesion lined with papillary epithelium and an associated mural nodule projecting into the cyst.

TAKE HOME POINTS

- Pancreatic cystic lesions are commonly identified incidentally on cross-sectional imaging.
- Differentiation of pancreatic cystic lesions is important to determine malignant potential.
- Signs/symptoms are often subtle, but their presence elevates malignant potential.
- Main pancreatic duct dilation and intracystic mural nodules both elevate malignant potential.
- Cytopathology is highly specific for malignancy, but has low sensitivity.
- Frozen section pathology should be obtained to guide intraoperative decision making.
- Side-branch IPMN are commonly multifocal. Operative resection, if indicated, should focus on removal of high-risk lesion(s) with preservation and surveillance of the pancreatic remnant.
- In IPMN, a positive main duct margin, high-grade dysplasia on initial pathology, or a new IPMN in a previously negative remnant that occurs during surveillance following segmental pancreatectomy are all risk factors for subsequent malignancy.
- Minimally invasive spleen-preserving distal pancreatectomy is the operation of choice for cystic lesions of the pancreatic body and tail.

SUGGESTED READINGS

Kooby DA, Gillespie T, Hawkins WG, et al. Left-sided pancreatectomy: a multicenter comparison of laparoscopic and open approaches. Ann Surg. 2008;248:438–446.

Merchant NB, Parikh AA, Kooby DA. Should all distal pancreatectomies be performed laparoscopically? Adv Surg. 2009;43:283–300.

Schmidt CM, White PB, Waters JA, et al. Intraductal papillary mucinous neoplasms: predictors of malignant and invasive pathology. Ann Surg. 2007;246(4):644–654.

Sohn TA, Yeo CJ, Cameron JL, et al. Intraductal papillary mucinous neoplasms of the pancreas: an updated experience. Ann Surg. 2004;239:788–797.

Waters JA, Schmidt CM. Intraductal papillary mucinous neoplasm—when to resect? Adv Surg. 2008;42:87–108.

32 Refractory Pain From Chronic Pancreatitis

SAJID A. KHAN and JEFFREY B. MATTHEWS

Presentation

A 43-year-old female presents with a 6-year history of progressively worsening upper abdominal pain, steatorrhea, and weight loss. She reports a history of chronic pancreatitis associated with heavy alcohol use in her 30s, although she has been abstinent for at least 2 years. Steatorrhea and weight loss have stabilized with encapsulated pancreatic enzyme therapy. Despite daily propoxyphene, her pain persists, interfering with work and other activities. She has insulin-dependent diabetes mellitus and smokes a half pack per day. There is no family history of pancreatic disease. She is thin but not cachectic, with no other significant physical findings.

Differential Diagnosis

Although the differential diagnosis for upper abdominal pain is broad, the chronic unrelenting nature of the pain, the presence of steatorrhea, and the association with heavy alcohol use narrows the diagnosis. The surgeon must consider disorders other than chronic pancreatitis that induce chronic pain, particularly those that often coexist with alcohol and tobacco abuse. These include peptic ulcer disease, hepatitis, and biliary tract disorders. Complications of chronic pancreatitis such as pseudocyst formation and pancreatic cancer must be considered. Symptoms secondary to duodenal or biliary obstruction due to chronic inflammation and fibrosis may occur. Chronic narcotic use may lead to dependency and drug-seeking behavior, as well as chronic constipation.

Workup

Chronic pancreatitis is an inflammatory disease characterized by progressive and irreversible destruction of gland parenchyma. Although excess alcohol consumption is the most common risk factor, chronic pancreatitis may also be associated with autoimmune disorders, pancreatic duct outflow obstruction due to traumatic stricture or pancreas divisum, and micronutrient deficiency (tropical pancreatitis). An estimated 20% to 30% of cases are hereditary or idiopathic. Hereditary pancreatitis is an autosomal dominant disorder often associated with germline mutations in the trypsinogen gene *PRSS1* and is estimated to increase the risk 15-fold for developing pancreatic adenocarcinoma. An increasing number of cases of otherwise idiopathic chronic pancreatitis have been linked to genetic variants in the cystic fibrosis gene *CFTR*, the protease inhibitor *SPINK1*, and chymotrypsin C.

There are several prevailing theories for the cause of pain. In some cases, an obstructed main pancreatic duct by stricture or stone is thought to increase intraductal pressure, causing pain and upstream ductal dilatation. In the so-called large duct disease, operations that achieve ductal decompression may be indicated. In other cases, it is thought that repeated inflammatory insults damage intrapancreatic and retroperitoneal sensory nerve pathways. Inflammation and calcification are often most pronounced in the pancreatic head and uncinate process. Pancreatic resection of this dominant disease focus may remove the "motor" of chronic inflammation, interrupting nociceptive signaling.

The pain of chronic pancreatitis typically presents as recurrent acute exacerbations of moderate to severe pain interspersed with periods of relative quiescence, but some patients experience persistent severe pain that causes significant incapacitation. Understanding the individual pattern of pain and the extent of chronic disability is important to selection of therapy. Current and past use of alcohol and tobacco should be documented. Some patients report pain that is more postprandial than steady, associated with gaseous distention, and localized in the midabdomen rather than the back or epigastrium. This type of pain may occur without overt steatorrhea and may be improved by pancreatic enzyme supplementation. Medical therapy with analgesics should be documented, and psychosocial support assessed. Endocrine insufficiency often occurs late in the course of the disease, usually many years after exocrine insufficiency.

Visualization of organ morphology, ductal anatomy, and possible involvement of surrounding structures is essential. The most useful initial imaging study is a triphasic IV contrast-enhanced computed tomography

(CT) with 2- to 3-mm slices. Key findings include areas of pancreatic ductal dilation, calcifications, focal areas of acute inflammation, dominant masses suspicious for neoplasia, dilation of the extrahepatic biliary tree, and complications such as pseudocyst or duodenal obstruction. This pancreas protocol CT may also show vascular complications such as splenic vein thrombosis.

Further detail of ductal anatomy may be visualized by endoscopic or magnetic resonance cholangiopancreatography (ERCP or MRCP) to identify main pancreatic duct strictures and intraductal stones, bile duct stricture, ductal communication with pseudocysts, and anatomic variations such as pancreas divisum. MRCP is generally preferred because it is noninvasive and avoids radiation exposure. Endoscopic ultrasound is useful to evaluate early disease and cystic lesions, and in tissue sampling for suspected neoplasia. In general, ERCP for diagnostic purposes should be avoided. Endotherapy may be selectively appropriate to achieve pancreatic or biliary decompression, dilate strictures, remove stones, or drain pseudocysts.

In the present patient, MRCP revealed a diffusely dilated main pancreatic duct with multiple intraluminal filling defects consistent with pancreatic duct stones **(Figure 1)**.

Diagnosis and Treatment

The most common indication for surgery is intractable pain. However, surgery is occasionally indicated to address pseudocyst, pancreatic ascites, bile duct or duodenal obstruction, or suspicion of neoplasia. Because the true basis of pain is often uncertain and the natural history of chronic pancreatitis is unpredictable, patients should be counseled that surgery provides long-term complete relief of symptoms in only approximately 85% of patients.

An operative strategy that drains the pancreatic duct system or resects the dominant focus of inflammation is more effective than therapy directed at interrupting the neural pathways. Celiac ganglion blocks and video-assisted thoracic splanchnicectomy only provide temporary pain relief. Pain recurrence within 3 to 6 months is common with such procedures, and they are recommended only as a bridge to more definitive therapy.

The choice of operation should be tailored to the individual anatomic circumstances and the most likely source of pain. Wherever possible, pancreatic parenchyma should be preserved to limit loss of endocrine and exocrine function. Significant ductal dilation and a dominant inflammatory mass are the two most important anatomic features that dictate the best choice of operation. Other important factors include symptomatic biliary or duodenal obstruction, pseudocyst, and mesenteroportal/splenic vein thrombosis.

Surgical Approach

Lateral Roux-en-Y Pancreaticojejunostomy (Puestow-type Procedure)

This drainage procedure is ideal to relieve pain associated with a pancreatic duct dilated ≥10 mm **(Table 1)**. A bilateral subcostal or midline laparotomy incision is used and the lesser sac is entered by separating the greater omentum from the transverse mesocolon. Adhesions between the posterior wall of the stomach and the chronically inflamed pancreas are taken down to widely expose the anterior surface of the pancreas. A generous Kocher maneuver to the level of the superior mesenteric vein (SMV) elevates and exposes the pancreatic head.

The main pancreatic ductal system is usually readily identifiable by palpation and an 18G needle (location confirmed when clear fluid is aspirated), although occasionally intraoperative ultrasound is useful. Cautery through the parenchyma overlying the needle widens initial access to the duct lumen, and then a right-angled clamp into the duct guides further unroofing, first toward the tail and then toward the ampulla. Intraductal stones are usually easily removed although occasionally they are deeply impacted within the head and uncinate process. It is not necessary to remove all stones provided that proximal drainage is achieved. The duct should be opened to within 2 cm of the tip of the tail. In the head of the gland, both the dorsal and ventral duct systems are unroofed to within 1 to 2 cm of the duodenal wall. This usually requires suture control of the anterior branches of the pancreaticoduodenal arterial arcade.

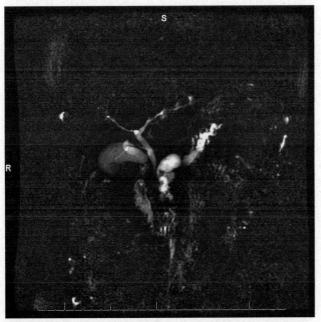

FIGURE 1 • MRCP showing dilation of main pancreatic duct.

TABLE 1. Key Technical Steps and Potential Pitfalls

I. Lateral Pancreaticojejunostomy (Puestow-type Procedure)
Key Technical Steps

1. Expose lesser sac through gastrocolic ligament and pancreatic head by Kocher maneuver.
2. Identify, expose and unroof main pancreatic duct.
3. Fashion retrocolic, Roux-en-Y conduit for drainage.

Potential Pitfalls

- Failure to remove impacted proximal intraductal stones.
- Hemorrhage from lack of suture control of pancreatico-duodenal arterial arcade.

II. Pancreaticoduodenectomy (Whipple Procedure)
Key Technical Steps

1. Expose lesser sac, pancreatic head and infrapancreatic IMV.
2. Carefully identify and divide GDA.
3. Develop tunnel behind neck of pancreas and assess resectability.
4. Remove gallbladder and divide bile duct.
5. Transect distal stomach (or proximal duodenum for pylorus preserving operation).
6. Take down ligament of Treitz, divide jejunum and its respective mesentery.
7. Transect pancreatic neck.
8. Carefully transect retroperitoneal margin posterolateral to SMV-PV confluence.
9. Fashion pancreatico-, choledocho- and gastro- jejunostomies.

Potential Pitfalls

- Failure to identify accessory and replaced arteries.
- Inadequate suture control of pancreaticoduodenal arterial arcade, venous tributaries from uncinate process, first jejunal venous tributary to SMV, and mesojejunum.
- Internal hernias from unapproximated mesenteric defects.

III. Duodenal Sparing Pancreatic Head Resections
Key Technical Steps

A. Beger procedure

1. Expose lesser sac, pancreatic head and infrapancreatic IMV, and form tunnel behind pancreas neck.
2. Spare the GDA and supraduodenal bile duct.
3. Transect pancreatic neck.
4. Resect pancreatic head 5 mm from duodenal wall while sparing intrapancreatic CBD.
5. Fashion Roux-en-Y anastomoses from pancreatic body and remnant head to jejunal limb.

B. Frey procedure

1. Expose lesser sac, pancreatic head and infrapancreatic IMV.
2. Core out pancreatic head.
3. Fashion longitudinal Roux-en-Y pancreaticojejunostomy.

Potential Pitfalls (Beger and Frey Procedures)

- Hemorrhage from lack of meticulous hemostasis (pancreaticoduodenal arcade, PV tributaries).
- Traumatic stricture to CBD.
- Duodenal ischemia.

A Roux-en-Y conduit is used for drainage. The jejunum is divided 20 cm distal to the ligament of Treitz using a 3.8-mm gastrointestinal (GIA) stapler. The limb should be at least 50 cm, and a stapled or hand-sewn side-to-side enteroenterostomy is performed. The Roux limb is advanced through the mesocolon to the right of the middle colic vessels and usually oriented with its proximal (stapled) end toward the pancreatic tail, although the reverse orientation may be used depending upon mesenteric flexibility. An enterotomy slightly smaller than the length of the pancreatic duct is made on the antimesenteric aspect. A single-layer, continuous, side-to-side anastomosis is then fashioned using double-armed absorbable monofilament suture. The jejunal sutures are full thickness or seromuscular; the pancreatic sutures should reach the duct lumen where possible but otherwise should include generous portions of fibrotic pancreatic capsule **(Figure 2)**.

Pancreaticoduodenectomy (Whipple Procedure)

Pancreaticoduodenectomy (PD) may be indicated in patients in whom inflammation and calcification are concentrated within the head and uncinate process (with or without upstream dilation of the main pancreatic duct), when there is a focal mass suspicious for neoplasm, or when there is biliary and/or duodenal obstruction. This procedure may include a distal gastrectomy ("classic" Whipple PD) or pyloric preservation (PPPD).

A midline or bilateral subcostal incision is used and a generous Kocher extended to mobilize the hepatic flexure. A cholecystectomy is performed, and the common bile duct is isolated at its insertion to the cystic

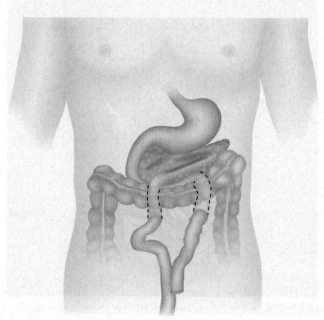

FIGURE 2 • A lateral Roux-en-Y retrocolic pancreaticojejunostomy.

duct. The gastroduodenal artery (GDA) is isolated and its identity confirmed by a persistent pulsation in the common hepatic artery after compression. An accessory or replaced right hepatic artery, if present, is usually palpable at the posterior aspect of the gastrohepatic ligament at the foramen of Winslow and should be preserved. The GDA is divided and underlying portal vein (PV) identified. A tunnel posterior to the neck of the pancreas is started. The lesser sac is entered via the gastrocolic ligament in an avascular plane, the right gastroepiploic vein is divided, and infrapancreatic SMV exposed. The tunnel behind the neck of the pancreas is completed, and a Penrose drain or umbilical tape is passed through it for traction. Once resectability has been assured, the bile duct is divided just proximal to the cystic duct insertion (if there is extrahepatic biliary dilation) or just distal to it (if there is not). The stomach is divided between two firings of a 4.8-mm GIA 60 stapler, starting from the greater curve near the junction of the right and left gastroepiploic arcades and ending at the lesser curve just proximal to the incisura angularis. The lesser omentum is divided, including the right gastric artery. The ligament of Treitz is taken down, the jejunum divided with a 3.8-mm GIA 60 stapler 20 cm distally, and the proximal mesojejunum and mesoduodenum are divided. The proximal jejunum is then advanced into the supracolic compartment by passing it posterior to the superior mesenteric vessels. Electrocautery divides the pancreatic neck between stay sutures. Resection is completed by carefully dividing small tributaries of the PV from the uncinate process and retroperitoneal tissues posteriorly.

The jejunum at the distal staple line is advanced through the transverse mesocolon to the right of the middle colic vessels. A number of acceptable techniques for pancreaticojejunostomy have been described, including a two-layered invaginating technique and a pancreatic duct-to-mucosa anastomosis with or without exteriorized transanastomotic stenting. Biliary–enteric continuity is restored by an end-to-side single layer interrupted or continuous anastomosis. Gastrojejunostomy is usually performed hand-sewn in two-layer fashion, with the afferent limb oriented toward the lesser curve.

Other Operations for Chronic Pancreatitis

PD carries significant postoperative morbidity and long-term digestive consequences even when performed by experienced surgeons. Duodenum-sparing pancreatic head resection (DSPHR) may be a safe and effective alternative for some patients and is indeed the preferred approach in many European centers. The Beger procedure has been advocated for patients with an inflammatory pancreatic head mass. In this form of DSPHR, after a generous Kocher, a

tunnel between the neck of the pancreas and the PV is developed as in a standard PD. However, the GDA and supraduodenal bile duct are spared. The neck is transected, the head retracted laterally, and tributaries to the PV controlled. The pancreatic head is resected 5 mm off the duodenal wall down to but sparing the intrapancreatic common bile duct. A Roux-en-Y pancreaticojejunostomy is fashioned to the left side of the pancreas (body and tail) and then tacked over the right-sided pancreatic head excavation. A modification of this approach (Berne variant) involves coring out the pancreatic head without formal transection of the neck. Patients with a dominant inflammatory focus in the pancreatic head and dilated main pancreatic duct may benefit from a Frey procedure that combines coring out of the pancreas head with longitudinal Roux-en-Y pancreaticojejunostomy.

Patients with hereditary chronic pancreatitis syndromes or who have failed previous operations may be candidates for total (or completion) pancreatectomy with or without autologous islet cell transplantation (AIT). AIT entails collagenase-based digestion of the resected pancreas followed by isolation of intact islets for infusion into the PV. This approach has been reported by several experienced centers, although indications and timing are somewhat controversial. Pain is durably relieved in approximately 70% of patients, and about 40% of patients will initially require no postoperative insulin therapy.

Outcomes of Operations for Chronic Pancreatitis

Comparison of surgical options for the treatment of chronic pancreatitis is hampered by the relative paucity of results from randomized, prospective clinical trials. Most reports include small numbers of patients, are nonrandomized, and are retrospective. There is no uniform method in reporting outcomes, and there is significant heterogeneity among patient populations and surgeon experience. Historically, PD has been viewed as the standard against which other procedures have been evaluated. In one review, PD was reported to achieve "pain relief" in 70% to 100% of patients. Comparison of various types of DSPHR to PD in several randomized trials has shown similar effectiveness with respect to pain relief, postoperative morbidity, new-onset postoperative diabetes, and quality of life. Comparisons between two variations of DSPHR (Beger vs. Frey procedures) have similarly shown no significant difference. Comparison between operative and endoscopic therapy for large duct chronic pancreatitis in randomized trials clearly indicates that surgical drainage is more effective than transampullary stenting and lithotripsy in terms of partial or complete pain relief and number of required procedures.

Postoperative Management

Postoperative management of patients with chronic pancreatitis should include attention to exacerbation of exocrine insufficiency (managed by pancreatic enzyme replacement therapy) and the development of endocrine insufficiency (initially managed by sliding scale insulin, and then adjusted with long-acting preparations as appropriate). Continued abstinence from alcohol and tobacco is important in prevention of symptomatic recurrence. Slow taper of narcotic analgesia is often required, and patients should be followed longitudinally for ongoing medical and psychosocial support.

Case Conclusion

The patient underwent Roux-en-Y lateral pancreaticojejunostomy for large duct disease without head predominance. She was discharged on postoperative day 5. She is currently 1 year from her operation, pain free, not requiring analgesics, and steatorrhea is controlled by pancreatic enzyme supplementation. She continues to be employed.

TAKE HOME POINTS

- Incapacitating pain is the most common reason for consideration of surgical therapy.
- IV contrast-enhanced CT should evaluate for pancreatic ductal dilation, dominant areas of inflammation and calcification, a focal mass suspicious for malignancy, and presence of complications such as pseudocyst or duodenal obstruction.

- Pancreatic duct anatomy and presence of areas of stricture or dilation should be delineated by MRCP or ERCP (if endotherapy or biopsy is indicated).
- The long-term goals for any of the operative approaches are pain relief and preservation of exocrine and endocrine function.
- The choice of operation should address anatomic abnormalities while preserving organ parenchyma, where possible.
- Treatment decisions should be tailored to individual clinical and anatomic circumstances as well as to the experience and preference of the surgeon.

SUGGESTED READINGS

Beger HG, Schlosser W, Friess HM, et al. Duodenum-preserving head resection in chronic pancreatitis changes the natural course of the disease. Ann Surg. 1999;230:512–523.

Cahen DL, Gouma DJ, Rauws EA, et al. Endoscopic versus surgical drainage of the pancreatic duct in chronic pancreatitis. N Engl J Med. 2007;356:676–684.

Diener MK, Rahbari NN, Fischer L, et al. Duodenum-preserving pancreatic head resection versus pancreaticoduodenectomy for surgical treatment of chronic pancreatitis. Ann Surg. 2008;247:950–961.

Schafer M, Mullhaupt B, Clavien P. Evidence-based pancreatic head resection for pancreatic cancer and chronic pancreatitis. Ann Surg. 2002;236:137–148.

Steer ML, Waxman I, Freedman S. Chronic pancreatitis. N Engl J Med. 1995;332:1482–1490.

Strate T, Taherpour Z, Bloechle C, et al. Long-term follow up of a randomized trial comparing the Beger and Frey procedures for patients suffering from chronic pancreatitis. Ann Surg. 2005;241:591–598.

33 Symptomatic Pancreatic Pseudocyst

MICHAEL G. HOUSE

Presentation

A middle-aged man with a history of alcohol abuse and several previous episodes of acute pancreatitis requiring hospitalization presents with vague upper abdominal pain, weight loss, and early satiety for the past several months. Physical examination reveals a nonpulsatile fullness in the epigastrium with minimal tenderness to palpation. A serum metabolic panel is unremarkable with the exception of a recorded albumin level of 2.5 g/dL. A computed tomography (CT) scan, enhanced with intravenous contrast, is obtained and demonstrates a 6- × 8-cm fluid collection compressing the posterior wall of the gastric body (Figure 1).

Differential Diagnosis

In the clinical setting of a patient with previous pancreatitis and a peripancreatic fluid collection, the differential diagnosis may be quite focused. Differentiation of a pancreatic pseudocyst from a peripancreatic fluid collection seen in acute pancreatitis is defined by the persistence of the lesion for 6 weeks or more from the time of the initial episode of acute pancreatitis. Other important lesions to distinguish from pancreatic pseudocysts include pancreatic mucinous cystic neoplasms (e.g., mucinous cystadenoma, intraductal papillary mucinous neoplasm), serous cystic tumors (e.g., serous cystadenoma), and visceral artery aneurysms (e.g., splenic artery aneurysm).

Workup

The mainstay of evaluation for patients with suspected chronic pancreatitis and a pancreatic pseudocyst is cross-sectional imaging. However, in addition to proper radiographic imaging, a careful evaluation of pancreatic endocrine and exocrine function should be conducted along with an overall nutritional assessment of the patient. Any clinical history of steatorrhea should be evaluated with formal fecal fat content studies. Daily fecal excretion of >7 g of fat is considered abnormal in the context of a regular balanced diet. Routine glucose monitoring and hemoglobin A1C testing can establish a diagnosis of diabetes mellitus. Patient nutritional status can be addressed globally (e.g., body mass index), but formal biochemical levels of nutritional status, including serum albumin, prealbumin, and transferrin, should be monitored.

High-resolution cross-sectional imaging with intravenous contrast, that is CT or magnetic resonance cholangiopancreatography (MRCP), will provide morphologic data on the size and structure of the pancreas, pancreatic ductal dilatation and calcifications, and the size and number of pancreatic pseudocysts (Figure 2). Relationship of the pseudocyst to the stomach, duodenum, spleen, transverse colon, and common bile duct can be addressed with either modality. Complications of pancreatitis and pseudocysts, including splenic, portal, or mesenteric vein thromboses; visceral artery pseudoaneurysms; and pseudocyst bleeding, can be identified with either CT or MRCP. Discriminating a mature pseudocyst from acute pancreatic necrosis can be difficult in some cases, particularly when the patient has suffered recurrent attacks of acute pancreatitis.

Distinguishing a pancreatic pseudocyst from a cystic neoplasm of the pancreas is crucial. Establishing a confident diagnosis is particularly important in patients who have no established history of pancreatitis and are being considered for nonresectional therapy (i.e., internal drainage procedures). Endoscopic ultrasound (EUS) can characterize a pancreatic pseudocyst by excluding internal septations that are frequently found in cystic neoplasms. EUS-guided fine needle aspiration of the cyst fluid can also help to discriminate these two diagnoses. Cyst fluid high in amylase but low in mucin content is consistent with a pseudocyst, whereas fluid enriched with mucin and carcinoembryonic antigen may be more suggestive of a mucinous cystic neoplasm.

Diagnosis and Treatment

Patients with symptomatic pancreatic pseudocysts should be considered for endoscopic internal drainage initially. In general, percutaneous external pseudocyst drainage is not advocated. Endoscopic retrograde cholangiopancreatography (ERCP) is helpful in determining whether a pseudocyst communicates with the main pancreatic duct and whether downstream strictures of the duct exist. Transpapillary internal drainage with stenting across the ampulla into the pseudocyst

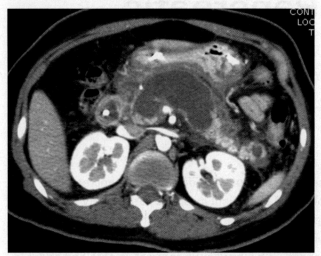

FIGURE 1 • CT scan enhanced with intravenous contrast demonstrates a 6- × 8-cm fluid collection compressing the posterior wall of the gastric body.

lumen is best suited for patients with mature pseudo-cysts containing thin fluid that communicate readily with the main pancreatic duct.

Pseudocysts that abut the posterior gastric wall can be drained internally via endoscopic cystogas-trostomy. The common technique for this procedure involves puncturing the common wall with a needle knife sphincterotome, serially dilating the orifice, and placing generous transgastric double-pigtail stents to prevent spontaneous closure. Endoscopic trans-duodenal drainage can be accomplished in a similar manner for pseudocysts located along the head of the pancreas. Pseudocysts that contain necrotic debris may require repeated endoscopic debridements across the transgastric orifice over several weeks. Relative con-traindications for endoscopic drainage include inter-vening perigastric varices, often observed in patients

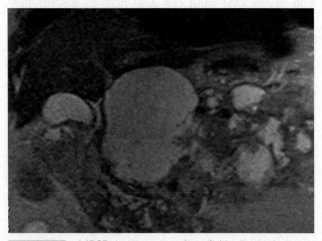

FIGURE 2 • MRCP demonstrates a large fluid collection in the region of the pancreatic head.

with splenic or portal vein thrombosis, and transmural distances to the pseudocyst lumen that exceed 1 cm. Operative therapy is recommended for patients who are not candidates for endoscopic drainage due to ana-tomic factors or those who have failed an initial endo-scopic attempt.

Surgical Approach

Cholecystectomy at the time of operation should be performed for patients who harbor gallstones, even if a history of biliary pancreatitis is not established. Most pseudocysts can be drained internally into the stom-ach, duodenum, or small bowel. Pseudocysts located along the tail of the pancreas, and those which can-not be discriminated from cystic neoplasms, may be approached with a regional pancreatectomy, for exam-ple distal pancreatectomy. In general, proximal and central pancreatectomies are not advocated for symp-tomatic pseudocysts located along the head or body of the pancreas, respectively, especially when a cystic neoplasm is considered unlikely.

Several factors need to be considered when deciding on an appropriate operation for a symptomatic pan-creatic pseudocyst. Pseudocysts that lie along the head of the pancreas and do not compress the ampulla or common bile duct can be approached with a cystoduo-denostomy; however, a Roux-en-Y cystojejunostomy is often more straightforward from a technical stand-point. Pseudocysts that project through the transverse mesocolon are best managed with a Roux-en-Y cystoje-junostomy with either an open or a laparoscopic tech-nique. Cystogastrostomy is the preferred operation for pseudocysts that abut and deform the posterior gastric wall on cross-sectional imaging. An open technique is summarized in **Table 1**, but laparoscopic and com-bined laparoscopic and endoscopic techniques have been described and are being used with greater fre-quency in recent years. Routine placement of perianas-tomotic drains is not employed.

Postoperative Management

Active nutritional therapy should be considered for most patients and should be initiated soon after opera-tion, that is, 24 to 48 hours. Enteral nutrition via a naso-jejunal tube, or direct jejunostomy placed at the time of operation, is preferred over parenteral nutrition. Antibiotic therapy is discontinued after the periopera-tive period even for patients who were found to have a large burden of necrotic debris within the pseudo-cyst. Nasogastric tubes may be considered to avoid early postoperative gastric distention. A liquid diet can be introduced early in the postoperative course and advanced when appropriate.

Chronic pancreatitis is associated with thrombo-embolism; thus, appropriate prophylaxis for deep venous thrombosis should be carried over into the

TABLE 1. Key Technical Steps and Potential Pitfalls in Open Cystogastrostomy for Pancreatic Pseudocyst

Key Technical Steps

1. Upper midline laparotomy.
2. Cholecystectomy ± intraoperative cholangiography.
3. Anterior gastrotomy (at least 5 cm) to expose posterior gastric wall.
4. Aspiration of pseudocyst to ensure location if bulge not apparent; culture fluid.
5. Electrocautery to open the posterior gastric and anterior pseudocyst walls.
6. Biopsy pseudocyst wall (frozen and permanent) to exclude epithelial-lined cyst.
7. Explore pseudocyst cavity and debride necrosis.
8. Anastomosis (at least 5 cm) completed with locking PDS or Vicryl suture.

Potential Pitfalls

- Bleeding from pseudocyst walls.
- Bleeding from injured splenic vessels during necrosectomy.
- Dehiscence of the gastric and pseudocyst walls.

postoperative period. Morbidity after cystogastrostomy or cystojejunostomy occurs in approximately 30% of patients and includes surgical site and deep organ space infection, anastomotic bleeding, ileus, and pseudoaneurysm formation.

TAKE HOME POINTS

- Treatment of pancreatic pseudocysts should be considered for symptomatic patients.
- Pancreatic pseudocysts can become complicated by infection, bleeding, and rupture.
- EUS can help secure a diagnosis of pancreatic pseudocyst over cystic neoplasm in patients without a clear history of pancreatitis.
- MRCP and ERCP can characterize pancreatic ductal anatomy and communication with pseudocysts.
- Endoscopic internal drainage procedures are first-line therapy for patients with chronic symptomatic pseudocysts containing thin fluid.
- Surgical cystogastrostomy and cystojejunostomy are indicated for symptomatic patients who either fail or are not candidates for endoscopic drainage procedures.
- Operative procedures and techniques are selected on the basis of pseudocyst location and adjacent anatomic relationships.

SUGGESTED READINGS

Cahen D, Rauws E, Fockens P, et al. Endoscopic drainage of pancreatic pseudocysts: long-term outcome and procedural factors associated with safe and successful treatment. Endoscopy. 2005;37:977–983.

Nealon W, Walser E. Main pancreatic ductal anatomy can direct choice of modality for treating pancreatic pseudocysts. Ann Surg. 2002;235:751–758.

Schlosser W, Siech M, Beger H. Pseudocyst treatment in chronic pancreatitis: surgical treatment of the underlying disease increases long-term success. Dig Surg. 2005;22:340–345.

Sharma S, Bhargawa N, Govil A. Endoscopic management of pancreatic pseudocysts: long-term follow-up. Endoscopy. 2002;34:203–207.

34 Cholecystoduodenal Fistula

PAUL PARK and ALI F. MALLAT

Presentation

A 75-year-old woman presents with possible small bowel obstruction. She is demented and resides at an extended care nursing facility. Over the past 6 days, she has had intermittent abdominal pain, confusion, and emesis. She was evaluated by the physician at her nursing facility 4 days ago, and she was treated empirically for a urinary tract infection. She continued to have episodic bouts of emesis, abdominal pain, and confusion over the ensuing days and was sent to the emergency room for further evaluation.

By her chart history, she has chronic obstructive pulmonary disease, diabetes mellitus, hyperlipidemia, Alzheimer's dementia, hypothyroidism, and cholelithiasis. She has had no prior abdominal surgeries.

On initial evaluation, she is found to be confused and somnolent. She is afebrile, mildly tachycardic at 102 beats per minute, and with a blood pressure of 116/78. On examination of her abdomen, she has no prior surgical scars. Her abdomen is moderately distended and tympanitic. She has diffuse, nonlocalized tenderness over her abdomen without involuntary guarding or signs of peritonitis. There are no palpable masses. She has no costovertebral angle tenderness. Her rectal exam reveals no masses or fissures, normal tone, and no fecal impaction.

Differential Diagnosis

This is a common presentation suspicious for bowel obstruction. The time course is not acute but rather one of progressive decline. Her differential will need to be broad, and her initial studies directed toward narrowing down her differential diagnosis rapidly (Table 1).

Workup

The initial workup should be directed toward narrowing the list of potential diagnoses quickly. In this case her history, clinical course, and examination are suspicious for potential obstruction, either mechanical or from an ileus. Her initial workup should include laboratory studies and imaging. A complete blood count, comprehensive metabolic panel, amylase and lipase, and urinalysis, along with multiview chest and abdominal radiographs would be an appropriate initial workup.

Her initial lab work reveals a mild leukocytosis at 11,000. Her creatinine is elevated to 2.4, and her chloride is low at 92. Her liver panel is within normal limits, and her amylase and lipase are normal. Urinalysis is normal. Her chest x-ray is unremarkable. On abdominal x-ray, she has diffusely dilated small bowel loops throughout her abdomen, with a paucity of gas in the colon (Figure 1). Careful inspection reveals a radiopaque density in the lower abdomen, consistent with an ectopic gallstone. Depending on the patient's clinical condition, further imaging may not be necessary before making the decision to intervene surgically. However, in cases where the physical exam and plain radiographs do not prompt immediate surgical intervention, computed tomography (CT) with enteric contrast can be helpful in establishing a diagnosis of bowel obstruction and in delineating other pathology in the abdomen.

In this case, CT showed evidence of a cholecystoduodenal fistula (Figure 2), with contrast from the duodenum filling the gall bladder. Images of the lower abdomen confirmed the presence of the calculus at a transition point in the small intestine (Figure 3).

Based on the abdominal imaging and clinical presentation, the diagnosis is of a bowel obstruction secondary to gallstone ileus. Only about 50% of cases are diagnosed preoperatively, which increases up to 77% with the addition of other imaging modalities, particularly CT, to elucidate the diagnostic picture. However, despite the improvement of radiologic imaging, clinical suspicion and upright and supine abdominal radiograph remain the most important components of the diagnostic evaluation.

Gallstone ileus accounts for < 1% to 4% of all mechanical small bowel obstructions. This incidence increases to 25% among episodes of small bowel obstruction in patients over 65 years old. The clinical picture is classically of an elderly woman presenting with recurrent intermittent episodes of obstruction. The clinical course is often subacute and indistinct, with progressive worsening over days prior to presentation at a hospital for evaluation. The average time prior to presenting at a hospital is 5 days. The average age of

TABLE 1. Differential Diagnosis

More likely	Must not miss
Appendicitis	Abdominal aortic aneurysm
Cholecystitis	Bowel obstruction
Constipation	Intestinal ischemia
Diverticulitis	Intestinal perforation
Gastritis	
Gastroenteritis	
Gastrointestinal malignancy	
Intestinal obstruction	
Pancreatitis	
Peptic ulcer disease	
Pyelonephritis	
Urinary tract infection	

patients with gallstone ileus is 70 years, with women affected much more frequently; therefore, this diagnosis needs to be kept in the differential particularly for this demographic. The patient population frequently has multiple comorbidities at baseline, with 86% noted to be in the American Society of Anesthesiology classification groups 3 or 4.

Using imaging, classic findings that may be found on plain radiographs of the abdomen comprise

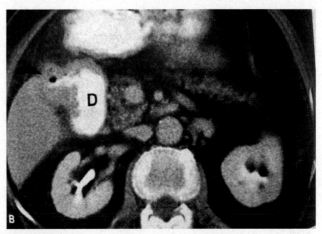

FIGURE 2 • Cholecystoduodenal fistula demonstrated via oral contrast CT. Contrast in the gallbladder is indicated by the arrow and appears to communicate with the duodenum (D).

Rigler's triad (pneumobilia, evidence of obstruction, and ectopic gallstone). The actual triad is uncommon to see on an abdominal radiograph due to the fact that most gallstones are radiolucent (only 15% of stones are radiopaque on abdominal films). While both pneumobilia and evidence of bowel obstruction occur in about 50% of these patients each, neither are diagnostic for gallstone ileus. Ultrasound may help visualize stone impaction, fistulas, as well as gallstones in the biliary system, but often imaging is limited due to body habitus and gas in the intestinal loops. CT scan may demonstrate gallbladder thickening, pneumobilia, intestinal obstruction with an identified transition point, or visualization of an ectopic gallstone. HIDA scans may allow visualization of a gallbladder fistula or perforation, although the sensitivity is only about 50%. Despite of these investigative modalities, diagnosis at the time of surgical exploration continues to be common.

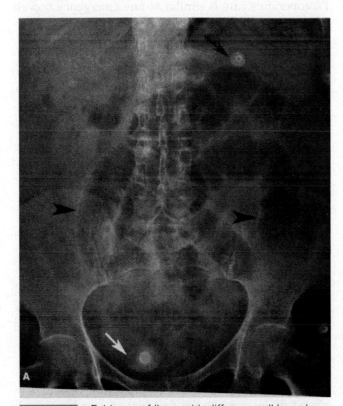

FIGURE 1 • Evidence of ileus with diffuse small bowel dilation (*arrowheads*), accompanied by an ectopic gallstone (*white arrow*) and pneumobilia (*black arrow*), is suggestive of gallstone ileus.

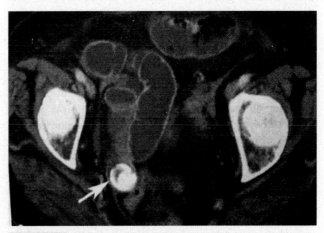

FIGURE 3 • CT scan demonstrating radiolucent calculus (gallstone, *white arrow*) in distal ileum.

Diagnosis and Treatment

The initial treatment of gallstone ileus, much like any intestinal obstruction, begins with appropriate resuscitation and stabilization, correction of electrolyte abnormalities, and surgical exploration. The surgical decision making depends on factors revealed during the workup along with information gathered during abdominal exploration.

Our patient has been adequately resuscitated but continues to vomit, remaining uncomfortable and distended despite nasogastric decompression. Her diagnosis is explained to her caregiver, and she is scheduled for urgent surgical exploration.

Surgical Approach

The primary goal of surgical management of gallstone ileus is to relieve the obstruction quickly and safely. While there have been reports in the literature of laparoscopic exploration and treatment for gallstone ileus, the standard approach would be an open exploration (Table 2). The intestinal tract should be fully evaluated for additional nonobstructing stones as well. The common locations for stones are in the distal ileum, followed by the jejunum and gastric outlet. The colon is an uncommon site of obstruction unless a history of medical or surgical illness suggests the presence of a colonic stricture. An enterolithotomy performed proximal to the obstructing stone is used to extract the stone in retrograde fashion. If there is any suggestion of bowel injury during the extraction, a formal bowel resection is warranted.

The patient is taken to the operating room where a midline laparotomy incision is used to explore the abdomen. The stone is located in the distal ileum, and an additional smaller stone is palpated in the midjejunum. Both are extracted atraumatically through an enterotomy, which is subsequently closed in a transverse orientation.

Special Intraoperative Considerations

The primary goal is to relieve the obstruction. The decision to perform a concurrent cholecystectomy and fistula closure is a controversial one as this will lead to significant increase in the operative time and increases the risk of morbidity and mortality. Therefore, addressing the obstruction alone is the most appropriate treatment strategy in the vast majority of patients. As gallstone ileus occurs most commonly in older debilitated patients, minimizing the length and complexity of the operative procedure is of paramount importance. Furthermore, the risk of recurrent gallstone ileus, or other complications related to persistence of the gallbladder and the cholecystoduodenal fistula, is relatively low.

In the unusual circumstance that gallstone ileus occurs in a stable patient without significant debilitation or comorbidity, concurrent fistula closure and cholecystectomy may be considered. Manual palpation of the gallbladder should be performed to determine if additional stones are present. The presence of stones in the gallbladder increases the risk of future ectopic stones. Patency of the extrahepatic biliary tree should also be established by preoperative laboratory studies and imaging. In general, a fistula without stones or concurrently obstructed biliary system can be expected to close spontaneously and generally should not have a concurrent cholecystectomy.

If cholecystectomy and fistula takedown are performed, the duodenal closure should be repaired using standard techniques for addressing duodenal injury. The most appropriate repair should be determined by the health of the tissue and the size of the defect. The techniques of primary repair, omental patch, pyloric exclusion, or duodenojejunostomy may each be appropriate depending on the severity of the duodenal defect, and surgeons should not approach cholecystoduodenal fistula takedown if not comfortable with these procedures. Cholecystectomy should be accomplished carefully, as the anatomy of the critical structures in the porta may be obscured by the inflammation surrounding the fistula. Closed suction drainage should be left following cholecystectomy and duodenal repair.

Postoperative Management

Postoperative care is similar to any emergency bowel operation on an elderly patient. The main source of morbidity and mortality will derive from the comorbidities of the patient and physiologic reserve to tolerate surgical exploration. Special consideration should be made to adequately resuscitate the patient. Aggressively correcting electrolyte imbalance and restoring acid–base equilibrium that may have occurred as a result of dehydration and emesis in advance of proceeding to operative intervention is preferred. A nasogastric tube for decompression until return of bowel function as well as a Foley catheter to assess adequacy of resuscitation should also be used.

In the case of patients who have undergone stone removal with or without bowel resection, the most concerning technical complication is enteric leak, and a high index of suspicion for this potentially devastating event has to be maintained in these frail and frequently malnourished patients. Prompt recognition and early surgical intervention for this complication is the only way to avoid a postoperative mortality.

In the case of patients who have undergone concurrent cholecystectomy and duodenal closure, leakage from either the cystic duct or the duodenal repair is possible. Concerning bilious drain output from operatively placed drains may be the first hint of a problem, and subsequent studies should be aimed at documenting the site of the leak. Measurement of amylase levels in the drainage may help to distinguish between a leak from

TABLE 2. Key Technical Steps and Pitfalls

Key Technical Steps

1. Full abdominal exploration with manual palpation for gallstones.
2. Localization of point of obstruction.
3. Proximal longitudinal enterotomy on the antimesenteric surface of the intestine.
4. Retrograde extraction of gallstones.
5. Transverse closure of enterotomy to prevent stricture.

Potential Pitfalls

- Attempting to extract the stone through an antegrade enterotomy or cecotomy often results in significant mucosal injury and is not recommended.
- Bowel resection should be performed if the stone cannot be removed or if excessive injury to the involved segment of bowel occurs during stone extraction.
- Failure to palpate for and extract all stones present in the intestinal tract is the most likely cause of early recurrent gallstone ileus after prior enterolithotomy, as 3%–16% of gallstone ileus patients have multiple gallstones present in the intestinal tract.
- Failure to evaluate the gall bladder for existing stones and evidence of biliary obstruction may predispose the patient to recurrent gallstone ileus.

the biliary tree versus the duodenum, although unfortunately, this is not a test with perfect accuracy. An upper gastrointestinal imaging (GI) with water-soluble contrast should be the first test, as a documented duodenal leak will likely require additional surgical intervention. If there is no duodenal leak, the cystic duct is the likely source. If the leak is of significant volume to prompt intervention, a percutaneous transhepatic cholangiogram and biliary drain placement should be considered, rather than attempting endoscopic retrograde cholangiography in the presence of a recent duodenal repair.

Once the patient has resumed bowel function and a diet, the drains can be removed provided there is no change in the quality and volume of effluent.

If cholecystectomy was not performed at the primary operation, interval cholecystectomy may be considered in patients who recover fully and remain reasonable operative candidates. An interval of at least 4 to 6 weeks following the initial surgery is recommended.

TAKE HOME POINTS

- Consider the diagnosis of gallstone ileus in an elderly patient with signs of bowel obstruction.
- No imaging gold standard exists for diagnosis although abdominal films, ultrasound, and CT scan are all useful adjuncts to clinical suspicion and serial examination. Rigler's triad, although diagnostic, is exceedingly uncommon.
- Surgical exploration should aim to clear all stones from the intestinal tract in order to treat the current obstruction and prevent early recurrent obstruction.
- Cholecystectomy and fistula takedown are rarely indicated at the time of the operation for bowel obstruction.

SUGGESTED READINGS

Ayantunde AA, Agrawal A. Gallstone ileus: diagnosis and management. World J Surg. 1994;31:1292.

Clavien PA, Richon J, Burgan S, et al. Gallstone ileus. Br J Surg. 1990;77:737–742.

Muthukumarasamy G, et al. Gallstone ileus: surgical strategies and clinical outcome. J Dig Dis. 2008;9:156–161.

Reisner RM, Cohen JR. Gallstone ileus: A review of 1001 reported cases. Am Surg. 1994;60:441.

Rigler LG, Borman CN, Noble JF. Gallstone obstruction: pathogenesis and roentgen manifestation. J Am Med Assoc. 1941;117:1753.

Rodriguez-Sanjuan JC, Casado F, Fernandez MJ, et al. Cholecystectomy and fistula closure versus enterolithotomy alone in gallstone ileus. Br J Surg. 1997;84:634–637.

35 Lower Gastrointestinal Bleeding

SCOTT E. REGENBOGEN

Presentation

A 53-year-old man presents to the emergency room with painless, bright red bleeding from the rectum. The bleeding is described as large volumes, occurring three times in the preceding 8 hours. His medical history includes hypertension and obesity. He takes a daily aspirin and occasional ibuprofen for back pain. He has never had a colonoscopy. He has no family history of colorectal cancer. His blood pressure is 90/55 and heart rate is 120 per minute. Abdominal exam is normal. There is blood in the rectal vault but no palpable mass.

Differential Diagnosis

Bright red rectal bleeding typically comes from the colon or the rectum, though in 10% to 15% of patients, brisk hematochezia results from upper gastrointestinal bleeding (UGIB), and another 10% to 15% originate in the small bowel. Diverticular hemorrhage is the most commonly identified source of major lower gastrointestinal bleeding (LGIB) in adults. Other common causes include inflammatory bowel disease and neoplasms, and in older adults, colonic angiodysplasia. In children and young adults, LGIB is most commonly caused by inflammatory bowel disease, Meckel's diverticula, or benign polyps. Minor intermittent bleeding in any age group may be related to anorectal disease, such as hemorrhoids or fissures. Ischemic colitis should be considered in patients with atherosclerotic disease, dehydration, or other causes of restricted mesenteric perfusion.

Workup

After obtaining large-bore venous access, a sample for blood type and crossmatch is sent. In this patient, his hematocrit is 18%, and his coagulation studies are normal. Nasogastric tube aspirate is bilious, without blood. Anoscopy reveals small, nonbleeding hemorrhoids. He is admitted to the intensive care unit, and resuscitated with isotonic fluids and transfused with packed red blood cells. His blood pressure normalizes, and the bleeding seems to subside.

A bowel preparation is administered, and colonoscopy the following day reveals extensive diverticulosis (Figure 1) and dark blood in the descending and transverse colon. Later that evening, he has another large bloody bowel movement and becomes hypotensive. Again, his blood pressure improves after transfusion. Urgent mesenteric angiography is performed. There is evidence of atherosclerotic disease, but no active bleeding is identified (Figures 2A and 2B).

Diagnosis and Treatment

Diverticular bleeding accounts for about half of acute LGIB hospitalizations in the United States, and an even greater share of cases among the elderly. Risk factors for bleeding among individuals with diverticulosis include systemic anticoagulation, hypertension, and use of nonsteroidal anti-inflammatory drugs or steroids. The bleeding can be massive and even life threatening, but it is often a diagnosis of exclusion, as the bleeding will cease spontaneously in 80% of cases, usually before the source can be identified. Recurrent bleeding will, however, occur in 15% to 30% of these patients.

Initial management is supportive, including close hemodynamic monitoring and, in appropriate cases, blood transfusion. Surgery is rarely required for management, except in cases with hemodynamic instability refractory to resuscitation and transfusion, or recurrent or ongoing bleeding that cannot be controlled by other means. When bleeding persists, all efforts should be made to localize the source, in an attempt to focus surgical resection and ensure that bleeding is indeed arising from the colon. A suggested algorithm for the evaluation of presumed diverticular LGIB is shown in **Figure 3**. Those with suspicion of UGIB (bloody nasogastric aspirate, history of peptic ulcer disease, recent NSAID use, cirrhosis, etc.) should undergo urgent upper endoscopy. Once an upper tract source has been excluded, the next test of choice may be either colonoscopy or angiography, depending on the patient's condition, and institutional preference.

For patients with brisk ongoing bleeding, many advocate urgent angiography for localization and embolization. In some institutions, tagged red blood cell scan is used as a screening test, because of its higher sensitivity, to decide which patients will undergo angiography. If a bleeding source is found

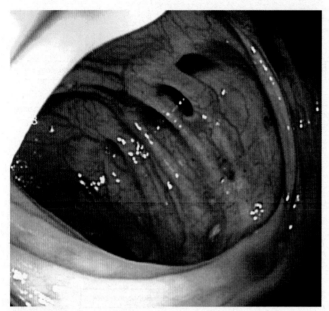

FIGURE 1 • Colonoscopy in a patient with LGIB, revealing diverticulosis, but no source of active bleeding.

on angiography, selective therapeutic embolization is attempted. If successful, patients can undergo elective colonoscopy after the bleeding episode has resolved. Colon resection in this setting is not obligatory because <20% of embolization patients will develop mucosal ischemia in the devascularized colon. If bleeding cannot be controlled with embolization, the angiographer can leave a catheter in the bleeding vessel to facilitate

localization at the time of surgery. In patients with recurrent intermittent bleeding and repeatedly negative angiograms, "provocative" angiography may be considered, using catheter-directed vasodilators, anticoagulants, or thrombolytics to reactivate a quiescent bleeding source. Provocative procedures should be performed only if urgent surgical intervention can be performed when needed.

Others advocate urgent colonoscopy for patients with ongoing bleeding, either with a "rapid-purge" bowel preparation with polyethylene glycol, or preparation by enema only. Rates of colonoscopy completion and of successful localization of bleeding in this setting vary widely in the literature. Some nonrandomized studies have suggested that urgent colonoscopy with endoscopic epinephrine injection, coagulation, and/or clipping reduces rates of rebleeding, as compared with delayed colonoscopy. The only randomized study on the topic (Green et al., 2005), however, found that urgent colonoscopy increased rates of localization, without reduction in mortality, length of stay, or need for surgical resection. In a hemodynamically stable patient, it is reasonable, therefore, to perform colonoscopy either promptly during the acute hospitalization, or electively after resolution of the bleeding episode. Regardless of timing, all patients with acute LGIB who have not had a recent complete colon evaluation should undergo colonoscopy to exclude neoplasm.

Despite all attempts, bleeding can be difficult to localize in patients with intermittent diverticular bleeding. Some patients may require surgery even in

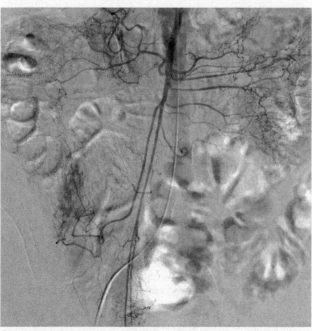 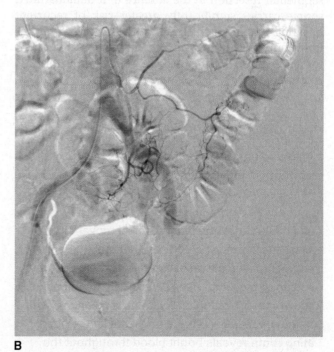

FIGURE 2 • Images from selective mesenteric angiogram revealing normal anatomy without evidence of active bleeding from the (**A**) superior mesenteric artery distribution and (**B**) inferior artery distribution.

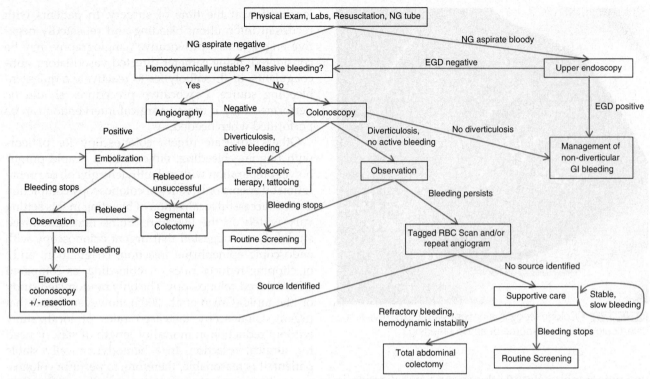

FIGURE 3 • A suggested algorithm for the evaluation and management of patients with acute LGIB presumed to be from bleeding colonic diverticula.

the absence of localization, due to repeated episodes of bleeding or acute hemodynamic instability. Because diverticulosis is most common in the sigmoid and descending colon, empiric left-sided resections were once advocated for such nonlocalized LGIB. However, segmental resection in the absence of a demonstrated source carries significantly greater risk of recurrent bleeding than total colectomy in this setting, and has fallen out of favor. Instead, when resection is required for unlocalized LGIB, total abdominal colectomy is recommended.

Presentation Continued

After angiography in our patient, his bleeding stops and the patient is transferred out of the intensive care unit. Two days later he has severe abdominal cramping, becomes hypotensive, and has a very large bloody bowel movement, associated with a 10% drop in hematocrit. Repeat angiography again fails to demonstrate a definite source of bleeding. He is persistently hypotensive, so with resuscitation ongoing, he is taken urgently to the operating room. Colonoscopy in the operating room reveals bright blood throughout the colon, but a discrete source cannot be identified.

TABLE 1. Key Technical Steps and Potential Pitfalls for Total Abdominal Colectomy

Key Technical Steps

1. Lithotomy position, or supine with split-leg position.
2. Exploration for source of bleeding (colonoscopy, enteroscopy, bimanual palpation).
3. Mobilize ascending colon and hepatic flexure, ligate ileocolic vascular pedicle, and divide ileum.
4. If preserving omentum, separate from transverse colon; if resecting omentum, divide and ligate outside the gastroepiploic arcade.
5. Mobilize sigmoid and descending colon, take down splenic flexure, and ligate inferior mesenteric and middle colic vascular pedicles.
6. Mobilize and ligate upper mesorectum, and divide across upper rectum.
7. Construct ileorectal anastomosis or ileostomy.

Potential Pitfalls

- Failure to identify an upper GI or small bowel source of bleeding.
- Ureteral injury, typically due to dissection into the retroperitoneum, or during ligation of the inferior mesenteric artery pedicle.
- Duodenal injury, due to dissection too far posteriorly on approach to the hepatic flexure.
- Avulsion of a middle colic vein due to excessive traction on the hepatic flexure.
- Splenic capsule laceration due to excessive traction on attachments to the splenic flexure.
- Hypogastric nerve injury during mobilization of the upper mesorectum.

Surgical Approach for Total Abdominal Colectomy

Patients with persistent unlocalized bleeding may require operation **(Table 1)**. After adequate resuscitation and correction of coagulopathy, all efforts should again be made to localize bleeding in the operating room before undertaking resection. The patient should be positioned in the lithotomy or split-leg position to permit access to the anus for colonoscopy and/or anastomotic leak testing. Exploration and resection are typically performed through a midline laparotomy but, in a hemodynamically stable patient without prohibitive intra-abdominal adhesions, may be performed laparoscopically with or without hand assistance by surgeons with expertise in laparoscopic colon surgery. Trocar arrangements for total colectomy vary, but we favor the use of an umbilical trocar for the camera and dissecting ports in all four quadrants. When using a hand-assist technique, a hand port is placed in the suprapubic position, through a Pfannenstiel or a lower midline incision. The specimen can be extracted through the hand port incision, or through a suprapubic, periumbilical, or stoma incision, depending on approach and anatomy. On-table colonoscopy, ideally with carbon dioxide insufflation, can be used to evaluate the colon intraoperatively. A colonoscope passed orally can often traverse the entire small intestine if the bowel is manually reduced over the scope. Bimanual palpation and transillumination of the intestine can identify mass lesions. If no convincing source can be identified, but bleeding is absent proximal to the ileocecal valve, total abdominal colectomy is recommended.

The colon is mobilized from the retroperitoneum by incision along the line of Toldt. On the right, the ureter and the gonadal vessels are identified and protected within the retroperitoneum, and the duodenum is swept posteriorly as dissection approaches the hepatic flexure. Care must be taken to avoid avulsing venous tributaries of the superior mesenteric vein as the flexure is elevated medially. The gastrocolic omentum can be preserved, by separating it from the transverse colon, or resected with the specimen by dividing it outside the gastroepiploic arcade. The transverse mesocolon is separated from the omentum, and then mobilized from the retroperitoneum through dissection in the lesser sac. At this point, division of the ileum and the ileocolic pedicle facilitates exposure for mobilization of the left and sigmoid colon. On the left, care is taken to avoid injury to the splenic capsule when taking down the flexure, and the ureter and the gonadal vessels must be identified and protected in the retroperitoneum during mobilization of the sigmoid colon and ligation of the inferior mesenteric artery pedicle. As dissection continues behind the upper rectum in the presacral space, the hypogastric nerves, which contribute to sexual function, are preserved by sweeping them down off the mesorectum. After ligating the remaining mesenteric vasculature, the bowel is divided across the upper rectum, either with a linear stapler or between bowel clamps, and the specimen is passed off the field. Intestinal continuity can be restored with an ileorectal anastomosis, or end ileostomy can be constructed and the rectal stump turned in and left closed.

Special Intraoperative Considerations

Because most LGIB is managed without surgery, those patients who require total abdominal colectomy in this setting typically will be either acutely unstable, or debilitated from protracted preoperative manipulations. In the presence of hemodynamic instability, malnutrition, major comorbidity, inflammatory disease of the terminal ileum or rectum, or poor anal sphincter function and fecal incontinence, ileorectal anastomosis should be avoided, and end ileostomy performed. Ileostomy and mucous fistula is also an option, but the divided rectum typically will not reach the abdominal wall, so the distal transection must occur above the rectosigmoid junction if mucous fistula is planned. The finding of an unexpected malignancy requires careful attention to an oncologically appropriate mesenteric lymphadenectomy. Other unexpected findings, such as inflammatory bowel disease, Meckel's diverticulum, arterial–intestinal fistula, or others, would require alteration of the operative plan and a focus on the source of bleeding.

Postoperative Management

Because of the extensive abdominal dissection, postoperative ileus after total abdominal colectomy is common. Total parenteral nutrition is often required, because patients who require surgery for LGIB may have suffered through extensive preoperative workup with prolonged restriction of oral nutrition. Routine prophylaxis for deep venous thrombosis should be used. Postoperative antibiotics are not typically necessary. After return of bowel function, stool output may be liquid and high volume, and the use of bulking agents plus antidiarrheal medications such as loperamide or diphenoxylate/atropine is often required to avoid dehydration. After the initial recovery period, most patients will continue permanently with several stools per day. Patients with good preoperative anal sphincter function will typically not suffer major deterioration in their continence.

Anastomotic leak rates after ileorectal anastomosis range from 2% to 5%. Leak can present as fever, pain, ileus, diarrhea, tenesmus, urinary retention, or fistula.

Depending on patient condition and the location, size, and spread of the leak, management might involve simple observation, percutaneous drainage, transanal repair, or reoperation with repair or resection of anastomosis and fecal diversion.

TAKE HOME POINTS

- Diverticular bleeding accounts for a majority of LGIB requiring hospitalization in adults.
- Diverticular bleeding is self-limited in 80% of cases, but 15% to 30% will have recurrent bleeding.
- Options for localization of LGIB include angiography, flexible endoscopy, capsule endoscopy, and nuclear scintigraphy.
- Indications for surgery in LGIB include recurrent refractory bleeding or hemodynamic instability.
- The operation of choice for unlocalized LGIB distal to the ileocecal valve is total abdominal colectomy, with ileorectal anastomosis or end ileostomy.

SUGGESTED READINGS

ASGE Standards of Practice Committee. An annotated algorithmic approach to acute lower gastrointestinal bleeding. Gastrointest Endosc. 2001;53:859–863.

ASGE Standards of Practice Committee. The role of endoscopy in the patient with lower-GI bleeding. Gastrointest Endosc. 2005;62:656–660.

Green BT, Rockey DC, Portwood G, et al. Urgent colonoscopy for evaluation and management of acute lower gastrointestinal hemorrhage: a randomized controlled trial. Am J Gastroenterol. 2005;100:2395–2402.

Hoedema RE, Luchtefeld MA. The management of lower gastrointestinal hemorrhage. Dis Colon Rectum. 2005;48:2010–2024.

Jensen DM, Machicado GA, Jutabha R, et al. Urgent colonoscopy for the diagnosis and treatment of severe diverticular hemorrhage. N Engl J Med. 2000;342:78–82.

Khanna A, Ognibene SJ, Koniaris LG. Embolization as first-line therapy for diverticulosis-related massive lower gastrointestinal bleeding: evidence from a meta-analysis. J Gastrointest Surg. 2005;9:343–352.

36 Splenic Flexure Colon Cancer

DANIEL ALBO

Presentation

An 83-year-old patient with known history of diabetes mellitus, hypertension, chronic renal failure, and congestive heart failure presents with a 2-week history of crampy abdominal pain following meals with thin-caliber bowel movements but no nausea and vomiting. His vital signs were normal. On physical exam, his abdomen was nontender, somewhat distended, with a palpable mass in the left upper quadrant of his abdomen. His rectal exam revealed guaiac-positive brown stool. His laboratory exams were significant for a hemoglobin of 10, a white cell blood count of 9, a creatinine of 2.9, and an albumin of 2.9.

Differential Diagnosis

An elderly patient presenting with symptomatic anemia, a high-grade partial bowel obstruction, and a palpable left upper-quadrant mass is highly suggestive of a distal colon cancer. However, the differential diagnosis is relatively broad and includes inflammatory conditions such as diverticulitis (less likely in this patient due to the lack of a fever and of left-sided abdominal tenderness on exam and with a normal white cell blood count), ischemic colitis (although he has risk factors for vascular disease, he did not present with bloody diarrhea, and he had a palpable left upper-quadrant mass), an enlarged spleen (such as seen in hematologic malignancies), and other neoplastic processes involving the left upper quadrant (gastric, pancreatic tail, adrenal or kidney cancer as well as retroperitoneal sarcomas).

Workup

The patient underwent a computed tomography (CT) scan of the abdomen and the pelvis (with oral contrast only due to his elevated creatinine), which revealed a large, obstructing mass in the splenic flexure of the colon (Figure 1), with a moderately distended cecum (<10 cm) and small bowel, with no evidence of liver metastases or carcinomatosis. A colonoscopy revealed a nearly completely obstructing mass at the level of the splenic flexure of the colon (Figure 2). The mass could not be traversed and they were unable to evaluate the proximal colon. A biopsy was obtained that showed a moderately to poorly differentiated adenocarcinoma. A carcino embrionic antigen (CEA) level was obtained and it was 34.6. This workup confirmed the diagnosis of an obstructing splenic flexure colon cancer.

Discussion

Carcinoma of the transverse colon (of which splenic flexure colon cancer is a subset) accounts for 10% of all colorectal cancers. Diagnosis is often delayed and complicated forms (perforation, fistulization, obstruction) occur in 30% to 50% of cases. The progression of symptoms is often insidious and tumors may be quite large by the time of diagnosis. These tumors can also extend or fistulize into adjacent organs. Distal transverse cancers may be small annular lesions, which are prone to obstruction.

From a surgeon's perspective, it is important to consider two types of complete colonic obstructions, those with a competent or with an incompetent ileocecal valve. In patients with an incompetent ileocecal valve, the pressure that builds up proximal to the splenic flexure tumor partially decompresses into the small bowel, allowing for preoperative stabilization of the patient (by nasogastric tube decompression, rehydration, and correction of underlying electrolyte disorders) and performance of a full workup, including a colonoscopy. Patients that present with a complete large bowel obstruction with a competent ileocecal valve, on the other hand, represent a true surgical emergency. In these patients, the pressure that builds up proximal to the splenic flexure tumor cannot decompress into the small bowel due to the competency of the ileocecal valve. In this situation, the proximal colon will progressively get more dilated and the tension on the proximal colonic wall will increase. According to Laplace's law, the increase in tension on the wall of the cavity will be directly proportional to the fourth potency of radius of the cavity. Therefore, the part of the proximal

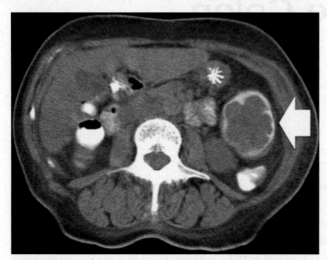

FIGURE 1 • CT scan of the abdomen showing a large, obstructing splenic flexure colon cancer (*arrow*). This CT scan was obtained with oral contrast only due to the patient's impaired kidney function.

colon with the largest radius, the cecum, will suffer the greatest increase in colonic wall tension. This increase in wall tension will lead to collapse of the intramural capillaries and ischemia, eventually producing a catastrophic cecal perforation. Patients with a complete colonic obstruction that present with right lower-quadrant abdominal pain should be operated on emergently, since this likely represent a sign of an impending cecal rupture. Colonoscopy in these patients is formally contraindicated, since it could lead to a critical delay before surgery, and the increase in intraluminal pressure due to insufflation during the colonoscopy could lead to a full-blown cecal perforation.

Workup

Clinical presentation permitting, the preoperative staging workup should include a CT scan of the abdomen and the pelvis with oral and intravenous contrast, a chest x-ray or a CT scan of the chest, a CEA blood level, and a full colonoscopy. In patients with bulky splenic flexure tumors in which it is not possible to evaluate the proximal colon by colonoscopy, a barium enema is indicated to rule out synchronous colon cancer in the proximal colon, although it frequently is either not feasible or reliable. Although the use of on-table colonoscopy through the appendiceal orifice has been described, this is often not practical. The incidence of a synchronous proximal colon cancer, though, is only about 5%, and only a subset of these synchronous tumors will not be detected by either preoperative CT scan or intraoperative palpation of the colon. Therefore, although evaluation of the full colon preoperatively by colonoscopy is preferred, in patients in whom evaluation of the proximal colon is just not possible, it is acceptable to perform surgery for the splenic flexure tumor and perform a short-interval colonoscopy postoperatively (6 months after surgery) to fully evaluate the reminder of the colon.

Surgical Approach

Colonic stenting is the best option either for palliation or as a bridge to surgery in patients with a complete bowel obstruction due to a splenic flexure colon cancer with a competent ileocecal valve. This approach reduces morbidity and mortality rate and it eliminates the need for temporary colostomy. Nevertheless, surgical management remains relevant as colonic stenting

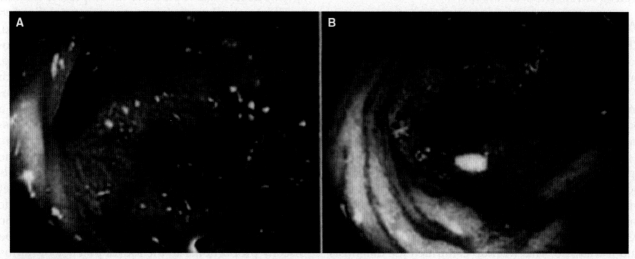

FIGURE 2 • Colonoscopy. **A:** Splenic flexure of the colon showing a large, fungating circumferential mass that is obstructing the lumen of colon. **B:** Descending colon, showing a normal colonic lumen distal to the splenic flexure mass and some evidence of bleeding from the tumor.

has a small rate of failure, and it is not always available. There are various surgical options for dealing with patients with obstructing splenic flexure colon cancer. One-stage primary resection and anastomosis is the preferred choice for low-risk patients. It is paramount to not only resect the bowel segment involving the splenic flexure of the colon with negative margins of resection, but to also include the entire lymphovascular pedicles associated with the splenic flexure of the colon (a minimum of 12 lymph nodes should be obtained). These include the left colic vessels, the left branches of the middle colic vessels, and the inferior mesenteric vein. Subtotal colectomy is useful in cases of proximal bowel damage (i.e., cecal perforation) or synchronous tumors. A two-stage procedure, with a resection and colostomy as a first step and colostomy takedown as a second step, should be reserved for high-risk patients. A three-stage procedure, with the creation of simple colostomy as a first stage, has no role other than for use in very ill patients who are not fit for any other procedure. The multistage approach is marred by a higher cumulative rate of perioperative morbidity and mortality and frequent failure to complete the planned sequence of operations and a resulting high permanent stoma rate (up to 40% of patients).

One of the most significant changes in colon surgery over the last decade has been the increased application

TABLE 1. Advantages of Minimally Invasive Surgery for Colon Cancer

- Smaller incisions
- Less pain
- Less use of narcotics
- Faster return to bowel function
- Shorter hospital stays
- Lower incidence of wound complications:
  - Wound infections
  - Incisional hernias
- Lower incidence of cardiopulmonary complications
- Faster recovery
- Potential decrease in overall cost of care

of minimally invasive surgery (MIS) techniques. MIS offers several key short-term patient advantages to open surgery **(Table 1)**, including less perioperative pain, smaller incisions **(Figure 3B)**, shorter hospital stays, faster recovery, and lower wound morbidity (including wound infections and incisional hernias). In elderly patients, and in patients with significant comorbidities, it may also reduce the incidence of postoperative pulmonary and cardiac complications. In addition, we believe that laparoscopic surgery offers a superior visualization in the left upper quadrant of the abdomen and an easier, more controlled mobilization of the splenic flexure versus open surgery **(Figure 3A)**.

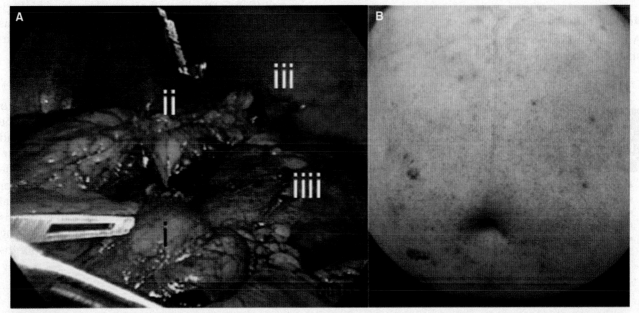

FIGURE 3 • **HALS** for colon cancer of the splenic flexure. **A:** Full mobilization of the splenic flexure showing the splenic flexure of the colon (i) fully mobilized to the midline, the tail of the pancreas (ii), the spleen (iii), and Gerota's fascia (iv). **B:** 10 days postoperatively, the extraction site (placed as small transverse suprapubic incision hiding in a skin crease) and the 5-mm umbilical port site are no longer visible. The 5-mm and the 12-mm right-sided port sites are noticeable only due to the Dermabond that we use to seal the incisions; after the Dermabond falls off, these ports will be barely noticeable.

Due to these advantages, for surgeons with the requisite skill and experience, we feel strongly that MIS should be considered the preferred approach to patients with colon cancer, including those with splenic flexure tumors.

Patients with large splenic flexure tumors can be particularly challenging even for advanced laparoscopic surgeons. The position of these tumors deep in the left upper quadrant and the close proximity to the spleen, the pancreas, and the stomach can make these cases extremely complex. As a result, surgeons tend to shy away from laparoscopic surgery in the management of these tumors. An alternative to conventional laparoscopic surgery is hand-assisted laparoscopic surgery (HALS). In this technique, the surgeon has the option of introducing a hand in the abdomen during surgery through a special port (called a Gelport) that can be inserted in the expected extraction site. This provides the surgeon with tactile feedback and allows for greater versatility during surgery. While preserving all the known short-term advantages of conventional laparoscopic surgery versus open surgery, HALS offers several key advantages over conventional laparoscopic surgery **(Table 2)**, including higher percentage of utilization of MIS, lower conversion to open rates, shorter operating times, and lower estimated blood loss rates. Key operative principles of MIS for the surgical management of splenic flexure colon cancer are summarized in **Table 3**.

Adjuvant Therapy

Adjuvant chemotherapy is reserved for patients with stage III (positive lymph nodes) and stage IV (distant

---

TABLE 2. Advantages of HALS Over Conventional Laparoscopy in the Management of Splenic Flexure Tumors

- Increased utilization of MIS
- Shorter operative times
- Lower conversion to open surgery rates
- Lower estimated blood loss
- Same short-term advantages over open surgery than conventional laparoscopy

---

TABLE 3. Key Technical Steps During HALS for Splenic Flexure Colon Cancer (HALS left hemicolectomy)

- Port placement: Gelport at extraction site (6-cm Pfannenstiel incision), 5-mm camera port (umbilicus), and two working ports, a 5-mm port in the right upper quadrant, and a 12-mm port in the right lower quadrant of the abdomen
- Step 1: Transect inferior mesenteric vein at the level of the ligament of Treitz.
- Step 2: Transect the left colic artery at the level of its origin from the inferior mesenteric artery.
- Step3: Complete medial to lateral mobilization of the splenic flexure of the colon.
- Step 4: Transect the white line of Toldt.
- Step 5: Transect splenocolic and gastrocolic ligaments.
- Step 6: Intracorporeal transection of the colon
- Step 7: Intracorporeal colo-colonic anastomosis

---

metastases) disease. Node-negative patients that may be considered for adjuvant chemotherapy include patient with high-risk characteristics, including lymphovascular invasion, perineural invasion, and lack of microsatellite instability. For patients with borderline lesions, genetic testing (such as Oncotype evaluation) is rapidly emerging as a potentially useful tool in determining which node-negative patients may benefit from additional therapy. Current adjuvant therapy protocols often times include oxalloplatin and 5-fluorouracil (FOLFOX) chemotherapy. The use of biological cancer therapy (such as Avastin) is also emerging as a potential treatment option in addition to more standard chemotherapy regimens.

Surveillance

Eighty five percent of colon cancer recurrences occur within 3 years of surgery, with the majority of the remaining recurrences occurring between years 3 and 5. The 2005 American Society of Clinical Oncology surveillance recommendations for colon cancer include an annual CT scan of the chest and abdomen for 3 years, a colonoscopy at 3 years, a history and physical examination and risk assessment every 3 to 6 months for the first 3 years and then every 6 months during years 4 and 5, and a CEA level checked every 3 months for at least 3 years after surgery.

Case Conclusion

The patient underwent a hand-assisted laparoscopic left hemicolectomy with a primary stapled midtransverse colon-sigmoid anastomosis. During surgery, we found a very large mass in the splenic flexure of the colon, with no direct extension into contiguous organs, and no evidence of synchronous colonic lesions in the right colon, liver metastases, or carcinomatosis. The estimated blood loss was <50 mL, and the operative time was 120 minutes. The patient recovered uneventfully and was discharged home on postoperative day 4, tolerating a regular diet, ambulating, with minimal incisional pain, and having bowel movements. The final pathology revealed an ulcerated, moderately differentiated adenocarcinoma involving the entire lumen of the colon that extended through the colonic wall and into the pericolonic adipose tissue with negative proximal, distal, and radial margins. There were 26 lymph nodes with no evidence of malignancy. There was no evidence of lymphovascular or perineural invasion. The tumor was positive for MLH-1, MSH-2, MSH-6, and PMS-2 by immunoperoxidase staining (microsatellite instability).

Due to the patient's advanced age, adequate lymphadenectomy negative for cancer, and lack of lymphovascular and perineural invasion, and the presence of microsatellite instability in the primary tumor, the medical oncologist decided that chemotherapy was not indicated in this patient.

TAKE HOME POINTS

- Diagnosis of transverse colon cancer is often delayed and complicated forms (perforation, fistulization, obstruction) occur in 30% to 50% of cases.
- Patients that present with a complete large bowel obstruction with a competent ileocecal valve represent a true surgical emergency.
- Clinical presentation permitting, the preoperative staging workup should include a CT scan of the abdomen and the pelvis with oral and intravenous contrast, a chest x-ray or a CT scan of the chest, a CEA blood level, and a full colonoscopy.
- Colonic stenting is the best option either for palliation or as a bridge to surgery in high-risk patients with a complete bowel obstruction due to a splenic flexure colon cancer with a competent ileocecal valve.
- In paitents undergoing surgery, it is paramount to not only resect the bowel segment involving the splenic fl exure of the colon with negative margins of resection, but to also include the entire lymphovascular pedicles associated with the splenic flexure of the colon (a minimum of 12 lymph nodes should be obtained). This should include include high ligation of the left colic vessels, the left branches of the middle colic vessels, and the inferior mesenteric vein.
- Subtotal colectomy is useful in cases of proximal bowel damage (i.e., cecal perforation) or synchronous tumors.

SUGGESTED READINGS

Comparison of self-expanding metal stents and urgent surgery for left-sided malignant colonic obstruction in elderly patients. Dig Dis Sci. 2011;56:2706–10.

Guo MG, Feng Y, Zheng Q, Di JZ, Wang Y, Fan YB, Huang XY. NCCN Clinical Practice Guidelines in Oncology: colon cancer. National Comprehensive Cancer Network. J Natl Compr Canc Netw. 2009 Sep;7(8):778–831.

Stipa F, Pigazzi A, Bascone B, Cimitan A, Villotti G, Burza A, Vitale A. Management of obstructive colorectal cancer with endoscopic stenting followed by single-stage surgery: open or laparoscopic resection? Surg Endosc. 2008;22:1477–81.

37 Anastomotic Leak After Colectomy

NEIL HYMAN

Presentation

A 64-year-old man with hypertension and mild chronic obstructive pulmonary disease is now 6 days after an elective sigmoid colectomy for recurrent diverticulitis. His initial postoperative course was unremarkable, but he developed confusion and agitation on the evening of postoperative day 4. His abdomen became more distended, but he did not have evidence of peritonitis. His morphine was stopped and a nasogastric tube was inserted. He seemed to improve somewhat initially, but then developed progressive tachypnea and a low-grade fever over the next 24 hours. He remained hemodynamically stable but required two fluid boluses to maintain adequate urine output. On postoperative day 6, his clinical status became acutely worse. At this point, he developed respiratory distress and tachycardia with a heart rate of 130. His lungs were clear with decreased breath sounds at the bases. He had marked abdominal distention and was tender across his lower abdomen with diffuse peritoneal signs.

Differential Diagnosis

Anastomotic leaks are perhaps the most dreaded complication of bowel resection. The reported incidence varies greatly based on definitions, indication for surgery, and anastomotic site. For a sigmoid colon resection, the anastomotic leak rate should be approximately 5%. Early postoperative leaks typically present in a dramatic fashion with severe abdominal pain, tachycardia, high fevers, and a rigid abdomen, often with hemodynamic instability. But leaks manifesting further along the postoperative course usually present far more insidiously, often with low-grade fever, ileus, and failure to progress. This latter presentation often mimics other infectious complications, such as pneumonia or urinary tract infection, or an early postoperative small bowel obstruction. Mental status changes and tachypnea are often the earliest signs of anastomotic leak, but these signs are nonspecific and could also suggest pulmonary embolism, pneumonia, atelectasis or an adverse drug reaction. In our patient scenario, the patient presents with symptoms that were initially nonspecific (fever, tachypnea, and tachycardia) and the differential diagnosis would include leak as well as other infectious complications.

But the patient eventually progresses to having a distended abdomen with peritonitis, which makes anastomotic leak the clear working diagnosis.

Workup

Patients with an early postoperative leak often have signs and symptoms of peritonitis and sepsis. In many circumstances, the diagnosis is clinically evident, and prompt return to the operating room is warranted. Too often, radiologic studies are wishfully obtained, when the indication for reexploration is clear. These studies should be limited to cases where there is some clinical uncertainty about the diagnosis. A water-soluble contrast enema will often rapidly confirm the presence of a leak in equivocal cases in the first few days after surgery (Figure 1). However, later in the postoperative period when the leaks that manifest themselves tend to be smaller and contained, this study becomes less reliable and a CT scan is preferable. In our experience, contrast enema failed to show a proven leak 60% of the time.

As described above, most leaks occurring later in the postoperative course are associated with a nonspecific presentation, and the diagnosis can actually be quite difficult to make. It must be recognized that a clouded sensorium or respiratory symptoms are often the presenting signs of a leak.

A chest x-ray and PE protocol chest CT scan may demonstrate pneumonia, lobar collapse, or pulmonary embolism. However, caution must be exercised in ascribing a downhill clinical course to subtle or minor abnormalities on these studies. Laboratory

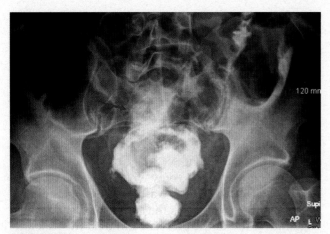

FIGURE 1 • Anastomotic leak: Contrast enema. *Arrow* indicates extravasation of water-soluble contrast from the colorectal anastomosis.

evaluation is generally nonspecific and often indicative of early multiorgan dysfunction. Plain abdominal films are not usually specific enough to make the diagnosis, but a large or an increasing amount of free intraperitoneal air is suggestive of a leak. The most helpful study in the setting of an occult leak is usually a CT scan of the abdomen and the pelvis with rectal contrast **(Figure 2)**. We have found that CT demonstrates the diagnosis almost 90% of the time; but it must be acknowledged that there is broad overlap in CT findings in postoperative patients with or without a leak. Free air may be present up to 10 days in patients without a leak and loculated air up to 30 days after surgery.

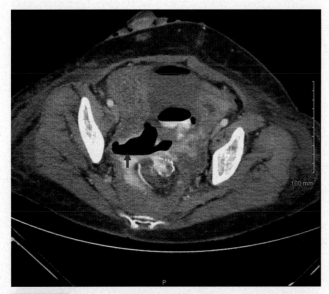

FIGURE 2 • Anastomotic leak: CT scan. *Arrow* denotes the interface between extraluminal air and extravasated rectal contrast.

Diagnosis and Treatment

Leaks occurring within the first few days after surgery almost invariably require operative exploration. Patients should be properly prepared for surgery with fluid resuscitation, administration of broad-spectrum antibiotics, and adequate intravenous access. A Foley catheter should be inserted as well as appropriate monitors such as a central line and an arterial line as needed. Of particular importance, patients should usually be marked for an intestinal stoma as this will often be required. Many ostomies created in the setting of a leak turn out to be permanent. Poor stoma siting (e.g., in a skin crease) can be a nightmare for the patient and be the difference in whether the patient can reassume self-care once they recover from surgery.

Contained leaks manifesting later on in the postoperative period in stable patients can often be managed nonoperatively with patience, antibiotics, and percutaneous drainage. Reoperation beyond 7 to 10 days after the initial procedure can be hazardous and may make things worse. Minor anastomotic disruptions may heal over time and obviate the need for any further operative treatment and an intestinal stoma.

Surgical Approach

The value and the importance of surgical planning when it comes to the management of an anastomotic leak cannot be overemphasized. Both the patient's physiologic condition and the nature of the leak are crucial to medical decision making. As a rule of thumb, the longer the interval between reoperation and the initial surgery, the more difficult the procedure is likely to be. Surrounding viscera will attempt to seal the leak off, incorporating the anastomosis into an inflammatory mass surrounded by friable bowel with an associated serositis. There is usually an associated ileus making the bowel distended and tense. As such, mobilizing the anastomosis without tearing the bowel or extending the anastomotic defect can be a challenge. In this setting, precision of purpose (e.g., having a clearly defined plan) and technical efficiency (e.g., avoiding unnecessary dissection) are the key elements to success.

The patient is usually positioned supine, but the lithotomy position is preferred in patients who have a colorectal anastomosis, so it can be tested with betadine or inspected endoscopically. The previous incision is utilized and extended as necessary. Using primarily gentle blunt maneuvers, the bowel is pinched off the abdominal wall to facilitate access and exposure. The peritoneal cavity is irrigated and suctioned to clear as needed, and a specimen obtained for Gram stain and culture. The anastomosis is gently exposed and inspected. In a hemodynamically stable patient, right-sided anastomoses (e.g., ileocolic) can be resected and redone as long as the ends are not ischemic. In patients with extensive local sepsis and hemodynamic instability, an end-loop stoma should be created whenever possible **(Figure 3)**. Although the surgeon's primary goal is control of sepsis, exteriorizing the distal end of the bowel will save the patient another major laparotomy down the line to restore gastrointestinal continuity. Resection with anastomosis and proximal loop ileostomy is another alternative.

Left-sided anastomotic leaks usually require fecal diversion. Again, preoperative stoma marking is vital, especially in obese patients. The anastomosis is inspected and the patient's hemodynamic status reviewed. Stable patients with a very small leak in an otherwise intact anastomosis, no ischemia, and minimal local sepsis can be treated with repair, omentoplasty, and loop ileostomy. Otherwise, ischemic anastomoses, major disruptions, or those associated with systemic sepsis should usually have the anastomosis resected and a Hartmann procedure performed. Resection with anastomosis and loop ileostomy is another option for stable patients. Most patients with leaking low colorectal anastomoses are best treated with fecal diversion

and drainage. The anastomosis is usually deep in the pelvis and attempts at exposure will usually worsen the defect. Endoscopic visualization to assure the anastomosis is not ischemic and to visualize the defect can provide the needed information for decision making without worsening the problem. A presacral drain is placed and the omentum is mobilized for placement over the anastomosis (or at least into the pelvis).

Common pitfalls are doing too much or too little at surgery. As noted above, the dissection should be restricted and focused to only what is needed to examine the anastomosis and washout the contaminated fluids. On the other hand, the surgeon must acknowledge the nature of the problem and treat the leak adequately. Anastomotic leaks exact a major emotional toll on the patient, their family, and the operating surgeon. It can be tempting just to suture the hole closed and hope, in lieu of creating an intestinal stoma ("perfuming the pig"). But if the patient had a leak under "ideal" or elective conditions, it is even more likely they will develop another leak in an emergency situation with local and systemic signs of sepsis. Patients who have already suffered a leak often cannot readily tolerate another septic insult. When in doubt, it is a good

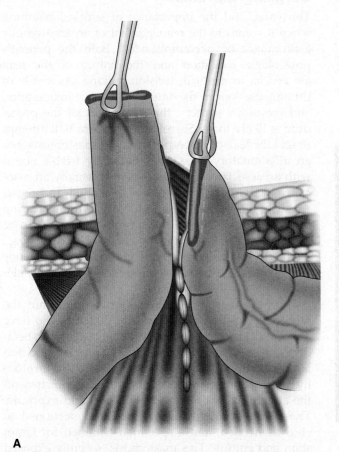

A

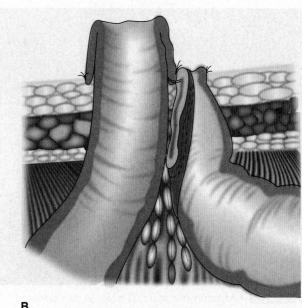

B

FIGURE 3 • End-loop stoma. The ileum and the proximal colon are exteriorized through the same hole to facilitate later closure without the need for laparotomy. **A**: The stapled ileum and the colon are delivered through the stoma site. **B**: A standard Brooke ileostomy is created. The antimesenteric edge of the colonic staple line is excised and sutured to the skin.

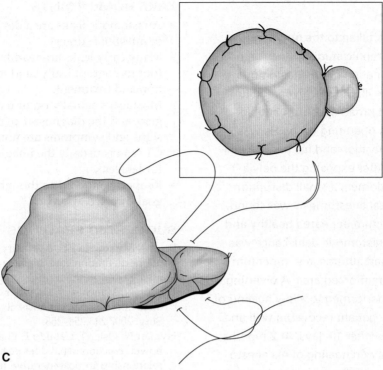

C

FIGURE 3 • *(Continued)* **C**: The end-loop stoma is completed.

time to "phone a friend" and speak with a trusted and experienced colleague **(Table 1)**.

Special Intraoperative Considerations

Special mention is made of the obese patient with a leak. Although the principles of management are the same, there are a few additional considerations. First, most obese patients have a much thinner upper than lower abdomen wall, where most of the pannus resides. Bringing out an ostomy in the lower abdomen without

---

TABLE 1. Key Technical Steps and Potential Pitfalls to Surgical Management of an Anastomotic Leak

Key Technical Steps

1. Adequate resuscitation and stoma marking.
2. Clear and well-delineated preop plan.
3. Careful blunt dissection.
4. Gentle exposure of the anastomosis.
5. Assessment of the patient's hemodynamic status.
6. Resect and redo it on the right if stable.
7. End-loop stoma on the right if unstable.
8. Repair/redo and proximal diversion on the left if stable.
9. Resect and stoma on the left if unstable.

Potential Pitfalls

- Have a plan.
- Don't "perfume the pig."
- Phone a friend as needed.

---

undue tension or ischemia may be difficult or impossible. As such, strong consideration should be given to placing the stoma in the right (or left) upper quadrant. Further, a loop ileostomy is possible in almost any patient, whereas creating a colostomy in an obese patient with a leak may be a nightmare. The bowel is friable; there is marked distension from the associated ileus; and the mesentery may be rigid, inflamed, and unyielding. This is one scenario where either repair with diverting loop ileostomy or resection with anastomosis and proximal loop ileostomy may be the only option.

Postoperative Management

An anastomotic leak is associated with a mortality rate of 10% to 15%. The first step in postoperative management is to support the patient through the sepsis as needed with inotropes, ventilatory support, and modern intensive care. Unfortunately, patients who leak commonly required prolonged hospitalization, further reoperations, and aggressive rehabilitation. Antibiotics should be administered in a goal-directed manner (e.g., until afebrile with normal white blood cell count and ileus resolves) instead of continued indefinitely. Nutritional support, good enterostomal therapy, and careful wound management are usually cornerstones of supportive care. Patients who have been reoperated for a leak are at high risk for further complications such as wound infection or intra-abdominal abscess and often require postoperative imaging studies and percutaneous drainage of residual infected collections.

Case Conclusion

In our patient, he was taken to the operating room without radiographic studies, since he had a clear clinical presentation of an anastomotic leak and was severely ill. He was given additional intravenous fluid and broad-spectrum antibiotics while readying an operating room. He was placed in lithotomy position and his midline incision was reopened. After exposing the pelvis and irrigating the abdomen, a small disruption in the lateral colorectal anastomosis was found. The colon and the rectum appeared healthy and viable. The area of anastomotic dehiscence was reinforced with lembert sutures, and omentum was placed over the reinforced area. A diverting loop ileostomy was performed to allow healing of the anastomosis. The patient recovered well and was discharged home after 10 days. At 2 months, a contrast enema showed healing of his anastomosis without leak or stricture. His ileostomy was taken down electively 3 months after his initial surgery.

TAKE HOME POINTS

- Anastomotic leaks are a devastating complication of intestinal surgery.
- Many early leaks are readily diagnosed clinically (not radiographically) and require prompt reoperation and treatment.
- Most leaks actually occur 6 days or more after surgery, and the diagnosis can be very challenging as signs and symptoms are nonspecific.
- CT scan is usually the imaging modality of choice for late leaks.
- Reoperation requires thoughtful planning and a goal-directed approach.

SUGGESTED READINGS

Bruce J, Krukowski ZH, Al-Khairy G, et al. Systematic review of the definition and management of anastomotic leak after gastrointestinal surgery. Br J Surg. 2001;88:1157–1168.

Hyman N, Manchester TL, Osler T, et al. Anastomotic leaks after intestinal anastomosis: its later than you think. Ann Surg. 2007;245:254–258.

Hyman N, Osler T, Cataldo P, et al. Anastomotic leaks after bowel resection: what does peer review teach us about the relationship to postoperative mortality? J Am Coll Surg. 2009:208:48–52.

Power N, Atri M, Ryan S, et al. CT assessment of anastomotic bowel leak. Clin Radiol. 2007;62:37–42.

38 Large Bowel Obstruction from Colon Cancer

NOELLE L. BERTELSON and DAVID A. ETZIONI

Presentation

A 78 year-old female is evaluated in the emergency department with a 2-day history of worsening nausea/anorexia, abdominal pain, and obstipation. Her last bowel movement and flatus were 36 hours ago. She has no significant medical history and no prior abdominal or pelvic surgical procedures; her vital signs are normal. On examination, her abdomen is soft and nontender but is significantly distended. Her white blood cell count is 10.3.

Differential Diagnosis

This patient presents with signs and symptoms of a bowel obstruction. Generally speaking, the differential diagnosis of obstruction can be broadly classified as being infectious, inflammatory, or neoplastic in origin. One of the key elements of this patient's history is the absence of prior abdominal or pelvic operations. The most likely cause of this type of presentation varies widely depending on the population from which the patient emerges. In most developed countries, this patient should be considered to have a gastrointestinal malignancy—most commonly colon or rectal cancer—until proven otherwise.

Infectious causes may be related to a wide variety of organisms, none of which occur with great prevalence in the United States but include Ascaris species, Taenia species, tuberculosis, and Yersinia. Diverticulitis and inflammatory bowel disease, including Crohn's, ulcerative colitis, and sarcoidosis, can present with acute/subacute colonic obstruction and on radiologic investigation are indistinguishable from colon cancer. The most common neoplastic disorders of the colon are benign adenomas and their malignant counterpart, adenocarcinoma. Nonclonic carcinoma, either metastatic or extrinsically compressing, also may be involved with the colon. Other less common neoplastic disease entities including lymphoma and carcinoid, followed by sarcoma, plasmacytoma, melanoma, leukemic infiltration, neuroendocrine tumor, medullary carcinoma, and schwannoma are also potential causes of colonic obstruction. Nonneoplastic/noninfectious processes, most notably volvulus and intussusception, can cause acute large bowel obstruction, with volvulus causing 10% of colonic obstructions and intussusception occurring in 1% of all bowel obstructions.

Workup

Initial workup proceeds with a supine x-ray, demonstrating gaseous distention of the right and the proximal transverse colon, with a paucity of gas in the distal colon and rectum (Figure 1). It is worth noting that the small bowel loops are not prominent, and that there is no significant bubble of gastric air. Based on this plain film, a computed tomography (CT) of the abdomen/pelvis with oral and intravenous contrast is ordered (Figure 2). This scan shows an obstructing mass in/around the midportion of the transverse colon. The patient's liver and intraperitoneal structures (omentum, etc.) do not show any evidence of metastatic disease or ascites. Although contrast enemas (with water-soluble contrast) are performed less commonly, they can be useful in this setting. Contrast enemas can identify the location and evaluate the patency of an obstructing or a partially obstructing mass. Alternatively, a CT scan with the instillation of rectal contrast could be used to obtain this information.

Diagnosis and Treatment

Colon cancer is diagnosed in over 110,000 individuals in the United States per year, resulting in approximately 90,000 colectomies. While the vast majority of these undergo surgical treatment on an elective basis, a subset are discovered during evaluation for an acute bowel obstruction.

In the management of any patient with a bowel obstruction, a balance must be struck between the possibility of nonoperative resolution of the patient's problem, and the likelihood of progression to bowel compromise and perforation. The key prognostic feature of this patient's presentation is the presence of a closed loop obstruction. Nondilated terminal ileum

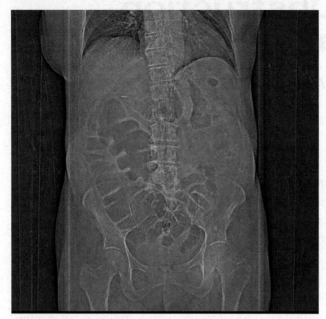

FIGURE 1 • Scout film.

immediately proximal to a distended cecum clearly indicates a competent ileocecal valve. The portion of colon between the ileocecal valve and the obstruction lesion in the transverse colon has no mechanism by which to decompress, and is therefore a closed loop. Any closed loop intestinal obstruction is an indication for *urgent/emergent* decompression.

As surgeons, we all develop a level of comfort with the initial nonoperative treatment of bowel obstructions. Although this approach may be appropriate for selected patients with partial small bowel obstruction, it is often not the right choice for patients with large

bowel obstruction. In this case presentation, without prompt intervention, this patient will progress quickly to compromise of her right colon and perforation. The absence of focal peritonitis or signs of significant systemic toxicity should not be considered reassuring.

Colon obstructions can be decompressed effectively using nonsurgical and surgical approaches. The only reasonable nonsurgical options would involve the endoscopic placement of a self-expanding metallic stent (SEMS). This stent would be used as a "bridge" to surgery, potentially allowing for the operation to be performed electively with a preoperative bowel preparation. Colonoscopic stenting is usually performed for left-sided lesions, but there is an emerging literature regarding their use for right-sided colonic tumors. In small series, they appear to be safe, but there is reason to be skeptical about the effectiveness of this approach: A recent trial examining stenting versus surgery for stage IV left-sided colorectal cancer was closed due to a high rate of serious complications in the stenting arm.

In considering the utility of a colonoscopic stent, it seems sensible to consider the risks of stent placement compared with the benefit (risk reduction) they might provide. In general, ileocolic anastomoses are robust and safe, with leak rates routinely reported at <2%. In this patient, the risks of a procedural complication from stent placement are almost certainly greater than any risk reduction that might be obtained in converting the operation from an urgent to a planned procedure.

What about problems related to the absence of a mechanical bowel preparation? The utility of a mechanical bowel preparation in elective colorectal surgery has been studied extensively. While the majority of the literature in this topic is of poor quality, the overall synthesis (including two large, well-conducted

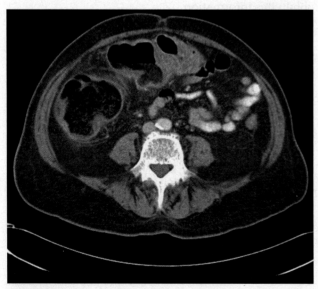

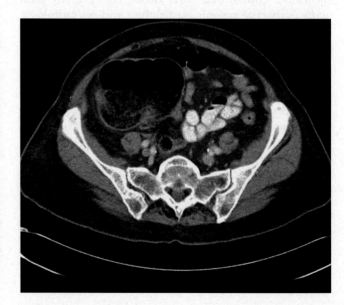

FIGURE 2 • CT scan of abdomen/pelvis.

trials) of existing knowledge is that these efforts provide little, if any, benefit. Placing a stent with the goal of being able to perform bowel preparation would not be justified. Furthermore, in this patient, the bowel (terminal ileum and descending colon) do not demonstrate fecal loading, thereby obviating any benefit of the preparation.

An important issue in planning for this patient is what efforts should be made to ensure that the portion of colorectum that will remain after the resection is free of neoplasia. Case series have documented a 6% to 10% rate of synchronous carcinoma in patients presenting with obstructing colonic tumors. While the proximal dilated portion will necessarily be removed with surgical resection, an intraoperative colonoscopy with minimal insufflation performed to the level of the tumor is a useful and important test.

The best treatment plan for this patient is to proceed to the operating room for intraoperative colonoscopy and subtotal colectomy.

Surgical Approach

The usual administration of prophylactic antibiotics and subcutaneous heparin should be performed. Patient positioning in a low lithotomy position will facilitate both the colonoscopy and the planned operation. While there has been a small case series of laparoscopically managed large bowel obstructions, the extent of distention of the dilation of proximal bowel generally precludes safe laparoscopic mobilization of the colon and should not be performed.

Once the abdomen has been explored through a generous midline incision, the right colon will be easily identified, usually tensely distended and potentially demonstrating early signs of impending perforation (discoloration, deserosalization, etc. **Table 1**). After placing a pursestring suture, a decompressive colotomy in the anterior surface of the proximal right colon will greatly facilitate the procedure. Careful attention to avoiding unnecessary stool spillage will minimize the potential risks from this maneuver.

With the right colon decompressed, dissection proceeds along the right paracolic gutter, moving toward the hepatic flexure. The dissection is carried medially to the level of the anterior surface of the second portion of the duodenum. Great care should be taken in retracting the colon medially, in order to avoid avulsion of the pancreaticoduodenal veins in this region. It is a generally accepted oncologic principle that the omentum is resected en bloc with any transverse colon carcinoma, so the omentum should be removed from the greater curvature of the stomach. This exposes the lesser sac and the transverse mesocolon. Continuing distally, the splenic flexure should be mobilized in order to facilitate an anastomosis between the descending colon and the terminal ileum.

TABLE 1. Key Technical Steps and Potential Pitfalls to Right Colectomy in Presence of Transverse Colon Obstruction

Key Technical Steps

1. Lithotomy positioning.
2. Midline incision, exploratory laparotomy (examine peritoneal surfaces, liver).
3. Decompressive enterotomy in the right colon (if necessary).
4. Mobilize the right colon from lateral to medial.
5. Enter lesser sac at hepatic flexure.
6. Remove greater omentum from stomach.
7. Mobilize splenic flexure.
8. Divide mesentery.
   - Ligate ileocolic vascular pedicle.
   - Ligate middle colic pedicle.
   - Ligate ascending branch of left colic artery.
9. Construct ileocolic anastomosis.
10. Close mesenteric defect.
11. Irrigate and close abdomen.

Potential Pitfalls

- Spillage of stool when decompressing the dilated colon.
- Avulsion of pancreaticoduodenal veins when mobilizing the right colon.
- Leak from an anastomosis due to a splenic flexure (watershed) anastomosis.

The distal extent of the resection is controversial, but for tumors distal to the midtransverse colon, a resection that encompasses the ascending branch of the left colic artery is prudent. An anastomosis to the splenic flexure of the colon is potentially risky because of potential problems with blood supply in this watershed area, especially in older patients or those with known vascular disease. The descending colon is a preferred location for the ileocolic anastomosis.

Once the colon is mobilized, the mesentery is divided and a high ligation is performed for all feeding vessels (ileocolic, middle colic, ascending branch of left colic). An anastomosis is then constructed between terminal ileum and descending colon. There are several options for reconstruction. A hand-sewn end-to-end anastomosis with an inner layer of running absorbable 3-0 (e.g., vicryl) suture and an outer layer of 3-0 interrupted silk sutures is a commonly employed technique. A stapled side-to-side/functional end-to-end anastomosis may also be performed. There are no good data to support one technique as preferred. There is some evidence that leak rates are lower in stapled ileo-transverse anastomoses after right colectomy, but it is uncertain whether this finding can be applied to ileo-descending anastomoses.

After anastomosis, the mesenteric defect may be approximated, and the abdomen is irrigated, and the fascia and skin closed.

Special Intraoperative Considerations
Perforation

In the setting of cecal perforation secondary to distention and ischemic compromise of the bowel wall, resection of the ischemic segment of bowel as well as the tumor is mandatory—in this case, the subtotal colectomy as planned. If the patient is unstable secondary to intra-abdominal sepsis from the perforation, judgment must be exercised in deciding whether to construct an anastomosis. A double-barreled stoma, incorporating the terminal ileum and a corner of the proximal colon, will avoid the risk of anastomotic leakage and allow for stoma reversal in the future without a formal laparotomy.

Duodenal/Pancreatic Invasion

Rarely, a transverse colon carcinoma may involve the duodenum or the head of the pancreas. Intraoperatively, any points of adherence between a known carcinoma and adjacent structures should be considered invasion and mandate consideration for en bloc resection. The magnitude of benefit compared with risk of such a resection needs to be considered on a case-by-case basis. Pancreaticoduodwenectomy can be performed in the setting of invasion into the pancreatic head, and there does appear to be some long-term survival in some patients with small case series quoting up to 55% 5-year survival. Duodenal invasion usually does not require a pancreaticoduodenectomy. When feasible, resection with primary repair should be performed. In cases of more extensive resection, a Roux-en-Y reconstruction with a duodenojejunostomy may be required.

Metastatic Disease

At the time of surgery, it is not uncommon to discover metastatic disease that was not clearly detected on preoperative imaging studies. Metastatic disease should not be considered a contraindication to a palliative resection, though the presence of gross peritoneal disease or a significant burden of hepatic disease may prompt an end stoma or intestinal bypass over anastomosis. In the setting of unexpected hepatic disease, intraoperative ultrasound can assist in further characterizing and identifying lesions. In an otherwise stable patient, isolated metastases amenable to simple wedge resection can reasonably be addressed at the time of the initial operation. However, in an unstable patient, metastatic disease should be noted, confirmed with biopsy, and addressed at a later date. Though outcomes are similar for synchronous resection of colon malignancy with liver metastases, unexpected necessity for a major liver resection of multiple segments or a lobectomy should be discussed with the patient and is likely to great of a physiologic stressor at the time of operation for obstruction.

Postoperative Care

Patient who demonstrate hemodynamic instability in the operating room or who experience unexpected massive fluid shifts/blood loss may require an intermediate level of care; most other patients should not need elevated levels of care. Nasogastric decompression is unnecessary. While early feeding has been associated with some improved outcomes and shorter hospital stays in elective cases, the obstructed patient may have a prolonged ileus, such that feeding should be delayed until the abdomen is flat and the patient is without nausea or emesis. There is no role for routine postoperative antibiotics beyond a 24-hour perioperative period. Prophylaxis for deep venous thromboembolism should be employed routinely, including subcutaneous heparin injections and sequential compression devices for the legs. Discharge can be expected when the patient is tolerating oral feeding and has had a bowel movement. Inpatient oncology consultation and outpatient surveillance are elements of care, which are also part of the standard of care for these patients.

TAKE HOME POINTS

- Obstructing colon cancer is a surgical emergency, especially in the presence of a competent ileocecal valve (closed loop obstruction); clinical findings of focal peritonitis and/or systemic toxicity are late findings.
- Self-expanding metallic stents have no role in the treatment of tumors that are within the scope of a subtotal colectomy (tumors proximal to splenic flexure).
- Intraoperative colonoscopy is an important exam in the stable patient and may lead to changes in the operative plan.
- Primary ileocolic anastomosis should be performed except in cases of hemodynamic instability and gross feculent peritonitis.

SUGGESTED READINGS
Bat L, Neumann G, Shemesh E. The association of synchronous neoplasms with occluding colorectal cancer. Dis Colon Rectum. 1985;28(3):149–151.

Brehant O, Fuks D, Bartoli E, et al. Elective (planned) colectomy in patients with colorectal obstruction after placement of a self-expanding metallic stent as a bridge to surgery: the results of a prospective study. Colorectal Dis. 2009;11(2):178–183.

Choy PY, Bissett IP, Docherty JG, et al. Stapled versus handsewn methods for ileocolic anastomoses. Cochrane Database Syst Rev. 2007;(3):CD004320.

Contant CM, Hop WC, van't Sant HP, et al. Mechanical bowel preparation for elective colorectal surgery: a multicentre randomised trial. Lancet. 2007;370(9605):2112–2117.

Dronamraju SS, Ramamurthy S, Kelly SB, et al. Role of self-expanding metallic stents in the management of malignant obstruction of the proximal colon. Dis Colon Rectum. 2009;52(9):1657–1661.

Etzioni DA, Beart RW Jr, Madoff RD, et al. Impact of the aging population on the demand for colorectal procedures. Dis Colon Rectum. 2009;52(4):583–590; discussion 590–591.

Fujiwara H, Yamasaki M, Nakamura S, et al. Reconstruction of a large duodenal defect created by resection of a duodenal tubulovillous adenoma using a double-tract anastomosis to a retrocolic roux-en-y loop: report of a case. Surg Today. 2002;32(9):824–827.

Gash K, Chambers W, Dixon A. The role of laparoscopic surgery for the management of acute large bowel obstruction. Colorectal Dis. 2009.

Gordon PH, Nivatvongs S. Principles and Practice of Surgery for the Colon, Rectum, and Anus. 3rd ed. New York, NY: Informa Healthcare USA, Inc, 2007.

Jemal A, Siegel R, Ward E, et al. Cancer statistics, 2007. CA Cancer J Clin. 2007;57(1):43–66.

Jung B, Pahlman L, Nystrom PO, et al. Multicentre randomized clinical trial of mechanical bowel preparation in elective colonic resection. Br J Surg. 2007;94(6):689–695.

Lee WS, Lee WY, Chun HK, et al. En bloc resection for right colon cancer directly invading duodenum or pancreatic head. Yonsei Med J. 2009;50(6):803–806.

Lustosa SA, Matos D, Atallah AN, et al. Stapled versus handsewn methods for colorectal anastomosis surgery. Cochrane Database Syst Rev. 2001;(3):CD003144.

Moug SJ, Smith D, Leen E, et al. Evidence for a synchronous operative approach in the treatment of colorectal cancer with hepatic metastases: a case matched study. Eur J Surg Oncol. 2010;36(4):365–370.

Saiura A, Yamamoto J, Ueno M, et al. Long-term survival in patients with locally advanced colon cancer after en bloc pancreaticoduodenectomy and colectomy. Dis Colon Rectum. 2008;51(10):1548–1551.

Slim K, Vicaut E, Launay-Savary MV, et al. Updated systematic review and meta-analysis of randomized clinical trials on the role of mechanical bowel preparation before colorectal surgery. Ann Surg. 2009;249(2):203–209.

van Hooft JE, Fockens P, Marinelli AW, et al. Early closure of a multicenter randomized clinical trial of endoscopic stenting versus surgery for stage IV left-sided colorectal cancer. Endoscopy. 2008;40(3):184–191.

Vitale MA, Villotti G, d'Alba L, et al. Preoperative colonoscopy after self-expandable metallic stent placement in patients with acute neoplastic colon obstruction. Gastrointest Endosc. 2006;63(6):814–819.

39 Colonic Vovulus

ARDEN M. MORRIS

Presentation

A 28-year-old woman presents to the emergency department with complaints of recurrent, severe upper abdominal pain for the third time in 1 month. Prior to her recurrent symptoms of crampy abdominal pain, nausea, and vomiting, the patient had a normal 8-month intrauterine pregnancy and was nonobese and otherwise healthy except for longstanding constipation.

Presentation

Colonic vovulus is a rare cause of bowel obstruction in the developed world, with an estimated annual incidence of about 3/10,000 in the United States. Although volvulus is unusual, it is the most common cause of bowel obstruction in pregnant women and the third leading cause of colonic obstruction after cancer and diverticulitis. Patients present with symptoms of excruciating abdominal pain out of proportion to the clinical examination, absence of flatus, and an empty rectal vault. Often, minimal distension is present during early volvulus that increases dramatically over time.

The mechanical etiology of volvulus is axial rotation of the colon, resulting in a closed loop obstruction. Axial rotation usually arises in one of two alternative mechanisms. First, in the case of a congenitally unfixed or partially unfixed colon, any portion of the colon—particularly the cecum—is at risk. During peristalsis, an unfixed ileocecal area on a narrow mesentery can twist, resulting in initial right lower-quadrant pain and symptoms of small bowel obstruction with minimal distension. Second, in an acquired fashion, the sigmoid colon may elongate due to chronic constipation and then twist on the relatively narrow mesentery. Major risk factors for sigmoid volvulus are advanced age, neurologic and psychiatric disease, lifelong high-fiber diet, and other causes of chronic constipation or elevated intraluminal pressure. Patients with compromised communication, such as those with dementia, previous stroke, or psychiatric disorders, are particularly susceptible to a delayed diagnosis.

If colonic volvulus does not self-reduce or otherwise resolve, the increased luminal pressure, thinning colon wall, and compromised venous outflow will lead over time to ischemic compromise of the bowel wall with necrosis and perforation.

Differential Diagnosis

Colonic obstruction should be considered cancer until proven otherwise. Other items in the differential diagnosis are pseudo-obstruction, constipation, obstipation, diverticulitis, intussusception, external compression by adhesions, and external compression by an extraluminal mass. Rarely, patients may present with late symptoms of volvulus including colonic ischemia, necrosis, and perforation. Therefore, the differential diagnosis of late volvulus includes the conditions listed above as well as mesenteric ischemia.

Workup

The diagnosis of volvulus is usually based on history and physical examination and confirmed radiologically. Volvulus pain can be intermittent, with initial self-reducing episodes of partial torsion. The pain tends to be diffuse and crampy in nature, which may differ from the constant pain of obstructing rectal cancer. Most patients present with symptoms several times before they are diagnosed. Important history and physical exam findings include elderly, infirm, or chronically institutionalized patients, the presence of longstanding constipation, vague recurrent discomfort, signs of obstruction, and no stool in the rectal vault on digital examination. The exception to this general picture is the young, otherwise healthy pregnant woman with intermittent bouts of increasing abdominal pain and obstructive symptoms during progression into the third trimester.

Laboratory tests are not diagnostic but may indicate secondary sequelae of obstruction such as electrolyte abnormalities, nonanion gap acidosis, and an elevated white blood count. High lactic acid levels are rare and indicate a more advanced disease process.

Radiologic imaging is the key to the diagnosis, starting with a flat and upright abdominal x-ray.

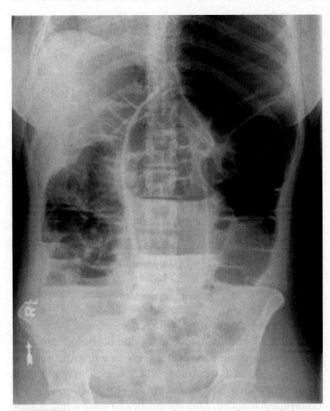

FIGURE 1 • Abdominal x-ray displaying a distended sigmoid in an inverted U, directed superiorly, with loss of haustral folds and proximal distended bowel. (Image supplied courtesy of Charles O. Finne.)

The classic appearance of sigmoid volvulus on x-ray is a "bent inner tube sign," with an inverted, distended sigmoid loop absent the normal Haustral folds and pointing toward the right upper quadrant **(Figure 1)**. If the patient is stable and there is any doubt about the diagnosis based on regular abdominal x-ray, a water-soluble radio-opaque enema may be performed. Barium is contraindicated in this setting due to risk of perforation. The classic finding on contrast enema of a "bird's beak" appearance to the bowel lumen **(Figure 2)** should result in resuscitation, colonic decompression, and elective operation. If a contrast enema is nondiagnostic or not feasible, a CT scan with intravenous contrast should be performed. Skipping the contrast enema and going immediately to a CT scan is also a reasonable practice. The CT scan can help to identify alternative diagnoses and can demonstrate the sine qua non "swirl sign" indicating a torsed mesentery. Rigid or flexible lower endoscopy can play either a diagnostic or more often a therapeutic role for the patient with volvulus.

Diagnosis and Treatment

If free intraperitoneal air is present on abdominal radiographs, no further studies are needed. The patient and family should be warned that this is an ominous sign and, after obtaining informed consent,

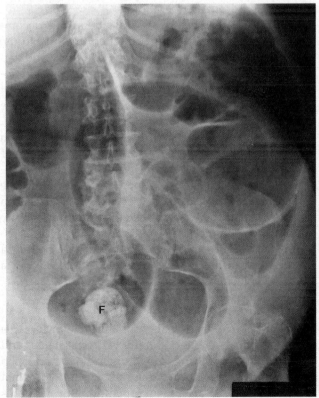

A

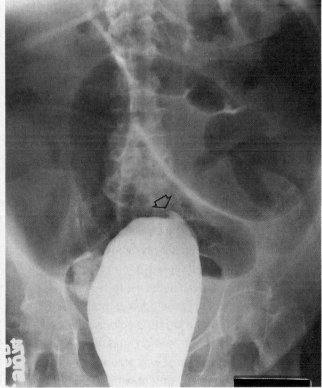

B

FIGURE 2 • Radio-opaque enema displaying the classic "bird's beak" of narrowed lumen at the distal site of torsion, without contrast (**A**) and with contrast (**B**).

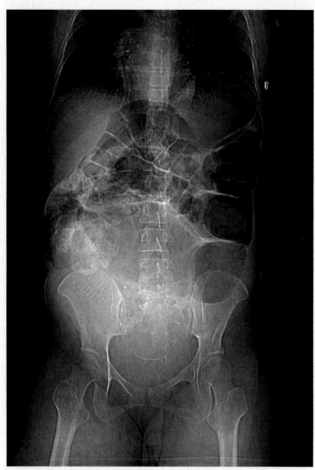

FIGURE 3 • Abdominal radiograph of patient displaying distended sigmoid colon with loss of Haustral markings and proximal distension, as well as a third-trimester fetus.

the patient should be resuscitated with normal saline or lactated ringers and electrolyte repletion before urgently performing an open exploratory celiotomy with Hartmann procedure and peritoneal irrigation.

Presentation Continued

In the scenario described above, the patient was clinically stable and her diagnosis remained in doubt despite a suggestive abdominal x-ray **(Figure 3)**. The abdominal x-rays showed a severely distended colon and an empty rectum but no characteristic signs. Therefore, lower endoscopy was performed, revealing a combination of spiral narrowing of the sigmoid colon with associated mucosal erythema, edema, and ulcerations **(Figure 4)**. The endoscopist was able to advance the scope beyond this segment without significant effort, revealing proximal colonic dilation.

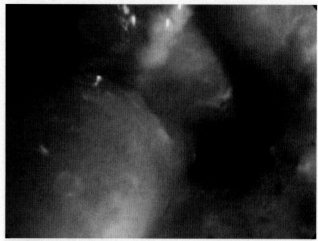

FIGURE 4 • Endoscopic appearance of the sigmoid mucosa with a swirl pattern confirming volvulus and ulcerations and erythema consistent with ischemia.

If *no* free intraperitoneal air is present and the patient is clinically stable, she can be resuscitated and the colon decompressed preferably with a flexible or rigid sigmoidoscope. Particularly in frail or elderly patients, rigid sigmoidoscope is preferable due to lower risk or colonic perforation and the ability to pass a rectal tube through the scope lumen to continue proximal decompression for several days. After supportive care and resolution of symptoms, an elective operation should be undertaken within 3 months as up to 70% of cases will recur without an operation.

In the case of an unsuccessful attempt at decompression, the patient should be taken urgently to the operating room for an exploratory celiotomy and sigmoid resection. The decision to perform an anastomosis versus colostomy will depend upon the presence of ischemia, stool spillage, and the general health of the patient.

Although sigmoid volvulus is the most common cause of colon obstruction during pregnancy, fewer than 100 cases have been reported in the literature. The consensus based upon these is that, in the absence of peritonitis, nonoperative decompression is preferred in the first trimester, sigmoid colectomy based upon these cases is preferred in the second trimester, and nonoperative treatment is again preferred in the third trimester until delivery. After delivery, a sigmoid colectomy is recommended.

Surgical Approach

As noted above, if the patient is unstable or has free intraperitoneal air, she should be resuscitated and taken to the operating room urgently for an open exploration **(Table 1)**. Laparoscopic exploration is not judicious during an urgent operation for volvulus given the extensive dilated bowel and negligible working space. A laparoscopic or an open approach could be used for a patient who has undergone successful endoscopic decompression.

For sigmoid volvulus, the appropriate operation is a sigmoid colectomy. For cecal volvulus, the definitive operation is a right colectomy with primary anastomosis. In both cases, intraoperative judgment should inform the decision for an ostomy versus primary anastomosis. Cecopexy to the right lower quadrant also has been described as a way to speed the operation and limit anastomotic complications. However, this advantage may be undone when placing suture in a distended, thinned cecal wall. Additionally, cecopexy for volvulus has historically been associated with a high recurrence rate. Placement of a cecostomy tube is also described for extremely frail patients.[1] Advantages are the avoidance of an abdominal wound and tethering of the cecum that theoretically prevents recurrent torsion.

For the most part, the key technical steps in operating urgently for sigmoid volvulus also apply to a resection for cecal volvulus. Fist, a midline laparotomy and full abdominal exploration are performed with the goal of identification of potential areas of

TABLE 1. Key Technical Steps and Potential Pitfalls in Operating for Sigmoid Volvulus

Key Technical Steps

1. Midline laparotomy and full exploration, examining for viability of bowel.
2. Place warm saline-soaked laparotomy sponges on any dusky-appearing bowel and recheck periodically for improving perfusion.
3. Identify areas of torsed mesentery and redundant bowel and prepare to resect, including areas of nonresolving ischemia.
4. Identify an appropriate proximal and distal anastomotic site and divide the sigmoid vessels and the intervening mesentery *without detorsing.*
5. Divide the bowel proximally and distally, passing off the specimen.
6. Perform anastomosis if clinical parameters are suitable (cardiovascular function, nutritional status, absence of bowel necrosis or gross contamination) and remaining bowel appears healthy and without tension.
7. If the clinical parameters for an anastomosis are not suitable, perform an end ostomy and mucus fistula.
8. If an anastomosis was performed, examine it closely for evidence of adequate perfusion, anastomotic patency, and absence of leaks if possible.

Potential Pitfalls

- Inflammatory cytokines or bacteria released to the circulation during detorsion of twisted mesentery.
- Nonresolving venous congestion.
- Placement of suture in distended, thinned colonic wall during a pexy procedure.

bowel ischemia or other causes of obstruction. Warm saline-soaked sponges are applied to any dusky bowel. Identify areas of torsed bowel as well as areas of ischemia extending beyond the obvious torsion. *Before* detorsing, identify appropriate proximal and distal sites for current or future anastomosis. Divide the mesentery prior to detorsing in order to avoid exposing the circulation to accumulated cytokines or bacteria in the ischemic segment. Divide the bowel proximally and distally and remove the specimen from the field.

Intraoperative judgment regarding whether to anastomose the bowel or to create an end ostomy and mucus fistula depends upon the patient's cardiovascular function, nutritional status, and absence of bowel necrosis or gross contamination. As well, the remaining bowel must be healthy-appearing and the ends must come together without tension. If an anastomosis is performed, it should be scrutinized for adequate perfusion, patency, and if possible undergo a leak test prior to closing the abdomen. A leak test can be performed for a sigmoid resection but is problematic for a right colectomy. A straightforward approach to the leak test is to fill the pelvis with sterile saline, gently compress the bowel proximal to the anastomosis, and insufflate the rectum with air using a rigid sigmoidoscope. The presence of bubbles indicates a leak. Other options for leak test include instillation of betadine or indigo carmine in the rectum and a search for discoloration of surrounding lap sponges applied to the anastomosis.

Special Intraoperative Considerations

Occasionally, a severely demented or otherwise noncommunicating patient with severe colonic distension and radiographic free air will undergo celiotomy and no evidence of perforation can be identified. If the bowel appears pink and viable and no evidence of a perforation site, sucus, purulence, or other spilled bowel contents can be identified, resection is not warranted. If the colon can be decompressed endoscopically, this may be advantageous but will likely be temporary.

Postoperative Management

Patients who have undergone a bowel resection for colonic volvulus should be managed expectantly with intravenous hydration, electrolyte repletion, and bowel rest until the return of peristalsis. Intravenous nutrition should be considered if the patient is initially malnourished or if more than a week passes without oral intake. Routine postcolectomy care is appropriate in the absence of clinical instability. For patients with an end ileostomy, waiting at least 6 to 12 weeks before performing an ostomy closure is prudent.

Case Conclusion

After decompression of the colon, patient A.B. was initially taken to the operating room for a transverse loop colostomy by the emergency surgery service. Six weeks later, she had a normal spontaneous vaginal delivery of a healthy baby. At 6 weeks postpartum, she underwent an uneventful closure of the transverse colostomy closure and resection of approximately 18 inches of sigmoid colon with a primary anastomosis through a small Pfannensteil incision by the colorectal surgery service.

TAKE HOME POINTS

- Colonic volvulus, an axial rotation of the colon resulting in a closed loop obstruction, can occur at any nonfixed portion of the colon, most commonly in the sigmoid colon and cecum.
- Conditions such as chronic constipation or treatment for neurologic or psychiatric conditions are associated with chronically increased intraluminal pressure and ultimately elongation of the sigmoid colon, resulting in greater risk of volvulus.
- Colonic volvulus is typically diagnosed based on radiographic studies, including upright abdominal radiograph ("bent inner tube sign" or "coffee bean sign"), radio-opaque enema ("bird's beak"), or computed tomography ("swirl sign").
- The first line of treatment for volvulus in a stable patient is endoscopic decompression and placement of a decompressing rectal tube, followed by supportive hydration and electrolyte correction.
- Patients who cannot be treated successfully with endoscopic decompression or who exhibit worsening clinical signs should be taken to the operating room for an open procedure.
- Prior to intraoperative detorsion of the volvulus, the mesentery should be divided to prevent circulation of inflammatory cytokines or septicemia.
- Even among stable, successfully decompressed patients, an elective laparoscopic or open sigmoidectomy is recommended due to recurrence rates ranging from 30% to 70%.

SUGGESTED READINGS

Alshawi JS. Recurrent sigmoid volvulus in pregnancy: report of a case and review of the literature. Dis Colon Rectum. 2005;48(9):1811–1813.

Ballantyne GH, Brandner MD, Beart RW Jr, et al. Volvulus of the colon. Incidence and mortality. Ann Surg. 1985;202(1):83–92.

Renzulli P, Maurer CA, Netzer P, et al. Preoperative colonoscopic derotation is beneficial in acute colonic volvulus. Dig Surg. 2002;19(3):223–229.

40 Complicated Diverticulitis

SEAN T. MARTIN and JON D. VOGEL

Presentation

A 65-year-old man presents to the emergency room with a 3-day history of severe, constant, worsening left lower-quadrant pain, with associated diarrhea, anorexia, and a fever of 102°F. His medical history is significantly for hypertension, mild angina pectoris, and hypothyroidism. Medications include hydralazine, aspirin, and levothyroxine. He lives alone but is independent and active.

He is febrile and tachycardic, at 110 beats per minute, with hypotension of 95/55 mm Hg. On clinical examination, he has generalized abdominal tenderness with signs of localized peritonitis in the left lower quadrant. His mucus membranes are dry and he is diaphoretic. He has no prior history of diverticulitis and has never had a colonoscopy.

Differential Diagnosis

This 65-year-old man presents with acute-onset left lower-quadrant abdominal pain. In this age group, the most likely diagnosis is acute diverticulitis, with an associated abscess or perforation. Important differential diagnoses, particularly in older patients with cardiovascular comorbidity, are intestinal ischemia and aortoiliac aneurysmal disease. Other diagnoses that should also be considered are perforated colon cancer, colonic volvulus, stercoral perforation of the colon, and acute manifestations of inflammatory bowel disease.

Diverticular disease, in the form of diverticulosis, is very common, affecting approximately 60% of 50-year-olds. However, only 10% to 20% of people with diverticular disease will develop diverticulitis, and of these, only 10% to 20% requires hospitalization. Of those hospitalized, 20% to 40% of patients will require operative intervention for "complicated diverticulitis," defined as perforation of the colon with resultant abscess, pneumoperitoneum, or peritonitis; colonic obstruction; or fistulization of the diseased portion of the colon.

Workup

This gentleman presents with evidence of sepsis and possible early septic shock. The initial goal, after taking an accurate history and performing a focused clinical examination, is resuscitation. Adequate intravenous access is obtained and aggressive fluid resuscitation is pursued. A bladder catheter is inserted to monitor urinary output. Supplemental oxygen may be required and intravenous opioid analgesia is administered as necessary. Given the clinical picture and suspicion of intra-abdominal infection, intravenous broad-spectrum antibiotics are given to the patient. Once resuscitation is underway, the next step is to proceed with investigations that will aid diagnosis and guide treatment.

Laboratory investigations in this patient reveal a leukocytosis of $24 \times 10^3/\text{mm}^3$, BUN of 30 mg/dL, and creatinine of 1.2 mg/dL. Amylase and lipase were within normal range. In patients with an acute abdominal presentation, plain film radiographs of abdomen and chest are of value in determining the presence of free intraperitoneal gas or concomitant pathology such as small bowel obstruction. Barring clear evidence of free air on abdominal radiograph, the diagnostic investigation of choice is a triple contrast (intravenous, oral, and rectal contrast) computed tomography (CT) of the abdomen and pelvis. Caution must be exercised when administering intravenous contrast to patients with renal compromise. The advantage of CT is that in addition to imaging all abdominal and pelvic organs, it can also facilitate therapeutic intervention; CT-guided drainage of a diverticular abscess allows control of sepsis, converting a potentially emergent scenario to an elective one.

In this case, plain abdominal radiograph showed no evidence of free air, and the abdominopelvic CT reveals sigmoid diverticulosis and an inflammatory phlegmon and associated mesenteric fat stranding in the region of the sigmoid colon, with extravasation of the rectally administered contrast, and free intraperitoneal gas **(Figure 1)**. These findings are consistent with a diagnosis of perforated diverticular disease of the sigmoid colon.

Discussion

A diverticulum is a sac-like protrusion in the colonic wall that develops as a result of herniation of the mucosa and submucosa through points of weakness in the muscular bowel wall. Colonic diverticulae may be acquired or congenital. Acquired diverticulae are commonly seen in the sigmoid colon, and are considered "false diverticulae" as they are mucosal herniations through the muscle wall. Congenital diverticulae contain the full thickness of bowel wall, and are therefore considered "true diverticulae." Classically, congenital diverticulosis affects the entire colon; right-sided and transverse colonic diverticulosis in isolation is rare.

Diverticular disease is relatively common in the western world. While the true prevalence is difficult to measure because most individuals are asymptomatic, it is estimated that in the United States, diverticulosis occurs in approximately one-third of the population older than age 45 and in up to two-thirds of the population older than 85 years. Incidence increases with age, and males and females are equally affected. A diet high in red meat and sugars but low in fiber (cereals, fruit, vegetables, brown bread) and water is postulated to be etiologic in acquired diverticulosis. With passage of hard, constipated stools, the intraluminal pressure in the sigmoid colon increases, causing segmentation. As a result, mucosal herniation occurs at the weakest point in the colonic wall, which is the point of entry of blood vessels and nerves supplying the colonic mucosa, between the mesenteric and antimesenteric teniae.

Men often require surgery for complicated disease earlier than women. Young men tend to develop fistulating disease; older male patients develop bleeding diverticulosis. In contrast, young women often present with perforated diverticulitis and older women with stricturing disease. Emergency surgery is typically indicated for management of perforated diverticulitis, which tends to occur on the index admission. In the elective setting, sigmoid colectomy may be required for recurrent episodes of uncomplicated diverticulitis (2 to 3 episodes) or a single episode of complicated diverticulitis, including micro perforation with abscess, sigmoid stricture, or the development of a colovesicle or colovaginal fistula.

Presentation Continued: Diagnosis and Treatment

Emergency surgery is required for this patient with perforated diverticulitis. The basic tenet of managing perforated diverticulitis is control of intra-abdominal sepsis with excision of the septic focus (e.g., source control), where possible. Firstly, appropriate resuscitation is required for this patient with septic shock and acute renal injury. Once resuscitation is underway, we proceed to surgery. The surgical options are diverse and varied; but typically in this situation, resection of the diseased segment of colon, with or without primary anastomosis, is favored.

Surgical Approach to Perforated Diverticulitis

The surgical procedure of choice in the management of perforated diverticulitis is dependent on the clinical condition of the patient at the time of emergency surgery. This patient has septic shock secondary to intra-abdominal sepsis following a diverticular perforation. Historically, a Hartmann's procedure was performed in this setting, by conventional open surgery or more recently using a minimally invasive approach. In this case, this 65-year-old man is significantly compromised by his condition and will benefit from an expeditious open operation. Additionally, in the setting of hypotension and shock, laparoscopy may further impair venous return and worsen hypotension.

The patient is placed on the operating table in the modified lithotomy position, facilitating transanal access to the rectum should it be required. Access to the peritoneal cavity is gained via a low midline laparotomy, extending from the umbilicus to pubic symphysis. Although it may be possible to complete the operation through this relatively small incision, if access is limited the incision can be extended cephalad. A wound protector is used to minimize risk of postoperative wound infection. The operation begins with a general laparotomy in which the four quadrants of the abdomen are inspected systematically. The stomach and duodenum are visualized for signs of perforation; the small bowel is palpated from the ligament of treitz to the ileocecal valve. Lastly, the colon and rectum are inspected. Frequently in this scenario, purulent or feculent peritonitis is encountered on entering the peritoneal cavity. In

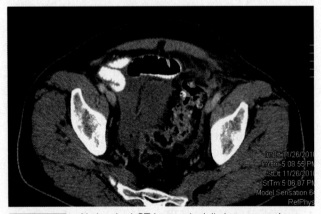

FIGURE 1 • Abdominal CT image (axial) demonstrating perforated sigmoid diverticulitis. Note the extravasation of rectal contrast into the peridiverticular cavity. Also free gas is visible in the abdominal cavity (*arrow*), indicating a perforation.

that setting, contaminants of the peritoneal cavity are thoroughly lavaged with warm sterile saline.

At laparotomy, an inflammatory phlegmon is noted in the region of the sigmoid colon and a perforation is visible in a diverticulum of the diseased bowel. The diseased sigmoid colon is adherent to the pelvic sidewall. It is critical to have optimal access to the diseased segment of colon, and packing the small bowel into the right upper quadrant with large moist packs before inserting a Balfour retractor can improve visualization and access to the colon. Surrounding tissues are typically quite friable and bleed easily. Sharp dissection in the area of the inflammatory segment is not advisable as the normal anatomical planes between the sigmoid mesentery and the retroperitoneum are obliterated. The left ureter may be pulled anteriorly into the inflammatory phlegmon and is in danger of iatrogenic injury particularly at the pelvic brim. The dissection should commence proximally, at a portion of nondiseased left colon by dividing the white line of Toldt, where the mesocolon fuses with the lateral abdominal wall. This can be carried out with electrocautery or Metzenbaum scissors. This allows the proximal colon to be mobilized and the correct anatomical plane to be entered between the mesocolon and the retroperitoneum. In this plane, we identify the left ureter and follow its course down toward the pelvis. As we approach the diseased phlegmon from above, the anatomical planes lose definition. We follow the course of the ureter and ensure it is not involved in the diseased segment of colon that will be excised. Should the ureter be adherent, we dissect it from the inflammatory phlegmon under direct vision using a combination of blunt and sharp dissection. At this point in the operation, with the ureter identified, we utilize blunt fingertip dissection to "pinch" the sigmoid colon from the pelvic sidewall. Once the sigmoid colon has been mobilized from the pelvis, we confirm the site of the perforation and decide how much colon to resect. At this point, a pitfall in the emergency setting is to attempt to resect the entire sigmoid colon with the aim of definitive treatment of the diverticular disease. This approach often requires mobilization of the splenic flexure to form a descending colostomy or both splenic flexure mobilization and entry into the pelvis for creation of a colorectal anastomosis. These extra steps should be avoided as they will increase the extent of the surgery, prolong the operation, and will expose previously unaffected tissue planes to the infectious process and the potential for a postoperative abscess.

After confirming the position of the left ureter, the sigmoid mesocolon is divided close to the bowel wall between hemostats, leaving the inferior mesenteric vein, inferior mesenteric and superior rectal arteries undisturbed. Next, we divide the colon proximal to the perforation with a linear stapling device. Distally, the sigmoid colon is divided above the pelvic brim,

again using a linear stapling device, and the specimen is extracted. The distal staple line is reinforced with a hemostatic stitch. A marking, nonabsorbable stitch may be placed on the distal segment to facilitate identification of the stump when we return to close the colostomy at a later date. Proximally, a tension-free colostomy is passed through the rectus muscle and positioned at the apex of the infraumbilical fat pad. It may be necessary to mobilize the left colon proximally, particularly in obese patients, to facilitate formation of colostomy, but mobilization of the splenic flexure is rarely required. At the end of the procedure, we repeat a thorough peritoneal lavage. The abdominal wall is closed, the subcuticular fat and skin are irrigated, and the skin is closed with staples. The colostomy is then matured with interrupted rapidly absorbable suture.

Alternative Approaches to Perforated Diverticulitis

Several alternative approaches to perforated diverticulitis are available. Data exist to support performing a primary colorectal anastomosis after emergency sigmoid colectomy for perforated diverticulitis. However, this typically adds 40 to 60 minutes to the procedure as the splenic flexure is freed, the entire sigmoid colon is removed, and an anastomosis between the descending colon and the rectum is created. This one-stage procedure may be considered for fit patients with Hinchey grade 1 and 2 diverticulitis **(Table 1)**, who are hemodynamically stable throughout the operation; there is minimal contamination of the operative field, and the surgery is completed without difficulties. The advantage of a one-stage procedure is that it obviates the need for a temporary stoma, which may be beneficial considering that up to 40% of patients having a two-stage procedure will elect not to have their stoma closed. Formal sigmoid resection with colorectal anastomosis may also be considered for select patients with Hinchey grade 3 and 4 diverticulitis (purulent and fecal peritonitis); however, we believe it is prudent to protect the anastomosis with a defunctioning loop ileostomy, which can be closed at a later date. In unusual situations, with patients who are unstable during the operation or with severe pericolinic inflammation that results in complete obliteration of tissue planes, it may be necessary to perform a proximal stoma, leaving the diseased segment in situ, with placement of appropriate drains to control the sepsis. Lastly, laparoscopic peritoneal lavage has been reported for treatment of Hinchey 3 diverticulitis (purulent peritonitis) with encouraging results. The obvious advantage of this technique is that it saves the patient an open operation, colonic resection, and possibly a stoma. However, this novel therapeutic strategy requires validation in a properly designed clinical trial. Key technical points of the various

TABLE 1. Intraoperative Hinchey[a] Classification of Perforated Colonic Diverticulitis

- Hinchey I—localized peridiverticular abscess (pericolic)
- Hinchey II—pelvic abscess (away from inflamed phlegmon)
- Hinchey III—purulent peritonitis (the presence of pus in the abdominal cavity)
- Hinchey IV—feculent peritonitis

[a]Proposed by Hinchey EJ, Schaal PG, Richard GK. Treatment of diverticular disease of the colon. Adv Surg. 1978;12:85–109.

surgical approaches to managing perforated diverticular disease are summarized in **Table 2**.

Special Intraoperative Considerations

On occasion, at emergency laparotomy for sigmoid perforation, we encounter a perforated sigmoid colon cancer. This unsuspected finding will alter the

TABLE 2. Key Technical Steps and Potential Pitfalls to Approaching Perforated Diverticulitis

Key Technical Steps

1. Position patient in the modified lithotomy position.
2. Lower midline laparotomy, have low threshold for extending cephalad to optimize exposure.
3. Use a wound protector.
4. Perform thorough peritoneal lavage upon entering the peritoneal cavity.
5. Full general laparotomy, inspecting four quadrants of the abdomen and pelvis.
6. Isolate the sigmoid colon by packing the small bowel into the right side of the abdomen. A Balfour retractor is often helpful.
7. Enter the correct anatomical plane proximal to the diseased segment of colon and identify the left ureter. Follow the course of the left ureter and ensure it is not involved in the inflammatory segment.
8. Bluntly free sigmoid phlegmon from pelvis by finger fracture.
9. Avoid unnecessary mobilization of the colon.
10. Ligate mesenteric vessels close to bowel wall.
11. Resect only the perforated segment of the colon ("perferectomy") and create an end colostomy.
12. Repeat peritoneal lavage prior to closing the abdomen.

Potential Pitfalls

- Full mobilization of the colon with entry into unaffected tissue planes with resultant increased risk for remote abdominopelvic abscess.
- Omission of a defunctioning stoma in cases in which a colorectal anastomosis is performed.
- Collateral damage (to the left ureter, bladder, or iliac vessels) in cases in which the inflammatory mass obliterates tissue planes. In this situation, a colostomy and drainage of the inflamed should be considered.

operative approach as it necessitates the performance of an oncologic resection (i.e., high ligation of the inferior mesenteric artery) rather than the more limited sigmoid resection described above. In this situation, the surgeon should consider which operation will result in the greatest benefit to the patient while minimizing the potential for risk. A sigmoid colectomy with end colostomy and closure of the rectal stump will eliminate the risk of anastomotic leak and may decrease the risk of postoperative abscess, both of which would interfere with or delay the use of chemotherapy. As with all cancer resections, any structure that is adherent to the perforated tumor mass (e.g., small bowel) must be resected en bloc to ensure radical clearance of all disease. We also lavage the peritoneal cavity with sterile water or dilute alcohol, in an attempt to eradicate any tumor cells that may have escaped from the area of perforation.

Another infrequently observed finding in association with sigmoid diverticular perforation and phlegmon is a right-sided colonic perforation. The inflammatory mass surrounding the perforated diverticulum compresses the colon, eventually obstructing the lumen. In the presence of a competent ileocecal valve, a closed loop obstruction ensues, with perforation occurring at the cecum as it is the portion of the colon with the thinnest wall. Classically, this patient presents with a history and clinical findings consistent with large bowel obstruction initially, or peritonitis at a later stage. In this setting, we perform a total abdominal colectomy with end ileostomy. Alternatively, in select fit patients with minimal peritoneal contamination and an uneventful operation, an ileorectal anastomosis with a proximal defunctioning ileostomy may be considered.

In the setting of a sigmoid colon perforation against a background of Crohn's colitis, the surgical options depend on the extent of the colonic and rectal disease and the condition of the patient. In general, the surgical options in this setting are to perform a limited resection of the perforated colon with end colostomy, total abdominal colectomy with end ileostomy, or total abdominal colectomy with ileorectal anastomosis and proximal diverting loop ileostomy.

Postoperative Management

Most patients with perforated sigmoid diverticulitis will benefit from an initial stay in the Surgical Intensive Care Unit (SICU). Intravenous broad-spectrum antibiotics should be continued until culture results and sensitivities are available, after which time the antimicrobial regimen should be tailored according to the causative organisms. The duration of antibiotic therapy is determined by the patient's clinical course. Both mechanical and pharmacologic venous thromboembolism prophylaxes are beneficial. For nutrition, the enteral route is favored. For patients who are alert and can protect their airway, a diet is started in the early postoperative period. Parenteral nutrition is reserved for patients who cannot tolerate enteral feeding for a prolonged postoperative period. Postoperative complications in the setting of intra-abdominal sepsis include intra-abdominal or pelvic abscess. Suspicion for abscess formation should be aroused by the occurrence of a prolonged ileus, nonfunctioning stoma, persistent fever, or leukocytosis. CT-guided drainage of intra-abdominal abscesses is typically successful in managing sepsis. Wound infections are common after a Hartmann's procedure and are managed by removing clips from the wound and expressing underlying pus. If the skin defect is large, a vacuum-assisted closure device may be applied. Following laparotomy for intra-abdominal sepsis, abdominal compartment syndrome can occur. Increasing inotropic and ventilatory requirements with signs of impaired organ perfusion (oliguria or anuria) should alert the clinician to the diagnosis, and prompt measurement of intra-abdominal pressure via a transducer inserted into the bladder. Severe abdominal compartment syndrome warrants emergent laparostomy.

Case Conclusion

The patient undergoes a successful Hartmann's procedure and is extubated in SICU the following day. His stoma functions on day 2 and he recommences diet on the fourth postoperative day. He spends 7 days in the hospital and is discharged well, without sequelae. He has his proximal colon assessed endoscopically prior to successful reversal of Hartmann's procedure 6 months later.

TAKE HOME POINTS

- A small proportion (1%) of patients requires surgery for complications of diverticular disease.
- Complicated sigmoid diverticulitis that results in generalized peritonitis and hemodynamic instability requires prompt resuscitation, the administration of broad-spectrum antibiotics, and urgent surgical exploration.
- The standard of care for patients with complicated sigmoid diverticulitis who require urgent surgery is resection of the perforated segment of the colon with creation of an end colostomy.
- In select patients with complicated sigmoid diverticular disease who present with a pericolonic abscess (Hinchey 1) or abdominal/pelvic abscess (Hinchey 2), sigmoid colectomy with colorectal anastomosis and proximal diversion, may be considered.
- In patients with complicated sigmoid diverticular disease and purulent (Hinchey 3) or feculent (Hinchey 4) peritonitis, the current standard of care is open resection of the perforated segment of colon with end colostomy and closure of the rectal stump.
- In rare cases of complicated sigmoid diverticular disease, due to severe inflammation of the colon or the surrounding structures, or in patients who are unstable during the operation, it is necessary to perform a proximal diversion, without resection, leaving abdominal and pelvic drains to control sepsis.
- During surgery for suspected complicated sigmoid diverticular disease, the surgeon should be alert for the unsuspected finding of cancer or Crohn's disease and modify the surgical approach accordingly.

SUGGESTED READING

Thorson AG, Beaty JS. Diverticular disease. In Beck DE, Roberts PL, Saclarides TJ, Senagore AJ, Stamos MJ, Wexner SD. The ASCRS textbook of colon and rectal surgery. New York: Springer, 2011:375–395.

41 Ischemic Colitis

MUNEERA R. KAPADIA and ANN C. LOWRY

Presentation

A 75-year-old man with a history of diabetes and hypertension presents with sudden onset of left-sided abdominal pain. He complains of bloody diarrhea for the last few hours and anorexia without nausea or emesis. On examination, he is mildly tachycardic with a low-grade fever, but otherwise his vitals are normal. He is mildly distended and tender in the left lower quadrant of his abdomen but does not have diffuse peritoneal signs. Rectal examination is normal but his stool is heme positive.

Differential Diagnosis

Ischemic colitis should be considered when a patient presents with sudden-onset abdominal pain with associated bloody diarrhea. The most common entities in the differential diagnosis are infectious colitides, inflammatory bowel disease, radiation enteritis, diverticulitis, and malignancy; a more complete list can be found in **Table 1**.

Ischemic colitis typically develops in patients over 65 years but can occur in younger patients as well. Risk factors include cardiac or vascular comorbidities such as diabetes or hypertension. Typical presenting symptoms include cramping abdominal pain of sudden onset followed by bloody diarrhea. Some patients also experience fecal urgency as well as nausea and vomiting secondary to an ileus. The abdominal examination is usually significant for tenderness over the affected area of colon but can include peritoneal signs in more severe cases.

Workup

In the patient presenting above, serum laboratory values reveal hemoglobin of 14.2 g/dL, a white blood cell count of 15.5, and a lactic acid level of 0.8 mEq/L. A CT scan shows mild descending and sigmoid colonic thickening **(Figure 1)**. Endoscopy demonstrates erythematous mucosa with superficial ulcerations in area of the splenic flexure **(Figure 2)**. Stool cultures are negative.

During the workup of ischemic colitis, blood tests and abdominal imaging are frequently obtained, but the findings are often nonspecific. The white blood cell count and the lactate level may be elevated, and metabolic acidosis may be present. Stool cultures and *Clostridium difficile* toxin studies should be obtained to rule out infectious colitides. Abdominal radiographs are generally not helpful unless severe ischemic colitis is present; in that case, plain films may demonstrate free air, pneumatosis, or portal venous gas. CT scans may demonstrate colonic wall thickening but are most useful for excluding other conditions. Barium enema may show the classic sign, "thumbprinting," which represents submucosal hemorrhagic nodules. Colonoscopy with biopsies of the affected area confirms the diagnosis. Angiography is rarely indicated unless acute small intestinal mesenteric ischemia is suspected.

The diagnostic test of choice is an unprepped colonoscopy unless there is evidence of peritonitis on examination. It allows for direct visualization of mucosal changes, and biopsies can be obtained. Ischemic colon can be fragile, and colonoscopy should be performed with care to avoid overdistension of the colon. The distribution of findings depends on the vascular insult sustained, and the mucosal changes can be variable. In mild to moderate ischemic colitis, the mucosa may appear erythematous hypers and edematous with petechiae. Additionally, ulcerations and hemorrhagic nodules, which represent submucosal bleeding, may be seen. In severe ischemic colitis, the mucosa may appear gray or black indicating transmural infarction. If this is encountered, the colonoscopy should be terminated due to significant risk of perforation. If peritonitis is present on examination, a colonoscopy should be avoided and laparotomy should be performed.

TABLE 1. Differential Diagnosis of Sudden-Onset Abdominal Pain and Bloody Diarrhea

Ischemic colitis
Infectious colitis
Diverticulitis
Radiation enteritis or colitis
Inflammatory bowel disease
Solitary rectal ulcer
Malignancy
Microscopic colitis
Eosinophilic colitis
Neutropenic enterocolitis (Typhlitis)
Drug-induced colitis
Collagen vascular–associated colitis

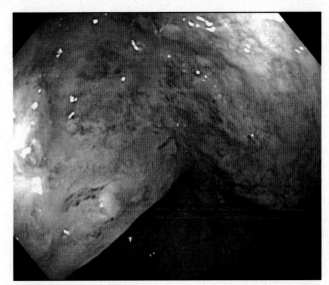

FIGURE 2 • Endoscopic image of moderate ischemic colitis.

Discussion

Etiologic factors are numerous **(Table 2)**; however, in most cases, a specific cause cannot be identified. Frequently the predisposing event, such as an episode of acute illness, has resolved by the time the patient presents.

Ischemic colitis can be divided into two categories: nongangrenous and gangrenous. Accounting for approximately 80% to 85% of cases, the nongangrenous type can be further subdivided into transient and chronic forms. Transient ischemic colitis typically involves the mucosa and submucosa and typically resolves in 1 to 2 weeks. The chronic nongangrenous form is characterized by injury to the deeper layers of the colonic wall. Healing may result in fibrosis in the colonic wall and development of a stricture. The gangrenous form with acute severe transmural injury results in perforation and/or

sepsis and requires surgical resection of the compromised colon.

Typically segmental, ischemic colitis may involve any area of the colon and rectum. The splenic flexure, descending colon, and sigmoid colon are most commonly affected, which can be explained by the vascular anatomy. The blood supply to the colon and rectum occurs through the superior mesenteric artery, the inferior mesenteric artery, and the superior hemorrhoidal artery. Watershed areas, regions dependent upon collaterals between the inferior and the superior mesenteric arteries (e.g., the splenic flexure and the descending colon), are especially susceptible to ischemic injury in low flow states **(Figure 3)**.

TABLE 2. Causes of Ischemic Colitis

Hypoperfusion
Sepsis
Cardiac failure
Hypovolemia

Occlusive Disease (Thrombotic or Embolic)
Hypercoagulable states
Cardiac embolus

Small Vessel Disease
Atherosclerosis
Vasculitis
Radiation

Iatrogenic
Abdominal aortic aneurysm repair
Previous colon resection
Drugs

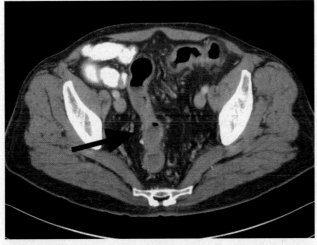

FIGURE 1 • CT scan: The sigmoid colon is thickened (*arrow*).

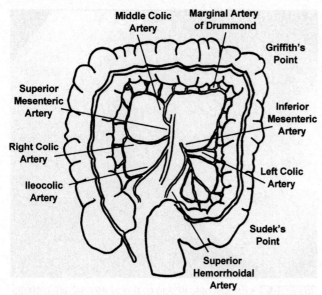

FIGURE 3 • Colonic bloody supply is derived from the superior mesenteric (SMA), inferior mesenteric (IMA), and superior hemorrhoidal (SHA) arteries. "Watershed" areas lie between two of the arteries and are susceptible to ischemia. Griffith's point is located at the splenic flexure, between the SMA and IMA. Sudek's point is located at the rectosigmoid junction, between the IMA and SHA. While these two points are particularly susceptible to ischemia, any portion of the colon and rectum can be affected by ischemic colitis.

Diagnosis and Treatment

Once the diagnosis is established, the treatment varies depending on the etiology and the severity of disease. Most patients can be managed expectantly with intravenous fluids, bowel rest, and broad-spectrum antibiotics. Restoration of adequate intravascular volume is important. If a symptomatic ileus is present, the patient may benefit from nasogastric decompression. Additionally, any specific causal agent should be addressed. If a patient has peritonitis, evidence of perforation, or deteriorates clinically with conservative medical management, laparotomy is warranted. Patients with right-sided ischemic colitis or ischemic colitis without hematochezia have been shown to need surgery more frequently and have worse outcomes. Additionally, if a patient develops a stricture or chronic colitis following ischemic colitis, colonic resection may be indicated.

Surgical Approach

In our clinical scenario from above, after 48 hours of medical management, the patient becomes acutely febrile and tachycardic. On examination his abdomen is diffusely tender. Given the patients clinical decline, emergent laparotomy is undertaken.

When operative intervention is warranted, a laparotomy should be performed through a midline incision. The abdomen is explored and the compromised segment of colon is identified. The extent of ischemic

TABLE 3. Key Technical Steps and Potential Pitfalls to Operative Management of Ischemic Colitis

Key Technical Steps

1. Midline abdominal incision.
2. Determine extent of gangrenous colon.
3. Mobilize and resect nonviable colon.
4. Check for brisk bleeding at the resection margins.
5. Creation of anastomosis or stoma depending on patient and bowel status.
6. Close abdomen.

Potential Pitfalls

- Inadequate resection leaving nonviable bowel.
- Anastomosis should be avoided in hemodynamically unstable patients.

colon can be usually be easily assessed by a visual inspection. If there is doubt, the combination of intraoperative colonoscopy, palpation, doppler assessment of the colonic vessels, and intravenous fluorescein can be helpful. Once the involved region is determined, all nonviable colon should be resected. There should be brisk bleeding at the resection margins. If the remaining bowel appears viable and healthy and the patient is stable, it is reasonable to perform a primary anastomosis. If the patient is hypotensive or there is significant surrounding inflammation, a primary anastomosis should be avoided and instead an end stoma created. If there is a question about viability, the resected colonic ends are brought out as a stoma and mucous fistula. In an unstable patient, the ends may be stapled and left discontinuous, and a second look laparotomy performed after 24 to 48 hours (Table 3).

Special Circumstance

Ischemic Colitis Following Aortic Surgery. Ischemic colitis is a well-described complication of aortic surgery. The overall incidence of ischemic colitis is about 2%; however, the incidence among patients requiring emergency surgery for ruptured aortic aneurysms is significantly higher. The underlying etiology is usually related to disruption of the inferior mesenteric artery, but additional contributory factors can include prolonged cross-clamping of the aorta and hemodynamic instability. Reimplantation of the inferior mesenteric artery may be necessary to prevent ischemic colitis if the superior mesenteric artery is stenotic and collateral bloody supply is inadequate to support the left colon. Symptoms of ischemic colitis develop in the first few days after aortic surgery and can include pain, fever, distention, and diarrhea. Diagnosis and treatment should proceed as previously discussed. If colonic resection is deemed necessary, a primary anastomosis should be avoided as an anastomotic leak risks graft contamination.

Postoperative Management

Depending on postoperative hemodynamic stability, patients may require a stay in the intensive care unit with close monitoring of urine output and volume status. A nasogastric tube is unnecessary unless the patient suffers a significant ileus. Dietary advancement should be as tolerated. If a primary anastomosis is created, patients should be monitored for evidence of an anastomotic leak. Return of bowel function should occur prior to discharge. If colonic diversion is deemed necessary at the initial operation, ileostomy or colostomy takedown can be considered at 3 to 6 months following the initial operation, depending on the patient's overall health status.

TAKE HOME POINTS

- Sudden-onset abdominal pain followed by bloody diarrhea should prompt suspicion of ischemic colitis.
- Colonoscopy is the test of choice for diagnosis of ischemic colitis.
- Ischemic colitis most commonly involves the splenic flexure, descending and sigmoid colon.
- Most patients can be treated effectively with hydration, bowel rest, and broad-spectrum antibiotics.
- Peritonitis, evidence of perforation, or clinical deterioration should prompt immediate surgical intervention.
- Operative management should include resection of compromised colon, followed by either primary anastomosis or creation of a stoma depending on the overall status of the patient.

SUGGESTED READINGS

Brandt LJ, Boley SJ. Colonic ischemia. Surg Clin North Am. 1992;72:203–229.

Brandt LJ, Feuerstadt P, Blaszka MC. Anatomic patterns, patient characteristics, and clinical outcomes in ischemic colitis: a study of 313 cases supported by histology. Am J Gastroenterol. 2010;105:2245–2252;quiz 53.

Montoro MA, Brandt LJ, Santolaria S, et al. Clinical patterns and outcomes of ischaemic colitis: results of the Working Group for the Study of Ischaemic Colitis in Spain (CIE study). Scand J Gastroenterol. 2011;46(2):236–246. [Epub 2010.]

Mosele M, Cardin F, Inelmen EM, et al. Ischemic colitis in the elderly: predictors of the disease and prognostic factors to negative outcome. Scand J Gastroenterol. 2010;45:428–433.

Paterno F, McGillicuddy EA, Schuster KM, et al. Ischemic colitis: risk factors for eventual surgery. Am J Surg. 2010;200:646–650.

Perry RJ, Martin MJ, Eckert MJ, et al. Colonic ischemia complicating open vs endovascular abdominal aortic aneurysm repair. J Vasc Surg. 2008;48:272–277.

Scowcroft CW, Sanowski RA, Kozarek RA. Colonoscopy in ischemic colitis. Gastrointest Endosc. 1981;27:156–161.

Steele SR. Ischemic colitis complicating major vascular surgery. Surg Clin North Am. 2007;87:1099–1114, ix.

Sun MY, Maykel JA. Ischemic colitis. Clin Colon Rectal Surg. 2007;20:5–12.

West BR, Ray JE, Gathright JB. Comparison of transient ischemic colitis with that requiring surgical treatment. Surg Gynecol Obstet. 1980;151:366–368.

42 Medically Refractory Ulcerative Colitis

SAMANTHA HENDREN

Presentation

A 28-year-old man with a history of ulcerative colitis (UC) diagnosed 13 months ago presents to the emergency department with bloody diarrhea and abdominal pain. His symptoms worsened 2 weeks ago, and his outpatient gastroenterologist started him on Prednisone 40 mg daily, in addition to his usual medications, pentasa and azathioprine. He is now having about 12 to 15 bloody bowel movements every 24 hours. This is his third hospital admission since diagnosis, with the most recent 3 months ago. Laboratory testing reveals hemoglobin of 9.8 g/dL, erythrocyte sedimentation rate (Westergren) of 43 mm/h, C-reactive protein of 12.06 mg/dL, and albumin of 2.8 g/dL.

Differential Diagnosis

This patient presents with an exacerbation of UC, superimposed on a relatively aggressive disease course since diagnosis. While medically refractory disease is the most likely diagnosis, it is important to remember that superimposed infectious colitis including *Clostridium difficile* colitis affects up to 30% of UC patients presenting with acute exacerbations of their disease. As such, ruling out superimposed infection and optimizing medical therapy is an essential step prior to proceeding with surgical therapy. A misconception among surgeons is that surgical therapy is inevitable for severe UC. On the contrary, recent case series have shown colectomy rates as low as 20% at 2 years for patients with severe UC. Long term, about 30% of all UC patients undergo colectomy, although this is likely decreasing over time due to improvements in medical therapy.

The consulting surgeon has a responsibility to recognize and offer immediate surgical treatment for toxic megacolon, characterized by the following signs and symptoms: abdominal distention, tenderness, fever, leukocytosis, more than 10 bowel movements per day, continuous bleeding, transfusion requirement, hypoalbuminemia, radiologic evidence of colonic wall thickening, and possible dilatation (not always present).

Workup

The patient is admitted to the medicine service, and the gastroenterologists perform a computed tomography scan (CT scan, **Figure 1**) and a colonoscopy. The colonoscopy reveals pancolitis with ulcerations, granularity, and distorted vascular pattern.

Stool samples were sent for *C. difficile* toxin and antigen, and biopsies for cytomegalovirus infection were obtained at colonoscopy; both these were negative. The patient was offered treatment with the anti-TNF agent,

infliximab, and surgery was also consulted to introduce the principles of surgical treatment to the patient. He did not have signs or symptoms of toxic megacolon.

As the surgical consultant, important features of the history and physical examination include the following: reviewing documentation of all prior colonoscopy, pathology, and radiologic testing to insure there is no evidence of Crohn's disease (such as small bowel disease), or dysplasia/malignancy that might alter the surgical approach. It is also essential to ask about any history of anorectal surgery or abscess-fistula disease, assessing continence (keeping in mind that some fecal incontinence during a severe flare is common), and quality of life related to disease activity and medical therapy. A patient who is unable to work due to frequent disease flares or toxic effects of medical treatments should be considered for surgery. Physical exam for signs of toxic colitis and for anal sphincter integrity and signs of any current or prior abscess-fistula disease are also essential.

Diagnosis and Treatment

Based on the workup, this patient has medically refractory UC. The principles of treatment include consideration of salvage medical therapy versus surgical treatment. The decision making between these two options should include a multidisciplinary approach, and the patient should always be introduced to the option of surgery at this point. The patient elected to proceed with infliximab treatment and was discharged after an improvement but not resolution of his symptoms on infliximab and high-dose steroids. Unfortunately his symptoms persisted at home, with bloody bowel movements, abdominal pain, and malaise. His gastroenterologist calls you and asks you to consider surgical treatment at this point.

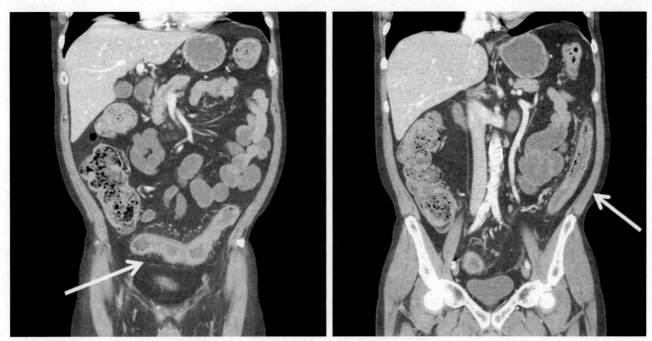

FIGURE 1 • Radiologic Appearance of Severe Ulcerative Colitis.

Surgical Approach

The goal of surgery for UC is removal of the entire colon and rectum, which can be immediately performed, or performed in a staged fashion. Both a total proctocolectomy with end ileostomy and reconstructive surgery with a pelvic pouch provide good quality of life, but most patients prefer reconstructive surgery to avoid a permanent ostomy. Since the 1980s, the most popular operation for medically refractory UC has been the ileal pouch anal anastomosis operation (IPAA, also called restorative proctocolectomy), usually with a J-pouch. This operation is associated with high but acceptable complication rates, good quality of life, and an overall success rate of about 90% long term **(Figure 2)**.

The decision of whether to perform UC surgery in 1-stage, 2 stages, or 3 stages is influenced by several factors: patient presentation, medications (especially anti-TNF agents and high-dose steroids, which may be associated with higher complication rates), nutritional status, comorbidities, and technical issues encountered at the time of surgery (such as the degree of tension on the pouch-anal anastomosis). For the patient in this scenario, a 2- or 3-stage approach beginning with a subtotal colectomy is probably the safest option, given recent administration of infliximab, malnutrition, and steroids—all of which may increase anastomotic leak rate if IPAA is performed immediately. An alternative of IPAA with diverting ileostomy could be considered.

A subtotal colectomy for UC can be performed laparoscopically or open. The key technical features include preoperative marking of the ileostomy site with the patient sitting and supine (avoiding folds and scars), and avoiding pelvic dissection to maintain the virgin tissue planes for the next stage of surgery. For severe colitis in which rectal stump leak is a concern, consider a mucus fistula of Hartmann's pouch, suturing the pouch to the abdominal wound so a leak can drain via the wound, or placing a temporary draining rectal tube to minimize pressure in the stump.

The steps of the routine IPAA procedure are outlined in **Table 1.** These include resection of the entire or the remaining colon and rectum, mobilization of the small bowel and its mesentery, creation of a 15- to 20-cm long J-pouch, suturing or stapling the pouch to the anus, and performing a diverting loop ileostomy in most cases. In the case of a double-stapled technique, the rectum is stapled and divided at the level of the levator ani muscles, and then the pouch is stapled to the anal canal using the EEA stapler. In the case of the hand-sewn pouch-anal anastomosis, the distal rectum is divided, the mucosa above the dentate line is stripped transanally, and the pouch is pulled through the rectal cuff and hand sutured at the dentate line **(Figure 3)**.

Special Intraoperative Considerations

The key intraoperative problem for which the surgeon must be prepared is the possibility that an ileal J-pouch will not reach to the anal canal for anastomosis. This is a particular problem for tall or obese male patients. In these cases, maneuvers to create length must be performed, including division of peritoneum overlying the mesentery and selective ligation of the mesenteric vessels with transillumination to ensure there are collateral pathways for blood flow to the entire small bowel. Usually, ileocolic artery ligation will result

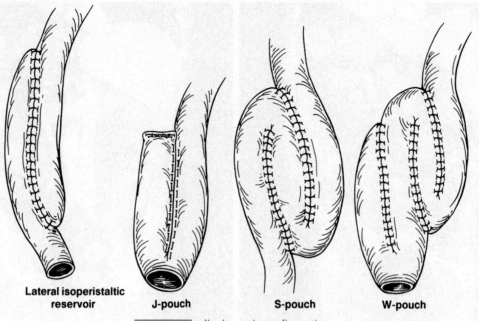

Lateral isoperistaltic reservoir   **J-pouch**   **S-pouch**   **W-pouch**

FIGURE 2 • Ileal pouch configurations.

in sufficient length, but if not consider temporary occlusion of vessels (e.g., with a bulldog clamp) prior to selective ligation. If reach is still a problem an S-shaped or W-shaped pouch may be considered, as these may reach better depending on the individual's mesenteric vascular anatomy.

Another pitfall is the finding of evidence of Crohn's disease at the time of surgery. While IPAA for highly selected Crohn's colitis patients is performed in specialty centers, small bowel or anal Crohn's disease is a contraindication to IPAA. Ileorectal anastomosis or ileostomy should be performed. Patients must be informed about these potential pitfalls prior to surgery.

TABLE 1. Key Technical Steps and Potential Pitfalls in Ileal Pouch Anal Anastomosis (IPAA)

Key Technical Steps

1. Patient is placed in the modified lithotomy position with access to the anus.
2. Perform total proctocolectomy or completion proctectomy, dividing the mesentery near the bowel, unless cancer is a concern.
3. Staple and divide the terminal ileum, preserving the ileocolic artery initially.
4. For double-stapled technique, use a TA-30 or other suitable stapler to staple the anorectal junction at the level of the levator muscles.
5. Mobilize the small bowel and its mesentery, including full lysis of adhesions and separation of the superior mesenteric a. pedicle from the third portion of the duodenum.
6. If reach is insufficient, perform lengthening procedures including divide peritoneum, selective vascular ligation, and/or consideration of alternate pouch shape.
7. Create a 15- to 20-cm long J-pouch by stapling the distal two limbs of ileum together with GIA stapler and inserting anvil of EEA stapler, if double-stapled technique is planned.
8. Perform stapled or hand-sewn anastomosis.
9. Perform diverting loop ileostomy.

Potential Pitfalls

- Injury to the small bowel mesentery during maneuvers to create length.
- Failure to separate the anal cuff from the vagina/prostate can result in fistula.

Postoperative Management

Complications are common after IPAA. The ACS-NSQIP database shows that 24% of patients had major complications and 17% had minor complications within 30 days after IPAA, most commonly superficial and organ space surgical site infections. The most feared early complication is anastomotic leak, for which management depends on the severity of presentation and whether or not ileostomy was performed at the original operation. Some combination of broad-spectrum antibiotics, percutaneous drainage, diverting ileostomy, and open washout may be required depending on the situation. While there is controversy about the value of diverting ileostomy with IPAA, most procedures are performed with diversion due to concern for increased risk of pelvic sepsis without diversion, and possible poor functional outcome after pelvic sepsis.

Long-term complications after IPAA include pouchitis, bowel obstruction, and female infertility. Long-term septic complications include anastomotic strictures and fistulas. Pouch failure occurs in approximately 10% of patients, due to septic complications, chronic pouchitis, or other complications. Frequent bowel movements are not a complication of IPAA, but rather the expected functional outcome. Five to seven loose bowel movements

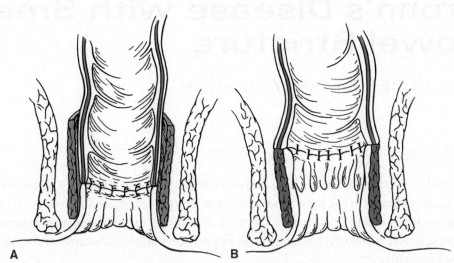

FIGURE 3 • Ileal pouch–anal anastomosis. (**A**) Sutured anastomosis at dentate line after mucosectomy. (**B**) Double-stapled anastomosis. There is a residual 1- to 2-cm cuff of rectal mucosa.

per day with at least one at night and some nighttime leakage is a reasonable functional result, and patients must be well informed preoperatively. Follow-up for dysplasia of the pouch-anal anastomosis is usually recommended beginning 8 to 10 years after onset of UC.

TAKE HOME POINTS

- Surgical treatment should be considered for medically refractory UC, and decision making is multidisciplinary.
- Prior to surgery, medical treatment should be optimized, including ruling out superimposed infectious colitis.
- Evaluate for signs and symptoms of toxic colitis and Crohn's disease.
- Consider a 3-stage approach with initial subtotal colectomy for ill patients.
- Ileal pouch anal anastomosis is the most common surgical treatment for UC.
- Be prepared with lengthening procedures and alternative pouch configurations for cases in which the pouch will not reach the anus.
- Diverting ileostomy is usually performed.
- Complications are common after IPAA, but there are 90% long-term success rates.

SUGGESTED READINGS

Andersson T, Lunde OC, Johnson E, et al. Long-term functional outcome and quality of life after restorative proctocolectomy with ileo-anal anastomosis for colitis. Colorectal Dis. 2011;13(4):431–437.

Aratari A, Papi C, Clemente V, et al. Colectomy rate in acute severe ulcerative colitis in the infliximab era. Dig Liver Dis. 2008;40:821–826.

Berndtsson I, Lindholm E, Oresland T, et al. Long-term outcome after ileal pouch-anal anastomosis: function and health-related quality of life. Dis Colon Rectum. 2007;50:1545–1552.

Bret A, Lashner M, Aaron Brzezinski M. Medical treatment of ulcerative colitis and other colitides. In: Victor W. Fazio M, James M. Church,Conor P. Delaney eds. Current Therapy in Colon and Rectal Surgery. 2nd ed. Philadelphia, PA: Elsevier Mosby, 2005.

Cottone M, Scimeca D, Mocciaro F, et al. Clinical course of ulcerative colitis. Dig Liver Dis. 2008;40(suppl 2):S247–S252.

Farouk R, Dozois RR, Pemberton JH, et al. Incidence and subsequent impact of pelvic abscess after ileal pouch-anal anastomosis for chronic ulcerative colitis. Dis Colon Rectum. 1998;41:1239–1243.

Fazio VW, O'Riordain MG, Lavery IC, et al. Long-term functional outcome and quality of life after stapled restorative proctocolectomy. Ann Surg. 1999;230:575–584; discussion 584–586.

Fleming FJ, Francone TD, Kim MJ, et al. A laparoscopic approach does reduce short-term complications in patients undergoing ileal pouch-anal anastomosis. Dis Colon Rectum. 2011;54:176–182.

Hahnloser D, Pemberton JH, Wolff BG, et al. Results at up to 20 years after ileal pouch-anal anastomosis for chronic ulcerative colitis. Br J Surg. 2007;94:333–340.

McMurrick PJ, Dozois RR. Chronic ulcerative colitis: surgical options. In: Victor W. Fazio, James M. Church, Conor P. Delaney, eds. Current Therapy in Colon and Rectal Surgery. 2nd ed. Philadelphia, 2005.

Michelassi F, Lee J, Rubin M, et al. Long-term functional results after ileal pouch anal restorative proctocolectomy for ulcerative colitis: a prospective observational study. Ann Surg. 2003;238:433–441; discussion 442–445.

Ricciardi R, Ogilvie JW Jr, Roberts PL, et al. Epidemiology of Clostridium difficile colitis in hospitalized patients with inflammatory bowel diseases. Dis Colon Rectum. 2009;52:40–45.

Tjandra JJ, Fazio VW, Milsom JW, et al. Omission of temporary diversion in restorative proctocolectomy–is it safe? Dis Colon Rectum. 1993;36:1007–1014.

43 Crohn's Disease with Small Bowel Stricture

HUEYLAN CHERN and EMILY FINLAYSON

Presentation

A 19-year-old otherwise healthy woman presents with abdominal pain and diarrhea. The abdominal pain is described as sharp and constant in the right lower quadrant. She denies melena or bloody diarrhea. She reports postprandial nausea and bloating without emesis. She denies recent travel history and her family history is unremarkable. Her menstrual cycle has been regular. On abdominal examination, her right lower quadrant is tender to palpation.

Differential Diagnosis

Differential diagnoses for right lower-quadrant abdominal pain include appendicitis, inflammatory bowel disease, Meckel's diverticulum, urinary tract infection, and infectious enterocolitis. *Campylobacter* and *Yersinia* infection from poor handling of food can affect the ileocolic region and mimic Crohn's ileocolic disease. In women, gynecologic causes such as ovarian torsion, tubal ovarian abscess, pelvic inflammatory disease, and ectopic pregnancy need to be considered as well.

Workup

The patient undergoes CT scan of the abdomen and pelvis with IV and oral contrast that reveals an inflamed, narrowed segment of terminal ileum (**Figure 1**). Serum laboratory values include hemoglobin of 11 g/dL, an albumin level of 3.3 g/dL, and a C-reactive protein level of 86 g/dL.

Discussion

Crohn's disease (CD) is a chronic inflammatory intestinal disease that can be unremitting and is incurable. It can affect any part of the gastrointestinal tract. The distribution is usually discontinuous with segments of uninvolved intestine. The inflammation in CD is transmural involving the full thickness of the bowel wall from the mucosa to serosa. The etiology for CD remains uncertain. CD has a bimodal age distribution with the first peak occurring between the ages of 15 to 30 years and the second between 60 and 80 years. The most common anatomic pattern in patients with CD is ileocolic disease occurring in 40%, followed by

small intestinal disease, isolated colonic disease, and gastroduodenal disease. The disease behavior is classified into three categories: inflammatory, stricturing, and fistulizing. However, the anatomic distribution and behavior can change in any given Crohn's patient over time.

The keys to evaluation of CD are determining extent and location of involved intestines and obtaining tissue for diagnosis. Several imaging modalities such as contrast studies, computed tomography (CT), and magnetic resonance imaging (MRI) have been used to evaluate CD. In the acute setting, CT of the abdomen and pelvic with contrast is a good choice to look for acute complication such as abscess, obstruction, or perforation and also to eliminate other causes for acute abdomen. CT is also helpful in looking for thickened intestine, stricture, adjacent organ involvement, fistulas, phlegmon, and abscess (**Figure 2A**). CD complicated by enterovesical or colovesical fistulas will present with air or oral contrast within the bladder (**Figure 2B**).

Contrast studies such as small bowel follow through are helpful for evaluation of Crohn's when small bowel proximal to terminal ileum is involved. CT enterography, MRI enterography, and capsule endoscopy are other modalities used to diagnose proximal small bowel disease. MRI enterography has recently gained popularity because it avoids radiation exposure in a typically young patient requiring imaging over lifetime for followup or diagnosis. Furthermore, unlike contrast studies, it has the ability demonstrate both extraluminal and intraluminal pathology.

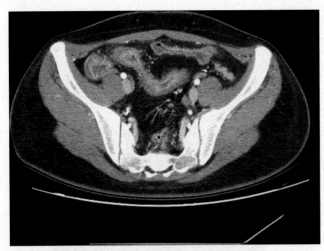

FIGURE 1 • Terminal ileum stricture.

Endoscopy is critical in workup, surveillance, and management of CD. Both colonoscopy and esophagogastroduodenoscopy are essential for demonstrating mucosal inflammation and obtaining tissue for diagnosis. The terminal ileum should be intubated and examined whenever possible during colonoscopy. The classic endoscopic findings for Crohn's include aphthous ulcers, patchy erythema, linear serpiginous ulcers, deep "bear claw" ulceration, and strictures. However, the risk of perforation from colonoscopy in acute inflammation is high. Therefore, colonoscopy is generally avoided in an acute setting. A limited endoscopy such as flexible sigmoidoscopy can be considered if results will alter management in the acute setting.

Diagnosis and Treatment

Medical Therapy

In this patient with newly diagnosed CD and a stricture that is likely inflammatory in nature, medical therapy is the most appropriate initial approach. In general, medical treatment is the initial and primary therapy for CD. Medication frequently used includes aminosalicylates, antibiotics, steroids, thiopurines, cyclosporines, and antibodies to tumor necrosis factor. Very few patients will require surgery at initial disease presentation. Patients presenting with obstructive symptoms can be managed with bowel rest and nasogastric tube. The fact that this patient has an elevated C-reactive protein level suggests that her stricture is most likely inflammatory in nature (not fibrostenotic). Intravenous steroid can be used to treat the acute inflammation. Patients presenting with an associated intra-abdominal abscess can undergo percutaneous drainage. Surgery if indicated for persistent symptoms can then be delayed and performed in an elective setting when inflammation is not as severe and overall condition more stable. The goal of staged resection is to avoid bleeding associated with acute inflammation and to preserve bowel length.

Surgical Therapy

If this patient has persistent pain and obstructive symptoms despite medical therapy, surgical resection is indicated. In general, surgical therapy is reserved for failed medical therapy or an acute, severe complication of CD **(Table 1)**. Because CD is not curable, operative intervention is only intended to address complication and alleviate symptoms to improve quality of life.

The most common indication for operation is obstruction from stricture. Several options exist including resection with or without anastomosis, strictureplasty, and bypass. What operation to perform depends on factors such as nutritional status, number of prior bowel resections, the length and number of strictures, surrounding inflammation, and immunosuppression status. Resection, strictureplasty, and

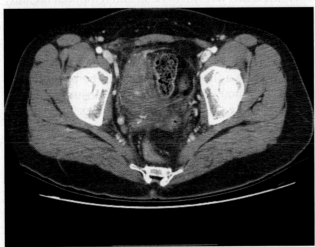

A
FIGURE 2A • Right lower-quadrant phlegmon.

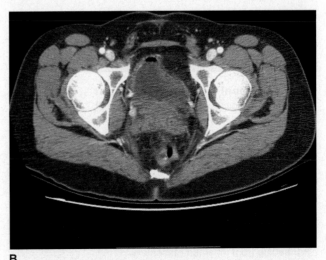

B
FIGURE 2B • Air in the bladder indicating fistula to the gastrointestinal tract.

TABLE 1. Indications for Surgery

- Medically refractory disease
- Medication-related complication
- Massive hemorrhage
- Free perforation
- Acute obstruction
- Neoplasia
- Abscess not amenable to percutaneous drainage
- Symptomatic fistula

bypass techniques may be used in one operation to treat multiple strictures. In this patients with a long, isolated segment of strictured terminal ileum, ileocolic resection is the recommended option.

Surgical Approach for Ileocolic Crohn's Disease

Laparoscopic resection by experienced surgeons can be done safely in inflammatory bowel disease **(Table 2)**. Preoperative imaging is essential to assess the entire gastrointestinal tract. If performed laparoscopically, one camera port and three working ports are typically necessary **(Figure 3)**. The entire small bowel is examined to assess the full extent of disease. Nondiseased intestines may be drawn into the inflammatory process, and they should be freed and preserved. A medial to lateral approach can be sometimes be difficult in ileocolic Crohn's because of associated inflammation, phlegmon, or abscess. However, if the duodenum can be identified and the ileocolic vessels can be appreciated, scoring underneath the ileocolic vessels may allow entry into the avascular plane between the mesentery and the retroperitoneum. If not, a lateral to medial dissection can be started by dividing along the

TABLE 2. Key Technical Steps and Potential Pitfalls of Ileocolic Resection

Key Technical Steps
1. Laparoscopic port placement **(Figure 3)**.
2. Visual evaluation of entire small bowel.
3. Lateral to medial or medial to lateral mobilization of the ascending colon and mesentery.
4. Identification of the duodenum.
5. Ligation and division of the ileocolic vessels.
6. Division of the bowel proximal and distal to grossly diseased intestines.
7. Anastomosis of the ileum to the ascending colon.

Potential Pitfalls
- Bleeding from inflamed mesentery.
- Injury to the duodenum.
- Injury to the ureter.

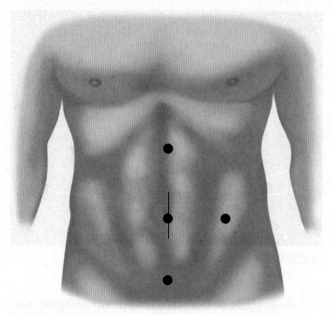

FIGURE 3 • Common port placement for a laparoscopic ileocolic resection.

line of Toldt. The terminal ileum, the right colon, and the hepatic flexure need to completely mobilized. Once the ileocolic vessels are ligated and divided, grossly abnormal bowel is resected. The bowel is divided and an anastomosis is constructed ensuring correct orientation, without tension, and with good blood supply. The anastomosis can be performed with stapled technique, handsewn technique in a side-to-side or an end-to-end fashion. The abdomen cavity is washed out and the fascia closed.

Intraoperative Considerations

When operating for CD, caution should be exercised in dividing the mesentery. Mesentery in CD is typically thickened with fat deposit and lymphadenopathy making division difficult. Rapid spread of mesenteric hematoma can result in further loss of intestinal length. Nondiseased intestine can also be drawn into the diseased process and involved in fistula formation or inflammatory adhesion. Care should be taken to preserve all normal intestines. Primary closure of the fistula after wedge resection in the unaffected intestine is usually sufficient. Wider margins do not decrease postoperative recurrence, and it is not necessary to achieve microscopic negative margins. Therefore, to preserve bowel length, the margins can be determined by resection to macroscopically normal intestine.

Risk of Recurrence, Postop Surveillance, and Treatment

After resection, endoscopic recurrence can be as high as 80% at 1 year. Twenty percent of the patients may experience clinical relapse at 1 year. The risk of developing disease complications requiring surgery approaches 50% at 10 years. Aminosalicylates, antibiotics, and thiopurines are only modestly effective in preventing disease recurrence. The antitumor necrosis factor agent has been shown to be most effective in preventing recurrence and therefore should be considered in patients at high risk for recurrence. Smoking is a well-known independent risk factor for recurrence. Therefore, smoking cessation is encouraged.

Case Conclusion

A CT of the abdomen and pelvis was done and showed inflamed terminal ileum. She, however, continued to have significant obstructive symptoms on maximal medical treatment and eventually required a laparoscopic ileocolic resection.

TAKE HOME POINTS

- Crohn's disease (CD) is a chronic inflammatory panintestinal disease that relies on medical treatment and surgery is not curable.
- Emergent surgery is rarely necessary because acute complication such as obstruction and abscess can often be managed nonoperatively.
- Preservation of healthy bowel is essential when operating on patients with CD.
- Surgery is intended to address complications and alleviate symptoms to improve quality of life.

SUGGESTED READINGS

Lichtenstein GR, Hanauer SB, Sandborn WJ; Practice Parameters Committee of American College of Gastroenterology. Management of Crohn's disease in adults. Am J Gastroenterol. 2009;104(2):465–483.

Strong SA, Koltun WA, Hyman NH, et al. Standards Practice Task force of The American Society of Colon and Rectal Surgeons. Practice parameters for the surgical management of Crohn's disease. Dis Colon Rectum. 2007;50:1735–1746.

Yamamoto T, Fazio VW, Tekkis PP. Safety and efficacy of strictureplasty for Crohn's disease: a systematic review and meta-analysis. Dis Colon Rectum. 2007;50(11):1968–1986.

44 Fulminant *Clostridium difficile* Colitis

NATASHA S. BECKER and SAMIR S. AWAD

Presentation

The patient is a 78-year-old gentleman with a past history of hypertension, peripheral vascular disease, and diabetes. Two weeks ago, he underwent carotid endarterectomy and was recently treated as an outpatient with ciprofloxacin for a UTI. He presents back to the hospital with abdominal pain and profuse watery diarrhea. He describes this as 10 bowel movements a day and states that the stool is foul smelling. He denies nausea/vomiting, fever, melena, or hematochezia. He denies any unusual food intake or recent travel, and he drinks only city tap water. No one else in his household is sick. Upon exam, he is afebrile, mildly tachycardic, but normotensive. He appears dehydrated with tacky mucous membranes and dry skin. His abdomen is soft, mildly distended, and diffusely tender without peritoneal signs. He has no abdominal scars.

Differential Diagnosis

Acute onset of profuse diarrhea is most commonly from an infectious cause. Infectious causes include viral infections such as norovirus, rotavirus, and adenovirus. Bacterial infections usually cause more severe diarrhea and in adults are usually due to *Vibrio*, *Escherichia coli*, *Salmonella*, *Campylobacter* or *Shigella*. However, in patients with recent antibiotic use, *Clostridium difficile* infection should be considered. Parasitic infections are also possible and can be due to *Giardia lamblia*, *Cryptosporidium*, and *Entamoeba histolytica*. Noninfectious causes should be considered if no pathogen is found and if diarrhea persists for longer than 10 to 14 days. Noninfectious causes can include osmotic antibiotic-associated diarrhea, carcinoid syndrome, collagenous colitis, and pancreatic insufficiency.

Workup and Treatment

The patient in this scenario was admitted to the internal medicine service and is resuscitated and kept NPO. Initial lab work shows WBC count of 14, Cr of 1.5, and CO_2 of 15. Stool is sent for culture and ova and parasites. Enzyme immunoassay is sent for *C. difficile* toxin, and empiric PO metronidazole is started due to high clinical suspicion for *C. difficile* colitis. This test comes back positive on hospital day 2. On hospital day 3, the patient's diarrhea resolves, but he begins to complain of increasing abdominal pain and fever to 101.7. He becomes more tachycardic and hypotensive. His abdomen also becomes more distended. He is transferred to the ICU for more intensive monitoring. Plain films are obtained that show a distended ascending and transverse colon (7 cm) **(Figure 1)**. PO vancomycin and IV metronidazole are started, but after 24 hours, the patient remains unstable and is requiring norepinephrine support despite adequate fluid status. WBC count rises to 23 K, and CT of the abdomen is obtained, which shows pancolonic thickening with dilation to 7 cm **(Figure 2)**. A surgical consultation is called, and the patient is prepared for surgery.

C. difficile colitis most commonly presents as watery diarrhea with abdominal tenderness in a patient who has recently been on antibiotics. It is a gram-positive spore forming anaerobe bacteria that is most likely part of the normal colonic flora. Broad-spectrum antibiotics may disrupt the normal anaerobic flora and allow *C. difficile* to flourish. Certain strains of *C. difficile* produce toxins. Toxins A and B have been identified and are believed to cause glycosylation of proteins that normally maintain cell membrane integrity. Cell membrane breakdown then leads to secretory diarrhea. Recently, there have been more virulent strains of *C. difficile* identified that are believed to produce more toxins. These include the BI/NAP1/027 strain that causes more severe disease and higher mortality. There have also been reports of *C. difficile* colitis occurring in patients with no history of antibiotic use.

Diagnosis is based on clinical suspicion and history. It can be confirmed with stool toxin enzyme immunoassay that detects toxins A and B. Sensitivity of this test ranges from 63% to 94%, with a specificity of 75% to 100%. There are also enzyme immunoassays against glutamate dehydrogenase that is a common *C. difficile* antigen. Other diagnostic tests include cell-culture cytotoxic assays and *C. difficile* culture. More recently,

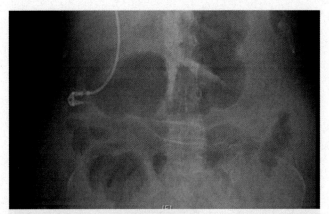

FIGURE 1 • Flat KUB showing distended colon.

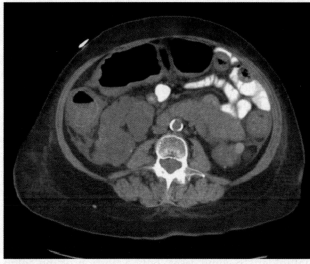

FIGURE 2 • CT scan showing thickened colon.

the use of polymerase chain reaction (PCR) for ampli-fication of *C. difficile* DNA in stool was approved by the FDA and can be performed in a few hours. PCR appears to be more sensitive than enzyme immunoas-says and also have high specificity. However, many individuals are asymptomatically colonized with *C. difficile*, so careful patient selection for this type of test-ing is very important. Endoscopy can also be used to diagnose *C. difficile* colitis; however, because of concern for bowel perforation, it is usually reserved for cases in which the diagnosis is in question.

Once a patient is diagnosed with *C. difficile*, or if there is high clinical suspicion, any broad-spectrum antibiotics should be stopped (if possible) and treat-ment started. Most cases can be successfully treated with metronidazole, although there are recent reports of treatment failures in more severe cases. PO van-comycin is also effective although more expensive, and there is concern about the development of vanco-mycin-resistant enterococcus. In patients with severe illness requiring ICU admission, IV metronidazole and PO vancomycin combination therapy should be started. In 95% of patients, this will be adequate treatment; however in 3% to 5%, fulminant colitis can occur.

Fulminant *C. difficile* colitis is defined as severe sys-temic toxic effects from infection resulting in toxic megacolon, need for ICU admission, need for colec-tomy, or death. Mortality rate is reported as 35% to 60% in most series. Surgical intervention may be curative in cases of fulminant colitis and is recommended if patients with signs of severe systemic toxicity fail to improve after 24 to 48 hours of maximal therapy. Other specific indications for surgery include organ failure, vasopressors requirement, worsening CT scan findings, and peritonitis. Some experts advocate ear-lier surgical intervention as mortality after colectomy for *C. difficile* is increased in patients in multisystem organ failure, those requiring vasopressors, and those requiring ventilatory support. As the disease process

involves the entire colon, the recommended surgery is total abdominal colectomy with end ileostomy.

Surgical Approach

The patient in our scenario is now intubated and requiring pressor support. As there is no improvement even with full intensive care unit support, consent is obtained from his family for exploratory laparotomy, total abdominal colectomy, and end ileostomy **(Table 1)**.

Patients with fulminant *C. difficile* colitis requiring surgery are often extremely ill and in multisystem organ failure. Total abdominal colectomy removes most of the diseased organ and toxin-producing bacteria and often results in dramatic improvement. Although the residual rectum may contain disease,

TABLE 1. Key Technical Steps and Potential Pitfalls for Total Abdominal Colectomy

Key Technical Steps
1. Proctoscopy.
2. Midline incision.
3. Abdominal exploration.
4. Colonic mobilization.
5. Transection of the mesentery.
6. Division of the ileum and rectum; removal of the colon.
7. Closure of the fascia and skin.
8. Maturation of the ileostomy.

Potential Pitfalls
- Damage to the dilated colon upon entry into the abdomen.
- Damage to the ureter during colonic mobilization.
- Failure to resect the sigmoid colon when ligating the sigmoidal vessels (predisposing to ischemia and stump dehiscence).
- Failure to resect the rectum if so diseased that stump cannot be securely closed.

most patients are too sick to allow for extensive pelvic dissection. Reanastomosis in this setting would be too risky given the patient's already tenuous state and likelihood of leak; therefore, end ileostomy is almost always preferred.

If possible, the patient is marked for ileostomy prior to being brought to the operating room. The patient is placed into modified lithotomy position to allow for proctoscopy. This may be performed prior to incision in order to evaluate the rectal mucosa. Exploratory laparotomy is conducted under general anesthesia through a midline incision. Care should be taken upon entry into the abdomen to avoid the dilated colon. Once in the abdomen, the colon should be inspected for any areas of perforation and the remainder of the abdomen should be quickly inspected for any other pathology. In some cases, only a portion of the colon will appear grossly diseased at laparotomy. However, given the high likelihood of pancolonic involvement and the poor condition of the patients, they will likely not tolerate a second laparotomy. Therefore, total abdominal colectomy should still be performed. The colon is then mobilized from its peritoneal attachments. The distal ileum is transected and the mesentery is divided with ligature of the ileocolic, right colic, middle colic, left colic, and sigmoid vessels. The distal colon is then divided at the pelvic brim with care taken to resect the whole sigmoid colon if the sigmoidal vessels have been ligated. The rectal stump may be oversewn. In rare cases, the rectum may be the source of bleeding or such severe disease that staples or sutures will cut through the bowel. In this case, further resection of the rectum or a total proctocolectomy should be considered. If gross spillage has occurred, the abdomen should be irrigated. The ileostomy is then brought through the abdominal wall, and after the fascia of the midline is closed, this is matured.

Special Intraoperative Considerations

If the colon is so dilated as to interfere with safe mobilization, consideration should be given to decompression either through the colon or through the ileum. If the patient is extremely unstable, a damage control operation may be performed in which the abdomen is left open after colon resection and the patient returns to the ICU for resuscitation. The patient is brought back to the operating room after 24 to 48 hours for closure and maturation of the ileostomy. In cases of colonic perforation where there is a large amount of contamination, the abdomen should be well irrigated after colon removal and the skin may be left open with wet to dry dressing changes.

Postoperative Management

Mortality rate after abdominal colectomy for *C. difficile* is very high (35% to 50%) and patients require intensive supportive care in the perioperative period.

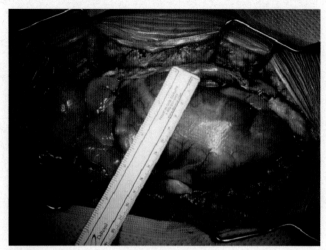

FIGURE 3 • Dilated colon seen at surgery.

Respiratory, cardiac, and renal support/replacement may be required. Postoperatively the patient is kept in the ICU until their hemodynamic stabilize. Antibiotic treatment against *C. difficile* is continued and the patient is kept NPO until bowel function returns. Recurrent *C. difficile* infection can occur in the residual rectum or in the small bowel, and this should be kept in mind if the patient relapses or continues to have symptoms of sepsis.

Case Conclusion

The patient is taken to surgery and dilated colon without signs of perforation or ischemia is found. Total abdominal colectomy with end ileostomy is performed. Postoperatively, his condition stabilizes and he is extubated on POD 2. His pressor requirements decrease and they are discontinued by postoperative day 2 also. He is transferred to the step down unit. He experiences a prolonged ileus and requires TPN support. On POD 13, his ileostomy begins to function and he is started on a diet. He tolerates this well and is discharged home on POD 16 **(Figure 3)**.

TAKE HOME POINTS

- *C. difficile* colitis should be considered in patents with profuse diarrhea, especially if they have received recent antibiotic therapy.
- Diagnosis can be confirmed through stool enzyme immunoassay or PCR testing.
- Most cases can be treated medically, but early consideration should be given to surgical intervention in patients with fulminant disease.

- Patients undergoing surgery for *C. difficile* colitis are very ill and usually in multiple organ failure. Perioperative mortality is very high.
- Given the pancolonic involvement and the poor health status of the patient, the procedure of choice is total abdominal colectomy with end ileostomy.
- The colon may grossly appear normal at colectomy but should still be removed in its entirety.

SUGGESTED READINGS

Ananthakrishnan AN. *Clostridium difficile* infection: epidemiology, risk factors, and management. Nat Rev Gastroenterol Hepatol. 2011;8:17–26.

Chan S, Ng K, Lyon D, et al. Acute bacterial gastroenteritis: a study of adult patients with positive stool cultures treated in the emergency department. Emerg Med J. 2003;20:335–338.

Couturier MR, Lee B, Zelyas N, et al. Shiga-toxigenic *Escherichia coli* detection in stool samples screened for viral gastroenteritis in Alberta, Canada. J Clin Microbiol. 2011;49(2):574–578.

Gash K, Brown E, Pullyblank A. Emergency subtotal colectomy for fulminant *Clostridium difficile* colitis–is a surgical solution considered for all patients? Ann R Coll Surg Engl. 2010;92:56–60.

Hall JF, Berger D. Outcome of colectomy for *Clostridium difficile* colitis: a plea for early surgical management. Am J Surg. 2008;196(3):384–388.

Jaber M, Olafsson S, Fung W, et al. Clinical review of the magagement of fulminant *Clostridium difficile* infection. Am J Gastroenterol. 2008;103:3195–3203.

Kufelnicka A, Kirn T. Effective utilizaion of evolving methods for the laboratory diagnosis of *Clostridium difficile* infection. Clin Infect Dis. 2011;52(12):1451–1457.

Kuntz JL, Chrischiles EA, Pendergast JF, et al. Incidence of and risk factors for communnity-associated *Clostridium difficile* infection: a nested case-control study. BMC Infect Dis. 2011;11:194.

Perera AD, Akbari RP, Cowher MS, et al. Colectomy for fulminant *C. difficile* colitis: predictors of mortality. Am Surg. 2010;76:418–421.

Rothenberger DA, Bullard KM. Surgery for toxic megacolon. In: Fischer JE, ed. Mastery of Surgery. Philadelphia, PA: Lippincott, Williams and Wilkins, 2007:1465–1474.

Sailhamer EA, Carson K, Chang Y, et al. Fulminant *Clostridium difficile* colitis. Arch Surg. 2011;144(5):433–439.

Sayedy L, Kothari D, Richards R. Toxic megacolon associated *Clostridium difficile* colitis. World J Gastrointest Endosc. 2010;2(8):293–297.

45 Appendiceal Carcinoid Tumor

WOLFGANG B. GAERTNER, ELIZABETH C. WICK and GENEVIEVE MELTON-MEAUX

Presentation

A 44-year-old female presents with a 2-day history of right lower-quadrant pain associated with anorexia and nausea. WBC is 12,000. An abdominal ultrasound shows a thickened appendix with minimal free fluid in the right lower quadrant. The patient undergoes an uneventful laparoscopic appendectomy and is discharged to home on postoperative day 1. Pathology returns 2 days later and shows a 1.5-cm carcinoid tumor located at the midappendix with invasion of the mesoappendix.

Differential Diagnosis

Appendiceal tumors are exceedingly rare with an age-adjusted incidence of 0.12 cases per 1,000,000 people per year. It is estimated that appendiceal cancer is found in 1% of all appendectomy specimens. In addition to being a rare form of cancer, the vast majority of appendiceal carcinomas are not diagnosed preoperatively; rather, they present with acute appendicitis or are detected as an incidental finding during operative exploration for another surgical disorder. Although carcinoid tumors were once considered the most common type of appendiceal tumor, the reported incidence has decreased since the 1970s and the incidence of appendiceal adenocarcinoma has increased.

Workup

The patient is further evaluated with a computed tomography (CT) scan of the abdomen and pelvis that shows postoperative changes in the right lower quadrant but no evidence of metastatic disease or enlarged lymph nodes. A chest X-ray is also performed and is normal. Further histologic evaluation reveals positive Ki67 staining and mitotic activity >2 cells/mm^2. The patient inquires if she needs further treatment.

Discussion

Neuroendocrine tumors (NETs) of the appendix occur in 1 of 100 to 300 patients undergoing appendectomy. Autopsy series report an overall incidence ranging from 0.009% to 0.17%, suggesting a natural degeneration of small benign lesions during later life. NETs (formerly known as carcinoids) originate from subepithelial neuroendocrine cells, usually present in the fourth decade, and favor the female gender. Some authors have ascribed a higher incidence in females to higher rates of laparoscopy and appendectomy among women. Crohn's disease has also been identified as a risk factor for gastrointestinal (GI) NETs overall. NETs comprise 32% to 57% of all appendiceal tumors.

They predominantly affect the small intestine (44.7%), followed by the rectum (19.6%), and the appendix (16.7%). Primary adenocarcinoma of the appendix, although also quite rare, has seen an increase in incidence over the past 20 years with reports of up to 26% of all appendiceal malignancies.

Diagnosis and Treatment

Most appendiceal NETs are asymptomatic and are found incidentally. Patients usually present with nonspecific abdominal pain at the lower right abdomen that leads to appendectomy. Although most patients undergo some form of abdominal imaging, a CT scan of the abdomen and pelvis should be performed whenever an appendiceal mass is suspected **(Figure 1)**. While CT is being increasingly used for the workup of abdominal pain, it is unlikely that the routine application of this imaging technique would be warranted with respect to associated cost and diagnostic yield. Appendiceal NETs occur more frequently at the appendiceal tip (60% to 70%), followed by the body (5% to 21%), and base (7% to 10%). With regard to size, 60% to 76% are <1 cm, 4% to 27% are 1 to 2 cm, and 2% to 17% are >2 cm in diameter. Tumors are graded as benign, borderline malignant, low-grade malignant, or high-grade malignant. The majority of reported metastasized GI lesions have been graded as low-grade malignant. Assessing the mitotic activity (>2 cells/mm^2) of so-called low-grade malignant lesions and the presence of proliferation marker Ki67 may be of prognostic value as well.

Tumors <1 cm in size require no staging unless identified as high-grade malignant. Patients with tumors between 1 and 2 cm may benefit from additional screening. Plasma chromogranin A is the most important tumor marker available, with 80% to 100% of patients with NETs having increased levels. Chromogranin A levels also correspond to tumor load and levels >5,000 µg/L correlate with poor outcomes.

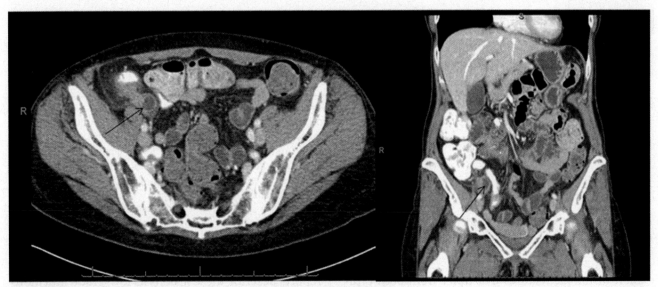

FIGURE 1 • CT of a patient with an appendiceal mucinous cystadenoma.

Patients with elevated chromogranin A levels require further imaging. In these patients, ^{111}In-labeled octreotide scintigraphy is the most sensitive imaging modality in the diagnosis and staging of metastatic disease. Patients with tumors >2 cm, incomplete resections, metastatic disease, or goblet cell tumors warrant further investigation including determination of plasma chromogranin A levels, 24-hour urinary levels of 5-hydroxyindoleacetic acid, CT scan of the abdomen and pelvis, and ^{111}In-labeled octreotide scintigraphy. A significant number of coexistent malignant tumors can be found in patients with appendiceal NETs (7% to 48%), primarily throughout the GI tract. Therefore, high-risk or symptomatic patients should be evaluated either endoscopically or with further imaging to assess the remainder of the GI tract.

All noncarcinoid appendiceal malignancies should undergo right colectomy, whereas the type of surgical intervention for NETs depends upon the tumor's size, histopathology, and location. As for all NETs, the risk of metastases increases with size. The risk of metastases in tumors <1 cm is virtually zero; tumors between 1 and 2 cm metastasize in 0% to 1%, and tumors >2 cm metastasize in 20% to 85%. These findings give the rationale for the hypothesis that patients with tumors >2 cm in diameter may benefit from an oncologic resection of the right colon.

Operative Treatment

NETs <1 cm in size, located at the body or tip of the appendix, and with no unfavorable histology or evidence of metastatic disease may undergo appendectomy. On the other end of the spectrum, patients with NETs >2 cm, goblet cell adenocarcinoid tumors of any size, positive mesoappendix or vascular invasion,

localization at the base of appendix, positive margins, or evidence of nodal metastasis should undergo right colectomy **(Table 1)**. With regard to NETs between 1 and 2 cm in size, one must take in account the operative risk. For patients with low risk and a NET between 1 and 2 cm with unfavorable histology (mitotic activity >2 cells/mm^2 or presence of proliferation marker Ki67), a right colectomy is required. For patients with high operative risk and a NET between 1 and 2 cm in size with favorable histology and located at the body or tip of the appendix, appendectomy is recommended.

With the widespread use of laparoscopic appendectomy, the question arises as if this technique is adequate for the treatment of appendiceal malignancies. Laparoscopic appendectomy for NETs seems to have a slightly higher rate of inadequate resection requiring further operative intervention. However, this has not been associated with a significantly worse prognosis compared to the open approach. The level of available evidence at present for recommendations with respect to use of laparoscopy is generally low for NETs in large part because of their low prevalence and often incidental detection.

Timing of a subsequent right colectomy should be within 3 months after appendectomy and can safely be performed laparoscopically. There are no data to support that a two-step approach may negatively affect prognosis. Adenocarcinoma of the appendix of any size should be treated with right colectomy due to the high rate of invasion and nodal metastases.

Special Considerations

Certain histologic characteristics should receive particular attention when treating appendiceal NETs. Goblet cell or crypt cell carcinoid (adenocarcinoid) tumors

TABLE 1. Treatment Recommendations for Appendiceal NETs

Tumor Size	Risk of Lymphatic Spread	Aggressive Characteristics to Tailor Therapy	Treatment
<1 cm	0%	Serosal invasion	Appendectomy
1–2 cm	0%–1%	Mesoappendiceal or vascular invasion, mitotic activity (>2 cells/mm^2), proliferation markers (i.e., Ki67), localization at base of appendix, positive margins.	Individual risk evaluation: appendectomy for high-risk (elderly) patient; right colectomy for low-risk (young) patient.
>2 cm	30%	None	Right colectomy
Goblet-cell histology (any size)	10%–20%	None	Right colectomy

exhibit histologic features that differ from both ordinary carcinoid and adenocarcinoma and have shown to be more aggressive than NETs **(Figure 2)**. Patients with these tumors tend to present at a later age (fifth decade), often present with a diffusely inflamed appendix on CT scan, and treatment should involve right colectomy regardless of the size of the tumor. While the role of proliferation markers such as Ki67 and mitotic activity (>2 cells/mm^2) is not precisely defined for appendiceal NETs, these parameters seem to indicate metastatic potential for other NET locations and might justify more extensive resection when present. Serosal involvement is present in approximately 70% of all malignant NETs but has not been related to outcomes in the published literature.

A variety of terms have been used to describe appendiceal mucinous lesions that are not frankly malignant, including cystadenomas, mucinous tumor of uncertain potential, disseminated peritoneal adenomucinosis, and malignant mucocele. Most reports describe these lesions as low-grade mucinous neoplasms. They have the potential to spread to the peritoneal cavity producing mucinous intraperitoneal ascites, resulting in pseudomyxoma peritonei and their malignant potential largely depends on the degree of cellular atypia. Perforated neoplasms or lesions ruptured intraoperatively result in pseudomyxoma peritonei. Lesions confined to the appendix with benign histology should be treated by appendectomy. Involvement of the base of the appendix requires cecectomy. Mucinous adenocarcinomas are more common in the appendix than the colon and account for 40% to 67% of all appendiceal adenocarcinomas. These tumors can also rupture and spread throughout the peritoneum causing pseudomyxoma peritonei and peritoneal carcinomatosis. Localized lesions should be treated with right colectomy, while selective ruptured lesions can benefit from cytoreductive surgery and hyperthermic intraperitoneal chemotherapy.

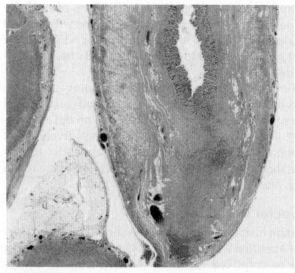 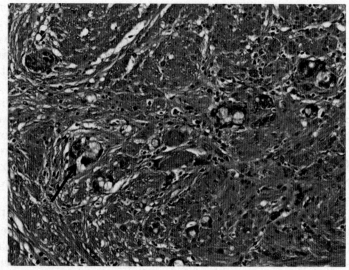

FIGURE 2 • Microscopic view of a goblet cell carcinoid tumor. High-power view shows a typical goblet cell (*arrow*).

The current treatment algorithm for appendiceal cancer best relies on a tissue diagnosis of carcinoid versus noncarcinoid histology. However, this requires a frozen section in the operating room, which could substantially delay an operation, and the results may differ from the final report anyway. Instead of relying on tissue diagnosis, some authors have proposed that all appendiceal malignancies should be treated with right colectomy. To further support this approach, reports have shown a decrease in NETs that would be appropriate for appendectomy alone and an overall underutilization of right colectomy in the treatment of appendiceal tumors. Other more recent reports have shown no difference in survival rates between right colectomy versus appendectomy alone, suggesting that appendectomy may be a viable treatment option even for larger tumors, therefore questioning the benefit of right colectomy with the currently available data. Although any cancer operation should be planned with curative intent, once advanced disease is present, right colectomy may be warranted to prevent complications such as bowel obstruction or endocrine-related syndromes. Although the role of cytoreductive surgery and hyperthermic intraperitoneal chemotherapy has become well established in properly selected patients for treatment of appendiceal adenocarcinoma, specifically the mucinous subtype, this form of therapy is not applicable to appendiceal NETs.

Postoperative Management

Patients with appendiceal NETs >2 cm, incomplete resections, and metastatic disease or goblet cell tumors require postoperative screening that includes serial plasma chromogranin A levels and abdominal CT. ^{111}In-labeled octreotide scintigraphy should be performed to stage patients with metastatic disease.

The calculated risk of metastases from tumors <1 cm is zero, while a definite increase occurs with a tumor size >2 cm, with a rate of metastases of 20%. Appendiceal NETs usually metastasize to the regional lymph nodes rather than to the liver. Five-year survival ranges from 80% to 89% for all stages. Patients with local disease have a 5-year survival rate ranging from 92% to 94%, those with regional metastases 81% to 84%, and those with distant metastases 31% to 33%. Surveillance for synchronous or metachronous tumors is warranted because the risk of a second primary malignancy in the GI tract is significantly increased in patients with NETs.

TAKE HOME POINTS

- NETs are common neoplasms of the appendix, occurring in 1 of 100 to 300 patients undergoing appendectomy.
- Patients with tumors >2 cm, unfavorable histology, incomplete resection, and metastatic disease or goblet cell tumors warrant further oncologic staging and postoperative screening.
- Small appendiceal NETs (<1 cm) have an excellent prognosis after appendectomy.
- NETs >2 cm, goblet cell adenocarcinoid tumors of any size, positive mesoappendix or vascular invasion, localization at the base of appendix, positive margins or evidence of nodal metastasis require right colectomy. Right colectomy should also be considered in NETs 1 to 2 cm in diameter with unfavorable histology.

SUGGESTED READINGS

Goede AC, Caplin ME, Winslet MC. Carcinoid tumour of the appendix. Br J Surg. 2003;90:1317–1322.

McGory ML, Maggard MA, Kang H, et al. Malignancies of the appendix: beyond case series reports. Dis Colon Rectum. 2005;48:2264–2271.

Murphy EM, Farquharson SM, Moran BJ. Management of an unexpected appendiceal neoplasm. Br J Surg. 2006;93:783–792.

46 Rectal Cancer

HYAEHWAN KIM and MARTIN R. WEISER

Presentation

A 62-year-old male presents to his primary care provider with complaints of bright red blood per rectum and thin-caliber stools for the past 2 months. His past medical history includes mild hypertension and hypercholesterolemia, and his current medications include Lopressor 25 mg daily, Lipitor 40 mg daily, and aspirin 81 mg daily. The patient denies any allergies. He had a right inguinal hernia repair at age 35. He quit smoking more than 20 years ago and drinks alcohol occasionally. His father died of complications related to a ruptured abdominal aortic aneurysm at the age of 80, and his mother was diagnosed with early-stage breast cancer at age 70. The patient has never had a colonoscopy. Digital rectal exam (DRE) in the primary care physician's office reveals a rectal mass, with gross blood on the examining finger. Serum laboratory studies show hemoglobin of 9.5 g/dL.

Differential Diagnosis

Although rectal bleeding and changes in bowel pattern can be associated with many benign conditions, rectal cancer is obviously the most likely diagnosis when an associated mass is identified on digital rectal examination. This is especially true of patients who present in the sixth or the seventh decade of life.

Workup

The patient is referred for colonoscopy, which was complete to the cecum. A 4-cm nonobstructing mass is noted in the rectum and biopsied. Additionally, a 1-cm transverse colon pedunculated polyp is completely removed. Pathology reveals an invasive, moderately differentiated adenocarcinoma of the rectum and an adenoma of the transverse colon. The patient undergoes a computerized tomography (CT) scan of the chest, abdomen, and pelvis with oral and intravenous contrast, which reveals a 2-mm nonspecific right upper lung nodule, a rectal mass consistent with the primary cancer, and no evidence of liver metastasis. Carcinoembryonic antigen (CEA) is within the normal range.

The patient is referred to a colorectal surgeon. On examination, DRE reveals the rectal mass to be tethered, but not fixed, and located 2 cm above the anorectal ring (i.e., 2 cm above the top of the external sphincter complex). On rigid proctoscopy, the lesion is 7 cm from the anal verge in the anterior position. It is ulcerated and occupies 40% of the bowel circumference. Endorectal ultrasound (ERUS) is performed and demonstrates that the rectal lesion extends to the muscularis propria and into the perirectal fat (uT3). There are two hypoechoic nodules in the mesorectum, adjacent to the tumor, measuring 4 and 5 mm, respectively.

These are consistent with mesorectal lymph node metastasis (uN1).

Discussion

Rectal cancer comprises nearly 30% of all colorectal cancers, approximately 41,000 new cases per year. Most rectal cancers present in patients in the sixth to the eighth decade of life. Synchronous adenomas and colorectal cancers are seen in 30% and 3% of cases, respectively. Thus, complete colonoscopy is necessary prior to surgery. Rectal cancer specifically refers to extraperitoneal lesions (i.e., lesions below the peritoneal reflection). Generally, these lesions are located <12 to 15 cm from the anal verge (as found on rigid proctoscopy). Lesions above the peritoneal reflection are usually treated as colon cancers.

The degree of tumor fixity in the pelvis is related to the depth of penetration of the primary lesion through the rectal wall. Mobile lesions are often limited to the mucosa, submucosa (cT1), or muscularis propria (cT2), whereas tethered lesions generally represent tumors extending into the perirectal fat or the mesorectum (cT3). Fixed tumors can extend into surrounding anatomic structures such as the prostate, seminal vesicles, or vagina (cT4). Many rectal cancer patients present without pain. However, when pain is present it indicates probable involvement of the sphincter by tumor. Tumors that are painful often extend into the external sphincter complex. ERUS **(Figure 1)** and phased array magnetic resonance imaging (MRI) **(Figure 2)** are currently the best imaging modalities for staging of rectal cancer, capable of accurately staging the primary lesion with up to 90% accuracy and locoregional lymph nodes with an accuracy of as much as 80%. ERUS is slightly

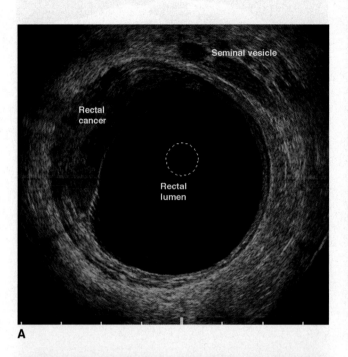

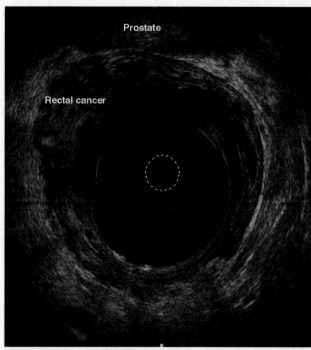

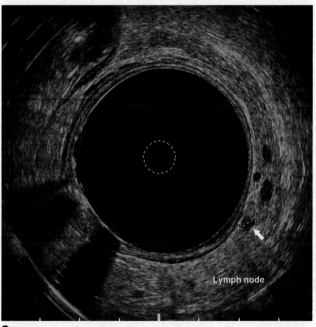

FIGURE 1 • ERUS demonstrating the hypoechoic primary rectal cancer at the level of the seminal vesicles (**A**) and the prostate (**B**) with invasion into the perirectal fat. Hypoechoic mesorectal lymph node indicative of nodal metastasis (**C**).

better than MRI in the staging of early lesions, while MRI is preferable for staging very bulky lesions with questionable invasion into surrounding organs (T4 lesions).

Pretreatment staging is critical to optimal patient care. Early lesions (stage I) are generally treated with surgery alone, while more advanced lesions (stages II and III) are treated with multimodality therapy including chemotherapy, radiotherapy, and surgery. Prospective randomized data have proven that chemoradiation is better tolerated and more effective if delivered preoperatively rather than postoperatively.

Rectal resection done in accordance with the proper technique of mesorectal excision is associated with local recurrence rates of <10%. Sharp dissection along the embryonic planes between the visceral and the parietal layers of the endopelvic fascia ensures complete removal of the locoregional lymph nodes in the mesorectum, preserves autonomic nerve function, and results in reduced blood loss.

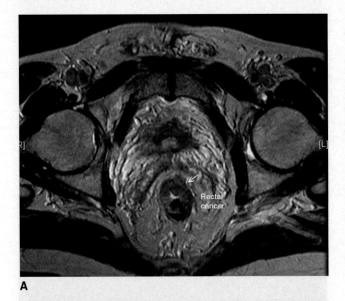

A

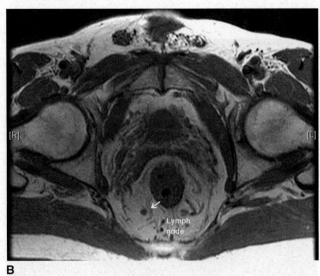

B

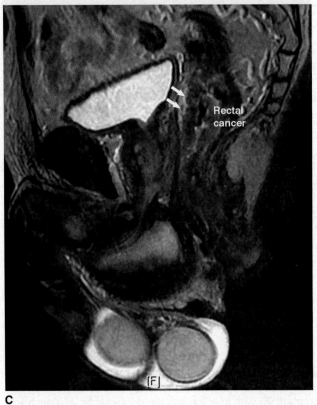

C

FIGURE 2 • MRI demonstrating the primary rectal cancer (**A**) and the mesorectal adenopathy (**B**) on axial imaging. (**C**) demonstrates the tumor in the sagittal plane.

Diagnosis and Treatment

In this patient, pretreatment staging indicates a uT3N1, stage III, mid-to-low rectal cancer. The patient should be treated with combined modality therapy (CMT), which most commonly includes 5 fluorouracil (5FU) administered as continuous intravenous infusion or as oral Xeloda, concomitant with 5,040 cGy delivered over the course of 25 to 28 daily fractions (Monday through Friday for 5.5 weeks). Following chemoradiation, repeat staging is done with a CT of the chest,

abdomen, and pelvis (with oral and intravenous contrast). Proctoscopy is also performed to assess for interval development of distant metastasis and evaluate the response of the primary tumor to therapy. As long as extensive distant metastases have not developed, the patient should proceed to surgical resection. Preoperative counseling should include a discussion regarding the possibility of a diverting stoma. The possibility of postoperative sexual and bladder dysfunction, as well as post low anterior resection (LAR) syndrome (which includes stool frequency, urgency, and clustering) should also be discussed. It is critical for the patient to understand that postoperative bowel function may take 12 to 24 months to plateau and may be permanently altered. Preoperative marking for a colostomy or an ileostomy in the office optimizes stoma location. Although the utility of bowel preparation has been questioned in regards to surgery for colon cancer, it remains useful in rectal cancer surgery.

Surgical Approach

In the operating room, the patient is placed in a modified lithotomy position. A bladder catheter is introduced. DRE and irrigation are performed to again assess the location of the tumor and remove any remaining stool from the rectum.

A midline incision is made, extending from the pubis to just above the umbilicus. Potential stoma sites must be kept in mind. Additional cephalad extension may be necessary to mobilize the splenic flexure. The abdomen is explored to search for metastatic disease in the liver or peritoneal surfaces and the small bowel packed in the upper abdomen. The patient is placed in a slight Trendelenburg position. Proper mobilization of the sigmoid is initiated by scoring the white line of Toldt followed. The left ureter and gonadal vessels are identified. The peritoneum is scored along the superior rectal artery to the base of the inferior mesenteric artery; this helps the surgeon maintain the sympathetic autonomic nerves in the retroperitoneum. The pedicle is ligated just distal to the takeoff of the left colic pedicle. High ligation of the inferior mesenteric artery is used selectively, as in the presence of bulky nodal disease; it has not been associated with improved oncologic outcome and can result in autonomic nerve injury. The mesentery is divided up to the left colon, which is divided with a stapler. The peritoneum is then scored bilaterally into the pelvis and around the anterior peritoneal reflection. The sigmoid mesentery is raised off the retroperitoneum again, with care taken to avoid injury to the autonomic nerves. With the rectum retracted anteriorly, the avascular plane between the visceral and the parietal layers of the endopelvic fascia is developed and characterized by loose areolar tissue. Posterior dissection is facilitated by use of the St. Marks retractor. It continues sharply through Waldeyer's fascia (rectosacral fascia that extends from S4 to the rectum/mesorectum). Blunt dissection should be avoided, as Waldeyer's fascia can tear at the presacral fascia, causing bleeding into the mesorectum resulting in an incomplete nodal dissection.

For mid to low rectal cancers, dissection is taken to the pelvic floor. Lateral dissection is also performed sharply with cautery, adjacent to the mesorectum, to avoid injuring the parasympathetic nerves. Pelvic sidewall dissection with en bloc removal of the parietal layer of the endopelvic fascia is performed, when necessary, to ensure clear circumferential margins. The anterior dissection is often developed last. In male patients, the dissection is continued through or anterior to Denonvilliers fascia and, if possible, both layers are removed from the seminal vesicles and the upper prostate, especially in the case of anterior lesions. At this point, the distal extent of the tumor and the transaction site are established. For tumors of the upper rectum, dissection continues 5 cm below the level of the mass. The mesorectum is then divided perpendicular to the intestine, to avoid "coning." For mid to low rectal cancers, dissection is completed to the pelvic floor, where the mesorectum ends. In the past, a 2-cm distal rectal margin has been recommended; however, numerous recent reports have shown that a 1-cm distal margin is sufficient, especially in the setting of preoperative chemoradiation. Once the distal resection line is identified, the rectum is clamped below the tumor and the distal rectum irrigated with a liter of saline to remove exfoliated cells and debris. Using a double staple technique, the rectum is stapled and divided with a linear stapler and the specimen is tagged and removed from the field.

The left colon, or occasionally the sigmoid (if it is supple and well vascularized), is used for reconstruction. Splenic flexure mobilization is often required. Additional maneuvers for obtaining length include dividing the inferior mesenteric vein adjacent to the ligament of Treitz and dividing the inferior mesenteric artery.

A circular stapler is then chosen, and the anvil placed within the opened bowel with purse-string stitch. After verification of hemostasis, the anvil is brought down to the stapler and connected; the staple is closed and anastomosis created (second staple line). After opening the staples, the tissues from the proximal and distal bowels are inspected to ensure that the two rings of tissue (donuts) are intact. Further verification of intact anastomosis is performed by proctoscopy, and while the rectum is insufflated the pelvis is filled with saline to assess for leakage of air.

Special Intraoperative Considerations

Patients with obstructing lesions may require colonic stenting or colostomy prior to beginning chemoradiation. The decision to intervene surgically before starting chemoradiation depends on the patient's symptoms as well as clinical examination. If an adult colonoscopy can be passed above the lesion, chemoradiation is often tolerated without further intervention.

For a very low anastomosis (<6 cm from the anal verge), a colonic J-pouch should be considered because it will improve bowel function in the short term. Limitations include a narrow pelvis or a descending colon of limited length.

For patients with bulky tumors and possible extension of tumor into surrounding structures (small intestine, ovary, bladder, vagina, prostate or seminal vesicle), en bloc resection should be performed. It is often not possible to identify a malignant fistula from a benign adhesion. Mere division, or "pinching," of tumor is not an acceptable surgical technique, as it may reduce the chance of cure.

Following creation of an anastomosis, an air leak test is performed to search for incomplete stapling. If the air leak test is positive, the anastomosis should be carefully evaluated by proctoscopy. Anastomotic takedown should be considered if large anastomotic defects are noted. Small defects can be repaired with sutures. In some situations, the leak is small and cannot be identified. In these situations, a diverting stoma should be strongly considered.

Postoperative Management

Nasogastric tubes are not routinely utilized postoperatively. Early mobilization and feeding can reduce ileus and hospital length of stay. Foley catheters are left in place for 4 to 5 days, as urinary retention (due to nerve edema associated with low dissection) can occur with early catheter removal. Anastomotic leak occurs in as many as 20% of patients and usually presents with fever, tachycardia, arrhythmia, tachypnea, or diffuse peritonitis within 4 to 7 days postoperatively. The incidence is higher in anastomoses within 7 cm from the anal verge, and in patients who have received antiangiogenic agent therapy (i.e., bevacizumab). Fecal diversion is commonly utilized in order to avoid the potential sequelae of an anastomotic leak. A meta-analysis study by Tan et al. evaluated data from four randomized controlled trials and 21 non-randomized studies (N = 11,429). They observed that lower clinical anastomotic leak rate (risk ratio [RR] = 0.39 and 0.74) and a lower reoperation rate (RR = 0.29 and 0.23) was associated with use of a diverting stoma in both randomized control trials and nonrandomized studies. Temporary fecal diversion should be considered in those patients thought to be at high risk for leak.

Long-term complications include sexual and bladder dysfunction associated with pelvic sidewall dissection, preoperative chemoradiation and abdominoperineal resection. Most patients opt for sphincter-sparing LAR over a permanent stoma. However, the rate of incontinence following LAR is reportedly as high as 60%, and patients must be counseled thoroughly regarding their options and the likely outcomes.

While preoperative CMT has been found to be beneficial, the role of adjuvant chemotherapy is not as clear. Randomized trials to determine the necessity of postoperative adjuvant chemotherapy are not available; thus, adjuvant chemotherapy currently remains the standard of care in the United States for Stage III rectal cancer.

Long-term rectal cancer follow-up includes serum CEA and physical examination, including DRE and proctoscopy, every 3 to 6 months for 2 years and then every 6 months for an additional 3 years. CT scan of the chest, abdomen, and pelvis is performed yearly for 3 years. Colonoscopy is performed 1 year from surgery and then 3 years later if no additional polyps are seen.

TAKE HOME POINTS

- Rectal cancer often presents in asymptomatic patients in the sixth to the seventh decade of life. When it is symptomatic, bright red blood per rectum, with or without a change in bowel pattern, is most common.
- Full colonoscopy is required to rule out synchronous lesions. If this is not possible due to obstruction, virtual colonoscopy or barium enema should be considered. Otherwise, colonoscopy within 3 months of surgery is recommended.
- Rectal cancer workup includes CT scan of the chest, abdomen, and pelvis to determine extent of disease. The primary lesions should be staged with ERUS/MRI and evaluated by proctoscopy.
- The standard of care for mid to low rectal cancer extending into the mesorectum, or involving locoregional lymph nodes, includes chemoradiation followed by mesorectal excision.
- Preoperative chemoradiation is better tolerated than postoperative treatment. It results in less local recurrence and is associated with fewer complications than postoperative treatment.
- Mesorectal excision is the standard surgical approach for mid to low rectal cancers and involves dissection along the areolar plane between the visceral and the parietal layers of the endopelvic fascia. Sharp mesorectal excision reduces rectal cancer–associated postoperative morbidity by preserving the superior and the inferior hypogastric nerve plexus.
- Postoperative complications following rectal surgery include sexual and urinary dysfunction, and anastomotic leak.
- Diverting ileostomy should be considered for low anastomosis, especially in the setting of preoperative chemoradiation.
- Serum CEA, DRE, and proctoscopy are performed every 3 to 6 months for 2 years after surgery and then every 6 months for an additional 3 years. CT scan of the chest, abdomen, and pelvis is performed annually for 3 years. Colonoscopy is performed after the first year; if no additional polyps are seen, it can subsequently be performed 3 years later.

SUGGESTED READINGS

Edelman BR, Weiser MR. Endorectal ultrasound: its role in the diagnosis and treatment of rectal cancer. Clin Colon Rectal Surg. 2008;21(3):167–177.

Fazio VW, et al. A randomized multicenter trial to compare long-term functional outcome, quality of life, and complications of surgical procedures for low rectal cancers. Ann Surg. 2007;246(3):481–488; discussion 488–490.

Minsky BD. Chemoradiation for rectal cancer: rationale, approaches, and controversies. Surg Oncol Clin N Am. 2010;19(4):803–818.

NCCN Guidelines, v. 2011 02/15/2011; Available from: http://www.nccn.org

Nelson H, et al. Guidelines 2000 for colon and rectal cancer surgery. J Natl Cancer Inst. 2001;93(8):583–596.

Sauer R, et al. Preoperative versus postoperative chemoradiotherapy for rectal cancer. N Engl J Med. 2004;351(17): 1731–1740.

Weiser MR, et al. Sphincter preservation in low rectal cancer is facilitated by preoperative chemoradiation and intersphincteric dissection. Ann Surg. 2009;249(2): 236–242.

47 Anal Carcinoma

A.V. HAYMAN and A.L. HALVERSON

Presentation

A 68-year-old female presents to her primary care physician (PCP) with complaints of anal pain and itching. Her past medical history is notable for a history of cervical dysplasia. Ten years prior, she underwent a hysterectomy for uterine fibroids. Her last colonoscopy was 18 years ago. Five months ago, the patient started experiencing anal pain with bowel movements and itching. Her PCP diagnosed her with an anal fissure and she was started on stool softeners and psyllium husk powder. A month later, the patient returned to her PCP with worsening symptoms, and she was prescribed topical nifedipine cream. A month later, the patient returned with no relief. Her PCP then referred patient to your clinic with the presumptive diagnosis of a chronic, nonhealing anal fissure.

Differential Diagnosis

Anal pathology is common in the general population. A thorough history can help differentiate between the most common problems, such as internal or external hemorrhoids, anal fissure, anal fistula, and pruritus ani. Anal fissures present primarily with sharp pain during defecation and are often associated with spotting of bright red blood on the toilet paper. Internal hemorrhoids may cause painless rectal bleeding. Thrombosed external hemorrhoids cause a constant pain that persists for several days. Pruritus ani may be caused by rectal mucosal prolapse or irritation from external hemorrhoidal skin tags. Pruritus has also been attributed to dietary irritants, such as citrus, caffeine, spicy foods, tomatoes, or milk. In the absence of other contributing pathology, the treatment for pruritus ani is supportive and includes avoidance of exacerbating factors.

Anal symptoms are often attributed to "hemorrhoids" without further workup, potentially leading to a delay in therapy for an undiagnosed malignancy. Any anal complaint in a high-risk patient, that is, age 50 or older, HIV seropositivity, history of anal or gynecologic human papillomavirus (HPV) or colorectal adenomas, or a relevant family history, should prompt endoscopic evaluation to rule out malignancy. For average-risk individuals, symptoms that persist more than 6 weeks with diet and/or medical therapy warrant endoscopic examination. Initial evaluation should include a complete history and physical exam, including digital rectal exam and anoscopy. Examination under anesthesia should be performed in individuals with persistent symptoms who are unable to tolerate anoscopy in the office.

For the patient in our scenario, during her appointment, you identify a 2-cm area of induration in the anal canal on digital rectal exam. Anoscopy identified ulceration overlying the area of induration. The ulcer was biopsied, and histology confirmed squamous cell carcinoma.

Workup

The patient should undergo a thorough physical examination. Particular attention should be paid to inguinal lymph node evaluation. Any lymphadenopathy should prompt a fine needle aspiration to rule out regional lymph node involvement. Indication for colonoscopy should be based on established colorectal cancer screening guidelines, beginning at age 50 (or earlier if a first-degree relative has a history of colon cancer or polyps) or if the patient is symptomatic.

In order to assess for distant metastases, the patient should undergo an abdominal/pelvic CT (or MRI) and a chest radiograph (or chest CT), although it should be noted that most lymph node metastases are small and may not be able to be detected by cross-sectional imaging. In some cases, a PET-CT may be obtained. HIV status should be ascertained. Evaluation for gynecologic dysplasia should be performed in females as well, since the same pathogen, the HPV, is implicated in both neoplastic processes (Table 1).

The patient in our scenario underwent computed tomography of the abdomen and the pelvis, which showed no evidence of regional or distant metastases. There was no inguinal lymphadenopathy detected on physical examination. Colonoscopy revealed only hyperplastic polyps.

Diagnosis and Treatment

Initial treatment for squamous cell carcinoma of the anal canal is nonsurgical, and consists of combined chemotherapy and radiation. Initial nonsurgical treatment is the standard of care because of the high response rate and the high rate of sphincter preservation. The standard protocol consists of 45 Gy in 25 fractions over 5 weeks to the primary cancer. 5-fluorouracil (5-FU) is infused on days 1 to 4 and 29 to 32 with mitomycin C bolus on days 1 and 29. Systemic treatment for metastatic disease consists of 5-FU and cisplatin.

TABLE 1. Staging of Anal Canal Carcinoma

Stage	T	N	M
	T1: <2 cm T2: 2–4.9 cm T3: 5+cm	N1: Perirectal Nodes N2: Unilateral Internal Iliac or Inguinal Nodes N3: Perirectal and Inguinal Nodes or Bilateral Internal Iliac or Inguinal Nodes	0: No Distant Mets 1: Distant Mets
	T4: Invades Adjacent Organs		
I	T1	N0	M0
II	T2–3	N0	M0
IIIA	T1–3	N1	M0
IIIB	T4	N1	M0
	T any	N2	M0
IV	T any	N any	M1

It is important to distinguish between squamous cell carcinomas of the squamous epithelial-lined anal canal (proximal to the anal verge), which are approached as outlined above, as opposed to the epidermis-lined anal margin (distal to the anal verge). For anal margin cancers, superficial, localized lesions (T1) are treated initially by wide local excision with negative margins. If margins are positive, reexcision is recommended if anatomically feasible; otherwise, the patient should be referred for adjuvant therapy as above. All other therapies follow the above guidelines.

For the patient in our scenario, given the absence of distant metastases, the patient was referred for chemoradiation, which she successfully completed. The patient returned 6 weeks after completion of chemoradiation. Due to residual anal pain, the patient was taken for an examination under anesthesia. The exam identified an area of residual induration. Biopsy of this area revealed residual squamous cell cancer.

Residual tumor may continue to regress for up to 12 weeks following completion of chemoradiation. Repeat examination with biopsy of any residual mass should be performed at 12 weeks to confirm residual disease. If progression of disease is identified at the first follow-up examination, proceeding directly to surgery is appropriate.

The patient in our scenario returns for repeat examination 6 weeks later, 12 weeks after completion of chemoradiation. Residual cancer is confirmed by biopsy of a persistent mass. The patient is recommended to undergo an abdominoperineal resection.

Preoperative Consideration

1. Stoma marking by a certified stomal therapist
2. Perioperative antibiotics
3. Venous thromboembolism prophylaxis

Surgical Approach

When performing an abdominoperineal resection in patients who have been treated with pelvic radiation,

a myocutaneous flap should be considered to facilitate wound healing (Table 2). The procedure is commonly performed with the patient in the lithotomy position. Mobilization of the distal colon and rectum and division of the mesentery may be performed using an open technique or laparoscopically when a rectus abdominus muscle flap is not being used. The surgical approach should include careful dissection to maintain the anatomic planes and preserve the peritoneal envelope around the mesorectum. Careful dissection avoids nerve injury that may result in sexual dysfunction. The mesentery should be divided at the proximal superior mesenteric vascular pedicle. Once the pelvic floor is reached, dissection is performed from the perineal approach continuing cephalad to meet the intraabdominal portion of the dissection. Care should be taken to maintain a wide dissection through the levator muscles. Grossly close margins may be sent for frozen section evaluation. After resection of the specimen, the muscle flap is placed into the pelvis. The perineal defect is closed in several layers with absorbable suture, including absorbable suture in the skin to avoid uncomfortable suture or staple removal postoperatively.

An alternative approach is to perform the abdominal portion of the procedure in the supine position. After creation of the colostomy and closure of the abdominal incision, the patient is turned prone for the completion of the perineal portion of the procedure. Inguinal node dissection should be considered for residual disease in the inguinal lymph nodes.

Postoperative Management

All anal canal cancer patients should be examined every 3 to 6 months for 5 years. Surveillance examination should include inguinal node examination and anoscopy. Anoscopy with topical acetic acid should be considered to survey for recurrent HPV-related dysplasia. For T3+ or N1+ lesions, annual chest/abdominal/pelvis imaging is also recommended for the first 3 years.

TABLE 2. Key Technical Steps for Surgical Management of Anal Cancer

Key Technical Steps

1. Consider myocutaneous flap when performing radical resection.
2. Maintain anatomic planes, that is, total mesorectal excision, to facilitate dissection and ensure adequate resection.
3. Continue wide dissection around the anal canal to obtain wide margins.

Special Intraoperative Considerations

If metastatic disease in encountered at the time of surgery, proceeding with abdominoperineal resection may be appropriate for palliation of symptoms from local disease.

TAKE HOME POINTS

- Anal bleeding that does not respond to medical management should be assessed via anoscopy and/or colonoscopy.
- The first-line treatment for nonmetastatic anal canal carcinoma is nonsurgical.

- Allow up to 12 weeks for regression of lesion after chemoradiation prior to proceeding with surgical resection.
- Abdominoperinal resection is indicated if combined chemoradiation fails.

SUGGESTED READINGS

Abbott DE, Halverson AL, Wayne JD, et al. The oblique rectus abdominal myocutaneous flap for complex pelvic wound reconstruction. Dis Colon Rectum. 2008;51(8):1237–1241.

Garrett K, Kalady MF. Anal neoplasms. Surg Clin North Am. 2010;90(1):147–161.

Hojo K, Vernava III AM, Sugihara K, et al. Preservation of urine voiding and sexual function after rectal cancer surgery. Dis Colon Rectum. 1991;34(7):532–539.

Meyer J, Willett C, Czito B. Current and emerging treatment strategies for anal cancer. Curr Oncol Rep. 2010;12(3):168–174.

NCCN GuidelinesTM Version 2.2011 ACC. www.nccn.org. Accessed June 17, 2011.

48 Perianal Abscess

RICHARD E. BURNEY

Presentation

A 40-year-old woman comes to your office for an urgent visit complaining of severe anal pain and tenderness that has developed over the past 2 days. She has no history of prior rectal complaints or change in bowel habit. There is no history of abdominal pain, diarrhea, or blood in her stools. On examination, she appears healthy and is afebrile. Examination of the perianal area reveals an erythematous, tender area about 1.5 cm in diameter at the posterior anal verge. It appears fluctuant. Gentle palpation is exquisitely painful precluding further rectal examination.

Differential Diagnosis

In evaluating the patient with acute pain and swelling in the perianal and buttock region, one must keep in mind both the possible etiologies and the anatomy of the region, in particular the various locations or spaces where infection and abscess can arise and be manifest. There are many possible etiologies of perianal and perirectal infection, ranging from anal gland infection, to defecation-related anal canal trauma, to inflammatory bowel disease. The specific etiology, however, is not of immediate concern at the time of acute presentation when prompt diagnosis and surgical management of abscess take precedence.

The first step in the differential diagnosis of acute anal pain and swelling is to distinguish between perianal abscess, which is painful but unlikely to cause serious illness or sequelae, and perirectal or ischiorectal abscess, which can be highly morbid and life threatening if treatment is delayed or inadequate **(Figure 1)**.

Perianal abscess is limited in extent and location to the perianal tissues and intersphincteric plane, the avascular space between the internal and the external sphincter muscles. Perianal abscesses are small and do not penetrate laterally through the anal sphincter into the ischiorectal fossa tissues or upward into the supralevator space. The swelling of a perianal abscess is usually readily visible and easily palpable at the anal verge and does not give rise to signs of systemic infection **(Figure 2)**.

Closely related to perianal abscess, and possibly its precursor, is intersphincteric abscess. An intersphincteric abscess is also small, and so named because it develops in the avascular plane between the internal and the external sphincter. Unlike perianal abscess, which is usually visible under the perianal skin, it causes no outward visible signs. It causes pain and tenderness more so in the anal canal than on the surface. Tenderness is usually exquisite and elicited during rectal examination by palpation in the anal canal. The diagnosis of intersphincteric abscess can be difficult because the signs are subtle. Intersphincteric abscess

if untreated may simply evolve into a perianal abscess, which is easier to diagnose, but it could also extend upward or outward leading to a much more serious supralevator or ischiorectal abscess.

Ischiorectal abscess develops when infection, which originates in the intersphincteric space, penetrates through the external sphincter and enters the larger, fat-filled space of the ischiorectal fossa where a much larger abscess can develop **(Figure 3)**. Patients with ischiorectal abscess will usually have fever, elevated white blood cell count, and may have signs of sepsis. The medial buttock will be erythematous, swollen, and tender. Because the abscess may be quite deep, more than 2 to 3 cm under the skin, obvious fluctuance is not always present. On rectal examination, one may feel a ballotable mass between the buttock and the lower rectum, which is more obvious when done under anesthesia. Perirectal abscesses are easily seen on CT, but CT should not be needed to make this diagnosis in most patients.

High intersphincteric or supralevator abscesses are rare and are the most difficult to diagnose and treat. Patients will have had rectal pain, with or without fever, usually for several days or more. External examination is unrevealing. On careful rectal examination, one may be able to feel a fluctuant mass high in the anal canal at the level of the levator or anorectal ring, but physical findings can be quite subtle. WBC count may be elevated. CT imaging of the pelvis, which is being done with increasing regularity in situations such as this, where one has a patient with unexplained rectal pain and signs of infection, can be very helpful in identifying the presence and exact location of these occult abscesses.

Patients can also develop simple perianal carbuncles, or simple abscesses involving the perianal or buttock skin and superficial subcutaneous tissues, which have no etiologic relation to anal canal structures **(Figure 4)**. Pilonidal abscess is usually located in the buttock cleft, well away from the anus. Sinus tracts arising from pilonidal cyst on occasion find their way to the perianal buttock tissues and when this happens can mimic

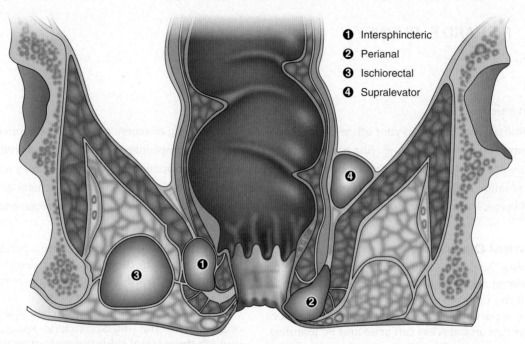

① Intersphincteric
② Perianal
③ Ischiorectal
④ Supralevator

FIGURE 1 • Schematic drawing showing typical locations of perianal and perirectal abscess. Locations of abscesses can be variable and do not necessarily conform to these locations.

ischiorectal abscess. Sebaceous cysts in the perianal skin can become infected and lead to abscess in the perianal region. When this happens, the patient may give a history of having had a lump there for some time that has suddenly become more tender and swollen. Finally, perianal hidradenitis suppurativa can cause anal pain and swelling. These patients rarely have disease limited to the perianal region, however, and almost always give a history of chronic pain, swelling, and drainage.

The differential diagnosis of patients with anal pain also includes such entities as acute hemorrhoidal inflammation, acute thrombosed hemorrhoid, acute anal fissure, anorectal inflammatory bowel disease

flare, and neoplasm. None of these entities will cause fever or WBC count elevation. Patients with anorectal inflammatory bowel disease usually have other visible abnormalities and tissue distortion in the perianal area that is characteristic **(Figure 5)**. Nevertheless, they may have local swelling and abscess, or ulceration that mimics abscess in its symptoms. Acute hemorrhoidal swelling and thrombosed hemorrhoids

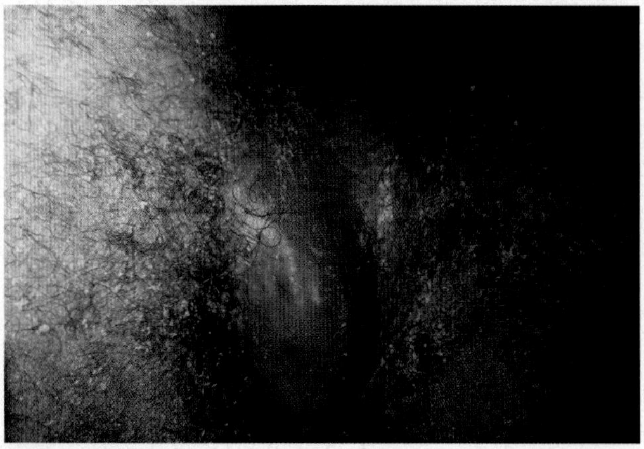

FIGURE 2 • Perianal abscess.

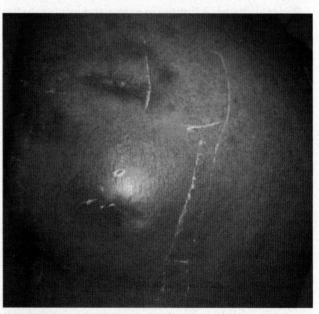

FIGURE 3 • Appearance of ischiorectal abscess. Scar is from I&D of previous abscess.

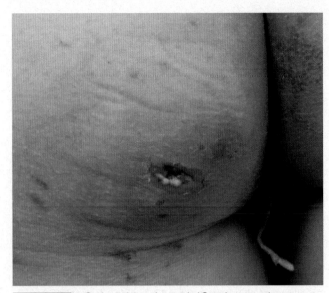

FIGURE 4 • Carbuncle on buttock (*Staph aureus*).

are visible and should be easily identified on external examination. By history, patients with anal fissure have anal bleeding and pain with defecation, followed by a burning or "razor blade" sensation that can last for up to an hour or more. Anal fissure can be identified most easily by simply stretching the perianal skin to expose the fissure in the anal canal. There is no swelling and tenderness is limited to the site of the fissure itself.

Patients with fistula in ano will most often give a history of chronic perianal drainage or intermittent, recurrent swelling and drainage from a perianal location, usually within 3 to 4 cm of the anal verge. Acute pain and swelling may be intermittently felt, but are not prominent symptoms of anal fistula. A small nubbin of granulation tissue may be present at the external fistula opening. A small proportion of patients who have undergone drainage of perianal

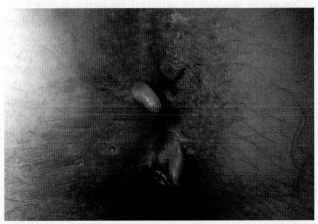

FIGURE 5 • Anal inflammation from Crohn's disease showing inflammatory tags, edema, and ulceration.

abscess may later be found to have an associated or underlying fistula in ano, but in my experience these fistulae are rarely evident at the time of surgical incision and drainage. There is no need to spend extra time looking for a possible fistula if it is not obvious at the time of initial surgical incision and drainage. If an underlying fistula is present, it will become apparent in time. Most patients with fistula in ano do not initially present with an abscess; most patients with abscess do not go on to develop fistula in ano.

Workup

The most important parts of the workup for anal pain and swelling are a complete history and a careful physical examination. The history should define the exact time course of symptoms and their specific nature. Temperature and pulse rate may give a clue as to depth and extent of abscess. Physical examination must include careful inspection and palpation of the buttock and perianal region, preferably with the patient in a knee-chest position on a sigmoidoscopy or similar table, under good lighting. In this setting, the diagnosis is frequently obvious with only simple observation and gentle palpation. Examination in lateral position in the usual exam room with poor lighting is inadequate. Lack of tenderness on rectal examination is reassuring that a high and/or deep abscess is not present.

When the diagnosis is not clear, and certainly if the patient has unexplained fever and/or elevated WBC count in conjunction with deep, unexplained rectal pain, pelvic CT is in order. Endorectal ultrasound examination might also show an abnormality, but will be more uncomfortable for the patient and probably less readily available as well.

Anorectal pain, tenderness, and swelling for which there is no good explanation may require urgent or emergent examination under anesthesia. An alternative is to closely monitor the patient and reexamine for progression of signs and symptoms in 24 to 48 hours, but close observation is mandatory. Treatment is emergent not elective and should not be delayed if abscess is suspected.

Diagnosis and Treatment

The treatment of perianal or intersphincteric abscess is surgical drainage. Whether the drainage procedure is done in the office, in the ED, or in the operating room is a judgment that must be made based on the size and location of the abscess, the cooperativeness and willingness of the patient, the skill and experience of the surgeon, and the resources available, such as instruments, lighting, and assistance. As a general rule, incision and drainage should be performed in the operating room unless the abscess is quite small and superficial.

When an abscess is suspected, the incision for drainage is best made over the point of maximal tenderness and swelling. Attempts to identify the presence or location of a perianal or an intersphincteric abscess by exploration and aspiration with an 18-gauge needle are frequently misleading or unrewarding. While it is possible that the abscess may be small and hard to hit with a needle, more often this maneuver fails because the pus is so thick that it does not flow through the needle and cannot be aspirated. Moreover, if one does happen to find the abscess and aspirates most of the pus from it, this will make it harder to locate after an incision is made.

In making an exploratory incision, knowledge of the perianal anatomy and how to identify the sphincters and intersphincteric plane is important. Sometimes, an incision is made and no abscess can be found. This is acceptable and preferable to missing an abscess. Close follow-up in such instances is recommended because a small abscess may have been missed.

Surgical Approach

Perianal abscess, if superficial, small and obvious, may be drained in the office or emergency department under local anesthesia, with or without sedation. 1% lidocaine with epinephrine 1:100,000 or 1:200,000 is infiltrated into the dermis (not the subcutaneous tissue) over and around the abscess. A lanceolate or an elliptical incision oriented either radially or tangentially to the anus is made over the abscess. This incision will remove a segment of overlying skin. Excision of the skin overlying the abscess helps to completely unroof it and drain it adequately **(Figure 6)**. Cruciate incision is both ugly and inadequate and does not provide good drainage. A small wick of moistened plain cotton gauze is placed into the abscess cavity and removed in 48 hours. Iodoform gauze is harsh, painful, and necrosis inducing and in my opinion should never be used. Rayon or polyester-based packing strip should be avoided as well.

If the abscess is deeper, larger, or more extensive, having expanded laterally in the intersphincteric plane and partially encircled the anal sphincter to form a horseshoe, a different approach is needed. In general, in this situation, one should avoid large or deep radial incisions, which might divide anal sphincter muscle. Tangential or circumferential incisions are preferred. In the case of horseshoe abscess, multiple small incisions are made through which a drain, such as a small Malecot catheter, rather than packing can be placed and secured with suture. Simple packing can be placed alongside the drains and removed in 24 to

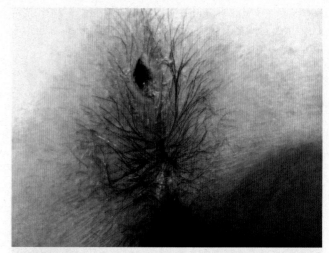

FIGURE 6 • Appearance 2 days after incision and drainage of intersphincteric abscess demonstrating good drainage. An ellipse of skin was removed by using a lanceolate incision at time of I&D.

48 hours, leaving the Malecot or equivalent drains in place for a much longer period as the abscess cavity closes.

If the patient does not have an acute abscess, but rather has intermittent drainage, the surgical approach is to evaluate the patient under anesthesia, looking for a fistula in ano. Fine silver or lacrimal duct probes are needed. Hydrogen peroxide solution injected through a fine cannula into an external opening can be helpful in identifying an occult internal opening. If a fistula is found, treatment will depend on the depth and characteristics of the fistula. In this situation, prior measurement of the anal sphincter length by careful rectal examination prior to induction of anesthesia can be critical. If there is acute inflammation or an underlying occult abscess, or if sphincter length is unknown, the best approach is to place a seton through the fistula for drainage and allow the inflammation to subside. One should never do a fistulotomy in the face of an acute abscess or without knowing the sphincter length. Sphincter length cannot be determined under anesthesia, but rather only by examination in an awake patient. It is done by palpation of the posterior anal canal with one's finger and measuring the distance from the levator ring at one's fingertip to the anal verge. Normal sphincter length is from 2 to 5 cm. One should try to preserve at least two and preferably 2.5 cm of anal sphincter when doing an I&D or fistulotomy.

It is possible for a patient to have recurrent buttock abscesses as a result of unrecognized fistula in ano **(Figure 7)**. If the abscesses are subcutaneous rather than deep (i.e., in the ischiorectal fossa), one should look for an underlying fistula **(Table 1)**.

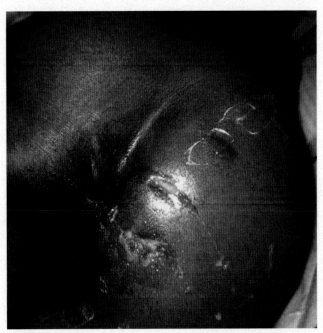

FIGURE 7 • This patient had undergone repeated I&D procedures for buttock abscess before an underlying posterior fistula in ano was sought, found and treated.

Special Intraoperative Considerations

The position of the patient on the operating table can be a matter of personal preference. In general, my preference is to do evaluation under anesthesia in the prone position under spinal or caudal anesthesia, unless the patient has a contraindication to this, such as extreme obesity. If general anesthesia is needed in an obese patient, lithotomy position is preferred to avoid the added anesthetic risk of general anesthesia in the prone position. I position the patient prone with hips over the kidney rest, which I elevate several inches prior to flexing the table. Gel pads to support the pelvis and chest are not needed if spinal anesthesia is used unless the patient has a very obese abdomen. Pulling the buttocks apart with 3-inch adhesive tape angled about 30 degrees toward the head improves exposure of the perianal region.

Prep solutions may obscure the skin erythema that provides a clue as to the location of the abscess. Marking the site with permanent skin marker before prepping obviates this problem. If an intersphincteric abscess is suspected, the intersphincteric plane must be identified and opened bluntly to gain access to and drain the abscess. A tangential incision parallel to the sphincter muscle is helps prevent unwittingly dividing muscle unnecessarily.

If an exploratory incision is made and no pus is found, do not suture the wound closed or pack it open. Simply place a dressing over the unclosed wound. If pus is found, culture is not usually helpful in otherwise healthy individuals. Aerobic and anaerobic cultures can be obtained if you have reason to suspect resistant organisms and if the patient has immune compromise, is in poor general health, or appears septic because of high fever and WBC count.

As mentioned above, avoid the use of Iodoform gauze, which has no proven benefit, causes pain, and impairs wound healing. Simple saline- or plain water-moistened plain cotton gauze works quite well.

TABLE 1. Key Technical Steps and Potential Pitfalls

	Key Technical Steps	Potential Pitfalls
Physical examination	Prone, knee-chest position Proper lighting and assistance	Inadequate examination failure to identify subtle signs
Exam under anesthesia	Exploratory aspiration with 18-gauge needle	Failure to identify abscess with thick pus unless incision is made
Incision and drainage	Adequate anesthesia and proper positioning: Spinal or general anesthesia, prone or lithotomy positioning is matter of surgeon preference	Subtle abscess will be missed unless there is good exposure and muscle relaxation allowing adequate exam.
	Excise an ellipse of skin over the abscess. Cruciate incision is inadequate. Open and explore abscess cavity widely.	Incision is too small leading to inadequate drainage and/or premature closure of skin over abscess cavity. Complex abscess (horseshoe) extensions may be missed.
	Leave moist gauze packing for 48 h to stabilize wound opening.	Once removed, packing may be difficult or impossible to replace.
	Avoid fistulotomy in face of acute abscess; place seton if fistula is found.	Dividing sphincter at the same time as incision and drainage leads to wide retraction of the divided sphincter muscle and can cause incontinence if too much sphincter is divided.

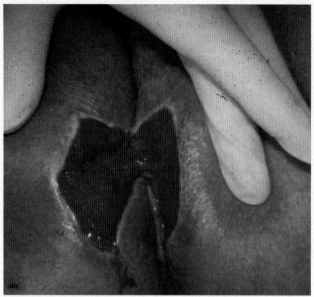

FIGURE 8 • Appearance of large perianal wound 2 weeks after incision and drainage of superficial horseshoe abscess. Wound care consisted of plain water-moistened gauze dressings changed three times a day.

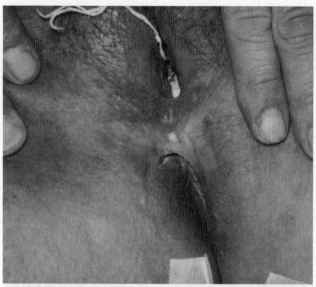

FIGURE 9 • The wound contracted and healed completely with minimal residual scar.

Postoperative Management

Sitz baths are traditional for comfort and to promote drainage. The initial packing can be left in place for 48 to 72 hours. If the patient has a simple perianal abscess, the packing once removed does not have to be replaced if a small ellipse of skin has been removed by the lanceolate incision because the skin edges will not close prematurely. Antimicrobial therapy can be discontinued after a brief period unless cellulitis is present.

If the abscess is larger, more complex, and deep, it is best to use Malecot or a similar catheter for drainage and to leave it in place for days or weeks. The wound can be irrigated two to three times a day through the drainage tube. The tube can be downsized as the cavity closes. If the wound is superficial but extensive and/or partially circumferential, wound care consisting of shower irrigation and water-moistened plain gauze dressings changed three times a day leads to good healing (Figures 8 and 9).

TAKE HOME POINTS

- Acute anal pain and swelling is not a trivial problem and demands urgent attention.
- Examination under anesthesia should be done if there is any question of occult or complicated abscess.
- Pelvic CT is not usually needed, but is indicated if supralevator abscess is suspected. Failure to aspirate pus through a needle does not mean an abscess is not present.
- Incision should be generous, with removal of overlying skin to promote adequate drainage.
- Do not attempt fistulotomy in the face of acute inflammation; place a seton if a fistula is obvious. Use plain, moist gauze packing and leave initial packing for 48 hours.
- If abscess is large and/or deep, place a Malecot or equivalent drain sutured in place.

49 Thrombosed Hemorrhoids

RICHARD E. BURNEY

Presentation

A 49-year-old obese male presents to the emergency department with a complaint of severe anal pain for the past 24 hours. He has not had this problem before. Over-the-counter pain medication has not helped. He has a history of constipation and recently returned from a business trip. Past medical history includes type 2 diabetes, hypertension, hyperlipidemia. He reports being compliant with medications prescribed for these conditions, including an oral hypoglycemic agent, aspirin, a statin agent, and a beta-blocker. On examination, he is afebrile. He has an exquisitely tender, swollen, edematous mass at the anal verge, with bluish discoloration, about 1.5 to 2 cm in diameter. There is no apparent cellulitis or erythema. He does not allow digital rectal examination.

Differential Diagnosis

The most likely diagnosis in this man is an acutely thrombosed external hemorrhoid **(Figure 1)**. Other possibilities in decreasing order of probability include (1) prolapsed edematous internal hemorrhoid **(Figures 3–5)**; (2) acute hemorrhoidal inflammation and edema brought on by constipation **(Figure 2)**; (3) perianal abscess; (4) prolapsed, strangulated internal hemorrhoid; (5) inflamed anal tag with or without associated inflammatory bowel disease; (6) infarcted hemorrhoid without prolapse; (7) prolapsed anal polyp; and (8) acute anal fissure, with an edematous sentinel tag.

Workup

Additional questions regarding patient's normal bowel habit, management of his chronic constipation, and medications are warranted. It is important to determine if he regularly strains when moving his bowels. The diagnosis is almost always made on the basis of physical examination. To do a good examination, the patient is best placed in prone jackknife position on a sigmoidoscopy table and examined under good light with the buttock spread apart. If a sigmoidoscopy table is not available, the patient can be placed in prone, jackknife position by lying face-down over rolled blankets placed under the hips to elevate the buttocks. Laboratory and imaging studies are rarely helpful unless the patient has a fever or at the time of examination, anal abscess is a distinct possibility. On rare occasion, examination may have to be facilitated by sedation or local anesthetic injection or evaluation under spinal or general anesthesia done in the operating room.

Diagnosis and Treatment

The diagnosis in this patient, based on history and physical examination, is thrombosed external hemorrhoid. This condition, although painful, is self-limited. Although surgical treatment, consisting of incision and evacuation of clots, is possible, it is not required. This is particularly true if the thrombosis is more than 48 to 72 hours old, by which time the acute inflammation and swelling are beginning to abate. With observation and attention to a proper diet, the hemorrhoidal thrombosis will reabsorb and the swelling will subside, leaving no sequelae. There is a common misconception that thrombosed hemorrhoids are an indication that there is some kind of underlying hemorrhoidal or other disease. This is not true.

Surgical Approach

If the acute thrombosis is <48 hours old and/or is quite large, such that one can anticipate it will take weeks for the swelling to subside, surgical treatment may be offered. The simplest and most efficacious, as well as expedient, surgical treatment is incision and evacuation of clot **(Figures 6–8)**.

This procedure can be done under local anesthesia in the office, clinic, or emergency department. 1% lidocaine with epinephrine is infiltrated through a very fine needle slowly into the dermis overlying the hemorrhoid. Infiltrating the subcutaneous tissue is not effective. The skin will blanch as this is done. It is not usually necessary to do a deeper block. After the local anesthetic has taken effect, an ellipse of skin is excised over the area of thrombosis, oriented to give the best exposure to the underlying thrombus. Simple, linear incision does not provide adequate exposure. The thrombi are intravascular, in small hemorrhoidal veins, and there are usually three to six vessels present containing thrombi. Thrombi are evacuated with a fine hemostat. The skin incision is left open. A longer-acting local anesthetic agent such as bupivacaine may

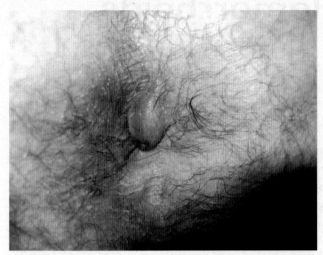

FIGURE 1 • Thrombosed external hemorrhoid: characteristic appearance.

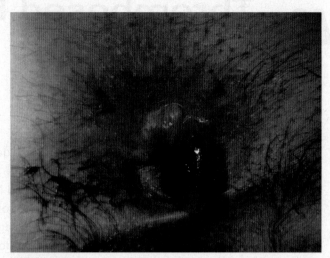

FIGURE 2 • Acutely inflamed hemorrhoid with thrombosis and ulceration. This was treated by hemorrhoidectomy in the operating room.

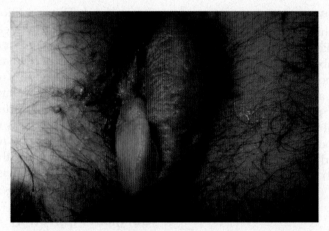

FIGURE 3 • Chronically prolapsed mixed internal/external hemorrhoid. Bluish discoloration in places suggests underlying thromboses, but do NOT try to I&D this.

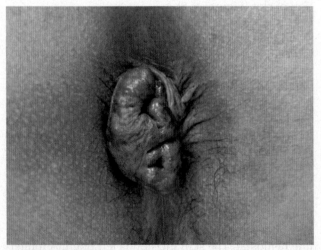

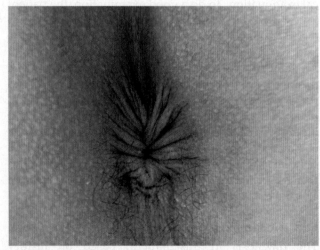

FIGURE 4 and 5 • Chronically prolapsed left lateral internal hemorrhoid. This is NOT a thrombosed external hemorrhoid. It was manually reduced under local anesthesia.

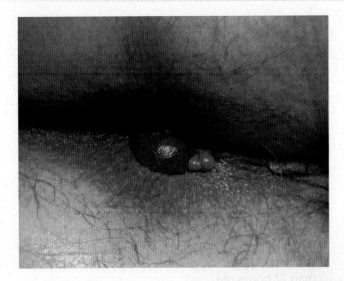
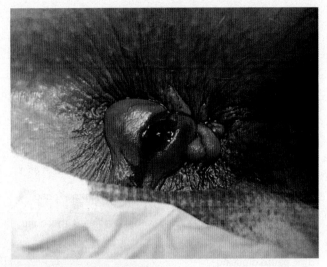
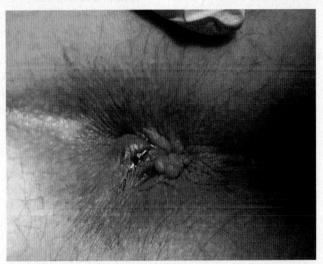

FIGURE 6-8 • Incision and drainage of thrombosed external hemorrhoid. Note that ellipse of skin has been excised over the thrombosis giving good exposure. After thrombectomy, there is still residual swelling. No sutures are required.

be infiltrated as well. Postoperative care consists of an outer dressing to absorb any drainage, sitz baths or moist applications, and nonsteroidal pain medications. Antibiotics are not needed.

The chief potential pitfall is failure to make the correct diagnosis. Prolapsed, thrombosed, or strangulated internal hemorrhoids have been mistaken for thrombosed external hemorrhoids, leading to painful errors in management **(Figures 2–4)**. Thrombosed (external) hemorrhoids are covered with dry, keratinized normal-appearing skin **(Figure 1)**. If this is not observed, consider another diagnosis. Other potential pitfalls are failure to have adequate lighting, assistance, and exposure, which will make the procedure more difficult. Other common pitfalls include the following: failure to adequately anesthetize the skin overlying the thrombosed hemorrhoid, or to wait long enough for the local

anesthetic to be effective (at least 2 minutes); failure to make an elliptical or a lanceolate incision that exposes all the thrombosed veins; and failure to carefully evacuate thrombus from each vein individually **(Table 1)**.

Special Intraoperative Considerations

If you find after gaining good exposure and lighting that you are not dealing with a thrombosed external hemorrhoid, but rather with prolapsed, strangulated internal hemorrhoids or other condition, **(Figure 2)** the patient may need to be evaluated in the operating room under better anesthesia, such as subarachnoid block.

Postoperative Management

No special postoperative management is needed. The patient may keep a slightly moistened gauze dressing

TABLE 1. Key Technical Steps and Potential Pitfalls of Incision and Evacuation of Hemorrhoidal Thrombi

Key Technical Steps

1. Arrange good exposure and good light. Have an assistant present.
2. If sedation is used, appropriate monitoring of blood pressure, pulse oxygen, and cardiac rhythm must be in place.
3. Infiltrate local anesthetic with epinephrine slowly and widely into the overlying dermis observing the skin as it blanches.
4. Excise a generous ellipse of overlying skin to expose the thrombi.
5. Extract thrombi individually with fine pointed, mosquito hemostat.
6. Do not close the incision; cover with slightly moistened gauze dressing.
7. Add additional long-acting local anesthetic if desired.

Potential Pitfalls

- Incorrect diagnosis.
- Inadequate lighting, assistance, and/or exposure.
- Inadequate local anesthesia.
- Incision that does not expose all thrombi.
- Failure to extract thrombi individually from hemorrhoidal veins.

over the operative site, which usually closes within a day or two. It will, however, be painful when the local anesthetic wears off and remain so for several days. It is a good idea to explain this to the patient. Stool softener and instructions for high-fiber diet should be given. There is no reason to subject the patient to additional examinations, such as colonoscopy. Thrombosed external hemorrhoids are rarely associated with underlying pathology of any kind, including internal hemorrhoids.

TAKE HOME POINTS

- First, be sure you have the right diagnosis. Remember that not all thrombosed hemorrhoids need surgical treatment; the majority of patients do not.
- Treatment does not lead to rapid resolution of symptoms, especially if the thrombosis is more than 72 hours old.
- If you do decide to evacuate thrombi, have adequate positioning, light, and assistance. Infiltrate local anesthetic slowly but widely into the skin. Take an ellipse of overlying skin and extract all the thrombi individually.
- Explain to the patient that there will be continued pain and swelling for several days or longer despite what you have done.

50 Palpable Breast Mass

TRAVIS E. GROTZ, SANDHYA PRUTHI and JAMES W. JAKUB

Presentation

A 40-year-old female presents with the complaint of a lump in her right breast. She has noted the mass for the past month, and it has not changed in size after her recent menstrual cycle. There is no associated pain. She has not had prior mammograms. She denies a history of breast trauma, breast surgery, or prior breast biopsies and is otherwise healthy. Her medications include oral contraceptives and multivitamins. Her mother was diagnosed with breast cancer at the age of 74 and is alive and well. On clinical breast examination (CBE), the breasts are symmetric, nipples everted, and there is no overlying skin retraction, erythema, or nipple discharge. A well-demarcated, firm, irregular mass, measuring 2 × 2 cm is palpated at the 10-o'clock position, 4 cm from the nipple. It is mobile and not fixed or attached to the overlying skin or the chest wall. She has no axillary or supraclavicular lymphadenopathy. The left breast examination is normal, and the remainder of the history and examination is negative.

Differential Diagnosis

The presentation of a breast mass is a common symptom. Although the majority of women who present with a palpable mass will have a benign finding however; as many as 10% will have an underlying malignancy. It is prudent therefore that a diagnostic evaluation be performed to exclude a cancer. The differential diagnosis includes cyst, fibroadenoma, fat necrosis, or carcinoma. Benign changes of the breast can be confused with a breast mass on self-exam including fibrocystic changes, prominent breast lobules, focal dense breast tissue, lipoma, or concentric thickening of the inframammary crease. Fibroadenomas are the most common benign breast lesions and are well circumscribed, firm, rubbery, mobile, and painless. They can present as single or multiple nodules and measure up to 5 cm in size. Cysts are round, well-circumscribed, smooth, mobile masses. They can often fluctuate with the menstrual cycle and are the result of obstruction and dilation of intramammary ducts. Cysts can enlarge and if under tension, can be painful. Both of these benign findings have classic breast ultrasound (US) characteristics. Even if the breast exam is suggestive of these benign etiologies, further evaluation with imaging and or biopsy/aspiration is required to assess clinical suspicion for a new breast mass. Fibrocystic changes are often bilateral, poorly localized, thickened symmetrical plaques of glandular parenchyma. These fibrocystic plaques are most prominent in the upper outer quadrants and can cause cyclical pain that can radiate to the axilla and also fluctuate in size with the menstrual cycle. Fat necrosis often presents with a firm, smooth, irregular mass that is occasionally tender and is associated with a history of trauma, reduction mammoplasty, or prior breast surgery. It may be associated with inflammation, pain, skin thickening, and nipple retraction mimicking carcinoma. The most common features of a primary breast carcinoma include a firm mass with poorly defined margins, associated with skin retraction, asymmetric and discrete when compared to the surrounding parenchyma and the contralateral breast. However, the clinical findings can be insidious, and one must be on guard against offering false reassurance for subtle changes without further diagnostic evaluation. Any new breast change reported by a patient typically deserves a confirmatory test before giving a benign diagnosis.

Workup

The CBE should be a standardized thorough inspection and palpation of the entire breast. During examination, both breasts should be palpated in a systematic fashion. The CBE is a diagnostic tool in the initial workup of a breast complaint. Upon inspection, the presence or absence of erythema, overlying skin or nipple retraction (including with the arms raised over the patient's head), dimpling, nipple discharge, asymmetry, or previous scars should be noted. Assessment includes fibroglandular consistency, discrete or distinct masses that are asymmetrical relevant to the contralateral breast, and nipple and areolar abnormalities. Clinically benign lesions tend to be smooth, well circumscribed, and mobile. Clinically worrisome masses are often firm and poorly defined; fixation to the chest wall or associated with skin changes are uncommon findings, but strongly suggestive of a malignant process. However, none of these findings in and of themselves are 100% reliable.

The next step after the CBE in the evaluation of a palpable and dominant mass is to obtain diagnostic breast imaging (**Figure 1**). It is critical to specify these imaging studies as diagnostic and not screening in the orders; this will alert the radiologist that there is an issue of concern and is a vital component of the workup. It is important to communicate to the radiologist the location using the clock face and the distance from the nipple of the palpable mass or apply a radioopaque skin marker over the area of concern. A negative mammogram in the face of a clinically suspicious breast exam is not adequate to offer reassurance. Relying on this as the sole method of evaluation is a common cause of delayed diagnosis and litigation.

In women <30 years of age who present with a focal area of concern, directed US evaluation is the initial preferred study, because of the low sensitivity of mammography in this setting. If the US findings are suspicious a diagnostic mammogram maybe obtained at the radiologists discretion. For women over 30 years of age, a diagnostic bilateral mammogram and directed US is indicated. The radiologist will most often obtain additional imaging that includes spot compression or magnification views. For a dominant mass, a focused exam in concert with a focused US will typically provide the most information. US can further assess the size of the mass, if it has cystic or solid features, and can often add clarity to benign lesions such as prominent lobules and focal areas of dense breast tissue. Magnetic resonance imaging is an expensive imaging modality with excellent sensitivity but low specificity that may be considered in high-risk patients with a clinically intermediate suspicion palpable mass and a normal or an indeterminate US and mammogram.

If findings on history, CBE, or imaging are suspicious for malignancy, a tissue diagnosis should be obtained. The sensitivity of fine needle aspiration (FNA) is 93% compared to 98% to 99% for core needle biopsy (CNB) and excisional biopsy. A CNB provides histologic architecture and yields more tissue for definitive diagnosis compared with an FNA, and is associated with a

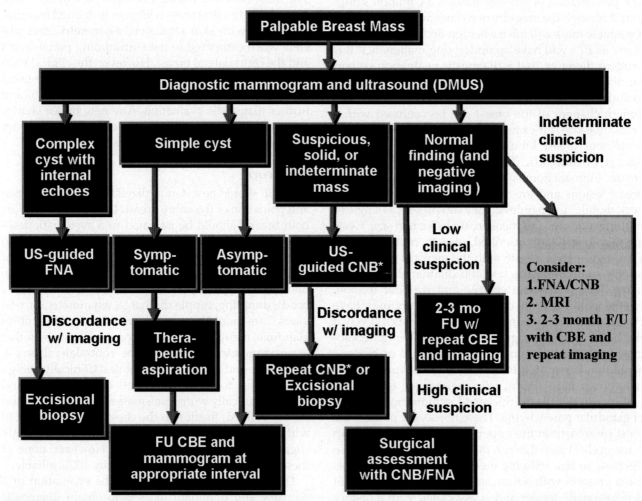

FIGURE 1 • Palpable breast mass diagnostic algorithm adapted from Pruthi S. Detection and evaluation of a palpable breast mass. (Reprinted from Mayo Clin Proc. 2001;76(6):641–648, with permission.) FNA can be used as an acceptable alternative to CNB if high-volume cytopathologists are available and comfortable with interpretation follow-up (FU).

lower incidence of complications compared to excisional biopsy. As supported by the American Society of Breast Surgeons consensus statements, image-guided biopsies are preferred over surgical biopsies. An image-guided biopsy is as accurate as a surgical biopsy, is associated with less risk and lower cost, and has less long-term implications on cosmetics and radiographic surveillance. Surgical excisional biopsies as an initial biopsy tool are strongly discouraged as 80% of suspicious lesions following radiographic evaluation are benign and a surgical procedure can be avoided. A core biopsy that results in a diagnosis of malignancy allows one oncologic operation to be performed and affords the patient an opportunity to be well educated on the diagnosis and treatment options prior to surgical intervention. It is paramount that the radiologist, surgeon, and pathologist are in communication after the breast biopsy results to assess for concordance between the clinical, mammographic, US, and pathology findings. If the findings are discordant, a surgical excision is often recommended for histologic diagnosis. If the comprehensive imaging is negative and the palpable abnormality cannot be confirmed on imaging, then further workup is directed based on the level of clinical suspicion. For a clinically suspicious palpable lesion, a tissue diagnosis is required. If the lesion is of low clinical suspicion by exam and negative on diagnostic imaging, short-term follow-up with repeat CBE and US versus an FNA to complete the triple test can be performed. If the CBE, imaging, and cytology are consistent with a benign etiology—more commonly known as the "triple test"—this is associated with an almost 100% accuracy of a diagnosis of a benign breast lesion. FNA is only useful if there is a dedicated cytopathologist with experience differentiating benign from malignant cytologic pathology.

Diagnosis and Treatment

Our patient had a bilateral diagnostic mammogram and directed US. The mammogram revealed a spiculated lesion measuring 2 cm in the right upper outer quadrant. US confirmed an irregular, solid mass with posterior acoustic shadowing in the 10-o'clock position, 4 cm from the nipple. An US-guided CNB was performed on the same day with clip deployment. Pathology revealed a grade III invasive ductal carcinoma. The tumor cells were negative for the estrogen and progesterone receptors and did not overexpress human epidermal growth factor receptor 2 (HER2/neu). As part of the diagnostic evaluation, an US of the axillary lymph nodes (LNs) was negative for lymphadenopathy. If there was ultrasonographic suspicious features, an FNA of the LN would be performed preoperatively. Staging the axilla preoperatively by this method has been shown to be cost effective and when positive avoids an unnecessary sentinel lymph node

(SLN) biopsy. If there is clinical suspicion of distant disease, a fluorodeoxyglucose-positron emission tomography scan or computed tomography should be obtained to assess for metastatic disease. If there is no clinical suspicion of distant disease, baseline preoperative laboratory and imaging tests should be those routinely required for a general anesthetic. The value of searching for occult distant metastatic disease in asymptomatic patients with clinical stage I-II disease is not beneficial.

The preoperative consultation for newly diagnosed breast cancer has become more complex and frequently requires a multispecialty approach. The discussion begins with a review of the breast pathology and breast imaging findings. The patient should be counseled about the options of breast-conserving treatment (BCT) versus mastectomy. This discussion entails understanding of the individual patient's breast to tumor size, medical history of contraindications to radiation, patient compliance to undergo radiation, and her personal values. BCT most often is followed by whole-breast irradiation over 4 to 6 weeks, is well tolerated, and begins 3 to 4 weeks after BCT. In select situations, the patient may be a candidate for a 5-day course of partial-breast irradiation.

Patients presenting with locally advanced breast cancer and are considering BCT, are candidates for neoadjuvant chemotherapy. Neoadjuvant chemotherapy has been employed for patients with operable breast cancers who desire BCT but are not candidates based on the initial size of the tumor in relation to the size of the breast. Neoadjuvant therapy can be given in the form of systemic cytotoxic therapy or hormonal therapy, and the decision is based on the individual case. In one study, 81% of patients who were candidates only for mastectomy became eligible for BCT after neoadjuvant chemotherapy.

If the patient is interested in a mastectomy and breast reconstruction, they should meet with a plastic surgeon preoperatively to discuss their options. The discussion entails immediate-versus-delayed reconstruction as well as reconstruction with tissue expanders and implants-versus-autologous tissue. If undergoing reconstruction, some patients may be eligible for preservation of the nipple-areolar complex. The eligibility criteria are evolving and not necessarily limited to traditional criteria such as small breasts and small tumors more than 4 cm from the nipple. A radiation oncologist may be consulted preoperatively for patients who will be considered for postmastectomy radiation based on the patients age, tumor grade, size, hormonal and LN status. Invasive ductal or lobular carcinomas should be considered for axillary staging; specifically, lymphatic mapping, and SLN biopsy if the preoperative axillary US and clinical exam is negative for pathologic lymphadenopathy. Completion axillary lymphadenectomy is not advised if the SLN is negative and new evidence suggests that a complete axillary lymph node dissection (ALND) can even be safely avoided in certain node-positive situations.

Surgical Approach

Our patient has a single focus of cancer within her right breast, and the axillary US was negative for lymphadenopathy; she is wishing to proceed with BCT and SLN biopsy.

SLN Biopsy: For lymphatic mapping, most institutions utilize a dual agent method and that is what is described here. Lymphatic mapping is performed preoperatively with radiolabeled colloid injected into the breast. Peritumoral, intradermal over the lesion, or subareolar injection techniques are appropriate based on institutional preference. For axillary staging, a lymphoscintigraphy is not needed for a primary breast cancer. SLN biopsy can be performed under conscious sedation and local anesthesia; however, general anesthesia is our preferred approach. At the time of surgery, blue dye (dilute methylene blue or isosulfan blue) is injected typically in a sub- or periareolar distribution. The injection site is vigorously massaged for 5 minutes. When performed in conjunction with a mastectomy, the SLN is typically harvested near the completion of the procedure through the mastectomy incision; when performed in concert with a lumpectomy, almost always a separate incision is utilized. A small curvilinear incision is made two-finger breaths below the hair baring line in the ipsilateral axilla and taken down through clavipectoral fascia. A blue lymphatic channel is identified and traced to a SLN **(Figure 2)**. The lymphovascular supply is clipped, and the SLN is removed and submitted for pathologic analysis. A search is made for any other SLNs. If a blue channel is not identified, then the search is guided by the gamma probe. Any blue LNs, LNs with blue lymphatic channels leading

to them, LNs with counts ≥10% of the hottest node, or LNs that are suspicious by palpation are submitted as "SLNs." It must be remembered that the goal is to find a LN with metastatic cancer if present and not to find a blue or hot node. Background radioactivity is obtained to ensure there are no remaining focal hot spots and that all SLNs have been removed. The axilla should then be palpated for any clinically suspicious lymphadenopathy prior to closure. On average, two to three SLNs are identified. Removing more than one SLN has been associated with a lower false-negative rate, stressing a search should be made to remove all SLNs and to not just stop when the first is found. This does not imply that if only one SLN is found, another normal LN in the field should be harvested. If only one SLN is found after careful search, it is appropriate to stop. In the unusual situation when there are more than five SLNs, and the hottest node was removed, it is safe to stop at five. The SLNs should be individually dissected out and removed as opposed to a section of fatty axillary tissue with the SLN and other nodes present in the section **(Table 1)**.

Special Intraoperative Considerations

One of the potential pitfalls when performing axillary staging is failure of lymphatic mapping. Fortunately, the inability to identify a SLN is rare. Some features that have been associated with failure to identify a SLN include increasing patient age and body mass index; but of most importance is surgeon experience. When proceeding to SLN biopsy, consider prior ipsilateral breast and axillary procedures. If the patient has had a recent excisional biopsy, then the lymphatics crossing this incision will be disrupted. Injection in a subareolar

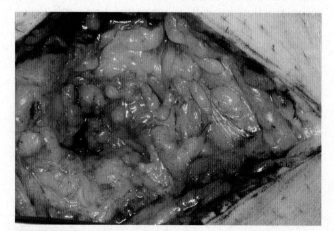

FIGURE 2 • Afferent lymphatic channels stained with methylene blue dye leading to a SLN in the axilla.

TABLE 1. Key Technical Steps and Potential Pitfalls in Sentinal Lymph Node (SLN) Biopsy

Key Technical Steps
1. Dual agent mapping.
2. Meticulous dissection once clavipectoral fascia is scored to identify the blue channel.
3. Trace the blue channel to a SLN or guided by the gamma probe if blue channel not visualized.
4. Be deliberate with gamma probe to focus on the exact location to minimize unnecessary dissection.
5. Remove all "hot," blue, or suspicious LNs (5 max).

Potential Pitfalls
- Making the incision too high in the axilla. This risks leaving behind a low-lying SLN and adds difficulty finding SLN due to "shine-through" from the injection site, by pointing the gamma probe toward the breast.
- Stopping at the first SLN without searching for additional SLNs.
- Aggressive dissection leading to disruption of numerous lymphatic channels or en bloc removal of a cluster of LNs increasing the risk of lymphedema.

location will fail to map in the setting of a recent upper outer-quadrant surgical scar. In this case, intradermal injection on the axillary side of the incision would be prudent **(Figure 3)**. Other breast operations (augmentation, reduction, surgical biopsies) and time from prior surgery need to be considered. Subareolar injection will reliably map the breast in cases of a primary tumor and allow consistent axillary staging. However, in a patient with prior breast cancer treatment, if attempting to map a recurrence or new primary in the same breast, we strongly favor a peritumoral injection with imaging to identify aberrant drainage outside the axilla, which is much more common in this situation. Mapping failures are also much more frequent in this scenario and predictive factors include extent of axillary surgery and prior radiation therapy that can ablate the lymphatic drainage. The standard answer for failed mapping of a primary breast cancer is to perform an axillary lymphadenectomy.

Postoperative Management

SLN biopsy is typically an outpatient procedure when combined with a lumpectomy. We also utilize a same-day

outpatient mastectomy protocol for our unilateral cases without reconstruction. Postoperatively, the patient is seen back in the clinic to assess wound healing and review the final pathologic results. The exam is focused on cellulitis, wound infection, seroma, hematoma, flap necrosis, and early lymphedema (extremity or breast). We attempt to coordinate a same-day postoperative visit with medical oncology, radiation oncology, and lymphedema clinic if a complete ALND was performed. A multidisciplinary team is utilized to discuss the risks and benefits of adjuvant treatment, including adjuvant systemic and hormonal therapy and radiation.

An individualize approach is the preferred method to determining the role of adjuvant therapy. Simplistic approaches such as tumor size >1 cm or node-positive disease are no longer the only factors to consider when deciding on adjuvant therapy options. In the era of targeted therapies and individualized medicine, patients and their medical oncology team together participate in the decision-making process. The patient should be informed of her risk of recurrence and death with and without adjuvant therapy as well as potential short- and long-term toxicities of

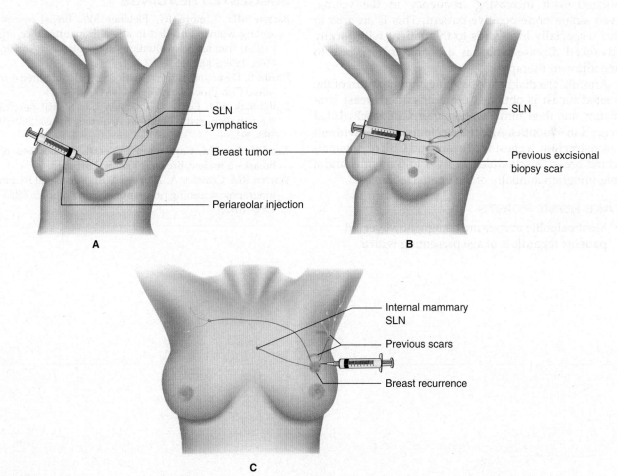

FIGURE 3 • **(A)** Lymphatic mapping of primary breast cancer using a subareolar injection technique **(B)** Lymphatic mapping of primary breast cancer after a previous excisional biopsy. The injection is intradermal on the axillary side of the incision **(C)** Lymphatic mapping of recurrent breast cancer using a peritumoral injection technique.

treatment. The tumor biology (predictive markers) as well as the tumor size, node status (prognostic factors), and patient's life expectancy without cancer death are factors that are considered when deciding who should receive adjuvant systemic therapy. Oncotype DX® can be a useful tool, and after hormonal status, it is one of the first tests employed as part of the available individualized tools to help identify patients who may be able to avoid chemotherapy. Oncotype DX® is introduced into the assessment postoperatively for postmenopausal, estrogen-receptor (ER)-positive cases with borderline tumor characteristics to assess the benefit of chemotherapy. It should only be ordered after thoughtful discussion if the results will influence the treatment decision and as a rule; therefore, should be ordered by the individual who will utilize the results to alter treatment decisions. Patients with triple-negative tumors (ER negative, progesterone-receptor negative, and HER2/neu negative) will likely be offered adjuvant systemic chemotherapy. Postmastectomy radiation has been shown to improve survival and decrease recurrence risk in patients with ≥4 metastatic LNs, extracapsular extension and ≥5 cm primary tumor. It is being utilized with increasing frequency in the young, even single node-positive patient. This is an area in flux, especially in regards to the patient with locally advanced disease who has a complete response to neoadjuvant therapy.

After BCT, a diagnostic baseline mammogram of the treated breast is obtained 6 months after breast irradiation and then annually thereafter; CBE is scheduled every 4 to 6 months. After mastectomy with or without reconstruction, a chest wall exam and CBE of the unaffected breast is scheduled every 4 to 6 months and a mammogram annually of the unaffected breast.

TAKE HOME POINTS

- Most palpable masses are benign; however, all patients regardless of age presenting with a palpable breast mass require an evaluation to exclude or confirm malignancy.
- Tissue diagnosis with CNB is often indicated unless the mass can clearly be attributed to an objective benign etiology.
- Concordance between the CBE, breast imaging, and CNB is of utmost importance in determining recommendations for further surgical excision and follow up.
- CNB provides preoperative histologic assessment and in most cases allows a one-stage surgical procedure. CNB has a high degree of accuracy as well as identifying benign lesions that can be followed safely.
- Excisional biopsy as a first step approach to a breast mass should be dissuaded.
- All excised breast specimens should be oriented.
- Preoperative assessment of the axilla with US and clinical assessment. If suspicious, FNA is useful, and if it confirms malignancy, ALND is performed.
- Remove only SLNs while preserving lymphatics and other neurovascular structures.

SUGGESTED READINGS

Barton MD, Elmore JG, Fletcher SW. Breast symptoms among women enrolled in a health maintenance organization: frequency, evaluation, and outcome. Ann Intern Med. 1999;130(8):651–657.

Pruthi S. Detection and evaluation of palpable breast mass. Mayo Clin Proc. 2001;76(6):641–647.

Pullyblank AM, Davies JD, Basten J, et al. Fat necrosis of the female breast – Hadfield revisited. Breast. 2001;10(5):388–391.

Tan PH, Lai LM, Carrington EV, et al. Fat necrosis of the breast – a review. Breast. 2006;15(3):313–318.

Warren RM, Crawley A. Is breast MRI ever useful in a mammographic screening programme? Clin Radiol. 2002;57(12):1090–1097.

51 Suspicious Mammographic Abnormality

CATHERINE E. PESCE and LISA K. JACOBS

Presentation

A 54-year-old female with a history of hyperlipidemia presents for her annual mammogram. She has never had an abnormal mammogram in the past, but she does have a family history of breast cancer in her mother who died in her 70s. On breast exam, there are no masses palpable in either breast or axilla. She does her own self-exams regularly. On review of her mammogram, she is found to have new calcifications in the upper outer quadrant of the right breast.

Differential Diagnosis

While calcifications can be overt invasive carcinoma, several other benign and premalignant lesions of the breast must also be considered.

- **Sclerosing adenosis** is a proliferation of the stroma and the smallest tubules within the terminal duct-lobular unit. It may mimic carcinoma clinically, radiologically, and histologically. The presence of myoepithelial cells confirms the benign nature of the lesion.
- **Atypical lobular hyperplasia** is a proliferation of the epithelium lining the lobules and is associated with an increased risk of future carcinoma.
- **Ductal hyperplasia** is proliferation of the ductal epithelial lining cells and may be of the usual or atypical type. It may have varying degrees of risk for future cancer.
- **Fibrocystic breast disease** is the single most common disorder of the breast. The condition is diagnosed frequently between the ages of 20 and 55 and decreases progressively after menopause. It encompasses a group of morphologic changes that often produce palpable lumps and are characterized by various combinations of cysts, fibrous overgrowth, and epithelial proliferation.
- **Columnar cell change** involves dilated terminal duct-lobular units, which are lined by uniform, ovoid-to-elongate, nontypical columnar cells, and these frequently exhibit prominent apical snouts. If associated with atypia, it is often associated with atypical ductal proliferations and *in situ* carcinomas.
- **Lobular carcinoma *in situ*** (LCIS) is a marker for increased risk of developing invasive carcinoma. Risk is equal for both breasts, and subsequent carcinoma may be either ductal or lobular.
- **Ductal carcinoma *in situ*** (DCIS) consists of malignant cells confined within the basement membranes

of ducts without invasion of the surrounding stroma.

Workup

When obtaining the history from the patient, certain risk factors must be obtained including the patient's age, history of pain, menstrual history, any skin changes over the breast, changes in the nipple-areolar complex, presence or absence of nipple discharge, personal history of previous masses or biopsies, and family history of breast cancer.

On physical exam, pertinent findings include the location of the mass, size, mobility, tenderness, fluctuance, any skin changes, nipple discharge, prior scars, and/or lymphadenopathy in the axillary, supraclavicular, or infraclavicular basins.

Mammography is the best screening test for the early detection of breast cancer for most women **(Figure 1)**. Ultrasound is currently not used for screening but is an excellent diagnostic tool for further evaluation of an abnormal mammogram or clinical breast complaint. MRI is used for screening women at high risk for breast cancer and to evaluate the extent of disease in the ipsilateral and contralateral breast in a patient with a new diagnosis of breast cancer. MRI is superior to mammography and ultrasound in determining the size of the tumor, the presence of multifocal or multicentric disease, and the presence of contralateral disease.

Palpable breast lesions are amenable to biopsy by fine needle aspiration (FNA), core biopsy, or surgical biopsy techniques. Fine needle aspirations can be performed in the office by either the surgeon or the pathologist. Proper and rapid fixation is imperative on an FNA specimen, and if the surgeon is to perform the procedure in the office, coordination with and assistance from the laboratory are important.

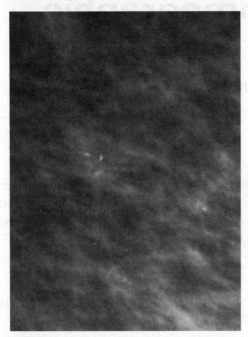

FIGURE 1 • Mammographic image of calcifications

Needle core biopsy offers greater sampling accuracy than FNA because the architecture of the area of concern is preserved, and this allows the pathologist to assess whether invasion is present. The National Comprehensive Cancer Network (NCCN) guidelines now recommend *core* biopsy before surgery.

Biopsy of nonpalpable breast lesions requires an image-guided biopsy technique. Many modalities exist to biopsy these lesions including stereotactic biopsy, ultrasound-guided biopsy, MRI-guided biopsy, and surgical excisional biopsy with image localization. Needle or wire localization of an image abnormality is the most common method for directing the surgeon to the target lesion. After needle placement, a mammogram is performed in the medial–lateral view as well as the cranial–caudal view to provide the operating surgeon with a three-dimensional location of the lesion. The surgical incision should be placed as close to the lesion as possible, while still trying to create an incision that can be incorporated into a mastectomy incision if that proves necessary in the future. The dissection is then performed down to the wire and along its course to the site of the lesion **(Figure 2)**.

After a biopsy is complete, the pathology results must be compared to the radiographic and physical examination findings. If the pathologic diagnosis cannot account for the other findings, then this biopsy is considered discordant and should either be repeated or excisional biopsy should be done. This involves the complete removal of the entire lesion.

Diagnosis and Treatment

The primary surgical options for the breast are mastectomy or breast conservation. Mastectomy has historically been indicated for tumors larger than 5 cm. A more patient-specific criterion is applying mastectomy when the tumor is large for the size of the remaining breast and when an oncologically acceptable lumpectomy would not leave a cosmetically acceptable outcome.

For the patient at hand, DCIS is the leading diagnosis and breast conservation would be appropriate. It must be emphasized that when breast conservation is performed, radiation is required postoperatively to achieve local recurrence rates similar to mastectomy. Relative contraindications to breast conservation include tumors >5 cm, large tumor-to-breast-size ratio, and pregnancy. Absolute contraindications include T4 tumors, multicentric disease, collagen vascular disease, previous history of breast radiation, and inability to access radiation therapy.

Sentinel lymph node biopsy is the initial axillary staging procedure of choice for women with clinically node-negative invasive breast cancer. It should be considered in women undergoing mastectomy for DCIS. Patients with micrometastases <0.2 mm on sentinel node biopsy are considered node negative (N0mic) and should not be considered for completion dissection or adjuvant chemotherapy based on their nodal status. Patients with metastases larger than 0.2 mm should continue to be treated as node positive and formal axillary lymph node dissection should be discussed.

Surgical Approach

The same surgical principles of the breast are maintained during excisional biopsy, partial mastectomy, and mastectomy.

During excisional biopsy and partial mastectomy, the incision is placed along Langer lines for the best cosmetic result. If possible, a periareolar incision should be used if the lesion is centrally located because the scar then blends in with the pigment change. In the lower half of the breast, radial incisions for malignant lesions are usually used. Even though the breast may be slightly

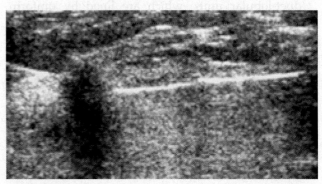

FIGURE 2 • Needle localization under ultrasound guidance

narrowed by a radial incision in the lower half of the breast, incisions along Langer lines in the inferior pole can cause more cosmetic deformity by shortening the distance between the areolar complex and the inframammary fold. A biopsy, as opposed to a partial mastectomy, has the surgical goal of obtaining a diagnosis by removing the lesion while minimizing excessive tissue loss. Therefore, wide margins are not appropriate for a diagnostic procedure. During partial mastectomy, however, a rim of surrounding normal tissue needs to be excised.

Mastectomy is usually required for women with multiple tumors in the same breast, diffuse malignant-appearing calcifications, T4 tumors, women who cannot receive radiation therapy, or positive margins after attempts at breast conservation. When positive margins occur after partial mastectomy, repeat local excision can be attempted. However, if margins remain positive when as much breast tissue as possible has been removed, mastectomy is required.

During mastectomy, the borders of the breast must be appreciated. These include the clavicle superiorly, the lateral border of the sternum medially, the latissimus dorsi laterally, and the inframammary fold inferiorly. All breast tissue, the nipple-areolar complex, and the fascia overlying the pectoralis major are removed, but the muscle is left intact.

When immediate reconstruction is planned, a skin-sparing mastectomy is preferred. This procedure involves performing an oncologically sound operation while leaving as much skin as possible. It includes removal of the nipple-areola complex, but some surgeons are pushing that boundary by using methods to preserve even the nipple and still reporting low local recurrence rates.

Sentinel lymph node biopsy entails the injection of technetium-99 m and/or isosulfan blue dye (Lymphazurin) in the breast. Nodal excision is typically performed through a small axillary incision, posterior to the lateral border of the pectoralis major muscle. Preoperative scanning with the gamma probe is often helpful in planning the incision. The incision should be easily incorporated in an incision for a subsequent axillary lymph node dissection. Nodes stained blue or with evidence of radioactivity on the gamma probe are excised intact and sent for pathologic review. In addition, nodes that are palpably firm or enlarged should also be excised. The procedure is considered complete after scanning with the gamma probe fails to reveal further radioactive counts >10% of the highest count detected (Table 1).

Special Intraoperative Considerations

Allergic reactions to the blue dye can happen in 1% to 2% of patients ranging from urticaria, blue hives, pruritis, bronchospasm, and hypotension. Allergic reaction should be considered in any patient experiencing hypotension in whom blue dye was used and is readily

managed with fluid resuscitation and short-term pressor support. A spurious decline in pulse oximetry readings occasionally occurs after injection of blue dye and does not represent hypoxemia.

When a sentinel node cannot be located via localization of blue dye or radioactivity or positive nodes are identified, a formal axillary lymph node dissection is usually recommended. This involves en bloc resection of the level I and level II lymph nodes. The axilla is anatomically defined posteriorly by the subscapularis and latissimus dorsi muscles, medially by the chest wall and the overlying serratus anterior muscle, laterally by the skin and subcutaneous tissue of the underarm area, and superiorly by the axillary vein. The fat pad defined by these areas is excised leaving the axillary vein, long thoracic nerve and the thoracodorsal nerve, artery, and vein intact.

Postoperative Management

Surveillance of breast cancer survivors is an integral part of their care, and its importance is growing with the increasing number of breast cancer survivors.

TABLE 1. Key Technical Steps and Potential Pitfalls

Key Technical Steps

Excisional Biopsy/Partial Mastectomy

1. Incision placed along Langer lines.
2. Biopsy: wide margins not necessary.
3. Partial mastectomy: rim of surrounding normal tissue required.

Mastectomy

1. Breast tissue, nipple-areolar complex, and pectoralis fascia removed.
2. Borders of the breast: clavicle, sternum, latissimus dorsi, inframmamary fold.
3. +/– reconstruction.

Sentinel Lymph Node Biopsy

1. Injection of technetium-99 m and/or isosulfan blue dye.
2. Axillary incision posterior to lateral border of pectoralis muscle.
3. Blue nodes or nodes with radioactivity excised intact.
4. Axilla scanned for remaining blue nodes or with >10% of highest count detected.

Axillary Dissection

1. En bloc resection of level I and II lymph nodes.
2. Borders of the axilla: subscapularis and latissimus dorsi, chest wall and serratus anterior, axillary vein, underarm skin and subcutaneous tissue.

Potential Pitfalls

- Positive margins after lumpectomy.
- Skin dimpling after closure.
- Injury to axillary vein, thoracodorsal nerve, or long thoracic nerve during axillary lymph node dissection.

Current standard of care for surveillance in patients with treated breast cancer constitutes scheduled history, physical examination, yearly mammograms, and breast self-exams. There is no good evidence supporting routine systemic imaging or laboratory testing such as tumor marker levels in breast cancer survivors.

Patients should be referred to genetic counseling if any of the following risk factors are present: Ashkenazi Jewish heritage, personal or family history of ovarian cancer, any first-degree relative diagnosed with breast cancer before age 50, two or more first-degree or second-degree relatives diagnosed with breast cancer, personal or family history of breast cancer in both breasts, and history of breast cancer in a male relative.

Postoperative management after breast surgery includes referral to medical and/or radiation oncology as is deemed appropriate. All women receiving breast conservation will be followed with radiation therapy. Adjuvant chemotherapy statistically can benefit most women with local–regional breast cancer, but the absolute benefit of chemotherapy must be balanced against the absolute risks of treatment to determine whether this intervention is worthwhile. All women with hormone receptor positive disease should be counseled regarding the benefits of antiestrogen therapy.

TAKE HOME POINTS

- One in 8 women will experience breast cancer in her lifetime, and 1 in 33 women will die of the disease.
- While calcifications can be overt invasive carcinoma, several other benign and premalignant lesions of the breast must also be considered.
- Mammography is the best screening test for the early detection of breast cancer for most women.
- Palpable breast lesions are amenable to biopsy by FNA, core biopsy, or surgical biopsy techniques, while biopsy of nonpalpable breast lesions requires an image-guided biopsy technique.
- The primary surgical options for the breast are mastectomy or breast conservation.

- When breast conservation is performed, radiation is required postoperatively to achieve local recurrence rates similar to those with mastectomy.
- Surveillance of breast cancer survivors should follow a care plan that includes the patient's surgeon, radiation and medical oncologists, as well as the primary care provider.

Acknowledgments

No funding was provided in this publication.

SUGGESTED READINGS

Arpino G, Laucirica R, Elledge RM. Premalignant and in situ breast disease: biology and clinical implications. Ann Intern Med. 2005;143(6):445–457.

Bellon JR, Come SE, Gelman RS, et al. Sequencing of chemotherapy and radiation therapy in early-stage breast cancer: updated results of a prospective randomized trial. J Clin Oncol. 2005;23(9):1934–1940.

Claus EB, Schildkraut JM, Thompson WD, et al. The genetic attributable risk of breast and ovarian cancer. Cancer. 1996;77(11):2318–2324.

Cox C, White L, Allred N, et al. Survival outcomes in node-negative breast cancer patients evaluated with complete axillary node dissection versus sentinel lymph node biopsy. Ann Surg Oncol. 2006;13(5):708–711.

Ellis IO, Elston CW, Poller DN. Ductal carcinoma in situ. In: Elston CW, Ellis IO, eds. The Breast. UK: The Bath Press, 1998:249–282.

Lee CH, Dershaw D, Kopans D, et al. Breast cancer screening with imaging: recommendations from the Society of Breast Imaging and the ACR on the use of mammography, breast MRI, breast ultrasound, and other technologies for the detection of clinically occult breast cancer. J Am Coll Radiol. 2010;7:18–27.

Lehman CD, Gatsonis C, Kuhl CK, et al.; ACRIN Trial of Investigators Group. MRI evaluation of the contralateral breast in women with recently diagnosed breast cancer. N Engl J Med. 2007;356(13):1296–1303.

Montgomery LL, Thorne AC, Van Zee KJ, et al. Isosulfan blue dye reactions during sentinel lymph node mapping for breast cancer. Anesth Analg. 2002;95:385–388.

NCCN guidelines for breast cancer screening, 2007. www.nccn.org/professionals/physician_gls/PDF/breast-screening.pdf, p4.

Parker SH, Stavros AT, Dennis MA. Needle biopsy techniques. Radiol Clin North Am. 1995;33:1171–1186.

52 Ductal Carcinoma In Situ

JESSICA M. BENSENHAVER and TARA M. BRESLIN

Presentation

A 50-year-old female presents with a new finding of clustered microcalcifications discovered on her annual screening mammogram. She has an unremarkable medical history and denies a history of previous breast biopsies or breast conditions. She reports a family history significant for breast cancer in a maternal grandmother and aunt. Her breast exam is unremarkable with symmetric, moderate-sized breast, without skin changes and with no erythema, dimpling, or nipple inversion. On palpation, there is no dominant mass or nipple discharge from either breast. She has undergone image-guided core biopsy and has a pathology report that reveals ductal carcinoma in situ (DCIS), nuclear grade 3 with associated comedonecrosis, estrogen receptor (ER) positive by immunohistochemistry.

Differential Diagnosis

DCIS falls along a spectrum of benign, preinvasive, and invasive breast histologies that include ductal hyperplasia, atypical ductal hyperplasia, DCIS, DCIS with microinvasion, and invasive carcinoma. Mammographic lesions can represent one of these conditions in isolation or different combinations.

Workup

This patient presented with new clustered microcalcifications on screening mammogram, a common presentation of DCIS. Further evaluation included in-depth history with risk assessment and thorough physical exam of BOTH breasts and lymph node basins.

A complete imaging evaluation consists of diagnostic mammography to address the characteristics (calcifications, soft tissue density) and extent (focal, multifocal, or multicentric) of ipsilateral disease, and rule out bilateral disease (Figures 1A and 2). Review of prior images is helpful for determining stability of probably benign findings. The information from these imaging studies is essential for planning surgery.

Diagnosis

Diagnosis requires tissue biopsy. Core biopsy is the preferred method. It is minimally invasive, accurate, and can be performed in office under local anesthesia. Image guidance, either stereotactic or ultrasound, is employed for accuracy and allows placement of a marking clip in the biopsy site. It must be noted that core biopsy represents just a portion of the lesion, and there is a 10% to 15% chance of associated invasive carcinoma being present with a core biopsy diagnosis of DCIS.

Treatment Principles

DCIS treatment is multimodal, including a combination of surgery, radiotherapy, and hormone therapy.

DCIS without invasive cancer is unlikely to cause death. Therefore, the focus of DCIS treatment is prevention of local recurrence, unlike most cancer treatments that focus on survival.

Surgical options include breast conservation (BC) or simple (total) mastectomy. BC is feasible if the following conditions are met: (1) the patient is a candidate for postpartial mastectomy radiation and (2) the size of disease allows for partial mastectomy with negative margins without sacrificing cosmesis. Simple mastectomy is indicated in cases of true multicentric disease or multifocal disease for which partial mastectomy would compromise cosmesis. Patient preference can play a role in choosing mastectomy in disease otherwise amenable to BC, usually seen in highly motivated women with genetic predisposition (BRCA mutation). These patients must understand that mastectomy offers a risk reduction benefit, but no survival benefit. Patients undergoing mastectomy should also be considered for reconstruction and undergo preoperative evaluation by a plastic surgeon.

Pathologic evaluation confirms diagnosis; addresses tumor size and extent; characterizes the nuclear grade, tumor architecture, and presence or absence of comedonecrosis; evaluates for microinvasion (focus of invasion <0.1 cm) or occult invasive disease; establishes receptor status; and assesses surgical margins with measurements. The optimal DCIS margin width is unknown, but a width of 1 mm or more is associated with a decreased chance of recurrence. DCIS is upstaged (from stage 0) by the presence of microinvasion or occult invasive disease and should be treated according to recommendation for invasive disease.

Radiotherapy is not routine after mastectomy, but is routine after BC as literature shows a 50% risk reduction in local recurrence with radiotherapy. However, no DCIS trial has ever demonstrated that radiation offers

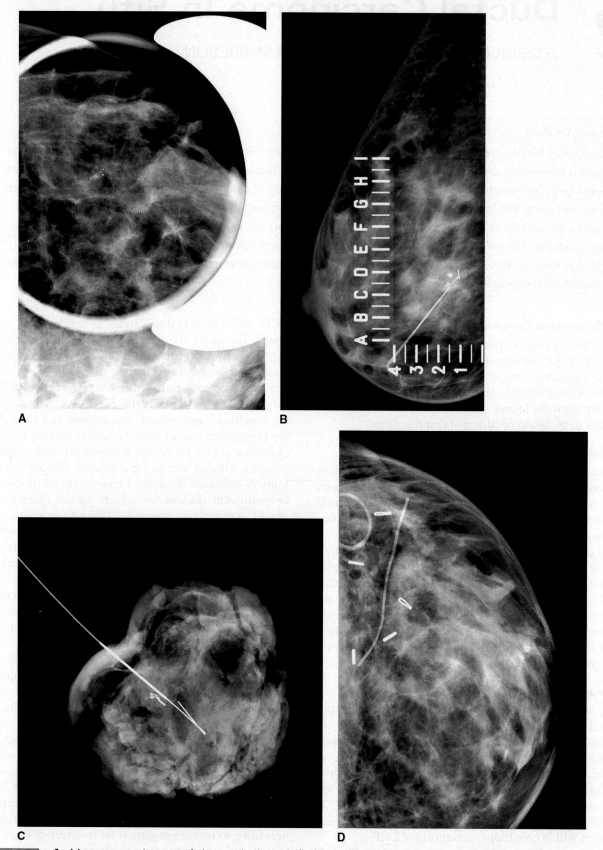

FIGURE 1 • **A:** Mammogram images of clustered microcalcifications. **B:** Wire localization image after core biopsy with clip placement. Note hooked portion of wire adjacent to biopsy clip. **C:** Intraoperative specimen radiograph. Note radiographic wide margins and calcifications and clip adjacent to reinforced portion of wire. **D:** Postsurgery comparison mammography showing complete removal of all calcifications. Note incision marker and metallic clips marking lumpectomy bed.

a survival benefit when compared with excision alone; therefore, omitting radiotherapy in low-risk patients is an area of active investigation. To date, however, there are no prospective trial data or established pathologic selection criteria for identifying appropriate patients.

Hormone therapy with tamoxifen has a role for risk reduction in patients with ER-positive DCIS. When used for 5 years, tamoxifen therapy reduces the risk of ipsilateral recurrence and contralateral disease. Therefore, noting no contraindications to tamoxifen exist, hormonal therapy should at least be considered for ER-positive DCIS.

Surgical Approach for BC

Partial mastectomy is performed with the patient supine, under general anesthesia or IV sedation **(Table 1)**. Wire localization is preformed preoperatively for nonpalpable lesions **(Figure 1B)**. Incision planning is strategic and based on lesion location and depth. It is preferable to plan the incision close to the lesion with an orientation (circumareolar, curvilinear, or radial) based on the breast anatomy, recognizing the possibility for future mastectomy if margin status is inadequate **(Figure 3)**. Include the skin overlying superficial lesions. Large skin excisions can affect

TABLE 1. Key Technical Steps and Potential Pitfalls of Breast Conservation (BC)

Key Technical Steps

1. Preoperative wire localization for nonpalpable lesions.
2. Strategically plan incision based on lesion location and depth.
   a. Orient incision recognizing possibility for future mastectomy if margin status is not adequate.
   b. Excise skin overlying superficial lesions.
   c. If the lesion is wire localized, include location of wire penetration if possible.
3. Excise the lesion with margins grossly appearing to be 1 cm.
4. Orient specimen and send to mammography for radiographic assessment.
5. Palpate lumpectomy cavity to ensure removal of suspicious tissue.
6. Ensure hemostasis and close.
7. Plan for postoperative mammogram (1–3 wk postoperative) to compare with preoperative film to confirm complete excision of area(s) of concern prior to the initiation of radiotherapy.

Potential Pitfalls

- Inadequate surgical margins requiring re-excision or mastectomy.

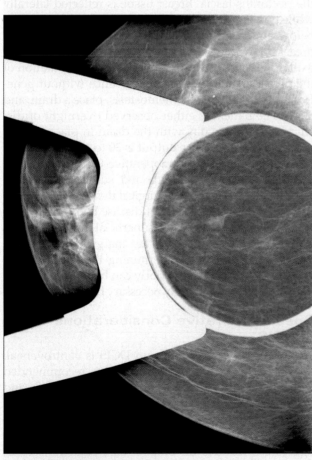

FIGURE 2 • Example of soft tissue density.

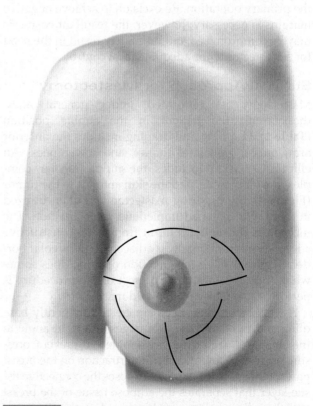

FIGURE 3 • Orientation of incisions for lumpectomy/partial mastectomy excision procedure. (From Bland KI, Klimberg VS, Master Techniques in General Surgery: Breast Surgery. Philadelphia, PA: Lippincott Williams & Wilkins, 2011.)

cosmesis by causing a mastopexy-type effect. If using wire localization, it is ideal to include the location of skin penetration by the wire with the incision, unless doing so will result in excessive tunneling during the dissection. If the incision does not incorporate the wire, be careful to note its location and then deliver it through the center of the incision once encountered.

In cases performed under IV sedation, local anesthesia is utilized prior to incision. The incision is made and dissection is aimed directly down to the lesion, avoiding thin skin flaps if possible. Excise the tissue around the specimen that creates margins grossly appearing to be around 1 cm. Amputate, orient the specimen, and sent it to mammography to confirm removal of the lesion, margins, radiopaque clip if placed at biopsy, and the localizing wire **(Figure 1C)**. Palpate the lumpectomy cavity to ensure removal of all suspicious tissue. Place marking clips on the borders of the specimen cavity (helpful for radiation planning and identification on future breast imaging). Ensure hemostasis and close.

The most common pitfall associated with partial mastectomy is inadequate margin status requiring re-excision or possibly mastectomy. Intraoperative specimen mammography and frozen section of the margins potentially avoids a second operation by providing an opportunity to identify and address margin issues at the primary operation. Re-excision to achieve negative margins is necessary; however, the resultant cosmesis may be compromised and ultimately result in the need for a mastectomy for adequate local control.

Surgical Approach for Mastectomy

Mastectomy is performed under general anesthesia with the patient in the supine position **(Table 2)**. Prepping and draping includes the anterior arm, breast, ipsilateral thorax, and lower neck. An elliptical incision includes the nipple–areolar complex, the biopsy site, and the skin anterior to the tumor **(Figure 4)**. Skin-sparing mastectomy is often utilized in cases with planned immediate reconstruction. The incision is chosen with input from the reconstructive surgeon and traditionally is adjacent to the areolar border **(Figure 5)**. This smaller skin opening does somewhat limit exposure, but the rest of the procedure is performed similarly to standard mastectomy.

After incision, skin flaps are created by gently handling and retracting the skin edges at a right angle to the chest wall (retractors are avoided to prevent pressure necrosis). Downward countertraction on the breast parenchyma toward the chest exposes the connective tissue layer that separates the adipose tissue of the breast and the adipose tissue of the skin. The skin flaps are developed along this connective tissue plane to the chest wall superiorly, inferiorly, and medially and laterally to the latissimus dorsi. Close attention to flap thickness

TABLE 2. Key Technical Steps and Potential Pitfalls of Mastectomy

Key Technical Steps

1. Elliptical incision oriented to include nipple–areolar complex, biopsy site, and skin overlying lesion.
2. Use electrocautery to develop the connective tissue plane.
3. Dissect along the plane superiorly, medially, and inferiorly to the chest wall, laterally to the latissimus dorsi.
4. Remove breast with the pectoralis fascia using electrocautery, traveling parallel to the pectoralis muscle fibers.
5. Amputate at the lateral aspect including the tail of Spence without penetrating into the axilla.
6. Ensure hemostasis, place a drain, and close.

Potential Pitfalls

- Adequate margin status in extensive, superficial disease requiring large skin resection.
- Wound closure in large resection specimens requiring subcutaneous undermining or skin grafting.

is important as overly thin flaps are at risk for necrosis and infection. Throughout dissection and removal, any encountered vessels should be isolated and ligated.

The breast is amputated from the chest wall with the pectoralis fascia. Breast tissue is reflected laterally while traveling parallel to the muscle fibers, so that just before amputation is complete, gentle tension on the breast allows visualization of the tissue plane of the axillary fascia. This technique results in amputation of the breast, including the tail of Spence without penetrating the axilla. Ensure hemostasis, place a drain, and close. The patient is either observed overnight or discharged the same day with the drain in place. Drains are often removed once output is 30 to 40 mL/d.

The most common intraoperative complications are inadequate surgical margins and subsequent wound complications. The goal of surgical therapy is local control with complete excision of disease both grossly and microscopically. If extensive superficial disease requires a large skin resection to ensure margins, skin closure can be compromised. Undermining the subcutaneous tissues inferiorly and superiorly can better mobilize the flaps. Skin grafting is rarely necessary but also an option.

Special Operative Considerations in DCIS

The role of axillary surgery in DCIS is controversial. Sentinel lymph node biopsy (SLNB) is recommended for women undergoing mastectomy for DCIS, and should be considered in women with lesions at higher risk for occult invasive disease including those that are clinically palpable, large (>4 cm on imaging), or have aggressive features on biopsy (e.g., comedonecrosis, microinvasion).

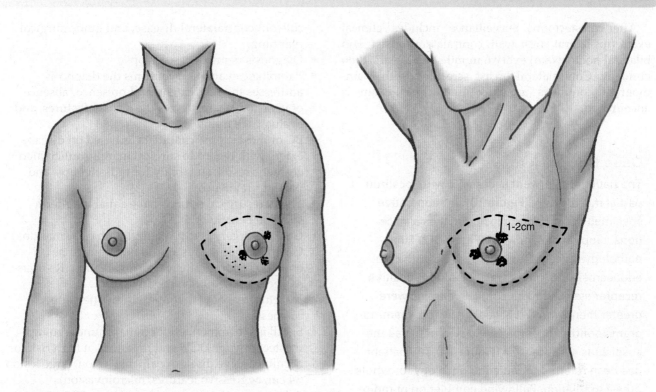

FIGURE 4 • Mastectomy incision. (From Bland KI, Klimberg VS. Master Techniques in General Surgery: Breast Surgery. Philadelphia, PA: Lippincott Williams & Wilkins, 2011.)

Oncoplastic surgical techniques are an emerging technology offering more choices for patients with tumor characteristics that would require generous partial mastectomy to achieve negative margins. These techniques are especially beneficial as an alternative to mastectomy in women with a generous amount of breast tissue. Contralateral reduction is often necessary for symmetry.

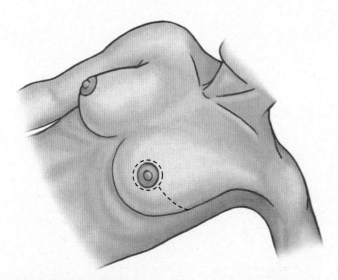

FIGURE 5 • Skin-sparing mastectomy incision. (From Bland KI, Klimberg VS. Master Techniques in General Surgery: Breast Surgery. Philadelphia, PA: Lippincott Williams & Wilkins, 2011.)

Postoperative Management

Common complications of both partial mastectomy and simple mastectomy are infection, hematoma, seroma, chronic incisional pain, and lymphedema. Preoperative prevention practices include prophylactic antibiotics especially in high-risk patients (obese, elderly, diabetic) and cessation of anticoagulants 10 to 14 days before scheduled surgery. Adequate postoperative counseling with PT/OT referral when necessary can address incisional pain and lymphedema. Although rare, brachial plexopathy from positioning can also occur. Two unique complications of BC are the rare potential for pneumothorax from wire placement and Mondor's disease. Postoperative flap necrosis can occur after mastectomy, seen most often with thin flaps and in smokers. This complication sometimes requires debridement and chronic wound management and/or delayed closure techniques.

Partial mastectomy follow-up starts with a postsurgical mammogram 1 to 3 weeks after surgery to compare with preoperative images and confirm complete excision of calcifications (Figure 1D). Surveillance mammography resumes 6 months after completion of radiation to evaluate treatment-associated changes and establish a new baseline. Annual bilateral screening is then reestablished. Clinical breast exam is recommended every 6 months for 2 years, then annually with screening mammography. Interim self–breast exam is always encouraged.

After mastectomy, surveillance includes clinical exam (ipsilateral chest wall, contralateral breast, and bilateral nodal exam) every 6 months for 2 years, then annually. Contralateral breast screening with mammogram continues annually. Interim self-exam is encouraged.

Case Conclusion

The patient underwent successful wire-localized partial mastectomy **(Figure 1B)**. Intraoperative specimen mammogram included the calcifications, biopsy clip, and wire **(Figure 1C)**. Final pathology revealed high-grade DCIS with comedonecrosis, no microinvasion, and ER-positive receptor status, and all surgical margins were greater than 2 mm. At 3 weeks post-op, mammogram confirmed complete excision of the all the suspicious calcifications **(Figure 1D)**. The patient has been referred to radiation oncology for whole breast irradiation. Following completion of radiotherapy, she will be evaluated for tamoxifen therapy for risk reduction due to her ER-positive DCIS.

TAKE HOME POINTS

- Screening mammography has increased the preclinical identification and overall incidence of DCIS.
- Preoperative diagnostic imaging is mandatory to evaluate the extent of ipsilateral disease, to rule out contralateral disease, and guide surgical planning.
- Diagnosis requires tissue biopsy.
- Pathologic evaluation confirms the diagnosis; addresses the size, extent, and presence/absence of invasion; characterizes the disease features; and evaluates margins.
- BC or mastectomy candidacy is based on disease extent with regard to surgical margin, anticipated cosmetic result, suitability for radiotherapy, and patient preference.
- The two surgical options have equal long-term survival benefits.
- Goal of surgery is local control with clear margins. Once the specimen is amputated, it must be oriented for appropriate margin evaluation. Re-excise as necessary to obtain negative margins, realizing that re-excision often affects cosmesis.
- SLNB is recommended for patients undergoing mastectomy for DCIS and in lesions at high risk for occult invasive disease (palpable lesion, large lesion >4 cm, aggressive features, microinvasion).
- Adjuvant radiation therapy results in 50% recurrence risk reduction in BC. Omission in low-risk patients treated with excision only is a controversial area of investigation.
- Adjuvant hormonal therapy with tamoxifen for 5-year duration should be considered for risk reduction in ER-positive DCIS patients.

SUGGESTED READINGS

Burstein HJ, Polyak K, Wong JS, et al. Ductal carcinoma in situ of the breast. N Engl J Med. 2004;350:1430–1441.

53 Lobular Carcinoma In Situ

LISA A. NEWMAN

Presentation

A 45-year-old African American female undergoes routine screening mammogram and is found to have scattered indeterminate microcalcifications bilaterally. One cluster in the lower left breast at the 6 o'clock position is particularly suspicious because it appears prominent and has a more branching pattern when compared to the patient's prior mammograms, which have been performed annually since age 40 years. She is referred to a surgeon for discussion of biopsy options. This patient's past medical history is noncontributory, but she does have a sister who was diagnosed with breast cancer at 40 years of age. Her clinical breast exam is negative for any skin abnormalities; there are no dominant or discrete palpable masses; there is no nipple discharge; and there is no suspicious adenopathy in either the axillary or supraclavicular nodal basins.

Differential Diagnosis

Mammographically detected microcalcifications can represent benign breast findings (fibrocystic hyperplasia, vascular calcifications, cystic hyperplasia, etc.), or they can represent a breast malignancy. Patients are routinely recommended to avoid use of talc-based deodorants or topical preparations, as these can create calcification artifact. Patients with history of prior breast surgery or radiation can also develop calcifications that are of a benign, inflammatory nature (fat necrosis). An experienced breast imaging team is necessary to distinguish the high-risk and frankly malignant patterns that require biopsy from the clearly benign patterns that can be monitored noninvasively.

Workup

Additional diagnostic mammographic views (compression and magnification images) will generally be necessary for the further evaluation of microcalcifications **(Figure 1)**. Calcifications that follow a linear and branching pattern, or that are associated with a spiculated density, will be considered more suspicious of a malignant etiology. Calcifications that layer out (e.g., "teacup" pattern) suggest benign cystic hyperplasia. Targeted breast ultrasound is indicated if there is any question of a coexisting mass density. Breast magnetic resonance imaging (MRI) will not be useful at this juncture because a normal MRI will not negate any mammographic indications for proceeding to biopsy. Any management decisions must be correlated with the clinical breast exam—a suspicious finding on breast exam (e.g., palpable breast mass or bloody nipple discharge) would be an indication to proceed with biopsy in order to obtain histopathologic information regarding the nature of the finding, regardless of whether or not the lesion has an imaging correlate.

This patient's additional imaging confirmed a dominant cluster of microcalcifications in the lower hemisphere of the left breast, and biopsy was recommended. Diagnostic biopsy options for nonpalpable, mammographically or sonographically detected breast abnormalities include image-guided fine needle aspiration (FNA), image-guided core needle biopsy, or wire localization surgical biopsy **(Table 1)**. A diagnostic surgical biopsy is the most definitive procedure because it yields the largest pathology specimen, and may result in complete extraction of the image-detected abnormality, but as a surgical volume-extracting procedure, it can result in cosmetic deformity and is less efficient compared to needle biopsy procedures. Image-guided needle biopsy procedures are generally preferred as the initial diagnostic maneuver, as they are less invasive and less costly. Core needle biopsy tends to have an improved diagnostic yield compared to FNA; false-negative/sampling error rates are usually <10% for core needle biopsies (especially if vacuum assisted) but can be as high as 30% with FNA biopsy. The FNA provides a cytologic sample only and therefore cannot distinguish in situ cancer from invasive cancer. Furthermore, while the spun-down cells from a cancerous FNA biopsy can be used for immunohistochemical evaluation of molecular markers (estrogen receptor, progesterone receptor and HER2/neu), it would not be known whether these markers were expressed on the invasive or the in situ component of the cancer.

Mammography can be used to guide a percutaneous needle biopsy (the stereotactic approach) or ultrasound may be used. Patient and image factors dictate the selection of image guidance. Microcalcifications usually require mammographic, stereotactic biopsy. While upright equipment is available, most stereotactic biopsies are performed on a specially designed table and require prone positioning of the patient. The affected

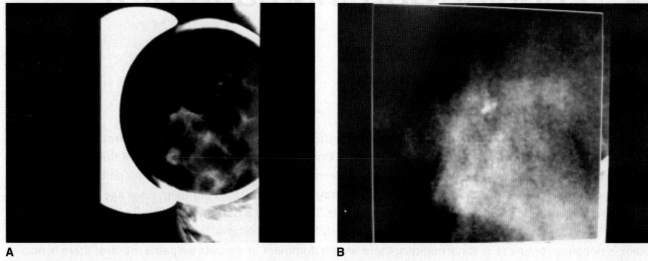

A   **B**

FIGURE 1 • **A,B:** Patient mammogram, revealing microcalcifications in left breast.

breast is fitted through an aperture facing the floor, and the ipsilateral arm must be raised above the head during the entire procedure. The biopsy needle is directed toward the target within the breast using stereotactic guidance, and a range of 5 to 12 core specimens are typically extracted under local anesthesia. Because of the positioning and table design prerequisites, some cases will not be amenable to the stereotactic biopsy approach: lesions that are adjacent to the pectoralis muscle, lesions that are too superficial or within the nipple, small breasts that compress to a thickness that is exceeded by the core needle trajectory, patients who cannot tolerate prone positioning for prolonged periods (half-hour or longer), and patients who exceed the weight limit of the biopsy table. Solid mass lesions that are sonographically visible can be biopsied with ultrasound guidance. A radiopaque marker should be left in place at the biopsy site to document the site that was sampled. In the event that a subsequent surgical procedure is needed (and the imaged target is no longer visible on postbiopsy films), the clip would serve as the target for a wire localization resection. The core biopsy specimens should be imaged to insure adequate sampling of the target, especially in cases of microcalcifications. Specific needle biopsy pathology results that mandate a follow-up surgical resection include the following: failed procedures, where the target is not adequately sampled; benign pathologic findings that are radiographically interpreted as being discordant with the target images; and "high-risk" pathology, such as lobular carcinoma in situ (LCIS), atypical lobular hyperplasia, and atypical ductal hyperplasia. These high-risk lesions are associated with an approximately 15% to 20% frequency of coexisting cancer (ductal carcinoma in situ and/or invasive cancer) when a follow-up diagnostic surgical wire localization biopsy is performed.

In this patient, the cluster of microcalcifications was not amenable to the percutaneous needle biopsy because of small breast size, and the patient therefore underwent a wire localization surgical biopsy. It is mandatory that a specimen mammogram be obtained for this type of procedure as well, and unfortunately in this case there were no calcifications visible in the excised breast specimen. Pathology evaluation nonetheless revealed a diagnosis of LCIS **(Figure 2)**.

Diagnosis and Treatment

The specimen mammography in this case documented a failed wire localization procedure. When this occurs, the surgeon can attempt to "blindly" resect or sample some breast fragments in the biopsy field, but once the wire has been extracted with the initial tissue specimen, it is extremely difficult to obtain an appropriate secondary specimen. Another option is to close the wound and await pathology results, and if these are negative for cancer, then the patient should undergo repeat mammography within the next few weeks (as chosen by the surgeon and patient in this particular case). A decision regarding any additional biopsy attempts would be made based upon the appearance of the follow-up mammogram.

In this patient, the surgical specimen revealed high-risk pathology in the form of LCIS. LCIS is identified in fewer than 5% of otherwise benign breast biopsies and is most commonly detected among women in their forties. It may be found coincidentally with other breast pathology in up to 25% of breast surgical cases. The magnitude of the increased future breast cancer risk for LCIS is approximately 1% per year, and this risk may be higher in women with a positive family history of breast cancer in addition to the LCIS. LCIS is perceived as a microscopic pattern of breast tissue that is present diffusely and bilaterally, but usually

TABLE 1. Key Technical Steps and Potential Pitfalls in Breast Biopsy Options for Nonpalpable, Screen-detected Abnormalities

Key Technical Steps

1. Image-guided percutaneous needle biopsy preferred as the most efficient maneuver.
2. Mammographically guided (stereotactic) or ultrasound-guided needle biopsy can be performed, depending on which study reveals best images of the target lesion. Core needle biopsies (14- or 16 guage) have lower false-negative rate compared to cytologic yield from FNA biopsy.
3. Radiopaque clip must be left in place to document site-sampled breast tissue.
4. When percutaneous image-guided needle biopsy technology is unavailable, or not feasible (body habitus too large or breast too small; patient unable to tolerate percutaneous procedure), then a follow-up wire localization surgical biopsy is necessary.
5. When needle biopsy reveals high-risk pathology such as LCIS, atypical ductal hyperplasia, or atypical lobular hyperplasia, then a follow-up wire localization surgical biopsy is necessary to rule out sampling error and coexisting cancer.

Potential Pitfalls

- Images of any needle biopsy and/or surgical biopsy specimens are mandatory to confirm inclusion of the target lesion.
- If needle biopsy specimen images demonstrate failed/nondiagnostic procedure or discordant findings, then surgical biopsy is necessary.
- If surgical diagnostic wire localization specimen images demonstrate failed procedure, then subsequent management is based upon pathology of any extracted specimen as well as follow-up, postoperative imaging.

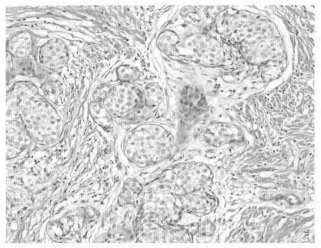

FIGURE 2 • Biopsy slide revealing LCIS.

well as postmenopausal women) or raloxifene (only approved for use in postmenopausal women), or bilateral prophylactic mastectomy. The surveillance options generally include annual or biannual clinical breast exam and annual mammography, and annual breast MRI may be considered as well. Chemoprevention can halve the future breast cancer risk and is usually prescribed for 5 years. Raloxifene may be used in selected postmenopausal women for longer periods if it is indicated in the control of osteoporosis. Premenopausal women must be advised to avoid pregnancy while taking tamoxifen. Both of these selective estrogen receptor modulators are associated with vasomotor symptoms (night sweats, hot flashes), thromboembolic phenomena, and uterine problems. Risk of uterine cancer is relatively greater in postmenopausal women taking tamoxifen. Patients opting for bilateral prophylactic mastectomy should meet with a plastic surgeon to assess their reconstruction options (immediate reconstruction vs. delayed; tissue expander/implant reconstruction versus autologous tissue reconstruction). Axillary staging surgery is not necessary for LCIS patients choosing prophylactic mastectomy.

Atypical hyperplasia (ductal or lobular) represents another high-risk pathology. Future risk of breast cancer is approximately four to five times that of the general female population with benign "usual" fibrocystic hyperplasia, and most of this risk is expressed within the initial 5 to 10 years after diagnosis. In contrast to the LCIS-associated breast cancer risk, atypia is more similar to a true cancer precursor lesion—subsequent breast cancers usually occur at the site where the atypia was identified (especially in cases of atypical ductal hyperplasia).

The patient in the scenario presented in this chapter underwent follow-up mammography imaging 3 months later that was unchanged, and the patient was offered the option of continued observation at that

without any clinical or radiographic correlate; it therefore tends to be detected as an incidental finding in women undergoing biopsy for some other reason. The future breast cancer risk is expressed equally in terms of laterality, and of those patients who do develop subsequent breast cancer, two-thirds will be diagnosed with ductal histopathology as opposed to invasive lobular cancer. LCIS is therefore a marker of increased risk and not an actual precursor lesion. When LCIS is detected incidentally at the time of lumpectomy for breast cancer, the margins do not need to be free of the LCIS histology.

Because LCIS is a marker of risk for either breast, the management options must address the bilateral breast tissue. These management options include close surveillance/observation alone, chemoprevention with either tamoxifen (appropriate for premenopausal as point because of the subtle/indeterminate appearance of her microcalcifications. She opted to undergo bilateral prophylactic with immediate reconstruction. Her final pathology revealed diffuse and bilateral LCIS (as expected) as well as extensive severe atypical ductal hyperplasia. Microcalcifications were identified in areas of atypical hyperplasia and also in areas of benign/usual hyperplasia.

Discussion Points/Special Considerations

Screening Mammography: This patient initiated annual screening mammography at age 40, despite ongoing controversy regarding whether surveillance mammography should begin prior to age 50 years. The American Cancer Society, the American College of Radiology, and the American College of Surgeons continue to advocate in favor of screening mammography beginning at age 40 years. Additional factors in this particular patient that support screening during the fifth decade of life include her positive family history, with breast cancer diagnosed at a young age in a second-degree relative, and her racial–ethnic identity. Lifetime incidence rates for breast cancer are lower for African American women compared to White American women, despite paradoxically higher mortality rates, and African American women have a younger age distribution. For American women younger than 45 years of age, breast cancer incidence rates are higher for African American compared to White American women.

Breast Cancer Risk Assessment: Individualized breast cancer risk is frequently estimated by use of the Gail model, a statistical tool that assesses likelihood of a woman being diagnosed with breast cancer over the following 5 years, and over her lifetime. Conventional thresholds for identifying "high-risk" women are based upon 5-year risk estimate that exceed 1.7%, or lifetime risk estimate >20% to 25%. The Gail model calculates risk probabilities by accounting for first-degree family history of breast cancer; reproductive history (age at menarche, age at first live birth); breast biopsy history (number of prior biopsies and whether or not any prior biopsy revealed atypical hyperplasia). The Gail model may underestimate risk in women with hereditary predisposition, since it does not account for the extended family history or

the paternal family history. The Gail model is not indicated for risk assessment in women with a personal history of breast cancer or a documented history of LCIS, as both of these features are associated with an established future new primary breast cancer risk that approximates 1% per year.

TAKE HOME POINTS

- Annual screening mammography in women with a normal breast exam should be initiated at age 40.
- The initial, preferred biopsy approach for a mammographically detected abnormality is via image-guided percutaneous core needle biopsy.
- High-risk pathology detected on needle biopsy specimens (LCIS, atypical hyperplasia) indicates the need for follow-up diagnostic surgical wire localization biopsy. This procedure will reveal coexisting cancer in approximately 15% of cases.
- LCIS is associated with an approximately 1% risk per year of subsequent breast cancer, affecting each breast equally and diffusely. Management options include surveillance (annual clinical breast exam, annual mammography, and possible annual breast MRI); chemoprevention; and bilateral prophylactic mastectomy.
- Atypical ductal hyperplasia is associated with an approximately four- to fivefold increased relative risk of breast cancer, with most of this risk expressed within the first 5 years after diagnosis, and mainly affecting the site where the atypia was detected. Management options include surveillance (as described above) and/or chemoprevention.

SUGGESTED READINGS

Kilbride K, Newman LA. Lobular carcinoma in situ. In: Harris JR, Lippman ME, Morrow M, et al., eds. Diseases of the Breast. 4th ed. Philadelphia, PA: Lippincott, Williams, and Wilkins, 2010.

Newman LA. Surgical management of high risk breast lesions. Probl Gen Surg. 2003;20:99–112.

Saslow D, Boetes C, Burke W, et al. American Cancer Society Guidelines for breast screening with MRI as an adjunct to mammography. CA Cancer J Clin. 2007;57:75–89.

Smith RA, Cokkinides V, Brooks D, et al. Cancer screening in the United States, 2011: a review of current American Cancer Society guidelines and issues in cancer screening. CA Cancer J Clin. 2011;61:8–30.

54 Advanced Breast Cancer

STEVEN CHEN and ERIN BROWN

Presentation

A 58-year-old woman with a newly found breast mass presents for further workup and treatment options. Six months ago, she discovered a palpable mass on her left breast during self-examination. Since this time, it has slowly increased in size. She denies any skin changes or nipple discharge. She has no significant medical history, and she has been in her normal state of health prior to presentation. She denies any personal history of breast cancer but notes that her mother was diagnosed with breast cancer at age 60. Her vital signs are normal. On physical exam, a left-sided breast mass is palpable and measures 5 cm in diameter. There are no overlying skin changes. The right breast is normal without palpable masses. Two palpable lymph nodes are present in the left axilla; the nodes are firm but mobile. There is no supraclavicular or right axillary lymphadenopathy.

Differential Diagnosis

A breast mass with palpable lymph nodes should be considered to be breast cancer until proven otherwise. However, the differential diagnosis also includes a number of benign breast lesions. A breast issue that may cause reactive lymph nodes such as abscess or injury may be a consideration in the right clinical setting. Additionally, other malignancies including malignant phyllodes tumors, angiosarcomas, or metastatic disease (e.g., melanoma) should remain in the differential.

Workup

A thorough history should be undertaken with an emphasis on breast cancer risk stratification. Important risk factors to include are age at menarche and menopause, age at first childbirth, history of breastfeeding, alcohol consumption, hormone use or exposure, family history of breast cancer, and personal history of breast cancer. If a strong family history is present, genetic testing should be considered. Factors that should prompt genetic testing include a first-degree relative diagnosed with breast cancer before the age of 50, three or more first- or second-degree relatives diagnosed with breast cancer at any age, breast cancer in a male relative, bilateral breast cancer in a first-degree relative, or a history of ovarian cancer in two or more first- or second-degree relatives. Prior to initiating genetic testing, counseling should be initiated to ensure that the risks and benefits of testing for the individual and her family are understood.

Due to the presence of a palpable mass in this patient, the next step is a bilateral mammogram in combination with ultrasound of the mass and the ipsilateral axilla. An MRI may be considered at this stage to evaluate the extent of the primary lesion (including invasion into the skin or deep structures), and to rule out

occult lesions in either breast or axilla. Needle biopsies should be obtained for histologic confirmation of the suspected diagnosis. Fine needle aspiration is most commonly used for biopsy of lymphadenopathy; however, core biopsy is the gold standard for biopsy of the breast mass because of its ability to preserve cell architecture. FNA should be avoided for biopsy of a solid breast lesion if a core is possible. The use of ultrasound or imaging to ensure proper sampling is encouraged, particularly if the tumor or lymph nodes are at all indistinct to palpation. Tissue specimens that demonstrate breast cancer are analyzed for ER, PR, and Her2/neu at a minimum. Consideration for distant metastases should also be entertained for those with locally advanced disease. Screening laboratory studies may include a CBC, liver function test, and alkaline phosphatase. In locally advanced breast cancer, a bone scan and CT chest and abdomen and pelvis should be obtained. PET/CT scan may also be substituted for the CT chest, abdomen, and pelvis.

This patient's workup confirms the left breast mass to be 5.2 cm in diameter based on imaging and is categorized as BI-RADS 5 (highly suggestive of malignancy). No radiographic abnormalities are noted within the right breast; however, two morphologically abnormal lymph nodes are detected in the left axilla. Biopsy reports reveal that both the breast and the lymph node biopsies are consistent with infiltrating ductal carcinoma. Tissue markers reveal an ER-positive, PR-positive, Her2-negative breast cancer. Metastatic workup is negative for any distant metastases.

Diagnosis and Treatment

The diagnostic workup is complete and consistent with the suspected diagnosis of locally advanced breast cancer. The tumor is 5.2 cm in diameter based on imaging without local extension (T3 provisionally), metastases to at least two lymph nodes (N1 provisionally), and no evidence of distant metastases (M0). This corresponds with a stage III breast cancer. For locally advanced breast cancer, two treatment options exist: primary surgical management followed by chemotherapy versus neoadjuvant chemotherapy followed by surgery. In either case, both would then be followed by radiation therapy and hormonal therapy in this case.

Surgical management may be either mastectomy or breast-conserving surgery (also known as lumpectomy, wide local excision, or partial mastectomy). Either surgical technique will also require complete axillary dissection in this patient due to the confirmed presence of palpable metastatic lymph nodes. In order to proceed with breast-conserving surgery (BCS), the surgeon must be able to remove the mass with negative margins while maintaining acceptable cosmetic results. Therefore, multiquadrant disease and large tumor size relative to breast size are traditionally considered relative contraindications to BCS. Furthermore, BCS for locally advanced cancer should always be accompanied by radiation therapy, so the patient must not have any contraindications to radiation such as prior history of radiation to the chest wall, connective tissue disease such as lupus and scleroderma, or active pregnancy during the planned time of radiation therapy. If a patient with locally advanced breast cancer desires BCS, but does not meet size criteria, has an inoperable tumor, or evidence of inflammatory breast cancer, neoadjuvant chemotherapy should be strongly considered.

The ultimate decision about BCS versus mastectomy should be made by a well-informed patient in consultation with the operating surgeon. When approaching the discussion with each patient, the surgeon must inform the patient of the risks and benefits of each surgical approach but should be prepared to provide guidance about the entire sequence of care. BCS benefits include preservation of the breast and a smaller operation; cons include increased rate of recurrence and risk of positive margins requiring further surgery. The pros of modified radical mastectomy include decreased recurrence and only one operation unless reconstruction is planned. However, the disadvantage of mastectomy is removal of the breast and the need for reconstruction if a breast mound is desired.

Neoadjuvant therapy involves chemotherapy or hormonal therapy prior to surgical therapy. The goal is to reduce the tumor burden in order to pursue breast conserving surgery or to pursue surgery in otherwise nonoperable or difficult to operate on tumors. Original concerns regarding induction chemotherapy included fear of decreased survival due to delaying surgery and increased surgical complication rates due to negative effects of chemotherapy on wound healing.

Studies report no difference in rates of seroma formation, wound infection, or delayed wound healing between neoadjuvant and primarily surgical groups. Additionally, multiple studies have shown equivalent survival rates among patients randomized to neoadjuvant chemotherapy in comparison to those randomized to primary surgical approach followed by postoperative chemotherapy. Furthermore, studies such as the NSABP trials have shown higher rates of BCS after preoperative chemotherapy due to significant reductions in tumor size.

Surgical Approach
Breast-Conservation Surgery
As described above, the goal of BCS is to remove the tumor with adequate margins as well as acceptable cosmetic results. In order to achieve this result, preoperative surgical planning is of the utmost importance. For the nonpalpable lesion, preoperative localization is essential. A wire localized technique using a preoperative wire placed by ultrasound or stereotactic methods can be helpful. Other potential localization technologies may include placement of a radioactive seed or biopsy hematoma directed surgery. This approach is usually not needed for an easily palpable mass such as the patient in this case. The incision should be made as close to the center of the breast as feasible while facilitating dissection to allow for future re-excision via mastectomy. Sharp or blunt dissection is used to remove the mass with the goal of 1-cm margins in all directions. After excision of the mass, many radiation oncologists prefer that the cavity walls be marked for potential radiation boost unless a balloon-based accelerated breast irradiation catheter is to be used. Margins of the specimen should be marked or separately submitted shave margins should be performed. Lastly, attention should be paid to hemostasis and closure of the defect. Simple closure is sufficient in many cases; however, complex closure may be necessary to prevent skin dimpling from a large cavity. For large excisions, an oncoplastic approach based on breast reduction principles may be beneficial to improve cosmesis and to facilitate wide margins while minimizing cosmetic impact to the shape of the breast. It is important, however, to ensure that the desire for an improved cosmetic outcome does not compromise the planned excision of the tumor and margins itself. Potential pitfalls of lumpectomy mainly relate to poor cosmetic effect and the possible need for further surgeries due to inadequate or grossly positive margins.

Complete Axillary Lymph Node Dissection
In the absence of clinically palpable nodes or previously biopsied lymph nodes negative for metastatic disease, sentinel node biopsy should be performed

in order to spare the morbidity of a complete axillary dissection. This may be performed before or after neo-adjuvant chemotherapy, although it is important to note that performing this after neoadjuvant chemotherapy slightly increases the false-negative rate. Most surgeons use a combination approach for locating the sentinel node that includes injection of both a blue dye (either methylene blue or isosulfan blue) and a radioactive tracer (typically technetium-99), although either can be used alone by experienced surgeons. The patient should be placed in the supine position, and the ipsilateral arm should be prepped and draped in order to allow manipulation of the arm during the procedure. Any radioactive and/or blue lymph nodes are dissected free and sent for pathologic examination. If negative for metastatic disease, no further dissection is required; however, positive metastatic disease is an indication to proceed with complete axillary dissection.

To proceed with complete axillary dissection, an incision is made just inferior to the axillary crease. First, the lateral edge of the pectoralis major and latissimus dorsi muscles are then identified. Beneath the pectoralis major is the pectoralis minor muscle, which defines the levels of axillary lymph nodes with level I nodes below, level II nodes posterior to, and level III nodes superior to the muscle. A complete axillary dissection involves the removal of all three levels of nodes. In the

absence of clinically positive nodes that extend into level III, only level I and II nodes are removed. To proceed with dissection, the interpectoral tissues, including Rotter's nodes, are dissected free. Next, the axillary vein is identified and the overlying fascia in incised; the tissue is freed with great care to spare the lymphatics superior to the vein. Care must be taken to identify and preserve several important structures during axillary dissection: the serratus anterior muscle, the thoracodorsal nerve, and the long thoracic nerve. Potential pitfalls for complete axillary dissection include over-skeletonization of the axillary vein, which may lead to increased risk of upper extremity lymphedema or injury to the axillary, long thoracic, or thoracodorsal nerves. Dissection above the axillary vein may also result in injury to the brachial plexus and should be avoided whenever possible **(Figure 1)**.

Modified Radical Mastectomy

As in BCS, the goal of modified radical mastectomy (MRM) is to remove the mass with adequate margins. In the case of locally advanced breast cancer, mastectomy is the most common surgical technique due to large tumor size even when neoadjuvant chemotherapy is pursued. To begin, an elliptical incision is made extending from just medial to the sternum to the midaxillary line, and skin flaps are created by dividing Cooper's

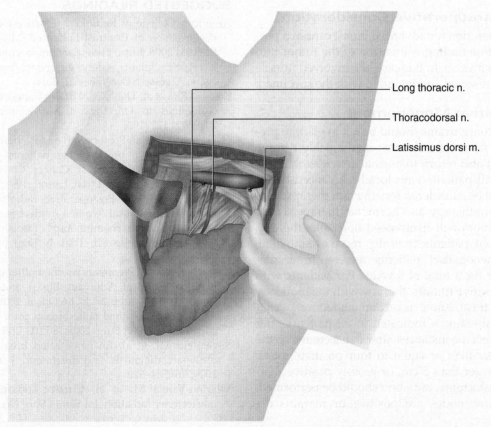

Long thoracic n.

Thoracodorsal n.

Latissimus dorsi m.

FIGURE 1 • Schematic of axillary lymph node dissection with preserved structures.

ligaments with the aid of countertraction. This is done by using electrocautery, sharp dissection, or a tumescent technique. The outer borders of dissection should extend to the lateral edge of the sternum medially, the latissimus dorsi laterally, the clavicle superiorly, and the inframammary fold inferiorly (which often takes one onto the rectus sheath). Care must be taken to completely excise the pectoralis fascia with the breast tissue. Technique varies depending on whether reconstruction is planned (either immediately following mastectomy or in the future). If reconstruction is planned, as much skin as possible should be preserved. In some select cases, the skin of the nipple-areola complex can be spared, but a complete excision of the underlying ductal tissue within the nipple papule should be performed. This is generally avoided in tumors that are close to the nipple for fear of tumor extension into the ducts within the nipple. In addition, biopsy of the tissue posterior to the complex should be obtained to ensure a negative margin. Without reconstruction, enough skin should be excised to allow closure without tension while avoiding skin overlap. Potential pitfalls include incomplete excision of the axillary tail leaving behind potentially cancerous cells, inappropriate thickness of the flaps (if too thick, potential for recurrence is increased, but if too thin, flap necrosis may occur), trauma to the flap causing skin breakdown and necrosis, and unnecessarily crossing the midline.

Special Intraoperative Consideration

During an operation for advanced breast cancer, a possible nonroutine finding is invasion of the tumor into the pectoralis muscle. In this case, the involved muscle must also be resected and included with the specimen.

Postoperative Management

After mastectomy, drains should be left in place to prevent seroma formation. Patients may quickly resume a regular diet and return to normal activities within a few weeks. All patients with locally advanced breast cancer should be considered for adjuvant therapy. This includes chemotherapy and hormonal therapy. Those with ER+ tumors will likely need hormonal therapy. Premenopausal patients typically receive tamoxifen, while postmenopausal patients receive an aromatase inhibitor for a total of 5 years. For patients with Her2/neu-positive tumors, therapy with the monoclonal antibody trastuzumab is recommended for 1 year.

Radiation therapy is indicated in all patients after BCS and in specific instances after mastectomy. In the case of greater than or equal to four positive nodes, tumor size larger than 5 cm, or grossly positive margins after mastectomy, radiation should be performed. If one to three nodes are positive or margins are inadequate, radiation should be strongly considered according to NCCN guidelines. The specific details of the various chemotherapy and radiation regimens are complex and beyond the scope of this chapter. This complexity emphasizes the importance of a team approach to breast cancer treatment involving a medical oncologist, radiation oncologist, surgical oncologist, and plastic surgeon.

Education regarding prognosis and surveillance are also crucial components of breast cancer treatment. The most important prognostic indicators for recurrence and death include age, comorbidities, tumor staging, and number of positive nodes. In general, stage I and II breast cancers have a 5-year disease-free survival between 65% and 92%. Stage III breast cancers have a 5-year disease-free survival of 44% to 47%, and a patient with a stage IV breast cancer diagnosis can expect a 5-year disease-free survival rate of 14%. Monitoring for recurrence is essential. Annual mammogram should begin 6 months after the completion of radiation and/or chemotherapy. Women should have a clinical breast exam performed by their physician every 4 to 6 months for the first 5 years and then annually thereafter. Finally, woman taking tamoxifen with an intact uterus should have a yearly pelvic exam due to increased risk of endometrial cancer.

SUGGESTED READINGS

American College of Radiology. Practice Guideline for the Performance of Contrast-Enhanced MRI of the Breast. Revised 2008. http://www.acr.org/SecondaryMainMenu Categories/quality_safety/guidelines/breast/mri_breast .aspx. Accessed: December 22, 2011.

Carlson RW, et al. The NCCN Breast Cancer Clinical Practice Guidelines in Oncology. J Natl Compr Canc Netw. 2009;7(2):122–192.

Overgaard M, et al. Postoperative radiotherapy in high-risk postmenopausal breast-cancer patients given adjuvant tamoxifen: Danish Breast Cancer Cooperative Group DBCG 82c randomized trial. Lancet. 1999;353:1641–1648.

Overgaard M, et al. Postoperative radiotherapy in high-risk premenopausal women with breast cancer who receive adjuvant chemotherapy. Danish Breast Cancer Cooperative Group 82b Trial. N Engl J Med. 1997;337: 949–955.

Rastogi P, et al. Preoperative chemotherapy: updates of National Surgical Adjuvant Breast and Bowel Project Protocols B-18 and B-27. J Clin Oncol. 2008;26(5):778–785.

Sabel MS, et al. Sentinel node biopsy prior to neoadjuvant chemotherapy. A J Surg. 2003;186:102–105.

Silverstein MJ, et al. Image-detected breast cancer: state-of-the-art diagnosis and treatment. J Am Coll Surg. 2009;7(6):504–520.

Vilarino-Varela M, et al. Current indications for post-mastectomy radiation. Int Semin Surg Oncol. 2009;6:5.

55 Inflammatory Breast Cancer

WALTER P. WEBER and MONICA MORROW

Presentation

A 49-year-old woman, G2 P2, age 30 at first birth with no family history of breast cancer, presents with a 1-month history of increasing redness, heaviness, and swelling of her right breast **(Figure 1)**. There was no antecedent history of trauma. Two weeks ago, she saw her primary care physician who made the diagnosis of breast infection and gave her a 10-day course of a cephalosporin. Her symptoms have not improved, and she was referred for surgical evaluation. On physical examination, there is diffuse erythema and edema of the right breast. The breast is diffusely firm compared to the left, but no discrete mass is palpable. There are no palpable supraclavicular or left axillary nodes. A firm, mobile, nontender 1-cm right axillary node is present.

Differential Diagnosis

In a nonlactating woman, erythema and edema over more than one-third of the breast that does not significantly improve with antibiotic treatment is inflammatory breast cancer (IBC) until proven otherwise. Bacterial infection, including mastitis and abscess, is the most common misdiagnosis. These infections, however, are rare in nonlactating women, and treatment with antibiotics tends to be of immediate benefit. Because IBC is not a true inflammatory process, it is not associated with symptoms such as fever, localized pain, or leukocytosis.

Workup

The patient undergoes bilateral mammography, which reveals only skin thickening and diffusely increased breast density on the right side **(Figure 2)**. Ultrasonography demonstrates increased vascularity and minor architectural distortions in the right breast, and confirms the presence of an enlarged 1.2-cm right axillary node with abnormal architecture. A punch biopsy of the skin, ultrasound-guided core biopsy of the architectural distortion in the breast, and fine needle aspiration cytology of the right axillary node demonstrate adenocarcinoma, thereby confirming the clinical diagnosis of node-positive IBC. The estrogen receptor (ER), progesterone receptor (PR), and HER2 are negative. Laboratory studies show that liver enzymes and lactate dehydrogenase are within normal limits. Further staging with a PET-CT scan reveals no signs of distant metastases.

Diagnosis and Treatment

IBC is a clinical diagnosis defined by the American Joint Committee on Cancer (AJCC) as "a diffuse brawny induration of the skin of the breast with an erysipeloid edge" and is designated T4d, Stage IIIB in the absence of distant metastases. Patients present with rapid enlargement of the breast, erythema and skin edema, often with an orange-peel appearance (peau d' orange), and induration or ridging over more than one-third of the breast. On palpation, the breast is warm and diffusely firm, although a discrete mass is often not palpable. In addition, physical exam often reveals palpable lymph nodes as more than 50% of IBC patients have nodal involvement at the time of diagnosis. Mammography with or without ultrasound is standard of care, even though imaging studies may be inconclusive. Classic mammographic features include skin thickening and increased breast density, and a discrete mass is evident in as many as 80% of cases in some reports. Ultrasonography demonstrates increased vascularity and architectural distortion in addition to mass lesions. Distant metastases are present in approximately 25% of patients at the time of diagnosis, and staging investigations should be performed on a routine basis. PET-CT is the imaging test of choice for the detection of distant metastases.

The inflammatory appearance of the breast is due to tumor emboli within the dermal lymphatics **(Figure 3)**. This finding can often be demonstrated on a full-thickness skin biopsy but is not necessary to make the diagnosis of IBC when the clinical signs are present and a biopsy reveals adenocarcinoma of any subtype. Core needle biopsy of any breast mass is the preferred method of diagnosis. In the absence of a discrete mass, core biopsy of any area of architectural distortion on ultrasound is usually diagnostic. The biopsy material should be sent for hormone receptor and HER2 determination.

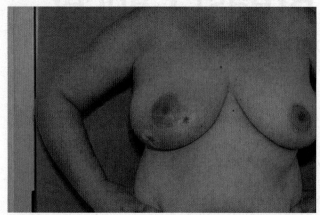

FIGURE 1 • The findings of diffuse erythema and edema of the enlarged right breast with adenocarcinoma on biopsy are diagnostic for IBC.

IBC is rare, accounting for <3% of breast cancer cases in the United States, but it is the most lethal form of primary breast cancer. Historically, mastectomy with or without radiotherapy was standard management, resulting on average 5-year overall survival rates of <5%. By the 1970s, the treatment paradigm for IBC had shifted to one involving chemotherapy followed by radiotherapy, which improved average 5-year overall survival rates to 30% or more. The use of surgery for IBC has increased again over the last two decades, but the timing of mastectomy has changed from initial cancer management to a postchemotherapy intervention,

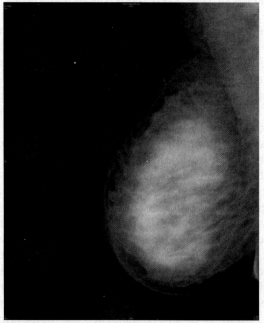

FIGURE 2 • Mediolateral oblique view of mammogram showing inferior skin thickening and diffuse increase in density from IBC.

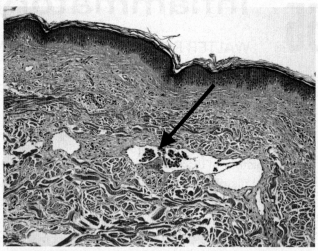

FIGURE 3 • Photomicrograph showing tumor in the dermal lymphatic spaces (*arrow*). This finding supports the diagnosis of inflammatory cancer, but tumor in dermal lymphatic spaces without clinical inflammatory changes is not IBC.

followed by radiotherapy in all cases and hormonal therapy in hormone receptor-positive disease. The advent of multimodality therapy has significantly improved survival, with 5-year survival rates of over 40% being reported. Hence, women diagnosed with IBC should be managed in a setting where such a specialized approach can be adequately provided.

Surgical Approach

The goals of surgery in IBC are to maintain local control and to improve survival in the absence of distant metastases. The current standard protocol for patients with IBC calls for initial treatment with neoadjuvant chemotherapy. Only patients who show complete resolution of all evidence of skin inflammation should undergo surgery. Surgery in the setting of residual inflammatory changes is associated with poor local control and survival.

The standard procedure in patients with IBC is modified radical mastectomy, which by definition includes total mastectomy with ipsilateral level I/II axillary lymph node dissection. Breast conservation is contraindicated in IBC. Skin-sparing and nipple-sparing mastectomies are contraindicated as well due to the diffuse nature of the tumor and the inability to reliably identify patients with pathologic complete response preoperatively. Moreover, sentinel lymph node biopsy is also contraindicated in patients with IBC. Even though increasing clinical experience suggests that sentinel node biopsy reliably stages the axilla after neoadjuvant therapy, the limited experience with sentinel node biopsy in IBC demonstrates that the false-negative rate of sentinel node biopsy in this setting is unacceptably high. Since many of the advantages of immediate reconstruction, such as the skin-sparing approach, are lost, and because postmastectomy radiotherapy is indicated for all patients, delayed reconstruction is generally preferred.

Mastectomy

The patient is placed supine, with the arm extended on a padded arm board. The arm should be prepped and draped separately to allow free rotation. The skin resection should encompass the nipple and areola, the surgical biopsy site (if present), and the excess skin of the breast. Skin flaps are then created with electrocautery or by sharp dissection with the scalpel or curved scissors. The skin flaps are raised in the plane between the subcutaneous fat and the breast tissue, and extend superiorly to the clavicle, medially to the sternal edge, laterally to the latissimus dorsi, and inferiorly to the rectus sheath. The next step is to remove the breast, which is most easily done from superior to inferior with the fascia of the pectoralis major as the deep margin of the resection. The internal mammary perforators should be ligated with clips or ties to avoid postoperative hemorrhage. The dissection is extended to the lateral aspect of the pectoralis major muscle, which is retracted, and the fascia overlying the pectoralis minor muscle is opened to allow placement of a retractor beneath the muscle. The axillary lymph node dissection is then carried out as described in detail below.

Lymph Node Dissection

Standard axillary dissection clears levels I and II (nodes lateral to the lateral border and posterior to the pectoralis minor muscle). A full level III dissection above the pectoralis minor muscle is carried out when there is gross nodal disease as described in this case. After the breast has been taken off the chest wall as described above, the latissimus dorsi muscle is followed proximally along its anterior surface until it turns tendinous, at which time it is crossed by the axillary vein. No important structures cross this plane of dissection, making it the safest approach to the axillary vein. The anterior surface of the axillary vein is then cleared of overlying fat from lateral to medial, with care being taken not to dissect superior to the vein or to strip the vein in the vascular plane, both of which promote lymphedema. When the vein is well visualized, dissection inferior to the vein is carried out, again working from lateral to medial, dividing the fat and controlling the branches of the axillary vein entering the specimen. The thoracodorsal neurovascular bundle is usually the first deep lateral branch identified after the superficial fat and the vessels have been divided. Once the thoracodorsal bundle is identified, the pectoralis minor is retracted and the level 3 nodes are dissected from the space below the axillary vein and against the chest wall. The axillary specimen is then retracted laterally; the long thoracic nerve is identified against the chest wall and dissected free from the specimen. The fat between the thoracodorsal and long thoracic nerves is then encircled with a clamp, divided, and bluntly swept inferiorly. Branches of the thoracodorsal vessels entering the specimen are controlled with clips, and the specimen is freed from its remaining attachments to the inferior chest wall. After hemostasis is obtained, two closed suction drains are inserted, one beneath the inferior flap and one in the apex of the axilla. The deep dermis is reapproximated with absorbable sutures, and the skin is closed with a running subcuticular stitch.

Special Intraoperative Considerations

Intraoperative findings that would change the operative strategy are rare after a patient has been

---

TABLE 1. Key Technical Steps and Potential Pitfalls to Mastectomy

Key Technical Steps

1. Plan the transverse elliptical incision to remove the nipple and areola and excess breast skin but allow tension free closure.
2. Create the skin flaps.
3. Dissect and remove the breast with the fascia of the pectoralis major muscle.

Potential Pitfalls

- Insufficient skin removal resulting in residual disease left behind in dermal lymphatics.
- Excessive skin removal resulting in tension on the wound delaying radiotherapy.
- Failure to raise flaps to the anatomic boundaries of the breast potentially resulting in residual disease left behind in the glandular tissue.
- Bleeding from internal mammary perforators.

TABLE 2. Key Technical Steps and Potential Pitfalls for Axillary Lymph Node Dissection

Key Technical Steps

1. Open axillary investing fascia lateral to pectoralis major and minor muscles.
2. Identify axillary vein by following the latissimus dorsi superiorly until it turns tendinous and is crossed by the vein.
3. Identify the thoracodorsal bundle and the long thoracic nerve and preserve.
4. Control vascular branches of thoracodorsal vessels entering the specimen.
5. Place suction drains.

Potential Pitfalls

- Injury to long thoracic nerve.
- Injury to thoracodorsal nerve.
- Bleeding from axillary vein or thoracodorsal branches.

adequately staged. If the cancer invades the pectoralis muscle, the involved muscle can be removed. There is no need for a classic radical mastectomy for limited muscle involvement, and extensive involvement is clinically evident preoperatively. If extensive axillary nodal metastases extending superiorly into the supraclavicular space are identified intraoperatively, they can be removed if they are mobile and this can be safely done. If residual disease is left behind, it should be marked with clips to assist in defining the radiotherapy fields.

Postoperative Management

The patient usually requires an overnight hospital stay. The drain should be removed when the drainage is <30 mL/24 h. A single dose of antibiotic is given prior to surgery, but ongoing prophylactic antibiotics when the drains are in place are not recommended. Postoperative complications other than seroma are infrequent and include bleeding and infection. Postoperative hemorrhage can result from failure to control internal mammary perforators, axillary vein branches, or thoracodorsal branches. Bleeding from these sites usually requires reexploration. Seroma formation can be minimized by removing drains when drainage is <30 mL/24 h rather than on some arbitrary day. If a seroma is clinically detectable, it should be aspirated since the mastectomy flaps cannot adhere to the chest wall in the presence of seroma fluid. The chest wall is anesthetic in 100% of patients post mastectomy. This is a side effect, not a complication, and patients should be educated about this preoperatively. Skin flap necrosis is another potential complication that results from closure under tension, technical error in cutting the skin flaps, or infection. Postmastectomy infections usually present as cellulitis, and any erythema of the wound should lead to prompt antibiotic treatment to avoid flap necrosis. If flap necrosis is suspected, it should be observed until clear demarcation is present and necrotic tissue debrided at that time. With proper incision planning, major full-thickness necrosis is rare, and most necrosis is superficial and limited extent, and will heal without surgical intervention.

Axillary lymph node dissection is associated with long-term morbidity, including chronic lymphedema (5% to 25%), and shoulder dysmobility (5% to 15%). Injury to the motor nerves in the axilla is rare (<1%). Injury to the long thoracic nerve results in a palsy of the serratus anterior muscle and, clinically, will create a winged scapula. Injury to the thoracodorsal nerve causes a palsy of the latissimus dorsi muscle, which may be evident during athletic activity or when trying to scratch in the midline of the back.

Case Conclusion

Following neoadjuvant therapy with dose-dense doxorubicin, cyclophosphamide, and paclitaxel with complete resolution of inflammatory skin changes, the patient underwent modified radical mastectomy and was staged pT4dpN2a, Stage IIIB. Pathology demonstrated scattered residual microscopic foci of tumor throughout the breast, with evidence of treatment effect in the remaining breast tissue. Five of fourteen nodes contained metastases, and the ER, PR, and HER2 remain negative. Adjuvant radiotherapy to the chest wall and supraclavicular, axillary, and internal mammary node fields is planned. She will be followed with clinical exam every 3 months for 2 years, then every 6 months for 3 years, and yearly thereafter, and with annual mammography.

TAKE HOME POINTS

- Prompt biopsy is required for inflammatory breast changes that do not resolve with antibiotics.
- IBC is a clinical diagnosis; histologic confirmation of tumor emboli in dermal lymphatics is not mandatory.
- Multimodality treatment consists of neoadjuvant chemotherapy, surgery, radiotherapy, and hormonal therapy if indicated.
- Surgery is reserved for patients with resolution of skin erythema during neoadjuvant chemotherapy.
- Modified radical mastectomy is standard of care; breast conservation and sentinel lymph node biopsy are contraindicated.

SUGGESTED READINGS

Chia S, Swain SM, Byrd DR, et al. Locally advanced and inflammatory breast cancer. J Clin Oncol. 2008;26(5):786–790.

Hance KW, Anderson WF, Devesa SS, et al. Large population-based epidemiological study of IBC: Trends in inflammatory breast carcinoma incidence and survival: the Surveillance, Epidemiology, and End Results program at the National Cancer Institute. J Natl Cancer Inst. 2005;97(13):966–975.

Merajver S, Iniesta MD, Sabel MS. In: Harris JR, Lippman ME, Morrow M et al., eds. Inflammatory breast Cancer. In: Diseases of the Breast. 4th ed. Philadelphia, PA: Wolters Kluwer/Lippincott, 2010:762–773.

Ueno NT, Buzdar AU, Singletary SE, et al. Combined modality treatment of inflammatory breast carcinoma: twenty years of experience at M.D Anderson Center. Cancer Chemother Pharmacol. 1997;40(4):321–329.

56 Breast Cancer During Pregnancy

JENNIFER E. JOH and MARIE CATHERINE LEE

Presentation

A 28-year-old female, with a history of type I diabetes mellitus, presents to her obstetrician for an initial prenatal evaluation. Her last menstrual period was approximately 12 weeks prior to this visit. The patient has had two prior pregnancies requiring cesarean delivery. She states that she has developed a palpable breast mass over the past 7 months. The mass has grown substantially over the past month. She underwent mammography and focused ultrasound a month after first noticing the mass. The imaging at that time was negative for suspicious lesions, and no further evaluation was initiated.

Differential Diagnosis

The differential diagnosis of a breast mass in young women includes many benign entities such as fibroadenoma, lipoma, phyllodes tumor, fat necrosis, fibrocystic disease, galactocele, cyst, abscess, or accessory breast tissue. Surgical excision is recommended for phyllodes tumors and fibroadenomas that are symptomatic or enlarging. Fat necrosis is usually a posttraumatic or postoperative finding. Galactoceles generally develop months after discontinuation of lactation. Breast abscesses are usually associated with skin erythema, induration, and/or fever. During pregnancy, accessory breast tissue may swell and present as an enlarging mass in the axillary tail or in the axilla. Breast cancer is an uncommon diagnosis in this age group, with only 0.3% of all breast cancers occurring in women between the ages of 20 to 29.

Presentation Continued

The patient has no prior history of breast masses or breast biopsies. She notes a history of mastitis with a prior pregnancy. She has had no prior surgery other than the two cesarean sections. She had one maternal grandmother diagnosed with breast cancer but denies any additional family history of cancer, including breast or ovarian cancer. On review of systems, she denies trauma to the breast, skin changes, nipple retraction, or nipple discharge. Breast examination reveals a mass in the upper outer quadrant. There is also ipsilateral palpable axillary adenopathy. The contralateral breast is unremarkable.

Workup

Focused imaging in the form of mammography and ultrasound are the initial diagnostic tests after a thorough physical examination. With appropriate abdominal shielding, mammography is considered safe in pregnancy. Digital mammography is the preferred modality in premenopausal patients or those with dense breasts. Breast density may be increased by both lactational changes and premenopausal status **(Figure 1)**. Masses, calcifications, and architectural distortion may all be visualized on mammography, despite the increased density of breast tissue seen during pregnancy and lactation. Focused ultrasound is used in conjunction with mammography for palpable breast masses to aid in the detection of solid versus cystic pathology. Sonography is more sensitive than mammography in the detection of breast cancer in pregnancy. In high-volume centers, ultrasound of the axilla may also help to detect the presence of axillary metastases. Evidence of axillary disease at initial diagnosis significantly affects recommendations for chemotherapy, surgery, and radiation therapy in patients with invasive breast cancer **(Figure 2)**. Fetal effects of gadolinium-enhanced breast magnetic resonance imaging during pregnancy are unclear. Considering the prone position and the concerns regarding fetal exposure to gadolinium, breast magnetic resonance imaging is not considered a safe modality in pregnant patients.

The current recommended modality for diagnosis of a breast mass is via image-guided, percutaneous biopsy with clip placement. Sonographically abnormal axillary lymph nodes should also undergo ultrasound-guided fine needle aspiration or core needle biopsy. In the case of a discordant breast biopsy result, surgical excision should be considered. Surgical excision in lieu of percutaneous biopsy is a feasible option but

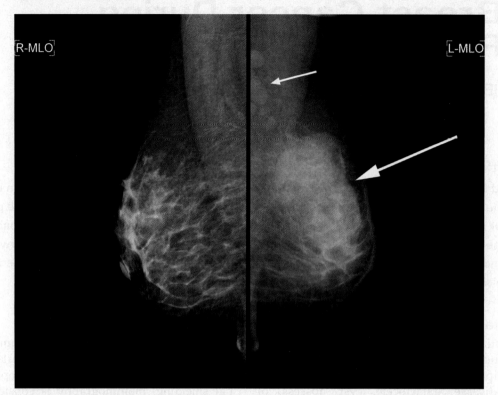

FIGURE 1 • Digital mammography of a lactating patient with a high-density, lobular mass in the left breast (*large arrow*) and multiple enlarged lymph nodes in the axilla (*small arrow*).

is outside the current recommended standard of care for initial tissue evaluation of a palpable breast mass. Furthermore, in the interest of minimizing risk to the pregnant patient as well as the fetus, avoidance of an additional surgical procedure is preferred.

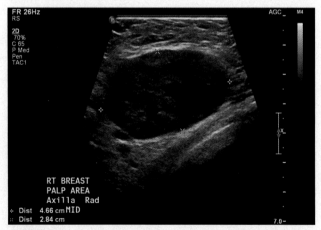

FIGURE 2 • Axillary ultrasound demonstrates a lymph node with metastatic disease. There is complete loss of normal nodal architecture.

Presentation Continued

In the 15th week of pregnancy, the patient had a focused breast ultrasound of the palpable mass. This demonstrated a 2.8-cm mass suspicious for malignancy. Ultrasound-guided core biopsy revealed invasive ductal carcinoma that was estrogen and progesterone receptor negative and HER2 negative. Ipsilateral axillary ultrasound also showed several abnormal lymph nodes; fine needle aspiration diagnosed metastatic disease on cytology. Both chest radiograph and ultrasound of the liver were negative for suspicious lesions.

Diagnosis and Treatment

Further evaluation and treatment of benign breast findings may be deferred until the postpartum period; however, a diagnosis of breast cancer during pregnancy warrants immediate attention. Invasive breast cancer is treated with multimodal therapy and may include surgery, chemotherapy, or radiation. For the pregnant patient, the timing and order of treatment is determined in part by gestational age as well as the stage of the cancer at diagnosis. Termination of the pregnancy does *not* improve outcome and should not be recommended to patients in the context of survival from breast cancer. Patients may maintain their pregnancy and safely undergo both local and systemic cancer treatment. Early delivery may be considered if felt to affect maternal oncologic outcome.

Pregnant patients with an invasive breast cancer diagnosis, particularly those with biopsy-proven axillary disease, should also have staging studies performed, in the form of chest radiograph and an ultrasound of the liver. Other imaging studies, such as computed tomography, bone, or positron emission tomography scans, should be deferred until the postpartum period. Any lesion suspicious for distant metastatic disease warrant a percutaneous biopsy, as patients with distant metastatic disease are not considered surgical candidates and should be initially treated with systemic chemotherapy.

Surgical Approach

For patients without evidence of distant disease, the goal is optimal curative treatment of the carcinoma without harm to the fetus; therefore, knowledge of all the treatment possibilities is important in deciding both the timing and type of operative procedure.

Systemic chemotherapy may be administered in the second and third trimesters of pregnancy safely. However, adjuvant radiation therapy is contraindicated in all trimesters of pregnancy due to the risk of teratogenesis. Patients who have surgically resectable disease and are clinically node negative at presentation are not candidates for neoadjuvant chemotherapy, and should be advised to proceed to primary surgery for accurate staging. An outline of the decision-making process is illustrated in **Figure 3**.

Key Considerations in Surgical and Treatment Decision Making:

1. Gestational age and associated surgical risk
2. Extent of breast and axillary disease
3. Need for and timing of systemic chemotherapy
4. Need for and timing of adjuvant radiation therapy

The second trimester is considered the optimum time period for surgery; organogenesis is complete, and the risk of preterm labor is low. Patients who present in the first trimester may undergo surgery without waiting until the second trimester; however, the potential effects of medications on organogenesis and the unquantifiable risk of spontaneous abortion in the

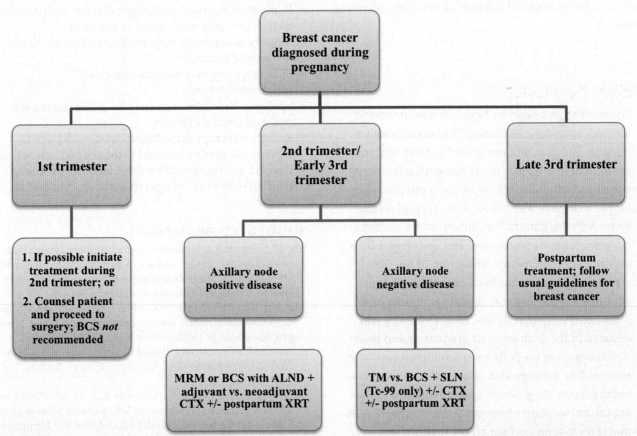

FIGURE 3 • Surgical decision-making tree for pregnant patients diagnosed with breast cancer. BCS, breast-conserving surgery; MRM, modified radical mastectomy; ALND, axillary lymph node dissection; CTX, chemotherapy; XRT, radiation therapy; TM, total mastectomy; Tc-99, technetium-99; SLN, sentinel lymph node.

first trimester mean that the overall risks incurred by surgery are poorly delineated. A detailed discussion of the potential risks is imperative. Women who present in the third trimester are generally recommended to defer surgery until the postpartum period due to the risk of preterm labor. General anesthesia is safe in pregnancy; however, local anesthesia or a paravertebral or a regional block is a safe alternative in all trimesters.

The extent of disease at presentation also plays a role in the decision for surgery. The traditional surgical choice for patients presenting with breast cancer during pregnancy is a modified radical mastectomy. However, breast conservation may be an option for patients presenting with limited in-breast disease in the third trimester or if chemotherapy is indicated and initiated during pregnancy. Decisions for breast-conserving surgery (BCS) require careful multidisciplinary planning due to the contraindications for radiation in pregnancy. Although blue dye mapping with lymphazurin or methylene blue is contraindicated, technetium-99 sulfur colloid for sentinel lymph node (SLN) surgery is safe and feasible in the second and third trimesters of pregnancy. In patients who have evidence of axillary disease on percutaneous biopsy, the SLN procedure is bypassed in lieu of an axillary node dissection at the time of breast surgery.

Case Conclusion

The patient was seen by high-risk obstetrics and medical oncology; because of her node-positive disease, she was recommended to have systemic chemotherapy. Based on the patient's gestational age at presentation, the decision to proceed with primary surgery was made. After several discussions with the patient, her family, and a multidisciplinary team of physicians, she underwent BCS and axillary lymph node dissection in her 18th week of pregnancy. Surgical pathology demonstrated a 2.4-cm invasive ductal carcinoma and 2 of 24 positive lymph nodes. Chemotherapy was initiated in the 20th week of pregnancy and then discontinued at week 32 for a scheduled cesarean section. The delivery was uncomplicated, and she proceeded to have whole-breast radiation following the completion of her systemic therapy. BRCA mutation testing performed postpartum was negative for a deleterious mutation.

Postoperative Management

Both tamoxifen and Herceptin (trastuzumab) are contraindicated in pregnancy but can be initiated safely in the postpartum period if indicated. All patients presenting with primary breast cancer before the age of 50 should be considered for genetic counseling and testing. BRCA1 and BRCA2 mutation carriers are advised to consider prophylactic bilateral oophorectomy and mastectomy due to their inherited risk of breast and ovarian carcinomas after completion of childbearing. In lieu of prophylactic surgery, increased annual screening with breast magnetic resonance imaging and pelvic ultrasound may also be considered for known mutation carriers. During follow-up, patients diagnosed with breast cancer at any age should have annual screening mammography of both breasts if mastectomy was not performed as long as they are in good health.

TAKE HOME POINTS

- A multidisciplinary approach is essential to caring for the pregnant patient with breast cancer.
- Mammography with abdominal shielding and focused ultrasound are the appropriate initial diagnostic tests.
- Axillary staging is important in multimodal planning of breast cancer treatment.
- Evaluate for distant metastatic disease with a chest radiograph and ultrasound of the liver.
- Surgery is safest for both mother and fetus during the second trimester.
- SLN mapping may be performed with technetium-99 only.
- Systemic chemotherapy may be given during second and third trimesters.
- Radiation therapy is contraindicated in all three trimesters but may be initiated in the postpartum period.
- Genetic testing should be discussed in any young woman (<50 years of age) diagnosed with breast cancer.

SUGGESTED READINGS

Abe H, Schmidt RA, Kulkarni K, et al. Axillary lymph nodes suspicious for breast cancer metastasis: sampling with US-guided 14-gauge core-needle biopsy—clinical experience in 100 patients. Radiology. 2009;250:41–49.

Ahn BY, Kim HH, Moon WK, et al. Pregnancy- and lactation-associated breast cancer: mammographic and sonographic findings. J Ultrasound Med. 2003;22:491–497.

American Cancer Society. Breast Cancer Facts and Figures, 2007–2008. Atlanta, GA: American Cancer Society, Inc., 2007–2008.

Anderson BO, Lawton TJ, Lehman CD, et al. Phyllodes tumors. In: Harris JR, Lippman ME, Morrow M, et al., eds. Diseases of the Breast. 3rd ed. Philadelphia, PA: Lippincott Williams & Wilkins, 2004:991–1003.

Behrman R, Homer M, Yang W, et al. Mammography and fetal dose. Radiology. 2007;243:605; author reply 605–606.

Berry DL, Theriault RL, Holmes FA, et al. Management of breast cancer during pregnancy using a standardized protocol. J Clin Oncol. 1999;17(3):855–861.

Brekelmans CTM, Seynaeve C, Bartels CCM, et al. Effectiveness of breast cancer surveillance in BRCA1/2 gene mutation carriers and women with high familial risk. J Clin Oncol. 2001;19:924–930.

Carlson R, Allred DC, Anderson BO, et al. NCCN Clinical Practice Guidelines in Oncology V.2.2010. Breast Cancer. 2010.

Cardonick EMD, Dougherty RMD, Grana GMD, et al. Breast cancer during pregnancy: maternal and fetal outcomes. Cancer J. 2010;16:76–82.

Chen M, Coakley F, Kaimal A, et al. Guidelines for computed tomography and magnetic resonance imaging use during pregnancy and lactation. Obstet Gynecol. 2008;112:333–340.

De Santis M, Cesari E, Nobili E, et al. Radiation effects on development. Birth Defects Res C Embryo Today Rev. 2007;81:171–182.

Gemignani ML, Petrek JA. Pregnancy-associated breast cancer: diagnosis and treatment. Breast J. 2000;6:68–73.

Gentilini O, Cremonesi M, Trifiro G, et al. Safety of sentinel node biopsy in pregnant patients with breast cancer. Ann Oncol. 2004;15:1348–1351.

Gentilini O, Cremonesi M, Toesca A, et al. Sentinel lymph node biopsy in pregnant patients with breast cancer. Eur J Nucl Med Mol Imaging. 2010;37:78–83.

Guillem JG, Wood WC, Moley JF, et al. ASCO/SSO review of current role of risk-reducing surgery in common hereditary cancer syndromes. J Clin Oncol. 2006;24:4642–4660.

Hinson J, McGrath P, Moore A, et al. The critical role of axillary ultrasound and aspiration biopsy in the management of breast cancer patients with clinically negative axilla. Ann Surg Oncol. 2008;15:250–255.

ICRP Publication 84. Abstract: pregnancy and medical radiation. Ann ICRP. 2000;30:1.

Kal H, Struikmans H. Pregnancy and medical irradiation; summary and conclusions from the International Commission on Radiological Protection, Publication 84. Ned Tijdschr Geneeskd. 2002;146:299–303.

Kanal E, Borgstede JP, Barkovich AJ, et al. American College of Radiology white paper on MR safety: 2004 update and revisions. AJR Am J Roentgenol. 2004;182:1111–1114.

Keleher AJ, Theriault RL, Gwyn KM, et al. Multidisciplinary management of breast cancer concurrent with pregnancy. J Am Coll Surg. 2002;194:54–64.

Khatcheressian JL, Wolff AC, Smith TJ, et al. American Society of Clinical Oncology 2006 update of the breast cancer follow-up and management guidelines in the adjuvant setting. J Clin Oncol. 2006;24:5091–5097.

Kok RD, de Vries MM, Heerschap A, et al. Absence of harmful effects of magnetic resonance exposure at 1.5 T in utero during the third trimester of pregnancy: a follow-up study. Magn Reson Imaging. 2004;22:851–854.

Krishnamurthy S, Sneige N, Bedi D, et al. Role of ultrasound-guided fine-needle aspiration of indeterminate and suspicious axillary lymph nodes in the initial staging of breast carcinoma. Cancer. 2002;95:982–988.

Kuczkowski KMMD. Nonobstetric surgery during pregnancy: what are the risks of anesthesia? Obstet Gynecol Surv. 2004;59:52–56.

Lee MC, Chau A, Eatrides J, et al. Consequences of axillary ultrasound in patients with T2 or greater invasive breast cancers. Ann Surg Onc. 2011;18:72–77.

Ní Mhuireachtaigh R, O'Gorman DA. Anesthesia in pregnant patients for nonobstetric surgery. J Clin Anesth. 2006;18:60–66.

Pisano E, Hendrick R, Yaffe M, et al. Diagnostic accuracy of digital versus film mammography: exploratory analysis of selected population subgroups in DMIST. Radiology. 2008;246:376–383.

Ring AE, Smith IE, Jones A, et al. Chemotherapy for breast cancer during pregnancy: an 18-year experience from five London teaching hospitals. J Clin Oncol. 2005;23:4192–4197.

Silverstein MJ, Recht A, Lagios MD, et al. Image-detected breast cancer: state of the art diagnosis and treatment. J Am Coll Surg. 2009;209:504–520.

Steenvoorde P, Pauwels EKJ, Harding LK, et al. Diagnostic nuclear medicine and risk for the fetus. Eur J Nucl Med Mol Imaging. 1998;25:193–199.

Tate J, Lewis V, Archer T, et al. Ultrasound detection of axillary lymph node metastases in breast cancer. Eur J Surg Oncol. 1989;15:139–141.

U.S. Preventive Services Task Force. Genetic risk assessment and BRCA mutation testing for breast and ovarian cancer susceptibility: recommendation statement. Ann Intern Med. 2005;143:355–361.

Yang W, Dryden M, Gwyn K, et al. Imaging of breast cancer diagnosed and treated with chemotherapy during pregnancy. Radiology. 2006;239:52–60.

57 Breast Reconstruction

JENNIFER F. WALJEE and AMY K. ALDERMAN

Presentation

A 42-year-old female presents to her primary care provider after noticing a firm, 2-cm mass in the upper outer quadrant of her left breast. She underwent ultrasound and mammography that revealed a spiculated 2-cm lesion in the upper outer quadrant of her breast with a BiRADs classification of 5. She underwent core needle biopsy revealing an invasive ductal carcinoma. Axillary ultrasound and clinical examination was negative for any suspicious lymph nodes.

She has no other past medical or surgical history. Her only medications include a proton pump inhibitor and an antidepressant. She is a nonsmoker with three children and is employed as a third grade teacher. She has no other relevant family or social history. She currently wears a C cup bra size and desires to remain the same size.

She has met with a surgical and medical oncologist prior to her consultation with plastic surgery. She is in the process of deciding between breast-conserving therapy including segmental breast resection with adjuvant radiation therapy or simple mastectomy. She will undergo sentinel lymph node biopsy at the time of her breast resection with a possible axillary lymph node dissection depending on the results of the biopsy. She presents today to discuss her options for breast reconstruction.

Discussion

In the modern era, many women diagnosed with breast cancer are candidates for breast reconstruction. Reconstruction following breast cancer resection is safe and does not delay adjuvant therapy or diagnosis of cancer recurrence. It is correlated with improved psychosocial functioning, body image, and mental health outcomes following cancer treatment. Nonetheless, prior research indicates that many women are not referred for reconstruction who may be appropriate candidates. Therefore, it is important to incorporate a routine discussion of breast reconstruction into preoperative surgical planning for women diagnosed with breast cancer. This chapter will discuss the current reconstructive options for breast reconstruction and will explain how to appropriately evaluate patients for these procedures.

Workup

Reconstructive surgery corrects anatomic deformities in order to re-create form, function, and symmetry. Breast reconstruction utilizes either autologous tissue flaps or breast implants, and can be performed either at the time of cancer resection or at a later date. Women who undergo either partial or complete mastectomy may be candidates for breast reconstruction. Therefore, breast reconstruction is an important component of multidisciplinary care, and a consultation with a plastic surgeon should be offered at the time of initial surgical decision making for any woman interested in breast reconstruction.

During the initial office visit, the surgeon should elicit a woman's understanding of breast reconstruction, her preference for type of reconstructive procedure and timing, and her expectations of the reconstructive process and outcome. It is helpful for women to review relevant literature with appropriate illustrations of different types of reconstructive options prior to the clinic visit in order to better guide the discussion and decision for surgery. Specifically, the surgeon should ask if a woman desires immediate or delayed reconstruction, and if she is interested in implant-based or autologous tissue reconstruction. The surgeon should also ascertain what breast size the patient would like to achieve with reconstruction. The surgeon should be aware if a unilateral or bilateral mastectomy is planned. If a unilateral mastectomy is planned, the surgeon should inquire if the patient has any aesthetic concerns regarding the contralateral breast that can be addressed with a symmetry procedure at a later time.

In addition to obtaining a complete history regarding the patient's breast disease and proposed treatment plan, a thorough evaluation of the patient's medical, surgical, and psychological history must be undertaken. Specifically, the surgeon should evaluate if there are any contraindications to general anesthesia, including significant cardiac or pulmonary disease.

Additionally, any condition that may impair wound healing, such as diabetes, collagen vascular disease, rheumatologic diseases, or renal failure, may be relative contraindications to elective reconstructive surgery. Morbidly obese patients also have an increased risk for surgical complications with both implant and autologous reconstruction. Nicotine use is a contraindication to reconstruction due to impaired wound healing, and patients should refrain from smoking for at least 1 month prior to any reconstruction procedure. Women who are actively smoking at the time of reconstruction suffer from an increased risk of mastectomy skin flap necrosis, infection, fat necrosis, flap loss, wound dehiscence, and donor site complications. Urine cotinine levels can be obtained to ensure that systemic levels have declined. The patient's medications should be reviewed, specifically for immunosuppressant medications or anticoagulants. Aspirin, nonsteroidal anti-inflammatory agents, and clopidogrel should be discontinued at least 7 to 10 days prior to surgery. Homeopathic medications such as garlic, ginseng, ginko biloba, ginger, St. John's wort, Echinacea, and other vitamin supplements should be stopped within 1 to 2 weeks of the operation as well due to the increased risk of bleeding.

The surgeon should obtain complete information regarding the patient's cancer diagnosis, including the type of mastectomy planned and the need for lymph node sampling or removal. For example, women with locally advanced cancers or clinically present nodal disease are likely to require radiation therapy. Radiation therapy can result in atrophy or fat necrosis of autologous reconstructive procedures and can result in delayed healing, capsular contracture, implant extrusion, and increased rates of infection for women undergoing expander/implant–based reconstruction. Additionally, the surgeon should ascertain if a woman has a strong family predisposition for cancer, such as presence of the BRCA gene, which may increase the possibility that she will undergo bilateral rather than unilateral mastectomy. Finally, the tumor biology is an important consideration, as women with certain diagnoses, such as lobular carcinoma in situ (LCIS), may be counseled toward bilateral rather than unilateral mastectomy.

On physical examination, the patient's blood pressure and heart rate should be examined, as postoperative hypertension may increase the risk of hematoma formation. The patient's body mass index (BMI) should be obtained, which may influence her reconstruction options. Obesity increases the risk of autologous flap loss, mastectomy skin flap necrosis, and donor site complications. The surgeon should examine both breasts for size, incisions, degree of ptosis, and symmetry. The chest wall skin should be examined for radiation therapy–related skin changes and evidence of pectoralis muscle atrophy. Potential autologous

tissue donor sites should be examined. The abdomen should be examined for the presence of any scars, abdominal wall laxity or rectus diastasis, and the presence of hernias. Paramedian and subcostal incisions may jeopardize the vascular supply of either the flap or the remaining abdominal wall skin. The chest wall should be examined for the presence of axillary or thoracotomy incisions that may damage the integrity of the latissimus dorsi muscle. The strength of the latissimus can be tested by asking the patient to adduct their arm against resistance.

For the patient in this scenario, on physical examination, she is awake, alert, and oriented. Her BMI is 28. Examination reveals pendulous breasts with grade 2 ptosis bilaterally and approximately C cup size. She has a small scar related to her core needle biopsy in the upper outer quadrant of her left breast. She has no abdominal wall scars, and no abdominal wall laxity, hernias, or rectus diastasis. She has normal strength in her upper extremities, and no evidence of pectoralis or latissimus dorsi atrophy.

Treatment Options
Types of Reconstruction
Breast Prostheses
Breast prostheses are ideal options for those women who are not appropriate candidates for breast reconstruction due to comorbid conditions or other factors, or who do not desire reconstruction. Breast prostheses are simple and convenient to obtain, and provide a satisfactory aesthetic result under most clothing options. These prostheses can be custom fit and are covered by insurance.

Breast Implant Placement Following Tissue Expansion
Permanent implant placement at the time of mastectomy is typically not possible as the skin flaps may be inadequate to cover the implant without tension, and the vascularity of the remaining skin may be tenuous with the trauma of mastectomy. Therefore, the risk of postoperative skin necrosis, dehiscence, and implant extrusion is high, and the long-term aesthetic appearance is poor related to contraction and scarring of the skin envelope. While immediate implant placement following mastectomies is occasionally performed, this option is typically limited to specialized centers in a small, select population of patients such as those undergoing nipple-sparing mastectomies

For the above reasons, permanent implant placement is accompanied by a period of tissue expansion prior to final implant placement in order to develop an appropriate skin envelope. Ideal patients are within the normal range of body mass index (BMI) who will undergo bilateral breast reconstruction and have not received or will not receive radiation therapy. It is more difficult to achieve symmetry in patients who will undergo unilateral reconstruction if the contralateral breast is ptotic. Reconstruction is typically performed in two phases. In the first phase, a tissue expander is placed underneath the pectoralis major muscle, with additional inferior coverage using either serratus anterior or acellular dermal matrix. The tissue expander is then sequentially inflated during postoperative visits in the office using sterile technique to the patient's desired volume, and then overexpansion is performed by 30%. The expander is then left in place for about 2 months, and then exchanged for a permanent saline or silicone implant. Tissue expanders are textured devices with an integrated valve, and are available in a range of shapes and sizes depending on the surgeon's preference and the patient's body habitus.

Indications for tissue expander reconstruction are those patients who desire a more expedient postoperative recovery and who are not candidates or do not desire autologous reconstruction due to donor site morbidity. Disadvantages include implant-related problems including contracture, rupture, and malposition. Additionally, implant reconstructions may have a less natural feel compared with autologous tissue, as well as appearance, including rippling of the implant. Contraindications to tissue expander and implant reconstruction include inadequate skin and pectoralis coverage to support expansion and implant placement. Radiation therapy has been correlated with higher rates of wound infection, implant extrusion, and capsular contracture. Therefore, women who have received radiation therapy will require additional muscle coverage using a latissimus dorsi myocutaneous flap on the radiated side if they desire implant-based reconstruction. This is typically performed once radiation therapy is complete and skin changes have stabilized.

Today, both saline and silicone implants are used for breast cancer reconstruction and both are equally safe. In 1992, the United States Food and Drug Administration placed a moratorium on the use of silicone implants due to the concern for increased risk for systemic illness related to the use of silicone. However, multiple studies have failed to show an increased risk of systemic illness, and these regulations have been discontinued. However, silicone implants are contraindicated in women younger than 22 years of age, and current guidelines suggest that women who receive silicone implants have a baseline MRI in 3 years following placement, and then every 2 years for the length of time that the implant is in place.

Autologous Tissue Reconstruction

Abdominal Wall Tissue Transfer. The transverse rectus abdominus myocutaneous flap, or TRAM flap, is the most commonly used flap for autologous breast reconstruction. In this approach, the infraumbilical skin and subcutaneous tissue is transferred to the chest wall defect, using the deep epigastric vessels through the underlying rectus muscle as the vascular supply. This procedure can be performed using a pedicled approach **(Figure 1A,B)**, a bilateral pedicled approach **(Figure 2)**, or microvascular techniques for free tissue transfer **(Figure 3)**. The pedicled TRAM flap is based on the superior deep epigastric vessel, and sacrifices the entire rectus abdominus muscle and overlying fascia during transfer. As the superior epigastric vessel is less robust compared with the inferior epigastric vessels, a delay procedure can be performed 2 weeks prior to flap elevation and inset by ligating the deep inferior epigastric system. This allows the vascular choke vessels to dilate to improve the vascularity and venous drainage of the

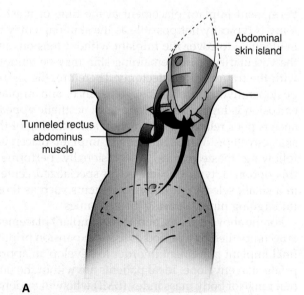

A

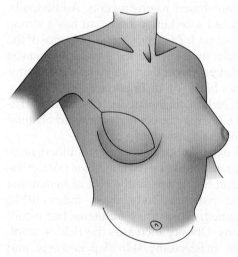

Breast scar may vary in appearance

B

FIGURE 1 • **A**: Design and inset of a pedicled unilateral transverse rectus abdominus myocutaneous (TRAM) flap. **B**: The final location of scars following a unilateral TRAM. (From the Section of Plastic Surgery, Department of General Surgery, University of Michigan, with permission.)

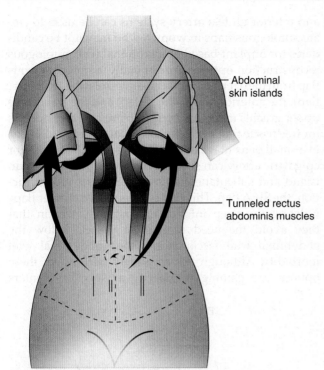

Abdominal
skin islands

Tunneled rectus
abdominis muscles

FIGURE 2 • Design and inset of a pedicled bilateral transverse rectus abdominus myocutaneous (TRAM) flap. (From the Section of Plastic Surgery, Department of General Surgery, University of Michigan, with permission.)

The deep inferior epigastric vessels are anastomosed using microsurgical technique to the thoracodorsal system in the axilla or the internal mammary vessels in the chest wall. Although there is a risk of complete flap loss with this approach, a minimal amount of rectus abdominus muscle and fascia is required with this approach, which minimizes donor site morbidity and abdominal wall weakness. Finally, the rectus muscle can be completely spared using the deep inferior epigastric perforator (DIEP) flap, in which the perforating vessels off of this vascular system are dissected completely from the rectus muscle and transferred to the chest wall defect as a free flap. These flaps have been shown to yield longer pedicle lengths and less abdominal wall morbidity, but have a risk of complete flap loss of around 1% depending on the surgeon experience and are technically demanding with long operating room times required.

Latissimus Dorsi Myocutaneous Flap. The latissimus dorsi muscle can be used as a myocutaneous, or a muscle-only flap for breast reconstruction in women who have undergone partial or complete mastectomy. The latissimus dorsi flap can be used without an implant in women who have undergone partial mastectomy with defects or asymmetry requiring reconstruction. The latissimus dorsi is typically used in conjunction with a permanent implant following a period of tissue expansion in women who undergo complete mastectomy **(Figure 4)**, with the exception of a small percentage of patients who undergo an "extended" technique. This technique incorporates the deep layer of subcutaneous fat beyond the borders of the muscle, which can provide sufficient volume to avoid the use of an

flap, and should be performed in high-risk patients such as those with diabetes, smokers, and obese patients. A "free" TRAM utilizes the deep inferior epigastric vessels, and allows for richer vascularity and a larger volume of tissue to be transferred as these vessels are more robust.

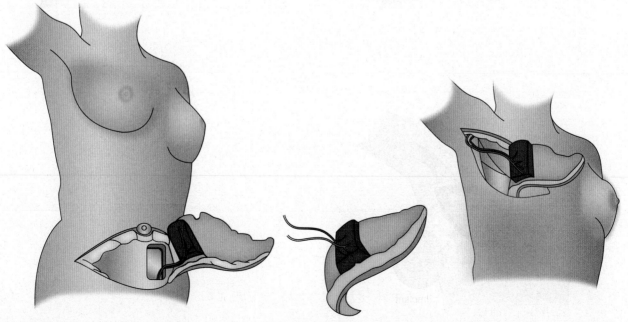

FIGURE 3 • The "free" TRAM technique by performing a microscopic anastomosis of the deep inferior epigastric vessels to the thoracodorsal artery and vein. (From the Section of Plastic Surgery, Department of General Surgery, University of Michigan, with permission.)

implant. Patients who have undergone prior thoracotomy are not candidates for this flap as the muscle has been divided, and patients who have previously undergone axillary node dissection should be considered for CT angiography to ensure the patency of the thoracodorsal artery. Sacrifice of the latissimus dorsi results in minimal functional deficit for women except in certain competitive athletes. The latissimus dorsi flap can be performed at the time of the mastectomy, can be used for bilateral reconstruction, and is ideal for women who may not be candidates for TRAM reconstruction due to abdominal wall obesity.

Other Perforator Flaps. The advent of microsurgery has allowed the development of a number of other perforator flap options for breast reconstruction. For example, perforators from the superior gluteal artery and inferior gluteal artery systems can be used to create autologous flaps in women who may not be candidates for implant-based or abdominal wall autologous reconstruction options. Additionally, a myocutaneous flap from the deep circumflex iliac vessels (the "Rubens" flap), the anterior lateral thigh flap, and the transverse upper gracilis myocutaneous flap are all other options for free tissue transfer for breast reconstruction. Finally, in a small percentage of women, the superficial inferior epigastric artery can support the lower transverse skin island and subcutaneous tissue for breast reconstruction, the SIEA flap. This flap is advantageous over flaps utilizing the deep inferior epigastric system in that they avoid the need to harvest vessels below the abdominal wall fascia, minimizing abdominal wall morbidity. Although not as widely performed, these options are gaining popularity at specialty centers

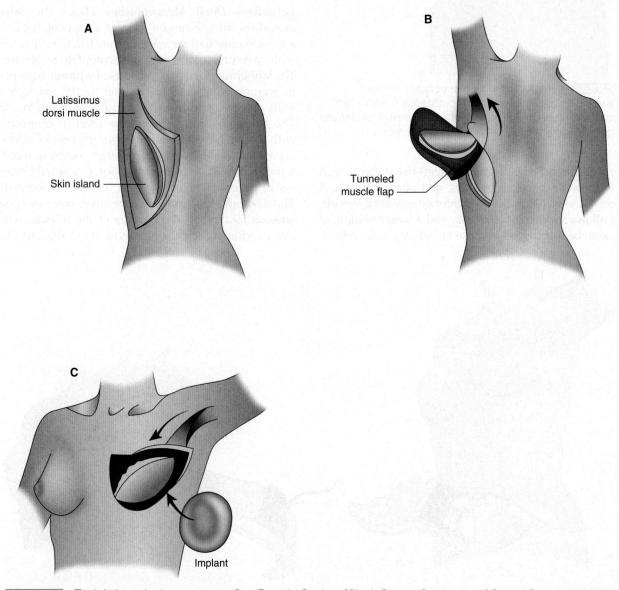

FIGURE 4 • The latissimus dorsi myocutaneous flap. (From the Section of Plastic Surgery, Department of General Surgery, University of Michigan, with permission.)

and are important options for women who cannot undergo implant or abdominal-based autologous reconstruction.

Surgical Decision Making and Approach

Timing of Reconstruction

Women who are not appropriate candidates for reconstruction or who do not wish to undergo the reconstructive process can be referred for breast prostheses, which can allow them to regain form in clothing without undergoing a surgical procedure. Women should be counseled that the process of breast reconstruction spans several months, and even years, and she should approach this journey fully informed of the risks, benefits, and limitations of reconstruction. Complete reconstruction, regardless of which type is selected, will require multiple operative procedures, each of which requires a postoperative recovery period of 3 to 12 weeks depending on the type of reconstruction selected. Thus, it is not a decision that should be taken lightly, and is often difficult for women to process the implications of reconstruction at the time of their diagnosis and initial decision for surgery. Therefore, some women may opt to defer reconstruction until a later time. The advantages of immediate reconstruction include fewer operative procedures, lower associated costs, and the ability to take advantage of skin-sparing mastectomy techniques. Immediate reconstruction occurs at the same procedure as the mastectomy, and can yield improved psychosocial functioning following the procedure due to less psychological distress. Furthermore, the aesthetic result may be better following immediate reconstruction due to less retraction of the skin envelope, although this is controversial. Immediate reconstruction is more efficient as the patient typically undergoes fewer operative procedures, the mastectomy defect does not require re-creation, and the risks of general anesthesia are minimized with fewer procedures. However, if postoperative complications occur, such as infection or delayed wound healing, these may delay adjuvant therapy until these issues have completely resolved. Immediate reconstruction may also be challenging if residual disease is identified in the surgical specimen, which may require reoperation or unplanned radiation therapy.

Delayed reconstruction can be undertaken any time after the mastectomy and adjuvant therapy is complete. Delayed reconstruction is advantageous in that the hematologic and immunologic effects of any chemotherapy are resolved. Some studies suggest that the overall complication rate following reconstruction is lower compared with immediate reconstruction and with a diminished need for blood transfusions. Finally, delayed reconstruction may be associated with improved postoperative quality of life and satisfaction with the aesthetic result, likely due to differences in psychological adjustment with the mastectomy defect.

Radiation therapy is historically considered to be a contraindication to implant-based reconstruction. Although there are some studies that suggest that implant-based reconstruction may be performed in an irradiated field, radiation increases the risk of capsular contracture, delayed wound healing, implant extrusion, and infection. Because of the skin changes related to radiation therapy, the overlying mastectomy flaps do not expand normally and can result in chest wall deformity due to noncompliance of the skin. Therefore, women who have or who are anticipated to have radiation therapy should be counseled toward delayed autologous reconstruction.

Technical Aspects

Tissue Expander/Implant Reconstruction (Table 1)

Preoperatively, the midline of the chest is marked, as well as the inframammary fold. The breast width is measured to select the expander of the appropriate base width. The skin envelope is examined following the mastectomy, or the skin flaps are re-created if the procedure is being performed in a delayed fashion. The tissue expander is placed in a subpectoral position (Figure 5). The lateral edge of the pectoralis major muscle is identified and elevated using cautery, and the muscle is elevated from the chest wall. Care is taken to identify perforators of the internal mammary vessels medially, which should be controlled with cautery to prevent a postoperative hematoma. Additionally, the vascular pedicle to the pectoralis major, the thoracoacromial vessels, is identified along the underside to the muscle at the midpoint of the clavicle. Care is taken to protect this structure. The pectoralis minor muscle is identified superiolaterally and is left adherent to the chest wall. Care is taken to avoid dissection outside of the boundaries of the breast, specifically laterally, medially, and inferiorly in order to prevent migration of the tissue expander. Excessive dissection medially can result in synmastia, and laterally can result in inappropriate expansion of axillary tissue. Violation of the inframammary fold can result in migration of the expander inferiorly and expansion of abdominal wall tissue. The pectoralis muscle is elevated off of the chest wall inferiorly, and the dissection is transitioned into the subcutaneous space down to the level of the inframammary fold. The expander should have complete coverage, which is accomplished via elevation of the medial aspect of the serratus anterior muscle, or by the placement of acellular dermal matrix (ADM). The selected tissue expander is then placed in the subpectoral pocket, and the pocket is closed using absorbable sutures to close the pocket in an interrupted fashion by closing the edge of the pectoralis muscle to the serratus anterior (or

TABLE 1. Key Technical Steps and Potential Pitfalls to Tissue Expander and Breast Implant Reconstruction

Key Technical Steps

1. Markings: sternal notch and midline, breast width, superior aspect of the breast, and inframammary fold.
2. Examine mastectomy skin flaps suitability for expansion, and pectoralis muscle for adequate coverage.
3. Elevate the lateral border of the pectoralis major muscle from the chest wall and enter the subpectoral space leaving the pectoralis minor adherent to the chest wall.
4. Develop the submuscular pocket for tissue expander placement based on the dimensions of the selected device for placement.
5. Divide the inferior border of the pectoralis major into the subcutaneous space up to the midline.
6. Elevate the anterior edge of the serratus insertions along the chest wall to create a complete submuscular pocket for lateral coverage of the tissue expander; can also consider the use of acellular dermal matrix for coverage of the expander as an alternative to serratus anterior flap.
7. Place tissue expander in pocket.
8. Close serratus anterior or acellular dermal matrix over the tissue expander with absorbable sutures to the inferior border of the pectoralis major.
9. Drains placed in the mastectomy pocket and/or the subpectoral pocket based on surgeon preference.
10. Skin closed in 2 layers.
11. Consider expansion at the initial operation based on the condition of the skin and the pectoralis muscle.

Potential Pitfalls

- Inappropriate tissue expander size or shape selection.
- Inadequate skin or muscular coverage over the expander.
- Hematoma in either the mastectomy pocket or the subpectoral pocket.
- Intraoperative bacterial seeding of the tissue expander.
- Distortion or obliteration of the inframammary fold or the medial attachments of the pectoralis muscle to the medial border of the sternum.

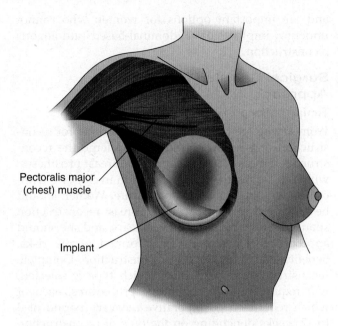

Pectoralis major (chest) muscle

Implant

FIGURE 5 • Placement of the tissue expander/implant into a subpectoral pocket. (From the Section of Plastic Surgery, Department of General Surgery, University of Michigan, with permission.)

ADM if this approach is selected). A drain is placed in the mastectomy pocket if immediate reconstruction has been performed or in the subpectoral pocket if delayed reconstruction is being performed. The pocket is irrigated with antibiotic irrigation and inspected for hemostasis. Fluid may be cautiously placed in the expander at the time of the operation if there is no tension on the muscle or skin closure. However, if there is any tension or concern for skin flap compromise, this should not be performed. Finally, the tissue expander has a magnetic port for postoperative filling, and the placement of this should be confirmed at the completion of the skin closure to make sure there is no difficulty with postoperative filling. Sterile tapes and a fluff dressing are placed over the incisions, but constrictive dressings are avoided to prevent compression on the skin flaps that could result in necrosis.

Tissue expansion can begin as an outpatient once the drains have been removed and the patient is steadily healing, at approximately 2 weeks postoperatively. This is performed in the office using sterile techniques, and the expanders are filled sequentially at weekly intervals depending on the patient's tolerance **(Figure 6A,B)**. The expanders are filled beyond the desired implant size by approximately 30%, and then left in place for about 2 months.

At that time, exchange can be performed of the tissue expanders for permanent implants. In the preoperative holding area, similar skin markings are used, and the chosen implants can be placed through the previous incisions. The skin is incised, and the subpectoral pocket is entered. The tissue expander is removed, and the pocket is inspected for constrictive scar bands. A capsule of scar will form around the tissue expander, and this is incised (capsuolotomies) or excised (capsulectomies) to release the skin envelope and allow for better skin draping over the implant. A temporary sizer implant is then placed in pocket and the patient is brought to a sitting position. The skin envelope is then readjusted using tailor-tacking techniques, and the breasts are inspected for symmetry in size, contour, shape, and position. The inframammary fold can be readjusted or defined using sutures, and the implant can be centralized along the chest wall by placing lateral sutures in the breast pocket. The pocket is then thoroughly irrigated, and the final implant is placed. The pocket is closed with absorbable suture, and the skin is closed in a layered fashion. Drains are not placed for the final implant exchange.

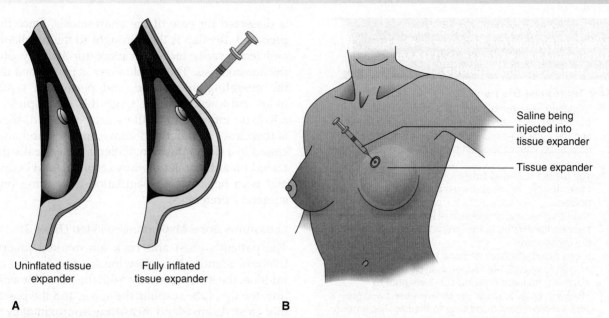

Uninflated tissue
expander

Fully inflated
tissue expander

Saline being
injected into
tissue expander

Tissue expander

A   **B**

FIGURE 6 • **A,B**: Accessing the tissue expander for inflation. (From the Section of Plastic Surgery, Department of General Surgery, University of Michigan, with permission.)

Transverse Rectus Abdominus Myocutaneous Flap (Table 2)

Preoperatively, the patient's chest wall is marked at the midline, as well as along the inframammary fold. The breast width is measured, and then an elliptical incision along the infraumbilical skin is created incorporating this width. A pinch test is used to ensure that this skin defect can be closed without tension. Elevation of the TRAM flap can be performed at the same time or following the mastectomy. The skin incisions are created, and the skin and subcutaneous tissue is elevated to the lateral row of perforators on the side of the muscle pedicle for a unilateral reconstruction. On the opposite side, the perforators are sacrificed and the dissection proceeds across the midline to the medial row of perforators of the muscle pedicle. The fascia overlying the rectus abdominus is divided sharply lateral to the perforators, and the inferior epigastric vessels are identified and ligated. The rectus muscle is carefully dissected out of the rectus sheath, taking care not to damage the rectus fascia, particularly at the tendinous inscriptions. The intercostal nerves are clipped and divided sharply. Once the rectus muscle has been circumferentially dissected inferiorly, the muscle is divided inferiorly and then the dissection proceeds superiorly to the costal margin to the superior epigastric vessels. These vessels are identified and protected. A subcutaneous pocket is created along the medial aspect of the inframammary fold for delivery of the flap with a width of approximately 4 fingerbreadths. The flap should fit easily through the tunnel without concern for strangulation of the vascular pedicle. The flap is then rotated 90 degrees into the mastectomy defect. The flap is then contoured to fit

the defect with respect for need for the skin defect and volume requirement. The flap is inset using absorbable sutures. The recuts sheath is closed using a running, large absorbable suture and may be reinforced with an overlay of mesh or ADM if there is excessive tension. The contralateral rectus sheath may be similarly plicated for symmetry. The abdominal incision is then closed by reapproximating Scarpa's fascia, the dermis, and the epidermis in three separate layers. The umbilicus is delivered through a U-shaped incision along the midline of the abdomen to lie at the level of the anterior superior iliac spines. The operating room table is placed in a flexed position to facilitate closure, and the patient is brought to a sitting position to facilitate inset of the TRAM flap.

If the flap is to be performed using microvascular techniques as a "free" flap, the deep inferior epigastric artery and vein are used as the dominant pedicle. Varying degrees of rectus abdominus muscle can be harvested with this flap, which can limit postoperative abdominal wall morbidity. The skin markings are designed as above, and the skin is incised along the ellipse. The initial flap dissection proceeds as above, but care is taken to meticulously dissect the deep inferior epigastric artery and vein without creating trauma to the vessel. These are dissected and ligated between clips as proximally as possible. The vessels are not ligated until the recipient site is completely dissected and prepared, so as to minimize warm ischemia time. The mastectomy pocket is dissected laterally into the axilla if the thoracodorsal vessels are selected as the recipient, or medially if the internal mammary vessels are selected. These vessels are circumferentially dissected using loupe magnification, and adequate length

TABLE 2. Key Technical Steps and Potential Pitfalls for Transverse Rectus Abdominus Myocutaneous (TRAM) Flap Breast Reconstruction

Key Technical Steps

1. Markings: the sternal notch, the anterior midline, the breast width, the anterior iliac spines bilaterally, and the pubic hairline. Elliptical incision designed across the lower abdomen to create the anterior breast skin.
2. The patient is placed supine on the operating room table, and the entire abdomen and chest is prepped and draped.
3. The designed abdominal skin resection is planned, and the skin is elevated to the lateral row of perforators on the chosen side.
4. If a pedicled approach is chosen: the deep inferior epigastric vessels are divided (can be performed as an elective outpatient procedure 2–3 wk prior to TRAM) in order to dilate the choke vessels and provide a more robust blood flow to the flap. The anterior abdominal wall is elevated up to the level of the xiphoid process, and a pocket is created between the mastectomy defect and the abdominal defect in order to allow for passage of the TRAM flap.
5. If a free approach is chosen: the deep inferior epigastric vessels are dissected to the external iliac and divided. A cuff of rectus abdominus and small area of fascia is harvested that incorporates the key perforating vessels to the overlying skin paddle. This is transferred as a free, composite flap of skin, subcutaneous tissue, with varying degrees of muscle and fascia to the chest wall. Either the thoracodorsal or the internal mammary vessels are selected as the recipient vessels. These vessels are dissected completely, and an end-to-end or end-to-side anastomosis is performed using the operating microscope.
6. The flap is inset with de-epithelialization of the unnecessary skin to fit the mastectomy defect.
7. The table is placed in the flexed position and the rectus sheath is closed using running absorbable suture. The contralateral rectus sheath is plicated for abdominal wall symmetry. Mesh or acellular dermal matrix placement as an overlay can be considered if abdominal wall plication appears tenuous.
8. Drains are placed in the breast pocket, and in the abdominal wall donor site.

Potential Pitfalls

- Inappropriate design of the skin paddle that is either inadequate to re-create the breast mound, or too generous to allow for abdominal wall closure.
- Injury to the medial row of perforating vessels or to the key perforating vessels to the overlying skin paddle.
- Inadequate closure of the abdominal wall fascia resulting in laxity or hernia.
- Thrombosis of the anastomosis in free tissue transfer resulting in partial or total flap loss.
- Distortion of the inframammary fold due to tunneling of the pedicled flap.
- Distortion of the umbilicus.

is dissected for ease of the anastomosis. Once this is prepared, the flap is then brought to the recipient site and temporarily tacked in place for stability during the anastomosis. The anastomosis is performed under the operating microscope, and performed typically in an end-to-end fashion. Once this is complete, and adequate inflow and outflow are confirmed, the flap is then inset as described above, and the abdomen is closed in a similar fashion. Patients are typically maintained on antiplatelet therapy (aspirin), and occasionally with heparin anticoagulation depending on the surgeon's preference.

Latissimus Dorsi Myocutaneous Flap (Table 3)

The patient's chest and back are marked preoperatively to identify the following landmarks: the chest midline, the inframammary fold, the posterior axillary line, the tip of the scapula, the spine, and the posterior iliac crest. A skin island measuring approximately 8 cm by 15 cm long can be designed in an oblique fashion, which can be concealed in most clothing. Flaps wider than 8 cm may be difficult to close without tension. The most posterior apical point of the axilla is used as a fulcrum to ensure that the flap will rotate into the mastectomy defect without difficulty.

The patient is placed in the lateral decubitus position with the shoulder abducted in order to provide adequate exposure of the posterior thorax and axilla. The latissimus dorsi muscle is a broad, flat, triangular-shaped muscle that measures approximately 25 × 35 cm. It originates from the thoracolumbar fascia, the posterior iliac crest, and the lower six thoracic vertebrae, and inserts on the intertubular groove of the humerus. The thoracodorsal artery and vein from the subscapular system are the primary vascular supply, but paraspinous perforators also supply the muscle posteriorly. The flap is raised by incising the skin paddle and dissecting down to the muscle fascia beveling away from the skin paddle. The skin and subcutaneous tissue is then elevated off the muscle by carrying the dissection inferiorly to the thoracolumbar fascia, medially to the paraspinous muscles, superiorly to the tip of the scapula, trapezius, and teres major. Posteriorly, the surgeon will encounter the perforating vessels at the paraspinous muscles, and these should be well controlled with cautery to prevent postoperative hematoma formation. The dissection is then carried anteriorly toward the edge of the latissimus, and the muscle is elevated from the serratus and the chest wall. The deep surface of the muscle is carefully dissected at the middle third, and progresses superiorly taking care to identify the thoracodorsal artery and vein and the serratus branch. The pedicle will enter the posterior surface of the muscle approximately 10 cm below its insertion on the humerus. The medial aspect of the muscle is then

TABLE 3. Key Technical Steps and Potential Pitfalls for Latissimus Dorsi Muscle Myocutaneous Flap Breast Reconstruction

Key Technical Steps

1. Markings: sterna notch, anterior and posterior midline, breast width, superior aspect of the breast, inframammary fold, posterior axillary line, tip of the scapula.
2. Measure the anticipated skin needed for reconstruction, which is oriented in an oblique fashion across the lower back centered over the lumbosacral perforators.
3. Patient is placed in the decubitus position on the operating room table with arm abducted at 90 degrees and both anterior and posterior midline exposed.
4. Examine mastectomy skin flaps suitability for expansion.
5. Anterior edge of latissimus is identified and elevated from the chest wall.
6. Thoracodorsal nerve, artery, and serratus branch are identified as the pedicle and preserved.
7. The skin and subcutaneous tissue is then elevated off of the posterior aspect of the latissimus dorsi to the posterior midline taking care to note the direction of the muscle fibers of the paraspinous muscle, teres major, external oblique, and trapezius in order to avoid elevation of these muscles.
8. Posterior skin flap is elevated to the level of the posterior iliac crest and the lumbosacral fascia.
9. The latissimus dorsi is then elevated off of the chest wall anteriorly taking care to avoid injury to the pedicle and identifying and ligating all intercostal perforators.
10. Latissimus dorsi is then divided as inferiorly as possible along the lumbosacral fascia and transposed anteriorly into the mastectomy defect. It is inset with absorbable sutures along the inframammary fold and the medial border of the pectoralis. The skin paddle is inset after tailoring to the mastectomy skin flap defect.
11. A tissue expander is placed below the pectoralis muscle in the new submuscular pocket.
12. Drains are placed in the latissimus dorsi donor site, the mastectomy pocket, and the submuscular pocket.

Potential Pitfalls

- Hematoma in the mastectomy pocket, the submuscular pocket, or the latissimus dorsi donor site.
- Seroma formation in the latissimus dorsi donor site.
- Tissue expander malposition or malfunction.
- Intraoperative bacterial seeding of the tissue expander.
- Distortion or obliteration of the inframammary fold or the medial attachments of the pectoralis muscle to the medial border of the sternum.
- Injury to the thoracodorsal artery or vein.
- Compression or torsion of the thoracodorsal artery and vein with inset.

dissected completely off of the chest wall, and divided as inferiorly as possible in order to allow for advancement of the muscle into the mastectomy pocket. The flap is then tunneled into the mastectomy defect and inset using absorbable sutures tacking the latissimus flap to the pectoralis fascia. A tissue expander is placed under the latissimus flap prior to completing the inset. A drain is placed both in the donor site along the posterior chest and in the mastectomy

pocket. The skin paddle of the flap is inset to the mastectomy flaps using absorbable suture in a layered technique, and soft dressing is applied taking care not to constrict the chest in any way and allowing for exposure of the skin paddle to monitor for ischemia or venous congestion.

Special Intraoperative Considerations

If breast reconstruction is to be performed immediately following mastectomy, it is imperative to closely examine the mastectomy skin flaps for signs of impending skin compromise. If there are signs that the mastectomy flaps may not survive, the surgeon should not proceed with reconstruction at that time, but instead wait until the skin flaps have completely declared themselves, as this may change the options for reconstruction.

The thoracodorsal artery and vein should be examined closely if an axillary lymph node dissection has been performed. If this is thrombosed or damaged, this may preclude creation of a latissimus dorsi flap or use of these vessels for free flap anastomosis. Finally, if a flap reconstruction has been performed, the skin paddle of the flap should be inspected closely for evidence of vascular compromise. If this is evidence the pedicle or anastomosis should be examined for evidence of kinking, twisting, or thrombosis, and the overlying skin tunnels should be examined to ensure that they allow for easy passage of the flap without constriction.

Postoperative Management

Following mastectomy and immediate placement of a tissue expander, women are usually discharged home on the day following surgery. Hospital stays are longer for women who undergo autologous tissue flaps, usually ranging from 3 to 5 days. The usual postoperative care is taken, with DVT mechanical and pharmacologic prophylaxis, and encouragement of early ambulation. Women are advised to refrain from driving, strenuous exercise, and household activities for a period of 6 to 8 weeks following reconstruction.

Early complications following breast reconstruction include hematoma, seroma, infection, flap loss, skin necrosis, and implant extrusion. The development of a postoperative hematoma typically warrants operative reexploration as it can increase the risk of skin or flap loss, infection, postoperative asymmetry, and capsular contracture. Infection is a feared complication following tissue expander/implant reconstruction and is treated promptly with antibiotics. Those infections associated with an abscess or who fail to improve on intravenous antibiotics should undergo implant or expander removal. Superficial skin necrosis can be managed conservatively with local wound care. Larger areas of skin necrosis may warrant operative debridement and implant or expander removal. Latissimus flap harvest can result in seroma formation in the donor site, and operatively placed drains may remain for 4 to 6 weeks until their output has dropped sufficiently for removal.

Late complications of breast reconstruction include asymmetry, implant wrinkling, malposition, implant rupture, capsular contracture, and donor site morbidity. Specific to TRAM reconstruction, abdominal wall weakness and hernias are important sources of donor site morbidity. Breast reconstruction revision and implant replacement can be undertaken to resolve these relatively common complications.

The process of breast reconstruction spans a period of months to years. Following reconstruction of the breast mound, further procedures may be desired to revise the shape of the breast, create a nipple, and achieve symmetry with the contralateral breast. Such procedures may include contralateral augmentation with implants or autologous fat grafting, reduction, and mastopexy to achieve symmetry. Finally, nipple reconstruction may be performed as early as 3 to 6 months following breast mound reconstruction, in order to allow for swelling to subside and the breast mound to achieve its final shape. Multiple local flap designs can be used for nipple and areolar reconstruction, and supplemented with tattooing for a more anatomic appearance.

TAKE HOME POINTS

- Many women are candidates for surgical breast reconstruction following partial or complete mastectomy for breast reconstruction.
- Breast reconstruction following mastectomy can improve psychological outcomes following breast cancer treatment and does not interfere with long-term surveillance for recurrence.
- Radiation therapy causes long-term skin changes that impair the ability to successfully expand the skin envelope. These patients should undergo reconstruction with autologous tissue transfer.
- Abdominal tissue transfer utilizing the rectus abdominus can result in hernia formation and truncal weakness. However, innovative perforator-based and muscle-sparing techniques can lessen donor site morbidity and increase reconstructive options for women.

SUGGESTED READINGS

Alderman AK, Collins ED, Schott A, Hughes ME, Ottesen RA, Theriault RL, Wong YN, Weeks JC, Niland JC, Edge SP. 2011. The impact of breast reconstruction on the delivery of chemotherapy. Cancer: 116(7): 1791–1800.

Alderman AK, Hawley ST, Waljee J, et al. Correlates of referral practices of general surgeons to plastic surgeons for mastectomy reconstruction. Cancer 2007;109: 1715–1720.

Alderman AK, Hawley ST, Waljee J, et al. Understanding the impact of breast reconstruction on the surgical decision-making process for breast cancer. Cancer. 2008; 112:489–494.

Alderman AK, McMahon L Jr, Wilkins EG. The national utilization of immediate and early delayed breast reconstruction and the effect of sociodemographic factors. Plast Reconstr Surg. 2003;111:695–703; discussion 4–5.

Alderman AK, Wilkins EG, Kim HM, et al. Complications in postmastectomy breast reconstruction: two-year results of the Michigan Breast Reconstruction Outcome Study. Plast Reconstr Surg. 2002;109:2265–2274.

Ascherman JA, Hanasono MM, Newman MI, et al. Implant reconstruction in breast cancer patients treated with radiation therapy. Plast Reconstr Surg. 2006;117:359–365.

Atisha D, Alderman AK, Lowery JC, et al. Prospective analysis of long-term psychosocial outcomes in breast reconstruction: two-year postoperative results from the Michigan Breast Reconstruction Outcomes Study. Ann Surg. 2008;247:1019–1028.

Chevray PM. Timing of breast reconstruction: immediate versus delayed. Cancer J. 2008;14:223–229.

Cocquyt VF, Blondeel PN, Depypere HT, et al. Better cosmetic results and comparable quality of life after skin-sparing mastectomy and immediate autologous breast reconstruction compared to breast conservative treatment. Br J Plast Surg. 2003;56:462–470.

Eberlein TJ, Crespo LD, Smith BL, et al. Prospective evaluation of immediate reconstruction after mastectomy. Ann Surg. 1993;218:29–36.

Forman DL, Chiu J, Restifo RJ, et al. Breast reconstruction in previously irradiated patients using tissue expanders and implants: a potentially unfavorable result. Ann Plast Surg. 1998;40:360–363; discussion 3–4.

Harcourt DM, Rumsey NJ, Ambler NR, et al. The psychological effect of mastectomy with or without breast reconstruction: a prospective, multicenter study. Plast Reconstr Surg. 2003;111:1060–1068.

Hu E, Alderman AK. Breast reconstruction. Surg Clin North Am. 2007;87:453–467, x.

Janowsky EC, Kupper LL, Hulka BS. Meta-analyses of the relation between silicone breast implants and the risk of connective-tissue diseases. N Engl J Med. 2000;342:781–790.

Kraemer O, Andersen M, Siim E. Breast reconstruction and tissue expansion in irradiated versus not irradiated women after mastectomy. Scand J Plast Reconstr Surg Hand Surg. 1996;30:201–206.

McCarthy CM, Mehrara BJ, Riedel E, et al. Predicting complications following expander/implant breast reconstruction: an outcomes analysis based on preoperative clinical risk. Plast Reconstr Surg. 2008;121:1886–1892.

Sigurdson L, Lalonde DH. MOC-PSSM CME article: Breast reconstruction. Plast Reconstr Surg. 2008;121:1–12.

Wilkins EG, Cederna PS, Lowery JC, et al. Prospective analysis of psychosocial outcomes in breast reconstruction: one-year postoperative results from the Michigan Breast Reconstruction Outcome Study. Plast Reconstr Surg. 2000;106:1014–1025; discussion 26–27.

Wilson CR, Brown IM, Weiller-Mithoff E, et al. Immediate breast reconstruction does not lead to a delay in the delivery of adjuvant chemotherapy. Eur J Surg Oncol. 2004;30:624–627.

58 Palpable Thyroid Nodule

HAGGI MAZEH and REBECCA S. SIPPEL

Presentation

A 42-year-old female, without any previous medical or surgical history, presents for routine physical examination. Her vital signs are within normal limits. On neck examination, she is noted to have a palpable nodule in the front of her neck. The nodule is located two finger breadth inferior to the cricoid cartilage and 1 cm to the right of the midline. The nodule measures about 2 cm in its greatest diameter; it is firm, mobile, and nontender. When the patient swallows, the nodule moves up and down with the thyroid cartilage. There are no palpable nodules on the left side of the neck, nor is there cervical of supraclavicular lymphadenopathy. The remaining physical examination is normal.

Differential Diagnosis

The description of the nodule suggests that it is located within the thyroid gland. Thyroid nodules may be of benign nature such as colloid-containing cysts, thyroid adenoma, hyperplastic nodules, or thyroiditis. Thyroid nodules may harbor malignancy including papillary, follicular, medullary, Hürthle cell, or anaplastic thyroid cancer. In rare cases, thyroid nodules may represent lymphoma, squamous cell carcinoma, or metastasis of other origin. The differential diagnosis of other neck masses is broad and is beyond the scope of this chapter.

Workup

At this point, it is important to identify whether the patient has any risk factors for malignancy. The two most important risk factors for thyroid malignancy are a history of neck radiation and a family history of thyroid cancer or other endocrine tumors. Specific attention must be paid to symptoms associated with local compression or invasion such as hoarseness, cough, dysphagia, or airway compressive symptoms. Rapid growth and new onset of hoarseness raise the suspicion for malignancy.

Thyroid function testing with a thyroid-stimulating hormone (TSH) level is recommended. If the TSH is abnormal, additional testing of thyroid function is warranted. If the TSH is elevated, serum concentrations of thyroperoxidase antibody should be checked. If the TSH is suppressed, a thyroid scintigraphy scan should be obtained to distinguish between Graves' disease and a toxic nodule. Currently, routine calcitonin testing is not recommended.

Ultrasound (U/S) is the imaging of choice for a newly diagnosed thyroid nodule. Ultrasound may assess nodule size, location, and other concomitant thyroid pathologies as well as the cervical lymph nodes.

Ultrasonic features suspicious for malignancy include hypoechogenicity, microcalcification, irregular margins, chaotic vascular patterns, as well as extracapsular invasion and lymph node involvement. **Figure 1** demonstrates the appearance of a malignant nodule on U/S.

Ultrasound-guided fine needle aspiration biopsy (FNAB) is the most important tool for evaluation of thyroid nodules. Possible FNAB results are nondiagnostic, benign, atypia or follicular lesion of undetermined significance, follicular neoplasm, suspicious for malignancy, and malignant (see **Figure 2**).

The patient's U/S demonstrated a 3.2-cm right thyroid lobe nodule. The nodule was hypoechoic and complex with some microcalcifications. In this patient, FNAB identified a follicular neoplasm.

Diagnosis and Treatment

Although the prevalence of thyroid nodules on ultrasound may exceed 50%, palpable thyroid nodules can be detected in 10% of women and 2% of men. Fortunately, most nodules are of benign nature and only 5% harbor malignancy. In the last two decades, FNAB of thyroid nodules has become the "gold standard" of thyroid nodule workup. In an attempt to develop uniform terminology of FNAB reports, six categories were defined as mentioned above.

Inadequate or nondiagnostic aspirates constitute 4% to 16% of FNAB results and should be reaspirated. If the repeated aspiration is not diagnostic, surgical excision is recommended. Benign results on FNAB are the most common finding (up to 70%) and may be treated expectantly. A follow up US should be obtained in 6 to 12 months to evaluate for interval growth. Malignant FNAB results should be treated with total thyroidectomy. Follicular neoplasms (FN) are identified in 15% to 20% of all FNAB and about 15% to 30% prove to be malignant. FNAB is unable to distinguish benign from

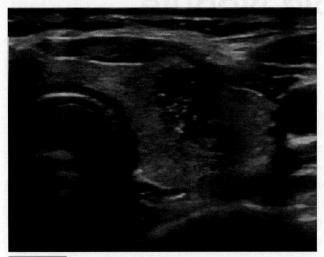

FIGURE 1 • A malignant thyroid nodule. The nodule appears heterogeneous, cystic, hypoechoic, irregular margins, and microcalcifications are present.

malignant FN; hence, surgical removal is required. **Figure 2** provides an algorithm for the evaluation of thyroid nodules.

Surgical Approach

The surgical approach to a patient with a follicular neoplasm result on FNAB requires an educated

decision by the patient. The appropriate surgical approach for a FN is a diagnostic lobectomy. If the final pathology reveals malignancy, then a completion thyroidectomy should be performed. Frozen section evaluation is usually not informative and is unnecessary unless there is a suspicion for papillary thyroid cancer. The advantages of thyroid lobectomy include avoiding possible injury to the contralateral recurrent laryngeal nerve (RLN) and parathyroid glands as well as avoiding the need for lifelong thyroid hormone replacement in the majority of patients. A major disadvantage of this approach is it involves the need for completion thyroidectomy if malignancy is identified on final pathology. This second procedure involves another admission and anesthetic. Patients with a history of radiation therapy to the neck, a positive family history for thyroid cancer, multinodular goiter, and those already on thyroid hormone replacement therapy may be best served with total thyroidectomy as the index procedure.

The patient in our scenario decided to undergo total thyroidectomy **(Table 1)**.

The procedure is usually performed under general anesthesia. The patient is positioned in a beach chair position and the neck is extended. A horizontal neck (Kocher) incision is performed and should be located just inferior to the cricoid cartilage, ideally

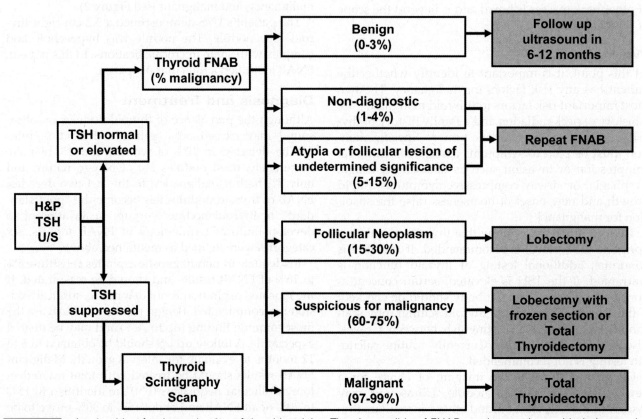

FIGURE 2 • An algorithm for the evaluation of thyroid nodules. The six possible of FNAB results are given with their associated risk of malignancy and the appropriate management. TSH, thyroid-stimulating hormone; FNAB, fine needle aspiration.

TABLE 1. Key Technical Steps and Potential Pitfalls of Thyroidectomy

Key Technical Steps

1. Position the patient with the neck extended.
2. Place your incision to enable access to both the upper and lower poles.
3. Elevate subplatysmal flaps and separate the strap muscles.
4. Take the upper pole vessels first.
5. Mobilize the lobe anteriorly and medially to facilitate RLN identification.
6. Carry all dissection as close as possible to the thyroid gland.
7. Always identify the parathyroid glands and preserve their blood supply.

Potential Pitfalls

- Nerve injury usually occurs close to the nerve insertion at the cricothyroid membrane.
- Inadvertently removed or devascularized parathyroid glands should be autotransplanted and implanted in muscle tissue at the end of the case.
- Postoperative expanding neck hematoma should prompt bedside wound exploration followed by return to the operating room.

in a neck crease. The platysma muscle is divided and subplatysmal flaps are elevated. The strap muscles are separated at the midline to offer access to the thyroid gland. At this point, it is preferable to begin the dissection on the side with the suspected lesion or tumor. It is important to dissect and retract the strap muscles off the thyroid gland in order to be in the correct plane. The middle thyroid vein should be divided. The upper pole of the thyroid is divided as close as possible to the thyroid gland in order to avoid injury to the superior laryngeal nerve and the upper parathyroid gland. Once the upper pole is divided, the thyroid lobe may be retracted medially and upward to assist further dissection. At this point, it is crucial to identify the recurrent laryngeal nerve (RLN) in the tracheoesophageal groove along its course to the cricothyroid membrane.

Parathyroid glands should be preserved with their native blood supply whenever possible. During the dissection, vessels can be divided with cautery, harmonic scalpel, clips, or ties according to surgeon preference. Once the lobe is mobilized, the isthmus is dissected off the trachea with cautery and the contralateral lobe is resected in a similar fashion. After hemostasis is assured, the strap muscles are reapproximated at the midline. The platysma muscle is sutured and the skin closed.

Special Intraoperative Considerations

- In cases of suspected malignancy or proven malignancy, special attention must be paid to the lymph nodes in the central compartment. Lymph nodes that are grossly involved should be resected and in such cases formal central lymph node dissection should be performed.
- Failure to identify and resect a pyramidal lobe can be the source of a significant thyroid remnant with radioactive iodine treatment. The pyramidal lobe may be elongated reaching above the thyroid cartilage. Special care must be taken to correctly identify and resect it as part of the thyroid gland.
- In order to identify and preserve the parathyroid glands, it is important to understand their anatomic location, especially in relationship to the recurrent laryngeal nerve. The upper parathyroid gland is located posterior and lateral to the RLN and the lower glands are located anterior and medial to the RLN. In cases when parathyroid glands are inadvertently resected, they should be autotransplanted in the sternocleidomastoid muscle.
- Identification of the RLN during thyroidectomy is essential to avoid injury. After dividing the upper pole of the thyroid gland, it is important to avoid further dissection inferiorly prior to the nerve identification because most nerve injuries occur close to the nerve entrance to the trachea. In rare cases, the nerve is entrapped within tumor tissue, and in such cases, the nerve should be sacrificed. Nerve-monitoring devices have a role in confirming the nerve is intact, especially in complicated cases.
- The role of intraoperative frozen section is controversial. Some surgeons use it to assist in deciding on the extent of surgery for lesions with no definite malignancy on FNAB. Frozen section is most helpful in cases that have an FNAB of suspicious papillary thyroid cancer. Frozen section is rarely able to distinguish follicular adenoma from follicular carcinoma, so it is probably not useful in most cases of FN.

Postoperative Management

Thyroid surgery may be performed in an outpatient setting or with a short admission (24 hours). Patients should be monitored for several hours after surgery to evaluate for the development of neck hematoma that may require emergent evacuation. Symptomatic transient postoperative hypocalcemia occurs in 10% to 20% of the patients that undergo total thyroidectomy and may be minimized with the use of oral calcium supplements. Measuring postoperative calcium and parathyroid hormone levels is used to identify patients that may require higher doses of calcium as well as calcitriol supplements. All patients that have the entire gland removed require thyroid hormone replacement therapy.

Follow-up varies according to the final histopathology results. Postoperative I ablation is administered for high-risk patients with differentiated thyroid carcinomas, especially those with gross residual disease, metastatic disease, or nodal involvement. In these patients, administration of levothyroxine at a suppressive dose (TSH < 0.1 mU) has been shown to improve disease-free survival. Serum thyrogobulin levels should be measured every 6 to 12 months for patients with differentiated thyroid cancer that underwent total thyroidectomy.

Case Conclusion

The patient undergoes uncomplicated total thyroidectomy as an outpatient. Postoperatively, she is treated with levothyroxine and calcium supplements, the calcium is discontinued after a week. On final pathology follicular thyroid carcinoma is identified, measuring 3.2 cm at greatest diameter with capsular invasion. The patient is treated with radioactive iodine ablation four weeks after surgery. Five years later, the patient is noted to have elevated thyroglobulin. Workup identifies a local recurrence that is removed surgically. At ten-year follow-up, she is free of disease.

TAKE HOME POINTS

- Palpable thyroid nodules are very common in up to 10% of the population.
- Most thyroid nodules are benign.
- The single most important test for palpable thyroid nodules is FNAB with an accuracy of up to 95%.
- Thyroid nodules should be managed according to FNAB results. Accurate terminology facilitates proper treatment.
- Follicular lesions on FNAB carry a 15% to 30% malignancy and require surgical intervention.
- The appropriate treatment for patients with a follicular neoplasm is at a minimum a thyroid lobectomy

SUGGESTED READINGS

American Thyroid Association (ATA) Guidelines Taskforce on Thyroid Nodules and Differentiated Thyroid Cancer, Cooper DS, Doherty GM, Haugen BR, Kloos RT, Lee SL, Mandel SJ, Mazzaferri EL, McIver B, Pacini F, Schlumberger M, Sherman SI, Steward DL, Tuttle RM. Revised American Thyroid Association management guidelines for patients with thyroid nodules and differentiated thyroid cancer. Thyroid. 2009;19(11):1167–1214.

Cibas ES, Ali SZ. The Bethesda system for reporting thyroid cytopathology. Thyroid. 2009;19(11):1159–1165.

Dean DS, Gharib H. Epidemiology of thyroid nodules. Best Pract Res Clin Endocrinol Metab. 2008;22:901–911.

Gharib H, Papini E, Valcavi R, et al. American Association of Clinical Endocrinologists and Associazione Medici Endocrinologi medical guidelines for clinical practice for the diagnosis and management of thyroid nodules. Endocr Pract. 2006;12:63–102.

59 Papillary Thyroid Carcinoma

GERARD M. DOHERTY

Presentation

A 42-year-old woman in good health, whose only medications are oral contraceptives, presents for evaluation of a central neck mass noted on health maintenance examination. Her neck examination shows a firm mass to the right of the larynx that moves up and down with swallowing. She has no palpable lymphadenopathy. She has no family history of thyroid disease and no personal history of radiation exposure.

Differential Diagnosis

A mass in the central neck that moves with swallowing is tethered to the larynx; the most common lesions are of the thyroid gland. Other possibilities include infectious or inflammatory lesions (lymphadenitis, abscess, or sarcoidosis), congenital lesions (thyroglossal duct lesions, branchial cleft cysts, cystic hygroma or laryngocele), or neoplasms of nonthyroid origin (salivary gland, subcutaneous lipoma, sebaceous cyst, carotid body tumor, laryngeal chondroma, soft tissue sarcoma, or metastatic lymphadenopathy). The thyroid lesions can be inflammatory (lymphocytic thyroiditis most common; others include acute thyroiditis, Reidels thyroiditis, or suppurative thyroiditis), benign neoplastic lesions (solitary or multiple adenomas, multinodular hyperplasia), or malignant lesions (papillary, follicular, anaplastic or medullary thyroid cancer, lymphoma or rarely metastatic lesions).

Workup

In this patient, point-of-care ultrasound shows a heterogeneous, mostly hypoechoic, irregularly shaped mass in the right thyroid lobe that measures 34 mm in maximum dimension (Figure 1). The left lobe of the thyroid gland appears normal. Measurement of thyroid function tests shows a normal TSH (thyroid-stimulating hormone) level of 1.37 mIU/L. Because of the suspicious ultrasound appearance, fine needle aspiration cytology under ultrasound guidance is performed and shows papillary thyroid carcinoma.

Discussion

Thorough initial evaluation includes ultrasound examination of the neck to clarify the physical examination findings. This can help to determine whether the lesion is thyroid in origin and what the characteristics of the thyroid lesion are (solid vs. cystic vs. complex; smooth vs. irregular borders; solitary vs. multiple; hyper-, hypo-, or isoechoic; degree of vascularity; presence or absence of microcalcification; and size). Thyroid nodules can be categorized based on these findings, and the clinical decision of whether to sample the lesion is informed by clinical management guideline. For example, any solid, hypoechoic nodule larger than 10 mm in diameter should be sampled, while mixed solid-cystic lesions without other suspicious findings should only be biopsied if larger than 20 mm.

Assessment of thyroid function is helpful, both to determine the potential need for thyroid hormone supplementation, and to guide the evaluation. Patients with an elevated TSH are more likely to have malignant nodules and may require thyroid hormone supplementation even if the thyroid nodule proves to be benign. Patients with a suppressed TSH may have an overactive thyroid nodule that is extremely unlikely to be malignant. A suppressed TSH in a patient with a thyroid nodule is the only situation currently in which a nuclear thyroid scintiscan is indicated. Other than this relatively uncommon situation, scintiscan is not useful. For these hyperthyroid patients, scintiscan can help to distinguish Grave's disease with a concomitant (potentially malignant) thyroid nodule from a solitary toxic adenoma (Figure 2).

Fine needle aspiration cytology is the gold-standard thyroid nodule assessment. This requires special expertise for interpretation but is very reliable. There are currently six standard categories for reporting of thyroid FNA results: nondiagnostic, benign, follicular lesion of undetermined significance, follicular neoplasm, suspicious for malignancy, and malignant. Nondiagnostic results usually prompt repeat FNA, Benign cytology is followed by interval follow-up evaluation, and suspicious or definitively malignant results are managed by operation. The indeterminate categories can be managed by diagnostic operation, repeat needle aspiration, or follow-up monitoring depending upon the associated characteristics of the patient and the nodule.

Diagnosis and Treatment

Preoperative cervical ultrasound to evaluate the central and lateral cervical lymph node compartments is

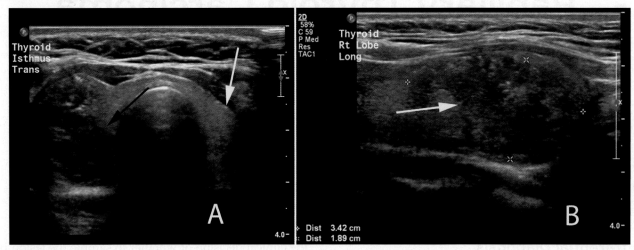

FIGURE 1 • Thyroid ultrasound demonstrating the suspicious right thyroid lobe mass. **A:** Transverse view of the thyroid gland. The left lobe (*white arrow*) appears normal. The right lobe contains a hypoechoic, irregular lesion suspicious for thyroid carcinoma (*black arrow*). **B:** Sagittal view of the right thyroid lobe showing the suspicious mass (*white arrow*) in the lower portion of the right lobe.

required prior to operation for thyroid carcinoma. This is necessary in order to identify involved lymph node compartments so that a thorough initial operation can be planned. If there is imageable lymphadenopathy in the lateral compartment, then fine needle aspiration of a lateral neck node with thyroglobulin measurement of the aspirate can determine the presence of metastatic papillary thyroid carcinoma and establish the need for therapeutic neck dissection in that basin. Selective neck dissection based upon the levels of the involved lymph nodes should include any compartment involved **(Figure 3)**.

For all but those with the very best prognosis (tumor <10 mm, normal lymph nodes, age < 45 years), patients

with papillary thyroid carcinoma should have an initial operation that includes removal of the entire thyroid gland. In addition, any lymph nodes involved by cancer based on preoperative or intraoperative assessment should be removed by complete compartmental dissection. The utility of prophylactic level 6 lymph node dissection for those patients with apparently uninvolved lymph nodes is more controversial, but may provide important prognostic information and potential therapeutic benefit.

In the patient in this scenario, ultrasound of the neck reveals a right level 3 lymph node with suspicious features **(Figure 4)**. Ultrasound-guided needle aspiration of the node shows cells consistent with metastatic

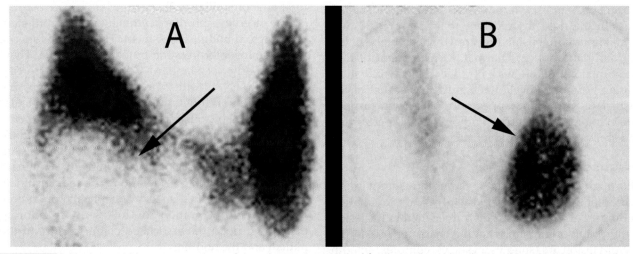

FIGURE 2 • Nuclear scintiscans are only useful, and are now reserved for, hyperthyroid patients with a thyroid nodule (low TSH). Ultrasound and cytology have replaced the routine use of scintiscan to evaluate thyroid nodules. However, hyperthyroid patients with a solitary thyroid nodule can fit one of two scenarios: Graves disease with a thyroid nodule that can be malignant (**A,** *arrow* on the cold right lower pole nodule) or a solitary toxic adenoma with suppression of function in the remainder of the thyroid gland (**B,** *arrow* on the hot left lower pole nodule)..

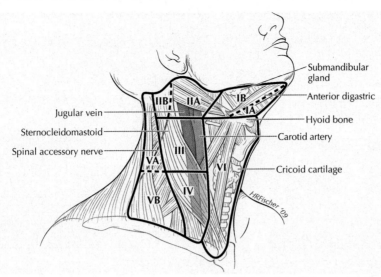

FIGURE 3 • Lymph node compartments separated into levels and sublevels. Level VI contains the thyroid gland, and the adjacent nodes bordered superiorly by the hyoid bone, inferiorly by the innominate (brachiocephalic) artery, and laterally on each side by the carotid sheaths. The level II, III, and IV nodes are arrayed along the jugular veins on each side, bordered anteromedially by level VI and laterally by the posterior border of the sternocleidomastoid muscle. The level I node compartment includes the submental and submandibular nodes, above the hyoid bone, and anterior to the posterior edge of the submandibular gland. The level V nodes are in the posterior triangle, lateral to the lateral edge of the sternocleidomastoid muscle. (From Cooper DS, Doherty GM, Haugen BR, et al. Revised American Thyroid Association management guidelines for patients with thyroid nodules and differentiated thyroid cancer.[see comment]. Thyroid. 2009;19(11):1167–1214, with permission).

papillary thyroid cancer and an aspirate thyroglobulin level of 934 ng/mL. Given these findings, the patient is scheduled for a total thyroidectomy with level 6 lymph node dissection, as well as a right level 2-3-4 lymph node dissection.

Surgical Approach

The extent of the planned operation is dictated by the location of disease. For this patient, with a significant papillary thyroid carcinoma and an involved right lateral neck node metastasis documented, the likelihood of level 6 lymph node involvement is high. The level 6 lymph nodes can be difficult to image by ultrasound when the thyroid gland is in place. The value of total thyroidectomy includes removal of potential multifocal disease in the thyroid gland and preparation for postoperative radioiodine therapy. If a thyroid lobectomy alone is used to manage a thyroid carcinoma, then radioiodine cannot be utilized. Similarly, the value of postoperative surveillance with thyroglobulin levels as a tumor marker is enhanced by total thyroidectomy.

This operation is best done under general anesthesia. Though many thyroid operations can be done using local anesthesia and sedation, the inclusion of central and lateral neck dissection makes this quite difficult. The key steps of the operation are listed in **Table 1**. Thyroidectomy can be complicated by infection, bleeding, and anesthetic reactions though these are quite unlikely. The more worrisome complications

of thyroidectomy are nerve injury and hypoparathyroidism, both because they are more common, and because they can cause permanent functional deficits for the patient.

The principles of the dissection are as follows:

1. Avoid dividing any structures in the tracheoesophageal groove until the nerve is definitively identified. Small branches of the inferior thyroid artery may seem like they can clearly be safely transected; however, the distortion of tumor, retraction, or previous scar may lead the surgeon to mistakenly divide a branch of the RLN.
2. Identify the nerve low in the neck, well below the inferior thyroid artery, at the level of the lower pole of the thyroid gland, or below. This allows dissection of the nerve at a site where it is not tethered by its attachments to the larynx or its relation to the inferior thyroid artery.
3. Keep the nerve in view during the subsequent dissection of the thyroid gland from the larynx.
4. Minimize the use of powered dissection posterior to the thyroid gland.
5. Treat each parathyroid gland as though it were the last one.
6. Autograft any parathyroid glands that have questionable viability.

The use of nerve stimulators and laryngeal muscle action potential monitors has been investigated as a tool

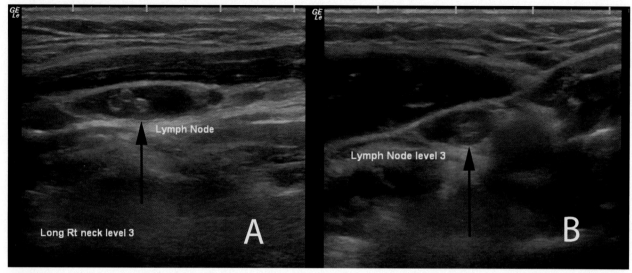

FIGURE 4 • Ultrasound examination of the right lateral cervical lymph nodes shows an abnormal right level 3 lymph node in the longitudinal (**A**) and transverse (**B**) images. The *arrows* denote the abnormal lymph node.

to try to limit or avoid nerve injuries. The data do not currently support the mandatory use of these devices. However, many experienced surgeons now routinely use a nerve monitoring system intraoperatively.

Management of Complications

Nerve Injury

The main nerves adjacent to the thyroid gland that can be deliberately or inadvertently affected include the recurrent laryngeal nerve immediately adjacent to the thyroid and the external branch of the superior laryngeal nerve. Damage to the RLN causes unilateral paralysis of the muscles that controls the ipsilateral vocal cord. Unilateral RLN injury changes the voice substantially in most patients, and also significantly affects swallowing. Bilateral RLN injury causes paralysis of both cords and usually results in a very limited airway lumen at the cords. These patients usually have a normal-sounding speaking voice, but severe limitations on inhalation velocity because of upper airway obstruction.

RLN paresis is usually temporary, and resolves over days to months. If a unilateral paresis proves to be permanent, then palliation of the cord immobility and voice changes can be achieved with vocal cord injection or laryngoplasty. These procedures stiffen and medialize the paralyzed cord, in order to allow the contralateral cord to appose the paralyzed cord during speech. If both cords are affected, then the palliative procedures are more limited and involve creating an adequate airway for ventilation; improvements in voice quality are not likely, as there is no muscular control of the cord function.

About 10% of patients have some evidence of RLN paresis after thyroidectomy, however, this resolves in most patients. About 1% or fewer patients have permanent nerve injury when total thyroidectomy is performed by experienced surgeons.

The external branch of the superior laryngeal nerve (EBSLN) courses adjacent to the superior pole vessels of the thyroid gland, before separating to penetrate the cricopharyngeus muscle fascia at it superior–posterior aspect. The nerve supplies motor innervation of the inferior constrictor muscles of the larynx. Damage to this nerve changes the ability of the larynx to control high-pressure phonation, such as high-pitched singing or yelling.

To avoid damaging this nerve, the dissection of the upper pole vessels should proceed from a space where the nerve is safely sequestered under the cricopharyngeal fascia, to the superior vessels themselves, thus safely separating the nerve from the tissue to be divided.

Parathyroid Gland Injury

The parathyroid glands are small, delicate structures that share a blood supply with the thyroid gland. Their size and fragility expose them to damage during thyroidectomy. Avoidance of permanent hypoparathyroidism is far more desirable than treatment of it. This can be accomplished by preservation of the parathyroid glands on their native blood supply, or autografting of parathyroid tissue to a muscular bed. If the parathyroid glands cannot be preserved on their native blood supply, then transfer of the gland to a convenient grafting site can maintain function. For normal parathyroid glands, transfer to the sternocleidomastoid muscle provides a convenient vascular bed for autograft. The parathyroid gland must be reduced to pieces that can survive on the diffusion of nutrients temporarily, while neovascular in-growth occurs over several weeks.

The symptoms of hypoparathyroidism are those of severe hypocalcemia. Patients have numbness and

TABLE 1. Key Technical Steps and Potential Pitfalls for Total Thyroidectomy

Key Technical Steps

1. Low collar incision within or parallel to natural skin lines.
2. Raise subplatysmal flaps.
3. Separate the strap muscles in the midline exposing the thyroid gland.
4. If using an intraoperative nerve monitoring system, expose the vagus nerve in the carotid sheath and confirm function of the monitor by stimulating the vagus nerve prior to exposure of the recurrent laryngeal nerve.
5. Separate the lateral border of the thyroid gland from the strap muscles and carotid sheath; enter the avascular plane medial to the upper pole without damaging the cricothyroid muscle fascia; isolate and divide the upper pole vessels.
6. Rotate the thyroid lobe anteriorly and identify the recurrent laryngeal nerve in the tracheoesophageal groove using the nerve monitoring system if available; dissect craniad along the nerve, separating from the thyroid, up to the cricothyroid muscle.
7. Divide the ligament of Berry anterior to the passage of the nerve into the larynx.
8. Separate the thyroid posterior surface from the trachea.
9. Identify and inspect the parathyroid glands; reimplant them if their vascularity is in question.
10. If using the nerve monitor, confirm unchanged function of the vagus nerve-recurrent laryngeal nerve-vocalis muscle system by stimulating the vagus nerve.

Potential Pitfalls

- Injury to the recurrent laryngeal or superior laryngeal nerves.
- Injury to the parathyroid glands.
- Tumor invasion into surrounding structures, such as larynx, trachea, esophagus, carotid sheath, or strap muscles.

tingling in the distal extremities and around the mouth or tongue in the earliest phases. For mild hypocalcemia with tingling, oral calcium supplements (calcium carbonate, 500 to 1,500 mg po, two to four times daily) are often sufficient to resolve the hypocalcemia. If supplementation beyond this level is necessary (as it is for most patients with severe hypocalcemia), then the addition of supplemental vitamin D (calcitriol 0.25 to 1.0 µg daily) increases the gastrointestinal absorption of calcium. Hypocalcemia not controlled by oral supplements, or accompanied by severe symptoms such as muscle cramping, is best managed by intravenous calcium administration. Intravenous calcium gluconate is the only option for intravenous calcium supplementation (calcium chloride should never be used).

Permanent hypoparathyroidism requires lifelong support with calcium supplements and vitamin D analogues. Missing doses of the supplements will usually produce symptoms, of varying severity, and which, while manageable, are often quite bothersome for patients.

In this clinical scenario, under general anesthesia, neck exploration shows a hard mass in the right lobe of the thyroid gland without evident extrathyroidal invasion. There are firm, small lymph nodes in level 6 adjacent to the thyroid gland; these are removed with the surrounding soft tissue. Both lower parathyroid glands are surrounded by abnormal lymph nodes, and so they are removed, minced into small pieces, and reimplanted into the right sternocleidomastoid muscle. The upper parathyroid glands are preserved on the native blood supply. The right level 2-3-4 lymph nodes are dissected free of the jugular vein with careful attention to preservation of the right vagus nerve

(cranial nerve X), phrenic nerve, spinal accessory nerve (cranial nerve XI), and hypoglossal nerve. The ansa cervicalis nerve and the omohyoid muscle are divided. At the completion of all dissection, EMG assessment of the bilateral vagus-recurrent laryngeal-vocalis muscle complex shows normal EMG signal with stimulation of the vagus nerve. There is no evidence of lymphatic leak, and no drain is placed.

Adjuvant Therapy

Papillary thyroid cancer typically retains the capability of concentrating iodine. This feature can be exploited by delivering radioactive iodine in doses that will damage the cells, and cause death over a period of several weeks. Iodine is also taken up by salivary gland tissue and gastric mucosa, and is excreted mainly through the kidneys. The radioiodine is most efficiently concentrated in the thyroid tissue when the TSH is elevated, stimulating any remaining normal thyroid cells or thyroid cancer cells, to concentrate the radioiodine. The patient can be prepared with elevated TSH either by removing the thyroid gland and leaving them free of exogenous thyroid hormone, or by administering exogenous recombinant TSH. Either approach appears to be effective in the adjuvant setting. Adjuvant radioiodine is typically reserved for patients with a moderate or high risk of recurrence.

After radioiodine therapy is completed, if indicated, or immediately if exogenous TSH is administered, the patient is treated with exogenous levothyroxine to replace their thyroid function, and to suppress their endogenous TSH. The degree of TSH suppression is determined by the risk of recurrence of the thyroid cancer. Low-risk patients can have the TSH maintained at about the lower limit of normal. Higher-risk patients may have the TSH suppressed further for several years.

In this scenario, the patient's postoperative recovery is unremarkable, with mild hypocalcemia for 1 week, and normocalcemia by the 2nd week follow-up. The voice is initially scratchy, but this resolves within 5 days. The final pathology shows a 35-mm papillary thyroid carcinoma with tall cell features, confined to the thyroid gland with negative margins. In level 6, 6 of 15 lymph nodes contain papillary thyroid carcinoma. In the level 2-3-4 dissection, 4 of 22 lymph nodes are involved. Because of the lymph node involvement, she subsequently receives 30 mCi of radioiodine under thyrogen stimulation. Her posttreatment radioiodine scan shows some uptake in the central neck consistent with residual thyroid tissue and no evidence of metastases. Her thyroglobulin at that time is <0.5 ng/mL. She will have regular follow-up including physical examination, thyroglobulin measurement, and ultrasound examination of the neck.

TAKE HOME POINTS

- Assessment of a central neck mass likely to originate in the thyroid gland should include ultrasound and possibly fine needle aspiration cytology.
- Papillary thyroid carcinoma has an excellent prognosis; thorough initial treatment including operation limits the long-term likelihood of recurrence and need for repeat therapy.
- Ultrasound evaluation of the lateral neck lymph nodes is important prior to operation in order to define the necessary extent of operation.
- Operation should include total thyroidectomy for most patients and compartmental dissection of any involved lymph node basins.

- Adjuvant radioiodine and TSH suppression with levothyroxine decrease the recurrence rate of papillary thyroid cancer.
- Follow-up management and surveillance algorithms are risk-based, and include monitoring of serum thyroglobulin levels and cervical ultrasound examination.

SELECTED READINGS

Cibas ES, Ali SZ. The Bethesda system for reporting thyroid cytopathology. Thyroid. 2009;19(11):1159–1165.

Cooper DS, Doherty GM, Haugen BR, et al. Revised American Thyroid Association management guidelines for patients with thyroid nodules and differentiated thyroid cancer.[see comment]. Thyroid. 2009;19(11):1167–1214.

Doherty GM. Prophylactic central lymph node dissection: continued controversy.[comment]. Oncology. 2010;23(7):603, 608.

Dralle H, Sekulla C, Lorenz K, et al. Intraoperative monitoring of the recurrent laryngeal nerve in thyroid surgery. World J Surg. 2008;32(7):1358–1366.

Hughes DT, White ML, Miller BS, et al. Influence of prophylactic central lymph node dissection on postoperative thyroglobulin levels and radioiodine treatment in papillary thyroid cancer. Surgery. 2010;148(6):1100–1106; discussion 1006–1107.

Kouvaraki MA, Lee JE, Shapiro SE, et al. Preventable reoperations for persistent and recurrent papillary thyroid carcinoma. Surgery. 2004;136(6):1183–1191.

Kouvaraki MA, Shapiro SE, Fornage BD, et al. Role of preoperative ultrasonography in the surgical management of patients with thyroid cancer. Surgery. 2003;134(6):946–954; discussion 954–945.

Olson JA Jr, DeBenedetti MK, Baumann DS, et al. Parathyroid autotransplantation during thyroidectomy. Results of long-term follow-up.[see comment]. Ann Surg. 1996;223(5):472–478; discussion 478–480.

60 Medullary Thyroid Cancer

BARBARA ZAREBCZAN and HERBERT CHEN

Presentation

A 27-year-old female presents to her primary care physician with a complaint of an enlarging neck mass. She first noticed this mass 2 months ago and comes in concerned because it has grown considerably larger. She denies having dyspnea, difficulty speaking, and dysphagia. She has no known medical problems and is currently not on any medications. She is adopted and does not know her family history. On physical examination, her vital signs are normal. She has a palpable, nontender neck mass, approximately 3 cm in diameter, to the left of midline just below the cricothyroid cartilage. No other masses are palpable, and the remainder of her exam is within normal limits.

Differential Diagnosis

A nontender neck mass has a wide differential that can be divided into three categories: neoplasms, congenital lesions, and inflammatory masses. Neoplasms presenting as a neck mass can be benign, such as lipomas and benign thyroid nodules, but in an adult, a neck mass should be considered a malignancy until proven otherwise. Some of the most common malignancies of the neck include thyroid cancers, laryngeal carcinomas, and lymphomas. Congenital masses can present at any age and include thyroglossal duct cysts and branchial cleft cysts, which usually become apparent when they become infected. Other congenital neck lesions include lymphangiomas, dermoid cysts, and thymic cysts. Enlarged lymph nodes resulting from a viral or bacterial illness are the most common inflammatory masses encountered.

Workup

The patient undergoes further evaluation of her neck mass with an ultrasound that demonstrates a 3-cm nodule in the left lobe **(Figure 1)** and suspicious lymph nodes in the central neck and near the left carotid artery. At this time, a fine needle aspiration (FNA) is performed and returns as being suspicious for medullary thyroid cancer.

The patient undergoes laboratory testing, which demonstrate an elevated serum calcitonin of 9,091 pg/mL (normal <5 pg/mL), an elevated carcinoembryonic antigen (CEA) level of 320 ng/L (normal <2.5 ng/mL), and a normal calcium of 9.3 mg/dL. The patient also undergoes RET gene testing, which comes back positive for a germline mutation. Given this finding, the patient undergoes additional testing to evaluate for tumors associated with MEN-2. Her parathyroid hormone, plasma normetanephrine, and plasma and urinary metanephrine levels are all normal.

Given the findings of suspicious lymph nodes on her ultrasound as well as her highly elevated calcitonin level, the patient undergoes a metastatic workup. Neck CT demonstrates the previously seen nodule and enlarged lymph nodes **(Figure 2A,B)**. A CT scan of her chest and abdomen demonstrates no metastatic disease.

Diagnosis and Treatment

Medullary thyroid cancer (MTC) represents 3% to 10% of all thyroid cancers. Similar to other thyroid cancers, many MTCs present as thyroid nodules, which should be evaluated with an ultrasound and FNA biopsy **(Figure 3)**.

MTCs arise from the parafollicular C cells of the thyroid, which produce calcitonin, a neuroendocrine tumor marker that is helpful in diagnosing the disease, as well as identifying recurrence. Approximately 50% of MTCs can also secrete CEA, which should also be obtained during preoperative evaluation. If the patient has evidence of lymph node metastases or a calcitonin level >400 pg/mL, a metastatic workup including CT scans of the neck, chest, and abdomen should be performed.

The majority of MTCs occur sporadically, but up to 20% are due to germ-line mutations in the RET proto-oncogene. Hereditary MTCs occur in multiple endocrine neoplasia (MEN) syndrome 2A and 2B and in familial MTC. According to the American Thyroid Association guidelines, all patients diagnosed with MTC should undergo RET gene testing. Screening for hyperparathyroidism and pheochromocytoma should also be performed, as a pheochromocytoma needs to be resected prior to thyroid resection.

The mainstay of treatment for MTC remains surgery. For patients with no evidence of lymph node and distant metastases, a total thyroidectomy and prophylactic central neck (level VI) dissection are recommended

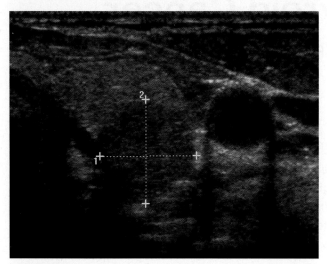

FIGURE 1 • Ultrasound demonstrating a 3-cm, hypoechoic left thyroid nodule.

by most surgeons. For those patients with lymph node metastases limited to the central neck compartment, a total thyroidectomy and central neck dissection are performed. Patients with suspected metastases to the lateral neck compartments should undergo a total thyroidectomy and central neck dissection, as well as a modified lateral neck (levels II, III, IV, V) dissection.

Surgical Approach

A total thyroidectomy begins with a transverse incision made just below the cricoid cartilage, ideally in an existing neck crease **(Table 1)**. In order to facilitate a modified radical neck dissection, this incision may be extended laterally or a hockey-stick incision may be made to allow for wider exposure. The total thyroidectomy should be completed in the usual manner with care taken to avoid injury to the recurrent laryngeal nerves and parathyroid glands.

Once the thyroid has been removed, attention can be turned to completing the central neck dissection. The recurrent laryngeal nerves are dissected out and all the fatty tissue between the carotid sheaths from the hyoid bone superiorly to the brachiocephalic vessels inferiorly, including the thymus, is removed.

The lateral neck dissection is then begun by dissecting the anterior triangle, containing level II, III, and IV lymph nodes. The submandibular gland is retracted superiorly, and the inferior margins of the digastric and omohyoid muscles are skeletonized defining the superior aspect of dissection. The internal jugular vein is exposed and the lateral branches are ligated or sealed, defining the medial border of dissection. The sternocleidomastoid muscle can then be retracted laterally and the tissue on its posterior surface can be dissected, with care taken to identify and preserve the spinal accessory nerve. Attention can then be turned to dissection of the posterior triangle, containing level V lymph nodes. Once the spinal accessory nerve has been identified, the posterior border of the sternocleidomastoid muscle can then be skeletonized down to the trapezius muscle, defining the lateral border of

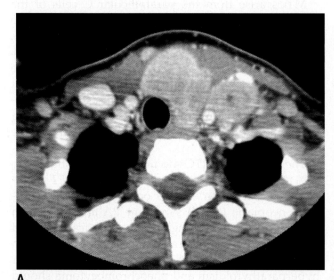

A

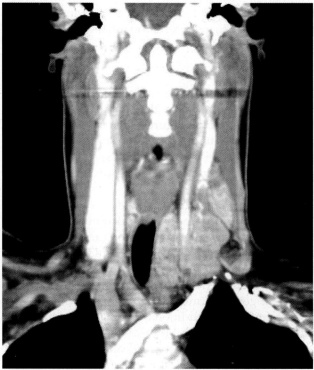

B

FIGURE 2 • **A:** CT of the neck with a cross-sectional image demonstrating a large, left thyroid nodule and left lateral lymph nodes. **B:** Coronal views of the same CT, redemonstrating the thyroid nodule and lymph nodes surrounding the left internal jugular vein and the carotid artery.

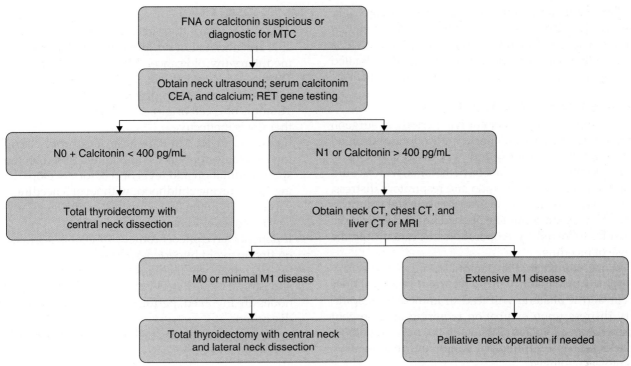

FIGURE 3 •Chart explains the workup of a patient with suspected medullary thyroid cancer, beginning with an ultrasound and FNA, followed by measurement of calcitonin and CEA levels. Operative management is based on the extent of nodal and metastatic disease.

dissection. The dissection proceeds down to the clavicle, which defines the inferior border of resection. Once the fatty tissue containing the lateral neck lymph nodes has been dissected free from all adjacent structures, it can be removed en bloc.

After the lymph node tissue has been removed, if required, a drain can be placed in the lateral neck. The medial aspect of the sternocleidomastoid muscle is then reapproximated to the lateral border of the sternothyroid muscle with interrupted sutures. The

platysma is reapproximated in the same manner. Finally, the skin is closed with a running subcuticular stitch.

Special Intraoperative Considerations

Due to the extent of the lymph node dissection, care should be taken to identify the thoracic duct as it enters the neck on the left. Most commonly, the thoracic duct empties into the left subclavian vein at its junction with the left internal jugular vein. Surgeons should be aware

---

TABLE 1. Key Technical Steps and Potential Pitfalls to Total Thyroidectomy with Central Neck Dissection and Modified Lateral Neck Dissection

Key Technical Steps

1. Make a transverse incision just below the cricoid cartilage and extend laterally or make a hockey-stick incision to facilitate lateral neck dissection.
2. Perform total thyroidectomy.
3. Central neck dissection is performed by dissecting out the recurrent laryngeal nerves and removing all fibroadipose tissue between the two carotid sheaths from the hyoid bone superiorly to the brachiocephalic vessels inferiorly.
4. Lymph node tissue from the anterior and posterior triangles, defined by the submandibular gland superiorly, the internal jugular vein medially, trapezius muscle laterally, and clavicle inferiorly is removed.
5. The medial aspect of the sternocleidomastoid muscle is reapproximated to the sternothyroid muscle, followed by the platysma, and then the skin.

Potential Pitfalls

- Injury to recurrent laryngeal or superior laryngeal nerves.
- Injury to or excision of parathyroid glands.
- Injury to the brachial plexus or phrenic nerves.

of aberrant ductal anatomy, with patients having a right thoracic duct, draining into the right subclavian vein. If the thoracic duct is inadvertently injured and a chyle leak is identified intraoperatively, it should be ligated with either nonabsorbable sutures and/or hemoclips.

Postoperative Management

In the immediate postoperative period, a surgeon should be aware of potential complications associated with total thyroidectomy and neck dissection. One of these complications is that of a hematoma, which could result in tracheal compression and respiratory distress. In the event of a hematoma causing tracheal compression, the incision should be opened immediately at the bedside, followed by reoperation to evaluate for the cause of bleeding.

As mentioned in the potential intraoperative pitfalls, inadvertent injury to the recurrent laryngeal does occur and if bilateral will lead to immediate respiratory distress upon extubation requiring an emergent tracheostomy. Unilateral injury of the nerve results in hoarseness and requires evaluation and treatment by an otolaryngologist.

Transient hypoparathyroidism, due to injury or removal of one or more parathyroid glands, is another complication of thyroidectomy and neck dissection, which requires short-term calcium supplementation. Rarely, this becomes permanent requiring, lifelong vitamin D and calcium supplementation.

Another complication of total thyroidectomy and neck dissection is that of a chyle leak, identified as a milky, white discharge high in triglycerides. Initially, this is managed by placing the patient on a fat-free diet, antibiotics, and application of a pressure dressing. If the chyle leak does not resolve, surgical exploration with ligation of the thoracic duct or application of a biologic sealant may be necessary.

Patients suffering from medullary thyroid cancer will also require long-term surveillance consisting of measurements of calcitonin and/or CEA levels every 6 months for 1 year and then annually thereafter. If the patient were to have an elevation in calcitonin and/or CEA levels, an ultrasound of the neck should be performed to evaluate for recurrent local disease.

Case Conclusion

The patient undergoes a successful total thyroidectomy with central and modified left lateral neck dissection. She is discharged on postoperative day 1 on thyroid hormone replacement. At 6 months, her calcitonin level is 3 pg/mL and her CEA is 0.5 ng/mL. At her 1-year visit, her calcitonin and her CEA levels are unchanged.

TAKE HOME POINTS

- 75% of medullary thyroid cancers are sporadic, and 25% are inherited in syndromes such as familial medullary thyroid cancer, MEN 2A, and MEN 2B.
- Tumors secrete calcitonin, CEA, serotonin, ACTH, calcitonin gene-related peptide (CGRP).
- Tumor is of C cell origin, so radioactive iodine therapy is ineffective.
- If patients are RET mutation carriers, prophylactic total thyroidectomy is recommended based on the specific mutation and level of risk for developing MTC during childhood, with level 3 needing surgery within the first 6 months of life, level 2 by age 5, and level 1 between ages 5 and 10.
- If patients have pheochromocytoma, it is operated on first to avoid hypertensive crisis.
- Surgical treatment includes total thyroidectomy and central neck dissection; if lateral neck lymph nodes are involved, perform modified lateral neck dissection.
- Long-term surveillance includes measurement of calcitonin and CEA.

SUGGESTED READINGS

American Thyroid Association Guidelines Task Force; Kloos R, Eng C, Evans D, et al. Medullary thyroid cancer: management guidelines of the American Thyroid Association. Thyroid. 2009;19:565–612.

Duh Q-Y, Clark OH, Kebebew E. Atlas of Endocrine Surgical Techniques. Philadelphia, PA: Saunders Elsevier, 2010.

Lal G, Clark OH. In F. Brunicardi, ed. Schwartz's Manual of Surgery. New York, NY: McGraw-Hill, 2006:943–988.

Pinchot S, Chen H, Sippel R. Incisions and exposure of the neck for thyroidectomy and parathyroidectomy. Operat Tech Gen Surg. 2008;10:63–76.

Shaha A. Complications of neck dissection for thyroid cancer. Ann Surg Oncol. 2008;15:397–399.

Sippel R, Kunnimalaiyaan M, Chen H. Current management of medullary thyroid cancer. Oncologist. 2008;13:539–547.

61 Primary Hyperparathyroidism

LESLIE S. WU and JULIE ANN SOSA

Presentation

A 75-year-old woman is brought to the emergency department from a nursing home with a 5-day history of worsening lethargy and confusion. From prior hospital records, her past medical history is notable for nephrolithiasis, gastroesophageal reflux disease, and hypertension. Her medications include hydrochlorothiazide, metoprolol, omeprazole, and aspirin. Physical examination reveals a frail-appearing woman, who is arousable to voice, and oriented only to person. She is afebrile and normotensive but mildly tachycardic with a heart rate of 100 beats per minute. Her neurologic exam is nonfocal. The remainder of her examination is significant only for poor skin turgor and dry mucous membranes. Laboratory studies are notable for a mildly elevated white blood cell count 11.2 thou/υL (normal, 4.2 to 9.9 thou/υL), mild hemoconcentration with hematocrit 42% (normal, 38% to 50%), blood urea nitrogen (BUN) 25 mg/dL (normal, 6 to 19 mg/dL), serum creatinine 1.3 mg/dL (normal, 0.5 to 1.3 mg/dL), serum calcium 14.7 mg/dL (normal, 8.6 to 10.4 mg/dL), and albumin 4.3 g/dL (normal, 3.4 to 5.4 g/dL). Urinalysis of cloudy urine is notable for pyuria, positive nitrites, and positive leukocyte esterase.

The patient is admitted to the hospital with a urinary tract infection and hypercalcemia. She is hydrated with intravenous crystalloid fluid and treated with the appropriate antibiotics. There is subsequent improvement of her mental status and a decline in calcium level. Additional laboratory evaluation is obtained, revealing an intact parathyroid hormone (iPTH) level of 250 pg/mL (normal, 10 to 65 pg/mL).

Differential Diagnosis

The most common reason for hypercalcemia in the outpatient setting is primary hyperparathyroidism (HPT), while hypercalcemia in the inpatient population often is secondary to malignancy. Population-based estimates reveal an overall incidence of approximately 25 per 100,000 in the general population, with 50,000 new cases identified annually. The peak incidence is in the fifth and sixth decades of life, with a female to male ratio of 3:1. Some studies have estimated the overall prevalence of primary HPT in the elderly at 2% to 3%, with approximately 200 cases per 100,000 population. Making the correct diagnosis requires careful clinical evaluation coupled with biochemical testing. After a thorough history and physical examination, laboratory measurements of fasting serum calcium, iPTH, creatinine, and vitamin D levels should be performed to determine if the hypercalcemia is non–parathyroid-mediated (in which serum iPTH levels are suppressed appropriately) or parathyroid-mediated (in which serum iPTH levels are elevated inappropriately). Etiologies of non–parathyroid-mediated hypercalcemia include malignancy (a parathyroid hormone-related protein, or PTHrP, level may be elevated), granulomatous diseases, endocrinopathies, medications, and immobilization. Parathyroid-mediated hypercalcemia is due to HPT, benign familial hypocalciuric hypercalcemia (BFHH), or lithium therapy. Primary HPT generally is caused by a benign, solitary parathyroid adenoma in 80% to 85% of patients. Approximately 5% of patients harbor two distinct adenomas ("double adenoma"), 15% to 20% have multigland parathyroid hyperplasia, and fewer than 1% of patients have parathyroid carcinoma (Table 1).

Workup

With the advent of routine serum calcium screening, the typical presentation of primary HPT has changed from a severe, debilitating illness to a disease with subtle symptoms and physiologic derangements. Common signs include nephrolithiasis, nephrocalcinosis, osteopenia, and osteoporosis; rarely, pancreatitis and peptic ulcer disease will occur. Hypertension frequently is present in patients with primary HPTH, and it appears to be most closely correlated with the degree of renal impairment seen in patients with hypercalcemia. In addition, there are many subtle abnormalities associated with primary HPT, including decreased cognitive function, anxiety and/or depression, lethargy/fatigue, myalgias and arthralgias, constipation, and urinary symptoms, such as increased thirst and urinary frequency (Table 2).

297

TABLE 1. Differential Diagnosis of Hypercalcemia

Parathyroid-Mediated	Non–Parathyroid-Mediated

Primary HPT
  Parathyroid adenoma (85%)
  Parathyroid hyperplasia (15%)
  Parathyroid carcinoma (<1%)
	Malignancy-associated hypercalcemia
	  Local osteolytic hypercalcemia
	  Humoral hypercalcemia of malignancy (PTHrP, calcitriol)

Secondary/tertiary HPT Benign familial hypocalciuric hypercalcemia Lithium therapy	Granulomatous disease (sarcoidosis, tuberculosis) Endocrinopathies (hyperthyroidism, adrenal insufficiency) Drugs (thiazides, vitamin D, calcium) Immobilization

The diagnosis of primary HPT typically is made by biochemical evidence of an elevated serum calcium concentration, usually in conjunction with an elevated or inappropriately high normal serum iPTH. The clinical entity termed "normocalcemic primary HPT" recently has emerged. It appears to be an early form of primary HPT in which patients have serum calcium levels in the high-normal range associated with an elevated serum PTH level and bone loss. When these patients are symptomatic, surgical intervention is appropriate. Approximately half of patients with primary HPT have hypophosphatemia. However, in the presence of significant renal impairment, serum phosphate levels may be elevated. Because of the effect of PTH on bicarbonate excretion in the kidney, patients with primary HPT often have a hyperchloremic metabolic acidosis. To distinguish patients with BFHH from those with primary HPT, a 24-hour urinary calcium excretion study should be performed; this measurement

TABLE 2. Symptoms and Associated Conditions in Patients with Primary Hyperparathyroidism

Symptoms
Weakness, exhaustion, fatigue
Bone pain, back pain, joint pain
Polyuria, nocturia, polydipsia
Loss of appetite, nausea, dyspepsia
Memory loss, depression, anxiety
Associated conditions
Weight loss
Bone fracture, joint swelling, gout
Nephrolithiasis, hematuria from passage of renal calculus
Gastric ulcer, duodenal ulcer, pancreatitis
Hypertension

is low (<40 mg per specimen; normal, 25 to 300 mg per specimen) in the setting of BFHH, and normal or elevated in primary HPT. Approximately 10% to 40% of primary HPT patients have elevated levels of alkaline phosphatase, which indicates some degree of increased bone turnover. Although osteitis fibrosis cystica, the classic form of parathyroid bone disease, is rarely seen today, even patients with mild disease can have biochemical or histologic evidence of bone involvement. Dual-energy x-ray absorption (DEXA) scanning of the lumbar spine, hip, and forearm has become the standard method for assessing bone density to diagnose osteoporosis in the setting of primary HPT.

Imaging modalities for the purposes of localization should be employed only after establishing the biochemical diagnosis of primary HPT. Imaging studies can be sorted into noninvasive and invasive techniques. The noninvasive studies include the following: nuclear medicine scans, such as methoxyisobutylisonitrile (sestamibi) studies, which can be combined with single photon emission computed tomography (SPECT) imaging; ultrasound **(Figure 1)**; computed tomography (CT) scans; and magnetic resonance imaging (MRI). The noninvasive localization study of choice is dependent largely on the availability and quality of imaging modalities at each institution. There is evidence to suggest that the best studies are technetium (^{99m}Tc)-sestamibi scan with SPECT, which results in a three-dimensional reconstruction that can delineate the location of an enlarged parathyroid gland in 85% of cases, as well as ultrasound by an experienced ultrasonographer (or surgeon). There are emerging data to suggest that four-dimensional CT (4D CT) also might afford excellent localization **(Figure 2A,B)**. Invasive techniques usually are reserved for reoperative cases, and include angiography and venous sampling for PTH gradients. Recently, the rapid PTH assay has been used in the ultrasound and angiography suites, as well as the operating room. It yields real-time feedback and has become invaluable in the development of minimally invasive surgical techniques.

Diagnosis and Treatment

Parathyroidectomy is the only effective long-term treatment for HPT. There is universal agreement that patients with clear symptoms and signs associated with primary HPT should undergo parathyroid surgery. However, controversy still exists about the management of patients with "asymptomatic" primary HPT. In 1990 and 2002, the National Institutes of Health (NIH) convened consensus conferences to delineate the surgical indications in patients with both symptomatic and asymptomatic primary HPT **(Table 3)** In 2008, an international workshop on HPT convened to review and update previous recommendations. Guidelines

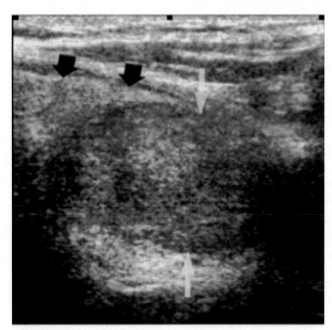

FIGURE 1 • Parathyroid adenoma. Sagittal ultrasound shows a parathyroid adenoma *(white arrows)* behind the lower pole of the right thyroid lobe *(black arrows)*.

also were created for the management of patients with asymptomatic primary HPT who did not undergo surgery, including biannual serum calcium, annual serum creatinine measurements, and annual bone density measurements. It has been suggested, however, that the NIH criteria for parathyroidectomy in asymptomatic patients are too limited, and that all patients with primary HPT should be referred for surgical therapy.

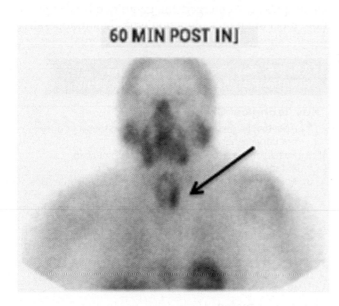

FIGURE 2A • Scintigraphic image from ^{99m}Tc-sestamibi depicting a left inferior parathyroid adenoma *(arrow)* in a patient with primary HPT.

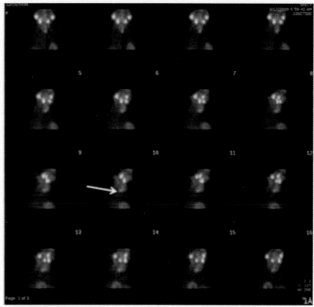

FIGURE 2B • Scintigraphic images from sestamibi single-photon emission tomography of the same patient presented in Figure 3A depicting multiple rotational tomographic planes. The posterior location of the parathyroid adenoma *(arrow)* is consistent with an ectopic superior parathyroid gland in an inferior retroesophageal location.

There is no long-term effective pharmacologic treatment for primary HPT. There are several pharmacologic agents that can transiently lower the serum calcium level **(Table 4)**. These can limit further loss of bone by reducing the activation of new remodeling units in the skeleton. Estrogen replacement, salmon calcitonin, bisphosphonates, and more recently, calcimimetics (cinacalcet) have been used to treat primary HPT in patients with complex comorbid medical conditions who either are unwilling or considered unfit for surgery. In addition, glucocorticoids and calcimimetics can be employed during refractory hypercalcemia of metastatic parathyroid

TABLE 3. Surgical Indications in Patients with Primary Hyperparathyroidism

All symptomatic patients, including those with significant bone, renal, gastrointestinal, or neuromuscular symptoms typical of primary HPT
In otherwise asymptomatic patients:
• Elevation of serum calcium by 1 mg/dL or more above the normal range (i.e., >11.5 mg/dL in most laboratories)
• Decreased creatinine clearance (reduced to <60 mL/min)
• Significant reduction in bone density of more than 2.5 standard deviations below peak bone mass at any measured site (i.e., T-score < –2.5)
• Consistent follow-up is not possible or is undesirable because of coexisting medical conditions.
Age younger than 50 y.

carcinoma. However, these therapies are not definitive, and with adequate preoperative parathyroid localization, high-volume parathyroid surgeons may employ minimally invasive techniques with excellent outcomes.

Parathyroidectomy has a high rate of success (>95%) with few complications when performed by experienced parathyroid surgeons. Complications associated with parathyroidectomy include recurrent laryngeal nerve injury, transient or persistent hypocalcemia, postoperative hemorrhage, and pneumothorax. Despite this, the specific operative approach has continued to evolve through the influence of a number of synergistic factors, including improvements in preoperative localization studies, rapid intraoperative PTH measurements, and adjunctive surgical technologies such as handheld gamma detection probes and improved videoscopic equipment. The net result has influenced patient selection, such

that the majority of parathyroid explorations are very well tolerated. However, a small fraction of these explorations remain challenging, especially those with atypical gland location or previously operated fields. Therefore, any surgeon performing parathyroidectomy must be facile with standard four-gland parathyroid exploration. In fact, experienced parathyroid surgeons today achieve cure rates of up to 98% with both minimally invasive and conventional techniques.

Surgical Approach

The conventional technique for parathyroid exploration requires bilateral cervical access and four gland exploration. This operation is usually performed under general anesthesia, although it can be performed under bilateral regional superficial cervical block. The goal is to identify all normal and abnormal parathyroid glands, thus distinguishing single-gland from multigland disease. Patients who have a single parathyroid adenoma undergo curative resection once the gland is removed. In the instance of multigland hyperplasia, a subtotal parathyroidectomy (leaving a normal-sized remnant of one well-vascularized parathyroid gland *in situ*), or total cervical parathyroidectomy with immediate heterotopic autotransplantation of parathyroid tissue, typically into the brachioradialis muscle in the forearm, is required **(Table 5)**.

The conventional approach has been challenged with increasing frequency in recent years, and minimally invasive parathyroid exploration now is performed routinely in a growing number of institutions. Three techniques have emerged: image-guided local exploration, most often in conjunction with the intraoperative

---

TABLE 4. Pharmacologic Treatment for Primary Hyperparathyroidism

Pamidronate/Bisphosphonates

Dosage	60–90 mg as a single dose
Adverse effects	Leukopenia, fever, myalgia
Contraindications	Hypersensitivity
Special points	Onset 1–2 d with long half-life

Chronic Oral Sodium Phosphates

Dosage	1–3 g daily
Adverse effects	Extraskeletal calcifications
Contraindications	Serum calcium >12 mg/dL, serum phosphorus >3 mg/dL
Special points	Not indicated in acute hypercalcemia

Calcitonin

Dosage	4–8 U/kg every 6–12 h
Adverse effects	Nausea, glucose intolerance
Contraindications	Allergic reactions
Special points	Effective within 2 h; can be used to lower serum calcium while awaiting effect of bisphosphonates

Furosemide

Dosage	20–40 mg up to 3 times daily
Adverse effects	Electrolyte imbalance
Contraindications	Anuria, hepatic coma, hypovolemia
Special points	Hydration is essential

Cinacalcet[a]

Dosage	30–90 mg daily
Adverse effects	Nausea, vomiting, diarrhea
Contraindications	Hypersensitivity, hypocalcemia
Special points	

[a]Off-label use in primary HPTH except parathyroid carcinoma

---

TABLE 5. Key Technical Steps and Potential Pitfalls to Parathyroidectomy

Key Technical Steps

1. Anesthesia: general endotracheal anesthesia or anterior cervical nerve block.
2. Positioning: semi-Fowler position with neck in extension.
3. Kocher incision and development of subplatysmal flaps.
4. Early identification of recurrent laryngeal nerve.
5. Identification of abnormal parathyroid gland(s); careful excision without breaching parathyroid capsule.
6. Intraoperative rapid iPTH monitoring if available.
7. Meticulous hemostasis within operative field.
8. Neck incision closure.
9. Overnight hospital observation or outpatient discharge to home.

Potential Pitfalls

- Injury to the recurrent laryngeal nerve.
- Injury to normal parathyroid glands.
- Inability to localize or identify abnormal parathyroid gland.

rapid PTH assay; intraoperative gamma probe-guided exploration after sestamibi injection; and image-guided video parathyroidectomy.

Image-guided local exploration has emerged as the most commonly employed minimally invasive technique. It is dependent on high-quality preoperative imaging, usually in the form of sestamibi scans, ultrasound studies, or, less commonly, 4D CT. This technique is appropriate even for patients who have had multiple previous explorations, as long as the preoperative imaging is adequate. When performed by an experienced parathyroid surgeon well-versed in minimally invasive techniques, this surgical procedure can be performed on an outpatient basis and can avoid the increased risks associated with bilateral neck exploration and general anesthesia.

Gamma probe exploration involves preoperative administration of ^{99m}Tc sestamibi to localize the abnormal parathyroid gland. The probe is then used in the operating room to find the area of increased radioactivity. In addition, the gamma probe can be used to measure radioactivity after tumor extraction to confirm the adequacy of resection. Although this technique has not gained widespread acceptance, the curative rates are comparable to the previously described technique.

Image-guided video parathyroidectomy has been employed by several investigators. Like other minimally invasive techniques, preoperative imaging is required to locate the adenoma. The procedure usually requires general anesthesia with or without carbon-dioxide insufflation to aid the dissection. There may be very select patients in whom this technique is indicated; however, this modality has not assumed a dominant role in parathyroid surgery in the United States.

Regardless of the chosen technique of parathyroidectomy, the key steps remain constant. Parathyroidectomy can be performed under general anesthesia or under anterior superficial cervical block with mild sedation. Proper positioning of the patient on the operating table is of paramount importance. The patient should be placed in a semi-Fowler position with the patient's neck extended dorsally to provide optimal access to the anterior neck. The arms of the patient should lie alongside the body to allow the surgeon and assistant to stand on both sides of the neck. All appropriate pressure points should be padded for protection. A symmetric Kocher incision is made, preferentially in a natural skin crease, approximately 3 to 4 cm cranially to the suprasternal notch. Flaps are developed in the subplatysmal plane, and dissected upward to the level of the thyroid cartilage and inferiorly to the suprasternal notch. Early identification of the recurrent laryngeal nerve expedites the exploration and is invaluable in protecting the nerve. Throughout the procedure, the operative field should be kept as bloodless as possible to prevent discoloring the parathyroid glands, which may impede their identification.

In patients with a solitary enlarged parathyroid gland, the vascular stalk of the tumor should be ligated and the tumor removed. During dissection of the parathyroid tumor, the capsule of the gland should not be opened to prevent seeding of parathyroid tissue, which can cause recurrent HPT due to parathyromatosis. In the case of multigland disease, a subtotal parathyroidectomy should be performed, leaving a well-vascularized remnant of approximately 30 mg *in situ*, which corresponds to the dimensions of a normal gland. An alternative to subtotal parathyroidectomy is total parathyroidectomy with immediate heterotopic autotransplantation of parathyroid tissue into the sternocleidomastoid muscle or the brachioradialis muscle of the nondominant forearm. This alternative procedure often is combined with cryopreservation of some parathyroid tissue. In multigland syndromic disease, the thymus should be removed bilaterally by a transcervical approach, as supernumerary parathyroids are located in the thymus in 3% to 5% of all patients.

In 1994, Irvin et al. reported the use of intraoperative PTH monitoring to determine when all hypersecreting parathyroid tissue has been removed. A decrease in intraoperative PTH from a baseline established prior to incision by over 50% following excision indicates sufficient removal of hyperfunctioning parathyroid tissue. When the PTH value fails to drop by 50%, this suggests that either the hyperfunctioning gland has not been removed or the patient has multigland disease. This modality may be employed as a surgical adjunct to confirm removal of all hypersecreting parathyroid tissue.

After completion of the parathyroidectomy, the operative field is checked thoroughly to achieve meticulous hemostasis. The raphe between the strap muscles and the platysma are reapproximated with absorbable suture. The skin is closed with optimal cosmesis.

Special Intraoperative Considerations

Parathyroid carcinoma is a rare cause of primary HPT, accounting for <1% of cases. Parathyroid carcinoma should be suspected in patients who demonstrate a rapid and sustained rise in both their serum calcium and iPTH levels, which can reach very high levels. A palpable neck mass sometimes may be appreciated, whereas a parathyroid adenoma is rarely, if ever, palpable on physical examination. In addition, sestamibi scan demonstrates a hyperintense focus that correlates with the lesion. If parathyroid carcinoma is suspected preoperatively or is found incidentally at the time of operation, *en bloc* resection with the ipsilateral thyroid lobe and central compartment lymph nodes is appropriate. Although these tumors are slow-growing, they have a high propensity to recur locally, and recurrent disease is difficult to eradicate. Patients with recurrent and metastatic disease often suffer from severe, debilitating hypercalcemia, control of which may involve palliative surgical resection and the use of drugs, including bisphosphonates and calcimimetics, to lower the serum calcium level. Chemotherapy and radiation therapy rarely are effective.

An enlarged parathyroid gland can remain undiscovered after routine exploration of the neck. It is of great importance to identify the normal parathyroid glands during the exploration, because a parathyroid missed at its normal localization can help the surgeon predict the site of the migrated enlarged parathyroid. One must identify correctly whether a superior or inferior gland is missing. In the circumstance in which three normal parathyroid glands have been identified but a superior gland is missing, the retroesophageal space should be explored, and the carotid sheath opened from the level of the carotid bifurcation to the base of the neck. In the situation in which three normal parathyroids have been identified but an inferior gland cannot be identified, the thymus on the side of the missing gland should be exposed. The retrosternal thymus can be mobilized by gentle traction on the thyrothymic ligament, and a transcervical thymectomy can be performed. If the missing inferior gland is not contained within the mediastinal portion of the thymus, an intrathyroidal parathyroid tumor should be considered. In the circumstance in which four normal parathyroid glands have been visualized but increased levels of intact PTH exclude another cause of hypercalcemia, one must consider a hypersecreting supernumerary parathyroid gland, most commonly located within the thymus. Bilateral thymectomy is indicated.

If the abnormal parathyroid tumor cannot be identified at the time of neck exploration and the patient has persistent HPT, additional imaging techniques may need to be employed to localize the ectopic gland. These modalities include thorough neck ultrasonography with potential fine needle aspiration identification of parathyroid tissue, neck and chest 4D CT or MRI studies, sestamibi scans, or selective jugular venous sampling for iPTH differential gradient. The operative note and pathology report from the patient's initial exploration should be reviewed, and the patient should undergo indirect laryngoscopy prior to remedial exploration to assure the integrity of the recurrent laryngeal nerves. Most missed glands (~40%) are located in eutopic positions. The thymus (~10%) and the anterior mediastinum (~13%) also are common locations for missed adenomas. Remedial parathyroidectomy is associated with increased risks of hypoparathyroidism and recurrent laryngeal nerve injury, and should be performed by experienced parathyroid surgeons.

Postoperative Management

For patients with severe bone disease, often evidenced by markedly elevated preoperative blood alkaline phosphatase levels, subsequent "bone hunger" often necessitates postoperative treatment with calcium supplementation and calcitriol. Normocalcemia generally is restored within the first 24 hours after a successful parathyroidectomy, and this may be accompanied by mild paresthesias circumorally and/or in the extremities. Symptoms may occur while the serum calcium level is within the normal range, reflecting the rapidity of change; however, this is usually transient and does not require treatment. Symptomatic hypocalcemia is more common in the elderly, in those with more severe preoperative primary HPT, or in patients with evidence of high-turnover bone disease. Restoration of normocalcemia can be achieved with calcitriol in combination with supplemental calcium. It is sufficient to maintain the serum calcium within the lower part of the reference range in order to control symptoms.

The rationale for parathyroidectomy is supported by evidence that in about 80% of patients, the clinical manifestations of primary HPT improve after successful parathyroidectomy. Thus, fatigue, weakness, polydipsia, polyuria, bone and joint pain, constipation, nausea, and depression regress in most patients. This is also true for associated conditions—renal stones usually stop forming, osteoporosis stabilizes or improves, pancreatitis becomes less likely, and peptic ulcer disease often resolves. In most patients, fracture risk and weakness also improve, and objective increase in muscular strength has been documented. In addition, neurocognitive impairments, confusion, spatial learning deficits, and depression have been shown to improve after successful operative intervention. Patients can resume a regular diet with or without calcium supplementation, and hypercalcemia is not a concern when these patients are hospitalized for other medical conditions.

Another important reason for recommending parathyroidectomy is that patients with primary HPT appear to be at risk for premature death primarily because of cardiovascular disease and cancer. More importantly, the increased death rate, even in patients with mild primary HPT, can be reversed by successful parathyroidectomy. Patients between the ages of 55 and 70 years seem to receive the greatest survival benefit.

Case Conclusion

After appropriate medical management of acute hypercalcemia, including intravenous hydration, bisphosphonate and furosemide therapy, the patient's serum calcium decreased to 10.8 mg/dL and her mental status returned to baseline. She underwent a sestamibi scan with SPECT, which revealed increased uptake in the right inferior anterior neck. After adequate medical evaluation, she underwent a minimally invasive parathyroidectomy with excision of a right inferior parathyroid adenoma. Intraoperative rapid PTH measurement documented adequate resection with a decline from her baseline of 250 to 35 pg/mL at ten minutes postresection. The patient returned home the following day with a normal serum calcium level of 9.8 mg/dL, and a postoperative regimen of oral calcium supplementation. At 6 months postoperatively, she remained eucalcemic and did not have any further episodes of nephrolithasis.

TAKE HOME POINTS

- In the outpatient setting, primary HPT is the most common reason for hypercalcemia. In the inpatient population, hypercalcemia often is secondary to malignancy
- Imaging modalities to localize hyperfunctioning abnormal parathyroid glands should be undertaken only after the diagnosis of primary HPT has been confirmed biochemically.
- An understanding of the embryology of the parathyroid glands and the ability to distinguish between a normal and an abnormal parathyroid gland are essential for successful parathyroid surgery. A systematic approach knowing the routine and unusual locations for parathyroid glands results in successful parathyroidectomy in more than 95% of patients with primary HPT.
- Permanent hypoparathyroidism, injury to the recurrent laryngeal nerves, and postoperative bleeding (with possible airway compromise) are some of the more serious complications that occur after parathyroidectomy.
- The increased death rate associated with primary HPT can be reversed by successful parathyroidectomy. In the hands of a high-volume parathyroid surgeon, cure rates of up to 98% have been documented with both minimally invasive and conventional techniques.

SUGGESTED READINGS

Adami S, Marcocci C, Gatti D. Epidemiology of primary hyperparathyroidism in Europe. J Bone Miner Res. 2002;17(S2):N18–N23.

Akerstrom G, Rudberg C, Grimelius L, et al. Causes of failed primary exploration and technical aspects of re-operation in primary hyperparathyroidism. World J Surg. 1992;16:562–568.

Bilezikian JP, Potts JT Jr, Fuleihan GEH, et al. Summary statement from a workshop on asymptomatic primary hyperparathyroidism: a perspective for the 21st century. J Clin Endocrinol Metab. 2002;87:5353–5361.

Bonjer HJ and Bruining HA. Technique of parathyroidectomy. In: Clark OH, Duh QY, Kebebew E, eds. Textbook of Endocrine Surgery. 2nd ed. Philadelphia, PA: Elsevier Saunders, 2005:439–448.

Cannon J, Lew JI, Solorzano CC. Parathyroidectomy for hypercalcemic crisis: 40 years' experience and long-term outcomes. Surgery. 2010;148:807–813.

Chen H, Mack E, Starling JR. Radioguided parathyroidectomy is equally effective for both adenomatous and hyperplastic glands. Ann Surg. 2003;238:332–338.

Diamond TW, Botha JR, Wing J, et al. Parathyroid hypertension: a reversible disorder. Arch Int Med. 1986;146:1709–1712.

Hedback G and Oden A. Increased risk of death from primary hyperparathyroidism – an update. Eur J Clin Invest. 1998;28:271–276.

Hruska KA, Teitelbaum SL. Renal osteodystrophy. N Engl J Med. 1995;333:166.

Irvin GL, Prudhomme Dl, Deriso GT, et al. A new approach to parathyroidectomy. Ann Surg. 1994;219:574–579.

Lew JI and Solorzano CC. Surgical management of primary hyperparathyroidism: state of the art. Surg Clin North Am. 2009;89:1205–1225.

Lo Gerfo P. Bilateral neck exploration for parathyroidectomy under local anesthesia: a viable technique for patients with coexisting thyroid disease with or without sestamibi scanning. Surgery. 1999;126:1011–1014.

Lowe H, McMahon DJ, Rubin MR, et al. Normocalcemic primary hyperparathyroidism: further characterization of a new clinical phenotype. J Clin Endocrinol Metab. 2007;92:3001–3005.

Miccoli P, Bendinelli C, Vignali E, et al. Endoscopic parathyroidectomy: report on an initial experience. Surgery. 1998;124:1077–1079.

Mittendorf EA and McHenry CR. Persistent parathyroid hormone elevation following curative parathyroidectomy for primary hyperparathyroidism. Arch Otolaryngol Head Neck Surg. 2002;128:275–279.

NIH Consensus Development Conference Panel. Diagnosis and management of asymptomatic primary hyperparathyroidism: consensus development state. Ann Intern Med. 1991;114:593–597.

Norenstedt S, Ekbom A, Brandt L, et al. Postoperative mortality in parathyroid surgery in Sweden during five decades: improved outcome despite older patients. Eur J Endocrinol. 2009;160:295–299.

Peacock M, Bilezikian JP, Klassen PS, et al. Cinacalcet hyperochloride maintains long-term normocalcemia in patients with primary hyperparathyroidism. J Clin Endocrinol Metab. 2003;90:135–141.

Rodgers SE, Hunter GJ, Hamberg LM, et al. Improved preoperative planning for directed parathyroidectomy with 4-dimensional computed tomography. Surgery. 2006;140:932–941.

Rodgers SE, Lew JI, Solorzano CC. Primary hyperparathyroidism. Curr Opin Oncol. 2008;20:52–58.

Rodgers SE, Perrier ND. Parathyroid carcinoma. Curr Opin Oncol. 2006;18:16–22.

Roman SA and Sosa JA. Psychiatric and cognitive aspects of primary hyperparathyroidism. Curr Opin Oncol. 2007;19:1–5.

Roman SA, Sosa JA, Mayes L et al. Parathyroidectomy improves neurocognitive deficits in patients with primary hyperparathyroidism. Surgery. 2005;138:1121–1128.

Roman SA, Sosa JA, Pietrzak R, et al. The effects of serum calcium and parathyroid hormone changes on psychiatric and cognitive function in patients undergoing parathyroidectomy for primary hyperparathyroidism. Ann Surg. 2010 (in press).

Sheldon DG, Lee FT, Neil NJ, et al. Surgical treatment of hyperparathyroidism improves health-related quality of life. Arch Surg. 2002;137:1022–1028.

Silverberg SJ, Lewiecki EM, Mosekilde L, et al. Presentation of asymptomatic primary hyperparathyroidism: proceedings of the Third International Workshop. J Clin Endocrinol Metab. 2009;94:351–365.

Solorzano CC, Carneiro-Pla DM, Irvin Gl. Surgeon-performed ultrasonography as the initial and only localizing study in sporadic primary hyperparathyroidism. J Am Coll Surg. 2006;202:18–24.

Sosa JA, Power NR, Levine MA, et al. Profile of a clinical practice: Thresholds for surgery and surgical outcomes for patients with primary hyperparathyroidism: a national survey of endocrine surgeons. J Clin Endocrinol Metab. 1998;83(8):2658–2665.

Tamura Y, Araki A, Chiba Y, et al. Remarkable increase in lumbar spine bone mineral density and amelioration in biochemical markers of bone turnover after parathyroidectomy in elderly patients with primary hyperparathyroidism: a 5-year follow-up study. J Bone Miner Metab. 2007;25:226–231.

Udelsman R. Primary hyperparathyroidism. Curr Treat Options Oncol. 2001;2:365–372.

Udelsman R, Aruny JE, Donovan PI, et al. Rapid parathyroid hormone analysis during venous localization. Ann Surg. 2003;237:714–721.

Udelsman R, Lin Z, Donovan P. The superiority of minimally invasive parathyroidectomy based on 1,650 consecutive patients with primary hyperparathyroidism. Ann Surg. 2011;253(3):585-591.

Udelsman R, Pasieka JL, Sturgeon C, et al. Surgery for asymptomatic primary hyperparathyroidism: Proceedings of the Third International Workshop. J Clin Endocrinol Metab. 2009;94:366–372.

Uludag M, Isgor A, Yetkin G, et al. Supernumerary ectopic parathyroid glands: persistent hyperparathyroidism due to mediastinal parathyroid adenoma localized by preoperative single photon emission computed tomography and intraoperative gamma probe application. Hormones. 2009;8:144–149.

62 Persistent Hyperparathyroidism

JAMES T. BROOME

Presentation

A 57-year-old man with a history of peptic ulcer disease is referred for management of persistent hypercalcemia. He initially presented to his primary care physician for routine physical examination where a basic metabolic panel revealed serum calcium elevated at 12.1 mg/dL. Subsequent workup demonstrated an ionized calcium of 6.61 mg/dL (normal, 4.48 to 5.28), serum calcium of 12.4 mg/dL (normal, 8.5 to 10.5), parathyroid hormone (PTH) level of 248 pg/dL (normal, 10 to 65), and a total 25 OH vitamin D level of 39 ng/mL (normal, 30 to 80). Preoperative sestamibi documented a right-sided abnormality (**Figure 1**). However, ultrasound was not done. He went to the operating room 6 months prior to presentation for exploration. During surgery, he underwent exploration and subsequent partial right thyroid lobectomy after failure to identify a parathyroid adenoma. Postoperatively, he has remained hypercalcemic prompting referral for persistent hyperparathyroidism.

Differential Diagnosis

Primary hyperparathyroidism is by far the most common cause of hypercalcemia. Other less common causes include malignancy, granulomatous disease(s), milk-alkali syndrome, and many others. Hypercalcemia with concurrent hyperparathyroidism (elevated PTH levels) has a much narrower differential diagnosis including sporadic primary hyperparathyroidism, familial isolated hyperparathyroidism, multiple endocrine neoplasia type 1 (MEN 1), multiple endocrine neoplasia type 2a (MEN 2a), medication-induced (lithium, HCTZ), secondary hyperparathyroidism (end-stage renal disease, hypovitaminosis D), and familial hypocalciuric hypercalcemia (FHH). In the patient in whom initial surgery for presumed primary hyperparathyroidism has failed to produce biochemical cure, a systematic approach must be undertaken to verify the diagnosis and indications for further intervention(s).

Workup

The patient undergoes further workup to delineate the cause of his hyperparathyroidism. Repeat serum calcium and PTH levels are 11.9 mg/dL and 225 pg/dL, respectively. Ionized calcium is elevated at 6.3 mg/dL, renal function is normal, and his total 25 OH vitamin D level is normal at 40 ng/mL. The patient is not taking any confounding/contributing medications and denies any known family history of calcium disorders. A 24-hour urine collection for calcium demonstrates his urine calcium to be 239 mg of calcium in 24 hours (normal, 100 to 300 mg/24 h) which rules out FHH.

Based on this workup, he continues to have a picture consistent with primary hyperparathyroidism.

The pathology report documents removal of an inferior parathyroid gland attached to the outer surface of the right thyroid lobe. The operative note describes identification of the right recurrent laryngeal nerve from its appearance under the subclavian artery up to its insertion into the cricopharyngeal joint. No visual confirmation was reported of the right superior gland, and the right inferior gland was removed at the time of thyroid lobectomy. There was no mention of exploration of the carotid sheath, removal of the cervical thymus, or exploration of the tracheoesophageal groove. The surgeon did not explore the left side of the neck during the first operation.

Although preoperative localization may be bypassed at initial operation, successful reoperative parathyroid surgery demands an exhaustive search for the pathologic gland. Ideally, two concordant localization studies should be obtained prior to proceeding with reexploration. Routine ultrasonography should be performed for all reoperative parathyroid patients. Ultrasound not only evaluates for the typical perithyroidal cervical adenomas but can also detect intrathyroidal lesions that may represent intrathyroidal parathyroid adenomas or thyroid nodular disease necessitating concurrent treatment at the time of reoperation. A detailed ultrasound should also include evaluation of both carotid sheaths from above the bifurcation of the common carotid artery down to the anterior mediastinum as allowed by body habitus. Fine needle aspiration

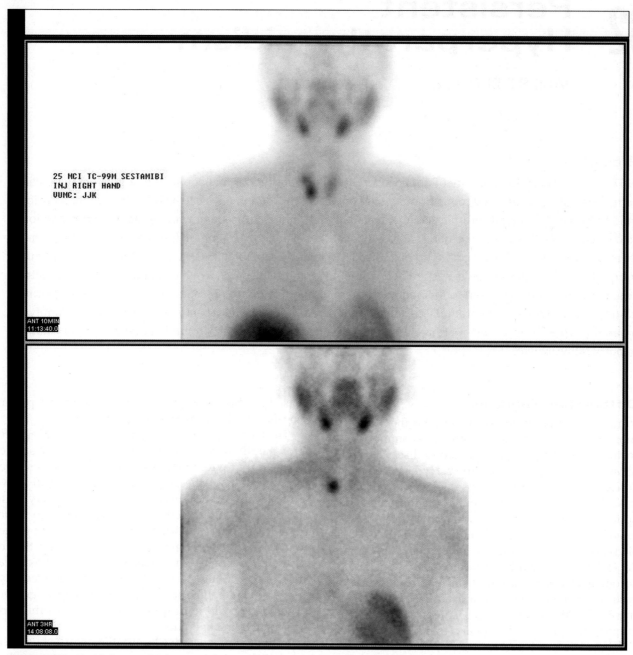

25 MCI TC-99M SESTAMIBI
INJ RIGHT HAND
VUMC: JJK

ANT 10MIN
11:13:40.0

ANT 3HR
14:08:08.0

FIGURE 1 • Tc-99 Sestamibi documenting persistent uptake in right cervical position.

of suspicious lesions can be sent for PTH washings/ measurements to confirm parathyroid tissue prior to surgery. Ultrasound is not a good imaging test for identifying mediastinal lesions or those ectopic adenomas located posterior to the larynx, trachea, or esophagus.

Routine imaging should also include repeat technetium-99 Sestamibi scanning, preferable with single-photon emission computed tomography (SPECT) for added anatomic detail. The sensitivity of sestamibi is decreased in reoperative surgery, but it has the advantage of evaluating deep structures in the neck (retrotracheal, retrolaryngeal) as well as identifying potential mediastinal adenomas.

High-resolution computed tomography (CT) scanning, either with computed tomography angiography (CTA) or 4D-CT, plays an important role in localization of missing glands. Adenomas will typically "light up" on arterial-phase imaging, and these modalities have essentially replaced percutaneous angiography for parathyroid localization. Accurate CT scan interpretation demands familiarity with the cervical anatomy and knowledge of the common locations for missing adenomas. Thin slice (2 to 3 mm) scans provide detailed examination of the carotid sheath, retrotracheal, retroesophageal, and mediastinal locations of adenomas. Institutional preferences and protocols should be considered when deciding between CTA versus 4D-CT scans. Other potential imaging utilizing MRI or C11 Methionine PET/CT for localization may be considered if other modalities have failed to demonstrate a missing adenoma.

Selective venous sampling (SVS) of the cervical and thoracic venous system provides another potential technique for localization. This demands a high level of technical skill from the interventional radiologist. SVS consists of multiple detailed measurements of PTH values from various locations within the cervical–thoracic venous system. Subsequent diagrams of the venous system mapped with the corresponding PTH values help to determine laterality to the parathyroid adenoma as well as demonstrate evidence of mediastinal drainage. Detailed anatomic information is difficult to extrapolate from SVS data.

Diagnosis and Treatment

The diagnosis of primary hyperparathyroidism can be difficult to make in some patients, and accuracy is of vital importance in the case of persistent hyperparathyroidism. A thorough understanding of the relationship of serum calcium to PTH levels can help the clinician look for common errors in diagnosis and confirm the etiology of the hypercalcemia. A detailed clinical history should be able to rule out specific disorders related to ingestion of supraphysiologic doses of supplements containing calcium, vitamin D, or excessive dietary intake of calcium and vitamin D foods. Specific attention must be paid to the family history in an attempt to screen for underlying genetic disorders related to calcium homeostasis. A strong family history of calcium disorders may suggest an undiagnosed MEN syndrome, FHH, or familial isolated hyperparathyroidism. Young patients (<30 years old) with hypercalcemia should raise suspicion of an unrecognized familial form of hyperparathyroidism. The diagnosis rests upon accurate measurements of concurrent serum calcium, ionized calcium, albumin, and PTH levels.

Once primary hyperparathyroidism is confirmed biochemically, the surgeon must next reexamine the indications for surgical intervention. Reoperative parathyroid surgery carries increased risk of injury to the recurrent laryngeal nerve, permanent hypoparathyroidism, as well as an increased rate of failure to cure the hyperparathyroidism. Before undertaking these risks, careful delineation of the indication for surgery must be outlined. The indications for reoperative surgery are no different than those for an initial exploration and generally follow the National Institute of Health guidelines. Laboratory and radiologic evidence of end-organ damage related to the hyperparathyroidism must be documented. All symptomatic patients with osteoporosis, osteofibrosis cystica, Brown's tumors,

kidney stones, or life-threatening episodes of hypercalcemia should undergo operation. The "asymptomatic" patients with severe hypercalcemia (>1 mg/dL above normal), hypercalcuria (>400 mg/24 h), osteoporosis (T-score less than −2.5 at any site), prior low-impact fracture, decreased kidney function (creatinine clearance <60 mL/min), or age <50 years should also be considered for reoperation.

Surgical Approach

Prior to any reoperative neck surgery, flexible laryngoscopy should be performed preoperatively to document vocal cord dysfunction from unrecognized recurrent laryngeal nerve injury.

As with any reoperative surgery, a thorough understanding of what has been done before is essential. Prior operative reports should be obtained and carefully reviewed. Particular attention should be paid to key structures visualized during the first operation (e.g., were the recurrent nerves identified? was any thyroid arterial supply ligated and where?). Visual identification of parathyroids and their location, even by trusted surgeons, should be viewed with skepticism. Even the most experienced surgeon can incorrectly identify a parathyroid gland intraoperatively. Pathologic confirmation of identified glands either by biopsy, excision, or aspiration for PTH levels is needed to feel confident the glands were correctly identified during prior surgery. The surgeon must also note which glands have been removed and anticipate what functional glands may remain, keeping in mind that biopsy of glands at previous exploration may have rendered them nonfunctional. Once the surgeon has convincing evidence suggesting a location for the missing adenoma, surgical approach can be determined (Table 1). A standard anterior approach the central neck is commonly used and has the advantage of familiarity for most surgeons. Scar from prior surgery and loss of normal tissue planes increase potential complications as well as limiting the success of "blind" exploration. A standard collar (Kocher) incision should be made roughly overlying the isthmus of the thyroid gland. Full mobilization of the strap muscles from their origin to insertion allows generous access to the central neck. If the lesion has been accurately localized or lateralized preoperatively, then a lateral approach to the central neck may provide an alternative exposure that avoids previously disrupted tissue planes and minimizes the impact of prior surgical scarring. This approach involves separating the medial border of the sternocleidomastoid muscle from the lateral border of the strap muscles allowing access to the central neck while also avoiding the scarring present along the midline. From this approach, the surgeon can access the inferior thyroidal artery, accurately identify

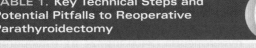

TABLE 1. Key Technical Steps and Potential Pitfalls to Reoperative Parathyroidectomy

Key Technical Steps

1. Two concurrent preoperative localization studies reviewed by the surgeon and at least one showing anatomic detail.
2. Consider intraoperative recurrent laryngeal nerve monitoring.
3. Baseline PTH levels drawn intraoperatively.
4. Cervical collar (Kocher) incision with creation of subplatysmal flaps.
5. Midline vs. lateral approach to central neck based on imaging studies and intraoperative findings.
6. Identification of adenoma and ligation of arterial supply.
7. Repeat PTH levels at 10 min postexcision and use institution-specific intraoperative cure criteria.
8. Be prepared for an extended exploration of central neck (as indicated by PTH levels).
9. Autotransplantation/cryopreservation of parathyroid tissue (as indicated).
10. Reapproximation of strap muscles (midline or lateral), platysma, and skin closure.

Potential Pitfalls

- Ectopic location of adenoma or parathyromatosis.
- Failure of PTH levels to decline >50% (need for further exploration in the presence of intense scarring).
- Resection of all functioning parathyroid tissue (need for autotransplantation).
- Postoperative compressive hematoma.
- Damage to recurrent laryngeal nerve.
- Permanent hypoparathyroidism.

and preserve the recurrent laryngeal nerve, as well as allow exposure of the carotid sheath and tracheoesophageal groove. Regardless of the approach used, a suspected parathyroid(s) should be sent for frozen section to confirm an accurate pathologic diagnosis and prevent misidentification. Intraoperative PTH monitoring should also be utilized to confirm removal of all hyperactive parathyroid tissue. Failure of PTH levels to drop >50% 10 minutes after removal of the gland should prompt further central neck exploration for another hyperactive gland when feasible.

The surgeon must also be familiar with the common and uncommon locations of "missing" parathyroid glands. Knowledge of the embryologic formation and descent of the parathyroids will aid in an educated search for missing glands. The most common location for a "missing" parathyroid adenoma is routine/regular anatomic locations. Inferior parathyroid glands are typically located within a 2-cm² area around the inferior pole of the thyroid gland. Superior glands are also typically located within 2 cm superior to the recurrent laryngeal nerve as it crosses the inferior thyroidal artery. The most common ectopic location of missing inferior adenomas is the cervical thymus. Inferior glands may also be located within the ipsilateral thyroid lobe,

carotid sheath, or anterior mediastinum. Median sternotomy is inappropriate during a search for a missing adenoma unless preoperative imaging demonstrated a mediastinal location. Superior glands may be located high along the path of the superior thyroid pedicle, deep along the prevertebral fascia, as well as within the tracheoesophageal groove. Mobilization of the trachea and esophagus will allow evaluation for retrolaryngeal or retroesophageal glands. Often, enlarged superior glands "descend" behind the inferior thyroidal artery and recurrent laryngeal nerve to lie inferior to these structures within the tracheoesophageal groove.

In this case, after surgeon's review of the prior operative note, pathology report, localization studies and biochemical confirmation of primary hyperparathyroidism, the patient underwent repeat sestamibi scanning and ultrasonography. Surgeon-performed ultrasound demonstrated a diminutive right thyroid lobe, no intrathyroidal lesions within the right or left thyroid lobes, as well as no suspicious/hypoechoic lesions in the bilateral central neck or within the carotid sheaths bilaterally. Sestamibi/SPECT was consistent with a left superior abnormality located just behind the superior pole of the left thyroid lobe **(Figure 2)**. CTA of the neck and mediastinum was then performed, demonstrating a hypervascular mass located in a retrolaryngeal position next to the left superior thyroid lobe **(Figures 3 and 4)**. There was no evidence of a mediastinal adenoma on either sestamibi or CTA. Decision was made to take him to the operating room for PTH-guided parathyroidectomy of a suspected left superior parathyroid gland.

Special Intraoperative Considerations

Several scenarios must be considered intraoperatively even in those patients in whom a single adenoma is suspected by history and localization studies. Multiglandular disease (MGD), either from sporadic hyperplasia or a familial syndrome, may still be present. In those patients in whom MGD is confirmed, the surgeon should proceed with complete cervical exploration, excision of parathyroid tissue, and reimplantation of approximately 30 to 40 mg of morselized parathyroid tissue into the nondominant brachioradialis muscle. Individual surgeon experience and preference ultimately determine between autotransplantation versus creation of an appropriate *in situ* parathyroid remnant. Cryopreservation of residual parathyroid tissue should be performed if available at the institution. Bilateral exploration may not be possible due to intense scarring and consideration should be given to the use of intraoperative recurrent laryngeal nerve monitoring in these difficult cases.

The surgeon must also be prepared to encounter parathyromatosis. In this situation, abnormal parathyroid tissue released during a prior exploration has

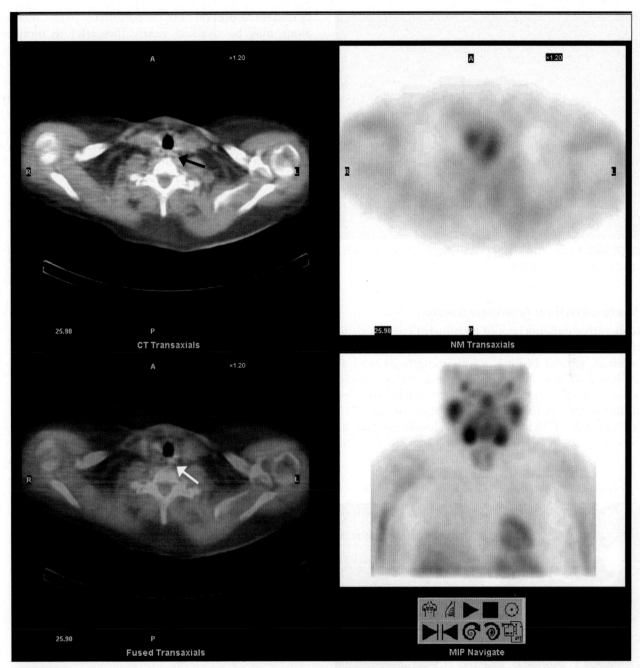

CT Transaxials

NM Transaxials

Fused Transaxials

MIP Navigate

FIGURE 2 • Fused sestamibi-SPECT axial images—*arrows* demonstrate left superior adenoma.

implanted into surrounding contiguous structures leading to diffuse seeding of hyperactive parathyroid tissue. Although difficult to achieve permanent normocalcemia, the surgeon should be prepared to perform a complete excision of all identifiable parathyroid implants including resection of involved strap muscles, thyroid lobe, as well as ipsilateral central lymph node dissection.

Finally, consideration must be given to the potential that resection of an adenoma will result in removal of all remaining functional parathyroid tissue. This scenario can be anticipated after detailed review of prior operative notes and pathology reports. If suspected, then utilization of PTH monitoring may demonstrate a precipitous drop in PTH levels confirming the absence of residual functional tissue. The surgeon must save a portion of the histologically confirmed hypercellular parathyroid for morselization and reimplantation. If PTH levels remain detectable but suspicion of hypoparathyroid is high, then cryopreservation of parathyroid tissue for possible reimplantation later should be performed.

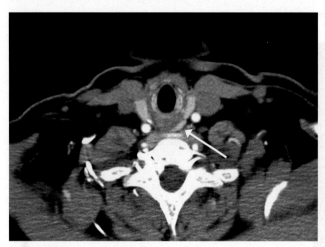

FIGURE 3 • Axial CTA images—*white arrow* indicates left-sided parathyroid adenoma.

Postoperative Management

Reoperative patients should be brought back to clinic in 1 to 2 weeks for postoperative evaluation for hypocalcemia, wound healing, vocal strength, as well as resolution of any symptoms present preoperatively. Serum calcium and PTH levels should be checked to document biochemical normalization of the PTH-calcium axis. Calcium and PTH levels should be rechecked at 6 months postoperatively to confirm

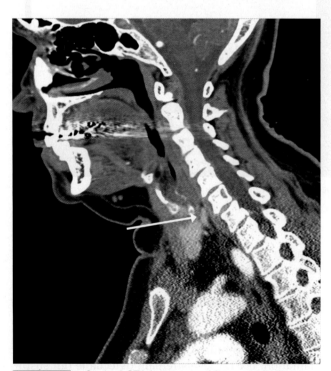

FIGURE 4 • *Sagittal CTA images—white arrow indicates* posterior location of left superior adenoma.

persistent resolution of hyperparathyroidism. Calcium alone may be checked yearly thereafter to monitor for long-term recurrence, which should be <5% after 10 years. Hypoparathyroidism with hypocalcemia can be treated surgically with reimplantation of cryo-preserved parathyroid tissue if available or medically with oral calcium supplements and activated 1,25 OH vitamin D. Those patients with insufficient or deficient 25 OH vitamin D levels should receive a course of ergocalciferol for supplementation in addition to calcium and 1,25 OH vitamin D.

Case Conclusion

The patient was taken to the operating room where he underwent a lateral approach the left central neck. Exploration of the space just posterior the left superior pole demonstrated a large, 2.1-cm left superior parathyroid adenoma. The gland weight 1.34 g. Intraoperative PTH levels dropped from 530 pg/mL down to 87 pg/mL 10 minutes after division of the single vascular pedicle to the adenoma. The patient was discharged home the same day after a brief period of observation in the postanesthesia care unit.

The patient's repeat serum calcium at 2 weeks postoperatively was 9.4 mg/dL with a concurrent PTH of 24 pg/mL. There was no clinical evidence of hypocalcemia or vocal cord paresis/paralysis. He described marked improvement in energy levels, mood, and resolution of esophageal reflux symptoms. At 6 months, the patient remained normocalcemic with serum calcium of 9.3 mg/dL.

TAKE HOME POINTS

- Biochemical reconfirmation of the diagnosis of hyperparathyroidism along with consideration of familial/genetic etiology should be conducted.
- Reoperative central neck surgery carries two to three times higher than baseline risk of complications including recurrent laryngeal nerve paralysis and permanent hypoparathyroidism.
- The surgeon must review of prior operative reports, pathology reports, localization studies and have a thorough understanding of parathyroid embryology and anatomy.

- Preoperative localization should involve at least two concordant imaging studies progressing from noninvasive to more invasive studies as necessary. At least one study should give anatomical detail.
- Most "missing" adenomas are found in standard locations around the thyroid gland.
- Reoperative surgery should be performed by a surgeon who is experienced in parathyroid surgery and reoperative cervical explorations.

SUGGESTED READINGS

Henry JF. Reoperation for primary hyperparathyroidism: tips and tricks. Langenbecks Arch Surg. 2010;395:103–109.

Powell AC, Alexander R, Chang R, et al. Reoperation for parathyroid adenoma: a contemporary experience. Surgery. 2009;146:1144–1155.

Richards ML, Thompson GB, Farley DR, et al. Reoperative parathyroidectomy in 228 patients during the era of minimal-access surgery and intraoperative parathyroid hormone monitoring. Am J Surg. 2008;196:937–943.

Incidental Adrenal Mass

63

BRIAN D. SAUNDERS and MELISSA M. BOLTZ

Presentation

A 42-year-old woman was referred for evaluation of a 2.3-cm, left, homogeneous adrenal mass discovered when a computed tomography (CT) scan was obtained on a visit to the emergency room for complaints of nausea and vomiting. During her ER visit, she was noted to have a blood pressure of 160/95. She reported a history of high blood pressure over the past year for which she had been on multiple antihypertensive medications. All laboratory data were normal at that time except for low serum potassium.

Differential Diagnosis

An adrenal incidentaloma is an asymptomatic adrenal tumor found on abdominal imaging performed for another indication. The frequency of incidentalomas is rising with the increased use of CT scanning and other imaging modalities. Currently, between 1% and 4% of all abdominal imaging studies will reveal an incidental adrenal tumor. In adults, incidental adrenal masses have a broad differential diagnosis (**Table 1**). Adrenal masses may be nonfunctional or functional (hormonally active), and malignant or benign. Although most incidentalomas are benign, a primary adrenocortical carcinoma is one of the most aggressive cancers, and thus this diagnosis must be considered in the differential diagnosis of any adrenal mass. Additionally, approximately 20% of incidentalomas are hormonally functional (albeit many with subclinical phenotypes), and although histologically benign, failure to diagnose and treat these patients results in avoidable morbidity.

Workup

The two major issues in managing a patient with an incidental adrenal mass are to evaluate for autonomous adrenal hormone production and to assess the malignant potential, both of which are indications for operative resection. **Figure 1** depicts a suggested algorithm for the workup of incidentalomas beginning with a complete history and physical examination with specific reference to history of prior malignancies and signs and symptoms of adrenal hormone excess.

An adrenal protocol CT scan is ideal when assessing adrenal masses. An adrenal protocol CT scan starts with a noncontrast study. The noncontrast scan is followed by the rapid injection of contrast agent, and 60 seconds later, a contrast enhanced CT scan is performed. Then, a delayed contrast (washout) scan is obtained 15 minutes after the initial contrast images. The relative percentage of contrast washout is calculated from the Hounsfield unit values of the contrast and delayed contrast CT scans. Benign adrenal cortical adenomas typically have CT attenuation values of <10 Hounsfield units on noncontrast imaging or washout >60%, which indicates a lipid-rich mass. Tumors with Hounsfield values >10 Hounsfield units are not necessarily malignant. An abdominal MRI is an increasingly utilized and acceptable imaging modality, especially in those patients with contrast allergies or reduced glomerular filtration rates. Review of imaging should account for features that would indicate malignancy, including large tumor size (>4 cm), irregular tumor margins, heterogeneity, hyperdensity, invasion into adjacent structures, lymphadenopathy, or presence of metastasis. **Figure 2** shows a 2.3-cm left adrenal mass found on CT scan in this patient.

Regardless of radiographic appearance, all patients with an incidental adrenal mass should undergo biochemical testing to determine functional status. A comprehensive screening panel should include serum potassium, plasma aldosterone concentration, plasma renin activity, fasting AM cortisol, ACTH, dehydroepiandrosterone sulfate (DHEAS), and plasma-free metanephrines and normetanephrines. Other measures to assess increased cortisol include 24-hour urinary-free cortisol and measurements of salivary cortisol. Urinary catecholamine measurements can also be used to screen for adrenal medullary hyperfunction. If the biochemical workup indicates the tumor is nonfunctional, the size of the tumor and the patient's medical condition determine further management.

Diagnosis and Treatment

As stated in the case above, this patient had significant and uncontrolled hypertension, concomitant with decreased serum potassium. Further biochemical workup revealed an elevated plasma aldosterone with concurrent low plasma renin activity suggesting aldosteronoma. Additionally, cortisol, DHEAS, and

TABLE 1. Classification of Adrenal Masses

Functional	Nonfunctional
• Cortical adenoma (aldosterone/cortisol/androgen)	• Cortical adenoma
	• Cortical carcinoma
• Pheochromocytoma	• Neuroblastoma
• Cortical carcinoma (any adrenal hormone)	• Ganglioneuroma
	• Metastasis
	• Cysts (true or pseudocysts)
• Congenital adrenal hyperplasia	• Hematoma
• Nodular hyperplasia (Cushing's disease)	• Myolipoma
	• Lipoma
	• Granuloma
	• Amyloidosis
	• Infiltrative disease

catecholamines were normal. Therefore, adrenalectomy is indicated in this patient with a homogeneous, 2.3-cm, functional adrenal mass.

The use of laparoscopic techniques in surgery of adrenal glands has replaced the traditional open approach and is the preferred procedure for all small, benign tumors. The mortality with the laparoscopic approach is low at 0.2% 1 month after surgery. The overall morbidity rate averages 9% with a higher rate in pheochromocytoma and Cushing's syndrome. Due to the benefits associated with laparoscopic surgery, open adrenalectomy should be reserved for tumors >8 cm, as well as tumors with obvious findings consistent with malignancy on preoperative imaging.

Prior to operative intervention, medical preparation may be indicated, based on functional status of the tumor. Preoperative control of hypertension in the patient with a pheochromocytoma is necessary. Alpha-adrenergic blockade is achieved using phenoxybenzamine for 7 to 10 days prior to the procedure. In addition, beta-adrenergic blockade is used after alpha-blockade to treat tachycardia and unopposed alpha-blockade. Patients with Cushing's syndrome should receive stress-dose steroids due to suppression of the hypothalamic–pituitary–adrenal (HPA) axis of the contralateral adrenal gland. For patients with severe hypercortisolism, consideration can be given to administration of an adrenolytic agent, such as ketoconazole or mitotane. In this patient with an aldosteronoma, blood pressure and hypokalemia should be controlled with a competitive aldosterone antagonist such as spironolactone or eplerenone. These agents block the mineralocorticoid receptor, promote potassium retention, and reduce extracellular fluid volume controlling blood pressure.

Surgical Approach for Laparoscopic Adrenalectomy

In patients undergoing laparoscopic left adrenalectomy (Table 2), general anesthesia is induced and an orogastric tube and Foley catheter are inserted with the patient in supine position. Afterward, the patient is placed in the lateral decubitus position with the ipsilateral side up. The table is flexed to widen the angle between the costal margin and iliac wing. Laparoscopic access is obtained with the camera port placed slightly superior and to the left of the umbilicus. The other two working ports are placed two fingerbreadths inferior to the subcostal margin and triangulated with the camera port.

After laparoscopic access is obtained, attention is directed toward mobilizing the splenic flexure of the colon and dividing the lateral peritoneal attachments of the spleen and lienophrenic ligament until the fundus of the stomach is in view. The spleen is then reflected medially with mobilization of the tail of the pancreas. A plane medial to the adrenal gland and lateral to the aorta is bluntly created. Then, the inferior phrenic vessels and central adrenal vein are dissected and divided. The inferior and lateral attachments of the adrenal gland are divided to mobilize the gland out of the suprarenal fossa, exposing the capsule of the superior renal pole. The adrenal gland is then placed in a specimen retrieval bag and removed from the abdomen via the camera port site. Maintaining insufflation, the suprarenal fossa is inspected for adequate hemostasis. The ports are then removed, followed by fascial closure of the camera port site, and skin closure.

Should the patient have needed a laparoscopic right adrenalectomy (Table 3) patient setup and positioning is the same as stated above, except the camera port is now located slightly superior and to the right of the umbilicus. After laparoscopic access has been obtained, the lateral attachments of the liver to the diaphragm (triangular ligament) are divided and the right lobe of the liver is retracted medially. Then, a separate medial port is placed to accommodate a laparoscopic retractor for the liver. The peritoneum overlying the medial aspect of the adrenal gland is opened inferior to superior and a plane medial to the adrenal gland and posterolateral to the vena cava is bluntly developed. The remainder of the procedure is performed as outlined for the laparoscopic left adrenalectomy.

Sometimes, the adrenal gland is difficult to visualize due to perinephric fat, which is more common in men, obese patients, and those with small tumors. Intraoperative ultrasound may be useful in this situation to determine gland location. In addition, the gland should always be dissected with a rim of fatty tissue attached to its surface. This allows for manipulation of the gland without grasping it, which may tear the gland, causing bleeding. During laparoscopic right adrenalectomy, liver injury can easily occur during retraction

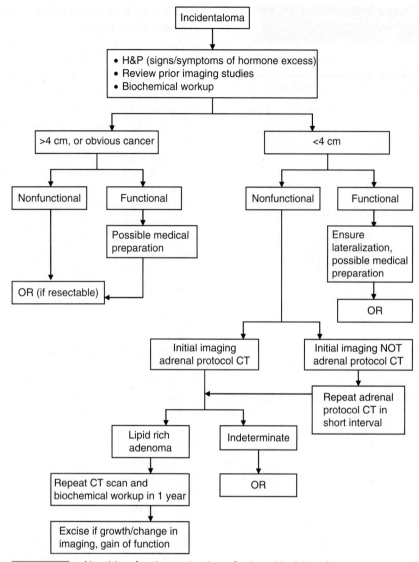

FIGURE 1 • Algorithm for the evaluation of adrenal incidentalomas.

causing large hematomas, which may make it impossible to proceed laparoscopically. Additionally, vena cava and other vascular injuries account for up to 7% of the complications of laparoscopic adrenalectomy, necessitating conversion to the open procedure. Consideration should also be given to the possibility of an aberrant adrenal vein, which drains into the right renal vein.

Special Intraoperative Considerations

Unexpected finding such as unusual retroperitoneal feeding vessels and tumor invasion into surrounding structures encountered at the time of laparoscopic adrenalectomy would raise the concern of a primary adrenal cancer and therefore, conversion to open adrenalectomy should be performed. Proceeding with the laparoscopic procedure would risk violating the tumor capsule. In addition, tumor manipulation during laparoscopic surgery causes aerosolization of cancer cells

via the pneumoperitoneum and leads to seeding of the peritoneal cavity and port sites, which is known as the "chimney effect."

Surgical Approach for Open Adrenalectomy

Should the patient have findings indicating the need for an open adrenalectomy, either a vertical midline incision or a subcostal incision is made. For conversion from laparoscopic to an open procedure, generally a subcostal incision is made with the patient in the lateral decubitus position. For a left adrenal mass resection via an open anterior approach, the lesser sac is entered. The splenic flexure of the colon is reflected caudad, and the spleen and tail of the pancreas are mobilized to expose the adrenal gland. The inferior phrenic vessels and central adrenal vein are dissected and divided with the remaining soft tissue attachments

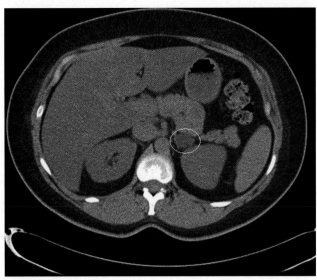

FIGURE 2 • Axial cut of a CT scan with white circle indicating a 2.3-cm diameter left adrenal mass. Radiodensity of the mass on unenhanced images shows a Hounsfield unit of 0.

to complete the adrenalectomy. For adrenocortical cancers, en bloc splenectomy, distal pancreatectomy, nephrectomy, or partial diaphragmatic resection may be necessary.

An open anterior right adrenalectomy requires mobilization of the hepatic flexure of the colon with a partial Kocher maneuver to expose the infrahepatic

TABLE 2. Key Technical Steps and Potential Pitfalls to Laparoscopic Left Adrenalectomy

Key Technical Steps

1. General anesthesia induced with patient in supine position.
2. Place patient in lateral decubitus position, ipsilateral side up.
3. Obtain laparoscopic access.
4. Mobilize splenic flexure of colon.
5. Divide lateral peritoneal attachments of spleen and lienophrenic ligament.
6. Reflect spleen medially and mobilize pancreatic tail.
7. Bluntly create a plane medial to adrenal gland and lateral to aorta.
8. Dissect and divide the inferior phrenic vessels and central adrenal vein.
9. Mobilize adrenal gland by dividing inferior and lateral attachments.
10. Remove adrenal gland from abdomen.
11. Inspect suprarenal fossa for hemostasis.
12. Close port sites.

Potential Pitfalls

- Inability to visualize the gland.
- Vascular injuries.
- Pancreatic injury resulting in pancreatic leak.

TABLE 3. Key Technical Steps and Potential Pitfalls to Laparoscopic Right Adrenalectomy

Key Technical Steps

1. General anesthesia induced with patient in supine position.
2. Place patient in lateral decubitus position, ipsilateral side up.
3. Obtain laparoscopic access.
4. Retract right lobe of liver medially.
5. Open peritoneum overlying adrenal gland inferior to superior.
6. Bluntly create a plane medial to adrenal gland and lateral to vena cava.
7. Dissect and divide the central adrenal vein (clip or linear stapler).
8. Mobilize adrenal gland by dividing inferior and lateral attachments.
9. Remove adrenal gland from abdomen.
10. Inspect suprarenal fossa for hemostasis.
11. Close port sites.

Potential Pitfalls

- Inability to visualize the gland.
- Liver injury resulting in hematomas and conversion to open procedure.
- Vascular injuries.
- Aberrant adrenal vein.

vena cava. The right lobe of the liver is mobilized by dividing the triangular ligament and retracting it medially to expose the adrenal gland. The lateral and inferior margins of the adrenal gland are then mobilized. The central adrenal vein is divided and controlled with the remaining of the soft tissue attachments divided as well. Large or invasive tumors may require a thoracoabdominal incision to obtain suprahepatic vena caval control. If adrenalectomy is performed for a large adrenal cancer, en bloc resection of the right hepatic lobe, right kidney, or portion of the vena cava or diaphragm may be required.

Postoperative Management

Postoperatively, patients who undergo laparoscopic adrenalectomy typically require less fluid replacement than those undergoing open procedures. Incentive spirometry should be used to prevent postoperative atelectasis and pneumonia. In addition, pharmacologic deep venous thrombosis prophylaxis should be started. A regular diet should be resumed as soon as possible, and the Foley catheter may be discontinued when the patient's hemodynamics, urinary output, and electrolytes are stable.

In patients with an aldosteronoma, potassium supplementation should be stopped postoperatively and antihypertensives weaned. Patients with a pheochromocytoma should be monitored in an ICU for signs of postoperative hypotension from vascular relaxation as well as hypoglycemia. Alpha blocking medications may be discontinued immediately, beta blockers weaned, and glycemic control initiated if necessary. Patients who underwent adrenalectomy for Cushing's syndrome should be placed on pharmacologic doses of corticosteroid replacement with a plan to wean to physiologic doses. The HPA axis should be intermittently interrogated with a cosyntropin stimulation test. In the initial postoperative period, they should also be assessed for hypotension, decreased urine output, hyponatremia, hyperkalemia, hypoglycemia, and fever.

Case Conclusion

The patient undergoes successful laparoscopic left adrenalectomy and she is discharged on postoperative day 1. Postoperatively, her oral potassium supplement medications were discontinued immediately and antihypertensives slowly weaned over 2 months. The final pathology report showed the tumor to be a benign cortical aldosteronoma.

TAKE HOME POINTS

- Approximately 20% of adrenal incidentalomas are hormonally functional, and although histologically benign, failure to diagnose and treat these patients results in unnecessary morbidity.
- Adrenal incidentalomas, regardless of radiographic appearance, should be screened to determine their functional status.
- Laparoscopic adrenalectomy is the procedure of choice for small tumors (functional or not) without evidence of malignancy. Open adrenalectomy is indicated for masses >8 cm or obvious radiologic evidence of malignancy.
- The adrenal gland should always be dissected with a rim of fatty tissue attached to its surface so as not to tear the gland, which may cause bleeding that is difficult to control or seed tumor cells.
- Unexpected findings concerning for a primary adrenal cancer during laparoscopic adrenalectomy necessitates conversion to an open procedure.

SUGGESTED READINGS

Nieman LK. Approach to the patient with an adrenal incidentaloma. J Clin Endocrinol Metab. 2010;95(9):4106–4113.

NIH State-of-the-Science Statement on management of the clinically inapparent adrenal mass ("incidentaloma"). NIH Consens State Sci Statements. 2002;19(2):1–23.

Shen WT, Sturgeon C, Duh QY. From incidentaloma to adrenocortical carcinoma: the surgical management of adrenal tumors. J Surg Oncol. 2005;89(3):186–192.

64 Adrenal Cancer

DAVID T. HUGHES and PAUL G. GAUGER

Presentation

A 69-year-old female was found to have an incidental 6.2 × 4.0 × 3.8 cm left adrenal mass on noncontrast CT scan of the abdomen obtained for abdominal pain. The patient has a recent history of new-onset hypertension, 25-lb weight loss and complaints of fatigue, muscle weakness, poor appetite, emotional lability, and insomnia. She has no significant family history of endocrine disease and no prior history of malignancy.

Differential Diagnosis

Nearly 4% of abdominal CT scans obtained for another indication demonstrate an incidental adrenal mass. Adrenal tumors can also be detected clinically due to manifestations of tumor hormone production. Of all adrenal masses, 80% are nonfunctional adenomas, while 15% are functional with laboratory evidence of hormonal overproduction. Functional tumors include pheochromocytomas, aldosteronomas, and cortisol-producing adenomas. In patients with a previous or present history of malignancy, adrenal metastasis should be considered in the differential. Adrenal cortical cancer (ACC) is a rare disease that can also be functional but should be considered on the differential of any adrenal mass, especially tumors larger than 4 cm. Less common benign masses include myelolipoma/lipoma, ganglioneuroma, epithelial cyst, and pseudocyst.

Workup

Key questions are (1) Is the tumor hormonally active? (2) Does it have radiologic characteristics of malignant lesion? (3) Does the patient have a history of previous malignancy?

On physical examination, evaluate for signs of hormonal excess including virilization, cushingoid appearance, and hypertension, which suggest functional tumors. Large, advanced ACC can present with a palpable abdominal mass or an enlarged liver due to metastases.

Laboratory Tests for Adrenal Incidentaloma

1. Plasma fractionated metanephrines or 24-hour urine metanephrines—must rule out pheochromocytoma for any adrenal mass; pheochromocytomas generally demonstrate metanephrine levels >2 times the upper limit of normal; ACC does not produce catecholamines in high amounts.

2. Serum potassium and aldosterone and plasma renin activity—rare cases of ACC are aldosterone producing; aldosterone to renin ratio >20 for aldosterone-secreting tumors.

3. 24-hour urinary-free cortisol or dexamethasone suppression test (1 mg DM at 11 PM, serum cortisol at 8 AM). Degree of hypercortisolism cannot distinguish benign from malignant tumor. Low ACTH level will confirm corticotropin-independent hypercortisolism.

Additional Laboratory Tests for Concern of Adrenal Cancer

4. DHEA-S—high levels can be associated with ACC; virilization is the clinical manifestation of androgen overproduction

Imaging Studies

1. CT—adrenal protocol CT with thin cuts through the adrenals; includes noncontrast phase, contrast-enhanced phase at 60 seconds postcontrast and delayed phase at 10 minutes or 15 minutes postcontrast (depending on specific protocol)

Adenoma (Typical characteristics)
- Low attenuation (<10 Hounsfield units on noncontrast phase)
- Rapid washout (>60% washout at 15 minutes postcontrast)
- Smooth borders

ACC (Typical characteristics, **Figure 1**)
- Size >4 cm
- High attenuation (>10 Hounsfield units on noncontrast phase)
- Enhancement on contrast-enhanced phase
- Delayed contrast washout (<50% washout at 10 minutes postcontrast)
- Calcifications
- Irregular shape
- Central necrosis

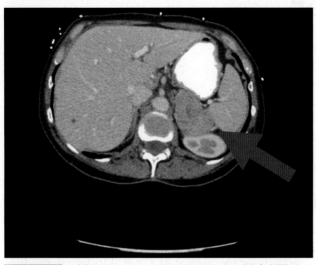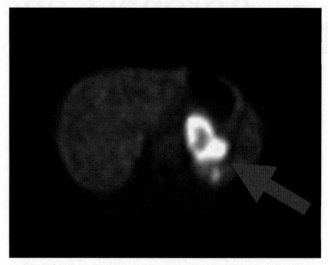

FIGURE 1 • CT with oral and IV contrast and FDG-PET demonstrating left adrenocortical cancer with central necrosis.

2. MRI—useful in distinguishing between adenoma (lipid rich—signal intensity loss on out-of-phase sequences), pheochromocytoma (high intensity on T2 images) and ACC (central necrosis, hemorrhage, calcification, local invasion, IVC tumor thrombus)
3. FDG-PET—pheochromocytoma and ACC are FDG-avid (adrenal to liver max SUV ratio >1.45) **(Figure 2)**; also helpful in evaluating for metastatic disease

This patient's laboratory studies showed elevated 24-hour urine cortisol (240 µg/24 h [normal 20 to 90 µg/24 h]) and nonsuppressible cortisol level with low-dose Dexamethasone (12 µg/dL [normal suppression <2 µg/dL]). Adrenal protocol CT demonstrated a left adrenal mass 6.2 × 4.0 × 3.8 cm that was heterogeneous with irregular borders and central necrosis as well as two 1-cm low attenuation liver lesions. FDG-PET was obtained to further characterize the hepatic lesions, which demonstrated an intensely FDG-avid left adrenal mass with no FDG avidity in the liver lesions and no distant metastases.

Diagnosis and Treatment

Adrenal tumors with evidence of hormone production or suspicion of ACC should be considered for adrenalectomy. Large adrenal masses, those with evidence of liver or pulmonary metastasis, virulizing tumors or those with imaging characteristics outlined above should be considered high risk for ACC. Percutaneous biopsy is contraindicated given risk of tumor seeding and lack of additional information provided, except when there is a question of metastatic adrenal mass in a patient with a history of extra-adrenal malignancy. Prognosis for ACC is dependent on treatment at an early stage and complete surgical excision with negative margins. In patients with hormone-producing tumors with metastatic disease, surgical debulking can provide palliation from hormone-related symptoms. This not typically considered if >90% of the tumor burden cannot be removed with the palliative operation. In nonfunctioning tumors with metastatic disease or those where >90% resection is not possible, primary treatment with systemic chemotherapy and external-beam radiation is indicated.

This patient had no evidence of local invasion or distant metastasis on preoperative imaging studies. There was high suspicion for cortisol-producing ACC given imaging and biochemical characteristics. Open left adrenalectomy was discussed with the patient and was scheduled after a thorough preoperative evaluation.

Cut edge of triangular ligament

Right adrenal vein

Adrenal tumor

Mobilized liver

FIGURE 2 • Right adrenalectomy. (Illustration courtesy Lippincott Williams & Wilkins, from Surgical Endocrinology by Gerard M. Doherty and Britt Skogseid.)

Surgical Approach to Adrenalectomy

Adrenal masses that are at all suspicious for ACC based on clinical presentation or imaging characteristics should *not* be approached laparoscopically given higher rates of early local recurrence due to inadequate margins and tumor implants. The goals of surgical management include complete tumor resection with negative margins and control of tumor hormone production. Patients should be prepared for an en bloc resection of large tumors with consideration of bowel preparation and evaluation of renal function. Preoperative administration of splenectomy vaccinations should be considered for left-sided tumors. Potential for IVC resection, tumor thrombectomy, or hepatic resection should be considered. Cortisol-producing tumors should be treated with perioperative glucocorticoid supplementation due to suppression of HPA Axis. Hypokalemia and hypertension with aldosterone-secreting tumors should be treated with spironolactone preoperatively **(Table 1)**.

Special Intraoperative Considerations

Discovery of invasive characteristics or suspicion of ACC during laparoscopic adrenalectomy for a

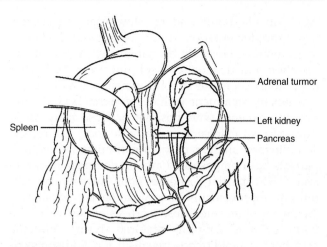

FIGURE 3 • Left adrenalectomy. (Illustration courtesy Lippincott Williams & Wilkins, from: Surgical Endocrinology by Gerard M. Doherty and Britt Skogseid.)

suspected adrenal adenoma or benign tumor should prompt conversion to open technique to obtain adequate resection margins. Right-sided ACC can invade into the IVC and require IVC resection or tumor thrombectomy. Conversion to thoracoabdominal incision to obtain supradiaphragmatic control of the IVC or cardiopulmonary bypass maybe required for extensive IVC involvement.

The patient underwent uneventful open left adrenalectomy via a subcostal incision after preparation with splenectomy vaccines and perioperative "stress-dose" hydrocortisone. The tumor was well localized without surrounding organ invasion. Final pathology demonstrated a 6-cm ACC with capsular invasion, focal extra-adrenal extension, negative margins and was classified as low grade (8/50 mitoses per high powered field). By AJCC staging, the patient was classified as having Stage III (pT2N0M0) because of extra-adrenal extension **(Table 2)**.

Postoperative Management

Routine postoperative management should include monitoring for hypoadrenalism manifesting as nausea, vomiting, abdominal pain, hypotension not responsive to fluid resuscitation, hypoglycemia, or hyperkalemia. Following complete resection, cortisol-producing

---

TABLE 1. Key Technical Steps and Potential Pitfalls to Open Adrenalectomy for ACC

Key Technical Steps

1. Obtain adequate central venous access and arterial blood pressure monitoring given potential need for large-volume resuscitation.
2. Subcostal or midline laparotomy with full exploration for metastatic disease.
3. Divide triangular ligament to mobilize liver medially for right adrenalectomy **(Figure 2)**. Mobilize spleen and tail of pancreas medially for left adrenalectomy **(Figure 3)**.
4. Open posterior peritoneum to enter retroperitoneal space.
5. Dissect and ligate central adrenal vein, which originates from IVC for the right adrenal and from the renal vein for the left adrenal. Additional venous supply comes superiorly from the inferior phrenic vascular pedicle (especially apparent on the left).
6. Arterial supply to the adrenal is via multiple small vessels entering posteriomedially originating from the aorta and renal arteries.
7. Include wide margins of retroperitoneal tissue.
8. En bloc resection of kidney, IVC, diaphragm, adjacent organs, or venous tumor thrombectomy is sometimes required for locally invasive tumors.

Potential Pitfalls

- Laparoscopic removal of ACC is associated with high recurrence rates due to inadequate margins or tumor implants and is *not* recommended when cancer is suspected or likely.
- Tumor rupture or positive margins leads to local recurrence.
- Be prepared for vascular resection and reconstruction.

TABLE 2. Adrenal Cortical Cancer AJCC Staging System

I   <5 cm, N0, no regional extension
II   >5 cm, N0, no regional extension
III any size with regional extension; N1
IV   any size; +/– regional extension with N1; invasion into surrounding organs; M1

ACC patients should undergo slow wean of glucocorticoid supplementation over a prolonged period of 12 to 18 months. However, in patients with incomplete resection and residual cortisol-producing ACC after operation, exogenous steroids may not be necessary.

Adjuvant treatment includes external-beam radiation for patients with positive or close margins or extra-adrenal extension to decrease local recurrence. A multistudy analysis of the use of mitotane for ACC patients has demonstrated an 11% complete response and a 52% partial response rate; however, no significant improvements in survival have been shown. Treatment with high-dose corticosteroids (>50 mg hydrocortisone daily) is required during mitotane treatment to avoid hypoadrenalism and Addison's crisis due to its nonspecific adrenal suppressive effects. Cytotoxic chemotherapy regimens including doxorubicin, 5-fluorouracil, Adriamycin, and methotrexate are used for treatment of metastatic disease.

Recurrence occurs in two-thirds of patients typically in the first 1 to 2 years following surgical resection. Prognosis is based on stage of disease with Stage I and II patients having a 50% 5-year survival, while Stage III and IV patients or those with positive margins have a mean survival of 8 to 10 months. Postoperative surveillance initially includes chest/abdomen/pelvis CT every 3 months. FDG-PET is useful for restaging purposes and to delineate metastases, which typically have high standardized uptake values (SUV).

The patient in this scenario was recommended external-beam radiation and adjuvant mitotane therapy given the presence of extra-adrenal extension and Stage III disease but refused given concern for side effects. She elected to undergo routine CT imaging surveillance every 3 months.

TAKE HOME POINTS

- Virilizing features, mixed cortisol and aldosterone hypersecretion, and heterogeneous or large adrenal tumors (>4 cm) should raise suspicion of ACC.
- Percutaneous biopsy of adrenal tumors is not recommended except for suspicion of metastatic adrenal tumors in patients with a history of previous malignancy after biochemically ruling out pheochromocytoma.
- Laparoscopic adrenalectomy is NOT recommended for ACC given higher local recurrence rates due to positive or close margins.
- Complete resection often requires en bloc resection of kidney, spleen, pancreas, liver, or IVC for negative margins.
- Overall prognosis remains poor with overall 5-year survival of 25%.

SUGGESTED READINGS

Allolio B, Fassnacht M. Clinical review: adrenocortical carcinoma: clinical update. J Clin Endocrinol Metab. 2006;91(6): 2027–2037.

Broome JT, Gauger PG. Surgical techniques for adrenal tumors. Minerva Endocrinol. 2009;34(2):185–193.

Clark OH, Benson AB, Berlin JD, et al. NCCN clinical practice guidelines in oncology: neuroendocrine tumors. J Natl Compr Canc Netw. 2009;7(7):712–747.

Dackiw AP, Lee JE, Gagel RF, et al. Adrenal cortical carcinoma. World J Surg. 2001;25:914–926.

Rodgers SE, Evans DB, Lee JE, et al. Adrenocortical carcinoma. Surg Oncol Clin N Am. 2006;15(3):535–553.

65 Cortisol-secreting Adrenal Tumor

HARI R. KUMAR and JUDIANN MISKULIN

Presentation

A 53-year-old obese female presents with a diagnosis of new-onset diabetes that has been difficult to control, requiring multiple oral medications and insulin. She notes an overall change in appearance including thinning of her skin and striations, increased facial hair, and a redistribution of her body habitus with more central adiposity. A workup initiated by her primary care physician reveals an elevated serum cortisol with a suppressed adrenocorticotropic hormone (ACTH) level.

Differential Diagnosis

The most common cause of hypercortisolism is administration of exogenous glucocorticoids. Steroid medications, such as prednisone, are often used to treat a variety of ailments due to their anti-inflammatory and immune-modulating effects. Once synthetic sources have been eliminated, endogenous causes can then be explored. Among endogenous causes, excess secretion of ACTH from the pituitary (Cushing's *disease*) accounts for over half of cases, with adrenal tumors, bilateral adrenal hyperplasia, and ectopic ACTH-producing tumors accounting for most of the remaining cases.

Discussion

Cortisol is a steroid hormone manufactured in the zona fasciculata layer of the adrenal cortex. As a member of the glucocorticoid family, cortisol mediates the stress-induced "fight or flight" response whose effects involve the cardiovascular, metabolic, immunologic, and other systems.

Serum levels of cortisol demonstrate diurnal variation with the peak occurring around 8 am and the nadir at midnight. The overall daily production of cortisol ranges from 10 to 30 mg a day but in times of stress may exceed 300 mg a day.

Cortisol synthesis is tightly regulated by a feedback loop consisting of the hypothalamus, pituitary, and adrenal gland (HPA axis). Corticotropin-releasing hormone is secreted by the hypothalamus, which stimulates release of ACTH from the anterior pituitary. ACTH then precipitates the release of various products from the adrenal cortex, including cortisol. Cortisol, in turn, inhibits further production from the hypothalamus and the pituitary.

Elevated levels of cortisol produce a constellation of symptoms known as Cushing's syndrome, named after the American neurosurgeon who first described the case in 1912. Symptoms include asymmetrical weight gain (truncal obesity, "buffalo hump," "moon facies"), hyperglycemia, hypertension, skin changes (striae, fragility, impaired wound healing), osteoporosis, mood lability, and sexual hormone imbalance (hirsutism, menstrual irregularities, decreased libido/impotence).

Workup

The initial step in diagnosing Cushing's syndrome is to establish the presence of hypercortisolism. Conventional methods include 24-hour urine cortisol measurements or failure to suppress endogenous cortisol with a low-dose (1 mg) dexamethasone test. Emerging methods include measurement of midnight plasma or salivary cortisol levels.

Once the presence of excess cortisol has been confirmed, the next step is to measure serum ACTH level to determine whether this production is ACTH-dependent or ACTH-independent. Normal to high levels of ACTH suggest a pituitary or an ectopic etiology. Low levels of ACTH suggest an adrenal source. Our patient's ACTH level was significantly below the normal level, which would indicate an adrenal source.

Imaging of the adrenal gland will then help to differentiate an adrenal tumor from bilateral adrenal hyperplasia. If on CT a discrete tumor is visualized, specific CT protocols can be used to further distinguish a benign adenoma from a malignant adrenocortical carcinoma. Benign adrenal tumors tend to have low attenuation on unenhanced images due to high

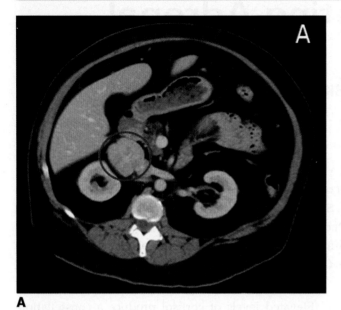
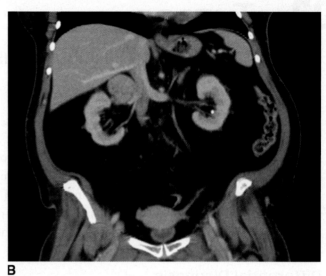

FIGURE 1 • **A:** CT scan of the abdomen demonstrating a contrast-enhancing mass in the right adrenal gland (circled). **B:** Coronal reformatting depicting the relationship of the mass to the right renal vein and the inferior vena cava.

lipid content. Both benign and malignant tumor will enhance with IV contrast; however, after a 10-minute post-contrast administration period, washout in excess of 50% is seen in benign lesions. In our patient, CT scan of the abdomen demonstrated a 5.3-cm contrast enhancing mass in the right adrenal gland **(Figure 1)**.

A biopsy of the adrenal to provide a tissue diagnosis is not warranted unless the patient has a history of cancer in some other organ system. In that case, a biopsy can help rule out the presence of metastatic disease. Otherwise, once the diagnosis of a functional adrenal lesion has been made, the patient should proceed toward surgical treatment.

Surgical Approach

The location of the adrenal gland within the retroperitoneum allows it to be accessed by multiple surgical routes. Open anterior, posterior, flank, and thoracoabdominal approaches have all been described. The enthusiasm for laparoscopic surgery has enabled for the conversion of several of these approaches to minimally invasive procedures.

For most patients with adrenal tumors, a laparoscopic adrenalectomy is the preferred method of resection. It is associated with shorter hospitalization, less pain and morbidity, quicker recovery, and fewer incisional hernias. An absolute contraindication to laparoscopic adrenalectomy is extension of the tumor into nearby structures. A relative contraindication is tumor size as controversy exists as to whether tumors >6 cm should be resected laparoscopically due to increased chance of local recurrence. From a practical standpoint, tumors of this size can be difficult to mobilize and manipulate and

more often result in conversion to an open procedure. In patients with local invasion, and perhaps those with large tumors, an open approach should be undertaken.

The following sections describe the most common methods of adrenalectomy: the laparoscopic transabdominal technique and the open transabdominal technique.

Laparoscopic Transabdominal Technique

The patient is placed on a beanbag in the lateral decubitus position. The table is flexed in order to open up the space between the costal margin and the pubis. Careful attention must be paid to safely padding the arms and positioning them in gentle anterior flexion to avoid nerve injury. The ports are placed in a line that approximates the standard subcostal incision. A 12-mm camera port is placed in the middle with two 5-mm working ports placed on either side. Some surgeons advocate moving the camera port off the subcostal line and more toward the umbilicus in order to reduce instrument collision during the operation.

For right-sided lesions, a fourth port is placed medially in order to facilitate retraction of the liver by an assistant. In order to mobilize the liver, the right triangular ligament is taken down using cautery or ultrasonic shears. The dissection begins laterally and proceeds medially until the inferior vena cava is identified. Retraction of the liver in an anterior and lateral fashion will appropriately expose the retroperitoneal space where the adrenal gland lies so that Gerota's fascia can then be opened. Blunt dissection between inferior vena cava and the medial aspect of the adrenal gland will identify the central adrenal vein that is then divided with either endoscopic clips or a laparoscopic stapling device. The inferior phrenic pedicle is then divided in a similar fashion. The remaining small vessels can usually be controlled with cautery or ultrasonic shears. Once the adrenal gland is freed from the surrounding structures, it is placed in an endoscopic specimen bag and removed.

For left-sided lesions, the port placement is similar, though a fourth port may not be necessary. The spleen and splenic flexure of the colon are taken down from their lateral attachments using cautery or ultrasonic shears. Once the spleen has been mobilized medially, the plane of dissection continues posterior to the pancreatic tail until the left adrenal is identified in proximity to the aorta. The dissection should begin between the junction of the adrenal and left renal vein. The left central adrenal vein empties into the left renal vein, and although this junction does not necessarily need to be identified, the central vein should be ligated close to the adrenal to avoid injuring the left renal vein. The central vein and inferior phrenic pedicle can be divided using clips or a laparoscopic stapling device. The gland can then be mobilized circumferentially with cautery or ultrasonic shears and removed in an endoscopic specimen bag.

Open Anterior Technique

The patient can be placed in the supine position or with the flank slightly elevated to provide exposure. Either a subcostal or a midline incision can be utilized. The anatomic details and step of the procedure mirror the laparoscopic approach **(Table 1)**. The key difference is that additional exposure is often needed in the open approach due to the large nature of the tumors or invasion of nearby structures. Any structure grossly involved with the tumor must be removed en bloc.

On the right side, additional exposure can be gained by further mobilization of the duodenum through a Kocher maneuver. If invasion through the liver is found, a nonanatomic partial hepatectomy can be performed. If the inferior vena cava is involved, it may be resected and reconstructed using a synthetic graft.

On the left side, a splenectomy can be performed to gain additional exposure. If the adrenal gland cannot be approached from the lateral aspect, then an anterior approach can be used. The gastrocolic ligament is divided and the lesser sac is entered. The inferior border of the pancreas can be elevated to find the left adrenal, which lies just posterior.

Postoperative Management

Adrenalectomy for hypercortisolism is a well-tolerated procedure with most patients leaving the

TABLE 1. Key Technical Steps and Potential Pitfalls

Left Adrenalectomy
1. Dissect right triangular ligament of liver to level of hepatic vein.
2. Retract liver anteriorly and laterally.
3. Dissect plane between adrenal gland and inferior vena cava.
4. Identify central adrenal vein and inferior phrenic pedicle and divide close to the adrenal gland.
5. Mobilize adrenal gland circumferentially.

Right Adrenalectomy
1. Release lateral attachments of spleen and splenic flexure to mobilize spleen, tail of pancreas and colon medially.
2. Dissect plane between adrenal gland and left renal vein.
3. Identify central adrenal vein and inferior phrenic pedicle and divide close to the adrenal gland.
4. Mobilize adrenal gland circumferentially.

Potential Pitfalls
- Injury to right hepatic vein.
- Injury to inferior vena cava.
- Injury to renal veins.
- Extension of tumor into nearby structures.

hospital within a few days. In addition to the routine infectious complications associated with most every surgery, when taking care of these patients, clinicians should specifically be monitoring for an Addisonian crisis. Symptoms to be wary of include weakness, mental status changes, hypotension, and hypoglycemia. These symptoms occur because chronic suppression of the HPA axis leads to a state of relative hypocortisolism. The day of operation and then postoperatively, patients must be supplemented with stress doses of steroids (hydrocortisone 100 mg three times daily) followed by a taper regimen to maintenance doses. This steroid replacement regimen should be continued until the HPA axis can recover.

While physical recovery from surgery is usually limited to a few weeks, resolution of symptoms and biochemical recovery often takes much longer. The median interval to discontinuation of steroid replacement therapy is between 12 and 30 months after a unilateral adrenalectomy. In a similar fashion, most of the physical and physiologic effects of hypercortisolism do improve after surgery, but the progression takes several months to years. Around three-quarters of all patients experience dramatic improvement in their physical features as well as significant decreases in their hypertension and diabetes.

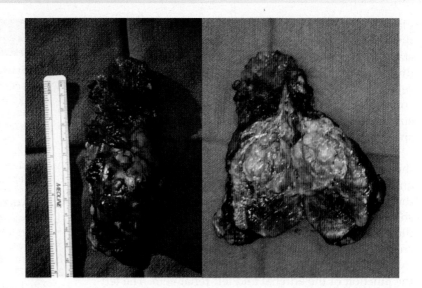

FIGURE 2 • The excised right adrenal gland (left) which was subsequently opened on the back table of the operating room (right) to reveal the large adrenal tumor.

Case Conclusion

The patient was taken to the operating room where a laparoscopic right adrenalectomy was attempted. The tumor was not able to be separated from the right renal vein safely and the case was converted to an open approach in order to complete the resection. Pathologic examination of the tumor revealed a large adenoma **(Figure 2)**. Postoperative testing showed resolution of the patient's hypercortisolism, but the steroid weaning and improvement in symptoms took place gradually over 12 months.

TAKE HOME POINTS

- Elevated with cortisol with suppression of ACTH production indicates an adrenal source of hypercortisolism.
- All biochemically functional adrenal masses should be resected.

- A laparoscopic transabdominal approach is the preferred method of resection unless the tumor is large or involves nearby structures, which then mandates an open approach.
- Postoperative management must include a steroid supplementation regimen due to suppression of the HPA axis.
- Biochemical recovery and resolution of symptoms is gradual.

SUGGESTED READINGS

Brunt LM, Doherty GM, Norton JA, et al. Laparoscopic adrenalectomy compared to open adrenalectomy for benign adrenal neoplasms. J Am Coll Surg. 1996;183:1–10.

Doherty GM, Nieman LK, Cutler GB Jr, et al. Time to recovery of the hypothalamic-pituitary-adrenal axis after curative resection of adrenal tumors with Cushing's syndrome. Surgery. 1990;108:1085–1090.

Findling JW, Raff H. Diagnosis and differential diagnosis of Cushing syndrome. Endocrinol Metab Clin North Am. 2001;30:729–747.

Shen WT, Sturgeon C, Duh QY. From incidentaloma to adrenocortical carcinoma: the surgical management of adrenal tumors. J Surg Oncol. 2005;89:186–192.

Primary Hyperaldosteronism

BARBRA S. MILLER

Presentation

A 45-year-old female is seen in her primary care physician's office with complaints of muscle cramps, fatigue, headaches, polyuria, polydipsia, and nocturia. She has a 10-year history of hypertension requiring four medications to achieve adequate blood pressure control. She also has long-standing hypokalemia, thought to be due to her diuretic, which is being treated with 60 mEq daily of supplemental oral potassium. She denies symptoms of chest pain, shortness of breath, or abdominal pain. She has had no episodes of flushing, tachycardia, tremors, or anxiety. Her vital signs are normal other than a blood pressure of 150/90. Her physical examination is unremarkable other than mild peripheral edema.

Differential Diagnosis

Difficult-to-control hypertension should prompt investigation of secondary causes for hypertension. These include renal artery stenosis, hyperaldosteronism, hyperthyroidism, intrinsic renal dysfunction, hypercortisolism, pheochromocytoma, sleep apnea, medications, and other supplements.

Workup

A thorough history and physical examination should be completed, including specific questions related to symptomatology and family history of cardiac disorders, sudden death, or genetic syndromes leading to hypertension. Laboratory studies to evaluate secondary causes of hypertension include a complete metabolic profile, serum aldosterone and renin levels, and fractionated plasma metanephrines. Certain antihypertensives may confound laboratory results. Antihypertensives such as spironolactone, eplerenone, angiotensin-converting enzyme inhibitors, and diuretics affect renin–aldosterone regulation and should be discontinued for 4 to 6 weeks in advance of testing if possible. Alpha blockers may be substituted. Antidepressants and beta blockers may affect plasma metanephrine levels, which should be considered when ruling out pheochromocytoma. Misdiagnosis of a pheochromocytoma and inadequate preoperative alpha blockade can lead to intraoperative complications and death. Diagnosis of primary hyperaldosteronism is confirmed with an elevated aldosterone level, suppressed renin level, and an aldosterone:renin ratio >20:1. Additional testing should be pursued when initial testing is equivocal. Recognizing the inability to suppress aldosterone secretion after sodium loading or administration of captopril can be helpful in this setting.

If evidence of primary hyperaldosteronism is identified, biochemical evaluation should be followed by radiologic evaluation of the adrenal glands. Imaging should not be obtained first without biochemical confirmation of the diagnosis, as many inconsequential "incidentalomas" are discovered on imaging studies. The adrenal glands are best evaluated by adrenal protocol computed tomography (CT). Thin cuts through the adrenal glands show small abnormalities and allow for assessment of tumor/nodule characteristics if present. Concern for an aldosterone-producing adrenocortical carcinoma, which is extremely rare, can usually be ruled out based on size criteria and calculation of Hounsfield units (HU) of the tumor/nodule and washout characteristics. Magnetic resonance images or NP-59 scans are alternative imaging modalities that may be requested.

Selective venous sampling of the bilateral adrenal veins should be obtained in all patients to confirm imaging findings (Figure 1). Venous sampling allows differentiation of unilateral from bilateral excess aldosterone production from the adrenal glands regardless of imaging findings, as CT and MRI findings tend not to correlate well with venous sampling results. Criteria suggesting unilateral excess aldosterone production are shown in Table 1.

Diagnosis and Treatment

Primary hyperaldosteronism is most commonly due to an aldosterone-producing adenoma or adrenal hyperplasia leading to difficult-to-control hypertension, volume excess, and hypokalemia (40% to 50%). Patients who develop hypertension at a young age or those requiring more than three antihypertensive medications for blood pressure control should be investigated for secondary causes of hypertension. Those patients found to have primary hyperaldosteronism due to unilateral excess aldosterone production are offered

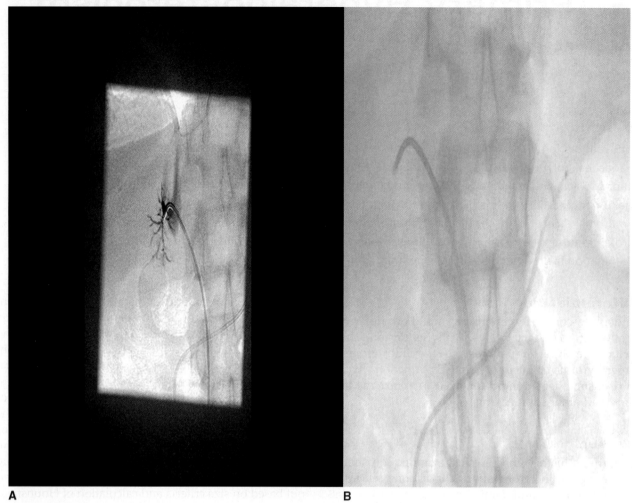

FIGURE 1 • **A:** Contrast injection of right adrenal vein to confirm catheter placement prior to selective venous sampling. **B:** Catheters placed in bilateral adrenal veins.

surgery for cure, while those found to have bilateral production of excess aldosterone are managed medically with aldosterone receptor antagonists, as the risks of iatrogenically induced Addison's disease after bilateral adrenalectomy (despite steroid replacement) outweigh the risks of continued medical management. Selective venous sampling of the adrenal veins is imperative, especially for those with bilateral normal- or abnormal-appearing adrenal glands but also for those with a single adrenal nodule, as cases are described in which a nonfunctioning incidentaloma is noted on imaging studies with excess production coming from the opposite normal-appearing adrenal gland. Selective venous sampling results should dictate which adrenal gland is removed rather than imaging results.

Laparoscopic resection of the affected adrenal gland has become the gold standard if malignancy

TABLE 1. Criteria Used to Confirm Unilateral Excess Aldosterone Secretion After Bilateral Adrenal Vein Sampling	
Adrenal Vein Sampling Aldosterone and Cortisol Ratios	Number
Confirmation of catheter placement in adrenal vein	
Pre-Cosyntropin adrenal vein C: IVC C	≥3
Lateralization	
Dominant A/C: Nondominant A/C	≥4
Supporting evidence	
Dominant A: Nondominant A	>3
Dominant A/C: IVC A/C	>1.5
Nondominant A/C: IVC A/C	<1

A, Aldosterone; C, Cortisol; A/C, aldosterone to cortisol ratio; IVC, inferior vena cava

is not suspected. Laparoscopic resection of primary adrenocortical malignancies has been shown to be associated with shorter time to local recurrence and a greater chance of margin-positive resections. Aldosterone-secreting adenomas seen on imaging studies are generally quite small with a median size <2 cm **(Figure 2)**. Larger aldosterone-secreting adenomas are rare, and concern for an aldosterone-secreting adrenocortical malignancy (even more rare) is raised in those nodules >3 to 3.5 cm having other concerning imaging characteristics (HU, washout characteristics, in-phase/out-of-phase changes). This size criterion for concern for malignancy is smaller than the 4- to 6-cm criteria normally used for assessment of other adrenal nodules.

Surgical Approach

The lateral transperitoneal approach to the adrenal gland is the most commonly employed when performing a laparoscopic adrenalectomy. Other approaches include anterior, lateral retroperitoneal, and posterior retroperitoneal. Open approaches (both anterior and posterior) may be used, but the laparoscopic approach has been shown to be associated with less pain, less morbidity, and shorter hospital stays.

Prior to operation, careful review of adrenal imaging should be undertaken to assess the position and course of the relevant vasculature including the adrenal veins, renal arteries and veins. On the left side, the surgeon should note the proximity of the splenic flexure of the colon, spleen, tail of the pancreas, and the splenic artery and vein. Patients with primary hyperaldosteronism should be prepared for surgery by correcting

volume, metabolic abnormalities, and hypertension. Aldosterone receptor antagonists, such as spironolactone or eplerenone, are most useful and help correct hypertension and hypokalemia and reduce the need for other antihypertensive medications.

Left lateral transperitoneal laparoscopic adrenalectomy requires placement of the patient in the right lateral decubitus position **(Table 2)**. Padding of pressure points is extremely important. The bed is extended to widen the space between the pelvis and the rib cage. The left arm is extended to the right side. The abdomen is accessed by an open Hasson technique at the junction of the lateral edge of the rectus muscle and the oblique musculature. Once the abdomen is insufflated and examined using a 30-degree laparoscope, at least two other ports are placed in a triangulated position. Using scissors, cautery, or ultrasonic instruments, attachments of the splenic flexure of the colon and the spleen are released and the spleen is rotated medially. The retroperitoneum is incised between the superiormedial aspect of the kidney and the inferior lateral aspect of the adrenal gland. Using cautery, ultrasonic shears and blunt dissection, the adrenal gland is mobilized from the retroperitoneal fat. At the superomedial aspect of the gland, the surgeon may encounter a branch from a phrenic vessel and should carefully ligate and divide this. Dissection at the inferior aspect

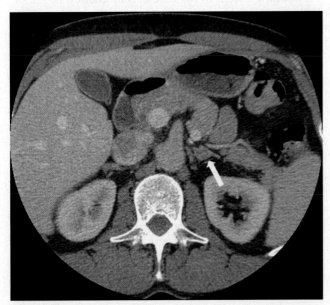

FIGURE 2 • Typical, small, benign-appearing aldosterone-secreting adenoma in the left adrenal gland.

TABLE 2. Key Technical Steps and Potential Pitfalls of Lateral Transperitoneal Laparoscopic Adrenalectomy

Key Technical Steps

1. Position patient on beanbag in lateral decubitus position at 45-degree angle with appropriate padding over pressure points, extending bed to widen distance between rib cage and pelvis.
2. Access peritoneal cavity at lateral edge of rectus muscle and place ports in triangulated fashion.
3. Release lateral attachments of viscera from peritoneum and side wall, rolling viscera medially. A paddle retractor may be helpful, especially on the right side.
4. Dissect circumferentially around adrenal gland, ligating and dividing adrenal vein when convenient.
5. Laparoscopic ultrasound can be helpful to identify the adrenal gland in obese patients.
6. Remove specimen and inspect to confirm presence of nodule, cortical, and medullary tissue.
7. Confirm hemostasis and close port sites.

Potential Pitfalls

- Bleeding from adrenal vein, renal vein, IVC on right, splenic vessels on left.
- Removal of periadrenal fat or pancreatic tissue instead of adrenal gland.
- Laceration of liver, spleen, or perforation of other nearby viscera.

should proceed cautiously to ensure no damage to the renal vessels. The adrenal vein will be found medially near a seven o'clock position draining into the renal vein. The adrenal vein should be ligated with clips and divided. The adrenal gland should be removed using an endo-bag and inspected to ensure complete removal of the gland prior to being sent to pathology.

Right lateral transperitoneal laparoscopic adrenalectomy proceeds in a fashion similar to the left side. A fourth port is usually required to retract the right lobe of the liver using a paddle retractor after mobilizing the triangular and coronary ligaments. The right adrenal vein drains directly into the vena cava. Meticulous dissection along the vena cava is required to prevent massive bleeding.

Special Intraoperative Considerations

It may be difficult to identify the adrenal gland in obese patients with large quantities of retroperitoneal fat. The adrenal gland has a golden-rod yellow color that is darker than the surrounding fat. Laparoscopic ultrasound can be extremely helpful in these situations as well and can help identify the adrenal veins and renal vessels. On the left side, lobulations of pancreatic tissue may appear similar to adrenal tissue and be mistakenly removed although the pancreas is usually lighter in color than the adrenal gland. The supposed adrenal gland should be carefully inspected after removal to ensure the characteristic cortical and medullary tissue is identified upon incision of the gland. If at any time malignancy is suspected, convert to an open procedure.

Postoperative Management

Patients generally do not require postoperative ICU management. Antihypertensive medications are held after surgery. Essential hypertension may necessitate reinstitution of some medications. Factors including age of onset of hypertension, length of time with hypertension, and number of medications required to control the blood pressure preoperatively allow for prediction of resolution of hypertension and hypokalemia after surgery. Hypertension due to hyperaldosteronism will resolve if patients have been evaluated appropriately (venous sampling used to differentiate between unilateral and bilateral excess aldosterone secretion) in the preoperative setting. Hypokalemia and need for potassium supplementation resolve within 24 hours and patients may become hyperkalemic for a short time. Autodiuresis of excess volume from hyperaldosteronism usually also occurs in the postoperative period. Most patients may be discharged on the first or second postoperative day.

Case Conclusion

The patient is found to have an aldosterone:renin ratio of 38. Computed tomography reveals a 1.4-cm lesion in the left adrenal gland. Selective venous sampling confirms unilateral excess aldosterone secretion with a dominant left A:C to nondominant right A:C ratio of 7. A left laparoscopic adrenalectomy is performed. Postoperatively, the patient's hypokalemia resolves; however, the blood pressure remains slightly elevated in the postoperative setting and she is reinstituted on beta-blocker therapy for the perioperative period. At the postoperative visit, her blood pressure is 124/68, potassium is 4.0 mEq/L, aldosterone is 8, and renin is 1.4.

TAKE HOME POINTS

- Secondary causes for hypertension should be sought in young patients or those with difficult to control blood pressure requiring more than three antihypertensive medications.
- Hypokalemia may not be present in all patients (40% to 50%).
- Diagnosis is by biochemical means, requiring an elevated aldosterone level and aldosterone:renin >20:1.
- Selective venous sampling of the adrenal veins is imperative to differentiate between unilateral and bilateral excess aldosterone secretion. Those with evidence of unilateral excess secretion should be offered surgery.
- Resection by a laparoscopic approach is the gold standard except in the case of malignancy.
- Resolution of hypertension is variable but predictable depending on age, severity of hypertension, and the degree to which essential hypertension contributes to the process.

SUGGESTED READINGS

McKenzie TJ, Lillegard JB, Young WF Jr, et al. Aldosteronomas—state of the art. Surg Clin North Am. 2009;89(5):1241–1253.

Nwariaku F, Miller B, Auchus R, et al. Primary hyperaldosteronism: effect of adrenal vein sampling on surgical outcome. Arch Surg. 2006;141(5):497–502;discussion 502–503.

White ML, Gauger PG, Doherty GM, et al. The role of radiologic studies in the evaluation and management of primary hyperaldosteronism. Surgery. 2008;144(6):926–933.

Zarnegar R, Young WF Jr, Lee J, et al. The aldosteronoma resolution score: predicting complete resolution of hypertension after adrenalectomy for aldosteronoma. Ann Surg. 2008;247(3).

67 Pheochromocytoma

ALEXIS D. SMITH and DOUGLAS J. TURNER

Presentation

A 52-year-old male with a history of poorly controlled hypertension is referred for evaluation of a 4.5-cm left adrenal mass. The mass was incidentally discovered during routine trauma computed tomography (CT) scans following a minor motor vehicle accident. History is significant for episodic headaches with blurry vision and occasional epistaxis, but he denies any chest pain, palpitations, shortness of breath, or diaphoresis. He denies any history of recent weight gain or loss. He has no personal history of cancer. He states his father died of sudden cardiac arrest in his 50s; his mother is alive and otherwise healthy. His antihypertensive regimen is currently nicardipine, lisinopril, metoprolol, and hydrochlorothiazide (HCTZ). On examination, blood pressure was 192/106 mm Hg; heart rate, 102 beats per minute; body mass index, 29. The remainder of his physical examination was normal.

Differential Diagnosis

Incidental discovery of adrenal masses is increasingly common. This is largely due to the widespread use of thoracic and abdominal cross-sectional imaging. Adrenal incidentalomas are present in up to 4% to 5% of all CT scans. In adults, an adrenal mass can represent an extensive differential diagnosis (Table 1). In order to determine the appropriate treatment of the mass, both biochemical testing and high-resolution imaging should be employed to differentiate between biochemically functional versus nonfunctional tumors and malignant versus benign tumors.

Workup

The patient subsequently undergoes initial evaluation of his adrenal incidentaloma with biochemical testing. Morning and 24-hour urinary cortisol levels are within normal limits. Additionally, plasma aldosterone: renin ratio is <20. Serum electrolytes are within normal limits. Subsequent 24-hour urinary-fractionated metanephrines and plasma-free metanephrines return elevated at 1,800 nmol/24 h and 2.6 nmol/L, respectively. This biochemical profile confirms the diagnosis of pheochromocytoma. The patient then undergoes an adrenal-protocol CT scan for localization of the tumor that demonstrates a 4.5-cm left heterogeneous adrenal mass with a 60% contrast washout after 15 minutes (Figures 1 and 2).

Discussion

Pheochromocytomas are catecholamine-producing neuroendocrine tumors derived from chromaffin cells of the adrenal medulla. Pheochromocytomas are rare, with a reported incidence of 2 to 8 per million individuals, occurring in 0.1% to 0.5% of hypertensive patients and in approximately 5% of patients with documented adrenal incidentalomas. However, the potentially lethal cardiovascular complications related to high levels of circulating catecholamines mandate biochemical testing in those found to have an adrenal incidentaloma as well as in patients with severe, episodic, or refractory hypertension. Historically, pheochromocytoma has been coined the "10% tumor" meaning that approximately 10% of cases are malignant, 10% extra-adrenal, 10% bilateral, and 10% associated with hereditary tumor syndromes. However, recent literature has demonstrated that those approximations largely underestimate the incidence of hereditary pheochromocytoma and paragangliomas (PG). Some studies have shown that up to 24% of cases are associated with familial tumor syndromes, including multiple endocrine neoplasia (MEN) types 2A and 2B, von Hippel–Lindau disease (VHL), neurofibromatosis type 1 (NF1), tuberous sclerosis, Sturge-Weber syndrome, and the familial pheochromocytoma–paraganglioma (PGL) syndrome.

Sporadic pheochromocytoma is most commonly diagnosed between the ages of 40 and 50, whereas hereditary types are usually diagnosed earlier, most often before 40 years of age. The classic triad of symptoms consists of paroxysmal hypertension, palpitations, and sweating. However, the true clinical presentation varies greatly, and it is often termed a great mimicker of many other clinical conditions. Hypertension, tachycardia, pallor, headache, and anxiety usually dominate the clinical presentation. Paroxysmal signs and symptoms are a hallmark of the clinical presentation and are due to the episodic nature of catecholamine release from the tumor. Extra-adrenal pheochromocytomas are termed PG and can be located anywhere along the sympathetic

TABLE 1. Differential Diagnoses for Adrenal Incidentalomas

Functioning Lesions	Nonfunctioning Lesions
Aldosteronoma	Cortical adenoma
Pheochromocytoma	Metastasis
Cortisol-producing adenoma (Cushing's disease)	Hemorrhage
Adrenocortical carcinoma	Cyst
Congenital adrenal hyperplasia	Infection: TB, fungal
	Myelolipoma
	Hemangioma

nervous system, but are most commonly found at the organ of Zuckerkandl.

Diagnosis and Treatment

All patients with suspected pheochromocytoma should undergo biochemical testing followed by high-resolution imaging for tumor localization and determination of the extent of disease. The preferred method of choice for biochemical assays remains a controversial topic. No current consensus exists on the best screening test and no prospective studies comparing test regimens have been published. However, current literature favors the measurement of plasma-free metanephrines and/or urinary-fractionated metanephrines as the most sensitive tests available for screening and diagnosis. However, these tests lack high specificity, and the common occurrence of false-positive results can

be attributed to external stressors as well as drug and dietary interferences related to catecholamine measurements. Some common interfering substances include coffee, nicotine, labetalol, tricyclic antidepressants, and monoamine oxidase inhibitors. A clonidine suppression test may be utilized to confirm diagnosis in those patients with equivocal results. Fine needle aspiration has no role in the diagnosis of PCC and should be avoided due to the risk of precipitation of a hypertensive crisis.

Once a biochemical diagnosis has been confirmed, tumor localization should be initiated in order to guide treatment planning. A CT scan of the abdomen, including pelvis (to below the level of the aortic bifurcation), is currently an appropriate initial imaging study with a >95% sensitivity for detecting adrenal pheochromocytoma.[4] Magnetic resonance imaging (MRI) is considered equally efficacious and is the procedure of choice in pregnancy and childhood. A major advantage of MRI is the lack of exposure to both radiation and iodinated contrast, which has the potential to elicit a hypertensive crisis in patients. Since no certain histologic criteria that distinguish benign from malignant tumors exist, a critical step in the radiologic evaluation is determination of malignancy, extra-adrenal extension, or bilateral disease. Malignancy is reported in 9% of sporadic pheochromocytoma and as high as 33% with extra-adrenal tumors. Tumors that secrete only dopamine have also been noted to be at increased risk of malignancy. Therefore, functional imaging in the form of metaiodobenzylguanidine (MIBG) scanning is warranted if there exists a high probability of malignancy

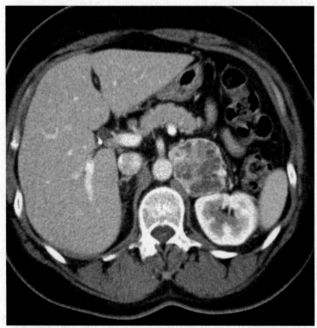

FIGURE 1 • Computed tomography (CT) scan of left pheochromocytoma.

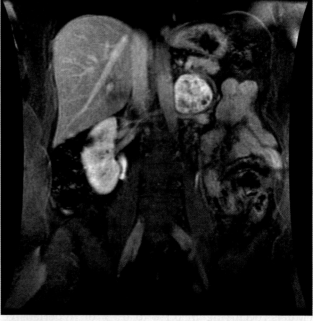

FIGURE 2 • Magnetic resonance imaging (MRI) of left pheochromocytoma.

noted by the presence of local invasion, metastases, adrenal lesions >5 cm, and contrast washout of <40% in 15 minutes on cross-sectional imaging.

Special Preoperative Considerations

Surgical resection is the only effective treatment for pheochromocytoma. Due to the high concentration of circulating catecholamines, cardiovascular lability is a frequent complicating factor during resection of these tumors. The likelihood of surgical success directly correlates to the degree of preoperative medical management. The goals of this regimen include correction of hypertension, restoration of intravascular volume, and control of dysrhythmias. The foundation of this regimen is alpha blockade, most typically phenoxybenzamine, a long-acting nonselective alpha antagonist initially dosed at 10 mg/d or twice daily with incremental increases to attain appropriate blood pressure control. A subsequent beta-blocker is added after adequate alpha blockade for heart rate control secondary to reflex tachycardia associated with alpha-blockade or for tachyarrhythmias. Monotherapy or initiation of therapy with a beta-blocker should be avoided due to the risk of a hypertensive crisis in the absence of β_2-adrenergic vasodilation. Calcium channel blockers may be utilized as a third agent for persistent hypertension. Some institutions prefer the use of shorter-acting selective alpha$_1$-blockers, such as prazosin, doxazosin, or terazosin, secondary to their avoidance of reflex tachycardia. However, no prospective head-to-head comparison trial has been done and phenoxybenzamine remains the mainstay for alpha blockade.

In addition to adequate preoperative blood pressure control, patients should be instructed about the importance of increased fluid and salt intake prior to surgery in order to assist with repletion of intravascular volume, which is low due to the vasoconstriction from high levels of circulating catecholamines.

Surgical Approach

Laparoscopic Adrenalectomy

The principles of successful surgical resection of a pheochromocytoma are minimizing tumor manipulation, avoidance of tumor spillage, complete extirpation of the tumor, early ligation of the adrenal vein, and close coordination with the anesthesiology team for tight control of intraoperative hemodynamics **(Table 2)**. Traditionally, an open approach was utilized due to the theory of an increased risk of catecholamine surge with insufflation and tumor manipulation during laparoscopic adrenalectomy. However, over the past decade, laparoscopy has evolved as the standard of care for surgical resection of pheochromocytoma.

Although multiple approaches to an adrenalectomy have been described, our institution prefers

---

TABLE 2. Key Technical Steps and Potential Pitfalls for Laparoscopic Adrenalectomy

Key Technical Steps

1. Pneumoperitoneum established with Veress needle.
2. Three or four ports placed between midclavicular line and midaxillary line, two finger widths below the costal margin.
3. Right adrenalectomy-right triangular ligament divided and mobilized cephalad. Left adrenalectomy-splenic flexure mobilized, lateral attachments of spleen and tail of pancreas mobilized medially.
4. Adrenal gland identified on superomedial aspect of kidney.
5. Adrenal vein identified at its junction with either the inferior vena cava (IVC) (right adrenal vein) or left renal vein (left adrenal vein).
6. Double-clip adrenal vein proximally and divide sharply.
7. Continue hemostatic division of remaining arterial branches and soft tissue attachments.
8. Endoretrieval bag for removal of specimen.

Potential Pitfalls

- Hypertensive crisis upon induction of anesthesia or excessive tumor manipulation.
- Bleeding secondary to adrenal vein, renal vein, or IVC injury.
- Hemodynamic instability following ligation of the adrenal vein.

---

the laparoscopic lateral transabdominal approach. Following induction of general anesthesia and placement of appropriate hemodynamic monitoring devices, the patient is placed in the lateral decubitus position and the operating table is flexed at the waist to optimize the space between the lower ribs and the iliac crest. A Veress needle is used to establish pneumoperitoneum. Three ports (four for right sided lesions) are placed between the midclavicular line anteriorly and the midaxillary line laterally, two finger widths below the costal margin. The abdomen is inspected for hepatic or peritoneal metastases. For a right adrenalectomy, the right triangular ligament is divided and the liver is mobilized from the diaphragm, retracting it cephalad with a fan or snake retractor; it is important to be able to visualize the IVC. It is rarely necessary to mobilize the hepatic flexure or duodenum. The adrenal gland is identified on the superomedial aspect of the kidney, and the right adrenal vein is identified at its junction with the IVC. Early identification and ligation of the adrenal vein is paramount. It is double clipped on the IVC aspect and divided sharply with endoscopic scissors. Division of the adrenal vein may also be accomplished with a vascular stapler. The vein is often on the posterior aspect of the vena cava, and occasionally there are accessory adrenal veins that require clipping. Hemostasis is difficult to achieve when the vein is injured, and retraction of the vein into the surrounding tissue may result in large-volume blood loss mandating conversion to an open procedure. The remaining arterial branches and soft tissue attachments are then divided hemostatically. The specimen is placed in an endoretrieval bag and brought through one of the port sites.

For a left laparoscopic adrenalectomy, patient positioning and port insertion are approached in a similar manner, although three ports often suffice on the left side. The retroperitoneum is opened by dividing the splenocolic ligament. The splenic flexure is mobilized. The lateral attachments of the spleen and the tail of the pancreas are divided for their medial mobilization. The adrenal gland is identified superior to the kidney under the mobilized pancreas and spleen. The left adrenal vein is identified when it emerges from the inferomedial aspect of the gland near to where it empties into the left renal vein. It is double clipped on the renal vein aspect and sharply divided. Any accessory adrenal veins should be handled in a similar manner.

Special Intraoperative Considerations

Hemodynamic fluctuations are a common intraoperative occurrence during resection of a PCC. Open communication with the anesthesia team is a critical component of surgical success. During induction of anesthesia, insufflation with carbon dioxide and tumor manipulation prior to ligation of the adrenal vein, the patient often experiences severe hypertension and tachyarrhythmias requiring intravenous medications such as nitroprusside, nicardipine, or esmolol. The anesthesiologists should be notified prior to ligation of the adrenal gland in order to anticipate and prepare for a precipitous drop in blood pressure following abrupt cessation of the catecholamine source with large-volume fluid resuscitation and vasoactive pressor support.

Postoperative Care

Postoperatively, patients require monitoring for hypotension and hypoglycemia. The average stay for patients following an uncomplicated laparoscopic adrenalectomy is approximately 2 days. Follow-up between 3 and 6 months is necessary to obtain a baseline plasma metanephrine level or 24-hour urine metanephrine level. Levels should be monitored every 3 months during the first year and then annually for at least 5 years. No consensus exists for extent of postoperative follow-up; however, the fact that recurrences and metastases may occur up to 20 years after curative resection argues for indefinite follow-up in sporadic PCC. Patients diagnosed with hereditary PCC should undergo yearly follow-up for their lifetime.

TAKE HOME POINTS

- Pheochromocytoma continues to be a rare catecholamine-producing neuroendocrine tumor responsible for a surgically correctable cause of hypertension.

Case Conclusion

The patient underwent a successful laparoscopic left adrenalectomy without any postoperative pressor requirement or intensive care unit admission. He was subsequently discharged to home on postoperative day 2. Surveillance plasma metanephrine taken 3 months following the operation was within normal limits. The patient opted for genetic testing secondary to his father's history of sudden cardiac death, but this test returned negative for any germline mutations.

- The incidence of hereditary pheochromocytoma is underestimated with recent studies demonstrating up to a 24% association with familial tumor syndromes including MEN2a, MEN2b, NF1, and VHL syndromes.
- Plasma metanephrine levels (sensitivity of 99%) can biochemically confirm the diagnosis and CT scans are utilized for tumor localization.
- Laparoscopic adrenalectomy has evolved as the standard of care for surgical resection of a pheochromocytoma.
- Surgical resection is the treatment of choice for malignant pheochromocytoma with curative intent for local disease and palliation in more advanced disease.

SUGGESTED READINGS

Amar L, Bertherat J, Baudin E, et al. Genetic testing in pheochromocytoma or functional paraganglioma. J Clin Oncol. 2005;23:8812–8818.

Barron J. Pheochromocytoma: diagnostic challenges for biochemical screening and diagnosis. J Clin Pathol. 2010;63:669–674.

Gagner M, Lacroix A, Bolte E. Laparoscopic adrenalectomy in Cushing's syndrome and pheochromocytoma. N Engl J Med. 1992;327:1033.

Harding JL, Yeh MW, Robinson BG, et al. Potential pitfalls in the diagnosis of phaeochromocytoma. Med J Aust. 2005;182:637–640.

Ilias I, Pacak K. Current approaches and recommended algorithm for the diagnostic localization of pheochromocytoma. J Clin Endocrinol Metab. 2004;89:479–491.

Inabnet WB, Pitre J, Bernard D, et al. Comparison of the hemodynamic parameters of open and laparoscopic adrenalectomy for pheochromocytoma. World J Surg. 2000;24:574–578.

Kalady MF, McKinlay R, Olson JA, et al. Laparoscopic adrenalectomy for pheochromocytoma: a comparison to aldosteronoma and incidentaloma. Surg Endosc. 2004;18:621–625.

Lenders JW, Eisenhofer G, Mannelli M, et al. Phaeochromocytoma. Lancet. 2005;366:665–675.

Lenders JW, Pacak K, Walther MM, et al. Biochemical diagnosis of pheochromocytoma: which test is best? JAMA. 2002;287:1427–1434.

Linos D, van Heerden JA, eds. Adrenal Glands: Diagnostic Aspects and Surgical Therapy. 1st ed. Germany: Springer, 2005:177–200.

Mellon MJ, Sundaram CP. Laparoscopic adrenalectomy for pheochromocytoma versus other surgical indications. JSLS. 2008;12(4):380–384.

Mittendorf EA, Evans DB, Lee JE, et al. Pheochromocytoma: advances in genetics, diagnosis, localization, and treatment. Hematol Oncol Clin North Am. 2007;21:509–525.

Neumann HP, Bausch B, McWhinney SR, et al. Germ-line mutations in nonsyndromic pheochromocytoma. N Engl J Med. 2002;346:1459–1466.

Petri BJ, van Eijck CH, de Herder WW, et al. Pheochromocytomas and sympathetic paragangliomas. Br J Surg. 2009;96:1381–1392.

Smith CD, Weber CJ, Amerson JR. Laparoscopic adrenalectomy: new gold standard. World J Surg. 1999;23:389–396.

Song JH, Chaudhry FS, Mayo-Smith WW. The incidental adrenal mass on CT: prevalence of adrenal disease in 1,049 consecutive adrenal masses in patients with no known malignancy. Am J Roentgenol. 2008;190: 1163–1168.

Turner DJ, Miskulin J. Management of adrenal lesions. Curr Opin Oncol. 2008;21:34–40.

Weingarter TN, Cata JP, O'Hara JF, et al. Comparison of two preoperative medical management strategies for laparoscopic resection of pheochromocytoma. Urology. 2010;76:508e6–508e11.

Weiss CA, Park AE. Laparoscopic adrenalectomy technique. Contemp Surg. 2003;59:26–29.

Zeiger MA, Thompson GB, Duh QY, et al. American Association of Clinical Endocrinologists and American Association of Endocrine Surgeons medical guidelines for the management of adrenal incidentalomas. Endocr Pract. 2009;15:1–20.

68 Pancreatic Neuroendocrine Tumors

STACEY A. MILAN and CHARLES J. YEO

Presentation

Case 1 A previously healthy 40-year-old nurse presents with complaints of an 18-month history of bouts of confusion, lightheadedness, diaphoresis, tremulousness, and occasional loss of consciousness. She reports a 20-lb weight gain over a similar time period. A recent episode required treatment in the emergency department, at which time her serum glucose (after an overnight fast) was 28 mg/dL (normal, 68 to 110 mg/dL). Her symptoms resolved with 10% dextrose intravenously.

Case 2 A 50-year-old female presents with a 6-month history of diarrhea. She first noted a change in her bowel habits from one or two formed stools daily to frequent loose stools of moderate volume. Over the next several months, her bowel movements became increasingly watery. She complains of mild abdominal pain, sometimes relieved with defecation, and tenesmus.

Case 3 A 54-year-old male was undergoing surveillance after surgery for prostate cancer. A CT scan identified a 2-cm mass in the head of the pancreas **(Figure 1)**. He had no symptoms of abdominal pain or obstructive jaundice, no past history of pancreatitis, and no family history of pancreatic neoplasia.

Differential Diagnosis

Case 1 The differential diagnosis of hypoglycemia includes reactive or postprandial hypoglycemia, surreptitious insulin or oral hypoglycemic use, noninsulinoma pancreatogenous hypoglycemia syndrome, acute hepatic failure, and uncommon tumors such as adrenocortical carcinoma, various sarcomas, and hepatocellular carcinoma.

Case 2 The differential diagnosis of a vasoactive intestinal peptide secreting tumor (VIPoma), which would present with watery diarrhea as this patient does, includes laxative abuse, villous adenoma of the rectum, celiac disease, inflammatory bowel disease, infectious and parasitic causes, gastrinoma, and carcinoid.

Case 3 Diagnoses of consideration when evaluating an incidentally discovered pancreatic mass include functional or nonfunctional pancreatic endocrine neoplasms, pancreatic adenocarcinoma, cystic pancreatic neoplasms (such as intraductal papillary mucinous neoplasm, mucinous cystadenoma or serous cystadenoma), solid pseudopapillary tumor, pseudocyst, metastatic lymphoma, sarcoidosis, or acinar cell carcinoma.

Workup

Pancreatic neuroendocrine tumors (PNETs) originate from multipotent stem cells in the pancreatic ductules and account for 1% to 2% of pancreatic neoplasms. They can be classified based on function: those associated with a functional syndrome due to ectopic secretion of a biologically active substance and those that are not associated with a functional syndrome. Functional pancreatic neuroendocrine tumors include insulinomas, gastrinomas, VIPomas, somatostatinomas, and glucagonomas **(Table 1)**. Less commonly, functional neuroendocrine pancreatic tumors may secrete adrenocorticotropic hormone, growth hormone–releasing hormone, parathyroid hormone–related protein, and calcitonin. Very rarely, neuroendocrine tumors of the pancreas may ectopically secrete leutinizing hormone, renin, IGF-2, or erythropoietin **(Table 2)**. Both functional and nonfunctional endocrine tumors of the pancreas frequently secrete a number of other substances including chromogranins (particularly chromogranin A), pancreatic polypeptide (PP), neuron-specific enolase, subunits of HCG or ghrelin, but these substances do not cause a specific hormonal syndrome.

Although there are prognostic implications to some of the functional categories (e.g., insulinomas are generally indolent), the biology of most functional pancreatic endocrine tumors is defined by the grade and size of the tumor. The World Health Organization (WHO) classification divides well-differentiated pancreatic endocrine tumors into well-differentiated endocrine neoplasms and well-differentiated carcinomas based upon their behavior **(Table 3)**. Local invasion beyond the pancreas or metastatic spread to lymph nodes

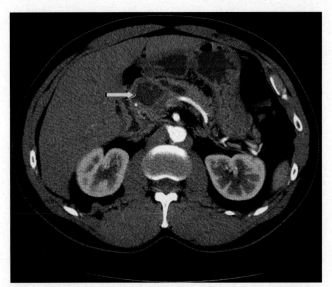

FIGURE 1 • Asymptomatic male presenting with pancreatic head mass (*arrow*) incidentally identified on surveillance CT scan of the abdomen and pelvis following treatment for prostate cancer.

and/or distant locations mandates classification as carcinoma.

PNETs occur both sporadically and with inherited disorders, including MEN-1, von Hippel–Lindau syndrome, neurofibromatosis 1, and tuberous sclerosis **(Table 4).** In MEN-1, the majority of patients develop nonfunctional PNETs, while gastrinoma is the most

common functional PNET, followed by (in order of decreasing frequency) insulinoma, glucagonoma, VIPoma, and somatostatinoma.

Diagnosis and Treatment

Patients presenting with symptoms from a functional pancreatic neuroendocrine tumor can present a diagnostic challenge, and patients are often misdiagnosed or disregarded for years before an accurate diagnosis is made. The clinical sequelae from hormone hypersecretion in functional pancreatic neuroendocrine tumors can be significant. Symptoms are often nonspecific, episodic, vary among individuals, and differ from time to time in the same individual.

Case 1 This scenario is consistent with symptoms of an insulinoma. The symptoms of hypoglycemia from an insulinoma can be divided into two categories: neuroglycopenic symptoms and neurogenic symptoms. Neuroglycopenic symptoms are due to central nervous system glucose deprivation and include behavioral changes, confusion, visual changes, fatigue, seizures, and loss of consciousness. Neurogenic symptoms are due to autonomic nervous system discharge caused by hypoglycemia and include hunger, paresthesias, sweating, anxiety, and palpitations.

Case 2 Patients with VIPomas, also known as Verner-Morrison syndrome or WDHA syndrome (watery diarrhea, hypokalemia, achlorhydria), may have diarrhea up to 20 times per day, as well as significant

TABLE 1. Well Recognized Functional Pancreatic Neuroendocrine Tumors

	Signs and Symptoms	Location in Pancreas	Malignant	Incidence
Insulinoma	Hypoglycemia Sweating Tachycardia Tremulousness Confusion Seizure	Evenly distributed head, body, tail	10%	4 per million
Gastrinoma	Gastric acid hypersecretion Peptic ulceration Diarrhea Esophagitis	Gastrinoma triangle Often extrapancreatic (duodenal) can be found anywhere in gland	50%	0.2–1 per million
VIPomas (Verner-Morrison Syndrome, WDHA)	Watery diarrhea Hypokalemia Achlorhydria (or acidosis)	Distal pancreas (body and tail) Often have spread outside pancreas	Most	0.05–0.5 per million
Somatostatinomas	Gallstones diabetes (Hyperglycemia) Steatorrhea	Pancreatoduodenal groove, ampullary, periampullary	Most	1 per 40 million
Glucagonomas	Diabetes (Hyperglycemia) Necrolytic migratory erythema Stomatitis Glossitis Angular cheilitis	Body and tail of pancreas Often large and have spread outside pancreas	Most	1 per 20 million

WDHA, watery diarrhea, hypokalemia, achlorhydria.

TABLE 2. Secretory Products of Rare Functional Pancreatic Neuroendocrine Tumors

Adrenocorticotropic hormone (ACTH)
Growth hormone–releasing hormone
Parathyroid hormone–related protein (PTH-rp)
Calcitonin
Leutinizing hormone (LH)
Renin
Insulin-like growth factor-2 (IGF-2)
Erythropoietin

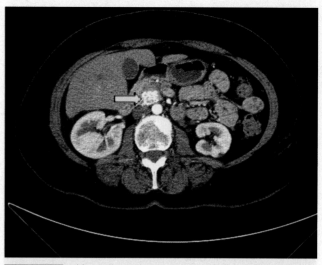

FIGURE 2 • Hyperdense appearance of a pancreatic neuroendocrine tumor (*arrow*) on arterial phase of CT scan.

dehydration and muscle weakness from water and electrolyte losses.

In working up patients with suspected functional tumors, the abnormal physiology or characteristic syndrome must be recognized. Well-described clinical syndromes exist for gastrinoma (not discussed in this chapter), insulinoma, glucagonoma, VIPoma, and somatostatinoma. Hormone elevation should be detected in the serum, and commercial assays are available for measuring insulin, VIP, somatostatin, and glucagon. The next step involves tumor localization and staging in preparation for operative intervention.

The initial imaging study used by most to identify and stage a PNET is a high-quality contrast-enhanced computed tomography (CT) scan. Pancreatic neuroendocrine tumors are typically hyperdense (i.e., enhance with contrast) and spherical on the arterial phase of imaging **(Figure 2)**. CT is useful in assessing the size and location of the pancreatic tumor, peripancreatic lymph node involvement, and the presence or absence of liver metastases for staging and surgical planning. Although dependent on the size of the tumor, the sensitivity and accuracy of CT approximate 94% and 82%, respectively.

MRI is increasingly used to detect pancreatic neuroendocrine tumors, especially small tumors. PNETs typically have high signal intensity on T2-weighted images **(Figure 3)**. The sensitivity of MRI has been reported to be between 74% and 100%.

Octreotide (somatostatin) scintigraphy may also be helpful in locating pancreatic endocrine tumors, as well as in assessing for extrapancreatic metastatic disease **(Figure 4)**. Neuroendocrine tumors often express large numbers of somatostatin receptors on the cell surfaces, and therefore the tracer preferentially identifies tumors. Octreotide scintigraphy performs well for gastrinoma, VIPoma, and glucagonoma, but less frequently localizes nonfunctional tumors and insulinomas.

Endoscopic ultrasound (EUS) is also useful in localizing pancreatic endocrine neoplasms, especially in the head of the pancreas. As with all ultrasound procedures, it is operator dependent. While EUS does not accurately evaluate for liver metastasis, it has been reported, in experienced hands, to be more accurate than CT or MRI in identifying lesions <1 cm in diameter.

When all other diagnostic measures fail to localize a functional pancreatic neuroendocrine tumor, either percutaneous transhepatic portal venous sampling or arterial stimulation with hepatic venous sampling may be useful. The first technique involves placing a venous catheter percutaneously through the liver into

TABLE 3. Who Classification of Pancreatic Neuroendocrine Tumors

Tumor	Size (cm)	Mitotic Count (per 10 hpf)	Ki-67 Index	Lymphovascular Invasion	Metastasis
Well-differentiated endocrine tumor					
Benign	<2	<2	<2%	Absent	Absent
Uncertain	≥2	2–10	≥2%	Present	Absent
Well-differentiated endocrine carcinoma		<10	≥2%	Present	Present
Poorly differentiated endocrine carcinoma		≥10	≥30%	Present	Present

TABLE 4. Inherited Disorders Associated with Pancreatic Neuroendocrine Tumors

Syndrome	Associated Clinical Features	Chromosomal Location	Pancreatic Neuroendocrine Tumor Type
MEN1	Primary hyperparathyroidism Pituitary tumors Less commonly Adrenocortical tumors Carcinoid tumors Nonmedullary thyroid tumors	11q13	Nonfunctional Gastrinoma Insulinoma Various
Von Hippel–Lindau Disease (VHL)	Pheochromocytoma (often bilateral) Retinal and cerebellar hemangioblastomas Renal cell carcinoma	3p25–26	Nonfunctional Various, including cystic tumors
Neurofibromatosis 1 (von recklinghausen disease)	Neurofibromas Café au lait spots Pheochromocytoma	17q11.2	Somatostatinoma
Tuberous sclerosis	Cardiac rhabdomyomas Renal cysts Angiomyolipomas	9q33.34 and 16p13.3	Insulinoma

the portal vein and sequentially sampling for hormone levels in the splenic vein, superior mesenteric vein, and portal vein, thus regionalizing the location of hormone production. Overall accuracy of this test ranges from 70% to 95%. The second technique (referred to by some as the Imamura test) is a doubly invasive test that involves selective visceral arterial injection of calcium with concurrent hepatic venous sampling for insulin. Calcium is serially injected at low doses through an arterial catheter into the splenic, gastroduodenal, and inferior pancreaticoduodenal arteries and samples are drawn from a hepatic vein catheter before and immediately after each injection, thereby allowing regionalization of the blood supply to the occult tumor.

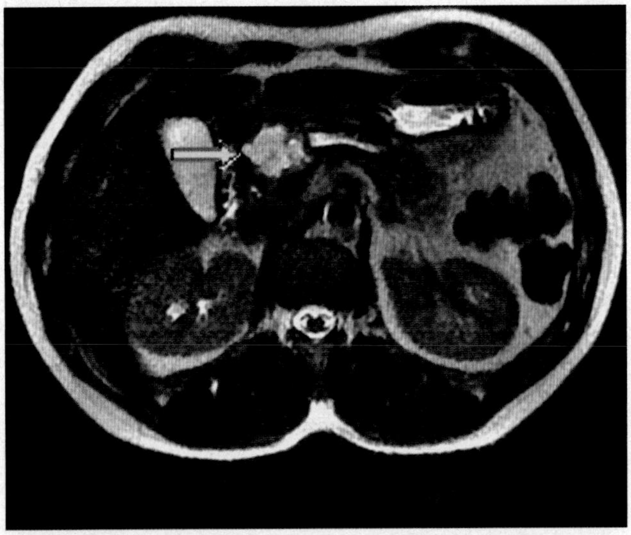

Specific Case Features

Case 1 Insulinomas are the most common functional pancreatic neuroendocrine tumor. Insulinomas often present with the classic syndrome recognized as Whipple's triad: symptoms of hypoglycemia, documented serum glucose of <50 mg/dL, and relief of symptoms after administration of glucose. This can be confirmed with a monitored in-hospital fast, during which glucose and insulin levels can be checked every 4 to 6 hours and at the time the patient becomes symptomatic. Serum insulin levels will be elevated, and C-peptides should be checked to rule out surreptitious insulin or oral hypoglycemic use. Patients with an insulinoma will have increased insulin, proinsulin, and C-peptide levels; those with hypoglycemia secondary to surreptitious insulin use will have increased insulin levels, but decreased levels of proinsulin and C-peptide. Urine tests for metformin and sulfonylurea can be performed to exclude surreptitious oral hypoglycemic use. Frequently small in size, insulinomas can be difficult to localize, although most are successfully localized with a combination of CT scan, EUS, and selective arteriography with venous sampling. In this case, a CT scan localized a 1-cm hypervascular mass in the midbody of the pancreas, with no other abnormalities.

Case 2 The classic features of a VIPoma include large-volume diarrhea (>5 L/d), severe hypokalemia with muscle weakness, and achlorhydria. Additionally, patients are often noted to be hyperglycemic. Further

FIGURE 3 • MRI demonstrating typical high signal intensity of pancreatic neuroendocrine tumor (*arrow*) on T2-weighted images.

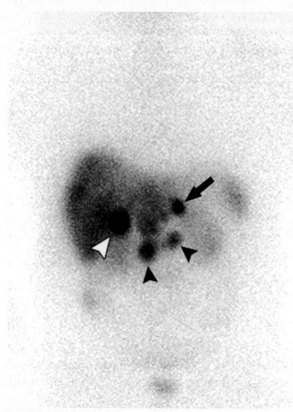

FIGURE 4 • Octreotide scan of a patient with a VIPoma with liver metastasis (*white arrowhead*) as well as regional lymph node metastasis (*black arrowheads*). (From Intenzo, et al. Scintigraphic imaging of body neuroendocrine tumors. Radiographics. 2007;27:1355–1369, reprinted with permission).

workup to exclude other causes of diarrhea in patient two includes stool samples that are negative for infectious causes of diarrhea and blood, and a colonoscopy that is normal. She notes muscle weakness and on routine labs has a potassium of 2.4 mmol/L as well as a metabolic acidosis. She has lost 25 lb in 6 months. CT scan demonstrates a large mass in the tail of the pancreas and multiple liver masses. Serum VIP was measured at 460 pg/mL (normal <50), and her serum gastrin was normal.

Case 3 Nonfunctional pancreatic neuroendocrine tumors are being increasingly detected due to increased usage of cross sectional imaging. A recent study by Lahat and colleagues found that 15.6% of pancreatic incidentalomas are neuroendocrine in origin. In contrast symptomatic, nonfunctional pancreatic neuroendocrine tumors are frequently large and at an advanced stage when first diagnosed, with 60% to 85% having liver metastasis in most series. Preoperatively, this patient was found to have elevated chromogranin A and pancreatic polypeptide levels in addition to the 2-cm mass in the head of the pancreas identified by CT.

Surgical Approach

Surgical exploration for pancreatic neuroendocrine tumors requires careful planning. The goals of the operation include eliminating or controlling the symptoms of hormone excess, safely resecting maximal tumor mass, and preserving maximal pancreatic parenchyma. Management strategies will vary for the different types of endocrine neoplasms, the location within the pancreas, and the presence of extrapancreatic disease. Surgical approaches include both laparoscopic and open procedures, and ranges from enucleation to pancreaticoduodenectomy, distal pancreatectomy or central pancreatectomy, with potential for debulking of metastatic disease, depending on the specific patient situation.

Case 1 Laparoscopic exploration confirmed an obvious 1-cm mass in the midbody of the pancreas. No other lesions were identified in the pancreas via visual inspection and intraoperative ultrasound, and the tumor was not intimately associated with the pancreatic duct. The tumor was successfully enucleated via the laparoscopic approach. In the postoperative period, she was noted to be euglycemic and was discharged from the hospital uneventfully on postoperative day 3. At 6-month follow-up, she remained euglycemic and had successfully lost 20 lb of excess weight.

Case 2 After discussion with the patient regarding the options of surgical debulking to control symptoms versus attempted long-term symptom control with somatostatin analog (octreotide), surgical debulking was elected. Preoperatively, the patient was commenced on octreotide and hospitalized for correction of dehydration and metabolic abnormalities. She underwent laparotomy, distal pancreatectomy, and en bloc splenectomy with careful attention to regional lymph nodes, and wedge resection of two peripheral liver metastases. A third intraparenchymal liver metastasis was treated with radiofrequency ablation to yield debulking of >95% of her disease. At 6-month follow-up, she was off octreotide, her diarrhea had completely resolved, her surveillance CT scan showed no evidence of imageable disease, and her serum VIP level was 53 pg/mL.

Case 3 After counseling and education, this patient underwent a pylorus-preserving pancreaticoduodenectomy, and pathology revealed a well-differentiated neuroendocrine carcinoma involving 2 of 16 resected lymph nodes. His postoperative course was complicated by a low-volume pancreatic fistula to an operatively placed drain that resolved with drain maintenance and somatostatin therapy. He was discharged from the hospital doing well, with one drain in place, on postoperative day 8. His drain was removed at his first postoperative office visit, and at 6-month follow-up, he was well. He was not advised to receive either chemotherapy or radiation therapy. His 6-month surveillance CT scan showed normal post-Whipple anatomy and no evidence of tumor.

Special Intraoperative Considerations

Approximately one-third of patients with malignant pancreatic neuroendocrine tumors have synchronous liver metastases at the time of diagnosis. While some of these patients remain asymptomatic and achieve long-term survival without aggressive therapy, overall 5-year survival for neuroendocrine tumors with liver metastases is <50%. In a selected subset of patients where surgical resection of >90% of tumor burden can be safely achieved, surgical debulking has shown a survival advantage, with 5-year survival rates of 60% to 75%. However, the value of surgical debulking has not been rigorously tested in a prospective, randomized trial setting.

Postoperative Management

Patients post pancreatic resection are typically managed in an intensive care unit (or well-monitored bed setting) for 1 to 2 days postoperatively, with attention to multisystem organ function, fluid balance, and pain control. Close postoperative attention must be paid to common complications of pancreatic resection, including pancreatic leak and or fistula, pneumonia, myocardial infarction, venous thromboembolism, postoperative bleeding, surgical site infection, and anastomotic dehiscence. Patients undergoing extensive pancreatic resection (where a considerable portion of normal pancreatic parenchyma is sacrificed) may experience abnormal endogenous blood sugar control and ultimately require insulin therapy.

For patients with hormonally active (functioning) pancreatic endocrine tumors associated with unresectable disease, further treatment is possible to ameliorate the symptoms of hormonal excess. In patients with metastatic insulinoma, diazoxide can reduce insulin secretion and raise glucose levels. Side effects include nausea and vomiting, hypotension, and hirsutism. Chemotherapy regimens for insulinoma are limited but often have included streptozocin, 5-fluorouracil, and doxorubicin in combination. Further work is ongoing in developing new anticancer regimens for metastatic neuroendocrine tumors, such as everolimus, capecitabine, and temozolomide, but have yet to become standard of care. Somatostatin can be useful in long-term management of symptoms in patients with insulinoma and VIPoma, although not all patients

respond to somatostatin and others may become refractory to it. Other treatments for metastatic pancreatic neuroendocrine tumors within the liver (not limited to insulinoma) such as hepatic artery chemoembolization and radiofrequency ablation may be useful in carefully selected patients.

TAKE HOME POINTS

- Pancreatic neuroendocrine tumors may present in a variety of ways, from the five well-described clinical hormone excess syndromes to incidental discovery during imaging for an unrelated issue.
- Clinical syndromes can be difficult to recognize and patients often elude diagnosis. Many patients experience a battery of tests over many months to years before the correct diagnosis is entertained and defined.
- Neuroendocrine tumors of the pancreas may occur sporadically or with familial syndromes such as MEN1, von Hippel–Lindau, neurofibromatosis 1, and tuberous sclerosis.
- Contrast-enhanced CT scan is the diagnostic modality of choice, but further testing may be needed to localize some tumors. EUS may be particularly helpful in identifying small tumors <1 to 2 cm in size.
- The surgical approach depends on the tumor location in the pancreas and extent of disease. In patients with liver metastases, surgical debulking to include resection of the primary lesion and either hepatic resection or ablation should be considered if ≥ 90% of the tumor burden can be eliminated.

SUGGESTED READINGS

House MG, Cameron JL, Lillemoe KD, et al. Differences in survival for patients with resectable versus unresectable metastases from pancreatic islet cell cancer. J Gastrointes Surg. 2006;10(1):138–145.

Imamura M. Recent standardization of treatment strategy for pancreatic neuroendocrine tumors. World J Gastroenterol. 2010;16(36):4519–4525.

Kennedy EP, Brody JR, Yeo CJ. Neoplasms of the endocrine pancreas. Greenfield's Surgery: scientific principles and practice. 5th ed. Philadelphia, PA: Wolters Kluwer and Lippincott Williams and Wilkins, 2010:857–871.

Kulke MH, Anthony LB, Bushnell DL, et al. North American Neuroendocrine Tumor Society Treatment Guidelines: well-differentiated neuroendocrine tumors of the stomach and pancreas. Pancreas. 2010;39(6)735–752.

69 Gastrinoma

GEOFFREY W. KRAMPITZ and JEFFREY A. NORTON

Presentation

A 22-year-old morbidly obese male with a history of peptic ulcer disease was referred to our clinic for epigastric pain. Over the past year, the pain has persisted despite a 3-month trial of proton pump inhibitor therapy. Prior esophagoduodenoscopy demonstrated a 1-cm nonhealing, solitary ulcer in the proximal duodenum with a workup that was negative for *Helicobacter pylori* infection. The patient's also describes chronic diarrhea over this same time interval. In our clinic, in addition to the chief complaints of burning epigastric pain and four to five large-volume loose bowel movements on a daily basis, the patient also divulged that he had been feeling increasingly fatigued over the last 3 years and his mood had become progressively depressed. He also complained of persistent bone and muscle pain that he attributed to his increasing weight. He also indicated that he had a soft mobile mass in his right inguinal region, similar to his prior lipomas. He had no fevers, chills, night sweats, weight loss, headaches, syncope, visual changes, galactorrhea, palpitations, shortness of breath, flushing, nausea, vomiting, hematochezia, melena, hematuria, or dysuria. His complete review of systems was otherwise negative.

His past medical history was significant for gynecomastia at the age of 16, the workup of which revealed elevated prolactin level >280 ng/mL and a 2.1-cm pituitary macroadenoma. He underwent a surgical reduction mammoplasty, and he was started on cabergoline therapy after which his prolactin level normalized. A recent prolactin level was normal at 40 ng/mL. A recent MRI showed slight reduction in tumor size, and visual field testing suggested no progression of his disease. He also had multiple lipomas excised over the past 5 years. He was diagnosed with hypogonadotropic hypogonadism for which he was prescribed transdermal testosterone with little improvement in symptoms, morbid obesity for which he was attempting dietary changes without success, and insulin resistance not requiring medications.

Family history was significant for his mother, now aged 54, who had amenorrhea at age 35, the workup of which revealed a prolactinoma that was managed medically. Several years later, she was diagnosed with parathyroid hyperplasia for which she underwent a subtotal (3 and ½ gland) parathyroidectomy. More recently, she had progressive epigastric discomfort for which she had yet to be evaluated.

The patient's physical exam was notable for morbid obesity (BMI, 56), undisturbed visual fields, nonfocal neurologic exam, and no expressible galactorrhea; heart exam revealed a regular rate and rhythm; lungs were clear to auscultation; abdomen was protuberant but soft, nontender, and nondistended; rectal exam showed a normal prostate and no masses or blood; normal external male genitalia; a 4-cm, soft, nontender, mobile soft tissue mass in the right inguinal region; and extremities with good pulses and without clubbing or cyanosis.

Differential Diagnosis

This patient has a constellation of symptoms classic for Zollinger-Ellison syndrome (ZES). The diagnosis of ZES is often delayed because it can mimic many other much more common conditions that result in peptic ulcers and/or hypergastrinemia. Ulcerogenic conditions with excessive gastric acid secretion include gastric outlet obstruction, retained gastric antrum after Billroth II reconstruction, and G-cell hyperplasia. Nonulcerogenic conditions without excessive gastric acid secretion include postvagotomy, postgastric bypass, pernicious anemia, atrophic gastritis, short gut syndrome after significant intestinal resection, renal failure, Helicobacter pylori infection, VIPoma, and stomach irradiation. Many of these conditions are associated with achlorohydria, in which stomach acid production is absent, resulting in hypergastrinemia, mimicking ZES. However, our patient had no obstructive symptoms, prior intra-abdominal operations, irradiation, renal failure, gastritis, or anemia. He had endoscopically proven peptic ulcers without *H. pylori* infection refractory to a standard trial of PPI therapy and in the presence of chronic diarrhea raising our suspicion for ZES.

Discussion

In 1955, Zollinger and Ellison first described a syndrome of severe peptic ulcers associated with pancreatic islet cell tumors that were refractory to conventional acid-reduction surgery. We now know that these tumors were gastrinomas causing gastrin hypersecretion and excessive gastric acid production, which in turn leads to intractable peptic ulcer disease. Gastrinoma has a yearly incidence of approximately 0.1 to 3 cases per million people, making it the second most common pancreatic neuroendocrine tumor overall. It is also the causative factor in approximately 0.1% to 1% of patients with peptic ulcer disease. In 80% of cases, ZES occurs sporadically. However, approximately 20% of patients with ZES have the familial form associated with multiple endocrine neoplasia type 1 (MEN-1). MEN-1 is a syndrome first described in 1954 by Wermer caused by mutations in a gene located on chromosome 11q13 encoding a tumor suppressor protein called menin. Patients with MEN-1 have asymmetrical parathyroid hyperplasia, duodenal and pancreatic neuroendocrine tumors and anterior pituitary tumors, lipomas, as well as thyroid and adrenocortical adenomas. Fifty percent of patients with MEN-1 have ZES, making gastrinoma the most common functional pancreatic or duodenal neuroendocrine tumor in MEN-1. Despite increased awareness of ZES and improvements in diagnostic methodologies, the mean time from symptom onset to diagnosis is 8 years in many studies, so that improvements in detection and awareness are still needed.

Workup

Any patient with peptic ulcer disease that is refractory, recurrent, atypical, requiring surgery, or in the absence H. pylori should undergo a workup for ZES. The presence of hyperparathyroidism, nephrolithiasis, or family history suggestive of MEN-1 should also raise suspicion for ZES. We begin our workup by obtaining a fasting serum concentration of gastrin. Hypergastrinemia occurs in almost all patients with ZES (99% sensitivity) and is defined as a serum gastrin concentration >100 pg/mL. Because PPI therapy can induce hypergastrinemia, we checked the patient's PPI for 1 week prior to the test. In this case, our patient's gastrin level was significantly elevated at 1,210 pg/mL. Basal acid output (BAO) was also elevated at 39 mEq/h (normal ≤15 mEq/h or <5 mEq/h in patients who have undergone previous acid-reducing operations). In addition, a gastric pH measured at 1.7 also indicated acid hypersecretion. Although less accurate than BAO, a gastric pH >3 essentially excludes ZES, whereas a pH ≤2 is consistent with ZES. However, many patients with ZES have gastric acid hypersecretion and minimally increased fasting serum gastrin concentrations (100 to 1,000 pg/mL).

For these patients, the secretin stimulation test is the provocative test of choice to establish the diagnosis of ZES.

Twenty percent of ZES cases occur in association with MEN-1, and ZES is the presenting symptom in 40% of cases of MEN-1. Thus during the initial workup for ZES, MEN-1 must always be excluded. This was particularly relevant in our patient who exhibited other signs and symptoms consistent with MEN-1, including pituitary adenoma, lipomas, as well as fatigue, depressed mood, and musculoskeletal pain. Our initial screen was a serum calcium measurement, exploiting the high penetrance of hyperparathyroidism in MEN-1, followed by serum parathyroid hormone (PTH) concentration, if necessary. In this case, our patient's serum calcium and PTH levels were elevated at 12 mg/dL and 146 pg/mL, respectively.

With a biochemical diagnosis of ZES established, the next step in the workup was to localize and characterize the gastrinoma to determine resectability and the best operative approach. Approximately 80% of gastrinomas are found within the gastrinoma triangle, the apices of which are bounded by the junction of the cystic and common bile ducts superiorly, the junction of the second and third portions of the duodenum laterally, and the neck of the pancreas medially. Gastrinomas associated with MEN-1 tend to be multiple, small, and usually originate in the duodenum.

In our case, a pancreatic protocol CT scan including PO and IV contrast with 5-mm cuts demonstrated a dominant 3-cm tumor in the superiomedial aspect of the head of the pancreas abutting the superior mesenteric vein (Figure 1). The sensitivity of CT is directly related to the size of the tumor. Tumors >3 cm are detected in 83% to 95% of cases, tumor 1 to 3 cm are detected in 30% of cases, whereas tumors <1 cm are not detectable. Another limitation of CT scanning in the setting of gastrinoma is that only 50% of liver metastases are detected.

We then obtained a somatostatin receptor scintigraphy (SRS, also called octreoscan) that revealed focal, intense tracer uptake in the region of the head of the pancreas corresponding to the 3-cm lesion seen on CT scan (Figure 2). In addition, SRS also demonstrated a 1-cm tumor in the neck of the pancreas on the anterior wall, a third 8-mm tumor in the inferior portion of the head of the pancreas abutting the duodenum, and no scintigraphic evidence of distant metastases. The additional findings seen on SRS demonstrate the increased sensitivity of this modality over CT. SRS has a sensitivity that surpasses all other imaging modalities combined, and in the setting of ZES has an overall sensitivity of about 90%, specificity of 100%, and positive predictive value near 100%. Nevertheless, the sensitivity of SRS is still limited when interrogating for very small tumors. The sensitivity of SRS for tumors

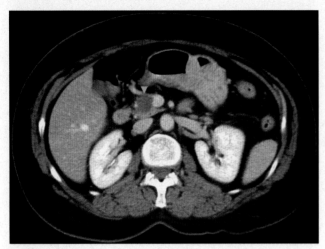

FIGURE 1 • Computed tomography scan demonstrating 3-cm gastrinoma at the head of the pancreas and abutting the superior mesenteric vein.

>2.2 cm is 96%, for tumors 1.1 to 2.2 cm is 64%, but for tumors <1.1 cm is only 30%. Because duodenal gastrinomas are usually subcentimeter in size, SRS fails to detect about 50% of these tumors.

The patient's constellation of signs including pituitary adenoma, hyperparathyroidism, multiple pancreatic gastrinomas, and lipomas, as well as similar finding of prolactinoma and hyperparathyroidism in his mother was strongly suggestive of MEN-1. The patient, his mother, and his two brothers underwent genetic testing for MENIN gene mutations. This testing revealed a T-278 mutation in the patient and the mother, but not in the siblings, thus establishing a genetic diagnosis of MEN-1.

Diagnosis and Treatment

The first principle of treating ZES associated with MEN-1 is to control symptoms medically. Following our diagnostic workup for ZES, we reinitiated PPI therapy for our patient and titrated the dose to obtain a BAO below 15 mEq/h, ultimately requiring 80 mg of pantoprazole orally twice per day.

The second principle of treating ZES associated with MEN-1 is to address parathyroid hyperplasia. Because ZES symptoms can be exacerbated by hypercalcemia resulting from hyperparathyroidism, the patient underwent a subtotal (3 and ½ gland) parathyroidectomy with a transcervical thyrmectomy. This allowed for decreased end-organ effect of hypergastrinemia and better medical control of ZES symptoms.

The third principle of treating ZES associated with MEN-1 is to determine if the patient is a candidate for operative intervention. Gastrinomas associated with MEN-1 have a propensity to spread to peripancreatic lymph nodes but are usually more indolent and less likely to metastasize to the liver when compared to sporadic tumors. Because hepatic involvement is the most important predictor of survival, ZES patients with MEN-1 have a more favorable long-term prognosis. Although surgery for MEN-1-associated disease is rarely curative (0% to 10%), resection may prevent liver metastases and thus affect long-term survival. Because tumor size >2 cm is predictive of progression to liver metastasis, surgery for ZES associated with MEN-1 is recommended only if there is an identifiable tumor larger than 2 cm. This is relevant to our patient because his main tumor was 3 cm in size.

Surgical Approach

Because of tumor multifocality (both in the pancreas and the duodenum) in MEN-1 patients, there is no biochemical cure. The goal of surgery is to prevent liver metastases and thus decrease tumor-related mortality. As such, we recommend operative approaches that focus on resecting tumor while preserving as much of the normal tissue as possible. In general, the operation should include resection of body and tail pancreatic tumors, enucleation of palpable pancreatic head tumors, duodenotomy with excision of duodenal tumors, and peripancreatic lymph node sampling. We do not favor routinely performing Whipple pancreaticoduodenectomy for attempted cure because long-term survival is excellent with the surgical approach described above, which has much less morbidity. Nevertheless, Whipple pancreaticoduodenectomy may be necessary with bulky tumors at the head of the pancreas, tumors involving the ampulla, or tumor invasion into major ductal or vascular structures. Our patient had multiple pancreatic tumors, the largest of which was a bulky tumor in the head of the pancreas abutting the superior mesenteric vein. Thus, we obtained informed consent for a possible Whipple procedure.

We entered the abdomen via bilateral subcostal incision and performed a full abdominal exploration. We inspected and palpated the liver without finding any evidence of hepatic metastases. In addition, there was no evidence of carcinomatosis or distant metastases. We then established exposure by placing a Thomson retractor and performed a cholecystectomy.

The next step was the portal dissection. The common hepatic artery was identified and protected. We identified the common bile duct that appeared normal in size and caliber. We also dissected out the common hepatic duct and placed a right-angled clamp and a Vessel loop around it. In between the common hepatic artery and the bile duct, we identified the portal. At the superior border of the pancreas, we identified the gastroduodenal artery, placed two 2-0 silk sutures around it, a 3-0 silk suture ligature on the side of the common hepatic artery, and divided it with a 15-blade. We were

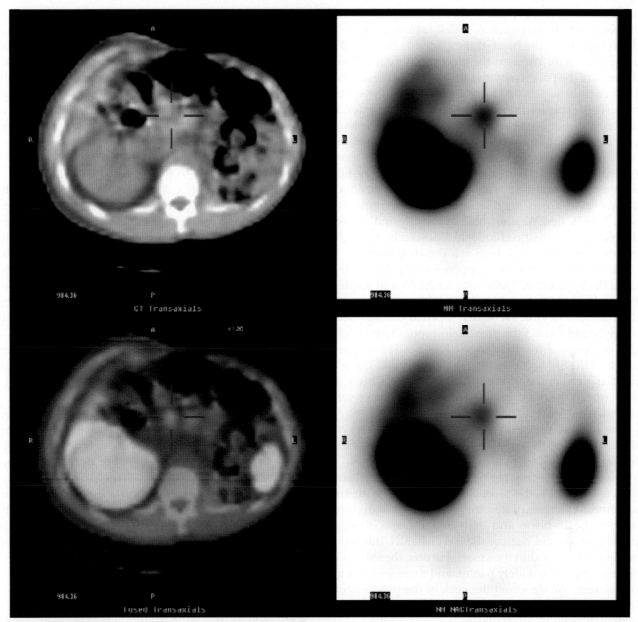

FIGURE 2 • Octreoscan demonstrating focal intense tracer uptake in the pancreatic head region corresponding to the 3-cm hypervascular lesion seen on CT.

then able to dissect underneath the neck of the pancreas toward the superior mesenteric vein.

In order to obtain adequate exposure of the pancreas, we mobilized the right colon and performed a Kocher maneuver. It was at this time we could clearly palpate the 1-cm tumor in the neck of the pancreas on the anterior wall, and as we did the Kocher maneuver, we could feel the 8-mm tumor in the more inferior aspect of the head of the pancreas abutting the pancreas and duodenum, as well as the larger 3-cm tumor in superiomedial aspect of the head of the pancreas, abutting the sidewall of the SMV. The remainder of the pancreas appeared and palpated normally.

We opened the lesser sac widely dividing the gastrocolic ligament and dissected along the inferior border of the body and tail of the pancreas from lateral to medial toward the superior mesenteric vein. We identified the superior mesenteric vein, the right sidewall of which was abutting the tumor. However, we were able to dissect underneath the neck of the pancreas and follow the anterior surface of the SMV toward the portal vein.

At this point, we felt that a Whipple operation was possible, but part of the sidewall of the SMV at the confluence of the SMV, splenic vein, and portal vein would have to be resected. We divided the duodenum 2 cm distal to the pylorus with a GIA 55-mm stapler. We elected to divide the pancreas initially rather than ligate the vessels from the head of the pancreas to the SMV and portal vein. We used the electrocautery to divide the neck of the pancreas with care to remove the second 1-cm pancreatic neuroendocrine tumor with the specimen. This exposed the confluence where the inferior mesenteric vein, superior mesenteric vein, and splenic vein combined to form the portal vein. We divided the bile duct with electrocautery and dissected the more superior aspect of the head of the pancreas and the bile duct off the portal vein. The superior pancreaticoduodenal vein was then identified and ligated in continuity with 2-0 silk ties. We were able to identify and dissect the inferior pancreaticoduodenal followed by the right gastric vein and ligated them in a similar fashion.

We divided the jejunum approximately 20 cm distal to the ligament of Treitz with a GIA 55-mm stapler. We took down the proximal jejunal mesentery with the LigaSure device. We widely opened the ligament of Treitz and passed the proximal jejunum to the right side of the abdomen. We dissected the head of the pancreas off the SMA, feeling the SMA pulse, and using a right-angle clamp and the LigaSure device. This was posterior to the SMV, but we were able to completely mobilize the head of the pancreas off the SMA.

The head of the pancreas was completely freed off the SMV except for approximately 8-mm aspect of the tumor that was adherent to the sidewall of the SMV. We used a TA-30-mm stapler with a vascular load and resected partially the sidewall of the SMV with the specimen. Once we placed the staple line, we divided it with the 15-blade and delivered the specimen to pathology. We did narrow the SMV slightly, but there was good flow within the vessel. Further, the IMV and splenic vein were widely patent, and there was a large portal vein. We dissected the neck of the pancreas off the splenic vein and IMV in order to mobilize it for the pancreaticojejunal anastamosis.

Next, we completed anastomoses of the jejunum to the pancreas, the common hepatic duct, and the duodenum. Because the pancreatic duct was not dilated (2 mm in diameter), we did a dunking anastomosis with 3-0 silk sutures, full thickness on the jejunum and capsule of pancreas such that 2 to 3 cm of the body of the pancreas was inverted into this area of jejunum. Approximately 6 cm distal to that anastomosis, we connected the common hepatic duct to the same limb of jejunum with interrupted 4-0 PDS sutures, such that the posterior row had the knots on the inside of the anastomosis while the anterior row had the knots on the outside. Next, we restored GI continuity by anastomosing the duodenum to the jejunum approximately 20 cm distal to the hepaticojejunostomy. This was done with a 3-0 silk seromuscular layer and a running full-thickness 3-0 PDS layer.

We irrigated saline solution and placed 10 mL of Tisseel fibrin glue on the pancreaticojejunostomy and the hepaticojejunostomy. We placed two No. 15 round JP drains to drain the right upper quadrant. We closed the fascia in two layers with looped No. 1-PDS. Finally, the skin was closed with a subcuticular 4-0 Monocryl. There were some lipomas in the subcutaneous tissue of the abdominal wall, and these were resected and sent to pathology **(Table 1).**

Special Intraoperative Considerations

The first intraoperative consideration is to confirm the presence or absence of tumor metastases seen on preoperative imaging. Hepatic metastases are the primary determinant of survival in ZES patients. Thus, tumors involving the liver would require appropriate debulking via wedge resection, sementectomy, or lobectomy depending on the extent and respectability of disease.

The second intraoperative consideration is to determine if the tumors seen on preoperative imaging indeed require a Whipple procedure or whether a more limited resection would be sufficient. As mentioned previously in this case, the tumor in the head of the pancreas was of a significant size that required a Whipple procedure.

The third intraoperative consideration is to determine whether involvement of vascular structures necessitates vascular reconstruction. Since the goal of the operation was not curative, but rather to prevent liver metastasis, microscopically negative margins are not as significant a consideration as in sporadic tumors. Thus, in this case, we decided to partially resect the sidewall of the SMV with the specimen since doing so would not compromise blood flow through the vessel

---

TABLE 1. Key Technical Steps and Potential Pitfalls for a Whipple Procedure

Key Technical Steps

1. Bilateral subcostal incisions and full abdominal exploration.
2. Mobilize the right colon and perform Kocher maneuver.
3. Open lesser sac and clear the anterior surface of the superior mesenteric vein.
4. Perform cholecystectomy, portal dissection, and ligation of gastroduodenal artery.
5. Divide proximal jejunum, duodenum, pancreas, and bile duct.
6. Dissect uncinate process from the superior mesenteric vein and artery.
7. Reconstruction with pancreaticojejunostomy, choledochojejunostomy, and gastrojejunostomy.

Potential Pitfalls

- Bleeding from the superior mesenteric or portal vein.
- Injury to the proper hepatic artery.

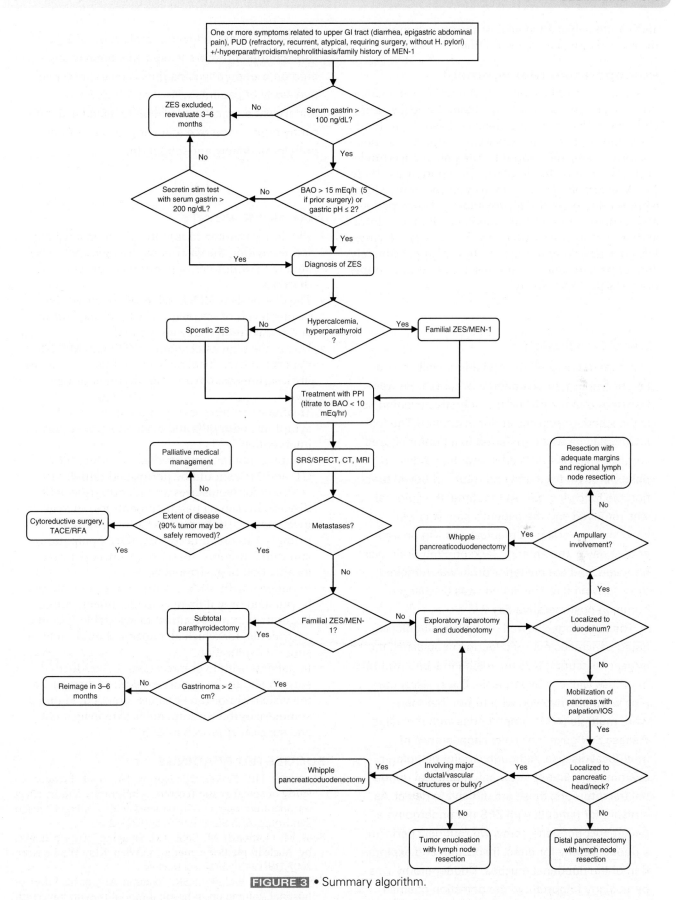

FIGURE 3 • Summary algorithm.

and would achieve the goal of the operation without the risks of vascular reconstruction.

Postoperative Management

The major complications of Whipple pancreatico-duodenectomy are death, anastomotic leaks, intra-abdominal abscesses, and delayed gastric emptying. With improvements in pancreatic surgery and postoperative care, the mortality for pancreaticoduodenectomy at most high-volume is reported as 2% to 6%. Anastomotic leaks, primarily at the pancreaticojejunostomy, occur in approximately 8% of patients and usually resolve with adequate drainage. Intra-abdominal abscesses occur in 5% to 10% of cases. Delayed gastric emptying occurs in approximately 30% of patients and usually resolves within a couple of weeks postoperatively.

Case Conclusion

Our patient tolerated the procedure well and had an uncomplicated postoperative course. He was transferred to the ICU on the operative evening as is the standard practice at our institution. The following day he was transferred to a nonmonitored surgical unit. He tolerated a clear liquid diet on postoperative day 3 and had return of bowel function the following day. At that time, the epidural was removed and the patient's pain was well controlled on oral pain medications. On postoperative day 5, the anterior Jackson-Pratt drain was removed, and the posterior drain was removed the following day. The patient was discharged home on postoperative day 7.

The pathology showed multiple well-differentiated pancreatic neuroendocrine neoplasms, the largest measuring 3.2 cm, arising in a background of diffuse islet cell hyperplasia. The surgical margins were not involved with tumor, but there were multiple (4/12) lymph nodes with metastatic disease that gave the clinical appearance of multifocal disease. Although careful pathologic examination did not show any multifocal duodenal microtumors, these are difficult to detect. As a result, for patients with ZES not undergoing a pancreaticoduodenectomy, we routinely perform a duodenotomy for direct inspection and exploration of the duodenal mucosa. Duodenotomy was particularly important in the detection of small duodenal tumors, allowing localization of 90% of subcentimeter tumors versus only 50% discovered on preoperative imaging. A recent prospective study of patients with sporadic ZES who underwent surgical exploration revealed a significantly higher cure rate following duodenotomy, both immediately and long term.

TAKE HOME POINTS

- ZES is a syndrome caused by gastrinoma usually located within the gastrinoma triangle and associated with symptoms of peptic ulcer disease and diarrhea.
- The diagnosis of ZES is achieved by measuring fasting levels of serum gastrin, basal acid output, and postsecretin challenge testing.
- Due to the high association of ZES with MEN-1, hyperparathyroidism must be excluded by obtaining a serum calcium and parathyroid hormone level.
- Treatment of ZES consists of medical control of symptoms with PPIs and evaluation for surgical intervention.
- Noninvasive imaging studies including SRS, CT, and MRI should be performed initially to evaluate for metastases and identify resectable disease. Invasive imaging modalities, such as EUS, may be performed to further evaluate primary tumors, if necessary. IOUS, palpation, and duodenotomy are used for intraoperative localization of gastrinomas.
- In patients with MEN-1, surgical resection should be pursued only if there is an identifiable tumor larger than 2 cm in contrast to resectable sporadic gastrinoma, for which all patients should undergo surgical exploration.
- In patients with liver metastases, cytoreductive surgery should be performed if more than 90% of the visible tumor can be safely removed. **Figure 3** summarizes the workup, medical management, and surgical approach to ZES.

SUGGESTED READINGS

Alexander HR, Fraker DL, Norton JA, et al. Prospective study of somatostatin receptor scintigraphy and its effect on operative outcome in patients with Zollinger-Ellison syndrome. Ann Surg. 1998;228(2):228–238.

Béhé M, Gotthardt M, Behr TM. Imaging of gastrinomas by nuclear medicine methods. Wien Klin Wochenschr. 2007;119(19–20):593–596. Review.

Birkmeyer JD, Finlayson SR, Tosteson AN, et al. Effect of hospital volume on in-hospital mortality with pancreaticoduodenectomy. Surgery. 1999;125:250–256.

Cisco RM, Norton JA. Surgery for gastrinoma. Adv Surg. 2007;41:165–176.

Diener MK, Fitzmaurice C, Schwarzer G, et al. Pylorus-preserving pancreaticoduodenectomy (pp Whipple) versus pancreaticoduodenectomy (classic Whipple) for surgical treatment of periampullary and pancreatic carcinoma. Cochrane Database Syst Rev. 2011;5:CD006053.

Eriksson B, Oberg K, Skogseid B. Neuro-endocrine pancreatic tumors: clinical findings in a prospective study of 84 patients. Acta Oncol. 1989;28:373–377.

Gibril F, Reynolds JC, Doppman JL, et al. Somatostatin receptor scintigraphy: its sensitivity compared with that of other imaging methods in detecting primary and metastatic gastrinomas. A prospective study (see comments). Ann Intern Med. 1996;125(1):26–34.

Howard TJ, Zinner MJ, Stabile BE, et al. Gastrinoma excision for cure. Ann Surg. 1990;211:9–14.

Imamura M, Komoto I, Ota S. Changing treatment strategy for gastrinoma in patients with Zollinger-Ellison syndrome. World J Surg. 2006;30(1):1–11. Review.

Li ML, Norton JA. Gastrinoma. Curr Treat Options Oncol. 2001;2(4):337–346.

Meko JB, Norton JA. Management of patients with Zollinger-Ellison syndrome. Annu Rev Med. 1995;46:395–411.

Norton JA. Gastrinoma: advances in localization and treatments. Surg Oncol Clin N Am. 1998;7(4):845–861.

Norton, JA. Neuroendocrine tumors of the pancreas and duodenum. Curr Probl Surg. 1994;31:77–164.

Norton, JA. Surgical treatment and prognosis of gastrinoma. Best Pract Res Clin Gastroenterol. 2005;19:799–805.

Norton JA, Fang TD, Jensen RT. Surgery for gastrinoma and insulinoma in multiple endocrine neoplasia type 1. J Natl Compr Canc Netw. 2006;4(2):148–153.

Norton JA, Fraker DL, Alexander HR, et al. Surgery to cure the Zollinger–Ellison syndrome. N Engl J Med. 1999;341:635–644.

Norton JA, Jensen RT. Resolved and unresolved controversies in the surgical management of patients with Zollinger-Ellison syndrome. Ann Surg. 2004;240(5):757–773. Review.

Norton JA, Venzon DJ, Berna MJ, et al. Prospective study of surgery for primary hyperparathyroidism (HPT) in multiple. Ann Surg. 2008;247(3):501–510.

Peterson DA, Dolan JP, Norton JA. Neuroendocrine tumors of the pancrease and gastrointestinal tract and carcinoid disease. In: Norton JA et al, eds. Surgery: Basic Science and Clinical Evidence. 2nd ed. New York, NY: Springer, 2008.

Pipeleers-Marichal M, Somers G, Willems G, et al. Gastrinomas in the duodenums of patients with multiple endocrine neoplasia type 1. N Engl J Med. 1990;322(11):723–727.

Pisegna JR, Norton JA, Slimak GG, et al. Effects of curative gastrinoma resection on gastric secretory function and. Gastroenterology. 1992;102:767–778.

Thompson NW, Vinik AI, Eckhauser FE. Micro-gastrinomas of the duodenum. Ann Surg. 1989;209:396–404.

Wank SA, Doppman HL, Miller DL, et al. Prospective study of the ability of computerized axial tomography to localize gastrinomas in patients with Zollinger-Ellison syndrome. Gastroenterology. 1987;92:905–912.

Wermer P. Endocrine adenomatosis and peptic ulcer in a large kindred: inherited multiple tumors and mosaic pleiotropism in man. Am J Med. 1963;35:205–212.

Wermer P. Genetic aspects of adenomatosis of endocrine glands. Am J Med. 1954;16(3):363–371.

Zollinger RM, Ellison EH. Primary peptic ulceration of the jejunum associated with islet cell tumors of the pancreas. Ann Surg. 1955;142:708–728.

70 Esophageal Cancer

MARK B. ORRINGER

Presentation

A 65-year-old man presents with a 3-month history of progressive low retrosternal dysphagia and a 15-lb weight loss. He has experienced heartburn and effortless regurgitation of gastric contents, worse when supine and after eating, for more than 15 years and treated with over the counter antacids. In the past 5 years, however, the heartburn has gradually subsided along with his need for antacid use. He has had no abdominal pain, hematemesis, or melena. Aside from mild chronic dehydration, his physical examination is entirely unremarkable.

Differential Diagnosis

The primary concern in an adult with new-onset dysphagia is esophageal carcinoma, and this symptom should never be attributed to a benign cause (e.g., gastroesophageal reflux disease [GERD]) without ruling out a gastrointestinal malignancy. In North America, adenocarcinoma of the esophagus has surpassed squamous cell carcinoma as the most common histologic type. The scenario of chronic reflux disease sets the stage for Barrett's metaplasia and the progression to dysplasia followed by adenocarcinoma. Barrett's mucosa is associated with a 30- to 40-fold increased risk for the development of esophageal carcinoma. The presence of high-grade dysplasia in a biopsy of Barrett's mucosa signals imminent malignant transformation and is the trigger for resectional therapy in appropriately selected patients. Not uncommonly, as in the presentation above, patients with Barrett's adenocarcinomas give a history of years of symptomatic GERD followed by a quiescent period as the squamous mucosa is replaced by metaplastic columnar mucosa, which is not acid sensitive, and then the development of dysphagia as obstruction from the carcinoma occurs. When taking a history in such a patient, finger point localization of the dysphagia ("sticking") to the low retrosternal area increases the likelihood of a distal esophageal mechanical obstruction. Other causes of dysphagia in the adult that need to be considered include a chronic reflux stricture due to recurrent esophagitis, neuromotor esophageal dysfunction (achalasia, diffuse spasm), reflux induced esophageal dysmotility, and an esophageal diverticulum.

Workup

There are few physical findings of esophageal carcinoma: signs of dehydration and recent weight loss from esophageal obstruction, an enlarged left supraclavicular (Virchow's) lymph node, and nodular hepatomegaly due to massive hepatic metastases. Laboratory studies showing anemia of chronic GI bleeding, hypoalbuminemia from impaired nutrition, and elevated liver enzymes due to hepatic metastases are uncommon in higher socioeconomic levels with access to medical care. In the adult who complains of new-onset dysphagia, two diagnostic studies are warranted: (1) a barium swallow examination (not a video fluoroscopic "swallow study" or an "upper GI series," which do not routinely image the thoracic esophagus), and (2) esophagoscopy and biopsy with brushings for cytology, which establish a diagnosis of carcinoma in 95% of cases. The barium swallow examination typically reveals an "applecore" constriction of the distal esophagus proximal to a sliding hiatus hernia **(Figure 1)**. Once the diagnosis of esophageal carcinoma has been established, the next order of business is "staging of the tumor," which dictates treatment. If a hard Virchow's node is palpated, a fine needle aspiration biopsy yielding metastatic carcinoma establishes a diagnosis of stage IV disease, which essentially eliminates the surgeon's role in the case and initiates referrals for chemotherapy and radiation therapy.

Diagnosis and Treatment

A complete, modern staging evaluation of esophageal carcinoma involves a CT scan of the chest and abdomen (to define the local extent of the tumor and obvious metastatic disease to mediastinal or upper abdominal lymph nodes or distant organs), a PET scan (to document that the tumor is localized and that there is no occult distant metastatic disease), and esophageal endoscopic ultrasonography (EUS) (to define the depth of intramural tumor invasion and the involvement of paraesophageal and upper abdominal lymph nodes) **(Table 1)**.

For patients with stage IA disease or those who are older than 75 years (and do not tolerate neoadjuvant treatment well), an esophagectomy is recommended. For those 75 years of age and younger with stage IB through III tumors, neoadjuvant chemoradiation therapy—typically with cisplatin and 5-FU and 45 to 50 Gy of radiation—is advised. Patients with stage IV

TABLE 1. TNM Staging of Esophageal Cancer

Definitions of TNM Primary Tumor (T)		Anatomic Stage/Prognostic Groups Squamous Cell Carcinoma					
TX	Primary tumor cannot be assessed	Stage	T	N	M	Grade	Tumor location
T0	No evidence of primary tumor	0	Tis (HGD)	N0	M0	1, X	Any
Tis	High-grade dysplasia	IA	T1	N0	M0	1, X	Any
T1	Tumor invades lamina propria, muscularis mucosae, or submucosa	IB	T1	N0	M0	2-3	Any
			T2-3	N0	M0	1, X	lower, X
T1a	Tumor invades lamina propria or muscularis mucosae	IIA	T2-3	N0	M0	1, X	Upper, middle
			T2-3	N0	M0	2-3	lower, X
T1b	Tumor invades submucosa	IIB	T2-3	N0	M0	2-3	Upper, middle
T2	Tumor invades muscularis propria		T1-2	N1	M0	Any	any
T3	Tumor invades adventitia	IIIA	T1-2	N2	M0	Any	Any
T4	Tumor invades adjacent structures		T3	N1	M0	Any	Any
T4a	Resectable tumor invading pleura, pericardium, or diaphragm		T4a	N0	M0	Any	Any
		IIIB	T3	N2	M0	Any	Any
T4b	Unresectable tumor invading other adjacent structures, such as aorta, vertebral body, trachea, etc.	IIIC	T4a	N1-2	M0	Any	Any
			T4b	Any	M0	Any	Any
			Any	N3	M0	Any	Any
		IV	Any	Any	M1	Any	Any

Regional lymph nodes (N)

NX	Regional lymph nodes cannot be assessed
N0	No regional lymph node metastasis
N1	Metastasis in 1-2 regional lymph nodes
N2	Metastasis in 3-6 regional lymph nodes
N3	Metastasis in seven or more regional lymph nodes

Adenocarcinoma

Stage	T	N	M	Grade
0	Tis(HGD)	N0	M0	1, X
IA	T1	N0	M0	1-2, X
1B	T1	N0	M0	3
	T2	N0	M0	1-2, X
IIA	T2	N0	M0	3
IIB	T3	N0	M0	Any
	T1-2	N1	M0	Any
IIIA	T1-2	N2	M0	Any
	T3	N1	M0	Any
	T4a	N0	M0	Any
IIIB	T3	N2	M0	Any
IIIC	T4a	N1-2	M0	Any
	T4b	Any	M0	Any
IV	Any	N3	M0	Any
	Any	Any	M1	Any

Distant metastasis (M)

M0	No distant metastasis
M1	Distant metastasis

Histologic grade (G)

GX	Grade cannot be assessed—stage grouping as G1
G1	Well differentiated
G2	Moderately differentiated
G3	Poorly differentiated
G4	Undifferentiated—stage grouping as G3 squamous

From the AJCC. Cancer Staging Manual. 7th ed. New York, NY: Springer-Verlag, 2010.

esophageal carcinoma (distant metastatic disease) are not candidates for esophagectomy.

Patient selection, careful preoperative evaluation, and preparation for surgery are key to a successful outcome after esophagectomy. Baseline pulmonary function tests (spirometry and diffusion capacity) are indicated in those with a history of cigarette smoking. Nuclear medicine assessment of myocardial perfusion and ventricular function is indicated in those with a cardiac history. Clinical judgment—taking into account the results of the above tests and one's assessment of the patient's ability to withstand the physiologic insult of an esophagectomy—dictates patient selection for surgery. The importance of adequate

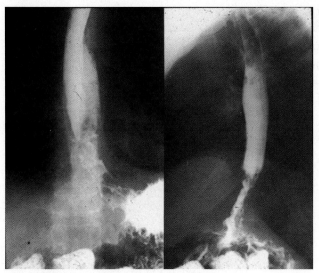

FIGURE 1 • Barium swallow study showing a typical "applecore" constriction of adenocarcinoma proximal to a sliding hiatal hernia This was an adenocarcinoma arising within Barrett's mucosa.

patient preparation for the operation cannot be over-emphasized: Patients *must* completely abstain from cigarette smoking and use an incentive inspirometer issued at their first consultation visit for a minimum of 3 weeks before the planned operation and walk 2 to 3 miles each day to condition themselves for early postoperative ambulation. Adequate preoperative hydration is key, particularly in those with radiation esophagitis, and may require insertion of a small caliber nasogastric feeding tube for administration of liquid diet supplements and water if swallowing is severely impaired. A gastrostomy tube is to be avoided since it complicates preparation of the stomach as an esophageal substitute and increases the rate of postoperative wound infections due to the proximity of the upper midline abdominal incision to the gastrostomy tube site. Patients are instructed to take sufficient fluids so that their urine is dilute; dehydration can lead to perioperative thromboembolic complications that require anticoagulation and delay the operation.

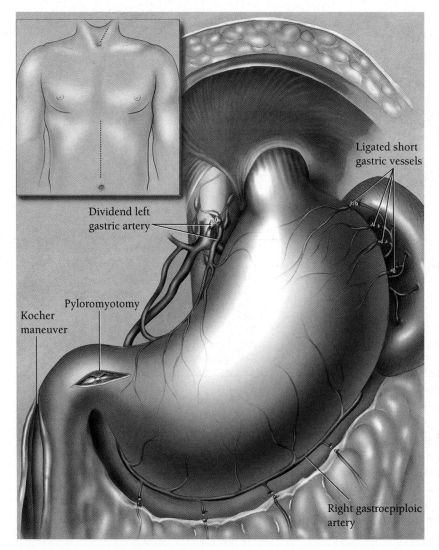

FIGURE 2 • THE is performed through a supraumbilical midline abdominal incision and a 5- to 7-cm long oblique left cervical incision that parallels the anterior border of the left sternocleidomastoid muscle (**inset**). Gastric mobilization involves division and ligation of the high short gastric and left gastroepiploic vessels along the greater curvature and the left gastric artery and vein along the lesser curvature. The right gastric and the right gastroepiploic vessels are preserved. A pyloromyotomy, Kocher maneuver, and insertion of the feeding jejunostomy tube complete the abdominal phase of the operation. (From Orringer MB. Transhiatal esophagectomy without thoracotomy. Oper Tech Thorac Cardiovasc Surg. 2005;10:63, with permission.)

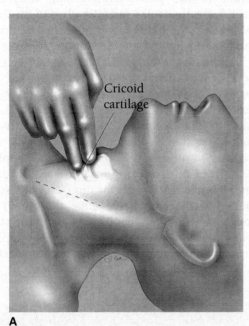 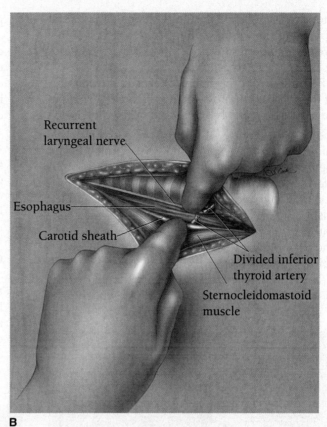

A

B

FIGURE 3 • **A:** The cricoid cartilage is palpated and marks the level of the cricopharyngeal sphincter. The most superior extent of the 5- to 7-cm incision extends no more than 2 to 3 cm superior to the cricoid cartilage. (From Orringer MB. Transhiatal esophagectomy without thoracotomy. Oper Tech Thorac Cardiovasc Surg. 2005;10:63, with permission). **B:** Only the surgeon's finger, no metal retractor, is placed against the recurrent laryngeal nerve in the tracheoesophageal groove. The cricoid cartilage is the anatomic landmark for localizing the inferior thyroid artery that occurs at the same plane but deeper in the wound. The sternocleidomastoid muscle and carotid sheath and its contents are retracted laterally, and the dissection proceeds posteriorly to the prevertebral fascia. After blunt finger dissection into the superior mediastinum, the cervical esophagus is encircled with a one-inch rubber drain carefully avoiding injury to the recurrent laryngeal nerve in the tracheoesophageal groove. (From Orringer MB. Transhiatal esophagectomy without thoracotomy. Oper Tech Thorac Cardiovasc Surg. 2005;10:63, with permission.)

Surgical Approach

There are a number of surgical approaches to esophagectomy: traditional open transthoracic, transhiatal, and minimally invasive video-assisted. The goals of esophagectomy are (1) achieving a complete (R0) resection and (2) restoring the ability to swallow comfortably. A transhiatal esophagectomy (THE) and cervical esophagogastric anastomosis (CEGA) offers advantages over the traditional thoracoabdominal Ivor-Lewis esophagectomy, including (1) avoidance of a thoracotomy (therefore fewer pulmonary complications) and (2) an intrathoracic esophagogastric anastomosis (therefore no mediastinitis from an anastomotic leak). There is little evidence that a mediastinal lymph node dissection at the time of a transthoracic esophagectomy confers a meaningful oncologic survival benefit over the lymph node dissection achieved with the transhiatal approach. Minimally invasive esophagectomy offers the advantages of a potentially more complete mediastinal lymph node dissection and less postoperative pain. However, the ability to fully mobilize the stomach and "straighten" it so that is readily reaches to the neck is compromised resulting in a higher incidence of cervical esophagogastric anastomotic leaks. The morbidity of esophagectomy is more a function of altered GI physiology and not the size or number of the incisions. THE and a CEGA is the author's preferred approach to resectable esophageal cancer.

Absolute contraindications to THE include (1) biopsy-proven distant metastatic (stage IV) disease; (2) tracheobronchial invasion by the tumor proven at bronchoscopy; (3) aortic invasion (documented on CT scan, MRI, EUS, or endovascular ultrasound); and most important, (4) the surgeon's assessment at the time of palpation of the esophagus through the diaphragmatic hiatus that there is too much esophageal fixation in the mediastinum to proceed safely with a THE.

A history of prior esophageal operations or radiation therapy more than 6 to 12 months before *may* signal the presence of periesophageal fibrosis that precludes a safe THE.

THE is not a random wrenching of the esophagus out of the mediastinum. The operation is performed in an orderly fashion and has four well-defined phases:

1. abdominal—**(Figure 2)** through a supraumbilical midline incision, exploration to exclude distant metastases and establish that the stomach is a satisfactory esophageal replacement; gastric mobilization, dividing and ligating the short gastric and left gastroepiploic vessels along the high greater curvature, the left gastric on the high lesser curvature, and preserving the right gastric and the right gastroepiploic vessels upon which the mobilized stomach is based; a Kocher maneuver; a pyloromyotomy; insertion of a feeding jejunostomy tube; opening the peritoneum overlying the hiatus and mobilizing the distal 5 to 10 cm of esophagus by blunt and sharp dissection;

2. cervical—**(Figure 3A,B)** through a 5- to 7-cm oblique low left neck incision along the anterior border of the sternocleidomastoid muscle, the carotid sheath is retracted laterally and the thyroid and trachea medially; the inferior thyroid artery is divided and ligated; the dissection stays posterior to the tracheoesophageal groove and the cervical esophagus is encircled with a Penrose drain;

3. mediastinal dissection—**(Figure 4)** posterior mobilization of esophagus from the prevertebral fascia using the hand inserted through the hiatus from "below" and a "sponge-on-a-stick" from above; **(Figure 5)** anterior mobilization of the esophagus away from the pericardium and tracheobronchial tree; **(Figure 6A,B)** mobilization and division of lateral esophageal attachments; **(Figure 7)** division of cervical esophagus with surgical stapler; delivering the stomach and attached esophagus out of the abdomen; inspecting low mediastinum

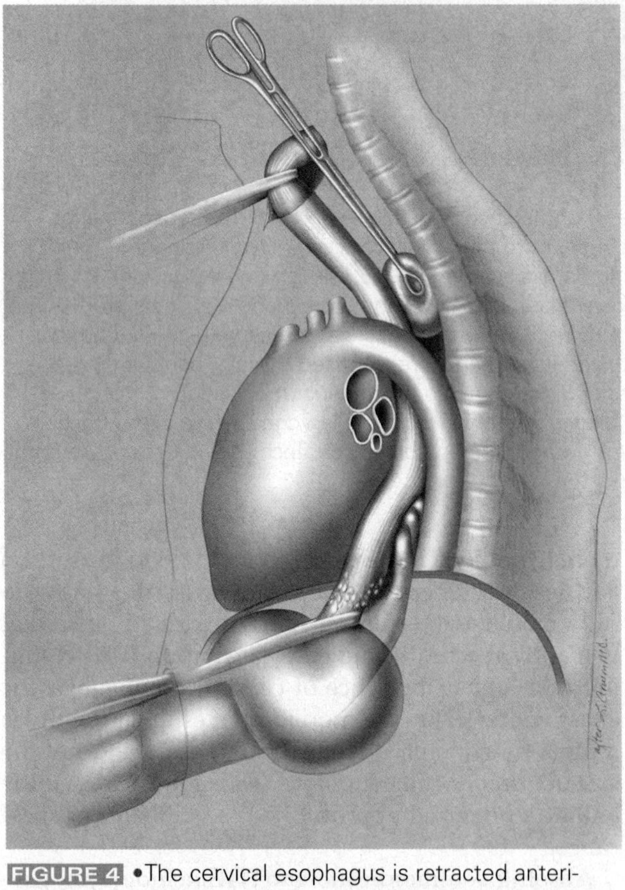

FIGURE 4 •The cervical esophagus is retracted anteriorly and to the right as a half sponge on a stick is inserted through cervical incision posterior to the esophagus and advanced downward through the superior mediastinum along the prevertebral fascia until it meets the hand inserted through the diaphragmatic hiatus. Blood pressure is monitored during the mediastinal dissection with a radial artery catheter to prevent prolonged hypotension. (From Orringer MB. Transhiatal esophagectomy without thoracotomy. Oper Tech Thorac Cardiovasc Surg. 2005;10:63, with permission.)

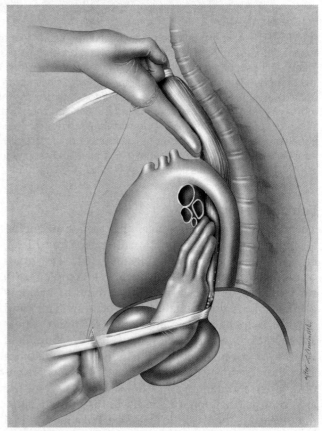

FIGURE 5 •The anterior esophageal dissection mobilizes the esophagus away from the pericardium and the posterior membranous trachea. (From Orringer MB. Transhiatal esophagectomy without thoracotomy. Oper Tech Thorac Cardiovasc Surg. 2005;10:63, with permission.)

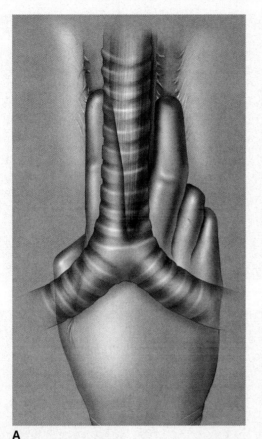
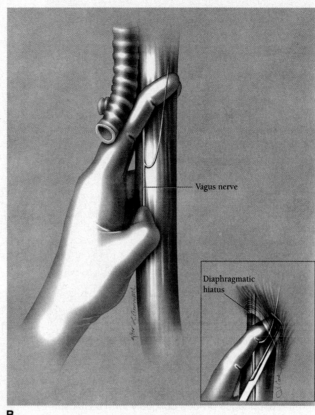

A

B

Vagus nerve

Diaphragmatic hiatus

FIGURE 6 • **A:** The hand inserted through the diaphragmatic hiatus along the anterior surface of the esophagus is advanced to the level of the circumferentially mobilized cervical esophagus. (From Orringer MB. Transhiatal esophagectomy without thoracotomy. Oper Tech Thorac Cardiovasc Surg. 2005;10:63, with permission). **B:** The esophagus is "trapped" against the prevertebral fascia between the index and the middle fingers, and a downward raking motion of the hand avulses the small remaining upper periesophageal attachments. Small vagal branches are avulsed. Larger vagal branches below the pulmonary hila may be delivered downward closer to the diaphragmatic hiatus, visualized, clamped, and either divided with electrocautery or ligated (**inset**). (From Orringer MB. Transhiatal esophagectomy without thoracotomy. Oper Tech Thorac Cardiovasc Surg. 2005;10:63, with permission).

through the hiatus for bleeding and pleural entry requiring a chest tube; packing the low mediastinum with a large abdominal gauze pack and the upper mediastinum with two narrow "thoracic" packs; **(Figure 8A,B)** preparing the gastric conduit by dividing the stomach with the linear surgical staple 4 to 6 cm distal to the esophagogastric junction; oversewing the gastric staple suture line; **(Figure 9)** transposing the "tubularized" stomach through the hiatus with one hand until the fundus can be palpated anterior to the spine with a finger inserted through the cervical incision; delivering 4 to 5 cm of gastric tip into cervical wound; bringing jejunostomy tube through the abdominal wall; abdominal closure;

4. CEGA—**(Figure 10A–F)** side-to-side stapled anastomosis using Endo-GIA surgical stapler; placement of nasogastric tube into intrathoracic stomach; cervical wound drainage (1/4 in Penrose) and closure.

Special Considerations

Unsuspected stage IV disease discovered during the operation (e.g., an omental implant of tumor, a small liver metastasis) contraindicates proceeding with an esophagectomy; the potential morbidity and mortality of an esophagectomy to palliate dysphagia in patients with such poor long-term survival is not justified. The most important contraindication to THE is the surgeon's assessment of the esophagus through the hiatus that there is so much tumor fixation or dense periesophageal fibrosis that the procedure is unsafe; to avoid an intraoperative "disaster" from persisting with a difficult transhiatal dissection, one should not hesitate to convert to a transthoracic approach if it is indicated. A full right posterolateral thoracotomy

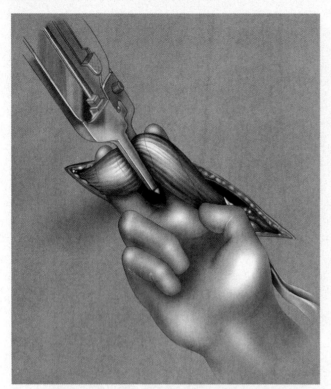

FIGURE 7 • Once the entire intrathoracic esophagus has been mobilized, 3 to 4 inches are delivered into the cervical wound and the esophagus divided obliquely with a GIA surgical stapler applied from front to back with the anterior tip slightly longer than the posterior corner. (From Orringer MB. Transhiatal esophagectomy without thoracotomy. Oper Tech Thorac Cardiovasc Surg. 2005;10:63, with permission).

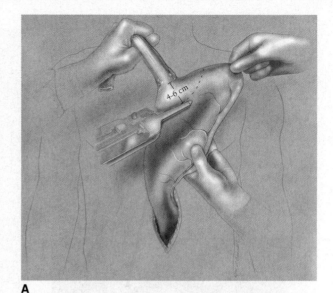

A

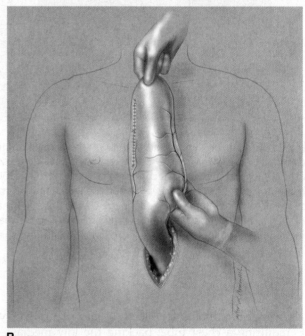

B

FIGURE 8 • **A:** Once the esophagus and stomach have been delivered out of the abdominal incision, the high lesser curvature of the stomach is cleared of fat and vessels at the level of the second "crow's foot" and the GIA stapler applied progressively toward the gastric fundus 4 to 6 cm distal to the esophagogastric junction, preserving as much gastric capacity and not "tubularizing" the stomach any more than necessary. (From Orringer MB. Transhiatal esophagectomy without thoracotomy. Oper Tech Thorac Cardiovasc Surg. 2005;10:63, with permission). **B:** After completing division of the upper stomach, the gastric staple suture line comes to rest toward the patient's right side. The gastric fundus readily reaches above the level of the clavicles. The staple suture line along the lesser curvature is oversewn with two running 4-0 monofilament absorbable sutures. (From Orringer MB. Transhiatal esophagectomy without thoracotomy. Oper Tech Thorac Cardiovasc Surg. 2005;10:63, with permission.)

through the 5th intercostal space provides the best access to the mid and upper thoracic esophagus; a left posterolateral thoracotomy is used to mobilize distal esophageal tumors.

Postoperative Management

Prior to extubation, a portable postoperative chest radiograph is obtained in the operating room to exclude an unrecognized hemo- or pneumothorax for which a chest tube is inserted. The routine use of epidural anesthesia facilitates extubation in the operating room. Use of the incentive inspirometer resumes within several hours of awakening from anesthesia, and ambulation begins the following morning. Ice chips for throat discomfort (not to exceed 30 mL/h) are permitted the evening of surgery. The nasogastric tube is typically removed on the 3rd post-op day. Diet is progressively advanced as tolerated, carefully assessing for ileus several times a day: clear liquids (day 4), full liquids (day 5), pureed diet (day 6), and soft diet (day 7). A barium swallow on day 7 documents integrity of the anastomosis, adequacy of gastric emptying, and absence of obstruction at

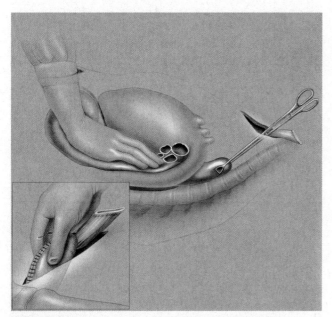

FIGURE 9 • The gastric fundus is gently manipulated through the diaphragmatic hiatus and advanced upward into the posterior mediastinum manually until the gastric tip can be palpated with the right index finger inserted through the cervical wound. The tip is then grasped with a Babcock clamp that is not ratcheted closed to avoid gastric trauma. The stomach is advanced upward more by pushing it through the mediastinum from "below" rather than pulling it upward from the neck incision. A 4 to 5 cm length of stomach is delivered above the level of the clavicles with the gastric staple line toward to the patient's right side (**inset**). (From Orringer MB. Transhiatal esophagectomy without thoracotomy. Oper Tech Thorac Cardiovasc Surg. 2005;10:63, with permission).

the jejunostomy tube site. Nocturnal jejunostomy tube feedings are administered if oral intake is inadequate. With an uncomplicated post-op course, discharge typically occurs on the 7th postoperative day. If it is no longer being used, the jejunostomy tube is removed 3 to 4 weeks after surgery. Should a cervical esophagogastric anastomotic leak occur, the cervical wound is opened in its entirety at the bedside and packing of the wound with saline moistened gauze begun. Nutrition is maintained with tube feedings. 36, 40, and 46 French Maloney esophageal dilators are passed at the bedside within 1 week of opening the neck incision to insure that swallowed esophageal contents pass preferentially down the esophagus and that an anastomotic stricture does not form; it is not uncommon for anastomotic leaks to close within 1 week of the esophageal dilatation. If the patient with an anastomotic leak remains febrile, has persistent purulent drainage from the neck wound, and there is an odor of putrid tissue, concern about gastric tip necrosis warrants a return to the OR for inspection of the wound with good lighting and retraction and fiberoptic esophagoscopy. Gastric tip necrosis generally requires takedown of the intrathoracic stomach through the hiatus, amputation of the devitalized stomach with a surgical stapler, and construction of an end cervical esophagostomy. Restoration of alimentary continuity is not undertaken for 6 to 12 months to see if the esophageal cancer recurs early. (Less than half of patients with esophageal cancer and gastric tip necrosis ever undergo reestablishment of alimentary continuity with a colon interposition.)

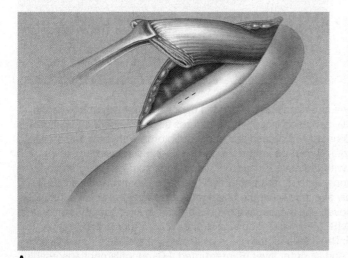
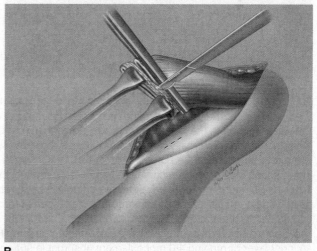

A   B

FIGURE 10 • **A:** The anterior surface of the gastric fundus is elevated out of the cervical wound with a 3-0 cardiovascular traction suture that is secured to an adjacent drape. A 1.5- to 2-cm vertical gastrotomy (*dotted line*) is performed on the anterior gastric wall. (From Orringer MB. Transhiatal esophagectomy without thoracotomy. Oper Tech Thorac Cardiovasc Surg. 2005;10:63, with permission). **B:** The stapled tip of the divided cervical esophagus is amputated distal to an occluding DeBakey forceps that serves as a guide for the transection. The amputated tip of the esophagus us submitted to pathology as the "proximal esophageal margin." (From Orringer MB. Transhiatal esophagectomy without thoracotomy. Oper Tech Thorac Cardiovasc Surg. 2005;10:63, with permission).

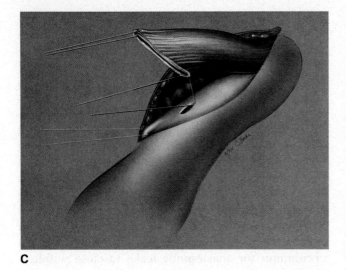

C

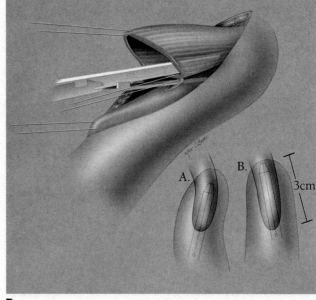

D

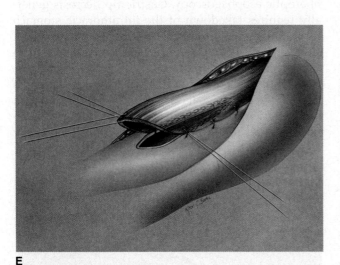

E

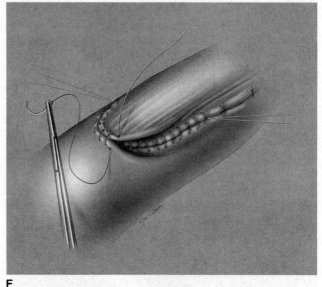

F

FIGURE 10 • (*Continued*) **C:** A stay suture is placed through the anterior tip of the divided esophagus and another through the upper end of the gastrotomy and the posterior tip of the divided esophagus. These sutures align the posterior wall of the esophagus with the anterior wall of the stomach. (From Orringer MB. Transhiatal esophagectomy without thoracotomy. Oper Tech Thorac Cardiovasc Surg. 2005;10:63, with permission). **D:** An Autosuture Endo-GIA 30-3.5 staple cartridge (United States Surgical Corporation, Norwalk, CT) is inserted with the anvil in the stomach and the staple-bearing portion in the esophagus. (From Orringer MB. Transhiatal esophagectomy without thoracotomy. Oper Tech Thorac Cardiovasc Surg. 2005;10:63, with permission). **E:** After firing the knife assembly and advancing the blade, a 3-cm long side-to-side esophago-gastric anastomosis has been constructed. The stapler is removed and a nasogastric tube inserted by the anesthesiologist and guided into the stomach by the surgeon. (From Orringer MB. Transhiatal esophagectomy without thoracotomy. Oper Tech Thorac Cardiovasc Surg. 2005;10:63, with permission). **F:** The esophagotomy and gastrotomy are closed in two layers, an inner layer of running 4-0 monofilament absorbable suture and an outer layer of interrupted 4-0 monofilament absorbable suture. (From Orringer MB. Transhiatal esophagectomy without thoracotomy. Oper Tech Thorac Cardiovasc Surg. 2005;10:63, with permission).

TABLE 2. Key Technical Steps and Potential Pitfalls to Transhiatal Esophagectomy and CEGA

Key Technical Steps

1. Upper midline laparotomy and abdominal exploration; assess suitability of stomach as esophageal replacement.
2. Divide triangular ligament; retract liver to right with table-mounted upper hand retractor.
3. Mobilize stomach by dividing and ligating high short gastric, left gastroepiploic and left gastric vessels while preserving the right gastric and right gastroepiploic vessels.
4. Perform generous Kocher maneuver.
5. Perform extramucosal pyloromyotomy.
6. Insert 14 French rubber jejunostomy feeding tube.
7. Open peritoneum overlying the hiatus and mobilize the distal 10 cm of esophagus under direct vision, clamping and ligating lateral attachments with long right-angle clamps and dissecting with electrocautery.
8. Through oblique left cervical incision anterior to the sternocleidomastoid muscle, mobilize and encircle cervical esophagus while *avoiding direct placement of metal retractors or instruments against the tracheoesophageal groove.*
9. Mobilize the thoracic esophagus from the posterior mediastinum with posterior, anterior and finally lateral dissections.
10. Retract 3–4 in. of esophagus into the cervical wound, divide it with a surgical stapler, and deliver the mobilized stomach and attached esophagus out of the posterior mediastinum.
11. Through the diaphragmatic hiatus, inspect the posterior mediastinum for bleeding and assess integrity of the mediastinal pleura and the need for chest tubes (place now if needed); place gauze packs into the posterior mediastinum through the hiatus from below and the neck incision from above to encourage hemostasis.
12. Divide stomach 4–6 cm distal to the esophagogastric junction, from lesser toward greater curvature, progressively straightening the stomach by traction on the gastric tip with each application of the stapler; remove the specimen from the field and assess need for frozen section on gastric margin.
13. Oversew gastric staple suture line and transpose stomach through posterior mediastinum until 3–5 cm of gastric tip is visible in cervical wound.
14. Loosely narrow diaphragmatic hiatus and suture stomach to edge of diaphragm and left lobe of liver against the hiatus.
15. Bring jejunostomy tube through left upper quadrant of anterior abdominal wall, suture tube site to anterior abdominal wall and tube to skin, close abdomen and cover the incision with a drape to prevent contamination by oral bacteria during performance of the CEGA.
16. Perform side-to-side stapled CEGA, place rubber drain adjacent to the anastomosis, and close cervical wound.
17. Obtain a portable chest radiograph in the operating room prior to extubation to identify and treat a previously unrecognized hemo- or pneumothorax.

Potential Pitfalls

- Abdominal, particularly if there is a hiatal hernia that displaces the greater curvature upward through the hiatus, division of the greater omentum away from the stomach may result in injury to the right gastroepiploic artery unless a conscious effort is made to pull the stomach down out of the hiatus prior to dividing any short gastric vessels to be certain this dissection is beginning high on the greater curvature; ischemic necrosis of the stomach by ligating the short gastric vessels too close to the gastric wall; splenic capsular tear due to excessive traction on the greater omentum and stomach during the gastric mobilization; inadvertent division of a "replaced left hepatic artery" because of failure to identify it in the gastrohepatic omentum; pyloroduodenal mucosal injury during pyloromyotomy (managed with several 5-0 monofilament sutures and a Graham patch and not requiring conversion to a pyloroplasty);
- Cervical-recurrent laryngeal nerve injury due to direct application of a metal retractor or instrument against the tracheoesophageal groove;
- Mediastinal dissection-hypotension (blood pressure monitored with routine radial artery catheter) from cardiac displacement as the hand goes into the mediastinum (the hand must consciously be kept as flat as possible parallel to the spine; hands with glove size 8 and above may not be appropriate for THE); pneumothorax from entry into one or both pleural cavities during the esophageal mobilization (assessed by direct inspection through the hiatus once the esophagus is out of the mediastinum; placement of chest tube(s) should be done before beginning preparation of gastric tube); bleeding from injury to the aorta or azygos vein (controlled initially by packing the mediastinum, and if unsuccessful, conversion to a thoracotomy for direct clamping/suturing); posterior membranous tracheal tear (managed by advancing the endotracheal tube down the left main bronchus and conversion to a right thoracotomy for suture repair if needed); chylothorax (with dense periesophageal adhesions), once esophageal mobilization is completed, do prophylactic "mass ligature" of thoracic duct through the hiatus with several 2-0 chromic sutures placed to the prevertebral fascia between the aorta and the azygos vein; gastric torsion (once the tip of the stomach has been delivered into the cervical wound, be certain that the gastric staple suture line is toward the patient's right side and that the right gastroepiploic vascular pedicle viewed through the hiatus is toward the patient's left side).
- CEGA leaks invariably have a cause, for example, tension due to insufficient mobilization of the stomach or excessive shortening of the cervical esophagus during its division; or trauma to the stomach during its mobilization so that it is contused and "blue" at the time of the anastomotic construction.

TAKE HOME POINTS

- The properly mobilized stomach virtually always reaches to the neck for construction of a tension-free CEGA.
- Gentle, atraumatic gastric mobilization—keeping the stomach "pink in the belly and pink in the neck"—is key to avoiding a cervical esophagogastric anastomotic leak.
- Fingertip retraction of the thyroid and trachea medially, avoiding placement of metal retractors against the tracheoesophageal groove, minimizes the chance of recurrent laryngeal nerve injury.
- Clinical judgment and experience determine when tumor fixation or periesophageal fibrosis preclude a safe THE; converting to a transthoracic approach is *not* a sign of weakness!
- A gastric drainage procedure (pyloromyotomy) is routine to avoid potential outlet obstruction (pylorospasm), which may follow the vagotomy and occurs with an esophagectomy.
- The cervical esophagus must not be divided too proximally in order to avoid tension on the subsequent anastomosis.
- The stomach should be divided 4 to 6 cm distal to the esophagogastric junction, preserving as much gastric volume and submucosal blood supply as possible, not "tubularizing" the stomach.
- To minimize trauma to it, the mobilized stomach is positioned in the mediastinum manually, not pulled by sutures or suction devices, and proper orientation (gastric staple line to the patient's right, right gastroepiploic pedicle to the patient's left) must be assured to avoid gastric torsion.
- The hiatus is closed loosely, the stomach sutured to the edge of the hiatus, and the left hepatic lobe secured back in place to avert late migration of intestine through the hiatus into the chest.
- A side-to-side stapled CEGA minimizes the incidence of cervical esophagogastric anastomotic leak.

SUGGESTED READINGS

Davis J, Zhao L, Chang A, Orringer, MB. Refractory cervical esophagogastric anastomotic strictures: management and outcomes. J Thorac Cardiovasc Surg. 2011;141:444–448.

Iannettoni MD. White RI, Orringer MB. Catastrophic complications of the cervical esophagogastric anastomosis. J Thorac Cardiovasc Surg. 1995;110:1493–1501.

Orringer MB. Transhiatal esophagectomy without thoracotomy. Oper Tech Thorac Cardiovasc Surg. 2005;10:63–83.

Orringer MB, Marshall B, Chang AC, et al. Two thousand transhiatal esophagectomies: changing trends, lessons learned. Ann Surg. 2007;246:363–372.

Orringer MB, Marshall, B, Iannettoni, MD. Eliminating the cervical esophagogastric anastomotic leak with a side-to-side stapled anastomosis. J Thorac Cardiovasc Surg. 2000;119:277–288.

71 Esophageal Perforation

ALYKHAN S. NAGJI and CHRISTINE L. LAU

Presentation

A 60-year-old man with a known history of alcohol abuse and binge drinking presents to the emergency department complaining of substernal chest pain after multiple episodes of vomiting. Initial vital signs reveal sinus tachycardia along with a systolic blood pressure of 85 mm Hg. The patient is also febrile to 39.1°C. On physical examination, the patient is found to have a systolic crunching sound heard at the left sternal border (Hamman's sign) along with subcutaneous emphysema. Laboratory tests demonstrate an elevated white blood cell count of 15,000/mm³ but are otherwise normal.

Differential Diagnosis

The combination of subcutaneous emphysema, vomiting, and chest pain comprises Mackler's triad, a pathognomonic sign for esophageal perforation. The potential causes of esophageal perforation include the following: iatrogenic (extra- or intraluminal), trauma (i.e., penetrating or blunt injury, barotraumas, and foreign body or caustic injury), malignancy, inflammation (i.e., gastroesophageal reflux, ulceration, and Crohn's disease), and infection. Though the most likely diagnosis in the case above is esophageal perforation secondary to barotrauma resulting in Boerhaave's syndrome, one must be careful to rule out other cardiac, vascular, or intrathoracic pathology that may contribute to this patient's presenting symptoms.

Presentation Continued

With respect to aforementioned case, the patient has suffered from an esophageal perforation secondary to Boerhaave's syndrome. This is a spontaneous esophageal perforation that occurs after an episode of vomiting. It is thought to occur from a series of events that culminate in a rapid increase in intraluminal esophageal pressure, such that a transmural rupture typically occurs in the left posterolateral wall of the esophagus approximately 2 to 3 cm proximal to the gastroesophageal junction. This area of the esophagus is inherently weak as the longitudinal fibers taper before passing onto the stomach wall.

Workup

The clinical presentation of esophageal perforation is highly dependent on the etiology and location. It is important that the diagnosis be made in a timely manner. Clinical suspicion combined with imaging (i.e., plain radiography, contrast esophagography, and computed tomography [CT] with oral contrast), laboratory analysis, and in some cases direct visualization (i.e., flexible esophagoscopy) serves to confirm or refute the diagnosis of perforation.

Radiographic studies play a significant role in the establishment of the diagnosis of esophageal perforation. In the case of cervical esophageal perforations, a plain film of the lateral neck may demonstrate air in the prevertebral fascial. If a thoracic or an abdominal esophageal perforation is suspected, an upright abdominal film along with a posteroanterior (Figure 1) and lateral chest radiograph should be obtained. It stands to reason that if plain films demonstrate a pleural effusion, pneumomediastinum, subcutaneous emphysema, hydrothorax, pneumothorax, or subdiaphragmatic air, the suspicion for esophageal perforation increases. However, if the plain film is normal after a suspected esophageal injury, further workup is required.

Contrast esophagography is the study of choice for the diagnosis of esophageal perforation. Two forms of contrast are available to decipher the presence and location of a perforation. Gastrograffin, being water soluble, has traditionally been the initial contrast of choice secondary to its rapid absorption after extravasation

Presentation Continued

After the initial assessment, history and physical examination were obtained, the patient had a posteroanterior/lateral (PA/lateral) chest radiograph that demonstrated a left pleural effusion along with mediastinal air. The patient undergoes a gastrograffin followed by dilute barium swallow, which demonstrates extravasation into the left chest consistent with a suspected esophageal perforation secondary to Boerhaave's syndrome (Figure 2).

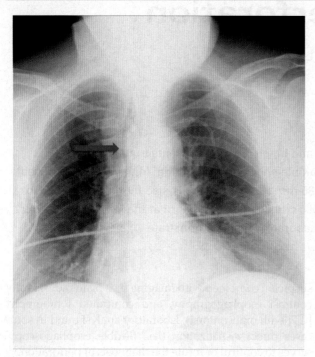

FIGURE 1 • Chest x-ray demonstrating pneumomediastinum (*arrow*).

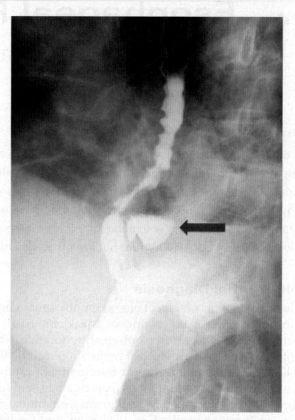

FIGURE 2 • Esophagogram demonstrating leakage of contrast (*arrow*) into the left chest secondary to distal esophageal perforation.

through the perforation **(Figure 2)**. In the event that no perforation is detected with a water-soluble agent, serial dilute barium esophagography should be performed. Dilute barium should be used exclusively in patients at high risk for aspiration or if a tracheoesophageal fistula is suspected. A negative result with suspicion of perforation requires repetition of barium contrast esophagography, and possibly a CT **(Figure 3)** and/or esophagoscopy. Flexible esophagoscopy provides direct visualization of the perforation.

Diagnosis and Treatment

Therapy for esophageal perforation is dependent upon the age and health of the patient, the damage to surrounding tissues, and the underlying esophageal pathology. The goals of treatment should include prevention of further contamination, elimination of infection, restoration of gastrointestinal integrity, and establishment of nutritional support. Management of a thoracic perforation requires the following: debridement and drainage of the pleural spaces, control of the esophageal leak, complete re-expansion of the lung, prevention of gastric reflux, nutritional support, and appropriate antibiotic treatment.

Surgical Approach

Surgical intervention includes the following strategies: primary closure with or without buttressing repair, esophagectomy with immediate versus delayed reconstruction, esophageal exclusion and diversion, T-tube placement and drainage, and drainage alone. The selection of the appropriate surgical approach relies heavily on the

location and degree of the perforation and the clinical situation. Though not addressed directly below, it should be noted that recently there has been an increase in both the use of esophageal stenting and occasionally nonoperative management of esophageal perforations. The intervention described below will reflect the patient in the clinical scenario who suffered a thoracic esophageal perforation.

Primary Repair

The surgical treatment of choice for an otherwise normal thoracic esophageal perforation is primary repair. The perforation in our case was approached using a left thoracotomy with the patient in the right lateral decubitus position and with single-lung ventilation. Single-lung ventilation is not required but helpful if the patient will tolerate. Once exposed, the esophagus needs to be mobilized and the necrotic esophagus is debrided carefully back to viable tissue. After proper exposure, a vertical esophageal myotomy should be performed, opening the longitudinal and the circular muscle layers to fully expose the mucosal injury. The esophageal defect is the esophageal mucosa and muscle is approximated in a two-layer closure, usually the mucosa is closed with vicryl and the muscle layer with interrupted silks. Reinforcement of the primary repair can be achieved using a variety of tissues (i.e., intercostal muscle, omental onlay graft, lattissimus dorsi, etc.), but it is imperative that the tissue be

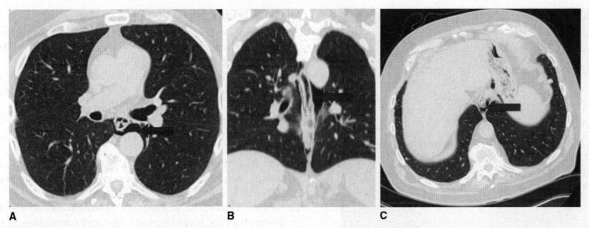

FIGURE 3 • **A:** Axial CT image demonstrating pneumomediastinum. **B:** Coronal CT image demonstrating pneumomediastinum. **C:** Axial CT image demonstrating air at the level of the distal esophagus and gastroesophageal junction.

well vascularized. A nasogastric tube is inserted to just above the repair, while the closure is submerged under saline. The repair is then tested by insufflating air and occluding the distal esophagus. The nasogastric tube is then advanced into the stomach. At this time, the surgeon may consider the need to obtain enteral access (i.e., gastrostomy or jejunostomy feeding tube placement) or perform additional procedures (i.e., fundoplication for significant reflux) **(Table 1).**

Presentation Continued

A left thoracotomy in the seventh interspace was used for exposure, during which an intercostal muscle flap was harvested. Care was taken to make sure the pleura and mediastinum were debrided and the distal esophagus was mobilized. The perforation was visualized and the esophagus was debrided. Subsequently, a myotomy was performed to expose the entire mucosal tear and a two-layer repair was performed. The repair was buttressed with an intercostal muscle flap. The thorax was irrigated and a chest tube was placed after which a feeding jejunostomy tube through a separate small upper abdominal incision was placed for enteral access.

Special Considerations

Resection and Diversion

When primary repair is not possible or the pathology makes it less desirable, surgical options include esophageal resection with immediate or delayed reconstruction, or exclusion and diversion. Resection should be considered when confronted with the following circumstances: megaesophagus from achalasia, esophageal carcinoma, caustic ingestion, or severe undilatable reflux strictures. The surgical approach to

an esophagectomy is dictated by the surgeon's experience and underlying pathology.

In patients with a severely devitalized esophagus or when a patient is unable to tolerate definitive repair, the surgeon should consider exclusion and diversion techniques. This includes closure of the perforation, esophageal diversion, and pleural drainage, along with the creation of a cervical esophagostomy for proximal diversion. Drainage can also be achieved via the placement of a T tube distal to the esophageal perforation with the long arm directed toward the stomach and the short arm in the esophagus proximal to the site of injury. The T tube is then brought out through a separate incision. In these circumstances, a jejunostomy should be placed for enteral access.

TABLE 1. Key Technical Steps and Potential Pitfalls for Primary Repair of Perforated Esophagus

Key Technical Steps

1. Thoracotomy (dependent on location of perforation).
   a. Proximal esophageal perforation—Left neck exploration (often just drainage performed and neck is left open and packed).
   b. Midesophageal perforation—Right thoracotomy in the 4th to the 6th intercostal space.
   c. Distal esophagus perforation—Left thoracotomy in the 7th intercostal space.
2. Harvest intercostal muscle flap—not required; decision must be made prior to thoracotomy.
3. Debridement of the pleura and mediastinum.
4. Mobilization of the esophagus.
5. Debridement of the esophagus.
6. Perform myotomy to expose entire mucosal injury.
7. Two-layer closure with or without buttressing of repair.
8. Enteral access (if deemed necessary).

Potential Pitfalls

- Inability to perform primary repair.
- Presence of a distal obstruction.
- Severe undilatable reflux strictures.

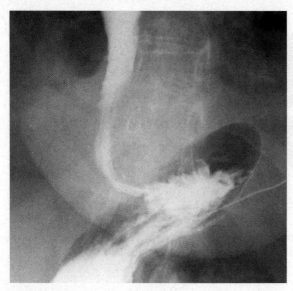

FIGURE 4 • Esophagogram demonstrating absence of leak after primary repair of esophagus.

Postoperative Management

Postoperative management of esophageal perforation is highly dependent upon the intervention taken. If a primary repair was attempted, a follow-up esophagogram **(Figure 4)** is needed to evaluate the repair. In the event that a leak is present, the chest tube placed intraoperatively should suffice for drainage. However, if not adequately drained, the surgeon should consider placement of a CT-guided pigtail. The thoracostomy tube(s) should be taken off suction, as long as the lung has completely re-expanded and a repeat swallow study should be performed in 5 to 7 days to show that the perforation has healed.

Case Conclusion

Postoperatively, the patient did well. The chest tube was taken off suction and the lung remained expanded. On postoperative day 5, the patient had an esophagogram that demonstrated no esophageal leak (Figure 4). The patient's nasogastric tube was removed and the patient was started on a liquid diet.

TAKE HOME POINTS

- Early identification of esophageal perforation is critical.
- Employment of proper imaging and direct visualization modalities are required.
- Surgical approach dictated by location of perforation
- Complete intraoperative exposure of mucosal injury and two-layer closure
- Intraoperative recognition of circumstances that prevent primary repair
- Postoperative imaging to confirm repair of esophageal perforation

SUGGESTED READINGS

Altorjay A, Kiss J, Voros A, et al. The role of esophagectomy in the management of esophageal perforations. Ann Thorac Surg. 1998;65:1433–1436.

Bladergroen MR, Lowe JE, Postlethwait RW. Diagnosis and recommended management of esophageal perforation and rupture. Ann Thorac Surg. 1986;42:235–239.

Brinster CJ, Singhal S, Lee L, et al. Evolving options in the management of esophageal perforation. Ann Thorac Surg. 2004;77:1475–1483.

Bufkin BL, Miller JI Jr, Mansour KA. Esophageal perforation: emphasis on management. Ann Thorac Surg. 1996;61:1447–1451; discussion 1451–1452.

Derbes VJ, Mitchell RE Jr. Hermann Boerhaave's Atrocis, nec descripti prius, morbi historia, the first translation of the classic case report of rupture of the esophagus, with annotations. Bull Med Libr Assoc. 1955;43:217–240.

Foley MJ, Ghahremani GG, Rogers LF. Reappraisal of contrast media used to detect upper gastrointestinal perforations: comparison of ionic water-soluble media with barium sulfate. Radiology. 1982;144:231–237.

Han SY, McElvein RB, Aldrete JS, et al. Perforation of the esophagus: correlation of site and cause with plain film findings. AJR Am J Roentgenol. 1985;145:537–540.

Lee SH. The role of oesophageal stenting in the non-surgical management of oesophageal strictures. Br J Radiol. 2001;74:891–900.

Menguy R. Near-total esophageal exclusion by cervical esophagostomy and tube gastrostomy in the management of massive esophageal perforation: report of a case. Ann Surg. 1971;173:613–616.

Morgan RA, Ellul JP, Denton ER, et al. Malignant esophageal fistulas and perforations: management with plastic-covered metallic endoprostheses. Radiology. 1997;204:527–532.

Nicholson AA, Royston CM, Wedgewood K, et al. Palliation of malignant oesophageal perforation and proximal oesophageal malignant dysphagia with covered metal stents. Clin Radiol. 1995;50:11–14.

Richardson JD, Tobin GR. Closure of esophageal defects with muscle flaps. Arch Surg. 1994;129:541–547; discussion 547–548.

Sabanathan S, Eng J, Richardson J. Surgical management of intrathoracic oesophageal rupture. Br J Surg. 1994;81:863–865.

Shaffer HA Jr, Valenzuela G, Mittal RK. Esophageal perforation. A reassessment of the criteria for choosing medical or surgical therapy. Arch Intern Med. 1992;152:757–761.

Urschel HC Jr, Razzuk MA, Wood RE, et al. Improved management of esophageal perforation: exclusion and diversion in continuity. Ann Surg. 1974;179:587–591.

White RK, Morris DM. Diagnosis and management of esophageal perforations. Am Surg. 1992;58:112–119.

Whyte RI, Iannettoni MD, Orringer MB. Intrathoracic esophageal perforation. The merit of primary repair. J Thorac Cardiovasc Surg. 1995;109:140–144; discussion 144–146.

Wu JT, Mattox KL, Wall MJ Jr. Esophageal perforations: new perspectives and treatment paradigms. J Trauma. 2007;63:1173–1184.

72 Achalasia

TYLER GRENDA and JULES LIN

Presentation

A 48-year-old male with an unremarkable past medical history presents to his primary care physician with a chief complaint of difficulty swallowing. He describes symptoms of progressive dysphagia to both solids and liquids over several years. He regurgitates undigested food daily and has lost 20 lbs over the past 9 months. He occasionally regurgitates when lying down at night and sometimes wakes up coughing. He denies any nausea, chest, or abdominal pain. His vital signs and physical examination are otherwise unremarkable.

Differential Diagnosis

There are several possible etiologies for this patient's progressive dysphagia. Painless dysphagia to both solids and liquids with regurgitation of undigested food is suggestive of achalasia. However, pseudo-achalasia, with obstruction secondary to a neoplasm in the distal esophagus or extraluminal compression, can present in the same manner and must be considered in the differential. Upper endoscopy is essential to evaluate for a tumor, stricture, or other esophageal or gastric pathology as the cause of his symptoms. The differential includes esophageal dysmotility, esophageal spasm, a peptic stricture, and Zenker's or epiphrenic diverticulum. Diffuse esophageal spasm results in simultaneous, frequent contractions. However, relaxation of the lower esophageal sphincter (LES) is normal, and patients complain more frequently of chest pain. Surgery is not indicated and is unlikely to resolve the patient's symptoms. Chagas' disease is clinically identical to achalasia but is caused by the parasite *Trypanosoma cruzi*, which destroys the myenteric plexus, and is common in South America.

Workup

The patient underwent a barium swallow, which reveals a dilated esophagus with a "bird's beak" narrowing at the gastroesophageal junction **(Figure 1A)**. An upper endoscopy is performed, which shows no evidence of a mass or stricture. The esophagus is dilated with retained fluid and food debris. The LES is tight with mild resistance when passing the endoscope. Laboratory values are obtained and are within normal limits. He also undergoes an esophageal manometry, which reveals an aperistaltic esophageal body with incomplete or absent relaxation of the LES on all wet swallows (WS) **(Figures 2 and 3)**.

Discussion

Achalasia is a primary esophageal motility disorder of unknown etiology that is characterized by an aperistaltic esophagus and a LES that fails to relax in response to swallowing. Due to neural degeneration from the dorsal motor nucleus to the myenteric plexus, vagal innervation is lost. Achalasia affects approximately 1 per 100,000 people in the United States and typically presents between the ages of 20 and 50, although it may present at any age. Failure of the LES to relax results in a functional obstruction at the level of the gastroesophageal junction.

Diagnosis and Treatment

Upper endoscopy must be performed to evaluate for pseudoachalasia caused by an esophageal carcinoma or a peptic stricture. Chest CT can also be useful to evaluate for extrinsic compression. A chest radiograph can suggest the diagnosis of achalasia with absence of a gastric air bubble or a dilated esophagus. The diagnosis is often confirmed on a barium swallow showing a dilated esophagus with an air-fluid level and narrowing of the gastroesophageal junction giving the classic "bird's beak" appearance **(Figure 1A)**. Manometry is an important tool in the diagnosis of achalasia and shows an aperistaltic esophagus and a LES that fails to relax with swallowing **(Figure 3)**. Given the findings present in this patient's workup, his symptoms are most likely secondary to achalasia.

The primary goal of treatment is palliation of the patient's symptoms by alleviating the distal esophageal obstruction present at the LES. None of the available treatments will return the esophagus to normal, and the esophageal body remains aperistaltic. In addition, a careful balance must be achieved between alleviating the obstruction and creating gastroesophageal reflux.

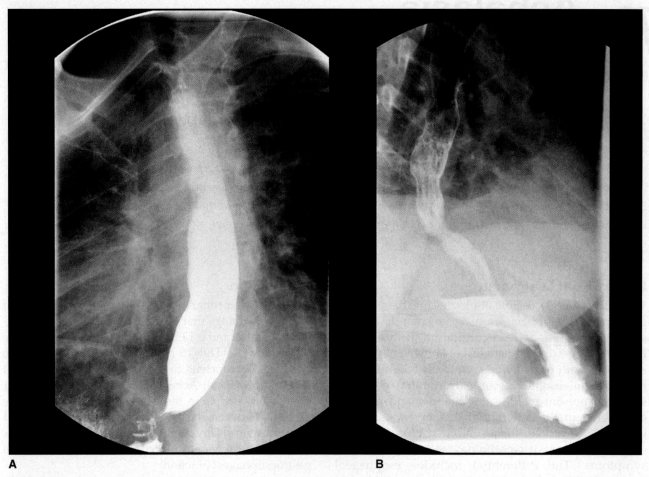

A   **B**

• On barium esophagram **(A)**, the distal esophagus is aperistaltic and mildly dilated. There is a bird's beak narrowing at the gastroesophageal junction with significant hold-up of contrast consistent with achalasia. Postoperative barium swallow **(B)** shows no leak and easy passage of contrast through the gastroesophageal junction.

Pharmacologic therapies, such as calcium channel blockers and nitrates, cause smooth muscle relaxation and decrease LES pressure. The effectiveness of these treatments is short-lived and often causes significant side effects. As a result, these should be reserved for temporizing therapy and for patients that are poor surgical candidates.

Endoscopic injection of botulinum toxin (Botox) into the LES relaxes the smooth muscle fibers. While this treatment can improve dysphagia, its effects often last <6 months and require repeat injections for continued relief of symptoms. Botox injections can also cause an inflammatory reaction, which can make a future myotomy more difficult. Therefore, Botox should be reserved for individuals that are poor candidates for endoscopy or surgery.

Pneumatic dilation disrupts the smooth muscle fibers of the LES and is successful in relieving dysphagia in 60% to 75% of patients after a single dilation and in up to 85% after multiple dilations. The risk of perforation associated with this procedure is approximately 3% to 5%. It is typically considered to be less effective in younger patients. Pneumatic dilation should be reserved for patients that are unable to undergo a laparoscopic esophageal myotomy.

Myotomy is the treatment of choice, particularly in patients younger than 40 years. Given this patient's degree of symptoms, findings consistent with achalasia, and limited comorbidities, a laparoscopic esophageal (Heller) myotomy with a Dor fundoplication would be the most appropriate treatment. While esophageal myotomy was performed through a thoracotomy or laparotomy in the past, it is now most commonly performed laparoscopically since the angle for the myotomy is easier and allows the addition of a fundoplication to prevent reflux. Laparoscopic myotomy relieves symptoms in 90% of patients and is more effective in providing prolonged symptom relief than endoscopic therapy with a low morbidity (6.3%) and mortality (0.1%). A partial fundoplication should be performed at the time of myotomy to reduce the incidence of gastroesophageal reflux (8.8% vs. 31.5%).

Since the esophagus remains aperistaltic, patients with a megaesophagus or a sigmoid esophagus with

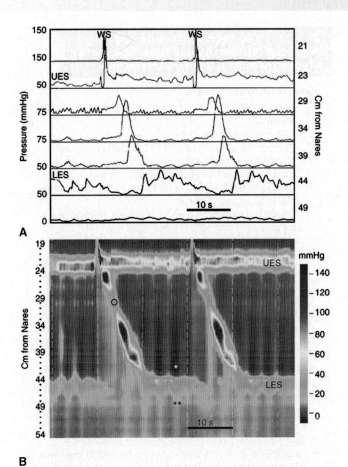

FIGURE 2 • Traditional esophageal manometry (**A**) and high-resolution manometry (**B**) show normal peristalsis and relaxation of the lower esophageal sphincter (LES) with each wet swallow (WS). UES, upper esophageal sphincter. (From Jee SR, et al. A high-resolution view of achalasia. J Clin Gastroenterol. 2009;43(7): 646.)

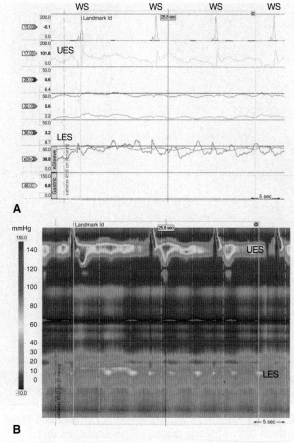

FIGURE 3 • Esophageal manometry (**A**) and high-resolution manometry (**B**) show aperistalsis of the esophageal body on all wet swallows (WS) with no relaxation of the lower esophageal sphincter (LES). UES, upper esophageal sphincter.

significant tortuosity or angulation **(Figure 4)** will continue to have poor emptying despite a myotomy and should undergo a transhiatal esophagectomy. In addition, patients who have had a previous myotomy should undergo esophagectomy unless there is concern that the previous myotomy was incomplete.

Surgical Approach

The patient is restricted to a clear liquid diet for 2 days prior to the operation. Since the dilated esophagus may contain large amounts of fluid and retained food, decompression with a nasogastric tube prior to induction of general anesthesia is critical to prevent aspiration. The patient is then placed in the supine position. A camera port is placed above the umbilicus, and pneumoperitoneum is established to 15 mm Hg. Four additional ports are placed under direct vision with two 5-mm working ports in the epigastrium. A 5-mm port is placed laterally on the right for the liver

retractor and a 5-mm port in the left abdomen to retract the stomach. The gastrohepatic ligament is opened, and the right crus is identified. The anterior aspect of the esophagus is bluntly dissected while the posterior planes are left intact unless there is a hiatal hernia.

The gastroesophageal fat pad is removed exposing the gastroesophageal junction. Care is taken to identify and preserve the anterior vagus nerve. The myotomy is started just above the gastroesophageal junction using the hook cautery. The longitudinal and circular muscle fibers are divided 6 cm onto the esophagus and 2 cm onto the stomach. The edges of the myotomy are bluntly separated from the mucosa for half of the esophageal circumference. The integrity of the esophageal mucosa is then tested with insufflation through the endoscope with the myotomy submerged under water. The location of the gastroesophageal junction is confirmed endoscopically to ensure that the myotomy extends at least 2 cm onto the stomach.

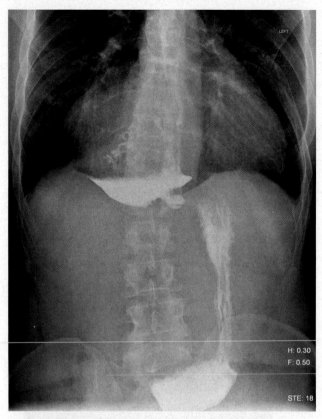

FIGURE 4 • Barium esophagram demonstrates end-stage achalasia with a grossly dilated megaesophagus up to 12 cm with minimal flow through the gastroesophageal junction 20 years after a previous esophageal myotomy.

TABLE 1. Key Technical Steps and Potential Pitfalls to a Laparoscopic Heller Myotomy with a Dor Fundoplication

Key Technical Steps
1. Place an NG tube prior to induction to prevent aspiration.
2. Five laparoscopic port sites.
3. Dissect the anterior aspect of the distal esophagus bluntly from the hiatus.
4. Expose the gastroesophageal junction by removing the gastroesophageal fat pad taking care to preserve the anterior vagus nerve.
5. Divide the longitudinal and the circular muscle fibers for at least 6 cm onto the esophagus and 2 cm onto the stomach.
6. Separate the edges of the myotomy from the underlying mucosa for half of the esophageal circumference.
7. Insufflate the esophagus under water to test for a leak from the myotomy site.
8. Perform an anterior (Dor) or a posterior (Toupet) fundoplication.
9. Close the laparoscopic port sites.

Potential Pitfalls
• Aspiration of retained food in the esophagus at the time of induction.
• Mucosal perforation particularly if there is scarring from previous Botox injections.
• Splenic injury due to retraction of the stomach.
• Incomplete myotomy due to failure to extend the myotomy adequately onto the stomach.

An anterior (Dor) or a posterior (Toupet) fundoplication is then performed after the myotomy is completed. The Dor fundoplication has the added benefit of buttressing the myotomy site and is constructed by placing two sutures on either side of the hiatus passing through the fundus, the divided esophageal muscle, and the crus.

Special Considerations

In separating the muscle fibers from the underlying mucosa, an esophageal perforation may occur particularly if there is scarring from previous Botox treatments. The procedure should be converted to a laparotomy if the surgeon is not facile at intracorporeal suturing. The mucosal perforation should be repaired with a 4-0 absorbable suture and the overlying myotomy closed with interrupted sutures to buttress the repair. A myotomy should then be performed on the contralateral aspect of the esophagus.

Postoperative Management

On postoperative day 1, an esophagram is obtained to evaluate for perforation **(Figure 1B)**. If no evidence of perforation is present, a clear liquid diet is started, and the patient is discharged home. Patients are typically advanced to a mechanical soft diet, which is maintained for 3 weeks, on postoperative day 3. Mild recurrent symptoms of dysphagia, heartburn, and regurgitation may occur in up to 40% to 50% of patients. However, few of these patients will require additional intervention other than initiation of a proton pump inhibitor or dietary modifications.

Case Conclusion

The patient successfully underwent a laparoscopic Heller myotomy with a Dor fundoplication. On postoperative day 1, his esophagram showed no evidence of leak with significant improvement in esophageal emptying. He is advanced to a clear liquid diet and discharged home. At his 6-month follow-up appointment, he is tolerating a regular diet without any symptoms of dysphagia or heartburn **(Table 1)**.

TAKE HOME POINTS

- Pseudoachalasia due to a carcinoma must be ruled out by upper endoscopy in a patient that presents with progressive dysphagia.
- Typical findings on esophageal manometry include an aperistaltic esophageal body with absent or incomplete relaxation of the LES.
- Botulinum toxin injection and pneumatic dilation are typically reserved for patients who are poor surgical candidates.
- Laparoscopic Heller myotomy is the standard surgical therapy for achalasia and is combined with a partial fundoplication to prevent reflux.
- Patients with megaesophagus and significant angulation or tortuosity of the esophagus should undergo a transhiatal esophagectomy.

SUGGESTED READINGS

Campos GM, Vittinghoff E, Rabl C, et al. Endoscopic and surgical treatments for achalasia: a systematic review and meta-analysis. Ann Surg. 2009;1:45–57.

Devaney EJ, Iannettoni MD, Orringer MB, et al. Esophagectomy for achalasia: patient selection and clinical experience. Ann Thorac Surg. 2001;72:854–858.

SSAT patient care guidelines. Esophageal achalasia. J Gastrointest Surg. 2007;11:1210–1212.

Williams VA, Peters JH. Achalasia of the esophagus: a surgical disease. J Am Coll Surg. 2009;208:151–162.

73 Solitary Pulmonary Nodule

JAMES HARRIS, ALICIA HULBERT and MALCOLM V. BROCK

[handwritten margin notes:
<3cm – SPN
>3 cm – mass
non-malignant
malig 75% - NSCLC
25%
45% adeno
20% SCC
25% large
cell
carcinoid
lymphoma
mets]

Presentation

A 65-year-old man with shortness of breath and tachycardia undergoes a spiral CT scan of the chest to rule out pulmonary emboli. The CT scan is negative for pulmonary emboli, but a noncalcified solitary pulmonary nodule (SPN) measuring 2.3 cm in diameter with spiculated borders is incidentally found in the right upper lobe of the lung. There is no mediastinal adenopathy on the CT scan. The patient has a past medical history significant for anxiety disorder (which he now admits usually presents with shortness of breath) and hypertension but denies a history of pulmonary disease. The patient has a 25 pack-year tobacco history without a family history of lung cancer or any other malignancies. His physical examination is unremarkable.

Differential Diagnosis

An SPN is classified as a single-lung parenchymal lesion that measures <3 cm, is surrounded by pulmonary parenchyma, and is without atelectasis or adenopathy. Lesions measuring >3 cm are classified as masses and are more likely to be malignant. The differential diagnosis of a SPN starts with the question of whether it is benign versus malignant. The range of incidences of cancer found in an SPN is quite wide, between 10% and 70%, largely because of varied patient characteristics. Of those SPNs found to be cancer, up to 75% are non–small cell lung cancer (NSCLC), with 50% being adenocarcinoma and 25% being squamous cell carcinoma. The remaining 25% of malignancies associated with SPN consist of large cell carcinoma, small cell carcinoma, carcinoid, lymphoma, and solitary metastatic lesions from extrapulmonary sources. Any patient with a known history of an extrapulmonary malignancy has a 25% chance of having an SPN pathologically consistent with a metastasis. SPNs that prove to be benign lesions are most often (80% of the time) consistent with infectious granulomas, while hamartomas make up a distant second at 10%. Other benign etiologies comprise the remaining 10% and are due to trauma, arteriovenous malformations, rheumatoid nodules, sarcoidosis, intrapulmonary lymph nodes, and plasma cell granulomas.

Workup

In order to establish an accurate diagnosis for an SPN found incidentally on a CT scan or a chest x-ray, the clinician must first perform a thorough history and physical exam along with a basic set of laboratory analysis to assess those patients at risk for malignancy versus those who may have a benign etiology. Probably the most important first question to an asymptomatic patient with an incidental radiographic finding concerns any previous chest x-rays or CT scans available for review. The existence of previous radiologic evidence of disease may be very helpful not only in assessing if the SPN is a new or preexisting lesion but also in establishing the tumor's doubling time. The latter can also be used as a rough predictor of the presence of cancer; lesions with a doubling time of <465 days are three to four times more likely to be malignant. One exception is a nodule doubling in <20 days, which usually suggests an acute inflammatory process.

Since cancer is a disease of aging, chronologic age has been shown to have a significant effect on the likelihood of an SPN harboring cancer; patients over the age of 70 years with an SPN are four times more likely to have cancer than those under the age of 70 years old. Any patient over the age of 60 years is considered high risk, those 40 to 59 years old are intermediate risk, and patients under 40 years are low risk. While one study found that only 3% of patients between the ages of 35 and 39 years old had SPNs found to be cancer, it is very important to evaluate each patient as other factors can significantly influence the likelihood of malignancy, regardless of age.

Importantly, tobacco use of 20 pack-years and greater has been associated with a high probability of cancer among patients with an SPN. Patients with less than a 20 pack-year history maintain an intermediate probability of cancer, while nonsmokers have a low probability. Other important factors that can significantly increase the likelihood of an SPN being cancer, even in nonsmokers, are exposure to second-hand smoke, asbestos, radon, a previous history of any malignancy, and a family history of cancer.

TABLE 1. Risk of Lung Cancer Based on Characteristics of Patient or Lesion

Characteristics of Patient or Lesion	Probability of Cancer		
	Low	Intermediate	High
Patient age (y)	<40	40–60	>60
Patient smoking history	Never smoked	<20 pack-y	≥20 pack-y
Lesion size (cm)	<1.0	1.1–2.2	≥2.3
Lesion margin	Smooth	Scalloped	Spiculated

From Pechet TT. Solitary Pulmonary Nodule. ACS Surgery: Principles and Practice. Chapter 5, 2010, with permission.

The radiographic characteristics of the SPN are very important in predicting the presence of cancer. Nodule size seems important with SPNs >2.2 cm having a high probability of being cancer. Lesions measuring 1.1 to 2.2 cm have an intermediate risk of malignancy, while those <1.1 cm are low risk. The shape of the SPN is also critical with nodules having spiculated borders with the highest risk of being cancer in comparison. One study by Gurney revealed that SPNs identified on CT scan with spiculated borders were five to six times more likely to be cancer in comparison to those without a spiculated border (Table 1).

Calcification patterns are another radiographic feature that can help to determine whether a lesion is benign or malignant. The most important characteristic of a benign nodule is the presence of calcification, such as the large central nidus, concentric calcification typical of a granuloma (Figure 1), or the diffuse speckled, "popcorn" pattern, typical of a hamartoma (Figure 2). Occasionally, however, a malignant nodule can exhibit a small "fleck" of calcification or it engulfs a nearby small granuloma during its growth (Figure 3). Metastatic osteogenic sarcoma may also have calcifications; thus, the presence of calcification alone does not ensure a benign diagnosis (Figure 4).

For any SPN with low clinical and radiographic likelihood of cancer, it is appropriate to monitor the patient with serial CT scans to ensure that there is no change in size or characteristics of the SPN that would warrant further evaluation. Patients with SPNs of intermediate cancer risk that measure 1 cm or more should receive positron emission tomography (PET) imaging, to help distinguish benign from malignant pulmonary nodules by measuring 18-fluorodeoxyglucose (FDG) and by showing increased FDG uptake and retention in malignant cells. FDG-PET scanning is a valuable, noninvasive tool with a 95% sensitivity for identifying malignancy and a specificity of 85% or greater; however, false-positive results may be obtained in lesions containing an active inflammatory process. FDG-PET scans lack sensitivity in SPNs

<1 cm; thus, lesions this size should be followed by serial CT scans. Although for SPNs that are considered clinically and/or radiographically high risk, it is appropriate to take patients with these lesions directly to the operative suite, tumor staging has been reported to be significantly better with integrated PET-CT rather than CT alone.

There are various recommendations in the literature regarding the appropriate timeline for CT scan follow-up; recommendations out of the Fleischner Society state that any SPN >8 mm should be monitored at 3, 9, and 24 months in patients over the age of 35 years, regardless of the risk status and less frequently in lesions <8 mm. For low-risk patients with lesions <4 mm, there is no need for further follow-up, and those with lesions between 4 and 8 mm should undergo increasing frequencies of surveillance CT scans based on the exact size of the lesion and the risk status of the patient.

In our 65-year-old heavy smoker, after appropriate questioning, the patient revealed the availability of an old CT scan from 12 months previously. The same SPN was evident, but with a diameter of 1.0 cm. Since the volume of a sphere is proportional to the square of the radius, this doubling of the CT diameter in a year suggests a very large increase in tumor volume. A PET/CT scan was ordered both to investigate the primary lung nodule and to render more accurate tumor staging. The PET/CT revealed a single focus of high FDG uptake in the right upper lobe. Given the radiologic evidence combined with the patient's age as well as the patient's substantial smoking history, the probability of a malignant process underlying this patient's tumor growth is very high.

Diagnosis and Treatment

All patients with an SPN who have a high clinical and/or radiographic probability of cancer, without evidence of malignancy outside of the area of surgical resection, should undergo surgical excision. Those individuals with an intermediate probability of a malignant SPN and negative PET scan findings should be followed

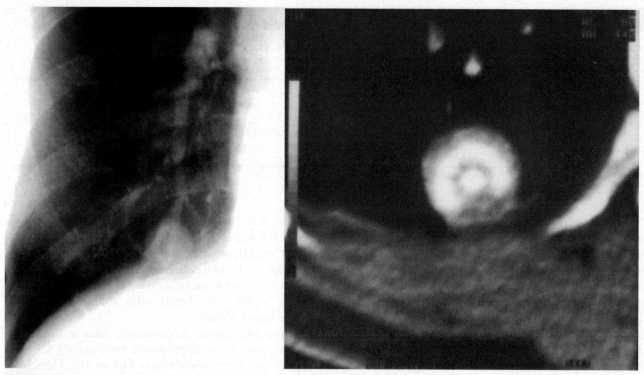

FIGURE 1 • Calcification in granuloma–benign. (Image provided by Dr. S. Siegelman, Johns Hopkins Hospital, Department of Radiology.)

with serial CT scans. Those with an SPN of intermediate probability and a positive PET scan should undergo surgical excision.

Although the definitive approach in most malignancies located outside of the chest cavity is to distinguish benign from malignant lesions with a tissue biopsy, often patients with a documented rapidly enlarging SPN are taken directly to the operating room without biopsy-proven carcinoma. The traditional argument has

been that benign lesions account for <10% of rapidly growing tumors in the chest, a figure that has recently been confirmed by prospective data from 31,567 asymptomatic patients screened with helical CT scans. With advances in fiberoptic bronchoscopy and image-guided transthoracic needle biopsy, however, many lesions are now amendable to these minimally invasive alternatives for obtaining tissue for diagnosis. Still, most thoracic surgeons adhere to the principle that SPNs with

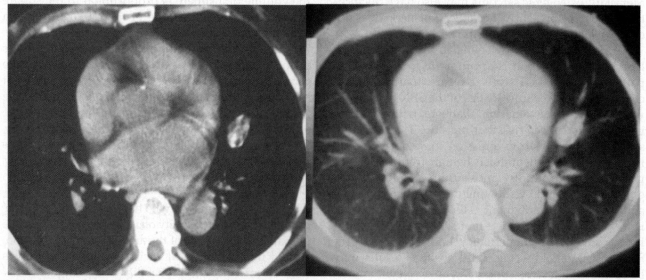

FIGURE 2 • Pulmonary hamartoma with "popcorn calcifications." (Image provided by Dr. S. Siegelman, Johns Hopkins Hospital, Department of Radiology.)

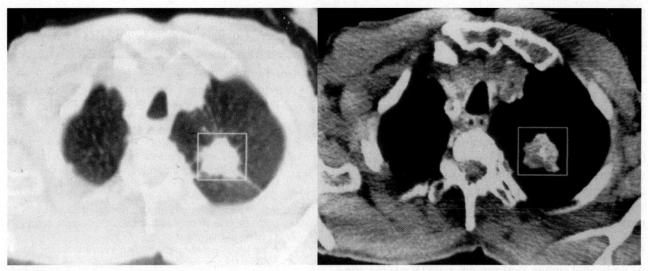

FIGURE 3 • Calcification in carcinoma. (Image provided by Dr. S. Siegelman, Johns Hopkins Hospital, Department of Radiology.)

an intermediate to high suspicion for cancer, which are not accessible to biopsy because of small size or location as well as high-risk SPNs with negative biopsy findings, should undergo excisional biopsy preferably via video-assisted thoracic surgery (VATS) with possibility of conversion to thoracotomy if indicated.

Surgical Approach

In patients with an SPN that is biopsy-proven NSCLC, but there is no evidence of mediastinal adenopathy (all mediastinal lymph nodes ≤1 cm), there is <10% prevalence of occult metastases. Although many thoracic surgeons perform mediastinoscopy routinely for appropriate staging, others prefer mediastinoscopy only for patients with radiologically evident mediastinal adenopathy. The exception is for those patients with small cell lung cancer (SCLC) found preoperatively within an SPN. All of these patients should undergo mediastinoscopy to rule out occult mediastinal metastases.

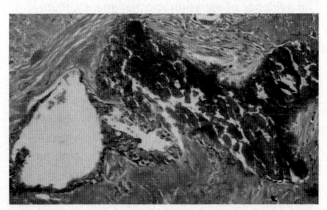

FIGURE 4 • Pathology specimen obtained from lesion seen in Figure 3. (Image provided by Dr. S. Siegelman, Johns Hopkins Hospital, Department of Radiology.).

The current recommendation by the National Comprehensive Cancer Network for patients, such as our 65-year-old man with suspected NSCLC (<4 cm) with node-negative lesions, is lobectomy alone. Five-year survival rates in such patients with SPN and NSCLC who undergo curative resection alone can be as high as 80%. For patients with node negative disease but larger tumors, the addition of adjuvant chemotherapy is encouraged. Multiple retrospective and prospective studies have shown that there is additional survival benefit in patients with stage 1 SCLC when treated with both lobectomy and adjuvant platinum-based chemotherapy.

In the operating room after a time out is performed and after induction of general anesthesia with subsequent placement of a double-lumen endotracheal tube, the patient is positioned with the nonoperative side down in the lateral decubitus position. Care is taken to pad and support all pressure points. It is then appropriate to ask the anesthesia team to begin one-lung ventilation, ventilating the nonoperative side so as to allow the lung with the SPN to collapse away from the chest wall. This will not only decrease risk of injury to the lung upon entry to the pleural space but also make smaller nodules more apparent to detection as the normal air-filled lung parenchyma collapses around the solid SPN.

Typically, three ports are placed between the fifth to the eighth intercostal spaces, depending upon the location of the tumor, in a triangulated position usually with placement of the camera first. Under direct vision, safe entry of the other two sites is attained. If the SPN is not apparent upon visual inspection, the lung can be indirectly palpated with a grasper or palpated directly as an alternate way of identifying a lesion before converting to thoracotomy.

If the SPN is identified, it is resected using a grasper and an endoscopic stapler device. If the specimen is small enough, it can be easily removed through the port; otherwise, it must be placed into an endoscopic specimen bag for removal so as to avoid seeding of tumor cells at the patients port site. If an SPN excised with a wedge resection is determined to be malignant on frozen section, and if the patient is thought to be a suitable candidate, a pulmonary lobectomy (either by VATS or open) is almost always warranted. Upon completion, an intercostal block can be performed under direct visualization along with chest tube placement through the thoracoscope port site.

Special Intraoperative Considerations

As indicated, when performing a VATS wedge lung resection on a patient, it is not only appropriate to consent for the possibility of conversion to open thoracotomy, but also to consent for the likely possibility of a more complete oncologic resection of the entire lobe if the specimen is found to be malignant. In preparation for such a scenario, pulmonary function tests should be performed on each patient to ensure that a lobectomy, if necessary, can be performed safely without significant postoperative morbidity or mortality as a result of preexisting pulmonary disease. In terms of technique during a VATS lobectomy for an SPN, perhaps the steepest learning curve is in understanding the 3-D anatomical relationships of the pulmonary vasculature and the bronchi, proper positioning and manipulation of the stapling devices as well as providing adequate exposure and traction for dissection during the procedure. The anatomy presents itself on the video monitor from an unfamiliar perspective if one has only been accustomed to open thoracotomy cases. The stapling devices are rigid instruments that must be manipulated deftly in the closed confines of the chest. Finally, an experienced first assistant is absolutely critical in enabling a risk-free procedure since good traction and exposure allow for meticulous dissection especially when there is dense hilar lymphadenopathy or a fused fissure. Conversion rates to open thoracotomy tend to decrease as the surgeon's experience with the VATS technique increases (Table 2).

Postoperative Management

Most patients undergoing a VATS lung wedge resection do fairly well postoperatively with very low morbidity and mortality. Most patients have their chest tubes removed on postoperative day 1 as long as they remain with low output and without an air leak and are sent home that same day. Increasingly, surgeons who are performing VATS lobectomies for malignant SPNs are reporting similar complication rates as the open thoracotomy equivalents.

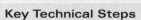

TABLE 2. Key Technical Steps and Potential Pitfalls to VATS Pulmonary Wedge Resection

Key Technical Steps

1. After positioning the patient in the lateral decubitus position, ask anesthesia to begin single-lung ventilation prior to prepping the patient so as to allow adequate collapse of the operative lung at time of entering the pleural space.
2. If the SPN cannot be visualized after adequate deflation of the lung, attempt to palpate the lung directly with a finger or indirectly using a grasper to localize the lesion that cannot be seen.
3. If the specimen is too large to remove through the port site, use an endoscopic specimen bag to avoid seeding of malignant cells.
4. If the lesion cannot be identified, convert to a thoracotomy for open palpation and SPN excision.
5. Perform an intercostal nerve block under direct visualization upon completion of surgery in order to diminish postoperative pain.

Potential Pitfalls

- Injury to the lung upon entry secondary to inadequate collapse of the operative lung and/or adhesions.
- Intraoperative hemorrhage due to poor positioning of stapling devices or inadequate visualization.
- Injury to the neurovascular bundle that runs under the rib, resulting in acute or delayed hemorrhage or a postoperative chronic pain syndrome from intercostal nerve injury.
- Inappropriate removal of the tumor specimen, resulting in recurrence of tumor at the port site.

From Flores RM. Video-assisted Thoracic Surgery. ACS Surgery: Principles and Practice. Chapter 10, 2005.

Case Conclusion

In this clinical scenario, with an isolated SPN and no evidence of extrathoracic malignancy, there is a high probability of this SPN being a cancer; especially given his age >60 years, tobacco history >20 pack-years, and the size/characteristics/doubling time of his SPN. It would be appropriate to take this patient straight to surgical excision by VATS or even thoracotomy if the SPN is not easily accessible for biopsy by transthoracic needle biopsy or bronchoscopy. He should undergo the appropriate preoperative medical clearance in addition to pulmonary function testing to ensure that a lobectomy, if required, can be performed safely.

TAKE HOME POINTS

- Among all SPNs found to be cancer, 75% are NSCLC.
- Among all SPNs found to be benign, 80% are infectious granulomas.
- Six important factors that significantly increase the likelihood of an SPN being cancer: (1) age >60 years, (2) tobacco history >20 pack-years, (3) prior history of cancer, (4) size >2 cm on chest x-ray or CT, (5) the presence of spiculations on chest x-ray or CT, (6) doubling size <465 days.
- Calcification patterns on CXR and/or CT of an SPN can be suggestive of a benign etiology but should not be used to exclude the diagnosis of cancer since some malignancies can also have the presence of calcifications.
- Patients with an SPN >1 cm who have an intermediate probability of cancer should have an FDG-PET scan to assess the need for surgical excision versus surveillance with serial CT scans.
- All patients with an SPN who have a high clinical and/or radiographic probability of cancer should undergo surgical excision.
- For patients with an SPN found to be stage 1a NSCLC, lobectomy alone is recommended.
- For patients with an SPN found to be stage 1 SCLC, lobectomy followed by platinum-based adjuvant chemotherapy is recommended.

SUGGESTED READINGS

Cahan WG, Shah JP, Castro EB. Benign solitary lung lesions in patients with cancer. Ann Surg. 1978;187:241.

Cronin P, Dwamena BA, Kelly AM, et al. Solitary pulmonary nodules: meta-analytic comparison of cross-sectional imaging modalities for diagnosis of malignancy. Radiology. 2008;246(3):772–782.

Dewan N, Shehan C, Reeb S. Likelihood of malignancy in a solitary pulmonary nodule. Chest. 1997;112:416–422. [A description of the possible role of PET scanning in the evaluation of the solitary pulmonary nodule.]

Ettinger D, Johnson B. Update: NCCN small cell and non-small cell lung cancer Clinical Practice Guidelines. J Natl Compr Canc Netw. 2005;3(suppl 1):S17–S21.

Flores RM. Video-assisted thoracic surgery. ACS Surgery: Principles and Practice. Chapter 10, B.C. Decker, 2005.

Gould MK, Fletcher J, Iannettoni MD, et al. Evaluation of patients with pulmonary nodules: when is it lung cancer?: ACCP evidence-based clinical practice guidelines (2nd ed.). Chest. 2007;132:108S.

Gurney GW. Determining the likelihood of malignancy in solitary pulmonary nodules with Bayesian analysis. Part I. Theory. Radiology. 1993;186:405–413.

Harris J Jr, Brock MV. Surgical treatment of small cell lung cancer. Lung Cancer: A Multidisciplinary Approach to Diagnosis and Management. Chapter 8. Demos Medical Publishing, 2010.

Henschke CI, et al. International Early Lung Cancer Action Program Investigators. N Engl J Med. 2006;355(17):1763–1771.

Lee PC, Port JL, Korst RJ, et al. Risk factors for occult mediastinal metastases in clinical stage I non-small cell lung cancer. Ann Thorac Surg. 2007;84(1):177–181.

Little AG, Rusch VW, Bonner JA, et al. Patterns of surgical care of lung cancer patients. Ann Thorac Surg. 2005;80:2051–2056.

MacMahon H, Austin JH, Gamsu G, et al. Guidelines for management of small pulmonary nodules detected on CT scans: a statement from the Fleischner Society. Radiology. 2005;237:395–400.

Ost D, Fein AM, Feinsilver SH. Clinical practice. The solitary pulmonary nodule. N Engl J Med. 2003;348:2535–2542.

Pechet TT. Solitary pulmonary nodule. ACS Surgery: Principles and Practice. Chapter 5, B.C. Decker, 2010.

Steele JD. The solitary pulmonary nodule: report of a cooperative study of resected asymptomatic solitary pulmonary nodules in males. J Thorac Cardiovasc Surg. 1963;46:21–39.

Tan BB, Flaherty KR, Kazerooni EA, et al. The solitary pulmonary nodule. Chest. 2003;123(suppl 1):89S–96S.

Trunk G, Gracey DR, Byrd RB. The management and evaluation of the solitary pulmonary nodule. Chest. 1974;66:236–239.

74 Spontaneous Pneumothorax

PIERRE THEODORE

Presentation

A 65-year-old man with a history of chronic obstructive pulmonary disease (COPD), hypertension, and a 50 pack-year history of smoking presents with acute-onset shortness of breath. He regularly has dyspnea on exertion but suddenly became short of breath at rest 1 hour ago. He has new right-sided chest pain, which he describes as knife-like and worse on inspiration. He has no history of pneumothorax, acute coronary syndrome, or stroke. He denies recent chest trauma. He smokes one pack of cigarettes per day. On physical examination, he is tachycardic, hypertensive, and tachypneic, and his oxygen saturation is 85% on room air. He has decreased breath sounds on the right side, decreased chest expansion on the right, and hyperresonance to percussion on the right. His trachea is midline.

Differential Diagnosis

Spontaneous pneumothorax in a young person is usually a rupture of a subpleural bleb in the lung apex without underlying lung disease and is known as primary spontaneous pneumothorax. Classically, patients are tall, young men who are light to moderate smokers and often physically active.

In the case patient, the pneumothorax is likely secondary to underlying lung disease. Other causes of secondary spontaneous pneumothorax include airway diseases, such as cystic fibrosis or asthma; significant lung infections, such as *Pneumocystis jiroveci* (*P. carinii*) pneumonia or tuberculosis; and other intrapulmonary diseases such as lung tumors, inflammatory lung disease, and connective tissue diseases of the lung. Pneumothoraces may also be due to trauma or iatrogenic causes such as subclavian line placement, percutaneous lung biopsy, chest tube clamping, or barotrauma such as deep-sea diving or mechanical ventilation.

In the elderly patient presenting with chest pain or shortness of breath, myocardial infarction, pulmonary embolism, aortic dissection, and pneumonia must be ruled out. The workup must include a physical examination with EKG, cardiac enzymes, chest x-ray, and a CT scan of the chest as directed by the findings.

In young women, two additional causes of pneumothorax are lymphangioleiomyomatosis (LAM) and catamenial pneumothorax. LAM, also known as pregnancy pneumothorax, is hormonally driven smooth muscle proliferation along lymphatic channels, which obstructs bronchioles leading to air trapping, bullae formation, and pneumothorax. Catamenial pneumothorax occurs in young women with endometrial tissue in the thorax; the endometriosis forms cysts that can rupture during menses.

Tension pneumothorax, resulting in a mediastinal shift and decreased venous return leading to circulatory collapse, should always be on the differential diagnosis. Any evidence of tracheal deviation on examination requires immediate needle decompression without waiting for a chest x-ray. Confirmation of the diagnosis is found in the audible escape of air under pressure from the thorax. Chest tube placement can then be performed electively. Patients with substantial pneumothorax who require intubation and ventilation should have a small chest tube placed first to prevent conversion to tension pneumothorax when positive pressure ventilation is initiated.

Workup

The patient in this case should first have supplemental oxygen administered and a peripheral intravenous catheter placed. An EKG and chest x-ray are performed that reveal the presence of sinus tachycardia without evidence of acute ischemia and a visible partial collapse of the right lung and pneumothorax without evidence of deviation of the mediastinum, respectively. His oxygen saturations were seen to improve with the administration of supplemental oxygen through nasal cannula. An urgent CT scan of his chest reveals a right-sided pneumothorax, emphysematous changes throughout both lungs, and no evidence of malignancy **(Figure 1)**.

Discussion

A pneumothorax can be most easily observed on upright chest x-ray **(Figure 2)**. An apex-to-cupola distance of <3 cm is considered a small pneumothorax. One possible error in chest x-ray interpretation is to confuse a skin fold for a pneumothorax. Skin folded against the x-ray cassette appears almost as a vertical

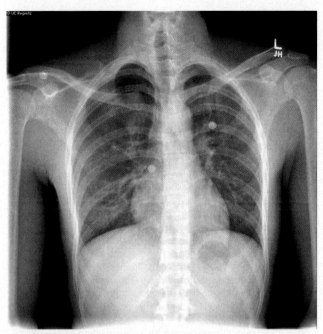

FIGURE 1 • Chest x-ray of right-sided spontaneous pneumothorax.

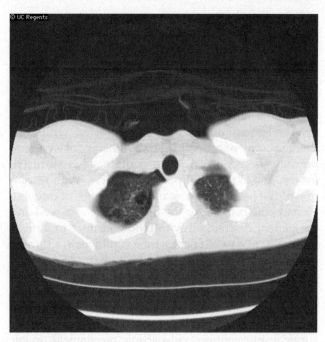

FIGURE 3 • CT Chest through the lung apex showing bulla.

line that does not follow the contour of the rib cage. A skin fold has a different radiographic density than a pneumothorax, and vascular markings may be seen lateral to the skin fold.

In the patient with preexisting lung disease, a CT scan of the chest can help differentiate among large bullae, cystic lesions, and pneumothoraces, which may appear similar on routine chest x-ray **(Figure 3)**. The CT scan can guide operative management by

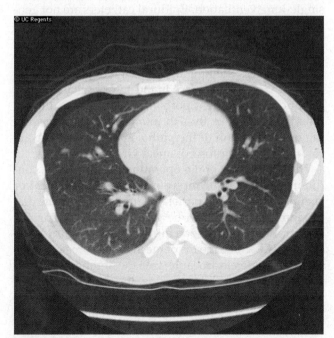

FIGURE 2 • CT Chest through the midlung showing pneumothorax.

providing information about underlying lung disease. A CT scan of the chest may be omitted for younger patients with a first presentation of primary spontaneous pneumothorax.

Diagnosis and Treatment

The American College of Chest Physicians published management guidelines in 2001; the goals of management are to treat the pneumothorax, and to reduce the risk of recurrence by achieving visceral and parietal pleural symphysis by means of pleurodesis or pleurectomy.

The risk of recurrence after a first episode of primary spontaneous pneumothorax is estimated at approximately 32%. These patients do not necessarily need surgical treatment or pleurodesis aimed at reducing recurrence unless they have bilateral pneumothoraces or are exposed to significant changes in transpulmonary pressure, such as pilots or divers. An additional indication for surgical management of primary spontaneous pneumothorax includes lack of access to advanced health care or periods of travel distant from adequate health services. The recurrence rate after spontaneous pneumothorax associated with underlying lung disease is approximately 43%, but these patients carry a higher risk of morbidity and mortality due to their baseline respiratory compromise. Operative management or pleurodesis is typically indicated at first presentation. For all patients, the risk of further recurrence increases with each episode. After the second pneumothorax, the recurrence risk is as high as 75% and exceeds 80% after the third pneumothorax. As such, most clinicians recommend intervention following a second episode of pneumothorax.

Clinically stable patients with small primary pneumothoraces can be observed; if the pneumothorax is radiographically stable over 6 hours and there is no progression of symptoms, they may be sent home with follow-up in 1 to 2 days. Most patients with large primary pneumothoraces will be treated with tube thoracostomy or a small "pigtail catheter" placed temporarily to suction. Water seal drainage is sufficient for the vast majority of pneumothoraces. With resolution of the pneumothorax and no evidence of ongoing air leak, the catheter or the tube may be removed and the patient discharged with follow-up in 1 to 2 days. Generally, a 16 to 24 Fr chest tube is sufficient, although patients with a large air leak or receiving mechanical ventilation may require larger chest tubes.

If an air leak persists for more than 3 days, the patient should be evaluated for persistent or recurrent pneumothorax. The patient should be considered for surgical intervention: videoscopic mechanical or talc pleurodesis, blebectomy, or a pleural tenting procedure. Another treatment option for persistent air leak is to perform a blood patch of 50 mL of the patient's own blood, drawn from the femoral vein, instilled through the chest tube under sterile conditions and flushed with saline. The tube is clamped for 30 minutes and then returned to water seal. This procedure should not be performed if the lung is incompletely re-expanded or if the patient has evidence of infection in the pleural space. The patient should be monitored for conversion to tension pneumothorax during the procedure, as this has been reported.

Patients with pneumothoraces in the setting of severe underlying lung disease should receive prompt evaluation, supplemental oxygen, and receive a small chest tube placed urgently. For loculated or complicated pneumothorax, placement of the chest tube under CT scan guidance may be required. The standard approach to surgical management of pneumothorax is video-assisted thoracoscopic surgery (VATS). In addition to shorter hospital stays, less pain and disability in comparison to open thoracotomy, VATS enjoys similarly high success rates of 95%. Patients who are poor surgical candidates or refuse surgery may be managed with tube thoracostomy and receive bedside pleurodesis through their chest tube.

A novel approach is the use of endobronchial valve technology to specifically obstruct the segmental orifice leading to the site of the classic air leak.

Chemical pleurodesis can be performed by direct instillation of talc or doxycycline into the pleural space. Talc pleurodesis is particularly effective and despite a chronic thickening of the pleura, very few long-term complications have been observed. Talc has rarely been associated with acute lung injury.

TABLE 1. Key Technical Steps for Video-Assisted Thoracosopic Bleb/Bullas Resection and Pleurodesis

Key Technical Steps

1. Prepare the patient with general anesthesia and a double-lumen endotracheal tube.
2. Commence the operation with a thorough bronchoscopy of the tracheobronchial tree.
3. For the resection, position the patient in the lateral decubitus position with single-lung ventilation.
4. Place the VATS camera port at the 5th intercostal space in the anterior-axillary line.
5. Depending on the location of the pathology, additional ports may be placed in the 4th intercostal space or the 7th intercostal space.
6. Similar to a wedge resection, grasp the affected tissue and apply the endoscopic stapler across the base of the bullae/bleb. Use a reinforced, linear GIA staple load.
7. After resection, abrade the parietal pleura through the VATS ports. This can be accomplished by using the electrocautery scratch pad, the electrocautery, or the argon beam coagulator.
8. Chemical pleurodesis can be accomplished by evenly distributing 1 to 5 mg of aerosolized sterile talc to the pleural space.
9. Upon completion of the procedure, remove the ports, and insert a single chest tube into the inferior VATS port.

Surgical Approach for Bullectomy and Pleurodesis Using VATS

The operation for bleb/bulla resection is similar to a standard wedge resection of the lung using videoscopic technique (**Table 1**). The patient is intubated with a double-lumen endotracheal tube, which permits single-lung ventilation. Epidural catheters are not generally necessary and the patient is placed in the lateral decubitus position. The operation commences with a thorough bronchoscopy of the tracheobronchial tree. In order to access the lung apex, a camera port is placed at the 5th intercostal space in the anterior-axillary line. Additional instrument ports may be placed in the 4th intercostal space or the 7th intercostal space depending on the location of the pathology. Apical bullae are resected using reinforced, linear GIA staple loads.

The second part of the operation is to create the conditions for pleural symphysis through mechanical or chemical means. The parietal pleura including the diaphragmatic surface can be gently abraded using the electrocautery scratch pad introduced through at VATS incision. Alternate means of mechanical abrasion of the pleura include electrocautery or the argon beam coagulator. Chemical pleurodesis is an important adjunct to mechanical pleurodesis and can be performed with 1 to 5 mg of aerosolized sterile talc evenly distributed to the pleural space.

Pleurectomy is an option for recurrent pneumothorax particularly in younger patients and can be performed through the VATS ports.

Intraoperative Complications

The main intraoperative complication is a large air leak after resection of the tissue. Prior to closure, the lung should be reinflated and examined for persistent air leak. Reinforcing the lung tissue with additional stapling, fibrin glue, or both may be necessary. Approved pulmonary sealants may reduce the risk of air leak. Bleeding and infections in the pleural space represent important potential complications. However, the most common concern is a persistent air leak following resection of diseased tissue.

Intraoperative management issues also include the approach to the "trapped lung." A lung incapable of expanding to reach the parietal pleural surface creates a judgment challenge for the clinician. If trapped by infection, decortication can be performed, often through open thoracotomy. Patients with trapped lung as a result of carcinoma often can be only managed with a pleural tent.

Postoperative Management

Postoperatively, patients should have a single chest tube, typically 24 or 28 French. The chest tube can be placed to water seal with resolution of the pneumothorax and can be removed on postoperative day 3 should there be no air leak.

If the patient has a persistent air leak after postoperative day 4, then the patient should be placed on to an outpatient suctionless device, such as a Heimlich valve. If the patient can tolerate this device for 24 hours without expansion of the pneumothorax or clinical deterioration, then they may be discharged home with the suctionless device with instructions to call the clinic for any worsening of symptoms. They should follow-up 2 weeks postoperatively; if they have remained asymptomatic on the outpatient suctionless device, they may have the chest tube removed even with a small persistent pneumothorax. Clamping the chest tube is not necessary prior to removal. The patient should have a chest x-ray in 4 hours to demonstrate stability of the pneumothorax.

Complications

Patients should be monitored for arrhythmias, air leaks, chest tube malfunction, or conversion to tension pneumothorax. Additionally, the presence of an air leak can lead to empyema, although this is not common. While empyemas can develop in as little as 2 weeks, the risk of empyema increases with the amount of time the chest tube remains in place. Antibiotics have not been shown to reduce empyema risk when given longer than 24 hours after surgery.

Fibrin deposition on an incompletely expanded lung can begin as soon as 7 days after lung collapse, creating a fibrous rind that may require decortication. Patients with infections of the pleural space are at risk of developing a trapped lung.

Particular attention to pain management is important as respiratory compromise, such as atelectasis or pneumonia, is common in patients with poor pain control and hypoventilation.

TAKE HOME POINTS

- A first presentation of a spontaneous pneumothorax should be managed based on size and clinical presentation with either observation or tube thoracostomy.
- All patients with pneumothorax due to significant underlying lung disease should be admitted and most should have operative management to reduce their recurrence risk.
- VATS is now the standard operative approach for bullectomy and pleurodesis.
- For nonoperative and postoperative patients, place chest tubes to water seal as soon as possible.
- Clinically stable patients with persistent air leaks postoperatively can be discharged home with an outpatient suctionless device and seen back in clinic in 2 weeks.

Acknowledgments

Our thanks to Dr. Brett Elicker, UCSF, for the radiographic images.

SUGGESTED READINGS

Baumann MH, Strange C, Heffner JE, et al. Management of spontaneous pneumothorax: An American College of Chest Physicians Delphi Consensus Statement. Chest. 2001;119:590–602.

Cerfolio RJ, Minnich DJ, Bryant AS. The removal of chest tubes despite an air leak or a pneumothorax. Ann Thorac Surg. 2009;87(6):1690–1694; discussion 1694–1696.

75 Pulsatile Abdominal Mass

PAUL D. DIMUSTO and GILBERT R. UPCHURCH Jr.

Presentation

A 70-year-old man with a history of hypertension, hyperlipidemia, and a 40 pack-year history of smoking presents for routine physical examination. His vital signs are normal. On abdominal exam, it is noted that he has a pulsatile mass in the epigastric region. In addition, he has a well-healed right lower-quadrant scar from a prior open appendectomy. He denies any symptoms of abdominal pain, back pain, or claudication. He is having normal bowel movements and denies melena. He has palpable femoral, popliteal, dorsalis pedis, and posterior tibial pulses bilaterally. The patient is retired, but active, able to work in his yard, and climb a flight of stairs without shortness of breath.

Differential Diagnosis

A pulsatile abdominal mass typically represents aneurysm disease of the arteries of the abdomen, most commonly of the aorta. Aneurysm disease may extend into the common iliac arteries in 20% to 25% of patients. Patients with an abdominal aortic aneurysm (AAA) have an approximately 15% risk of also having femoral or popliteal aneurysms; thus, all patients with AAAs should undergo duplex ultrasound screening for femoral and popliteal aneurysms.

Workup

The patient undergoes further evaluation of his pulsatile abdominal mass with a CT scan of the abdomen and pelvis with IV contrast, which reveals a 5.8-cm AAA that begins 2 cm below the renal arteries (Figure 1). The iliac arteries are not aneurysmal, with a diameter of 1 cm bilaterally. Femoral and popliteal aneurysm scan by duplex ultrasound does not reveal any evidence of aneurysm. Serum laboratory studies reveal a hemoglobin of 14 g/dL, a normal platelet count, and creatinine of 0.9 mg/dL.

Discussion

An AAA is defined as an aortic diameter of >50% larger than normal, with the normal abdominal aorta being 2 to 2.5 cm. Thus, a diameter of 3 to 3.5 cm is typically used to label the aorta aneurysmal. Men are affected approximately four times as often as women. Additional risk factors for AAA formation include smoking, hypertension, chronic obstructive pulmonary disease, atherosclerosis, and advanced age. AAAs are often discovered incidentally on imaging for workup of another disease, with only 30% to 40% of patients having abnormal physical exam findings.

Aortic diameter is used to determine the risk of rupture and the indications for repair. One-year rupture rate rises quickly with increasing diameter: 0.5% to 5% per year for 4 to 5 cm, 3% to 15% per year for 5 to 6 cm, 10% to 20% per year for 6 to 7 cm, and as high as 50% per year when they reach 8 cm in size. Other factors that increase the likelihood of AAA rupture at a given diameter are chronic obstructive pulmonary disease, female gender, rapid expansion rate on serial imaging, hypertension, and smoking. Most recommend that the average patient with an AAA < 5.5 cm in diameter be followed, unless rapid expansion is noted.

Diagnosis and Treatment

Aneurysm repair is indicated in this patient with a 5.8-cm AAA. Because of its lower operative risk, the endovascular aneurysm repair (EVAR) has become the preferred method of repair for patients who meet the appropriate anatomic criteria. The aneurysm neck (the area between the lowest renal artery and the top of the aneurysm) must be at least 1 to 1.5 cm in length and have an angulation of <60° to qualify for EVAR. Additionally, the iliac arteries must be of appropriate diameter (6 to 8 mm) and without significant tortuosity to allow for delivery of the device. This patient meets criteria for EVAR and this would be recommended.

Surgical Approach for Endovascular Aneurysm Repair

In order to choose an appropriate sized endograft and plan the operation, the patient will need a 3D reconstruction of his CT scan (Figure 2). The diameter of the graft should be oversized by approximately 10% to 20% based on the diameter of the proximal landing zone. Standard endograft configurations are bifurcated, terminating in the common iliac arteries bilaterally. This type of graft can be used if the common iliac arteries are not aneurysmal. If anatomically required to get a seal distally, an internal iliac artery can be coiled or occluded and the graft

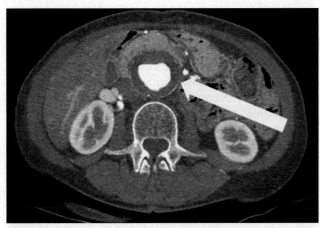

FIGURE 1 • Axial cut of a CT scan documenting an infrarenal AAA.

extended past the orifice of the internal iliac artery, as it is generally acceptable to exclude one internal iliac artery. If, however, both common iliac arteries are aneurysmal, most would agree that an external-to-internal iliac artery bypass be performed on one side in order to avoid debilitating pelvic pain and potential mesenteric ischemia.

EVAR is typically performed under general anesthesia for patients who are not of prohibitive risk **(Table 1)**. However, it can also be performed under regional or local anesthesia with sedation if necessary. The patient is supine on the angiography table with an arterial line and good peripheral intravenous access. The locations of the distal lower-extremity pulses are marked. The patient is prepped from the nipples to the toes,

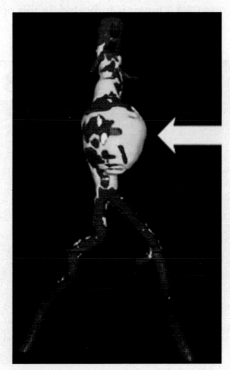

FIGURE 2 • 3D reconstruction of the patient's CT scan demonstrating an infrarenal AAA.

and draped so that both groins are exposed. Bilateral cutdowns exposing the common femoral arteries (CFAs) are performed. The patient is systemically heparinized and wires are placed into the thoracic aorta. Bilateral iliofemoral sheaths are introduced and a marking catheter is placed in the aorta at the level of the renal arteries. An aortogram is performed to define the location of the renal arteries and internal iliac arteries as well as to verify lengths obtained by computed tomographic angiography (CTA). The main body of the endograft is inserted over a stiff wire and deployed just below the renal arteries. Once the contralateral gate is opened, it is cannulated, and a stiff wire is introduced. The contralateral limb is then introduced over the wire, docked into the main body, and deployed. Balloon angioplasty is then performed at the upper and lower fixation sites, as well as at the graft joints, to smooth out any folds in the endograft. Completion angiography is performed to document the absence of endoleaks **(Table 2)** and

TABLE 2. Types of Endoleaks

- Type Ia—Failure of seal at proximal aortic neck
- Type Ib—Failure of seal at one of the iliac landing sites
- Type II—Continued flow into aneurysm sac via a branch artery, typically the lumbar artery or the inferior mesenteric artery (IMA)
- Type III—Leak at junction of the main body of the graft and the iliac limb
- Type IV—Pressure in the aneurysm sac due to leak from small holes in graft material
- Type V—Seroma or hygroma

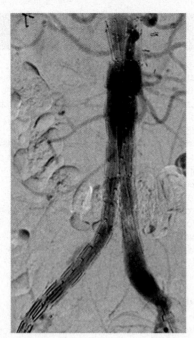

FIGURE 3 • Completion angiogram following EVAR.

confirm exclusion of the AAA **(Figure 3)**. Once the wires and sheaths are removed, the arteriotomies are closed, flow is confirmed distal to the artery closures, and protamine is administered to reverse the heparin. The groin wounds are closed in multiple layers. The distal extremity pulses are checked before leaving the endovascular suite. The patient's diet is quickly advanced following recovery from anesthesia, with patients typically discharged home on postoperative day 1 or 2.

Surveillance Following EVAR

A common complication following EVAR is development of an endoleak, documented during postoperative surveillance. Current recommendations are for an abdominal and pelvic CT scan with intravenous contrast at 1, 6, and 12 months following EVAR, and then annually thereafter assuming no endoleaks are noted. There are five types of endoleaks **(Table 2)**. Type I and III endoleaks are typically identified on completion angiogram at the time of the initial EVAR and should be immediately repaired, as the aneurysm is still subjected to arterial pressure. Type IV endoleaks typically resolve without intervention and are most often the result of small holes where the stent was sewn onto the graft material. Type V endoleaks result from porosity in the graft material leading to a seroma in the aneurysm sac. These were more common with early endograft materials and are rare when using the endografts currently on the market. Occasionally, an older endograft will need to be "relined" with a second endograft to stop a type V endoleak. Type II endoleaks, while not always visualized on completion angiogram, are often detected on postoperative surveillance CTAs in the delayed phase. Type II endoleaks associated with an increasing aneurysm sac size require intervention, most often with an endovascular approach **(Figure 4)**. Those that are associated with no change in sac size or a decreasing sac size can be followed with imaging.

Surgical Approach to Open Aneurysm Repair

Should the patient not be anatomically eligible for EVAR, open AAA repair is indicated. In this operation,

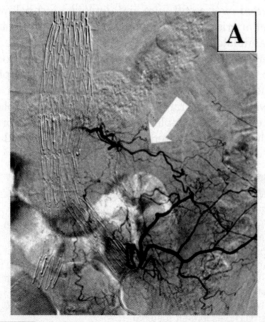
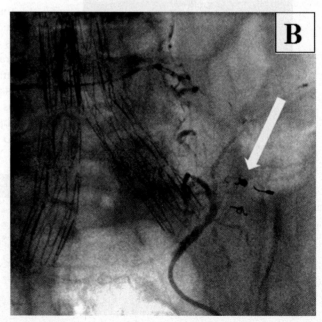

FIGURE 4 • **A:** Selective angiogram demonstrating a lumbar artery causing a type II endoleak (*arrow*). **B:** Angiogram following placement of embolic coils in the offending lumbar artery (*arrow*) demonstrating no flow in the vessel.

the abdomen is widely prepped and draped after marking the distal extremity pulses. Typically, a midline incision is made; however, a transverse or retroperitoneal incision may also be used. A retroperitoneal approach is particularly well suited for a patient with an aneurysm that involves the renal or visceral arteries, or who has a "hostile" abdomen from multiple prior abdominal operations. Multiple randomized trials have not shown a convincing difference in the incidence of postoperative complications between transperitoneal and retroperitoneal approaches.

The small bowel is reflected to the right, the transverse colon superiorly, and a self-retaining retractor is placed. After dissecting the duodenum off the aorta, proximal exposure of the aorta is obtained below the renal arteries, while distal exposure is obtained of the common iliac arteries. The left renal vein may be divided if necessary to provide appropriate exposure to the aorta. Brisk diuresis is established with mannitol and furosemide. Following heparin administration for an Activated Clotting Time (ACT) > 250, the iliac arteries are clamped distally, then the aorta proximally. The aneurysm sac is opened longitudinally opposite the inferior mesenteric artery (IMA) and aortic thrombus removed. All lumbar arteries are oversewn. The IMA may be ligated if there is good back bleeding from it, while a poor back bleeding IMA typically should be reimplanted onto the aortic graft at the end of the case (selective IMA implantation) in order to avoid colonic ischemia. A prosthetic graft is sewn in place proximally first, followed by distally, with monofilament suture. Blood flow is reestablished to the legs in a staged fashion. Once the graft is in place and the patient is hemodynamically stable, heparin is reversed, and the aneurysm sac is closed over the graft. The retroperitoneum is closed to prevent subsequent aortoduodenal fistula. The abdomen is closed in the standard fashion and the distal extremity pulses are checked prior to leaving the operating room **(Table 3)**.

Special Intraoperative Considerations to Open Repair

Several unexpected findings may be encountered at the time of open AAA repair. The discovery of a previously unknown colon cancer or other intra-abdominal malignancy is not uncommon. In this scenario, the most immediately life-threatening condition is treated first. Generally, it is ill advised to perform a contaminated procedure and aortic repair simultaneously given the risk of prosthetic graft infection. Typically, the AAA should be repaired first, followed by recovery and subsequent operation for resection of the malignancy 6 to 12 weeks later, unless a near obstructing colon cancer is discovered. If the malignancy is discovered on preoperative imaging and the patient is a candidate for EVAR, endovascular repair should be undertaken first

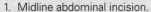

TABLE 3. Steps to an Open AAA Repair

1. Midline abdominal incision.
2. Reflect small bowel to right, transverse colon superiorly, insert self-retaining retractor.
3. Dissect duodenum off of aorta and define proximal clamp site.
4. Dissect distal aorta and proximal iliac arteries taking care to avoid sympathetic nerves.
5. Choose appropriate graft size; administer heparin, lasix, and mannitol.
6. Clamp iliac arteries followed by proximal aorta.
7. Open aneurysm sac opposite IMA, remove thrombus, and oversew back bleeding lumbar arteries.
8. Sew in graft starting proximally, followed by distally, with monofilament suture.
9. Reestablish blood flow through graft, administer protamine, and obtain hemostasis.
10. Close aneurysm sac and retroperitoneum over graft.
11. Close abdomen and check distal pulses.

Potential Pitfalls

- Embolus to lower extremities.
- Significant Aorto-iliac Occlusive Disease (AIOD).
- Aberrant venous anatomy.
- Ischemia-reperfusion injury to lower extremities.

followed by resection of the malignancy. Recovery from EVAR is typically much faster than from open repair and avoids the difficulties encountered from a repeat open abdominal operation.

Embolism to the lower extremities can occur from dislodgement of atheromatous plaque or mural thrombus from the aortic wall upon placement of vascular clamps or from concurrent aortoiliac occlusive disease (AIOD). Distal pulses should always be documented before and after an aortic operation to detect this problem. Placing vascular clamps on the iliac arteries before the proximal aortic clamp may help to decrease the incidence of embolism, although there is no strong evidence to support this. If an embolus causes significant hemodynamic compromise to the leg and foot, indicated by absent pulses and a cool or discolored extremity, embolectomy should be performed before leaving the operating room. If an embolus lodges in a small vessel, such as to a single toe, no further operative intervention is typically performed and antiplatelet therapy is indicated.

Ischemia-reperfusion injury may also occur following open AAA repair, as a result of the ischemic insult to the legs during the operation. Clinically, ischemia-reperfusion injury is typically manifest by hypotension, acute renal failure, and an increasing serum creatinine phosphokinase level. Minimizing ischemic time and restoring blood flow to the lower extremities in a staged fashion can help to reduce the incidence of this injury. Treatment is supportive, with fluids, maintaining adequate urine output, and renal replacement therapy if necessary.

Postoperative Management

Patients are typically cared for in the ICU for at least 1 to 2 days following open AAA repair depending on their clinical status and comorbidities. Patients' volume status and renal function should be closely monitored and managed in the postoperative period. Ischemia of the left colon can occur following AAA repair regardless if the IMA is reimplanted and is more common following ruptured AAA repair. Bloody bowel movements, abdominal pain out of proportion to exam, or unexplained elevated leukocyte count should prompt urgent evaluation of the colon by sigmoidoscopy. Resection is indicated if transmural necrosis of ischemic bowel is found.

Additionally, approximately 20% of patients who undergo open AAA repair will develop a ventral hernia. Patients should be counseled about this complication and examined for development of a hernia at their postoperative visits.

Case Conclusion

The patient undergoes successful EVAR and is discharged from the hospital on postoperative day 2. Surveillance CT scan at 1 month demonstrates a type II endoleak. The endoleak is still present at 6 months and there is now an enlarging aneurysm sac. The patient is returned to the endovascular suite where the offending vessel is successfully embolized via a transfemoral approach with selective coiling of an internal iliac artery branch supplying the aneurysm **(Figure 4)**. Repeat CT 1 month later shows no evidence of an endoleak and a shrinking aneurysm sac.

TAKE HOME POINTS

- Abnormal physical exam findings are only present in 30% to 40% of patients with AAAs.
- An AAA should be repaired when the diameter is larger than 5.5 cm, the aneurysm is rapidly expanding, or if the patient has unexplained or new back or abdominal pain.
- Endovascular repair has become the standard of care for older patients who have suitable arterial anatomy. Open repair is still perhaps more appropriate for younger patients or those that do not have suitable anatomy for EVAR.
- Patients need surveillance CT scans at 1, 6, and 12 months following EVAR and then regularly thereafter to check for endoleaks.
- Incisional hernia, colon ischemia, and aortoenteric fistula are some of the more serious complications that occur after aneurysm repair.

SUGGESTED READINGS

Chaikof EL, Brewster DC, Dalman RL, et al. The care of patients with abdominal aortic aneurysm: the Society for Vascular Surgery practice guidelines. J Vasc Surg. 2009;50(4 suppl):S2–S49.

Eliason JL, Upchurch GR. Endovascular abdominal aortic aneurysm repair. Circulation. 2008;117:1738–1744.

EVAR Trial Participants. Endovascular aneurysm repair versus open repair in patients with abdominal aortic aneurysm (EVAR trial 1): randomized controlled trial. Lancet. 2005;365:2179–2186.

Lederle FA, Freischlag JA, Kyriakides TC, et al. Outcomes following endovascular vs open repair of abdominal aortic aneurysm: a randomized trial. JAMA. 2009;302(14):1535–1542.

76 Ruptured Abdominal Aortic Aneurysm

ADRIANA LASER, GUILLERMO A. ESCOBAR, and GILBERT R. UPCHURCH Jr.

Presentation

A 65-year-old male smoker presents to the emergency room complaining of a sharp, continuous pain in his left back and groin starting earlier in the evening. His vital signs are significant for tachycardia and a decreased mental status. There was no associated trauma. He has a history of coronary artery disease and hyperlipidemia. He is taking aspirin and an HMG CoA reductase inhibitor daily. He smokes approximately one pack per day. On physical examination, the patient is neurologically intact but lethargic. He is in sinus tachycardia by EKG. On abdominal examination, he is obese with guarding, but no rebound tenderness. A pulsatile midabdominal mass is noted, and no hernias are identifiable. He has palpable femoral pulses, but decreased popliteal and dorsalis pedis pulses with livedo reticularis of bilateral lower extremities.

Differential Diagnosis

The incidence of ruptured abdominal aortic aneurysm (rAAA) in the United States is 1-3/100,000. Mortality from rAAA repair remains high despite advances in screening, medical therapy, operative technique, and postoperative management. The mean age for a patient with rAAA is 70.6 years in males and 77.3 years in females.

Presentation and therefore differential diagnosis of an rAAA are varied. If the AAA ruptures intraperitoneally, presentation is usually acute with hemodynamic instability. Cardiovascular collapse often ensues. An AAA can also rupture retroperitoneally, and the patient can present hemodynamically stable. Retroperitoneal rupture is most often posterior and can at least temporarily be contained via clotting, plugging by the aneurysm's mural thrombus being ejected, and tamponade by the retroperitoneal periaortic and perivertebral tissues. One study of 226 patients found that rAAA bleed into the retroperitoneum 85% of the time, the peritoneum 7%, the inferior vena cava (IVC) 6%, and enterically in 2% of cases.

Some studies report that up to three-quarters of patients are asymptomatic before rupture. Presentation, either with or without preceding symptoms, includes 45% of patients with hypotension, 72% with back and abdominal pain, and 83% with a pulsatile abdominal mass. Less than 50% of patients present with the classic triad of hypotension, abdominal pain, *and* pulsatile abdominal mass. Symptoms of rAAA can include those resulting from hematoma on adjacent structures or signs of hypovolemic shock, such as diaphoresis, emesis, syncope, pallor, flank ecchymosis, and vital sign abnormalities. Contained or sealed rupture can even exist chronically before being discovered. Chronic

ruptures can present with chronic lower back pain, lower-extremity neuropathy, or can be asymptomatic. Another complication of chronic rAAAs is IVC fistulae. These can occur in as many as 2% to 6% of patients with rAAA and can present as lower-extremity swelling, congestive heart failure, or a left varicocele. Atypical presentations of rAAA can include pain radiating to the groin, acute femoral neuropathy or thigh ecchymosis from femoral nerve compression, partial upper gastrointestinal (GI) obstruction (third part of duodenum), lower-extremity ischemia from emboli of mural thrombi or aortic thrombosis, visceral thromboembolism, aortic enteric fistula, trauma, and gross hematuria. The differential diagnosis of rAAA can be seen in **Table 1**.

Largely because many AAA patients are asymptomatic, it is believed that one-third to one-half of patients with rAAA die before arriving at the hospital. In hospitals, mortality can reach 40% including patients who die before repair or perioperatively. This brings the overall mortality of patients with rAAA to a reported range of 50% to 94% and essentially 100% for *untreated* true rAAA.

Predisposition to rupture of an existing AAA includes female gender, with a three- to fourfold higher risk when compared with males. Current smoking predisposes to rupture with a 2.7 odds ratio; current smoking is an independent predictor of rupture and greater than formerly smoking. Aortic morphology, such as an eccentric or a saccular shape leading to increased wall stress, less tortuosity, greater cross-sectional diameter asymmetry, and increased aortic compliance also predispose to rupture. Other factors that have been associated with an increased probability of rupturing an existing AAA include **(Table 2)** large size at initial diagnosis, rapidly progressing in

TABLE 1. Differential Diagnosis for rAAA

System	Differential Diagnosis
Gastrointestinal	Initial GI bleed, pancreatitis, cholecystitis, perforated ulcer or viscus, appendicitis, diverticulitis, acute strangulated hernia
Genitourinary	Ureteral obstruction, nephrolithiasis or renal colic, pyelonephritis
Vascular	Aortic rupture or dissection, symptomatic AAA, ruptured visceral or iliac artery aneurysm, myocardial infarction (MI), mesenteric ischemia
Musculoskeletal	Lumbar radiculopathy, vertebral fracture, paravertebral muscle spasm
Other	Lymphoma

size with an expansion rate >1 cm/y, chronic obstructive pulmonary disease (COPD) and a lower forced expiratory volume in one second (FEV_1) (independent risk factor), hypertension (independent risk factor), pain upon manual palpation of aneurysm, a mycotic AAA, family history, and uninsured status. It was also noted that more ruptures occur in winter, likely due to lower atmospheric pressure. Diabetes has been found to be associated with a greater risk of rupture of a small AAA, although it is negatively associated with the development of AAAs.

Once an AAA is diagnosed, size becomes one of the most important determinants for planning surgical repair. The VA Cooperative Natural History of Large Abdominal Aortic Aneurysms Study determined the incidence of rupture in patients with large AAA > 5.5 cm. One-year incidence of rupture by

TABLE 2. Risk Factors for Rupture

Risk Factors for Rupture	
Female Gender	
Smoking	
COPD	Low FEV_1
Hypertension	Uncontrolled
Aortic diameter	
AAA expansion rate	>1 cm/y
Aortic morphology	Saccular
	Less tortuosity
	Greater cross-section diameter asymmetry
Peak wall	Increased stress
	Increased tension
Decreased wall strength	Decreased stiffness, increased thickness
Increase in intraluminal thrombus	Thickness

initial aortic diameter was 9.4% for 5.5 to 5.9 cm, 20% for 6.5 to 6.9 cm, and 29.5% for ≥7.0 cm AAA. The annual rupture risk of observed small aneurysms (4 to 5.5 cm) was 0.6% per Aneurysm Detection and Management (ADAM) screening program and 3.2% per UK Small Aneurysm Trial (UKSAT). Other studies have also reported that one-third to one-half of all AAAs eventually rupture. Although the above factors describe who is at risk of rupturing an AAA, most are too prevalent and nonspecific to be used to identify patients for management or treatment. Risk of aneurysm rupture relates to hemodynamic stresses placed on a degenerative aortic wall and the capacity of the tissue to resist tensile stress. Berguer et al. numerically analyzed wall thickness, herniation of soft plaque through elastic coats of aneurysm, and local stress concentrators due to rigid calcium plaques using finite element analysis to determine that hemodynamic stresses are better than periodic diameter changes at predicting rupture. Although it is more time consuming, volume analysis is more sensitive than change in diameter alone in predicting rupture; however, diameter remains the predominantly used determinant of rupture risk clinically.

On a molecular level, the cause of AAA rupture involves many other complex processes. Choke et al. discovered increased angiogenesis at the rupture site and HIF-1-alpha up regulation with relative hypoxia at the aneurysm rupture edge. Other changes seen within the ruptured aortic wall are decreased elastin, changes in the extracellular matrix, such as increased collagen turnover, and an imbalance of matrix metalloproteinases and their inhibitors. Thrombosis-associated enzymes (tissue plasminogen activator), lipids (lysophosphatidic acid), and inflammatory mediators (c-reactive protein) may also be associated with AAA expansion and rupture.

Workup

If available, an unstable patient without a diagnosis can undergo ultrasound examination in the emergency room, especially when there is unclear etiology of hemodynamic instability. Contrast-enhanced computed tomography angiography (CTA) should be performed in all stable patients where rAAA is suspected to confirm the presence of an AAA and determine operative planning and suitability for endovascular aneurysm repair (EVAR). This will also make available evaluation of the iliac arteries and any venous anomalies, should open repair be undertaken. If ultrasound or CTA is unavailable, and the unstable patient has a history of an AAA or a current pulsatile abdominal mass, he should be taken to the endovascular hybrid suite directly for immediate endovascular or surgical repair based on angiography, recognizing that aortography often underestimates the true size of an AAA because laminated clot obscures the outer limit

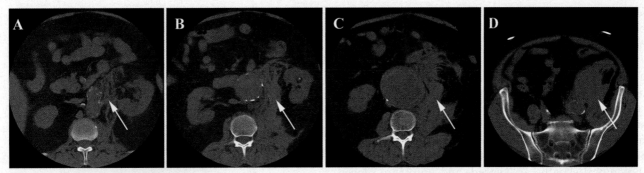

FIGURE 1 • Axial noncontrast CT image of a 60-year-old male with an rAAA preoperatively. **A:** Aneurysm is shown with left renal artery (*arrow*) and stranding. **B:** Further high attenuation stranding and retroperitoneal blood. **C:** Retroperitoneal blood contained. **D:** Extravasation of blood from the aorta.

of the wall. If the receiving facility is unable to perform surgical repair, then immediate transfer should be undertaken.

The patient was deemed stable for transport to CT. **Figure 1** shows an rAAA with an indistinct border on the left side and a likely site of rupture. There is left perinephric region stranding and a collection of increased attenuation in the retroperitoneum. The patient is believed to have suitable anatomy for EVAR.

Diagnosis and Treatment

Arrival to the endovascular suite or operating room should occur immediately because it is better to resuscitate there than in the emergency room. Fluids should be minimized, allowing for permissive hypotension, as blood pressure needs only to maintain cerebral and end-organ perfusion. Resuscitation beyond this can increase bleeding, and crystalloid dilutes the coagulation factors. Patient should have blood products type and crossed, labs drawn for a CBC and creatinine, placement of two large-bore peripheral intravenous catheters and an arterial blood pressure monitoring line, bladder catheter placement, and antibiotics given. A dedicated vascular operating room (OR) team should be involved from beginning to end of the case. The patient should be prepped and draped from chest to toes, and the surgical team should be ready to make an incision before anesthesia is induced since sudden hypotension can occur due to reversal of the tamponade, vasodilatation from the anesthetic agents, abdominal wall muscle relaxation, and decompression by the incision. Traditionally, open rAAA repair has been the only option with its attendant high mortality (44%) and morbidity (56%). EVAR is now becoming the preferred option for repair of rAAA at facilities where it is available on an emergency basis. Although only 8.8% of rAAA were repaired endovascular in 2003 (vs. 43% for unruptured AAA), a recent meta-analysis illustrated that 34% to 100% of patients presenting with rAAA met criteria for EVAR via CT. A 2010 study found

that implementing an algorithm favoring endovascular repair over open repair for rAAA significantly improved mortality. A significant mortality advantage, a reduction by 25%, was also found in another study of EVAR-suitable patients undergoing EVAR as compared with open repair, though follow-up was a short 6 months.

Surgical Approach

For open repair, a transperitoneal approach via midline incision is most commonly undertaken. The primary goal is to first control the inflow and limit hemorrhage, so rapid supraceliac aortic control can be undertaken by manual (or sponge-stick) aortic compression at the level of the diaphragm. This is complemented by dividing the gastrohepatic ligament and the left crus of the diaphragm and then bluntly dissecting through the crus and around the aorta to place a clamp. Then, the third and fourth portions of the duodenum are rotated to the right to expose the perirenal aorta for assessment of infrarenal clamping. Heparin is often omitted if the patient is actively bleeding, but lasix and mannitol are given. Distal control of the aorta is obtained by dissecting the iliac arteries free and clamping them. Then, the aneurysm can then be opened and any lumbar and inferior mesenteric arteries that are bleeding into the sac are ligated. If at all possible, a tube graft is selected to serve as the repair conduit as this configuration requires the least length of anastomosis (when compared to a bifurcated graft). The graft is anastomosed proximally with 3-0 monofilament suture. After checking this anastomosis, the distal anastomosis is created in an end-to-end configuration as well. Iliac clamps should be removed after informing the anesthesiologists and done one at a time to decrease hypotension from sudden perfusion to the lower extremities. The aneurysm sac is closed over the graft to decrease the risk of graft-enteric fistulae later on. Typically, the retroperitoneal hematoma is not decompressed. Distal pulses are checked before abdominal closure. There should be a low threshold for considering the patient at risk for abdominal compartment syndrome (ACS) and the abdomen may need to be left open.

EVAR can be performed under local, regional, or general anesthesia, depending on patient comfort, hemodynamic status, respiratory status, and level of consciousness. The patient should be placed supine on angio table, preferably in a hybrid OR. Prep should be from chest to toes. Bilateral femoral artery cut-downs are done before giving systemic heparin. Bilateral iliofemoral sheaths are placed, and wires are placed into the thoracic aorta along with a marking catheter. An angiogram of the aorta is performed using either iodinated contrast dye or carbon dioxide (to minimize injury to the kidneys) in order to identify the anatomy and location of the renal arteries. At this time, a decision is made regarding whether to use an aortouni-iliac (tube) or a modular, bifurcated endograft. Once this is done, the endograft body is inserted over a stiff guidewire and deployed below the renal arteries. Assuming a bifurcated graft is chosen, the contralateral gate is opened, cannulated, and a contralateral limb is docked into the endograft and deployed. Balloon angioplasty is performed at the proximal and distal fixation sites, as well as in the gate area. Completion angiogram is performed to confirm there are no leaks and ensure exclusion of the ruptured aneurysm. All wires and sheaths are removed and the femoral arteriotomies are closed. Flow is confirmed distal to the arteriotomy closures by handheld Doppler. Protamine is given to reverse the heparin if heparin was used. Groin incisions are closed in multiple layers, and lastly pulses are checked prior to leaving the endovascular suite. These steps are highlighted in **Table 3**. Conversion

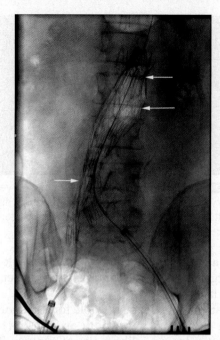

FIGURE 2 • Intraoperative angiography with CO_2 at completion of endograft placement for rAAA. Endograft successfully excluding aneurysm with no leaks (*arrow*).

to open repair may be necessary due to continuing blood loss, difficult access, graft migration, and other anatomic challenges.

The patient in this scenario underwent endovascular repair under general anesthesia. The postprocedure angiogram was undertaken with CO_2 angiography and no leaks were detected **(Figure 2)**. He was then transported to ICU in stable condition for recovery.

Special Intraoperative Considerations

If the patient is bleeding and hypotensive, rather than depend on open control of the aorta, an endovascularly placed aortic occlusion balloon catheter (inserted either transfemoral or transbrachial) can be utilized as an alternative for rapid proximal aortic control. It can also be used to minimize the acute drop in blood pressure during general anesthesia. Some institutions find that balloon occlusion is necessary in up to one-third of rAAAs treated. Care must be taken to minimize renal, mesenteric, and spinal ischemic time during all occlusions of the proximal aorta. Other scenarios that may be encountered intraoperatively are an infection that preceded the rupture, an aortoenteric fistula, or an aortic-IVC fistula. These are rare occurrences and in the acute setting may be treated as other rAAA, although higher morbidity and mortality are expected.

Endoleaks occur after elective and ruptured AAA repairs, and are the primary indication for

---

TABLE 3. Key Technical Steps and Potential Pitfalls for EVAR for rAAAA

Key Technical Steps

1. Expose bilateral common femoral arteries (or insert percutaneous closure devices).
2. Introduce wires and sheaths.
3. Perform aortogram.
4. Systemic heparin.
5. Main body of endograft inserted and deployed just below renal arteries.
6. Contralateral limb inserted and deployed.
7. Balloon angioplasty.
8. Completion angiogram.
9. Protamine.
10. Close arteriotomies, check pulses, and close wounds.

Potential Pitfalls

- Endoleak (Type I or III).
- Embolism.
- Dissection or rupture of iliac, femoral arteries.

reintervention. Type I, II, or III is seen in up to one-half of patients by 1 year after AAA repair. Endoleaks appear to be more common following rAAA repair; therefore, long-term follow up is mandatory.

Postoperative Management

Morbidity after rAAA repair has been documented at 61%, including respiratory failure, tracheostomy, renal failure, sepsis, MI, congestive heart failure, and bleeding. Less commonly seen postoperative complications are stroke, ischemic colitis, lower-extremity ischemia, and paraplegia. Late vascular complications are also higher after rAAA, 17% as compared with 8% after elective AAA repair. As well there is a high rate (20%) of secondary operations: 50% get laparotomy and 50% undergo other procedure. Complications, notably the prevalent respiratory and renal failure, are seen more frequently in open as compared with endovascular rAAA repair.

One of the most serious complications patients have for an increased risk of developing following rAAA repair, as compared with elective AAA repair, is sigmoid colon ischemia (presumable from ligation or covering of the inferior mesenteric artery during the repair). Ischemic colitis may present as hypotension, thrombocytopenia, bloody diarrhea, or metabolic acidosis. Sigmoidoscopy is performed at the bedside to evaluate for transmural ischemia. Mild cases may be treated with antibiotics and supportive care alone; however, severe cases may require resection. Bowel ischemia is described as occurring in 42% of patients after open rAAA repair and 22% after endovascular rAAA repair.

Another complication, abdominal compartment syndrome (ACS), can result if the abdomen is closed under excessive tension, or due to massive resuscitation attempts in the setting of EVAR or open repair for rAAA. ACS is defined as bladder pressure >25 when bladder volume is 50 to 100 mL. ACS may occur in the setting of an rAAA as a result of an expanding retroperitoneal hematoma, but it is not clearly defined if risk is greater from endovascular or open repair. Presumably, the risk of ACS after rAAA would be higher following EVAR as compared with open repair due to unligated aortic branch vessels causing an enlarging hematoma. However, a recent study found that rAAA treated with open repair had significantly higher postoperative intra-abdominal pressures than those undergoing EVAR. The state of shock associated with AAA-free rupture and the insult of an open repair also contribute to tissue edema via microvascular permeability alterations. Since increased abdominal pressure leads to bowel ischemia and respiratory, cardiac, and renal dysfunction, immediate intervention is required. This consists of intra-abdominal pressure monitoring, early recognition, and abdominal decompression, at the bedside, if the patient is unstable. In a recent study of rAAA, factors associated with increased risk of developing ACS included need for occlusion balloon, greater transfusion requirement, higher partial activated thromboplastin time, and higher use of aortouni-iliac grafts. These patients, and those with a massive bowel edema or a large retroperitoneal hematoma, should be considered intraoperatively for temporary abdominal closure with vacuum-assisted closure or mesh if undergoing open repair.

Mortality rates after rAAA open repair have been shown to be 35% to 65% (95% if present in extremis) and are not decreasing like the mortality rates of unruptured AAA. In contrast, elective AAA repair mortality is 2% to 5%. Consecutive patient series have found rAAA mortality to be associated with age >80 years, history of hypertension, angina, or MI, APACHE II score, low hematocrit, preoperative cardiac arrest or loss of consciousness, pre- or intraoperative hypotension, estimated blood loss ≥ 6 L or resuscitation with ≥ 12 L, and postoperative renal or respiratory failure. Traditionally, the majority of postoperative mortality is attributed to other cardiovascular diseases, such as coronary artery disease.

However, EVAR has become the new gold standard for rAAA. Veith et al. took patients with rAAA and, utilizing hypotensive hemostasis, performed arteriography. EVAR was undertaken if anatomy was deemed suitable. Supraceliac balloon occlusion was used if circulatory collapse ensued (10 of 29 patients required it). Operative mortality was only 13%. More recently, mortality was shown to be 33% for rAAA patients undergoing EVAR versus 41% for open repair. The advantage for rEVAR remained significant for patients >70 years old (36% vs. 47%, $p < 0.001$). Elevated operative risk for patients undergoing open repair of rAAA as compared with rEVAR has been attributed to aspects of the procedure. Both general anesthesia induction and sudden decompression of the aorta may lead to hypotension. Increased hypothermia and blood loss leading to coagulopathy are also often involved. Cost analysis for rAAA repair has been estimated at double that of elective repair, but more information is still needed contrasting open and endovascular repairs of rAAA.

Case Conclusion

The patient recovered uneventfully from his surgery except for mild renal dysfunction. He developed azotemia but did not require dialysis. He underwent CT imaging on postoperative day 2, which showed no endoleaks **(Figure 3)**. He had no neurologic sequelae, was eating a regular diet, had no signs of infection, and had adequate blood pressure control. He was able to be discharged home on postoperative day 5 with smoking cessation information and a follow-up visit in 1 month with CT.

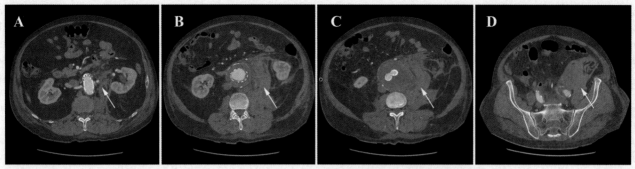

FIGURE 3 • Axial CT image with contrast enhancement of a 60-year-old male with an rAAA post-EVAR. **A:** Aneurysm is shown with endograft in place, stranding (*arrow*). **B:** Aneurysm sac around endograft with residual blood in the retroperitoneum (*arrow*). **C:** Retroperitoneal blood (*arrow*) with possible site of rupture. **D:** Residual blood in the pelvis (*arrow*).

TAKE HOME POINTS

- Rupture increases with age, female gender, and increased aortic diameter.
- Presentation is varied. However, patients uncommonly present with the classic triad of hypotension, abdominal pain, and pulsatile abdominal mass.
- CT imaging for stable patients, ultrasound or OR for unstable patients
- ACS and bowel ischemia are severe complications following rAAA repair.
- Endovascular repair shows morbidity and mortality advantage over open repair for rAAA.

SUGGESTED READINGS

Berceli SA. Ruptured Infrarenal Abdominal Aortic Aneurysm. Clinical Scenarios in Vascular Surgery. In: Upchurch GR, Henke PK, eds. Philadelphia, PA: Lippincott Williams & Wilkins, 2005.

Berguer R, Bull JL, Khanafer K. Refinements in mathematical models to predict aneurysm growth and rupture. Ann N Y Acad Sci. 2006;1085:110–116.

Bosch JAT, Teijink JAW, Willigendael EM, et al. Endovascular aneurysm repair is superior to open surgery for ruptured abdominal aortic aneurysms in EVAR-suitable patients. J Vasc Surg. 2010;52(1):13–18.

Boxer LK, Dimick JB, Wainess RM, et al. Payer status is related to differences in access and outcomes of abdominal aortic aneurysm repair in the United States. Surgery. 2003;134:142–145.

Brewster DC, Cronenwett JL, Hallett JW, et al. Guidelines for the treatment of abdominal aortic aneurysms. Report of a subcommittee of the Joint Council of the American Association for Vascular Surgery and Society for Vascular Surgery. J Vasc Surg. 2003;37:1106–1117.

Brown MJ, McCarthy MJ, Bell PR, et al. Low atmospheric pressure is associated with rupture of abdominal aortic aneurysms. Eur J Vasc Endovasc Surg. 2003;25(1):68–71.

Champagne BJ, Darling RC, Daneshmand M, et al. Outcome of aggressive surveillance colonoscopy in ruptured abdominal aortic aneurysm. J Vasc Surg. 2004;39(4):792–796.

Champagne BJ, Lee EC, Valerian B, et al. Incidence of colonic ischemia after repair of ruptured abdominal aortic aneurysm with endograft. J Am Coll Surg. 2007;204(4):597–602.

Cho JS, Gloviczki P, Martelli E, et al. Long-term survival and late complications after repair of ruptured abdominal aortic aneurysms. J Vasc Surg. 1998;27(5):813–819.

Choke E, Cockerill GW, Dawson J, et al. Hypoxia at the site of abdominal aortic aneurysm rupture is not associated with increased lactate. Ann N Y Acad Sci. 2006;1085:306–310.

Choke E, Cockerill GW, Dawson J, et al. Increased angiogenesis at the site of abdominal aortic aneurysm rupture. Ann N Y Acad Sci. 2006;1085:315–319.

Cowan JA Jr, Dimick JB, Henke PK, et al. Epidemiology of aortic aneurysm repair in the United States from 1993–2003. Ann N Y Acad Sci. 2006;1085:1–10.

Duong C, Atkinson N. Review of aortoiliac aneurysms with spontaneous large vein fistula. ANZ J Surg. 2001;71:52–55.

Fillinger MF, Marra SP, Raghavan ML, et al. Prediction of rupture risk in abdominal aortic aneurysm during observation: wall stress vs diameter. J Vasc Surg. 2003;37:724–732.

Fillinger MF, Racusin J, Baker RK, et al. Anatomic characteristics of ruptured abdominal aortic aneurysm on conventional CT scans: implications for rupture risk. J Vasc Surg. 2004;39:1243–1252.

Fillinger MF, Raghavan ML, Marra SP, et al. In vivo analysis of mechanical wall stress and abdominal aortic aneurysm rupture risk. J Vasc Surg. 2002;36:589–597.

Giles KA, Hamdan AD, Pomposelli FB, et al. Population-based outcomes following endovascular and open repair of ruptured abdominal aortic aneurysms. J Endovasc Ther. 2009;16(5):554–564.

Harkin DW, Dillon M, Blair PH, et al. Endovascular ruptured abdominal aortic aneurysm repair (EVRAR): a systematic review. Eur J Vasc Endovasc Surg. 2007;34(6):673–681.

Harris LM, Faggioli GL, Fiedler R, et al. Ruptured abdominal aortic aneurysms: factors affecting mortality rates. J Vasc Surg. 1991;14(6):812–818.

Hechelhammer L, Lachat ML, Wildermuth S, et al. Midterm outcome of endovascular repair of ruptured abdominal aortic aneurysms. J Vasc Surg. 2005;41(5):752–757.

Kimball EJ, Adams DM, Kinikini DV, et al. Delayed abdominal closure in the management of ruptured abdominal aortic aneurysm. Vascular. 2009;17(6):309–315.

Lambert ME, Baguley P, Charlesworth D. Ruptured abdominal aortic aneurysms. J Cardiovasc Surg (Torino). 1986;27(3):256–261.

Lederle FA, Johnson GR, Wilson SE, et al. Prevalence and associations of abdominal aortic aneurysm detected through screening. Aneurysm Detection and Management (ADAM) Veterans Affairs Cooperative Study Group. Ann Intern Med. 1997;126(6):441–449.

Lederle FA, Johnson GR, Wilson SE, et al. Rupture rate of large abdominal aortic aneurysms in patients refusing or unfit for elective repair. JAMA. 2002;287:2968–2972.

Markar RR, Badger SA, O'Donnell ME, et al. The effects of abdominal compartment hypertension after open and endovascular repair of a ruptured abdominal aortic aneurysm. J Vasc Surg. 2009;49(4):866–872.

Mehta M, Darling RC, Roddy SP, et al. Factors associated with abdominal compartment syndrome complicating endovascular repair of abdominal aortic aneurysms. J Vasc Surg. 2005;42(6):1047–1051.

Miani S, Mingazzini P, Piglionica R, et al. Influence of the rupture site of abdominal aortic aneurysms with regard to postoperative survival. J Cardiovasc Surg (Torino). 1984;25(5):414–419.

Nicholls SC, Gardner JB, Meissner MH, et al. Rupture in small abdominal aortic aneurysms. J Vasc Surg. 1998; 28(5):884–888.

Noel AA, Gloviczki P, Cherry KJ Jr, et al. Ruptured abdominal aortic aneurysms: the excessive mortality rate of conventional repair. J Vasc Surg. 2001;34(1):41–46.

Riesenman PJ, Farber MA. Endovascular repair of ruptured abdominal aortic aneurysm. In: Upchurch G, Criado E, eds. Aortic Aneurysms, Contemporary Cardiology. New York, NY: Humana Press, 2009.

Starnes BW, Quiroga E, Hutter C, et al. Management of ruptured abdominal aortic aneurysm in the endovascular era. J Vasc Surg. 2010;51:9–18.

The UK Small Aneurysm Trial Participants, Brown LC, Powell JT. Risk factors for aneurysm rupture in patients kept under ultrasound surveillance. Ann Surg. 1999;230:289–296.

Thomas PRS, Stewart RD. Abdominal aortic aneurysm. Br J Surg. 1988;75:733–736.

Veith FJ, Ohki T, Lipsitz EC, et al. Treatment of ruptured abdominal aneurysms with stent grafts: a new gold standard? Semin Vasc Surg. 2003;16:171–175.

Visser JJ, van Sambeek HM, Hamza TH, et al. Ruptured abdominal aortic aneurysms: endovascular repair versus open surgery—systematic review. Radiology. 2007;245(1):122–129.

Wakefield TW, Whitehouse WM Jr, Wu SC, et al. Abdominal aortic aneurysm rupture: statistical analysis of factors affecting outcome of surgical treatment. Surgery. 1982;91:586–596.

Lifestyle-Limiting Claudication

EDOUARD ABOIAN and PHILIP P. GOODNEY

Presentation

A 53-year-old male with a long history of smoking presents to the vascular clinic with complaints of pain in right leg with ambulation. This pain occurs reproducibly at 50 ft and is relieved with rest. His past medical history is significant for hypertension, hypercholesterolemia, and diabetes mellitus. He is a 1 pack per day smoker.

Differential Diagnosis

Lifestyle-limiting claudication is the most common manifestation of peripheral arterial disease (PAD) and most plausible in this individual. *Critical limb ischemia (CLI)* is a more advanced stage of peripheral arterial occlusive disease (PAOD) than intermittent claudication (IC). It is defined as rest pain (pain in the limb while at rest, unlike claudication, which occurs with activity) or tissue loss. *Venous claudication* results from proximal venous occlusion. Patient usually has a history of venous thromboembolism. The pain develops following ambulation as veins become engorged and tense, which causes a bursting sensation or pain that is then relieved with rest or leg elevation. *Diabetic neuropathy* can involve the forefoot and digits and is often described as a burning pain, hyperesthesia, or a "pins and needles" sensation. A careful history should permit differentiation between ischemic rest pain and neuropathy because neuropathic pain is constant and unrelieved by dependency.

Spinal stenosis results from compression of the spinal cord or its nerve roots. Symptoms usually are not consistently associated with activity and not rapidly relieved with rest.

Detailed History and Physical Exam

This patient reports a chronic history of the predictable onset of right calf pain with ambulation, occurring reproducibly at 50 ft, that is improved with rest. He reports progressive worsening of walking distance over last 3 months and is currently unable to complete his activities of daily living because of the pain in his right leg.

He tried to quit smoking several times in his life but has been unsuccessful. He reports no prior interventions or vascular operations on his lower extremities. His diabetes is poorly controlled with an average blood glucose level in the 200 mg/dL range, with a hemoglobin A1C of 9.4. He has not seen a doctor for several months. His blood pressure is reasonably controlled, on an angiotensin converting enzyme (ACE) inhibitor and Beta Blocker. He is not taking aspirin or statin at present.

On physical examination, he is in no acute distress. He has lack of skin hair on his right leg, with slight muscle atrophy. There is no tissue loss or ulceration. His carotid upstrokes are equal bilaterally, and there are no carotid bruits. His heart is regular, and his lungs are clear. There is no pulsatile abdominal mass. There are good femoral pulses bilaterally, but there are no appreciable popliteal or pedal pulses in either extremity.

Based on the history and physical examination, the most likely diagnosis is a lifestyle-limiting claudication.

Discussion

Overall Incidence of Claudication

PAOD currently affects approximately 10 million adults in the United States, and of these, nearly 4 million have IC. This disease process therefore is common among elderly patients, and it is estimated that 13.7% of men aged 70 and older are affected. PAOD is a common manifestation of systemic atherosclerosis, and has similar risk factors to this disease, such as smoking and diabetes.

PAOD as a Marker of Overall Cardiovascular Risk

PAOD is a sensitive marker for overall cardiovascular risk. For example, patients presenting with PAOD are at significantly higher risk for premature cardiovascular events, such as myocardial infarction (MI), stroke, and sudden death. PAOD is also a very specific indicator of systemic atherosclerosis. For example, normal ankle brachial indices (whereas PAOD is defined as an ankle-brachial index [ABI] of <0.9) are almost 100% specific in identifying healthy individuals.

Types of PAOD

Patients with symptomatic PAOD are generally divided into two categories: IC and CLI. It is important to distinguish these two groups of patients because of the dramatically different natural history of each of the two different disease states. In terms of the potential for limb loss, patients with IC demonstrate a benign natural course, with amputation rates of 1% to 7% at 5 years, and a relatively low lifetime risk of clinical deterioration of the limb in 25% of cases. However, studies suggest that 40% to 60% of untreated patients with CLI will progress to amputation within 12 to 24 months. Therefore, the need for intervention in patients with IC is based upon weighing the risks of intervention against the extent of the patient's symptoms. Those patients with "lifestyle-limiting" claudication often proceed with treatment, while those patients with more mild symptoms usually do not undergo invasive management, and are often treated with supervised exercise therapy and smoking cessation.

Presentation

The typical patient with IC presents with lower-extremity symptoms that occur in the muscles of the calf. The symptoms may range from muscle fatigue to aching while walking. The character of pain is usually burning, cramping, or aching, and these symptoms are relieved by rest. As the disease progresses, the distance to onset of claudication shortens, and symptoms become more frequent.

Location of the Disease

The affected muscle group is usually located below the level of hemodynamically significant stenosis or occlusion. Generally, the arterial tree can be divided into three levels: aortoiliac, femoropopliteal, and tibioperoneal. Stenosis or occlusion on one of these levels will typically result in IC. Occlusive lesions of infrarenal aorta or iliac vessels will result in buttock or thigh claudication, whereas superficial femoral artery disease will result in calf claudication. Patient risk factors can also be useful in identifying angiographic patterns of disease. For example, infrarenal and iliac arterial disease is associated more with cigarette smoking, whereas diabetes affects more small vessels at the tibioperoneal level.

Workup: Noninvasive Evaluation

Noninvasive studies are a useful adjunct to the history and physical exam, providing objective evidence of the extent and location of vascular disease with essentially no risk to the patient. The ABI, or ankle-brachial index, is a widely used noninvasive test to assess location and severity of the PAD. It samples blood pressure in lower extremity at different levels (thigh, calf, midfoot, and even the toes) and compares to pressure in upper extremity, often measured at the level of brachial artery. This quantitative data are supplemented with qualitative data of blood pressure wave form morphology, which informs of the level and extent of

disease. Toe pressures are especially helpful in diabetic patients, as the digital arteries may not be as calcified as the tibials and provide a more accurate assessment of the extent of lower-extremity PAD. Serial ABIs are useful in measuring the progression of disease, aiding in the timing of an intervention. This test can also be an effective measure postintervention result.

While the general extent and location of disease can be addressed by ABIs and toe pressures, duplex ultrasound provides the vascular surgeon with the most detailed information available in a noninvasive armamentarium. Interrogation of the arterial system with duplex ultrasound provides information on blood flow velocities in different arterial beds. These data can then be extrapolated to determine the degree and length of stenosis, and algorithms to establish these thresholds have been derived and published widely.

Lastly, transcutaneous partial pressure of oxygen or $TcPO_2$ is another useful adjunct in evaluating lower-extremity ischemia. While each of the tests has its limitations, when used in conjunction with a careful history and physical, it allows for quantitative assessment of the patient's symptoms and risks from their lower-extremity PAOD.

Physical examination reveals that the patient has a palpable right femoral pulse, but an absent popliteal pulse and nonpalpable pedal pulses. Patient's ABI is 0.65 on the right and 0.75 on the left. Duplex arteriography suggests an occlusion in the midportion of the superficial femoral artery.

Based on information provided, the importance of detailed history and physical examination is obvious, as the symptom complex (claudication) should match the anatomic findings (lack of infrainguinal pulses) and noninvasive findings (ABI of 0.65). While this patient in the stem has several risk factors, only a portion of them are modifiable. For example, smoking cessation is a modifiable risk factor. These strategies are discussed in detail in the next section.

Diagnosis and Treatment

Our working diagnosis at this point is a lifestyle-limiting IC. There are several therapeutic interventions for the vascular surgeon to consider.

Risk Factor Modification is the First Step in the Management of Claudication

Several aspects of this patient's care need careful attention in managing his claudication. First, smoking is a modifiable risk factor. Smoking cessation has been shown to reduce the risk of MI and death in patients with PAOD and to delay progression of lower-extremity symptoms. It is also important to emphasize that after lower-extremity revascularization, the incidence of graft failure is threefold higher in smokers than in nonsmokers.

Second, diabetes is widely prevalent in patients with PAOD and it has been estimated that for each percent increase in glycosylated hemoglobin, there is a 28% increase of PAD. While some debate in this regard persists, strict glucose control reduces microvascular complications and improves outcomes with revascularization.

Third, aspirin lowers the risk of MI, stroke, and death in patients with PAOD, and must be initiated in all patients after the diagnosis of PAOD has been established. It also enhances graft patency following peripheral bypass. However, there is no evidence that antiplatelet therapy directly improves symptoms of claudication, although it is widely recommended for primary prevention in patients with PAOD.

Finally, treatment of hyperlipidemia with statins is important to reduce progression of atherosclerosis. Currently, the American College of Cardiology—American Heart Association (ACC/AHA) guidelines recommend an low-density lipoprotein (LDL) cholesterol level of <100 mg/dL (2.59 mmol/L) in patients with PAOD and an even lower level (<70 mg/dL [1.8 mmol/L]) in high-risk patients with more generalized atherosclerosis.

Supervised Exercise Therapy: A Nonpharmacologic Intervention

A supervised walking program is supported by ACC/AHA guidelines and is I A recommendation. Supervised exercise should be made available as part of the initial treatment for all patients with PAD. The most effective programs employ treadmill or track walking that is of sufficient intensity to bring on claudication, followed by rest, over the course of a 30 to 60 minute session. Exercise sessions are typically conducted three times a week for 3 months, and, with persistence have shown consistently effective results. This treatment, along with a summary of medical management treatment options, is outlined in **Figure 1**.

Pharmacologic Management: A Noninvasive Treatment Option

Pentoxifylline was the first FDA-approved medication for the treatment of PAOD. It improved maximal walking distance by 12%. It is believed that pentoxifylline improves oxygen delivery by exerting rheolytic effect on red blood cell wall flexibility and deformability, ultimately reducing blood viscosity. Pentoxifylline is also believed to inhibit platelet aggregation. However, this finding appeared to be more statistically than clinically relevant in patients with claudication. In real-world clinical practice, some patients experience substantial long-term symptom relief with pentoxifylline, but others do not, and it is often difficult to predict patient response without a trial of the drug.

Cilostazol (Pletal) is another FDA-approved medication for treatment of PAOD. Results have shown increased maximal walking distances up to 50%, as well as significant improvements in quality-of-life (QoL) measures. There is also increasing evidence that cilostazol may modulate the synthesis of vascular endothelial growth factor, potentially stimulating angiogenesis in patients with chronic lower-extremity ischemia. However, headache, diarrhea, and

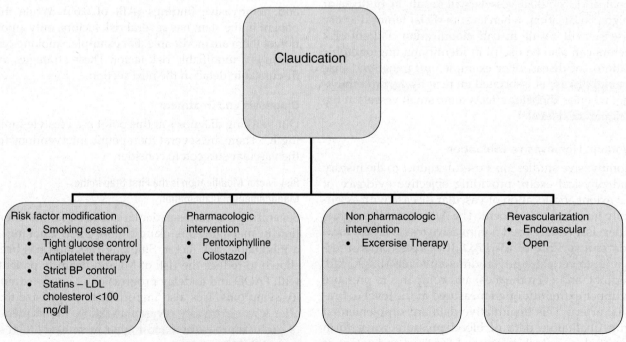

FIGURE 1 • Summary of management of claudication.

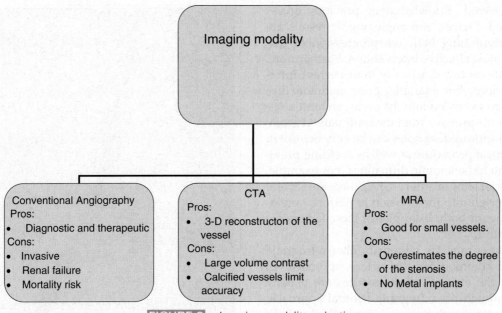

FIGURE 2 • Imaging modality selection.

gastrointestinal discomfort may develop. Cilostazol is contraindicated in patients with NY stage three to four congestive heart failure.

Revascularization Therapy: Open and Endovascular

If this patient's symptoms remain lifestyle limiting, and no improvement was observed with initial risk factor modification strategy, initiation of medical management, and institution of a supervised exercise program, consideration must be given for intervention. Detailed discussion with the patient should precede any intervention and all risks and benefits must be explained. It is important to emphasize the relatively benign nature of IC and a low risk of limb loss.

If the decision to intervene is made, then the next step is to visualize the arterial tree and to localize an arterial lesion with imaging modality. Conventional digital subtraction arteriogram, computed tomographic angiogram (CTA), and magnetic resonance angiogram (MRA) are commonly used modalities. Conventional digital subtraction arteriogram is the most commonly used imaging modality. The advantage of conventional arteriogram is the ability to intervene in the same setting. However, it is invasive and has potential complications, such as bleeding, thrombosis, renal failure, or infection, and even has a measurable mortality risk of 0.16%. CTA and MRA, in contrast, are noninvasive imaging modalities that allow visualization of the arterial tree. However, MRA may overestimate the degree of stenosis and is not suitable for patients with metallic implants and may require sedation in patients with claustrophobia. Further, CTA may not offer adequate precision to delineate patency of the tibial or pedal vessels. Further, CTA requires large-volume intravenous

contrast, which may cause or exacerbate renal failure. Additionally, in severely calcified small vessels, three-dimensional reconstruction may project occluded vessels as patent. Utility of each individual modality is summarized in **Figure 2**.

Right lower-extremity angiography shows a segmental occlusion of the superficial femoral artery, with above-knee popliteal reconstitution, as shown in Figure 3.

Endovascular Intervention: A Step-by-step Navigation

Prior to any endovascular intervention, all prior imaging of the lower-extremity arterial system should be

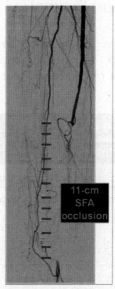

FIGURE 3 • Angiogram of mid-SFA occlusion.

carefully reviewed. Knowledge of previous access sites, deployed devices, and angiographic results are critical in determining both the progression of disease and the most effective intervention. Furthermore, past interventions can drastically limit current interventional options. For example, prior common iliac "kissing" stents extended into the aorta can limit a retrograde femoral approach from the contralateral groin. Review of prior procedure notes can be very helpful in planning a repeat procedure as well as avoiding previously encountered anatomic difficulties. For example, in the superficial femoral artery (SFA), there are several factors that weigh into the decision to perform angioplasty, stenting, or both. Examples of these factors are shown in **Table 1**.

Arterial access must be obtained either retrograde or antegrade common femoral artery approach. In our practice, the majority of procedures are usually performed through the retrograde femoral approach. A small diameter sheath is placed. Typically, 4 to 5 Fr sheath is sufficient for majority of diagnostic procedures and a 6 Fr sheath for most therapeutic procedures. Aortography and bilateral pelvic angiography is performed to ensure proper inflow. Selective arteriogram then is performed to define the arterial lesion and plan the intervention.

After review of the diagnostic imaging, the lesion is determined to be amenable to percutaneous intervention based on trans-atlantic classification (TASC) II classification. In general, class A and B lesions are amenable to percutaneous intervention, while class C and D lesions present more difficult technical challenges. Intervention often consists of angioplasty, and several studies demonstrate improved results when angioplasty is accompanied by stent placement, especially in the superficial femoral artery, as shown in **Figure 4**.

Preoperative Consideration in Open Revascularization

For open lower-extremity bypass, patients with active cardiac conditions should undergo preoperative evaluation. The list of conditions that require cardiac

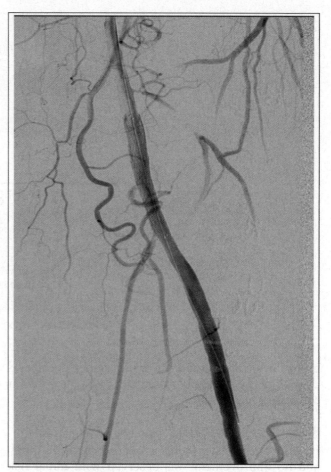

FIGURE 4 • Angiogram of stented SFA.

evaluation can be found in **Table 2**. Venous mapping must also be performed prior to intervention. Vein diameter and length are evaluated with duplex ultrasound, and patency of deep venous system is evaluated to assure adequate venous return following revascularization. Suitable vein for the bypass is ipsilateral greater saphenous vein usually 3 mm or more in diameter. The course of the saphenous vein is marked and length of suitable vein is measured to assure tension-free bypass to desired location. If no suitable veins were found in lower and upper extremities, then consideration must be given to alternative conduit, such as prosthetic material.

Infrainguinal bypass procedures need to arise from a patent and uncompromised inflow artery. If the infrainguinal bypass is constructed following an inflow procedure, anastomosis to a native artery rather than the inflow graft improves patency. Accordingly, the procedure, in a "step-by-step" navigation, is outlined below.

The lower abdomen and the affected extremity are prepped and draped in sterile fashion. Incision is made along the previously marked saphenous vein based on preoperative venous mapping. The vein is dissected and evaluated for quality and length for bypass

TABLE 1. Landing Zones and the Technical Considerations to Aid in Successful SFA Interventions

Lesion Location	Technical Consideration
Flush occlusion of the SFA	Complex recanalization versus surgery
Mid-SFA lesions	Do not take away future fem-above-knee (AK) popliteal options.
Lesions at the adductor canal	Limit stent extension into the popliteal artery.
Popliteal artery	Limit stent placement.

TABLE 2. Clinical Indications for Cardiac Evaluation Prior to Lower-extremity Revascularization

Symptom/Condition	Examples
Unstable coronary artery disease	Unstable angina, chest pain
Decompensated congestive heart failure	
Significant arrhythmia	Atrioventricular block, supraventricular tachycardia, newly recognized ventricular tachycardia
Severe valvular disease	Aortic stenosis with valve area <1.0 cm², symptomatic mitral stenosis

Adapted from Fleisher LA, Beckman JA, Brown KA, et al. ACC/AHA 2007 Guidelines on Perioperative Cardiovascular Evaluation and Care for Noncardiac Surgery: Executive Summary: A Report of the American College of Cardiology/American Heart Association Task Force on Practice Guidelines (Writing Committee to Revise the 2002 Guidelines on Perioperative Cardiovascular Evaluation for Noncardiac Surgery). Circulation. 2007;116(17):1971–1996.

procedure. The saphenofemoral junction is exposed. All venous tributaries are ligated and vein is harvested by transecting vein distally and proximally. The common femoral artery enters the femoral triangle slightly medial to the midpoint of the inguinal ligament. Within the femoral triangle, the common femoral divides into deep and superficial branches. To expose the common femoral artery, a vertical incision is placed in the groin over the pulse and extended one-third above the inguinal ligament and two-thirds below. The femoral artery is identified and exposed by opening the femoral sheath. Care must be taken not to injure femoral vein that lies medial to the artery. The distal target vessel is selected to provide inline flow to the foot. For patients

TABLE 3. Key Technical Steps of Femoral to Popliteal Bypass

1. Exposure of proximal vessel.
2. Mobilization of target vessel.
3. Preparation of conduit (vein harvest, angioscopy, vein preparation).
4. Tunneling.
5. Distal anastomosis.
6. Proximal anastomosis.
7. Completion arteriogram/duplex.

Potential Pitfalls

- Bleeding from the artery.
- Femoral vein injury with massive bleeding.
- Nerve injury.
- Tunneling problems, twisting of the conduit, technical issues at anastomosis.

with claudication, commonly the popliteal artery will be sufficient to provide flow to the foot. As the infrageniculate popliteal artery is less likely to be affected by atherosclerotic process, in our practice it is used more frequently for bypass. The popliteal artery is exposed by placing incision 1 cm behind the posterior border of the tibia. If the saphenous vein has not been harvested at this point in the procedure, care must be taken not to injure it in this location. The crural fascia is incised and the gastrocnemius muscle is retracted posteriorly. The popliteal artery is identified medial to the posterior tibial nerve and the popliteal vein. The popliteal vein must be retracted to gain access to more lateral artery. Bridging veins often times have to be divided to gain access to popliteal artery. It is carefully dissected free over a distance of 4 to 5 cm.

Decisions then need to be made in terms of how to route the conduit from the inflow to outflow artery. Reversed, nonreversed, and in situ vein conduits appear to work equally well, and each strategy has distinct advantages and disadvantages. In our practice, we most commonly perform in situ technique with intraoperative angioscopy and valve lysis.

After preparation of the vein conduit and establishing a tunnel site, the patient is systemically anticoagulated with heparin. Longitudinal arteriotomy is performed on popliteal artery and anastomosis is performed in running fashion with 6-0 prolene suture. After completion of the anastomosis, the suture line is tested for any evidence of leak or stenosis. The proximal anastomosis is then performed in similar fashion **(Figure 5)**. If there is significant calcification at the origin of profunda femoris, an endarterectomy is performed with a patch angioplasty and bypass graft is sutured to the patch. Upon completion of the bypass, duplex ultrasound interrogation or completion arteriogram should be performed to evaluate the technical adequacy of the bypass graft.

Postoperative Management

We routinely prescribe clopidogrel for all endovascular interventions performed below the inguinal ligament. Further, recent evidence suggests that cilastozol is also a helpful adjunct in preventing restenosis. Anticoagulation with coumadin is not routinely used unless the patient took this medication prior to the procedure, or unless the bypass is "compromised" in some way, such as poor conduit or outflow. This is typically restarted on the night of the procedure. Based on findings of better primary and secondary patency with statin agents, we routinely prescribe statin agents for all those undergoing SFA and tibial interventions. Whether there is more benefit in high-dose compared with low-dose statins remains unclear, and therefore in most patients we generally treat with low-dose statins.

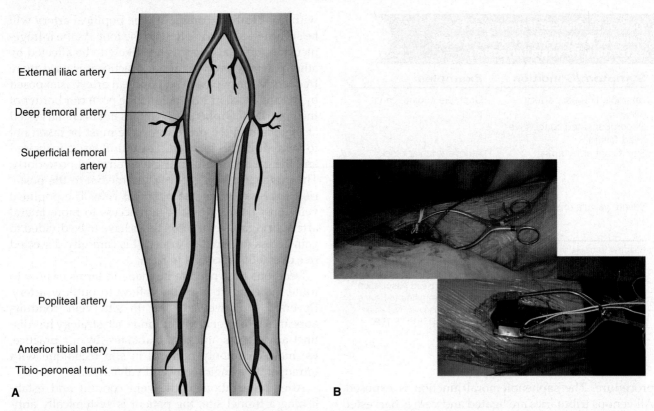

External iliac artery

Deep femoral artery

Superficial femoral artery

Popliteal artery

Anterior tibial artery

Tibio-peroneal trunk

A

B

FIGURE 5 • **A:** Diagram of femoral to below the knee popliteal bypass. **B:** Arterial exposures for femoral to below the knee popliteal bypass.

Surveillance duplex after open bypass is performed based on the type of bypass, prior duplex US findings, and the risk of bypass graft stenosis or thrombosis. Decisions about the timing and frequency of surveillance should be tailored to individual patient characteristics. In our practice, the first duplex surveillance typically is scheduled 3 to 4 weeks following the bypass, and follow-up occurs 6 months to yearly thereafter.

TAKE HOME POINTS

- Life-limiting claudication has low risk of limb loss but is a sensitive marker of overall patient-level cardiovascular risk.
- It is important to distinguish lifestyle-limiting claudication and CLI.
- Risk factor modification and supervised exercise therapy are key elements in the initial treatment of claudication.
- Careful preoperative planning of endovascular interventions and open lower-extremity bypass procedures is vital in achieving good outcomes.

SUGGESTED READINGS

Barnett AH, Bradbury AW, Brittenden J, et al. The role of cilostazol in the treatment of intermittent claudication. Curr Med Res Opin. 2004;20(10):1661–1670.

Criqui MH. Peripheral arterial disease—epidemiological aspects. Vasc Med. 2001;6(3 suppl):3–7.

Effect of intensive diabetes management on macrovascular events and risk factors in the Diabetes Control and Complications Trial. Am J Cardiol. 1995;75(14):894–903.

Fleisher LA, Beckman JA, Brown KA, et al. ACC/AHA 2007 Guidelines on Perioperative Cardiovascular Evaluation and Care for Noncardiac Surgery: Executive Summary: A Report of the American College of Cardiology/American Heart Association Task Force on Practice Guidelines (Writing Committee to Revise the 2002 Guidelines on Perioperative Cardiovascular Evaluation for Noncardiac Surgery): Developed in Collaboration With the American Society of Echocardiography, American Society of Nuclear Cardiology, Heart Rhythm Society, Society of Cardiovascular Anesthesiologists, Society for Cardiovascular Angiography and Interventions, Society for Vascular Medicine and Biology, and Society for Vascular Surgery. Circulation. 2007;116(17): 1971–1996.

Gardner AW, Poehlman ET. Exercise rehabilitation programs for the treatment of claudication pain. A meta-analysis. JAMA. 1995;274(12):975–980.

Hankey GJ, Norman PE, Eikelboom JW. Medical treatment of peripheral arterial disease. JAMA. 2006;295(5):547–553.

Hirsch AT, Hiatt WR. PAD awareness, risk, and treatment: new resources for survival—the USA PARTNERS program. Vasc Med. 2001;6(3 suppl):9–12.

Jonason T, Bergstrom R. Cessation of smoking in patients with intermittent claudication. Effects on the risk of peripheral vascular complications, myocardial infarction and mortality. Acta Med Scand. 1987;221(3):253–260.

Kannel WB, McGee DL. Update on some epidemiologic features of intermittent claudication: the Framingham Study. J Am Geriatr Soc. 1985;33(1):13–18.

Kannel WB, McGee DL. Diabetes and cardiovascular disease. The Framingham study. JAMA. 1979;241(19):2035–2038.

Malmstedt J, Wahlberg E, Jorneskog G, et al. Influence of perioperative blood glucose levels on outcome after infrainguinal bypass surgery in patients with diabetes. Br J Surg. 2006;93(11):1360–1367.

Moneta GL, Yeager RA, Antonovic R, et al. Accuracy of lower extremity arterial duplex mapping. J Vasc Surg. 1992;15(2):275–283; discussion 283–284.

Newman AB, Siscovick DS, Manolio TA, et al. Ankle-arm index as a marker of atherosclerosis in the Cardiovascular Health Study. Cardiovascular Heart Study (CHS) Collaborative Research Group. Circulation. 1993;88(3):837–845.

Norgren L, Hiatt WR, Dormandy JA, et al. Inter-society consensus for the management of peripheral arterial disease. Int Angiol. 2007;26(2):81–157.

Porter JM, Cutler BS, Lee BY, et al. Pentoxifylline efficacy in the treatment of intermittent claudication: multicenter controlled double-blind trial with objective assessment of chronic occlusive arterial disease patients. Am Heart J. 1982;104(1):66–72.

Samlaska CP, Winfield EA. Pentoxifylline. J Am Acad Dermatol. 1994;30(4):603–621.

Schillinger M, Sabeti S, Loewe C, et al. Balloon angioplasty versus implantation of nitinol stents in the superficial femoral artery. N Engl J Med. 2006;354(18):1879–1888.

Selvin E, Erlinger TP. Prevalence of and risk factors for peripheral arterial disease in the United States: results from the National Health and Nutrition Examination Survey, 1999–2000. Circulation. 2004;110(6):738–743.

Stewart KJ, Hiatt WR, Regensteiner JG, et al. Exercise training for claudication. N Engl J Med. 2002;347(24):1941–1951.

Waugh JR, Sacharias N. Arteriographic complications in the DSA era. Radiology. 1992;182(1):243–246.

78 Tissue Loss Due to Arterial Insufficiency

WILLIAM P. ROBINSON III

Presentation

A 74-year-old white male with a history of hypertension, diabetes mellitus (DM), tobacco abuse, coronary artery disease, atrial fibrillation, and end-stage renal disease on hemodialysis presented to the emergency department with a 3-week history of spontaneous ulceration of the left great toe and increasing rest pain in the left foot (**Figure 1**). Vital signs are normal. On physical exam, there was dry gangrene at that base of the left great toe with mild surrounding cellulitis. The patient had dry and hairless skin of the bilateral lower extremities. The patient has dependent rubor and elevation pallor of the left foot. Bilateral femoral and popliteal pulses were palpable. Pedal pulses were not palpable on either foot, but there was an audible Doppler signal at the left dorsalis pedis. The patient had intact strength and sensation of the lower extremities. The patient walks independently and performs his own activities of daily living.

Differential Diagnosis

Tissue loss due to arterial insufficiency most often affects the lower extremity due to the predilection of atherosclerotic occlusive disease to occur in the lower extremity. Trauma secondary to diabetic neuropathy and venous hypertension can also lead to lower-extremity ulceration or coexist with arterial insufficiency. Tissue loss secondary to arterial insufficiency typically occurs on the distal aspect of the extremity such as the digits and is often associated with underlying ischemic rest pain of the affected extremity. Tissue loss represents the most advanced form of ischemic secondary to arterial occlusive disease as perfusion is not adequate to maintain tissue integrity. Ischemic ulcerations usually begin as small, dry ulcers of the toes or heel area and progress to frankly gangrenous changes of the forefoot or heel with greater degrees of arterial insufficiency (**Figure 2**). Such progressive disease, affecting multiple levels of the peripheral vasculature tree, is more frequently encountered in the elderly. Patients with diabetes or renal failure are more susceptible to the development of ischemic pedal ulcers. Disease progression can be very rapid, as up to 50% of patients with critical limb ischemia (CLI) are asymptomatic 6 months before onset of pain or ulceration. The prevalence of peripheral arterial disease (PAD) is between 3% to 10% overall and 15% to 20% in those over age 70. Of those aged >50 with PAD, 1% to 3% will have critical leg ischemia in the form of rest pain or gangrene. The incidence of CLI ranges from 220 to 1,000 new cases per year in a European or an American population of 1 million people. The risk factors for infrainguinal occlusive disease are the same as those for the development of atherosclerosis in general and include age, male gender, hypertension, DM, smoking, dyslipidemia, family history, and homocysteinemia.

Because of the extremely high risk of limb loss, tissue loss from arterial insufficiency must be expeditiously and accurately diagnosed. Although clinical experience indicates that in some patients with CLI small ulcerations may heal with improved cardiac hemodynamics and optimal local wound care, significant tissue necrosis inevitably progresses to limb loss without revascularization. In addition, CLI is associated with an extremely high risk of mortality as it is a marker of advanced comorbidities and cardiovascular disease. Overall, approximately 25% of patients with CLI will die at 1 year, 30% will undergo major amputation, and 45% will be alive with two limbs. The rate of amputation is 10 times higher in diabetics than nondiabetics. The 5-year survival rate for patients with CLI is approximately 50% to 60%.

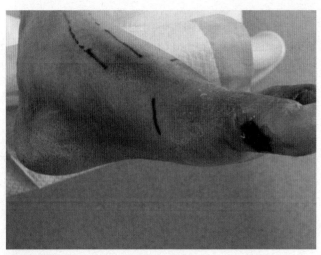

FIGURE 1 • Left foot with dry gangrene of great toe, dependent rubor, and erythema on dorsum of foot.

Workup

A careful physical examination can diagnose the extent of tissue loss and the presence of arterial insufficiency. A lack of a pedal pulse indicates abnormal arterial perfusion and, in the presence of ulceration or gangrene, warrants further investigation. An ankle-brachial index (ABI) is an essential part of the detailed vascular examination. An ABI of <1.0 is considered abnormal and <0.4 is generally considered consistent with the potential for tissue loss. Further workup can be conducted using noninvasive arterial testing, most often in a vascular laboratory. Segmental pressures measured at the level of the upper thigh, lower thigh, calf, ankle, and metatarsal level can diagnose the anatomic level

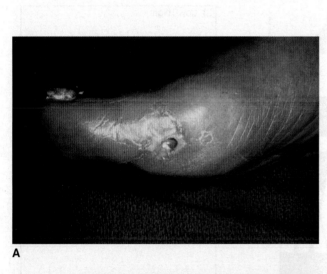

A

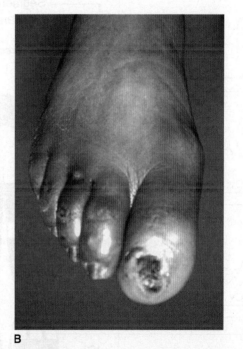

B

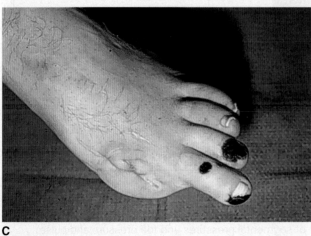

C

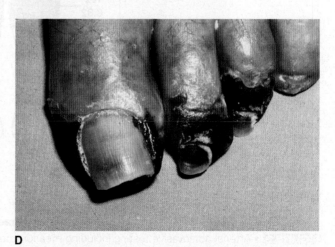

D

FIGURE 2 • Progressive stages of tissue loss from small ischemic ulcerations **(A,B)** to gangrene **(C,D)**.

of occlusive disease. If vessels prove noncompressible with the blood pressure cuffs inflated to pressures of 225 mm Hg, which is secondary to severe calcification of vessels in the setting of diabetes and end-stage renal disease, then the ABI and segmental pressure are not reliable indicators of perfusion. Pulse volume recordings, which measure the volume blood delivered to each segment of the lower extremity, are then utilized to assess perfusion. In addition, toe blood pressures remain a reliable indicator of distal perfusion. A toe-brachial index <0.3 or absolute toe pressure of <30 mm Hg is indicative of severe ischemia and strongly predictive of inability to heal a lower-extremity wound.

Presentation Continued

The patient was started on broad-spectrum intravenous antibiotics. Ankle-brachial indices and segmental pressures were not diagnostic due to noncompressible vessels. Pulse volume recordings were consistent with severe ischemia and indicative of disease at the tibial and pedal levels **(Figure 3)**. The patient had an absolute toe pressure of 0 mm Hg.

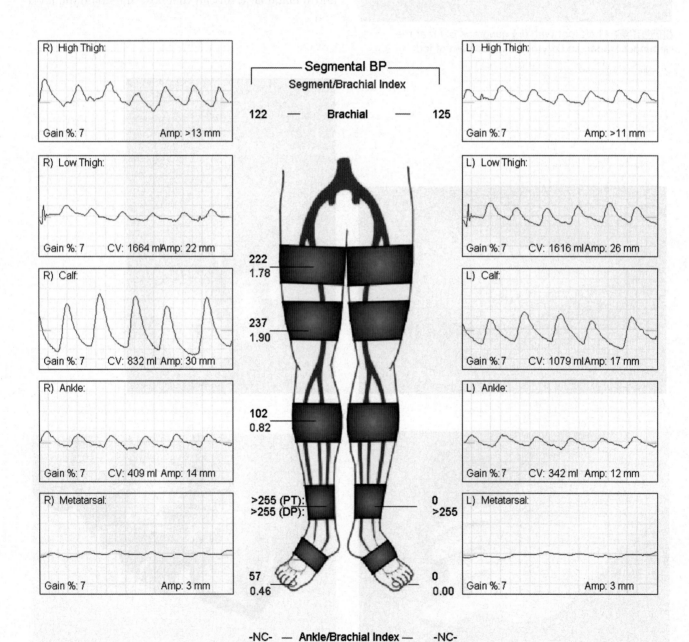

FIGURE 3 • Arterial noninvasive testing including measurement of segmental pressures and toe pressure and pulse volume recordings.

Diagnosis and Treatment

The diagnosis of tissue loss secondary to arterial insufficiency is based upon history, physical examination, and noninvasive arterial testing. The goal of arterial imaging is to plan revascularization and is only indicated if physiologic testing has indicated significant ischemia and the decision has been made to pursue revascularization. Imaging options include digital subtraction angiography, magnetic resonance angiography (MRA) and computed tomographic angiography (CTA). Although MRA and CTA are noninvasive, they are subject to artifact and may not provide the anatomic detail necessary to adequately plan infrainguinal bypass. Digital subtraction angiography provides optimal vessel detail and remains the gold standard. In addition, percutaneous endovascular therapy can often be performed at the time of diagnostic angiography if the patient and anatomy is deemed suitable.

Revascularization options for lower-extremity occlusive disease include percutaneous endovascular therapy, open surgical therapy, and combinations of the two modalities. The optimal treatment is dependent primarily upon the extent and location of occlusive disease and on the patient's operative risk. The goal of either mode of therapy is to establish inline flow to the affected extremity. Percutaneous endoluminal therapy is best utilized for those with less extensive lesions and high surgical risk. The technical success and the durability of endovascular therapy are best for iliac and superficial femoral artery lesions. Extensive popliteal and tibial disease can be treated via endovascular means, but their durability is quite limited. In addition, long segment stenoses and occlusions are less favorable for endovascular therapy than more limited lesions. Endovascular therapy avoids some of the morbidity and mortality associated open surgery, as general anesthesia is not required, and blood loss and wound issues are largely avoided.

Extensive occlusive disease at multiple levels of the circulation is generally required to develop tissue loss secondary to arterial insufficiency. Therefore, open surgical therapy in the form of endarterectomy and surgical bypass is often required. In particular, extensive tissue loss of the foot often requires the restoration of a palpable pulse in the foot for healing and limb salvage. Surgical revascularization provides durable results. For example, the 5-year results of infrainguinal saphenous vein graft using modern techniques have been excellent, with primary and secondary patency rates of up to 75% and 80%, respectively, and limb salvage rates as high as 90%.

Surgical Approach

Percutaneous Endovascular Therapy

Endovascular treatment of iliac disease is generally performed through ipsilateral retrograde femoral access. Infrainguinal lesions are generally treated via a sheath placed "up and over" the aortic bifurcation from the contralateral femoral artery. In general, the principle of endovascular therapy is to cross the diseased segment with a wire and then successively dilate the stenosis or the occlusion with balloon catheters and/or stents over the wire. Keys to success include stable placement of a sheath, which allows controlled wire and catheter manipulation in traversing lesions and accommodates the passage of balloon catheters and stents of adequate caliber for restoring flow. Potential pitfalls of endovascular therapy include atherothromboembolism to distal arteries, access site hematoma and pseudoaneurysm, and contrast-induced nephropathy.

Infrainguinal Bypass

The principle of successful bypass is to perform the shortest bypass possible to re-establish inline flow to the foot. The three principles of "inflow," "outflow," and "conduit" are repeatedly emphasized by vascular surgeons. First, flow must be unobstructed to the level of the proximal anastomosis. Second, a site distal to significant disease must be chosen for the distal anastomosis. In general, the target vessel should be the least diseased artery that is the dominant supply to the foot. Finally, the conduit for the bypass must be adequate to support pulsatile flow. For bypass to below the level of the knee, autogenous conduit, preferably ipsilateral greater saphenous vein, provides maximal durability. Prosthetic conduit is preferred for aortoiliac reconstruction and acceptable for femoral to above-knee popliteal bypass when autogenous conduit is not available.

Infrainguinal surgical bypass can be performed under general, spinal, or occasionally regional anesthesia. It is our practice to work from proximal to distal, first exploring the inflow artery and exposing the venous conduit. We then explore the site proposed for the distal anastomosis, as high-quality preoperative imaging has already defined a suitable target vessel. Having determined the suitable donor and target arteries, vein of sufficient length is then harvested and prepared for use by gentle distension and testing for leaks with heparinized saline solution. The proximal anastomosis is performed prior to the distal anastomosis. This allows confirmation of adequate inflow before the bypass is performed and allows the graft to be tunneled and tailored to appropriate length under arterial pressure. Prior to vessel occlusion for the proximal anastomosis, the patient is systemically anticoagulated with 5,000 to 7,000 units of intravenous heparin and additional heparin is given as necessary. Blunt tunneling with placement of umbilical tapes through the tunnels is completed before heparin is administered to prevent bleeding. Atraumatic vascular clamps are placed proximally and distally and the donor artery is incised. The vein is then spatulated and a beveled proximal anastomosis carried out. Typically, a 5-0 polypropylene is used for the femoral anastomosis and a 6-0 used at the popliteal level. If a nonreversed orientation is used, the vein valves are then lysed with a valvulotome under arterial pressure. The vein is carefully brought through the tunnel under pressure and pulsatile flow confirmed with brief release of the clamp. The graft is then tailored to appropriate length and the distal anastomosis is then completed after occluding the target vessel. 7-0 prolene suture is generally used at the tibial or pedal level. If extensive calcification of the vessel risks significant injury from clamping, bleeding can be controlled by occlusion balloons placed intraluminally. A pneumatic tourniquet is particularly advantageous for arterial control when sewing to diminutive distal tibial or pedal targets, where crush injury or plaque dislodgment could cause graft failure. Flow through the graft and the outflow arteries is assessed following completion of the bypass with a continuous-wave Doppler and pulse examination. An angiogram is performed by directly cannulating the proximal graft. This allows for immediate repair of any technical defects that are identified. Intraoperative completion duplex ultrasonography is an additional sensitive screen for hemodynamically significant abnormalities within the graft.

Pitfalls of infrainguinal bypass that lead to early graft failure include attempted anastomosis to highly calcified vessels inappropriate for anastomosis and use of inadequate conduit. Technical defects not corrected at time of operation are sure to precipitate early graft failure. In addition, adequate hemostasis and meticulous attention to wound closure are necessary to prevent hematoma and wound dehiscence, which incur significant morbidity and can precipitate graft failure. Key steps of infrainguinal bypass with ipsilateral saphenous vein are outlined in **Table 1**.

Special Intraoperative Considerations

Adequate preoperative planning based on high-quality angiography generally avoids unanticipated intraoperative findings. Occasionally, the necessity of improving the inflow to support an infrainguinal graft is determined intraoperatively, either by direct visual assessment of inflow at the desired donor site or by comparison of a transduced pressure tracing from the donor site with that of a systemic pressure tracing. Aortoiliac angioplasty and stenting is increasingly becoming the preliminary procedure performed to attain sufficient inflow prior to construction of a more distal bypass graft. At times, saphenous vein will be found to be inadequate on exploration despite appearing adequate on preoperative mapping. Alternative autogenous conduit, such as contralateral saphenous vein and arm vein, must then be available and utilized for bypass below the level of the knee.

Postoperative Management

The most common major complications of infrainguinal bypass surgery are cardiac in nature. These are best

TABLE 1. Key Technical Steps and Potential Pitfalls of Infrainguinal Bypass Graft with Nonreversed Saphenous Vein

Key Technical Steps

1. Expose inflow artery for proximal anastomosis and evaluate suitability for proximal anastomosis.
2. Expose target artery for distal anastomosis and evaluate suitability for distal anastomosis.
3. Expose saphenous vein of adequate length through skip incisions. Ligate side braches with fine silk and divide. Ligate and divide vein distally and at saphenofemoral junction.
4. Prepare vein for bypass with gentle distension of heparinized saline and repair any leaks. Excise proximal valves under direct vision.
5. Create bypass graft tunnel between donor and target arteries with blunt clamp or tunneler. Place umbilical tape through tunnel.
6. Systemically heparinize.
7. Perform proximal anastomosis
   - Clamp donor artery distally and then proximally.
   - Make arteriotomy.
   - Fashion proximal vein to match arteriotomy.
   - Perform anastomosis with running polypropylene suture.
8. Lyse valves in vein under arterial distension with valvulotome. Confirm pulsatile flow.
9. Bring graft through tunnel under arterial pressure. Confirm pulsatile flow.
10. Perform distal anastomosis
    - Occlude target artery (clamps or pneumatic tourniquet).
    - Make arteriotomy.
    - Trim vein under distension and fashion to match arteriotomy.
    - Perform anastomosis with running polypropylene suture.
11. Confirm flow though graft and outflow arteries with pulse exam and continuous-wave Doppler.
12. Perform completion angiography and/or duplex ultrasonography.

Potential Pitfalls
- Poor preoperative planning: donor and target arteries unsuitable for anastomosis.
- Use of conduit of inadequate quality or caliber.
- Poor hemostasis and wound closure.

prevented with perioperative optimization including use of beta blockade, statin therapy, and careful attention to volume status. Wound infection and dehiscence and skin flap necrosis can best be avoided by gentle tissue handling and careful avoidance of skin flaps during vein harvesting. Leg elevation in the early postoperative period minimizes leg swelling and healing complications. Aggressive mobilization and rehabilitation maximizes return to function. All patients are maintained indefinitely on aspirin or clopidogrel following surgical bypass. When a graft is at increased risk of failure, as in cases in which there is compromised outflow or only marginal conduit available, the anti-platelet agent may be supplemented with heparin and then warfarin. Serial duplex ultrasound scanning is necessary to identify hemodynamically significant stenoses within the vein graft that threaten graft patency. Duplex ultrasonography is generally done at 1, 6, and 12 months with yearly scans thereafter.

Debridement is avoided or deferred until after revascularization is complete unless infection necessitates it.

Small, uninfected ulcerations of the toe or foot often can be safely managed conservatively. However, larger, gangrenous lesions of the toe, forefoot, or heel usually require debridement of all necrotic tissue after revascularization. If the ischemia is particularly severe or infection is present, a toe or transmetatarsal amputation may be necessary in order to achieve a margin of healthy tissue. Pressure offloading is often necessary to facilitate healing.

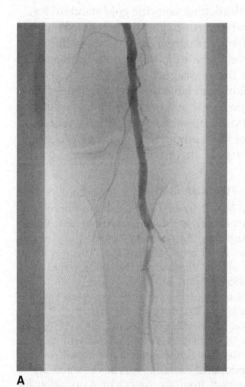
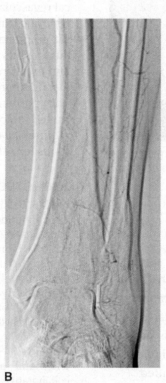
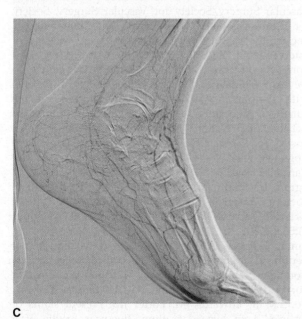

FIGURE 4 • Lower-extremity angiogram showing preservation of below-knee popliteal artery with posterior tibial and anterior tibial artery occlusion and single vessel runoff via the peroneal artery **(A)**, occlusion of the peroneal artery in the distal calf **(B,C)**, and reconstitution of the dorsalis pedis artery in the foot **(C)**.

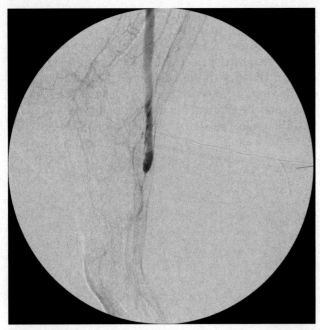

FIGURE 5 • Intraoperative completion angiogram demonstrating excellent result of below-knee popliteal to dorsalis pedis vein bypass graft.

Case Conclusion

The patient underwent left lower-extremity angiography via a right common femoral approach. There were no significant stenoses in the iliac, femoral, and popliteal vessels. There was severe tibial disease with single vessel run-off via a peroneal artery that was occluded in the distal leg **(Figures 4A,B)**. A dorsalis pedis artery was reconstituted in the foot with patent vessels in the pedal arch **(Figure 4C)**. He underwent below-knee popliteal to dorsalis pedis bypass with ipsilateral reversed greater saphenous vein. Intraoperative angiogram revealed no technical defects **(Figure 5)**. Bypass resulted in a palpable pulse in the dorsalis pedis artery distal to the graft and greatly improved perfusion of the foot. He was discharged on postoperative day 3 on ASA. The wound healed with gentle serial debridements done as an outpatient.

TAKE HOME POINTS

- The diagnosis of tissue loss due to arterial insufficiency is made based on patient symptomatology, physical examination, and noninvasive tests, such as segmental pressure measurements and pulse volume recordings.
- Patients with tissue loss secondary to arterial insufficiency are at high risk for limb loss and death.
- Tissue loss secondary to arterial insufficiency represents the most advanced form of CLI and mandates revascularization for limb salvage.
- Percutaneous endovascular therapy is often applied as first-line therapy in appropriate patients with limited extent of anatomic disease and/or prohibitive operative risk.
- Due to the extensive, multilevel atherosclerotic occlusions present in patients with tissue loss, open surgical revascularization remains the gold standard for restoring durable perfusion to the threatened limb.
- Infrainguinal bypass surgery performed with autogenous vein conduit offers durable patency and excellent limb salvage
- Debridement of nonviable tissue should be delayed until perfusion is restored to the limb unless uncontrolled infection is present. Many patients will require one or more adjunctive operative procedures for salvage of their foot.

SUGGESTED READINGS

Conte MS, Belkin M, Upchurch GR, et al. Impact of increasing comorbidity on infrainguinal reconstruction: a 20-year perspective. Ann Surg. 2001;233(3):445–452.

Criqui MH, Fronek A, Barrett-Connor E, et al. The prevalence of peripheral arterial disease in a defined population. Circulation. 1985;71(3):510–515.

Halperin, JL. Evaluation of patients with peripheral vascular disease. Thromb Res. 2002;106(6):V303–V311.

Hirsch AT, Haskal ZJ, Hertzer NR, et al. ACC/AHA 2005 guidelines for the management of patients with peripheral arterial disease (lower extremity, renal, mesenteric, and abdominal aortic): executive summary a collaborative report from the American Association for Vascular Surgery/Society for Vascular Surgery, Society for Cardiovascular Angiography and Interventions, Society for Vascular Medicine and Biology, Society of Interventional Radiology, and the ACC/AHA Task Force on Practice Guidelines (Writing Committee to Develop Guidelines for the Management of Patients with Peripheral Arterial Disease) endorsed by the American Association of Cardiovascular and Pulmonary Rehabilitation; National Heart, Lung, and Blood Institute; Society for Vascular Nursing; TransAtlantic Inter-Society Consensus; and Vascular Disease Foundation. J Am Coll Cardiol. 2006;47(6):1239–1312.

Norgren L, Hiatt WR, Dormandy JA, et al. Inter-Society Consensus for the Management of Peripheral Arterial Disease (TASC II). J Vasc Surg. 2007;45(Suppl S):S5–S67.

Selvin E, Erlinger TP. Prevalence of and risk factors for peripheral arterial disease in the United States: results from the National Health and Nutrition Examination Survey, 1999–2000. Circulation. 2004;110(6):738–743.

Taylor LM Jr, Edwards JM, Porter JM. Present status of reversed vein bypass grafting: five-year results of a modern series. J Vasc Surg. 1990;11(2):193–205;discussion 05–06.

Wengerter KR, Veith FJ, Gupta SK, et al. Prospective randomized multicenter comparison of in situ and reversed vein infrapopliteal bypasses. J Vasc Surg. 1991;13(2):189–197; discussion 97–99.

Wolfe JH, Wyatt MG. Critical and subcritical ischemia. Eur J Vasc Endovasc Surg. 1997;13(6):578–582.

Acute Limb Ischemia

PETER K. HENKE and JOHN W. RECTENWALD

Presentation

A 68-year-old active man presents to the emergency room (ER) with a 4-hour history of right limb pain and numbness. He had fallen out of bed and noticed worsening limb symptoms ever since. He notes no prior leg problems and no history of claudication. His past history is significant for a myocardial infarction 7 years ago and subsequent CABG. Past medical history includes tobacco use and hypertension but no diabetes or stroke. Medications include an aspirin, a calcium channel blocker, and a statin agent. He was able to ambulate with assistance into the car and ER but now has a difficult time moving his foot due to pain and neurologic impairment.

Differential Diagnosis

At this point, lower limb etiologies include direct trauma and possible fracture, deep vein thrombosis, spinal cord compression, and arterial ischemia.

Evaluation

Physical Examination

On exam, his cardiac rhythm is irregularly, irregular with a rate of 130, BP = 130/90, and RR = 20. His abdomen is soft and nontender. Pulse exam is +2/4 of radial, left femoral, and pedal pulses, right femoral +3/4, but 0/4 for right popliteal and pedal pulses. He has a normal neurologic exam on the left. He has diminished sensation below the knee on the right and decreased foot dorsiflexion, associated with coolness. No external trauma is noted, and no swelling is noted in either limb.

Laboratory/EKG

As comorbid diseases and conditions account for much of the mortality of ALI, it is important to evaluate for common problems that may compromise the patient acutely. These are primarily cardiac and renal diseases, including a potential for hyperkalemia, anemia, and acute myocardial infarction after ischemia reperfusion injury. Standard blood assessment includes CBC, electrolytes, BUN, creatinine, troponin, and CPK. A baseline CXR is optional.

Other Imaging and Noninvasive Tests

These should not delay definitive treatment, the urgency of which is dictated by the history and PE findings. If immediately available, duplex ultrasonography can image the arterial flow and demonstrate the location and extent of the occlusive embolus. An echocardiogram, if rapidly available, may also be useful for confirming presence of cardiac thrombus and overall function, but is not necessary preoperatively and should not delay revascularization. An ankle brachial index can be done as well, but in most cases of true ALI, is zero.

Therapy

Medical

Hydration with normal saline is standard practice. Urine output should be monitored, with a goal of at least 1 mg/Kg/h. An oral aspirin should be administered,

Presentation Continued

Acute limb ischemia (ALI) is a common vascular emergency that all physicians should be able to recognize and treat in a timely fashion (Figure 1). Delays in diagnosis and lack of anticoagulation are causes of limb loss in ALI. At this point, the history and PE give a clear picture of ALI. In this case, lack of external trauma, swelling, and DVT makes fracture less likely. Nerve root compression is possible but would usually be associated with a distinctly different neurologic exam usually involving a whole-leg motor deficit. The most significant finding suggesting ALI is that he has a total pulse deficit below the femoral artery on the symptomatic side but a normal exam on the nonaffected side. This patient has several of the "6" "P's" of ALI, namely parathesis, pulselessness, poikliothermia, and paralysis. According to the Society for Vascular Surgery (SVS) limb ischemia grading system, he has a level IIb ischemia and requires rapid revascularization to save his leg.

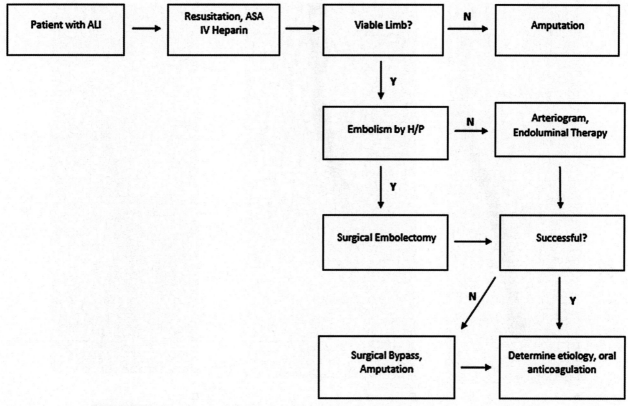

• Diagnostic and therapeutic algorithm for a patient who presents with ALI.

and a heparin bolus given, approximately 80 U/Kg, followed by 18 U/Kg/h continuous infusion for a goal aPTT 2 to 2.5× baseline. It is common for patients with ALI to have multiple acute medical problems that must be treated appropriately, and saving life before limb is paramount. First and foremost is evaluation and stabilization of cardiac issues, and ensuring adequate renal clearance.

Interventional

The most likely etiology of ALI in this case is a cardiac embolism, and the lower extremity is the most common site of origin in general. Other etiologies include thrombosis *in situ* (such as a graft thrombosis) or peripheral aneurysms, trauma, and aortoiliac dissection. Arteriography with thrombolysis is an option, but given the patient's classic history for an arterial thromboembolism (an antecedent cardiac event, lack of history of claudication, and normal vascular exam on his contralateral asymptomatic leg), this step may delay reperfusion achieved more readily with surgery. For cases where the etiology is not clear or points toward a nonembolic etiology (e.g., graft thrombosis or occluded aneurysm), proceeding to the arteriogram suite is best.

Procedural Basics

A longitudinal incision in the groin (or in the medial upper thigh, or below the knee, depending on the

clinical circumstances) is made and the femoral artery is exposed to include the common, deep, and superficial femoral artery. These are controlled with vessel loops. After ensuring the patient's ACT is >250, the loops are secured and the artery opened transversely if not significantly diseased. After adequate pulsatile arterial inflow is established by embolectomy, attention is turned to the distal thrombectomy. The use of the embolectomy catheter relies on the catheter traversing a thrombus, and pulling it out with gentle inflation of the balloon, in a continuous motion. The typical sizes are 4 and 5 for larger arteries, such as femoral and iliacs, and smaller with 2 and 3 size for distal arteries. After ensuring adequate back bleeding and having passed the catheter at least twice without retrieving thrombus, the arteriotomy is flushed with heparinized saline and closed with nonabsorbable suture in an interrupted fashion. Blood flow is reestablished to the distal limb, and Doppler signals are checked.

When the etiology of ALI is not clear by history and physical exam, arteriography with thrombolysis or catheter-assisted extraction is the best option **(Figures 2 and 3)**. Versatile equipment in well-outfitted endovascular, hybrid rooms includes over-the-wire embolectomy catheters, suction embolectomy catheters, and high-resolution C-arm fluoroscopy that allows concurrent endovascular and open techniques. This scenario will likely be the standard

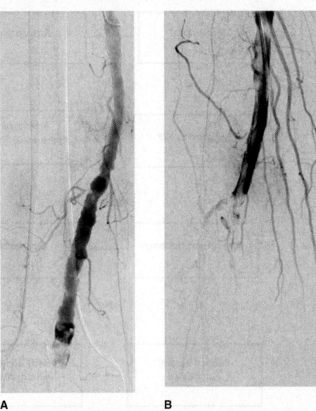
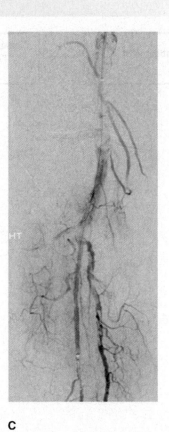

A   **B**   **C**

FIGURE 2 • **A:** Appearance of a patient with underlying mild peripheral arterial disease who presented with severe right lower ischemia. **B:** Later DSA arteriogram after 5 mg of tPA intra-arterially. **C:** Shows wire traversal and approximately 8 hours after thrombolytic started with opening of tibial vessels. This patient went on to have full resolution, with the underlying etiology thought to be a hypercoaguable state.

in the next 5 years. Proper case selection is essential, as failed lysis or frivolous persistence at endoluminal approaches confers a significantly increased risk of limb loss and death. Thrombolytic agents may cause a systemic fibrinolytic state and potentially release thrombus from the atrium or ventricle and may cause a stroke or other complications. Thus, an echocardiogram should be obtained prior to beginning thrombolysis if the suspected source of the embolus is intracardiac.

It is important to continue therapeutic heparin throughout the case, as well as maintain adequate hydration. Determining a postoperative CPK and urine myoglobin may aid with resuscitation. Consideration of a four-compartment fasciotomy to treat postreperfusion compartment syndrome should be given to any patient with ALI greater than 6-hour duration, as the morbidity is low. With good wound care, these can often be closed by delayed primary closure.

Routine follow-up with history and physical exam, but no specific imaging protocol, is needed for the affected and contralateral limb if palpable pulses returned. Standard cardiovascular risk factor modification therapies should be pursued.

Presentation Continued

Laboratory evaluation reveals a normal hematocrit (HCT) of 38, and a normal BUN/Cr, and potassium. An EKG shows atrial fibrillation with no obvious ST elevation or depression. Baseline CPK is elevated at 1,000. The patient also denies any chest pain and a rapid troponin I level is within normal limits. Thus, it is unlikely he has suffered a recurrent major myocardial infarction. His urine output is greater than 30 mL/h. If his blood pressure tolerates it, an intravenous (IV) beta-blocker or calcium channel blocker is reasonable with his tachycardia.

The embolic location is likely below the femoral artery as his femoral is normal (if not prominent), and no pulses or signals are present distally. The patient needs revascularization within 1 to 2 hours, as it is likely he has had approximately 4 hours of total ischemia, or

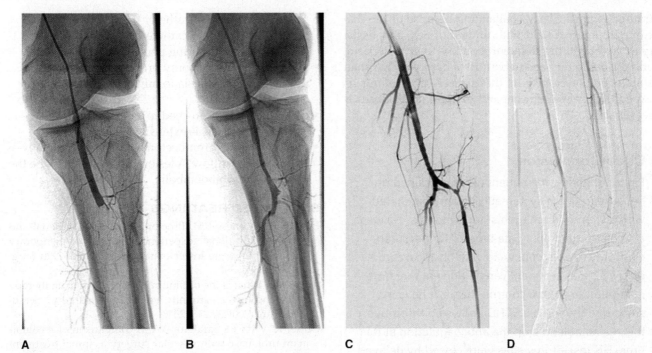

A   B   C   D

FIGURE 3 • This patient with modest bilateral PAD presented with ALI and underwent percutaneous suction catheter embolectomy for ALI. **A:** The arteriogram shows a complete thrombotic obstruction at the distal popliteal artery. **B,C:** A five French guide catheter is advanced into the thrombus with aspiration, followed by pulsed infusion of thrombolytic agent. Repeat arteriogram shows opening of the tibial-peroneal trunk and tibial vessels. **D:** Completion arteriogram with tibial vessels showing arterial patency and no evidence of distal thromboemboli.

he may suffer permanent muscle and nerve damage, rendering a nonsalvageable limb. As this patient has critical late ischemia, surgical embolectomy is the most appropriate means to rapidly restore limb blood flow, as compared with thrombolysis, which may take several hours before adequate reperfusion.

After cardiac rate control and heparinization, he is taken to the operating room and both lower extremities are prepped and draped to allow potential inflow site, as well as vein for conduit, should these be necessary. An open thromboembolectomy via a femoral approach under local anesthesia with IV sedation

is performed. Pedal signals are present at close. The patient undergoes four-compartment fasciotomy.

Discussion

Several important issues with ALI should be kept in mind; first, major errors occur with lack of timely diagnosis, anticoagulation, documentation of the exam pre- and postoperatively, and focusing too much on the limb salvage at the expense of the life **(Table 1)**. Second, the same principles hold if the patient presents with upper-extremity ALI. The operative approach is usually the medial distal brachial artery in the upper arm, or at the confluence of the radial and ulnar in the forearm. Third, recurrent on table or early recurrent ALI suggests an incomplete thrombectomy, or a persistent nidus of thromboembolism. For this, it is important to proceed with an on-table angiogram to visualize the inflow anatomy. Similarly, if no signals are present after reestablishing blood flow to the limb (after full embolectomy), an arteriogram is best for imaging the outflow. An intraoperative thrombolytic agent can be given (e.g., 10 mg tPA) intra-arterially and/or vasodilator, nitroglycerin (50 to 100 µg), may be helpful. Fourth, never force the embolectomy catheter in the artery, as dissection of the artery is a major problem that often requires endoluminal techniques or an open bypass to repair. Lastly, ALI in the setting of

---

TABLE 1. Acute Limb Ischemia Pitfalls

Choosing the wrong diagnosis and attempting an embolectomy in a patient with peripheral arterial disease in whom a catheter cannot be passed subsequently limits thrombolytic agent administration.

Be aware of reperfusion in patients with anuria, as fatal hyperkalemia may result. Communication with the anesthesiologist is critical.

Use fluoroscopy over the wire technique to traverse areas where stenosis may be present.

Thrombolectomize and embolectomize inflow first, flow followed by distal embolectomy.

Don't forget fasciotomies after reperfusion.

trauma is particularly challenging because of the disrupted operative field with limited, if any, soft tissue graft coverage, the frequent inability to give heparin, and the common need to perform a bypass rather than simple embolectomy. In these cases, proceeding as expeditiously without heparin or local small doses is reasonable.

Case Conclusion

Postoperatively, the patient was maintained on heparin and then systematically anticoagulated with a vitamin K antagonist for 3 months. He was also discharged on a beta-blocker for heart rate control with early follow-up with his local cardiologists. Reassessment can be done at that time in relation to source control; that is, if he is in sinus rhythm and his ECHO shows no thrombus, it is reasonable to stop the anticoagulation at this time. His fasciotomy sites were closed by delayed primary closure on his initial inpatient admission, and his mild foot drop has since resolved.

TAKE HOME POINTS

- Early recognition of ALI is critical.
- Determine the site of occlusion based on exam and ease of anatomical exposure.
- Don't limit your therapy options; consider contrast imaging intraoperatively if available.

- Start with the small catheter first, followed by a larger embolectomy catheter and don't force the catheter if encountering persistent obstruction.
- Any of the embolectomy procedures can be done under local anesthesia to minimize cardiovascular stress.
- Don't hesitate to proceed to a distal arterial exposure if thrombosis is extensive.
- Always pass a thrombectomy catheter proximally—regardless of inflow. A lesion proximally may be the source of thromboemboli.

SUGGESTED READINGS

Eliason JL, Wainess RM, Proctor MP, et al. A national and single institutional experience in the contemporary treatment of acute lower extremity ischemia. Ann Surg. 2003;238:382–390.

Henke PK. What is the optimum perioperative drug therapy following lower extremity vein bypass surgery? Semin Vasc Surg. 2009;22:245–251.

Ouriel K, Veith FJ, Sarahara AA. A comparison of recombinant urokinase with vascular surgery as initial treatment for acute arterial occlusion of the legs. N Engl J Med. 1998;338:1105–1111.

Palfreyman SJ, Booth A, Michaels JA. A systematic review of intra-arterial thrombolytic therapy for lower limb ischemia. Eur J Vasc Endovasc Surg. 2000;19:143–157.

Panetta T, Thompson JE, Talkington CM, et al. Arterial embolectomy: a 34-year experience with 400 cases. Surg Clin N Am. 1986;66:339–352.

Rutherford RB, Baker JD, Ernst C, et al. Recommended standards for reports dealing with lower ischemia: revised version. J Vasc Surg. 1997;26:517–538.

80 Asymptomatic Carotid Stenosis

PAUL D. DIMUSTO, JOHN E. RECTENWALD, and GILBERT R. UPCHURCH Jr.

Presentation

A 67-year-old man is referred to your office after a right-sided neck bruit was detected by the patient's primary care physician on routine physical examination. The patient has a past medical history significant for hypercholesterolemia and hypertension that are managed medically with a statin and a beta blocker. He also takes an aspirin daily. The patient has a 40 pack-year tobacco use history and continues to smoke 1 pack per day of cigarettes. The patient denies any neurologic symptoms, including difficulty with speech, sensory or motor deficits, or amarosis fugax. He denies any history of transient ischemic attack (TIA) or stroke. On physical exam, a right neck bruit is confirmed, and bilateral upper-extremity pulses are equal. There are no deficits on complete neurologic exam.

Differential Diagnosis

The most likely diagnosis in this case is asymptomatic internal carotid artery (ICA) stenosis given the patient's history of smoking and hypercholesterolemia. Other pathologies that could cause a neck bruit include a carotid aneurysm, dissection, carotid body tumor, or reversal of flow in the vertebral artery secondary to "subclavian steal." All of these can be detected on duplex ultrasound exam.

Workup

The initial diagnostic imaging test for suspected carotid artery stenosis is duplex ultrasound. This allows for gray-scale evaluation of the degree of stenosis along with Doppler estimation of the blood flow velocities in the area of stenosis. The peak systolic velocity (PSV) in the ICA and the estimate of the percent occlusion caused by the plaque are the primary factors involved in determining the degree stenosis (Table 1). The ratio of the ICA to common carotid artery (CCA) PSV and the ICA end diastolic velocity (EDV) are additional parameters that can be used to classify the stenosis. The degree of stenosis can be estimated as none, <50%, 50% to 69%, 70% to 99%, or total occlusion based on the duplex results. Occasionally, the extent of the lesion will not be able to be appropriately visualized with ultrasound, usually due to a high lesion. In this case, computed-tomography angiogram (CTA) is useful in defining the extent of the lesion and the degree of the stenosis (Figure 1). While the gold standard for measuring the degree of carotid stenosis is angiography, it is rarely used now given the reliable results from noninvasive duplex ultrasound scanning and CTA. Most surgeons will make operative decisions based on

ultrasound alone. However, angiography does have a role in carotid stenting.

The patient undergoes a carotid duplex scan (Figure 2) with the following results:

Right			Left	
PSV (cm/s)	EDV (cm/s)		PSV (cm/s)	EDV (cm/s)
56	10	Common (CCA)	67	16
52	9	Bulb	42	7
475	194	Internal (ICA)	69	29
87	14	External (ECA)	87	8
27	7	Vertebral	38	15
8.48		ICA/CCA Ratio	1.03	

RIGHT CAROTID DUPLEX:

Images:
CCA: Evidence of minimal and smooth heterogeneous plaque
BULB: Evidence of irregular calcific plaque with acoustic shadowing
ICA: Evidence of extensive calcific plaque with acoustic shadowing
ECA: Within normal limits.

Doppler:
CCA: Within normal limits
BULB: Within normal limits
ICA: 70% to 99% diameter stenosis
ECA: Within normal limits
Vertebral: Antegrade

IMPRESSION:
The right carotid reveals evidence of 70% to 99% stenosis involving the Bulb/ICA.

411

TABLE 1. Ultrasound Criteria for Diagnosis of ICA Stenosis

Degree of Stenosis (%)	ICA PSV (cm/s)	Plaque Estimate (%)	ICA/CCA PSV Ratio	ICA EDV (cm/s)
Normal	<125	None	<2.0	<40
<50	<125	<50	<2.0	<40
50–69	125–230	≥50	2.0–4.0	40–100
79–99	>230	≥50	>4.0	>100
Total occlusion	Undetectable	No detectable lumen	N/A	N/A

CCA, common carotid artery; ICA, internal carotid artery; PSV, peak systolic velocity; EDV, end diastolic velocity.
de Weerd M, et al. Prevalence of asymptomatic carotid artery stenosis in the general population: an individual participant data meta-analysis. Stroke. 2010;41:1294–1297.

LEFT CAROTID DUPLEX:
Images:
CCA: Within normal limits.
BULB: Evidence of minimal heterogeneous plaque
ICA: Evidence of minimal heterogeneous plaque
ECA: Within normal limits.

Doppler:
CCA: Within normal limits
BULB: Within normal limits
ICA: Within normal limits
ECA: Within normal limits
Vertebral: Antegrade

IMPRESSION:
The left carotid study reveals no hemodynamically significant disease.

Diagnosis and Treatment

Based on the carotid duplex results, this patient has a high-grade right ICA stenosis without significant disease on the left side. Given this patient's history, physical examination, and duplex ultrasound results, the diagnosis in this case is high-grade asymptomatic ICA stenosis. A right carotid endarterectomy (CEA) is recommended given the patient's relatively young age and the results of randomized controlled trials demonstrating a reduction in stroke risk over medical management alone. Smoking cessation, along with continuation of the patient's statin, beta blocker, and aspirin are also recommended.

The patient is quoted a risk of 3% for combined ipsilateral stroke and death, and a risk of 10% for cranial nerve injury (usually transient). The patient agrees to proceed with CEA. An EKG is obtained at his clinic

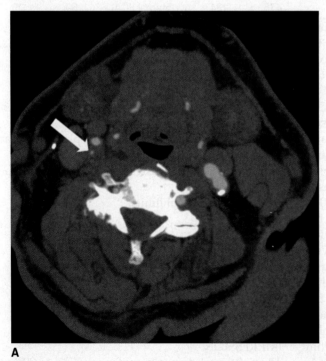
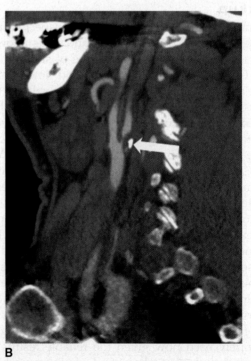

A   **B**

FIGURE 1 • CT angiogram demonstrating a patient with high-grade right carotid artery stenosis in (**A**) axial section (*arrow*) and (**B**) 3D reformat (*arrow*).

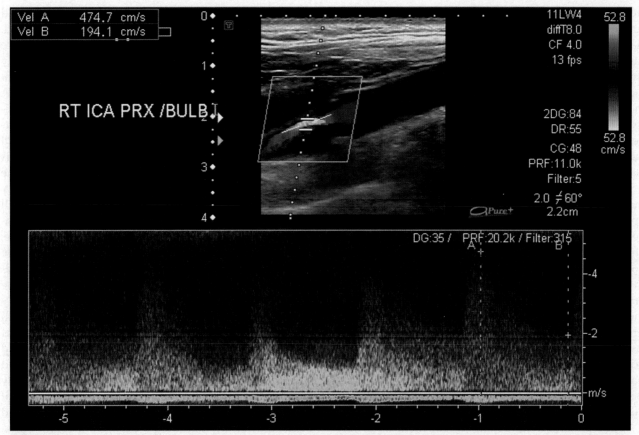

FIGURE 2 • Preoperative duplex scan demonstrating high-grade carotid stenosis with elevated peak systolic velocity and high EDV in right ICA.

visit that is normal. He has a good functional capacity, able to walk up two flights of stairs without becoming short of breath. No further cardiac testing is indicated given his young (<70) age, normal EKG, and good functional capacity.

Discussion

Stroke was the third leading cause of death in the United States in 2007, with 136,000 deaths attributed to stroke and cerebrovascular disease. The prevalence of severe asymptomatic carotid stenosis in the general population is approximately 0.1% in men <50 years old to 3.1% in men ≥80 years old. The prevalence in women ranges from 0% for those <50 to 0.9% for those ≥80. Moderate asymptomatic carotid stenosis is more common, ranging from 0.2% to 7.5% in men, and 0% to 5% in women.

The Asymptomatic Carotid Atherosclerosis Study (ACAS) compared the risk of TIA and stroke between best medical management and CEA in 1,662 patients from 39 sites across the United States and Canada. Patients with a carotid stenosis ≥60% by angiography (correlates to ~75% stenosis by ultrasound) were randomized to aspirin and risk factor counseling alone or aspirin and risk factor counseling plus CEA. The aggregate risk of ipsilateral TIA, stroke, or death in the perioperative period was 5.1% in the patients undergoing CEA versus 11.0% in patients receiving only medical management, for a 53% aggregate risk reduction for CEA.

The Asymptomatic Carotid Surgery Trial (ACST) was conducted in Europe and randomized 3,120 patients from 1993 to 2003 who had >60% ICA stenosis by ultrasound to medical management or medical management plus CEA. Ultimately the medical management was at the discretion of the treating physician but generally included antiplatelet therapy, antihypertensive treatment, and lipid-lowering therapy in the later years of the study. After 5 years, the stroke risk for CEA was 6.4% (including perioperative events) compared to 11.8% for medical management alone, again demonstrating a benefit for CEA.

These studies have been criticized for a relatively high stroke rate in the CEA group, and because medical management has improved since they were conducted, mostly due to the benefits of statins. Some claim that aggressive modern medical management can reduce the risk of stroke to at least that of the CEA group in the published studies, if not lower. This option of medical management alone may be best for patients who are at high operative risk; however, it has not been fully evaluated in modern randomized trials.

Additionally, carotid artery stenting (CAS) has become a third option for the management of carotid stenosis. However, trials have not shown CAS to be superior to CEA in terms of stroke outcomes, especially in most asymptomatic patients. Carotid stenting can be useful in patients with high-grade lesions with concomitant high-risk anatomic factors that would make open surgery difficult. These anatomic factors include previous CEA with recurrent stenosis, prior ipsilateral neck radiation, previous ablative neck surgery, common carotid stenosis below the clavicle, contralateral vocal cord paralysis, and the presence of a tracheostomy or stoma.

Until further trials can be completed comparing modern medical management including statin therapy, traditional CEA, and CAS, the issue of how to best manage a patient with high-grade asymptomatic carotid stenosis will continue to be debated. The Society for Vascular Surgery issued practice guidelines in 2008 for the management of atherosclerotic carotid artery disease to help guide physicians. They recommend best medical management, including blood pressure control, glucose control for diabetics, lipid reduction, and smoking cessation, for asymptomatic patients with a <60% stenosis. For asymptomatic patients with ≥60% carotid stenosis, CEA with medical management is recommended, as long as the perioperative risk is low. The committee recommended against CAS for patients with asymptomatic stenosis of any grade, with the possible exception of those patients with ≥80% stenosis with high-risk anatomy (defined above).

Surgical Approach

CEA can be performed under local or general anesthesia depending on surgeon's preference. The GALA trial, published in 2008, was a large randomized trial comparing the incidence of stroke, myocardial infarction, or death within 30 days between patients who had CEA under local anesthesia versus general anesthesia. No significant differences were found between the groups. An advantage of local anesthesia is that the patient's neurologic status can be monitored during the time of carotid artery clamping and a shunt inserted if needed. If the operation is done under general anesthesia, EEG monitoring or carotid stump pressure can be used to determine the need for shunting. Alternatively, routine use of a shunt can be employed.

The patient undergoes appropriate monitoring including a radial arterial line. A cervical block is placed. After prepping, an incision is made parallel to the anterior sternocleidomastoid muscle. The platysma is divided and the sternocleidomastoid muscle is retracted laterally. The carotid sheath is entered and from this point on in the operation, sharp dissection is utilized to reduce the risk of cranial nerve injury. The facial vein is identified, ligated, and divided. Carotid artery dissection is performed with as little

manipulation of the artery as possible. The vagus and the hypoglossal nerves are identified and protected. The CCA and the external carotid artery (ECA) are encircled with vessel loops. The patient is systemically heparinized (100 U/kg) and the ICA is encircled distal to the plaque. After 3 minutes, a test clamp of the ECA and ICA is performed. The patient remains neurologically intact; therefore, the CCA is clamped. An arteriotomy is made in the CCA and extended up the ICA until the top of the plaque is reached. The endarterectomy is begun in the CCA. An eversion endarterectomy of the ECA is performed with good back bleeding. A nicely feathering plaque is removed from the distal ICA. All debris is removed with heparinized saline, and a synthetic patch is sewn in with 6-0 monofilament suture. Prior to completing the patch, the ECA and the ICA are back bled and the CCA is forward bled. The patch is completed. Following patch closure, the clamp on the ECA is released first, followed by the CCA, and finally the ICA. An intraoperative duplex scan shows normal velocities (**Figure 3**) and no evidence of residual debris or stenosis. The incision is closed in layers, a closed suction drain is placed in the subplatysmal space, and the drapes are removed. The patient is neurologically intact and is transferred to the postanesthesia care unit where he receives an aspirin. The patient is monitored overnight for any neurologic changes or errant blood pressure. The drain is removed the following day prior to discharge (**Table 2**).

Special Intraoperative Considerations

It is critical to identify and protect the cranial nerves encountered during the operation to avoid even temporary paralysis. The vagus and hypoglossal nerves are the most commonly encountered; however, the glossopharyngeal can also be exposed, especially in high distal exposures. Care must be taken to not injure the vagus nerve when applying the carotid clamps.

It is also imperative to see the distal end of the plaque to ensure a smooth, feathered end to the endarterectomy. Occasionally, interrupted sutures will be needed to tack down the intima at the distal endpoint. If preoperative imaging suggests that the lesion is high and that adequate visualization of the distal endpoint may be difficult, subluxation of the mandible can be performed prior to the start of the operation to allow for better exposure. If high disease is unexpectedly encountered intraoperatively, the digastric muscle can be divided, the hypoglossal nerve mobilized, the styloglossus and stylopharyngeus muscles can be divided, and finally the styloid process can be fractured to provide adequate exposure.

Postoperative Management

Patients are typically monitored in a moderate-care setting with arterial line blood pressure monitoring overnight following a CEA as manipulation of the

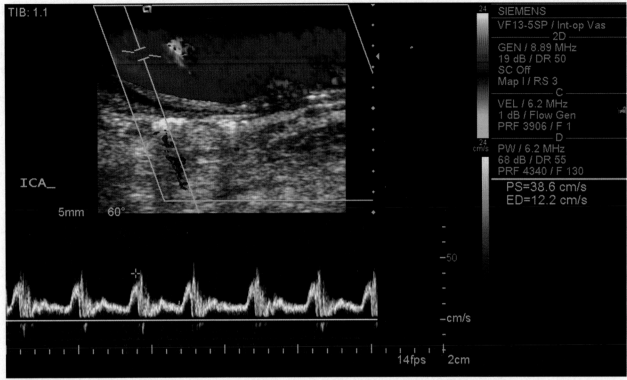

FIGURE 3 • Intraoperative duplex scan demonstrating no residual debris or stenosis in the right ICA.

carotid bulb and a change in the flow dynamics can cause variations in blood pressure. Changes in neurologic function should also be monitored as while rare, a patient could have a postoperative stroke related to

an embolus from thrombus formation at the operative site. Any new neurologic deficit within 24 hours of CEA should be presumed to be of an embolic origin, and the patient should be promptly taken back to the operating room for exploration and thromboembolectomy. Most patients however are discharged home the following day with aggressive blood pressure, glucose, and lipid control, as well as recommendations for smoking cessation if necessary.

The patient is seen in 2 weeks for an incision check and then in 3 months for a repeat carotid duplex to check for restenosis as well as monitor any contralateral stenosis that may be present. Up to 85% of patients with a moderate contralateral stenosis will progress to severe stenosis and require intervention. Therefore, yearly carotid duplex monitoring is recommended.

TABLE 2. Key Technical Steps and Potential Pitfalls to CEA with Patch Angioplasty

Key Technical Steps

1. Establish arterial line blood pressure monitoring and neurologic monitoring and position the patient.
2. Incise the skin and platysma, retract the sternoclydomastoid laterally, and ligate the facial vein.
3. Expose the CCA, ECA, and ICA with sharp dissection and minimal manipulation, identifying and preserving the vagus and hypoglossal nerves.
4. Administer heparin; clamp the ICA, CCA, and ECA; and insert shunt if needed.
5. Make arteriotomy starting on CCA and extending to ICA; perform the endarterectomy.
6. Flush with heparinized saline, assess the endpoints of endarterectomy, and place tacking sutures if needed.
7. Sew in prosthetic patch, back bleed ICA and ECA, and forward bleed CCA prior to completion of patch placement.
8. Unclamp ECA, CCA, and then ICA.
9. Assure hemostasis; perform duplex ultrasound scan.
10. Place closed suction drain in subplatysmal space and close incision in layers.
11. Recheck neurologic status; transport patient to recovery.

Potential Pitfalls

- Cranial nerve injury.
- Perioperative stroke.
- Perioperative myocardial infarction.

TAKE HOME POINTS

- Duplex ultrasound scan is best initial diagnostic test for asymptomatic carotid stenosis.
- Patients with high-grade asymptomatic carotid stenosis (70% to 99% by ultrasound) should undergo CEA along with aggressive medical management to reduce their risk of stroke.
- CEA can be performed under local anesthesia with neurologic monitoring, under general anesthesia with EEG or stump pressure monitoring, or with routine shunt use.
- CAS should be reserved for those patients with a stenosis ≥80% and high-risk anatomy.

SUGGESTED READINGS

Abbott A. Medical (nonsurgical) intervention alone is now best for prevention of stroke associated with asymptomatic severe carotid stenosis—results of a systematic review and analysis. Stroke. 2009;40:e570–e583.

de Weerd M, et al. Prevalence of asymptomatic carotid artery stenosis in the general population: an individual participant data meta-analysis. Stroke. 2010;41:1294–1297.

Grant E, et al. Carotid artery stenosis: gray-scale and Doppler US diagnosis—Society of Radiologists in Ultrasound Consensus Conference. Radiology. 2003;229:340–346.

Halliday A, et al. Prevention of disabling and fatal strokes by successful carotid endarterectomy in patients without recent neurological symptoms: randomised controlled trial. Lancet. 2004;363:1491–1502.

Hobson R, et al. Management of atherosclerotic carotid artery disese: clinical practice guidelines of the Society for Vascular Surgery. J Vasc Surg. 2008;48:480–486.

Lewis S, et al. General anaesthesia versus local anaesthesia for carotid surgery (GALA): a multicentre, randomised controlled trial. Lancet. 2008;372:2132–2142.

Toole J, et al. Edarterectomy for asymptomatic carotid artery stenosis. JAMA. 1995;273(18):1421–1428.

81 Symptomatic Carotid Stenosis

SARAH M. WEAKLEY and PETER H. LIN

Presentation

A 73-year-old man presents to the emergency room of a local hospital with a 5-day history of amaurosis fugax of the right eye. The patient reports that his eye symptoms have occurred two to three times daily since the initial onset of symptoms, with each episode lasting for approximately 10 minutes followed by spontaneous symptom resolution. The patient denies any residual ocular deficits or speech impairment after these episodes. The patient reports that he never loses consciousness or experiences any motor weakness or sensory deficits involving his arms or legs. His past medical history was significant for hypertension and coronary artery disease for which he underwent a coronary artery bypass 8 years ago. Regarding his medications, he takes an aspirin daily. On physical examination, a right neck bruit is confirmed, with symmetrical bilateral upper-extremity pulses. The patient does not have any neurologic deficits on physical examination.

Differential Diagnosis

The most likely cause of his transient ischemic attack (TIA) with clinical manifestations of amaurosis fugax is cerebral ischemia due to extracranial carotid artery disease. Other differential diagnoses in this patient with symptomatic cerebral ischemia include carotid aneurysm, carotid dissection, cardiac emboli, paroxysmal emboli, carotid coils or kinks, and fibromuscular dysplasia of the carotid artery. With his prior history of coronary artery atherosclerotic disease requiring coronary revascularization, one must consider carotid artery atherosclerotic disease as the most plausible cause of his symptoms.

Workup

The patient undergoes further evaluation with carotid duplex ultrasound that allows sonographic assessment of the severity of carotid stenosis using grayscale evaluation as well as blood velocity measurement at the level of carotid stenosis. The ultrasound study revealed high-grade right internal carotid artery (ICA) stenosis with greater 70% luminal stenosis, as well as proximal innominate artery stenosis. Due to his hemodynamically significant tandem lesions affecting the origin of the aortic arch vessels and the right ICA, a computed tomography angiography of the neck and the chest with intravenous contrast administration was performed that confirmed the presence of tandem high-grade stenosis involving the innominate artery origin and ipsilateral carotid artery at the level of the carotid bifurcation.

Diagnosis and Treatment

Since the patient's TIA symptoms can be caused by either the carotid stenosis or the innominate artery stenosis, revascularization of his carotid and innominate artery stenosis should be considered. While current literatures support the role of either carotid stenting or carotid endarterectomy (CEA) for high-grade symptomatic carotid artery stenosis, the presence of a high-grade supra-aortic vessel stenosis adds therapeutic challenges in this patient as it may potentially increase the risk of embolization for carotid stenting via a transfemoral approach. Although a proximal innominate artery stenosis can be treated surgically with aortoinnominate artery bypass via a median sternomy approach, his prior history of coronary artery bypass would make this treatment option a high-risk surgical procedure due to the repeat nature of an open chest operation. An ideal approach for these tandem carotid and supra-aortic trunk stenoses is to correct these two atherosclerotic lesions during one operative setting while minimize potential risk of cerebral embolization. Given these treatment considerations, a combined right CEA with synchronous retrograde innominate artery stenting is recommended.

Surgical Approach

In our patient with tandem lesions involving the carotid and innominate artery origin, a synchronous treatment approach with right CEA and retrograde innominate artery stent placement via the carotid arteriotomy site is planned. While CEA can be performed under various anesthetic options, including general anesthesia, local anesthesia, or cervical nerve block, we elect to perform CEA under local anesthesia without electroencephalic monitoring. A neck incision is made along the lateral border of the sternocleidomastoid muscle, which is followed by the exposure of the common carotid artery (CCA), external carotid artery, and ICA. The patient is given systemic heparin for anticoagulation. The ICA is test-clamped for 1 minute. If the patient does not demonstrate any neurologic changes, carotid shunting is not utilized. Proximal and distal vascular controls are established by placing vascular clamps in the common, external, and internal carotid arteries. A standard CEA is performed in which the carotid plaque is removed in it entirely. We routinely perform prosthetic patch angioplasty using Dacron graft to close the carotid arteriotomy site.

Following completion of the endarterectomy and closure of the arteriotomy, retrograde angioplasty and stenting of the proximal innominate artery is performed. The CCA is first clamped just proximal to the bifurcation. Next clamps on the internal and external carotid arteries are released, which allows retrograde flow from the external carotid artery (ECA) to perfuse the ICA during angioplasty and stenting. The placement of a CCA clamp also minimizes cerebral embolus during innominate artery angioplasty and stenting procedure. A Seldinger needle is used to cannulate the common carotid just proximal to the clamp, which is followed by the insertion of a 0.035-in guidewire under fluoroscopic guidance. An 8-F, 12-cm introducer sheath with radiopaque marker at the tip is next inserted over the guidewire whereby the introducer sheath is placed in a retrograde fashion toward the innominate artery origin. A short sheath is important since the endarterectomy is typically in close proximity to the site of angioplasty and stent placement. Following the sheath insertion, retrograde arteriogram of the innominate artery is performed to identify the location of the innominate artery ostial lesion. Next a premounted stainless steel balloon-expandable stent is inserted over the guidewire within the introducer sheath. The sheath should be advanced along with the stent well into the aorta, crossing the lesion first before positioning the stent at the deployment site. This maneuver minimizes the possibility of dislodging the stent from the balloon. The sheath is next retracted proximally to uncover the balloon-expandable stent. A retrograde innominate artery angiogram is performed followed by stent deployment under fluoroscopic guidance. We routinely extend the stent 1 to 2 mm into the aorta to assure ostial plaque coverage by the stent. Once the final angiogram is obtained to demonstrate adequate angioplasty and stent placement, a

5-0 prolene pursestring suture is placed around the introducer sheath site followed by the carotid sheath removal. Back bleeding from the sheath insertion site is allowed in order to flush out any embolic debris during the stenting procedure. Next the CCA clamp is removed, which restores the antegrade blood flow in the innominate and carotid artery.

Postoperative Management

Postoperative management following this combined treatment of CEA and retrograde innominate artery stent placement is similar to post-CEA patient care. Patients are monitored in either surgical intensive care unit or intermediate care unit with careful blood pressure monitoring. Additional attention should be focused on possible neck hematoma formation, which may compromise airway. Neurologic status should be monitored carefully. Any development of neurologic deficit should be assumed to be carotid artery thromboembolism caused by technical error, which should be explored surgically for possible thromboembolectomy. The patient should be given clear liquid diet following the operation. Most patients can tolerate dietary advancement and are discharged home the following day.

The patient should resume oral daily aspirin following the operation. Because of the innominate artery stent placement, postoperative therapy should also include 3 months of oral clopidogrel (Plavix), which has been shown to reduce platelet aggregation and decrease potential stent-related thrombosis.

Discussion

The presence of carotid tandem lesions involving the carotid bulb and its proximal vessel origin, located in either the left CCA or the innominate artery origin, represents a potential therapeutic dilemma and technical challenge. Studies have reported that such combined lesions can occur in 2% to 4% of patients undergoing diagnostic evaluations in preparation for CEA for a carotid bifurcation lesion. When a tandem lesion is detected, several treatment approaches can be considered, which include (a) CEA via neck incision and surgical revascularization of supra-aortic trunk lesion via median sternotomy, (b) endovascular stenting of both carotid and supra-aortic trunk lesion via transfemoral approach, (c) carotid stenting via transfemoral approach and surgical revascularization of supra-aortic trunk lesion via open chest approach, (d) CEA via neck incision and endovascular stenting of supra-aortic trunk lesion via transfemoral approach, or (e) CEA via neck incision and endovascular stenting of supra-aortic trunk lesion via retrograde carotid approach.

In patients with symptomatic carotid artery disease, CEA is effective in preventing future ipsilateral ischemic events, provided that the perioperative combined risk of stroke and death is not higher than 6%. Its effect is marked in patients with high-grade (>70%) stenosis, with eight patients needed to be treated to prevent one ipsilateral stroke in a 2-year period. The stroke-reduction benefit persists, although less significantly, in symptomatic patients with a moderate (50% to 75%) degree of stenosis, with 20 patients needed to be treated to prevent one ipsilateral stroke during a 2-year period.

The ideal treatment strategy for symptomatic carotid artery lesion has been thoroughly investigated in recent years as multiple prospective randomized studies have shown similar efficacy between percutaneous carotid artery stenting (CAS) and CEA. While transfemoral stent placement can be performed for both carotid and innominate lesions, in our patient, the risk of procedural-related embolization would undoubtedly be increased significantly due to the manipulation of endovascular devices across these tandem lesions. It has been shown that procedural-related embolization, caused by vessel plaque breakage due to endovascular device instrumentation, is a major risk factor for cerebral infarction during the carotid stenting procedure.

Considering various recent clinical trials comparing carotid stenting and CEA, it is noteworthy to highlight the Carotid Revascularization Endarterectomy versus Stenting Trial (CREST) study, which is the largest trial to date comparing outcomes in patients with symptomatic and asymptomatic carotid artery stenosis. The study enrolled 2,502 patients at 117 centers in the United States and Canada and compared the treatment outcome in prospective randomized fashion between CEA and carotid stenting. The primary end point for the study was any periprocedural stroke, myocardial infarction (MI), death, or postprocedural ipsilateral stroke up to 4 years after intervention. An embolization protection device was successfully used in 96% of carotid stenting patients. A unique outcome measured element in the CREST trial involves a patient of general health status with the use of the Medical Outcomes Study 36-Item Short-Form Health Survey (SF-36) at 2 weeks, 1 month, and 1 year after the procedure.

The study reported similar primary end point at a mean follow-up of 2.5 years between the two groups. However, the 30-day incidence of stroke or death was 4.4% and 2.3% for CAS- and CEA-treated symptomatic and asymptomatic patients, respectively, a difference that was significant. The incidence of MI was significantly higher in CEA-than in CAS-treated patients (2.3% vs. 1.1%). Interestingly, the SF-36 data indicate that the impact on quality of life by MI was not significant, whereas the impact of major or minor stroke was significant. No significant differences (CAS vs. CEA) in results were noted when the outcomes were examined by symptomatic status. A 4-year Kaplan-Meier curve examining freedom from the primary end point demonstrated no significant difference in the curves for CAS versus CEA treatment out to 4 years (risk reduction, <1% per year), showing that both methods result in durable benefit. The SF-36 subscale data at 1 year indicate that the increased incidence of cranial nerve palsy in CEA-treated patients has no significant impact on quality of life.

Regarding treatment approach for supra-aortic trunk lesions, direct aortic reconstructions via transthoracic approach have been reported as a durable treatment option. However, complication rates for these procedures can be as high as 23% which chylothorax, graft thrombosis, pneumothorax, phrenic nerve palsy, and Horner's syndrome being the most serious. Over the past decades, endovascular treatment with transluminal balloon angioplasty and stent placement of the brachiocephalic vessels has shown acceptable results with outcomes equal to surgery. These endovascular treatment strategy offers the advantages of reduced morbidity and mortality and decreased length of stay compared to the traditional open transthoracic aortic bypass procedures. In our patient who had undergone a prior coronary artery operation, endovascular treatment of his innominate artery stenosis offers significant advantage of reduced operative morbidities and expeditious recovery due to the avoidance of a redo open chest incision.

Taken together these various treatment considerations for tandem lesion involving carotid artery and supra-aortic trunk ostial lesion, it is our assessment that the best treatment strategy for this patient is to perform synchronous CEA and retrograde innominate artery stenting **(Table 1)**. We postulate that synchronous treatment strategy offers several advantages. The innominate stenting procedure is performed using a retrograde approach and employed temporary occlusion of the CCA to prevent distal embolization. Because CEA has already been completed prior to innominate stent placement, the placement of a CCA clamp during the innominate stenting procedure allows continual ICA perfusion via retrograde ECA circulation. Additionally, the retrograde approach allows a short distance access to the origin of the supra-aortic arch occlusive lesion, which reduces the hazards of guidewire manipulation through a diseased or tortuous aortic arch typically associated with a transfemoral approach. The short working distance between the supra-aortic trunk lesion and the carotid entry site permits precise fluoroscopic control for lesion location, guidewire manipulation, and stent deployment. Once the endovascular procedure is completed, back bleeding from the sheath insertion site prior to arteriotomy closure was performed, which permits flushing away of procedural-related embolic debris.

TABLE 1. Key Technical Steps and Potential Pitfalls to Performing CEA and Innominate Artery Stenting

Key Technical Steps
1. Perform CEA in a standard fashion with patching.
2. Clamp distal CEA so that the ECA retrograde fills the ICA.
3. Place innominate artery stent in a retrograde fashion.
4. Closure of arteriotomy.
5. Close incision.

Potential Pitfalls
- Embolization to brain following CEA or stent.
- Reperfusion syndrome following treatment of sequential lesions.

Several studies have reported the technical feasibility and the clinical efficacy of this synchronous treatment approach in patients with tandem lesion involving the carotid and the supra-aortic arch ostial lesions. Length of hospital stay was decreased substantially when compared to transthoracic bypass procedures for treatment of similar aortic arch occlusive lesions. The majority of patients were discharged after 23 hours of observation. This decreased length of stay resulted in decreased care costs because extensive bypass surgery was avoided and return to full activity occurred more quickly. Performing the endovascular portion of the procedure using a retrograde approach from the neck avoided potential vessel entry site complications that can be associated with a retrograde femoral approach.

TAKE HOME POINTS
- The most likely cause of TIA with clinical manifestations of amaurosis fugax is cerebral ischemia due to extracranial carotid artery disease.
- Carotid duplex ultrasound allows sonographic assessment of the severity of carotid stenosis using grayscale evaluation, as well as blood velocity measurement at the level of carotid stenosis.
- In patients with symptomatic carotid artery disease, CEA is effective in preventing future ipsilateral ischemic events, provided that the perioperative combined risk of stroke and death is not higher than 6%.
- CREST comparing CAS and CEA reported similar primary end point at a mean follow-up of 2.5 years between the two groups. However, the 30-day incidence of stroke or death was 4.4% and 2.3% for CAS- and CEA-treated symptomatic and asymptomatic patients, respectively, a difference that was significant.

- While there are various treatment considerations for tandem lesion involving carotid artery and supra-aortic trunk ostial lesions, it is our assessment that the best treatment strategy for most patients is to perform synchronous CEA and retrograde proximal CCA or innominate artery stenting.

SUGGESTED READINGS

Allie DE, Hebert CJ, Lirtzman MD, et al. Intraoperative innominate and common carotid intervention combined with carotid endarterectomy: a "true" endovascular surgical approach. J Endovasc Ther. 2004;11:258–262.

Arko FR, Buckley CJ, Lee SD, et al. Combined carotid endarterectomy with transluminal angioplasty and primary stenting of the supra-aortic vessels. J Cardiovasc Surg (Torino). 2000;41:737–742.

Gurm HS, Yadav JS, Fayad P, et al. Long-term results of carotid stenting versus endarterectomy in high-risk patients. N Engl J Med. 2008;358:1572–1579.

Lal BK, Brott TG. The Carotid Revascularization Endarterectomy vs. Stenting Trial completes randomization: lessons learned and anticipated results. J Vasc Surg. 2009;50:1224–1231.

Mordasini P, Gralla J, Do DD, et al. Percutaneous and open retrograde endovascular stenting of symptomatic high-grade innominate artery stenosis: technique and follow-up. AJNR Am J Neuroradiol. 2011;32(9):1726–1731.

Paraskevas KI, Mikhailidis DP, Nicolaides AN, et al. Interpreting the Carotid Revascularization Endarterectomy Versus Stent Trial (CREST): additional trials are needed. Vascular. 2010;18:247–249.

Ricotta JJ II, Malgor RD. A review of the trials comparing carotid endarterectomy and carotid angioplasty and stenting. Perspect Vasc Surg Endovasc Ther. 2008;20:299–308.

Rouleau PA, Huston J III, Gilbertson J, et al. Carotid artery tandem lesions: frequency of angiographic detection and consequences for endarterectomy. AJNR Am J Neuroradiol. 1999;20:621–625.

Sacco RL, Adams R, Albers G, et al. Guidelines for prevention of stroke in patients with ischemic stroke or transient ischemic attack: a statement for healthcare professionals from the American Heart Association/American Stroke Association Council on Stroke: co-sponsored by the Council on Cardiovascular Radiology and Intervention: the American Academy of Neurology affirms the value of this guideline. Stroke. 2006;37:577–617.

Safian RD, Bresnahan JF, Jaff MR, et al. Protected carotid stenting in high-risk patients with severe carotid artery stenosis. J Am Coll Cardiol. 2006;47:2384–2389.

Uurto IT, Lautamatti V, Zeitlin R, et al. Long-term outcome of surgical revascularization of supraaortic vessels. World J Surg. 2002;26:1503–1506.

Yadav JS. Carotid stenting in high-risk patients: design and rationale of the SAPPHIRE trial. Cleve Clin J Med. 2004;71(suppl 1):S45–S46.

82 Diabetic Foot Infection

JEFFREY KALISH and ALLEN HAMDAN

Presentation

A 65-year-old man with a history of hypertension, hyperlipidemia, and non–insulin-dependent diabetes mellitus presents with a 3-day history of pain in his left foot. He reports that his blood sugars, while normally very well controlled, have been very difficult to manage over the past day. His vital signs are normal. On physical examination, he has palpable femoral and popliteal pulses bilaterally but only dopplerable signals in the dorsalis pedis and the posterior tibial arteries. He has redness around the second toe, with a small 5-mm ulcer on the dorsal surface of the toe. The ulcer does not appear to probe deeply.

Differential Diagnosis

The lifetime risk of acquiring foot lesions (ulcers/gangrene) in diabetic patients has been estimated at 15% to 25%, with an annual incidence of approximately 1.0% to 4.1%. The clinical presentation of peripheral arterial disease (PAD) encompasses intermittent claudication, rest pain, and ulcers with or without gangrene. Diabetic patients may exhibit these typical symptoms, but more often they present with a wound that fails to heal or with pain at the site of a callus, pressure point, or other bony prominence. It is imperative to identify the presence of neuropathic ulcers, which arise at points of increased pressure and weight bearing, as well as the characteristic findings of a "Charcot foot."

Workup

The three pathologic components leading to diabetic foot complications (ischemia, neuropathy, and infection) frequently occur in combination as an etiologic triad. Thorough clinical examination of foot ulcers is necessary to evaluate the depth and extent of involvement, anatomic location, etiology, and presence of ischemia or infection. Diabetic patients typically suffer from tibial and peroneal arterial occlusive disease with relative sparing of the foot arteries, and ischemia results from both atherosclerotic macrovascular disease and microcirculatory dysfunction. Diabetic neuropathy has multiple manifestations in the foot because it encompasses sensory, motor, and autonomic fibers. Because of a blunted neuroinflammatory response, diabetic patients lack a crucial component of the body's natural first-line defense against pathogens and thus are more susceptible to an ensuing foot infection.

The typical inflammatory signs of infection may be absent or diminished (e.g., erythema, rubor, cellulitis, or tenderness). The usual systemic manifestations of infection (e.g., fever, tachycardia, or elevated white blood cell count) are frequently absent as well. Unexplained hyperglycemia should prompt an aggressive search for a source of infection because the elevated glucose may be the only sign of impending problems. Careful palpation of the foot for areas of tenderness or fluctuance is important in order to detect undrained abscesses in deeper tissue planes. All ulcers must be carefully inspected and probed, and superficial eschar unroofed, to look for potential deep space abscesses. Osteomyelitis occurs after the spread of superficial infection of the soft tissue to the adjacent bone or marrow. Although numerous expensive radiologic techniques are available to diagnose osteomyelitis (e.g., MRI, bone scan, tagged white blood cell scan), a simple sterile metallic probe will usually suffice; if this sterile probe hits bone, then osteomyelitis can be diagnosed with a sensitivity of 66%, a specificity of 85%, and a positive predictive value of 89%. Plain radiographs of the foot should be obtained in every patient with suspected foot infection. X-rays can reveal the presence of a foreign body, gas, osteolysis or joint effusion, as well as delineate anatomy for surgical planning.

A complete vascular exam is imperative in any patient reporting symptoms consistent with claudication or rest pain, and in any patient with extremity ulcers or gangrene. In those cases where the vascular status is unclear, noninvasive vascular laboratory studies (ankle brachial indices/pulse volume recordings [ABI/PVR]) are particularly useful. Patients with severe ischemia usually have ABI of <0.4, but many diabetic patients have noncompressible vessels with resulting artificially elevated ABIs so PVRs are required. Intra-arterial digital subtraction arteriography is the most accurate method to evaluate the lower-extremity arterial circulation. Although magnetic resonance arteriography had been used more frequently during the past decade in patients with marginal renal function, recent reports about nephrogenic systemic fibrosis have shifted clinical practice back to conventional arteriography. A carefully performed arteriogram must show the appropriate inflow source and outflow target artery, and it must incorporate the complete infrapopliteal circulation, including foot vessels.

Diagnosis and Treatment

In the absence of deep infection or necrosis, minor infections or ulcers may be managed conservatively with local wound care and/or antibiotics. Topical dressings, typically saline-impregnated gauze, should be aimed at maintaining a moist environment. The ulcer should be protected from excessive pressure by

Presentation Continued

The patient is admitted to the hospital and placed on an insulin drip. The ulcer and surrounding cellulitis worsen **(Figure 1)**, and he does not respond to the intravenous broad-spectrum antibiotics. An arteriogram shows patency of vessels to the level of the below-knee popliteal but long-segment occlusions in his anterior and posterior tibial vessels with a large reconstituted dorsalis pedis artery **(Figure 2)**.

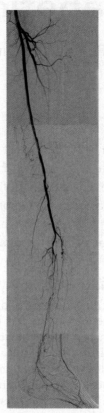

FIGURE 2 • Composite arteriogram of left lower-extremity revealing tibial artery occlusions with reconstitution of dorsalis pedis artery in foot.

placement of an accommodative pad around the lesion to distribute pressure to surrounding tissues. Patients with limb-threatening infections require immediate hospitalization, immobilization, and intravenous antibiotics. Cultures from the depths of the ulcer should be sent; wound swabs are unreliable and should not be performed. Empiric broad-spectrum antibiotic therapy

(dictated by institutional preferences, local resistance patterns, availability, and cost) should be initiated to cover the polymicrobial infections usually seen in diabetic patients. Although various trials have tried to compare various antibiotic regimens, they fail to focus on an inherent weakness of simply using antibiotics alone, that is, the reported "failure rates" in these

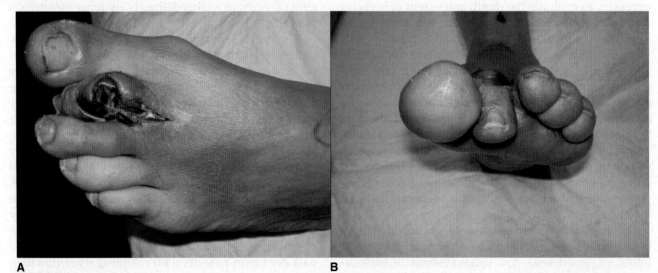

A   **B**

FIGURE 1 • **(A,B)** Left second toe ulcer and surrounding cellulitis.

trials of 11% to 12% for moderate infections and 19% to 30% for severe infections. Furthermore, the presence of PAD predicts a higher failure rate for healing any diabetic foot lesion after 1 year (31% failure vs. 16% failure). Mild infections usually require only 7 to 10 days of antibiotic therapy, whereas moderate and severe infections may require up to 3 weeks of treatment. Traditional therapy for osteomyelitis was accepted as 4 to 6 weeks of intravenous antibiotics, but recent studies have documented a >30% recurrence rate using this modality alone.

Surgical Approach

Debridement/Drainage Procedures

Presentation Continued

The patient undergoes an open second toe amputation, continues on intravenous antibiotics, and has resolution of the surrounding cellulitis. Vein mapping shows adequate ipsilateral greater saphenous vein for a planned below-knee popliteal to dorsalis pedis artery bypass.

Patients with abscess formation or necrotizing fasciitis must undergo prompt incision, drainage, and debridement including partial open toe, ray, or forefoot amputation. Tendon sheaths should be probed as proximally as possible and excised if infected. Despite fears to the contrary, long and extensive drainage incisions will heal when infection is controlled and foot circulation is adequate. It is imperative to make any necessary incision initially, but at the same time to contemplate the implications of those incisions on the potential completion amputation. Wounds should be packed open with saline-moistened gauze, and dressings should be changed two to three times a day. Wounds should be examined daily, and additional bedside or operative debridement should be repeated as needed. Adequate dependent drainage is crucial, and limited incisions with drains (closed-suction or penrose) should be avoided.

Patients with salvageable ischemic foot lesions and concomitant active infection need the infection controlled prior to vascular surgical intervention. In addition to instituting broad-spectrum antibiotics, options include open debridement and drainage or partial foot amputation. A short delay (usually <5 days) before revascularization in order to control active infection is justified; however, longer waits in order to "sterilize wounds" is inappropriate, and may result in further necrosis and a lost opportunity to save the foot.

Lower-Extremity Bypass

From a revascularization perspective, the most important difference in lower-extremity atherosclerosis in the patient with diabetes is the anatomic location or distribution of the arterial lesions. While patients with diabetes who abuse cigarettes may manifest iliac or femoral occlusive disease, diabetic patients typically have significant occlusive disease in the infrapopliteal arteries, while arteries of the foot are spared. This "tibial artery disease" requires a different approach to arterial reconstruction and presents special challenges for the surgeon (Table 1).

Each operation must be individualized, based on the patient's available venous conduit and arterial anatomy. In 10% of cases a foot artery, usually the dorsalis pedis artery, is the only suitable outflow vessel; in an additional 15% of patients, the dorsalis pedis artery will appear to be the best target vessel in comparison to other patent but diseased tibial vessels. Although pedal bypass represents the most "extreme" type of distal arterial reconstruction, it is almost always possible, particularly when the surgeon is flexible in terms of venous conduit and location of proximal anastomosis. Primary patency, secondary patency, and limb salvage rates approach 57%, 63%, and 78% at 5 years and 38%, 42%, and 58% at 10 years.

Endovascular Therapy

Although surgical reconstruction has traditionally been the gold standard for diabetic foot revascularization, endovascular intervention has become a viable

---

TABLE 1. Key Technical Steps and Potential Pitfalls to a Lower-extremity Bypass

Key Technical Steps

1. Identify greater saphenous vein and harvest with full-length leg incision.
2. Obtain control of proximal and distal anastomotic sites.
3. Create tunnels for bypass (subcutaneous or subfascial).
4. Dilate vein with heparinized saline, check for any holes requiring repair.
5. Heparinize patient systemically.
6. Perform proximal anastomosis, tunnel vein, and confirm pulsatile flow.
7. Perform distal anastomosis.
8. Confirm unobstructed doppler signal in distal artery and at anastomosis.
9. Reverse heparin with protamine.
10. Close incisions and confirm pulses or signals in foot prior to leaving OR.

Potential Pitfalls

- Inadequate caliber or length of vein.
- Inadequate hemostatic control of target vessels.
- Need to combine an open/endovascular hybrid approach to revascularization.

alternative. With the potential pitfalls accompanying traditional surgical approaches to limb salvage, as well as the overall poor health and life expectancy of patients with PAD, less invasive endovascular therapy can represent an attractive option. Balloon angioplasty and stenting are well suited to focal, short-segment iliac stenoses or occlusions, which exist in 10% to 20% of diabetic patients. With regard to outflow procedures, the morbidity of open surgery can be quite significant, and not simply limited to local wound complications or myocardial infarctions. Readmissions to the hospital, reoperations, slow time to healing, and time spent in rehabilitation must be factored into the risk-benefit analysis. In fact, the ideal outcome (patent graft, healed wound, no additional operations in a fully ambulatory patient who can sustain independent living) may only be obtainable up to 20% of the time. Although patency rates of bypass grafts have been shown to be equivalent in diabetics and nondiabetic patients, endovascular interventions may be associated with worse patency rates in diabetics due to their higher prevalence of limb-threatening ischemia as the presenting symptom.

The best scientific attempt to compare primary open and endovascular interventions was the bypass versus angioplasty in severe ischemia of the leg trial. Perioperative (30-day) morbidity was higher with surgery; all-cause mortality trended higher with surgery for the first 6 months but then trended lower for the next 6 months; amputation-free survival was similar in both groups. Two-year post hoc analysis revealed that surgery was associated with a reduced risk of future amputation and/or death. The trialists concluded that although the strategies are roughly equivalent at medium-term follow-up with regard to mortality and amputation-free survival, angioplasty should be used first for patients with significant comorbidities and with a life expectancy of <1 to 2 years. Moreover, longer-term results favor surgery over angioplasty if there is a "good" vein and a medically fit patient. More recent reviews have shown that after 2 years, tibial angioplasty requires repeat endovascular intervention in up to one-third of patients, and another 15% of patients go on to have a surgical bypass.

Amputation

The last alternative remains amputation. Closed minor amputations (toes or transmetatarsal) are practical following infection control and revascularization, and typically leave the patient with a functional foot for walking **(Figure 3)**. In situations involving extensive tissue loss precluding a functional foot, when there are nonhealing wounds in the setting of patent grafts, and for control of sepsis, amputation below the knee is necessary. Surgeons should strive to preserve the

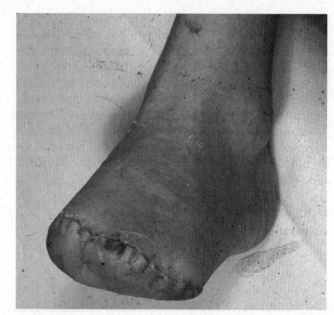

FIGURE 3 • Transmetatarsal amputation.

knee joint because of its functional significance for rehabilitation. Above-knee amputations are reserved for debilitated patients with severe tissue loss or with no capacity to ambulate. Because of modern advances in prostheses coupled with aggressive approaches to rehabilitation, amputation should be viewed as an acceptable modality to treat diabetic foot complications and not as a treatment failure.

Special Intraoperative Considerations

Several unexpected findings may be encountered during a lower-extremity revascularization procedure. If an artery is found to be too heavily calcified or does not have an adequate lumen, then the surgeon must reevaluate the preoperative arteriogram to find a more suitable target. If the venous conduit is not of suitable quality or length to perform the planned bypass, then the surgeon must consider splicing the greater saphenous vein with alternative venous conduits or using an alternative conduit altogether (such as contralateral greater saphenous vein, ipsilateral or contralateral lesser saphenous vein, basilic or cephalic arm veins, or even a composite sequential bypass with prosthetic and vein). Another current option involves hybrid procedures to achieve revascularization; this involves the combination of a shorter bypass with either an inflow or outflow endovascular procedure (such as a superficial femoral artery angioplasty/stent coupled with a popliteal to distal bypass, or a prosthetic femoral to popliteal bypass coupled with a tibial angioplasty/stent). Vascular surgeons have many tools and technologies available, and these should all be used in the efforts to achieve limb salvage.

Postoperative Management

Patients should be observed in a monitored setting overnight following lower-extremity revascularization, and neurovascular checks should be performed every 1 to 2 hours. Arterial lines and foley catheters can usually be discontinued after 1 to 2 days once blood pressures have stabilized, and urine output has been adequate. Patients should get out of bed to chair by postoperative day 1 and typically can ambulate on postoperative day 2. Physical therapy consults should be involved early in order to facilitate a patient's transition home or to rehabilitation. Because these vascular surgery patients typically have significant comorbidities, practitioners must be vigilant for postoperative complications such as myocardial infarction, pneumonia, wound infection, hematoma, etc.

Surveillance studies should typically be done on both lower-extremity bypass grafts and endovascular interventions in order to monitor for recurrent stenoses or impending failure. Exact algorithms are debatable, but the basic premise relies on surveillance duplex ultrasounds in regular intervals (such as every 3 months for 1 year, then every 6 months for 1 year, then yearly) in order to identify grafts that are at risk for failure. This allows for certain patients to undergo arteriograms to identify and treat potential areas of intimal hyperplasia or new atherosclerotic lesions.

Case Conclusion

The patient undergoes a successful bypass and is discharged to rehabilitation on postoperative day 5. His wound improves with local wound care, and he eventually granulates the wound and heals secondarily. Surveillance duplex shows a patent bypass graft with no areas of elevated velocities.

TAKE HOME POINTS

- The three pathologic components leading to diabetic foot complications (ischemia, neuropathy, and infection) frequently occur in combination as an etiologic triad.
- The typical inflammatory signs and systemic manifestations of infection may be absent or diminished in diabetic patients, and unexplained hyperglycemia may be the only indicator of a foot infection.
- Patients with salvageable ischemic foot lesions and concomitant active infection need the infection controlled for a short period (usually no more than 5 days) prior to vascular surgical intervention.
- Each lower-extremity bypass operation must be individualized, based on the patient's available venous conduit and arterial anatomy, with diabetic patients typically manifesting tibioperoneal disease with sparing of foot arteries.
- Although surgical reconstruction is the current gold standard for diabetic foot revascularization, endovascular intervention has become a viable alternative.

SUGGESTED READINGS

Adam DJ, Beard JD, Cleveland T, et al. BASIL trial participants. Bypass versus angioplasty in severe ischaemia of the leg (BASIL): multicentre, randomised controlled trial. Lancet. 2005;366(9501):1925–1934.

Gibbons GW, Eliopoulos GM. Infection of the diabetic foot. In: Kozak GP, Campbell DR, Frykberg RG, et al., eds. Management of Diabetic Foot Problems. 2nd ed. Philadelphia, PA: WB Saunders, 1995:121–129.

Mills JL, Armstrong DG, Andros G. Strategies to prevent and heal diabetic foot ulcers: building a partnership for amputation prevention. J Vasc Surg. 2010;52(3 suppl):1S–103S.

Pomposelli FB, Kansal N, Hamdan AD, et al. A decade of experience with dorsalis pedis artery bypass: analysis of outcome in more than 1000 cases. J Vasc Surg. 2003;37: 307–315.

83 Acute Mesenteric Ischemia

BABAK J. ORANDI and JAMES H. BLACK, III

Presentation

A 71-year-old woman with a remote but significant smoking history presents to the emergency department (ED) with 24 hours of abdominal pain, nausea, vomiting, and diarrhea. She was discharged from the hospital 1 week prior after an elective coronary artery bypass graft, which was significant only for an episode of new-onset atrial fibrillation, which resolved after administration of an amiodarone bolus. In the ED, her vitals are as follows: temperature: 38.1°C, heart rate: 101, blood pressure: 148/67, respiratory rate: 16, and 98% saturation on 2 L of oxygen via nasal cannula. On physical examination, she is clearly uncomfortable. She has a number of well-healed incisions on her abdomen, including a right subcostal incision from an open cholecystectomy, a left lower-quadrant incision from an open appendectomy, a Pfannenstiel incision from two prior cesarean sections, and a lower midline incision from a total abdominal hysterectomy. Her abdomen is obese, distended, and diffusely and impressively tender to palpation throughout. Rectal exam reveals no gross blood, but a stool sample is guaiac positive.

Differential Diagnosis

Acute abdominal pain can pose a diagnostic challenge to clinicians as the presenting symptoms for a variety of etiologies are often nonspecific and overlapping. The differential diagnosis includes acute pancreatitis, abdominal aortic aneurysm, aortic dissection, myocardial infarction, acute diverticulitis, small bowel obstruction, peptic ulcer disease with perforation, and gastroenteritis. Though not applicable to this patient given her past surgical history, the differential also includes cholecystitis and appendicitis.

Workup

The patient undergoes CT angiography (CTA) for further evaluation of her abdominal pain, which reveals an abrupt cut-off in the superior mesenteric artery (SMA), approximately 4 cm distal to the vessel's take-off from the aorta. The small bowel is dilated, the walls are thickened, and there is trace free fluid in the pelvis. Laboratory testing is significant for a serum lactate level of 2.8 mmol/L, a leukocytosis of 16,200 cells/mL, a serum bicarbonate level of 19 mEq/L, an INR of 1.1, a partial thromboplastic time (PTT) of 22 seconds, and a prothrombin time (PT) of 13 seconds.

CTA has become the most important diagnostic test for acute mesenteric ischemia (AMI). While angiography has been the historic gold standard and has the benefit of also allowing for simultaneous endovascular revascularization options, CTA has the advantages of being more readily available and rapid. It also permits simultaneous evaluation of the bowel and the vasculature, as well as allowing for a more thorough evaluation of the abdominal cavity, which may rule out other etiologies, as the diagnosis is often in question prior to performing the CTA.

A number of laboratory abnormalities are variably present in AMI. Unfortunately, no specific, rapidly available serum marker exists for AMI in the way that cardiac enzymes are available for myocardial ischemia, for example. Worse yet, most of the markers that do rise in AMI only do so after transmural bowel infarction has already occurred. AMI causes a significant elevation in the white blood cell count, and lactic acidosis and serum amylasemia are often seen later in the course of the disease.

Diagnosis and Treatment

AMI is a relatively uncommon diagnosis, accounting for <1 in every 10,000 admissions. However, maintaining a high index of suspicion is critical because mortality is very high with this disease process and a delay in diagnosis and treatment can be fatal. Even if diagnosed within 24 hours, the mortality rate is 50%, and it climbs to over 70% if the diagnosis is established after that. AMI is typically the clinical manifestation of one of four processes: embolism, thrombosis, nonocclusive mesenteric ischemia (NOMI), or mesenteric venous thrombosis (MVT).

An embolic event, usually to the SMA, is the most common cause of AMI, accounting for approximately half of all cases (Figure 1). Risk factors include atrial fibrillation, congestive heart failure, a history of prior embolic events, and a recent myocardial infarction. Emboli tend to lodge in the SMA distal to the takeoff of the middle colic artery, which causes ischemia of the distal jejunum through the ascending colon, with

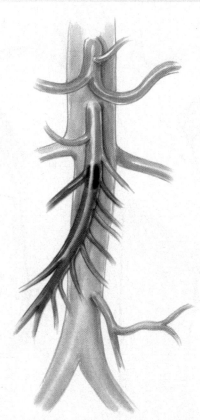

FIGURE 1 • Acute embolus to the SMA usually lodges in the region of the first branches of the SMA, with the length of small bowel ischemia less affected, usually only portions of the distal jejunum, ileum, and colon. (From Cameron JL, Sandone C. Atlas of Gastrointestinal Surgery. Vol. 2, 2nd ed. 2011, with permission from PMPH-USA, Ltd.)

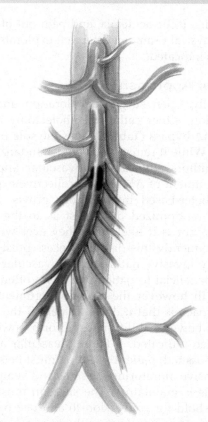

FIGURE 2 • Acute thrombotic occlusion of the SMA usually occurs secondary to a proximal atherosclerotic plaque, yielding extensive ischemia of the entire small bowel and large bowel. (From Cameron JL, Sandone C. Atlas of Gastrointestinal Surgery. Vol. 2, 2nd ed. 2011, with permission from PMPH-USA, Ltd.)

sparing of the proximal jejunum and the transverse colon.

Arterial thrombosis accounts for 20% of AMI cases. Many of these patients have extensive atherosclerotic disease in the mesenteric vasculature. A thorough history will often reveal abdominal pain after meals, weight loss, and food avoidance. Unlike in SMA embolism, which tends to occur slightly more distal, SMA thrombosis typically occurs at the origin of the vessel, which creates ischemia from the midduodenum to the splenic flexure **(Figure 2)**.

NOMI results from a relative low-flow state and vasoconstriction, creating an imbalance between mesenteric oxygen supply and demand. These patients typically have a heavy burden of atherosclerotic disease and are critically ill, which predisposes them to NOMI, though the celiac, superior mesenteric, and inferior mesenteric arteries are all usually patent. These patients' CTAs usually demonstrate narrowing of multiple branches of the SMA, alternating dilation and narrowing of the vessel, spasm of the SMA arcades, and impaired filling of intramural vessels.

CTA often will show a flattened inferior vena cava, consistent with the low-flow etiology of NOMI.

MVT is a less common cause of AMI. The ischemia is secondary to venous engorgement, which eventually impairs arterial inflow, which is why MVT has a more subtle onset than do arterial thrombotic and embolic events. Significant ascites is often appreciated on imaging. Many patients with superior mesenteric vein (SMV) thrombosis are asymptomatic, but patients with an occluded SMV on CT and abdominal findings on physical exam may have AMI.

In general, the cornerstones of treatment for AMI include fluid resuscitation, correction of electrolyte abnormalities, intravenous antibiotics, anticoagulation, immediate revascularization, and resection of irreversibly necrotic bowel. Patients with NOMI and MVT typically only require surgery for necrotic bowel. NOMI patients may benefit from intra-arterial infusion of arterial vasodilators, including papaverine. MVT patients require immediate anticoagulation. Given this patient's recent history of atrial fibrillation, cardiac disease, leukocytosis, low-grade fever, tachycardia, lactic acidemia, and pain out of proportion to physical exam, an emergent exploratory laparotomy is indicated.

Surgical Approach

Historically, open surgical exploration and revascularization, either catheter embolectomy or retrograde SMA bypass **(Table 1)**, was the sole treatment for AMI. While it remains the gold standard, a number of authors advocate endovascular approaches to the treatment of AMI as the collective experience with catheter-based interventions grows. No prospective, randomized data exist as to the optimal approach, nor is it likely that they ever will, given how infrequently this disease process presents. The minimally invasive nature of endovascular surgery may be beneficial to patients who are often already critically ill; however, the strongest argument against this approach is that it does not permit the surgeon to assess bowel viability and perform bowel resections when indicated. If an endovascular approach is to be pursued, patient selection must be stringent and intensive monitoring for signs and symptoms of peritonitis is mandatory. The surgeon must have a low threshold for conversion to an open operation. More often than not, even with successful endovascular revascularization, a laparotomy is still required to assess the bowel **(Figures 3–8)**.

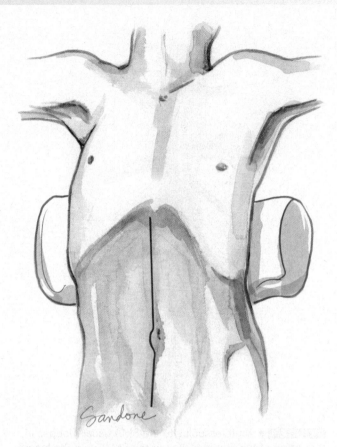

FIGURE 3 • A long midline incision is best used to evaluate the viscera and provide ample exposure to identify suitable targets for revascularization. The towel rolls lifts the costal margin upward and facilitates exposure of the supraceliac aorta, which is usually spared from significant plaque burden and thus may provide suitable inflow for SMA revascularization. (From Cameron JL, Sandone C. Atlas of Gastrointestinal Surgery. Vol. 2, 2nd ed. 2011, with permission from PMPH-USA, Ltd.)

TABLE 1. Key Technical Steps and Potential Pitfalls to SMA Revascularization (Figures 3–8)

Key Technical Steps

1. Liberal midline incision and full abdominal exploration.
2. Exposure of SMA by cephalad retraction of the transverse mesocolon, retraction of the small bowel to the right, and division of the ligament of Treitz.
3. Obtain proximal and distal control of the SMA and administer systemic heparin.
4. Perform an embolectomy via transverse arteriotomy and passage of a Fogarty catheter.
5. If inflow is reestablished, close the SMA utilizing a patch angioplasty if vessel narrowing is anticipated.
6. If inflow fails to be reestablished, the etiology is likely SMA thrombosis and a retrograde SMA bypass should be performed.
7. Create the distal anastomosis on the SMA first, ideally with saphenous vein graft.
8. Proximal anastomosis can be performed either on the infrarenal aorta or the iliac vessels.
9. Assess bowel viability after 30 min using visual inspection, Doppler probe, and/or fluorescein.

Potential Pitfalls

- Not adhering to "damage control" principles.
- Resecting too much bowel.
- Metabolic disturbances once the affected bowel has been revascularized.

Special Intraoperative Considerations

Many surgeons advocate a mandatory "second look" operation within 24 to 36 hours with minimal bowel resection at the time of the first surgery. While no data support or refute this approach, its supporters suggest that it minimizes the amount of bowel that must be removed as this waiting period after revascularization renders salvageable bowel that at first glance might have been removed. In addition, avoiding bowel resection and leaving the patient with an open abdomen permits a rapid return to the ICU for resuscitation and stabilization, as many of the patients are critically ill at the time of their operation. Other authors have reported the use of a selective second-look strategy.

Postoperative Management

Patients should be continued on systemic heparin therapy in the immediate postoperative period. All

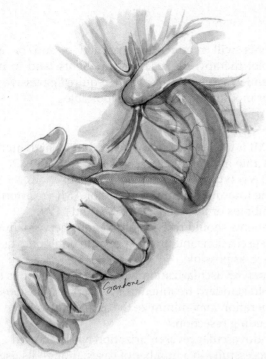

FIGURE 4 • Palpation of the root of the mesentery is the first step to determine the status of the mesenteric circulation. In thrombotic occlusion from proximal plaque, the pulse will be absent and a revascularization will be necessary. In acute embolus, a pulse will be palpable via transmission through fresh clot. (From Cameron JL, Sandone C. Atlas of Gastrointestinal Surgery. Vol. 2, 2nd ed. 2011, with permission from PMPH-USA, Ltd.)

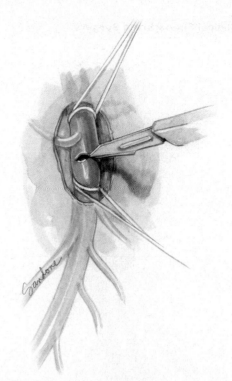

FIGURE 5 • A transverse arteriotomy on the mid-SMA in the region of the middle colic can be used to extract the clot. (From Cameron JL, Sandone C. Atlas of Gastrointestinal Surgery. Vol. 2, 2nd ed. 2011, with permission from PMPH-USA, Ltd.)

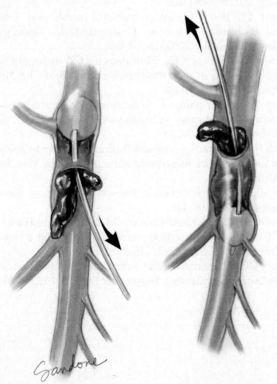

FIGURE 6 • A four to five French embolectomy catheter is used to clear the clot and restore inflow from the SMA. Distally, careful passes of a three to four French embolectomy catheter are used for clot extraction. (From Cameron JL, Sandone C. Atlas of Gastrointestinal Surgery. Vol. 2, 2nd ed. 2011, with permission from PMPH-USA, Ltd.)

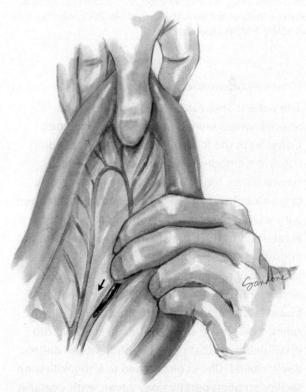

FIGURE 7 • Distant clot in the mesenteric arcade can be milked back to the arteriotomy to extract the clot burden. (From Cameron JL, Sandone C. Atlas of Gastrointestinal Surgery. Vol. 2, 2nd ed. 2011, with permission from PMPH-USA, Ltd.)

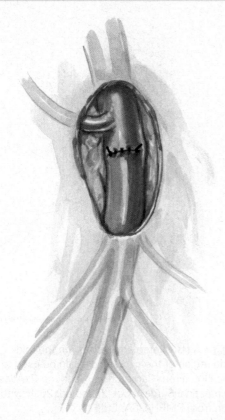

FIGURE 8 • Interrupted, nonabsorbable, monofilament closure of the arteriotomy is preferred to avoid narrowing the closed SMA. (From Cameron JL, Sandone C. Atlas of Gastrointestinal Surgery. Vol. 2, 2nd ed. 2011, with permission from PMPH-USA, Ltd.)

Case Conclusion

The patient undergoes an exploratory laparotomy, which reveals extensively threatened bowel from the jejunum through the ascending colon. An embolectomy is performed, which reestablishes blood flow after the removal of a large embolus. The patient's abdomen is left open with a wound vacuum system left in place. She is returned to the Surgical Intensive Care Unit for aggressive resuscitation. Approximately 36 hours later, she is returned to the operating room for a second look. Much of the previously threatened bowel has demonstrated significant improvement, though she still requires resection of the distal ileum. At that time, her abdomen is definitively closed. She is discharged to a rehabilitation facility on postoperative day seven, with warfarin anticoagulation, aspirin, a statin, and monthly vitamin B_{12} injections to compensate for the distal ileum resection.

patients will require anticoagulation and/or antiplatelet therapy. Because these patients tend to have systemic vascular disease, they require aggressive risk factor modification as much as possible.

TAKE HOME POINTS

- AMI is a relatively rare disease, but its high mortality rate mandates a low threshold for action.
- CTA is typically the diagnostic test of choice.
- The four most common causes of AMI are arterial embolus or thrombosis, NOMI, and MVT.
- Patients should receive intravenous heparin, fluid resuscitation, and broad-spectrum antibiotics as soon as possible.
- Open revascularization with bowel resection is the gold standard treatment for AMI. A second-look operation may minimize the amount of bowel needing resection.
- Endovascular revascularization has been used successfully in a number of cases, though its use does not preclude the need for a laparotomy to assess bowel viability and to resect if necessary.

SUGGESTED READINGS

Arthurs ZM, Titus J, Bannazadeh, et al. A comparison of endovascular revascularization with traditional therapy for the treatment of acute mesenteric ischemia. J Vasc Surg. 2011;53:698–705.

Brandt LJ, Boley SJ. AGA technical review on intestinal ischemia. American Gastrointestinal Association. Gastroenterology. 2000;118:954–968.

Horton KM, Fishman EK. Multidetector CT angiography in the diagnosis of mesenteric ischemia. Radiol Clin North Am. 2007;3(9):677–685.

Meng X, Liu L, Jiang H. Indications and procedures for second-look surgery in acute mesenteric ischemia. Surg Today. 2010;40:700–705.

Resch TA, Acosta S, Sonesson B. Endovascular techniques in acute arterial mesenteric ischemia. Semin Vasc Surg. 2010;23:29–35.

Sise MJ. Mesenteric ischemia: the whole spectrum. Scand J Surg. 2010;99:106–110.

Wasnik A, Kaza RK, Al-Hawary MM, et al. Multidetector CT imaging in mesenteric ischemia—pearls and pitfalls. Emerg Radiol. 2011;18(2):145–156.

Wyers MC. Acute mesenteric ischemia: diagnostic approach and surgical treatment. Semin Vasc Surg. 2010;23:9–20.

84 Chronic Mesenteric Ischemia

MAUREEN K. SHEEHAN, MATTHEW J. SIDEMAN and KEVIN E. TAUBMAN

Presentation

A 67-year-old woman is referred for evaluation of possible chronic mesenteric ischemia (CMI). She has a 10-month history of postprandial abdominal pain, which has led to a fear of food and a 30-lb weight loss. Her past medical history is significant for hypertension, hyperlipidemia, and a 60 pack-year smoking history. She has had multiple tests including an esophagogastroduodenoscopy (EGD), colonoscopy, barium swallow, computed tomography (CT) scan, abdominal ultrasound, and a HIDA scan. She underwent a laparoscopic cholecystectomy 4 months ago for biliary dyskinesia without improvement in her symptoms.

Differential Diagnosis

The diagnosis of CMI is usually made late in the course of the disease. Most patients have had multiple tests before the diagnosis is considered. Peptic ulcer disease, biliary disease, enteritis, colitis, and gastrointestinal tumors should all be ruled out before settling on a diagnosis of CMI. However, in the patient with classic symptoms and significant risk factors, a high index of suspicion for CMI should be maintained and explored.

Patients with CMI tend to have the same risk factors as other individuals with atherosclerosis including hypertension, dyslipidemia, and smoking. The classic CMI symptom is postprandial abdominal pain, which typically occurs 15 to 45 minutes after food intake with severity frequently linearly related to the size of the meal. The pain is most often dull and located in the midepigastrium but may have some radiation. Due to the postprandial pain, many patients will develop fear of food—avoidance of food to avoid pain. As a result, significant weight loss tends to be a prevalent symptom as well. Because symptoms are general and nonspecific, patients will frequently have undergone extensive workup and perhaps treatment for their abdominal pain prior to presentation to a vascular surgeon.

Physical exam of patients with CMI tends not to be significantly telling. Patients in general will be thin secondary to their ongoing weight loss. They may have other sequelae of peripheral vascular disease, such as carotid bruits or diminished lower-extremity pulses. Patients may have an abdominal bruit present but that is neither sensitive nor specific.

Discussion

CMI is a relatively rare disease. Estimates show mesenteric atherosclerosis to affect only 17% of patients over 65 years of age, with many of the affected patients having asymptomatic disease. Open intervention was first described in 1958 followed by percutaneous intervention in 1980. Since the introduction of endovascular treatment, there has been debate regarding the best treatment for CMI. Open bypass has longer durability but carries significant morbidity and mortality. On the other hand, endovascular treatment has significantly less morbidity and mortality but also increased restenosis rates. Therefore, treatment choice needs to be individualized to the patient.

Workup

Duplex ultrasonography is an excellent screening modality for mesenteric occlusive disease. As noted previously, patients tend to have an ongoing history of weight loss and tend to be thin if not near cachectic so that imaging the celiac artery and superior mesenteric artery (SMA) with the ultrasound probe is not as difficult as usual; however, there remain the challenges of intra-abdominal gas and respiratory variation. Moneta et al. have reported that a peak systolic velocity (PSV) of 275 cm/s or greater in the SMA detects a 70% or greater stenosis with sensitivity of 92% and specificity of 96%, while a PSV of 200 cm/s or greater in the celiac artery detects a 70% or greater stenosis with a sensitivity of 87% and specificity of 80%. In a separate study, Zwolak et al. found that an end diastolic velocity (EDV) of 45 cm/s in the SMA correlated with a >50% stenosis, while the same was true of an EDV of 55 cm/s in the celiac artery. However, each vascular laboratory needs to determine their own criteria for diagnosis of mesenteric artery stenosis with validation.

Angiography is the gold standard diagnostic test and allows for definitive planning. Complete angiography requires both anteroposterior and lateral aortic views and may require selective injections of the celiac, superior mesenteric, and inferior mesenteric arteries. Atherosclerotic disease in the celiac artery and SMA tends to be orificial and may result from "spillover" disease from the aorta (**Figure 1**). Presence of well-developed collaterals supports the diagnosis of

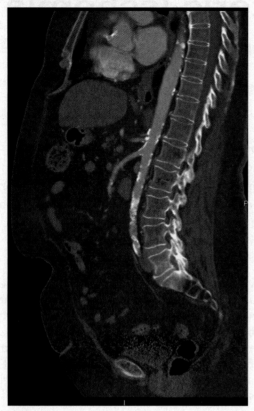

FIGURE 1 • Aortic atherosclerotic disease with mesenteric "spillover."

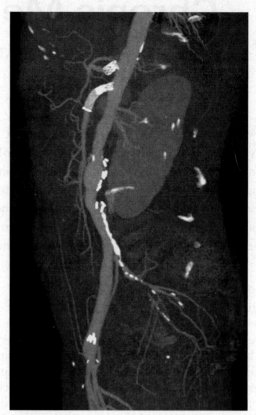

FIGURE 2 • Celiac and SMA stenting.

mesenteric ischemia. Generally, occlusion or significant stenosis of at least two of the vessels needs to be present for the patient to have symptoms; however, if the patient lacks adequate collateral pathways, symptoms may be present with disease of only one vessel.

general anesthesia. Benefits include the potential to reduce morbidity, mortality, length of hospital stays, and costs. Limitations of endovascular repair include questionable long-term durability. Restenosis within mesenteric stents is common **(Figure 3)**.

Presentation Continued

Computed tomography angiogram (CTA) of the patient showed atherosclerotic disease of the abdominal aorta with involvement of the visceral vessels. Lateral abdominal aortogram showed significant stenosis of the celiac and the SMA. Endovascular stents were place in the orifices of the celiac and SMA with resolution of abdominal pain and the patient was able to regain her weight **(Figure 2)**.

Diagnosis and Treatment

CMI can be treated endovascularly with angioplasty, or more commonly, stenting of the diseased vessels. This can be done for stenosis and occlusions, assuming that the occlusions can be crossed with a wire. Endovascular treatment is attractive because it is minimally invasive, can be performed at the same time as the diagnostic angiogram, and can be done without

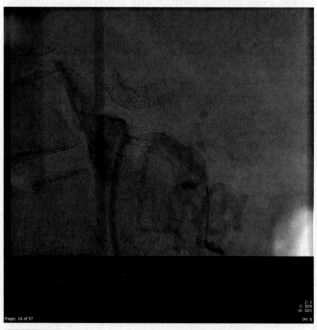

FIGURE 3 • In-stent stenosis of an SMA stent.

TABLE 1. Key Technical Steps and Potential Pitfalls to Endovascular Treatment of CMI

Key Technical Steps

1. Choose appropriate access site.
2. Insert sheaths and catheters.
3. Perform anterior–posterior and lateral abdominal aortogram.
4. Administer heparin.
5. Obtain wire access of mesenteric vessel.
6. Place long guiding catheter or long sheath into target vessel.
7. Chose appropriate type and appropriate-sized stent (consider IVUS to assist selection).
8. Treat addition mesenteric vessel as above if indicated.
9. Perform completion angiogram.
10. Surrender wire access and remove sheaths.
11. Consider use of closure devices.
12. Check distal pulses and monitor postoperatively.

Potential Pitfalls

- Access site complications.
- Inability to access target vessel.
- Distal embolization.

Technical considerations for endovascular repair include access site and stent choice **(Table 1)**. Femoral access can be used, but access of the mesenteric vessels can be difficult from this approach due to the angle of origin from the aorta of the celiac and SMA. A reverse curve angiographic catheter is used to access the orifice of the vessel, which can be difficult given the disease. Once the vessel is accessed, a stiff wire and either a guide or a long sheath should be advanced into the vessel to maintain access for the intervention. An easier approach is from the brachial artery, which yields a more direct access angle to the mesenteric vessels; however, sheath size needed for intervention must be taken into consideration in relation to the size of the brachial artery. If stenting is planned, a 6 Fr sheath will likely be required, which may be too large for a small brachial artery in an elderly female making brachial artery thrombosis post intervention an unacceptable risk or necessitating a brachial cutdown for sheath removal.

Once the diagnostic angiogram is completed, the decision made to intervene, and access to the target vessel accomplished, the distal vessel is assessed with angiogram and the appropriate-sized stent chosen. Intravascular ultrasound (IVUS) can be an extremely useful adjunct in choosing the appropriate-sized stent. Orificial lesions that are heavily diseased, and or calcified are best treated with balloon expandable stents given their superior radial force. If the disease extends beyond the bend in the SMA, consideration should be given to self-expanding stents to accommodate the tortuosity and motion of the artery. After successful deployment of the stent(s), a completion angiogram is performed and access surrendered. Closure devices for the access site are used at the discretion of the physician.

Success of the intervention is ultimately determined by symptomatic improvement in the patient. Function of the stents can be followed with duplex surveillance or by CT angiograms. Both modalities have their benefits and limitations. Duplex is inexpensive and noninvasive, but it is highly operator dependent and visualization of the stents can be problematic. CT is more reliable for imaging but is expensive and carries the risks of repeated radiation and contrast exposure.

Outcomes of endovascular treatment have shown good initial results but poor long-term patencies compared to open repair. Up to 30% of endovascular repairs will require secondary interventions for recurrent symptoms due to failing or failed stents. Despite these results, Medicare utilization studies have shown that mesenteric angioplasty/stenting has surpassed open surgical repair as the treatment of choice.

Surgical Repair of CMI

There are multiple options for surgical treatment of CMI **(Table 2)**. Since the disease is most often caused by "spillover" atherosclerosis of the aorta into the origins of the celiac and the SMA, one surgical treatment is endarterectomy. To perform this operation **(Table 3)**, a left-sided medial visceral rotation and retroperitoneal dissection is done to expose the abdominal aorta from the hiatus to the iliac bifurcation. The supraceliac aorta, infrarenal aorta, celiac, SMA, and left renal arteries are controlled with vessel loops. The patient is systemically heparinized and the vessels clamped. A "trap door" incision is made in the aorta by making transverse arteriotomies proximal to the celiac and distal to the SMA and then connecting them longitudinally on the left lateral side of the aorta. The anterior wall of the aorta with the visceral vessels is then reflected anteriorly and the atherosclerotic plaque removed from this segment as well as the celiac and SMA. The newly endarterectomized

TABLE 2. Surgical Options for Treatment of CMI

1. Aortomesenteric endarterectomy
2. Antegrade aortomesenteric bypass
   a. Conduit—autogenous or prosthetic
   b. Target—Single or multiple vessels
3. Retrograde bypass
   a. Inflow—Infrarenal aorta or iliac artery
   b. Conduit—autogenous or prosthetic
   c. Target—Single or multiple vessels

TABLE 3. Key Technical Steps and Potential Pitfalls to Surgical Treatment of CMI

Key Technical Steps

1. Midline abdominal incision.
2. Expose inflow vessel.
   a. Left medial visceral rotation for aortomesenteric endarterectomy.
   b. Through the lesser sac for antegrade bypass.
   c. Infrarenal aorta or iliac artery for retrograde bypass.
3. Expose target (outflow) vessel.
   a. Through lesser sac for celiac.
   b. Root of mesentery for SMA.
4. Confirm decision on number of vessels to revascularize.
5. Choose appropriate bypass conduit including type and size.
6. Systemically heparinize patient.
7. Clamp inflow vessel, perform arteriotomy, and complete proximal anastomosis with running monofilament suture.
   a. Alternatively, clamp aorta and mesenteric vessels; perform trapdoor incision and endarterectomized flap.
8. Clamp target vessel, perform arteriotomy, and complete distal anastomosis with running monofilament suture.
   a. Close trapdoor incision with running monofilament suture.
9. Reestablish blood flow through graft.
10. Assess mesenteric pulses and viability of the bowel.
11. Obtain hemostasis and consider reversal of heparin.
12. Close abdomen and transfer to ICU for postoperative care.

Potential Pitfalls

- Kinking of bypass graft.
- Ischemia-reperfusion injury to bowel.
- Significant aortoiliac occlusive disease.
- Distal embolic events.

portion of the aorta is then closed primarily with running monofilament suture and flow reestablished to the bowel.

The other surgical option for treatment of CMI is bypass. There are multiple options and configurations for bypass of the mesenteric arteries (Table 2). One option is an antegrade bypass with the inflow arising from the supraceliac aorta. The bypass can either be to one vessel or it can be a bifurcated graft to the celiac and SMA. If only one vessel is to be revascularized, the most important vessel to bypass is the SMA as it supplies the majority of the blood flow to the gut and has collaterals to the celiac and the inferior mesenteric distributions. For this operation (Table 3), a laparotomy is performed and the supraceliac aorta exposed through the lesser sac. The crura of the diaphragm are

dissected to gain full exposure of the aorta in this location. The distal targets are exposed and controlled. The celiac can be exposed through the lesser sac on the anterior surface of the aorta. The SMA needs to be exposed in the root of the mesentery. A tunnel is then created behind the pancreas connecting the exposed SMA in the root of the mesentery with the exposed supraceliac aorta. After completing the dissection, the patient is systemically heparinized and the vessels controlled. A side-biting aortic clamp can be used to partially occlude the supraceliac aorta and either a bifurcated graft or a solitary graft sewn with running monofilament suture. Autogenous venous grafts can be used instead of prosthetic if desired. The distal anastomoses are then completed in a standard fashion with running monofilament suture as well.

Another bypass option is a retrograde bypass to the mesenteric arteries (Table 2). In a retrograde bypass, the inflow is taken from either the infrarenal abdominal aorta or an iliac artery. Again, the bypass can be to a solitary mesenteric vessel or it can be bifurcated to two vessels. The operation is begun with a laparotomy and exposure of the inflow vessel with proximal and distal control (Table 3). The target vessel(s) are then exposed as described above. The patient is systemically heparinized and then the proximal and distal anastomoses are completed with running monofilament suture. Prosthetic graft material is generally used but autogenous grafts can be used as well. If vein is used for the bypass, it is preferable to make the length of the bypass as short as possible to prevent kinking of the graft. Care must be taken to measure the length and the angle to prevent this complication after the retractors have been removed and the bowel returned to its normal location. Again, if only one vessel is to be revascularized, the SMA is the most important vessel to bypass. A prosthetic graft has a theoretic advantage in this scenario. An externally reenforced polytetrafluoroethylene graft can be used in a gentle reverse "C" configuration from the infrarenal aorta (or iliac) to the SMA. The gentle curve allows the graft to lie within the bowel without kinking.

Regardless of the surgical approach to mesenteric revascularization, all patients need to be carefully monitored postoperatively for signs of visceral ischemia. Large-volume resuscitation may be necessary, especially if patients have sustained prolong bowel ischemia times. Lactate levels, urine output, and volume status all need to be closely monitored. The intensive care unit (ICU) setting is typically best suited for the initial postoperative care.

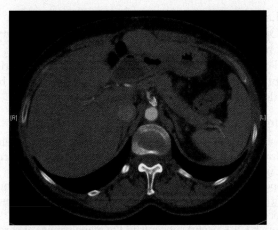

FIGURE 4 • Stenosis of celiac stent.

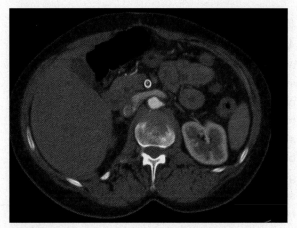

FIGURE 5 • In-stent stenosis of SMA stent.

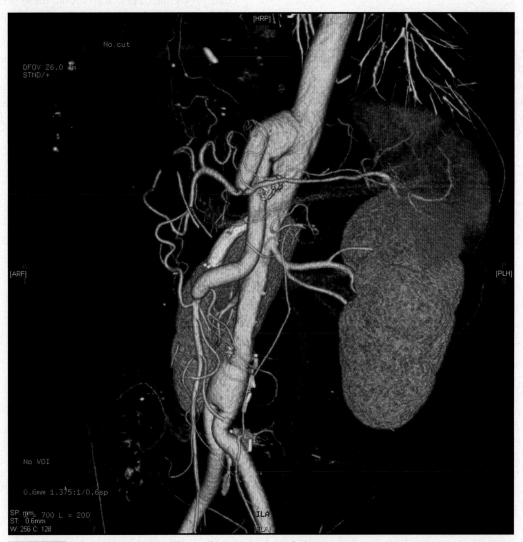

FIGURE 6 • Antegrade aortoceliac and aortomesenteric bypass.

Case Conclusion

Approximately 1 year after stenting of the celiac and SMA, the patient experienced recurrent symptoms of postprandial abdominal pain, fear of food, and weight loss. She continued to smoke heavily. CTA showed near occlusion of both stents (**Figures 4 and 5**). Conversion to surgical bypass was recommended. She underwent antegrade aortoceliac and aorto-SMA bypass without sequelae. She recovered well and had complete resolution of her symptoms. Postoperative CT scan showed good function of her bypass grafts (**Figure 6**).

TAKE HOME POINTS

- CMI is a rare disease.
- The triad of postprandial pain, fear of food, and weight loss must be present to entertain the diagnosis.
- Atherosclerotic disease with "spill-over" into the visceral vessel orifices is the main cause.
- Lateral aortogram is the gold standard test.
- Open surgical treatments include endarterectomy, antegrade bypass, and retrograde bypass.
- The SMA is the most crucial artery to revascularize.
- Endovascular treatment caries lower morbidity but also has lower long-term patency rates.

SUGGESTED READINGS

Ernst CB. Bypass procedures for chronic mesenteric ischemia. In: Ernst CB, Stanley JC, eds. Current Therapy in Vascular Surgery. 4th ed. Mosby, St. Louis, MO, 2001:682–685.

Moneta GL, Yeager RA, Dalman R, et al. Duplex ultrasound criteria for diagnosis of splanchnic artery stenosis or occlusion. J Vasc Surg. 1991;14(4):511–518.

Oderich GS. Current concepts in the management of chronic mesenteric ischemia. Curr Treat Options Cardiovasc Med. 2010;12(2):117–130.

Oderich GS, Malgor RD, Ricotta JJ II. Open and endovascular revascularization for chronic mesenteric ischemia: tabular review of the literature. Ann Vasc Surg. 2009;23(5): 700–712.

Schermerhorn ML, Giles KA, Hamdan AD, et al. Mesenteric revascularization: management and outcomes in the United States, 1988–2006. J Vasc Surg. 2009;50(2): 341–348.

Zwolak RM, Fillinger MF, Walsh DB, et al. Mesenteric and celiac duplex scanning: a validation study. J Vasc Surg. 1998;27(6):1078–1087.

85 Deep Venous Thrombosis

JUSTIN HURIE and THOMAS W. WAKEFIELD

Presentation

A 35-year-old man presents to the emergency department with a few days of left leg swelling and pain. The patient first noticed the swelling 3 days ago after returning on a long car trip from Florida. The patient describes his pain as an ache in his left leg and he has no prior episodes. The patient is otherwise healthy except that he smokes a half a pack of cigarettes a day. The patient takes no medications and has no family history of clotting and/or hypercoagulable conditions. The patient's physical examination is essentially normal other than extensive asymmetric left leg swelling that does not involve the foot. The patient's neurovascular examination is unremarkable, although pulses are only dopplerable and not palpable due to swelling.

Differential Diagnosis

In this scenario, the most likely diagnosis is deep venous thrombosis (DVT), which also carries the highest risk associated with a delay in diagnosis, given its association with pulmonary embolism. In an extreme form, phlegmesia cerulea dolens involves extensive DVT causing massive lower-extremity swelling and leg threat **(see Figure 1)**. The patient is relatively young without a history of trauma or use of anticoagulation, which if positive could indicate a hematoma as an underlying etiology. Another cause of leg swelling is lymphedema, which tends to include swelling on the dorsum of the foot. Although it may arise spontaneously, lymphedema may also be iatrogenic, after surgery or radiation therapy. Other possible causes of leg swelling include congestive heart failure or nephrotic syndrome, but these generally involve bilateral leg swelling.

Workup

Venous thromboembolism (VTE) is a common diagnosis encompassing deep vein thrombosis and pulmonary embolism, with a yearly incidence >900,000 in some estimates. The most widely utilized test to diagnose DVT is duplex ultrasound imaging with a sensitivity and specificity >95%. First, an ultrasound is performed using gray scale to image the external iliac, femoral, and popliteal veins. The veins below the knee are able to be imaged although with less reliability. Under direct vision, compression is applied, which causes normal veins to collapse completely indicating patency **(see Figure 2)**. When veins fail to collapse, either partially or completely, this indicates intraluminal material, usually either acute thrombus or chronic scar tissue **(see Figure 3)**. There are rough guidelines to distinguish acute from chronic clot, but none are definitive or absolute **(see Table 1)**. Acute clot generally appears echolucent and the vein that contains the clot may appear enlarged on ultrasound. As DVT becomes chronic, its ultrasound appearance changes and becomes echodense and heterogeneous, and the vein shrinks in size. Subacute thrombus generally represents a noncompressible vein with a combination of features of both acute and chronic clot.

The second component of duplex evaluation involves using color flow doppler. Color flow may give additional information regarding partial versus complete occlusion. In addition, color flow may give indirect evidence of occlusions not directly visualized. Lack of respiratory variation indicates an obstruction cephalad to the vessel that is being imaged. Flow augmentation is used to evaluate patency of caudad vessels.

Diagnosis and Treatment

The leading diagnosis is DVT and the main modality of treatment is anticoagulation. Initially, the patient may be treated with intravenous unfractionated heparin, subcutaneous low-molecular-weight heparin (LMWH), or fondaparinux. Patients with a reversible cause of DVT may be then treated with 3 months of anticoagulation using a vitamin K antagonist. An exception is patients with an active diagnosis of cancer who should be treated with 3 months of LMWH. In patients with an unprovoked DVT, the duration of treatment depends on the patient's underlying coagulability and should be at least 3 months. More details regarding duration of treatment are found in the CHEST guidelines (see suggested readings). Newer treatment modalities include the use of thrombolysis with the goal of reduction of clot burden. The goal of thrombolysis is to decrease the chance of developing one of the long-term sequelae of DVT, chronic venous insufficiency. Chronic venous insufficiency is due to longstanding venous hypertension, either due to valvular incompetence, obstruction or both. It occurs in up to 30% to 40% of patients 5 years after developing a DVT, with an even higher incidence in those with

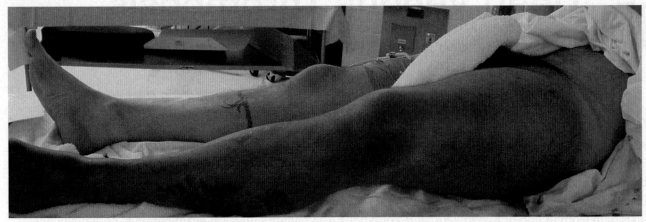

FIGURE 1 • Photograph of a patient with phlegmesia cerulea dolens.

iliofemoral DVT and those with ipsilateral recurrent DVT. Risk factors for chronic venous insufficiency include multiple DVTs, advanced age, cancer, recent surgery, immobilization or trauma, pregnancy, hormone replacement therapy, obesity, and gender.

In younger patients without a clear etiology, it is important to look for anatomic risk factors, such as the May-Thurner syndrome, defined as compression of the left iliac vein by the overlying right iliac artery, which forms an area of narrowing predisposing to thrombosis. Treatment of the May-Thurner syndrome includes venoplasty and stenting and, if thrombosis, thrombolysis, venoplasty, and stenting **(see Figure 4)**.

Surgical Approach

The primary determinant of the level of intervention is guided by the degree of symptoms. Systemic anticoagulation is the primary treatment for DVT. In patients that are unable to be anticoagulated, DVT is an indication for placement of an inferior vena cava filter. In patients with severe symptoms of leg swelling and extensive DVT, more aggressive intervention is indicated. In the most severe form, patients with phlegmesia cerulea dolens require venous decompression in order to decrease the chance of venous gangrene and the associated 20% to 50% amputation rate. One modality involves catheter-directed thrombolysis, which more quickly restores patency compared to anticoagulation alone. In patients that fail to respond to thombolysis, open venous thrombectomy remains a good option. There are a variety of adjunctive measures that may be required in order to correct any underlying anatomic abnormality. In severe cases with limb threat, fasciotomy after or simultaneous with thrombolysis or thrombectomy may be required to avoid amputation.

The patient should be placed on full anticoagulation involving heparin including a bolus (80 U/kg) or LMWH (1 mg/kg). Thrombolysis involves prepping the bilateral lower extremities circumferentially. The venous system may be accessed in the groin or

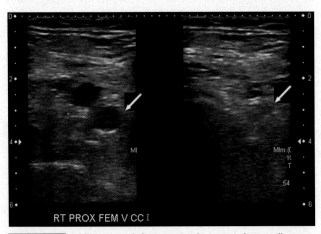

FIGURE 2 • Ultrasound demonstrating complete collapse with compression indicating a patent femoral vein.

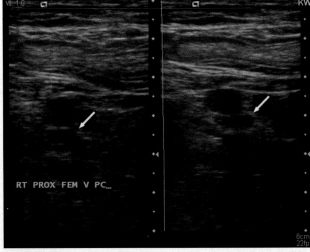

FIGURE 3 • Ultrasound demonstrating only partial collapse with compression indicating intraluminal thrombus.

TABLE 1. Acute Versus Chronic DVT

Acute	Chronic
Loss of compressibility	Loss of compressibility
Echolucency	Increased echogenicity
Lack of collateral vessels	Presence of collateral vessels
Venous distension	Shrunken fibrous cord
Surrounding inflammation	No inflammation

peripherally at the popliteal area. Once a guidewire is passed across the lesion and position confirmed within the distal vein, an infusion catheter may be placed with an infusion run overnight. Along with pharmacologic thrombolysis, today mechanical catheters are also used. These catheters use various physical principles to help obliterate thrombus, and when used in combination may decrease both the amount of thrombolysis needed and also the time thrombolysis is required (pharmacomechanical thrombolysis).

If these methods fail to reestablish outflow, open surgery may be indicated. The femoral vein is exposed through a groin incision. Cephalad and caudad control is obtained with vessel loops and a venotomy is made through the vein itself or a sidebranch. Five or six French venous thrombectomy catheters may be carefully passed in order to remove thrombus and reestablish venous flow. In patients with a chronic DVT, the femoral vein often contains webs (scar tissue) that requires removal. Once adequate flow is established, the venotomy may be closed with a polypropylene suture or with a patch of vein or polyester. A completion duplex is performed in order to evaluate for technical problems. In some patients, an additional venogram may be needed in order to confirm adequate clearance of clot.

Given the required use of postoperative anticoagulation, there is a significant risk of bleeding.

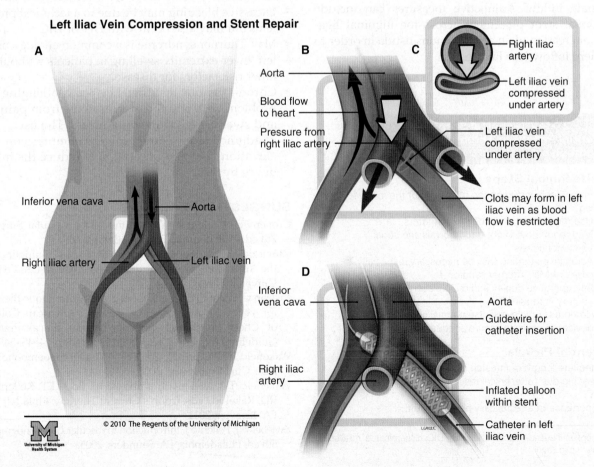

Left Iliac Vein Compression and Stent Repair

A
- Inferior vena cava
- Aorta
- Right iliac artery
- Left iliac vein

© 2010 The Regents of the University of Michigan

University of Michigan Health System

B
- Aorta
- Blood flow to heart
- Pressure from right iliac artery

C
- Right iliac artery
- Left iliac vein compressed under artery
- Left iliac vein compressed under artery
- Clots may form in left iliac vein as blood flow is restricted

D
- Inferior vena cava
- Right iliac artery
- Aorta
- Guidewire for catheter insertion
- Inflated balloon within stent
- Catheter in left iliac vein

FIGURE 4 • Depiction and treatment of May-Thurner syndrome, which is left iliac vein compression by the overlying right iliac artery.

This requires careful postoperative observation and adequate drainage. Another potential pitfall involves the unforgiving nature of venous interventions and a low-flow state. This requires the use of intraoperative duplex in order to evaluate for technical errors that may be easily remedied at the time of the initial procedure but may be catastrophic at a later point **(Table 2)**.

Special Intraoperative Considerations

As with most vascular cases, potential difficult situations will usually involve bleeding or the lack thereof. In terms of postoperative bleeding, one potential source is technical or another is generalized oozing due to ongoing anticoagulation. Additional causes of bleeding include the development of heparin-induced thrombocytopenia (HIT) or disseminated intravascular coagulation (DIC). HIT usually manifests 3 to 10 days after administration of heparin, although the time can be reduced with prior exposure. DIC can complicate thrombolysis and requires the serial measurement of fibrinogen levels. Finally, lack of flow can be just as detrimental predisposing the patient to vein and stent thrombosis. Outflow into pelvic veins can usually be treated using a combination of stenting and venoplasty. A more troubling problem can be lack of adequate inflow. Adjunctive measures can include additional stent placement across the inguinal ligament or creation of an arteriovenous fistula in order to augment inflow **(see Figure 4)**.

TABLE 2. Key Technical Steps and Potential Pitfalls in Thrombectomy/Thrombolysis

Key Technical Steps

1. Prep widely including the full extent of the involved leg.
2. Use mechanical thrombolysis catheters.
3. May require overnight thrombolysis and serial fibrinogen levels.
4. Adjunctive stenting may be necessary, especially in cases of May-Thurner syndrome.
5. Intraoperative duplex and drain placement if open surgery is required.
6. Compression/elevation/sequential compression devices in order to assure adequate inflow.

Potential Pitfalls

- Adequate length of infusion catheter to cross the lesion.
- Bleeding due to technical reason, anticoagulation, HIT, or DIC.
- Importance of a technically perfect result.

HIT, heparin-induced thrombocytopenia; DIC, disseminated intravascular coagulation.

Postoperative Management

The use of elevation, compression, and ambulation can reduce the incidence of chronic venous insufficiency (postthrombotic syndrome) by 50% and should be recommended to all patients with DVT along with adequate anticoagulation. In the case presented, the patient underwent thrombolysis and stenting for May-Thurner syndrome. The patient had resolution of her symptoms and improvement in her leg swelling. Postoperatively, the patient was treated with anticoagulation for 3 months and continues to wear compression stockings.

TAKE HOME POINTS

- VTE is common with an incidence of more than 900,000 cases per year.
- Duplex evaluation is the cornerstone for diagnosis of DVT.
- Evaluate for phlegmesia given the high rate of associated gangrene and amputation.
- Anticoagulation is a cornerstone for the treatment of DVT and duration of therapy depends on etiology.
- Consider thrombolysis for significant symptoms or limb threat in order to reduce thrombus burden.
- Excessive bleeding may be due to a technical problems but may also occur with HIT or DIC.
- May-Thurner syndrome is a common etiology of left lower-extremity swelling in patients without other risk factors for disease.
- Chronic venous insufficiency is a challenging problem with a range of symptoms from pain and swelling to nonhealing ulcers. The use of adjunctive measures, such as compression, elevation, and ambulation, may reduce the incidence by 50%.

SUGGESTED READINGS

Cronenwett JL, Johnston W. Rutherford's Vascular Surgery. 7th ed. Philadelphia, PA: Saunders, 2010.

Gloviczki P. Handbook of Venous Disorders. Guidelines of the American Venous Forum. 3rd ed. Oxford, UK: Oxford University Press, 2009.

Kearon C, Kahn SR, Agnelli G, et al. Antithrombotic therapy for venous thromboembolic disease: American College of Chest Physicians Evidence-Based Clinical Practice Guidelines (8th ed). Chest. 2008;133(6 suppl):454S–545S.

Wakefield TW, Caprini J, Comerota AJ. Thromboembolic disease. Curr Probl Surg. 2008;45(12):833–900.

Wakefield TW. Venous thrombosis. In: Bope ET, Kellerman RD, Rakel RD eds. Conn's Current Therapy. Philadelphia, PA: Elsevier, 2011.

Zwiebel WJ, Pellerito J. Introduction to Vascular Ultrasonography. 5th ed. Philadelphia, PA: Saunders, 2005.

86 Need for Hemodialysis Access

ALEXIS D. JACOB and THOMAS S. HUBER

Presentation

A 63-year-old female with a history of type II diabetes mellitus, hypertension, and chronic kidney disease (CKD) presents to the emergency room with shortness of breath and bilateral lower-extremity swelling. She states that she has not seen her primary care physician or nephrologist recently. She is hemodynamically stable but requires 2 L of oxygen by nasal cannula to maintain an oxygen saturation of >90%. Her physical examination is notable for bibasilar rales and pitting edema in both lower extremities. Her laboratory studies are remarkable for a blood urea nitrogen of 102 mg/dL, a serum creatinine 6.8 mg/dL, and a serum potassium of 6.1 mmol/L. An electrocardiogram demonstrates a normal sinus rhythm with slightly peaked T waves, and chest radiograph demonstrates findings consistent with fluid overload and congestive heart failure.

Diagnosis and Treatment

The patient appears to be in acute renal failure with the diagnosis based upon her generalized fluid overload, elevated blood urea nitrogen, and elevated potassium. She requires acute hemodialysis and needs dialysis access.

Discussion

The National Kidney Foundation Kidney Disease Outcome Quality Initiative (KDOQI) and the Fistula First Breakthrough Initiative (FFBI) have helped define the care of patients with CKD and end-stage renal disease (ESRD), emphasizing the role of autogenous hemodialysis access. These guidelines suggest that patients with stage 4 CKD (GFR < 30 mL/min) should be referred to an access surgeon for a permanent access well in advance of their anticipated dialysis initiation date. The guidelines recommend that autogenous arteriovenous access (AVF) should be constructed 6 months prior to initiation, while prosthetic access (AVG) should be constructed 3 to 6 weeks prior to initiation. Notably, the longer lead time for AVF allows for access maturation and any necessary remedial procedures. Additionally, patients with advanced CKD should be educated about the various options for renal replacement therapy (i.e., hemodialysis, peritoneal dialysis, transplantation) and engaged to preserve the veins on their nondominant arm for future access options. Despite national initiatives, the majority of patients in our country initiate dialysis with a catheter according to the United States Renal Data System. Although these dialysis catheters facilitate life-sustaining treatment, they are associated with a variety of complications including thrombosis, infection, and central vein stenosis/occlusion. The associated catheter patency rates are limited (i.e., primary patency rates 2 to 3 months), and the limited flow rates can lead to ineffective dialysis. Long-term catheter use is associated with increased mortality when compared to AVFs or AVGs, and the percentage of patients dialyzing through catheters is used as a marker of quality (or lack thereof) for the dialysis units. Noncuffed catheters are frequently placed in the urgent or emergent setting to facilitate the initiation of dialysis and should not be used for more than a week. Cuffed, tunneled catheters are more resistant to infection and can be used for time periods ranging from weeks to months. Both the noncuffed and the cuffed catheters should be inserted through the internal jugular vein opposite the side of the proposed permanent access. Notably, insertion of a dialysis catheter into the subclavian vein is associated with a significant risk of stenosis/occlusion that can preclude an ipsilateral permanent access.

Presentation Continued

A noncuffed hemodialysis catheter is placed in the emergency room and the patient is initiated on dialysis. The noncuffed catheter is replaced with a cuffed tunneled catheter after several dialysis sessions.

Diagnosis and Treatment

After the patient is "stabilized" on hemodialysis and her volume and electrolyte abnormalities are corrected, a permanent hemodialysis access should be constructed.

Discussion

As noted above, the KDOQI and the FFBI have emphasized the use of AVFs and have set ambitious national targets (AVF prevalence: KDOQI—65%, FFBI—66%). This strong emphasis on AVFs is based upon their improved patency rates **(Figure 1)**, reduced complication rates, reduced mortality rate, and lower cost when compared with both cuffed tunneled catheters and AVGs. However, not all patients have suitable veins for an AVF and there are some disadvantages with AVFs that include an obligatory maturation period that can last several months (frequently mandating the use of a cuffed tunneled catheter as a "bridge") and the need for remedial procedures to facilitate maturation. Although most providers would concede that a "mature" AVF is the optimal access, the ultimate goal should be a functional, durable permanent access rather than an AVF.

The evaluation of patients presenting for permanent hemodialysis access includes a focused history and physical examination in combination with noninvasive imaging. Special attention should be directed at documenting the access history including procedures, revisions, and associated complications. Physical examination should include a detailed pulse examination with an Allen's test to determine the forearm vessel responsible for the dominant arterial supply to the hand. The noninvasive testing in the diagnostic vascular laboratory includes examination of both the arterial and venous circulation. The arterial studies include blood pressure measurements of the brachial, radial, ulnar, and digital arteries along with the corresponding Doppler waveforms of all but the digital vessels **(Figure 2)**. Additionally, Allen's test is repeated and the diameters of both the radial and the brachial arteries are measured at the wrist and antecubital fossa, respectively. Venous imaging includes the interrogation of the cephalic and basilic veins from the wrist to the axilla complete with diameter measurements similar to the preoperative vein survey obtained prior to infrainguinal arterial revascularization **(Figure 3)**.

An operative plan is then generated, based upon the results of the history/physical and noninvasive imaging with a strong emphasis on autogenous access. Our objective has been to select the combination of the artery and vein that would most likely result in a successful AVF. We have not felt constrained by the usual conventions of using the nondominant > dominant extremity and the forearm > arm although we have followed these standard approaches when the choices are equivocal. The criteria for an adequate artery and vein include an adequate diameter, no hemodynamically significant arterial inflow stenoses, no venous outflow stenoses, and a peripheral vein segment of suitable length and diameter **(Table 1)**. Our preferences in descending order include the radiocephalic, radiobasilic, brachiocephalic, and brachiobasilic autogenous accesses prior to use of prosthetic material **(Table 2)**. Notably, these preferences are consistent with the current KDOQI guidelines. Contrast arteriography and venography can be used to confirm the preliminary access choice although these are usually reserved for select patients with suspected arterial inflow or venous outflow lesions respectively.

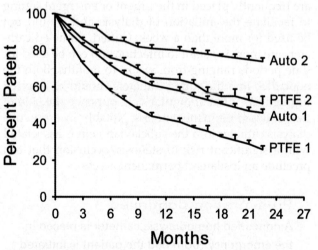

FIGURE 1 • The patency rates (percent patent) for the autogenous (*Auto*) and prosthetic (polytetrafluoroethylene [*PTFE*]) upper-extremity hemodialysis accesses are plotted against time (months) with the positive standard error bars. Both the primary (*Auto 1, PTFE 1*) and the secondary (*Auto 2, PTFE 2*) patency rates for the two access types are shown. The patency rates for the autogenous accesses were better than their corresponding prosthetic counterparts with the one exception of the initial (1.5 mos) time point for the primary patency comparison. (From Huber TS, et al. Patency of autogenous and PTFE upper extremity arteriovenous hemodialysis accesses: a systematic review. J Vasc Surg. 2003;38:1005–1011.)

Presentation Continued

The patient undergoes noninvasive imaging and is found to have a suitable basilic vein in the left upper arm for a possible AVF. Her brachial artery on the same side measures 3.5 mm at the antecubital fossa, and she has no evidence of arterial inflow stenosis based upon her Doppler waveforms and pressure measurements. Additionally, she has no evidence of venous outflow stenosis on either side.

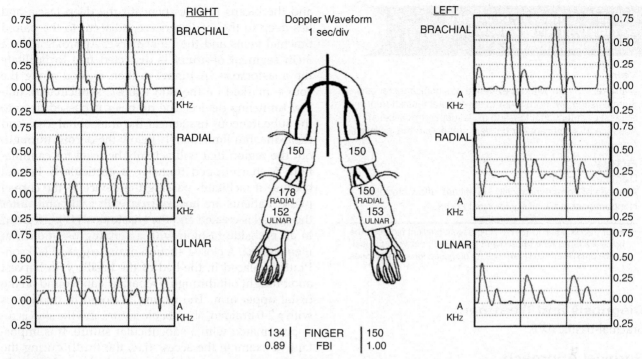

FIGURE 2 • Part of the preoperative noninvasive arterial imaging studies are shown. The brachial, radial, and ulnar arterial pressures (mm Hg) are shown on the diagram of the upper extremities, while the finger pressures are shown in the center of the figure at the bottom. The corresponding Doppler waveforms (sec/div) are shown for the brachial, radial, and ulnar arteries. The FBI denotes the finger/brachial index and is the ratio of the finger pressure to the ipsilateral brachial artery pressure. Note the symmetric brachial artery pressures and the corresponding normal appearing triphasic Doppler waveforms.

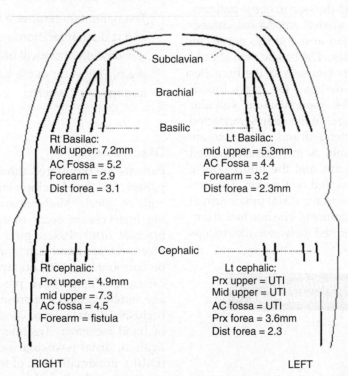

FIGURE 3 • Part of the preoperative noninvasive venous imaging studies are shown. The diameters (mm) of both the basilic and cephalic veins are shown on the diagram of the upper extremities. The diameters are reported for the corresponding anatomic segment (prx upper—proximal upper arm, mid upper—mid upper arm, ac fossa—antecubital fossa, dista forea—distal forearm). Note that the basilic vein segments in both upper arms and the cephalic vein in the right upper arm are suitable for autogenous access using the diameter criteria (≥3 mm). The cephalic vein in the left upper arm was unable to be imaged. Additionally, the patient has a patent access in the right forearm that was not imaged.

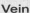

TABLE 1. Criteria to Determine Suitability of Artery and Vein for Autogenous Access

Vein

Diameter ≥ 3 mm without evidence of significant stenosis

Suitable segment from wrist to antecubital fossa (forearm access) or antecubital fossa to axilla (upper arm access)

Absence of significant central vein stenosis in the ipsilateral extremity

Artery

Diameter ≥ 2 mm

Absence of hemodynamically significant inflow stenosis[a]

Nondominant radial artery for wrist access

---

[a]Greater than or equal to 15-mm Hg-pressure gradient between the brachial arteries for proposed arm accesses or between the ipsilateral brachial and radial arteries for proposed forearm accesses.

Diagnosis and Treatment

Brachial-basilic AVF.

Surgical Approach

An incision is made in the upper arm over the basilic vein and this can be facilitated by having the course of the vein marked on the skin in the vascular laboratory during the preoperative evaluation. The basilic vein courses deep to the subcutaneous tissue and can actually be quite deep relative to the skin in obese patients. It courses adjacent to the medial antecubital cutaneous nerve in the distal upper arm and this nerve can actually serve as a landmark. The basilic vein should be dissected throughout its course and the branches ligated. We frequently suture-ligate the larger, broad-based branches with a 5-0 monofilament vascular suture. After the proximal end of the vein is transected (antecubital end), it is distended and all defects are repaired. The distended vein is then gently draped over the upper arm in an arc, and the future course of the transposed vein is marked on the skin. The brachial artery is dissected free in the distal upper arm at the site of the planned anastomosis. The brachial artery courses in the groove formed between the triceps

TABLE 2. Hierarchy for Permanent Hemodialysis Accesses Configurations

Autogenous radial—cephalic

Autogenous radial—basilic

Autogenous brachial—cephalic

Autogenous brachial—basilic

Forearm prosthetic

Upper arm prosthetic

and the biceps muscles beneath the deep fascia and lies deep to the median nerve, adjacent to the paired brachial veins and the ulnar nerve. Approximately a 3-cm segment of artery is dissected free to facilitate the anastomosis. A tunnel is then created along the course marked on the skin using a semicircular, hollow tunneling device. The tunneler is passed deep to the subcutaneous tissue near the antecubital fossa and the axilla, but immediately below the dermis throughout the region that will actually be used for cannulation. A sharp-tipped tunneler is particularly helpful because it facilitates passing the device in the correct plane. Patients are heparinized with 5,000 units after the tunnel is created and the anastomosis is performed in an end-side fashion with a running 6-0 monofilament suture. A closed suction drain (e.g., #10 Jackson-Pratt) is placed in the bed of the basilic vein harvest and brought out through a separate stab wound on the distal upper arm. The wound is closed in two layers with a 2-0 braided, absorbable suture and the skin is re-approximated with a subcuticular suture. It is important to examine the access (i.e., the thrill) during the closure to assure that it is has not been inadvertently narrowed or kinked.

Case Conclusion

The patient undergoes a left brachial-basilic AVF and is discharged home on her first postoperative day after removal of the closed suction drain. Follow-up to the vascular surgery clinic is arranged in 2 weeks.

Discussion

Patients are monitored throughout the postoperative period for the development of access-related ischemia or "steal." Moderate or severe symptoms requiring intervention occur in approximately 10% of the brachial artery-based procedures. The diagnosis of access-related hand ischemia is a clinical one that can be corroborated with noninvasive testing for equivocal cases. Preoperative predictors include advanced age, female gender, the presence of peripheral vascular occlusive disease, large conduits, and a prior episode of hand ischemia. Treatment options include access ligation, distal revascularization and interval ligation (DRIL), proximalization of the anastomosis, and limiting the flow through the access (e.g., "banding").

Patients are seen in the outpatient clinic 2 weeks after their operative procedure and at monthly intervals thereafter until their accesses are usable for dialysis. The KDOQI recommendations ("rule of 6's"—6 mm in diameter, 6 mm depth below the skin, 600 mL/min) are used to determine when the access is suitable for cannulation. Accesses that fail to dilate and those without a thrill are investigated with a catheter-based fistulagram to identify potential problems. Open surgical or endovascular procedures (e.g., balloon angioplasty, vein patch angioplasty) are performed as necessary based upon the fistulagram. When the accesses are ultimately deemed suitable for cannulation, the patients are provided with a diagram of their specific access configuration and instructions for cannulation while a similar facsimile is sent to their dialysis unit. The cuffed, tunneled catheter is removed when the AVF can be cannulated repeatedly.

TAKE HOME POINTS

• Patients with stage IV and V CKD should be referred to an access surgeon well in advance of their anticipated hemodialysis initiation date.
• Cuffed tunneled catheters should be inserted into the internal jugular vein contralateral to the site of the planned permanent access.
• A mature autogenous arteriovenous hemodialysis access is the best access option, but the primary goal is a durable, functional permanent access.

• Preoperative arterial and venous noninvasive imaging can help identify the optimal artery and vein combination for a permanent access.
• Patients should be followed in the surgical clinic until the access is suitable for cannulation and monitored closely for access-related hand ischemia.
• The construction and maintenance of hemodialysis access is a challenging problem that requires a lifetime plan and committed providers.

SUGGESTED READINGS

Fistula First Breakthrough Initiative: http://fistulafirst.org.

Huber TS, Carter JW, Carter RL, et al. Patency of autogenous and PTFE upper extremity arteriovenous hemodialysis accesses: A systematic review. J Vasc Surg. 2003;38:1005–1511.

Huber TS, Ozaki CK, Flynn TC, et al. Prospective validation of an algorithm to maximize native arteriovenous fistulae for chronic hemodialysis access. J Vasc Surg. 2002;36:452–459.

National Kidney Foundations KDOQI 2006 Vascular Access Guidelines. Am J Kidney Dis. 2006;48:S177–S322.

U.S. Renal Data System. USRDS 2010 Annual Data Report: Atlas of Chronic Kidney Disease and End-Stage Renal Disease in the United States, National Institutes of Health, National Institute of Diabetes and Digestive and Kidney Diseases, Bethesda, MD, 2010.

87 Emesis in an Infant

ERICA R. GROSS and ROBERT A. COWLES

Presentation

A 4-week-old, full-term male infant is brought to the emergency room by his parents at the instruction of the pediatrician. The mother reports that the baby has had several days of progressively worsening vomiting. The child acts hungry and drinks from a bottle without difficulty, but then, 30 to 60 minutes after eating, throws up most of his formula. The vomit is described as forceful and resembling formula. The baby is still having wet diapers, but not as frequently, and he is less active than usual. The pregnancy and the delivery were uncomplicated, and the infant is otherwise healthy and had been developing normally. Vital signs are remarkable for tachycardia. On physical examination, the baby is sleeping, but easily aroused. The anterior fontanelle is depressed. His abdomen is soft, nondistended, and appears nontender. No masses are palpable, but gastric waves are visible on the abdomen. No inguinal hernias are detected. A complete blood count and chemistry panel are ordered, and the results are given in **Table 1**. The patient is admitted for treatment of dehydration and electrolyte imbalance.

Differential Diagnosis

It is important to differentiate bilious from nonbilious emesis in a neonate. Bilious emesis raises suspicion for malrotation with volvulus, a true surgical emergency that must be ruled out. From the presentation above, however, this infant has nonbilious emesis, leading to the following differential diagnoses: formula intolerance, gastroesophageal reflux, pyloric stenosis, pylorospasm, antral or duodenal web, and gastroparesis. Recurrent emesis can also be associated with metabolic disorders, inborn errors of metabolism, or elevated intracranial pressure due to brain tumors; however, emesis is rarely the isolated symptom in these systemic or neurologic disorders. Based on the history provided by the caregiver, pyloric stenosis can often be identified by the report that the infant is hungry after emesis, that the emesis is forceful and nonbilious, and that the baby is otherwise well. As emesis persists over days, lethargy may develop secondary to hypovolemia.

Workup

The clinical history and the physical exam alone are sufficient to make a diagnosis of pyloric stenosis in the majority of infants with the condition. Electrolytes and an abdominal ultrasound **(Figure 1)** confirm the diagnosis and evaluate the severity of the associated electrolyte imbalance. Ultrasound is very sensitive and specific for the diagnosis of pyloric stenosis. It is quick, available, inexpensive, noninvasive, and does not expose the child to radiation. A pylorus is considered hypertrophied if the thickness is ≥4 mm and if the pyloric channel length is ≥16 mm. In addition to these static measurements, the radiologist can often assess whether fluid is able to pass from the stomach into the duodenum. In the uncommon situation that the diagnosis is not clear after physical exam and ultrasound, an upper gastrointestinal series can show a distended stomach that cannot empty due to pyloric obstruction ("shoulder sign") and a narrowed pyloric channel ("string sign") **(Figure 2)**.

Discussion

Pyloric stenosis is the most common cause of gastric outlet obstruction in the 1 to 2 month old infant and has an incidence of 1/500 live births. This disorder is most common in male Caucasian infants. No single etiology has been identified, but more than one family member can be affected.

Diagnosis and Treatment

The ultrasound of this patient showed that the pyloric muscle is 5 mm thick and the channel length is 20 mm. After receiving these results, the diagnosis of pyloric stenosis is confirmed. Pyloric stenosis is not a surgical emergency. What should be addressed urgently, however, are the infant's electrolyte abnormalities and hypovolemia. This child has a hypokalemic, hypochloremic metabolic alkalosis. Prolonged emesis results in dehydration, metabolic alkalosis, and hypochloremia. As dehydration worsens, aldosterone release stimulates the absorption of sodium and excretion of potassium in the urine in an attempt to maintain blood volume. Hypokalemia then causes the excretion of hydrogen and a paradoxical aciduria. In pyloric stenosis, the longer the duration of symptoms, the worse the electrolyte abnormalities become.

TABLE 1. Laboratory Values

Complete Blood Count		Chemistry Panel	
WBC	8.3	Sodium	136
HCT	38.6	Potassium	3.3
Hgb	13.7	Chloride	97
Platelets	301	Bicarbonate	30
		BUN	7
		Creatinine	0.4
		Glucose	93

It is important to re-hydrate these patients aggressively and correct their electrolyte derangement prior to surgery. All infants diagnosed with pyloric stenosis should receive a 20 mL/kg bolus of normal saline (NS). Closely monitor urine output and administer additional fluid boluses until adequate urine output is achieved (1.5 to 2 mL/kg/h). Intravenous (IV) fluids, D5 ½ NS, should be infused at 1.5 times maintenance rate. Potassium supplementation can be given after urine output is re-established. Emesis should cease once the infant is taking nothing by mouth and, therefore, a nasogastric tube (NGT) is not necessary.

Surgical Approach to Open Pyloromyotomy

After the electrolyte imbalances have been corrected, the surgeon must relieve the gastric outlet obstruction. Medical treatment with atropine and endoscopic dilation has been attempted, but these therapies are inferior to surgical treatment. The standard of care is a Fredet-Ramstedt pyloromyotomy. Classically, the

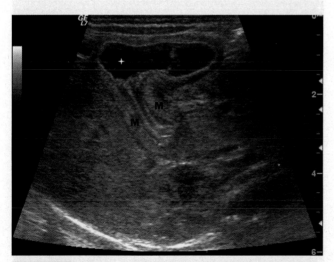

FIGURE 1 • Abdominal ultrasound of hypertrophied pylorus. The patient has taken Pedialyte® by mouth, and the stomach appears the density of water (*white asterisk*). Mucosa is radiopaque and is seen outlining the pyloric channel (*black asterisk*). The hypertrophied pyloric muscle (M) measures 5 mm in thickness and 20 mm in length.

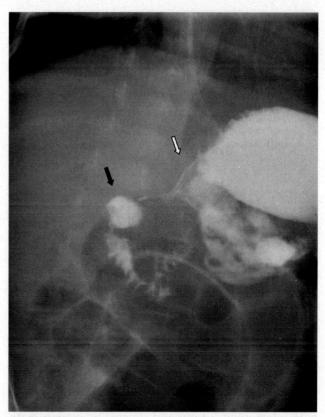

FIGURE 2 • Fluoroscopy after oral contrast. A string sign is seen between the antrum (*white arrow*) and the duodenal bulb (*black arrow*) indicating pyloric stenosis.

procedure was performed though a transverse right upper quadrant incision. A supraumbilical curvilinear incision is currently the preferred approach and will be described here (Table 2).

The infant is placed in a supine position on the operating table, an NGT is placed, and general anesthesia is induced. After the infant is relaxed, the pylorus should be palpable in the epigastric region. An incision is made over this area in the right upper quadrant or above the umbilicus and is carried down through the muscle and fascia. The omentum is retracted downward to lift the transverse colon and reveal the stomach. Then, the antrum and the pylorus are identified and brought through the incision. Holding the duodenum with the left index finger supporting the pylorus, the serosa is incised approximately 2 mm proximal to the pyloric vein extending onto the gastric antrum (Figure 3). A blunt instrument is then used to divide the remaining circular muscle fibers without injuring, or violating, the underlying mucosa. When separation is complete, bulging of the mucosa is often seen, and the two sides of the pyloric muscle can be moved independently. The anesthesiologist can then fill the stomach with air to assess for perforation. The pylorus is then placed back into the abdomen, and the fascia and the skin are closed.

TABLE 2. Surgical Approach to Open Pyloromyotomy

Key Technical Steps

1. Palpate the limits of the pyloric muscle. Identify the pyloric vein. Start the pyloromyotomy superficially, taking care to avoid the duodenum.
2. Extend the incision onto the antrum of the stomach
3. Bluntly separate the deep muscle fibers
4. Look for a bulge of the mucosa after completion of muscle separation
5. Test for duodenal perforation

Potential Intraoperative Pitfalls

1. Incomplete myotomy
2. Perforating the duodenal mucosa

TABLE 3. Surgical Approach to Laparoscopic Pyloromyotomy

Key Technical Steps

1. Avoid a shallow cut through the serosa with the arthrotomy knife

Potential Intraoperative Pitfalls

1. Incomplete myotomy
2. Perforating the duodenal mucosa
3. Prevent omentum from herniating through the trocar sites during closure of incisions

If the pyloric incision is not deep enough or long enough, the child may show signs of persistent pyloric obstruction and require re-operation. Incomplete myotomy commonly occurs proximally, close to the gastric antrum. If the incision is too deep, through the mucosa, leakage of gastric or duodenal contents will occur. This most commonly occurs at the distal aspect of the incision, on the duodenal bulb. If this is identified intraoperatively, the mucosa should be closed with interrupted sutures and covered by omentum. In the case of perforation, the NGT can be left for 24 hours after repair to ensure gastric decompression.

Surgical Approach to Laparoscopic Pyloromyotomy

The first laparoscopic pyloromyotomy was described by Alain in 1991. Studies have shown that the laparoscopic approach is safe and effective and offers shorter operative times and hospital stays **(Table 3)**.

General anesthesia is induced and the infant is placed transversely on the operating table. The monitor is placed at the baby's head, across from the operating surgeon, who stands at the infant's feet. An incision is made through the umbilicus or inferior to it. The Veress needle is then placed into the peritoneal cavity through this incision. A 4-mm trocar is inserted after inflation and a 4-mm, 30° scope is inserted. The abdomen is insufflated to 8 to 10 mm Hg. Two 3-mm trocars are then inserted in the right and left epigastrum under direct visualization. The proximal duodenum is grasped with the left hand and an arthrotomy knife is used to incise the serosa of the pylorus **(Figure 4)**. The same landmarks are used for the pyloric incision. A laparoscopic pyloric spreader is used to spread the deep muscular layers **(Figure 5)**. Again, the stomach should be insufflated with the duodenum occluded to evaluate for mucosal perforation. The carbon dioxide is then evacuated from the abdominal cavity, and the

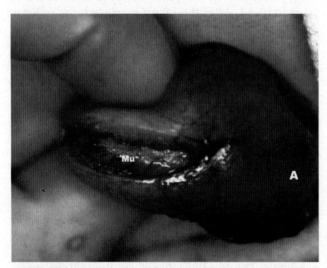

FIGURE 3 • Externalization of pylorus during open pyloromyotomy. The duodenum is being held, and the pyloromyotomy has been extended onto the gastric antrum. Mucosa (Mu) is seen ballooning through the completed incision.

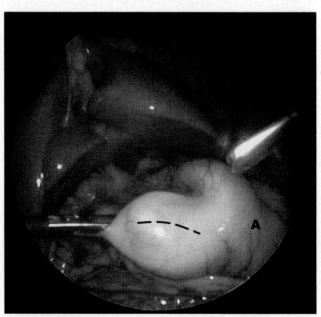

FIGURE 4 • Serosal incision on pylorus (*dashed line*) during laparoscopic pyloromyotomy, carried proximally onto the antrum of the stomach (A).

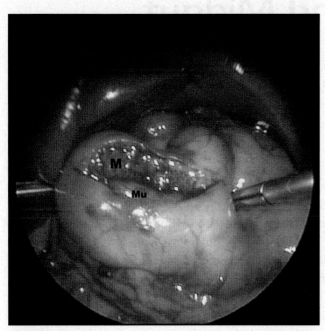

FIGURE 5 • The gastric mucosa (Mu) is seen ballooning through the completed laparoscopic pyloromyotomy (pyloric muscle, M).

umbilical fascia and the skin are closed. The epigastric incisions can be closed with steri-strips or Dermabond.

Special Intraoperative Considerations

While diagnostic error is unusual, a normal pylorus can be an unexpected intraoperative finding. This error in diagnosis is likely due to pylorspasm, a condition expected to resolve with bowel rest. When this occurs, patency of the stomach, pylorus, and proximal duodenum should be confirmed. This can be achieved by passage of an orogastric tube across the pylorus or by performing an intraoperative fluoroscopic gastric emptying study. In addition, other etiologies of upper gastrointestinal obstruction should also be ruled out.

Postoperative Management

Oral acetaminophen should provide adequate pain control. Oral intake can begin 4 to 6 hours postoperatively with small volumes of Pedialyte® and increased as tolerated. Once the infant is able to tolerate an adequate volume of Pedialyte®, he or she can be transitioned to breast milk or formula. It is common for an infant to vomit after surgery. If the infant vomits a feeding, allow 3 hours and re-attempt the same volume. Continue maintenance IV fluids until the infant is tolerating oral feedings well. Most patients are discharged 24 to 48 hours after surgery. Very few patients have long-term complications, such as gastric dysmotility. Any infant with persistent emesis 1 week after surgery should be evaluated for an incomplete myotomy or for severe gastroesophageal reflux.

Case Conclusion

The baby is adequately rehydrated, and electrolytes normalize over the first 36 hours. On hospital day 2, a laparoscopic pyloromyotomy is performed. Oral feeding with Pedialyte® is started 4 hours postoperatively and administered in increasing volumes every 3 hours. The baby has one episode of emesis, but does well, and is discharged home on the first postoperative day. At a 4-week follow-up appointment, the child is gaining weight appropriately according to growth curves.

TAKE HOME POINTS

- In any newborn, differentiate bilious from non-bilious vomiting. Bilious emesis is intestinal obstruction secondary to volvulus and a surgical emergency, unless proven otherwise.
- The morbidity associated with pyloric stenosis comes from the dehydration and electrolyte disturbances rather than the gastric outlet obstruction alone. The dehydration and hypokalemic, hypochloremic alkalosis require treatment with IV fluids and monitoring for correction prior to surgery.
- Postoperative vomiting is usually self-limited and does not indicate surgical failure unless it becomes persistent with failure to gain weight.
- Incomplete myotomy occurs proximally (gastric antrum). Perforation occurs distally (duodenal bulb).

SUGGESTED READINGS

Alain JL, Grousseau, Terrier G. Extramucosal pyloromyotomy by laparoscopy. Surg Endosc. 1991;5:174–175.

Aldridge RD, MacKinlay GA, Aldridge RB. Choice of incision: the experience and evolution of surgical management of infantile hypertrophic pyloric stenosis. J Laparoendosc Adv Surg Tech A. 2007;17(1):131–136.

Aspelund G, Langer JC. Current management of hypertrophic pyloric stenosis. Semin Pediatr Surg. 2007;16(1): 27–33.

Leclair MD, Plattner V, Mirallie E, et al. Laparoscopic pyloromyotomy for hypertrophic pyloric stenosis: a prospective, randomized controlled trial. J Pediatr Surg. 2007;42(4):692–698.

88 Malrotation and Midgut Volvulus

ADAM S. BRINKMAN and DENNIS P. LUND

Presentation

An 8-day-old male infant presents to the emergency department accompanied by his mother with concerns for feeding intolerance, weight loss, and several episodes of emesis. He was a full-term baby, born to a G1P1 healthy 29-year-old female. The labor was prolonged without distress to the fetus, but meconium was present at birth. He was discharged home on day of life two, afebrile, tolerating breast milk, having regular bowel movements with a discharge weight of 6 lb 14 oz. Over the past 2 days, he has had increasing episodes of nonprojectile emesis, slightly green in color both during and in between feedings. The infant's vital signs are temperature: 38.0, heart rate: 146, respiratory rate: 26, and systolic blood pressure: 86 mm Hg. He is alert but fussy and easily falls to sleep in his mother's arms with gentle rocking. His current weight is 6 lb 10 oz.

Differential Diagnosis

When evaluating a newborn with feeding intolerance and bilious emesis, the working diagnosis should be malrotation with midgut volvulus until proven otherwise. The classic presentation of malrotation consists of a previously healthy infant with sudden-onset bilious emesis, feeding intolerance, and failure to thrive. The differential diagnosis is included in **Table 1**. A newborn with feeding intolerance, irritability, and bilious emesis should be approached as a surgical emergency as outcome is largely time dependent.

Workup

While the true incidence of malrotation remains unknown, autopsy studies estimate it as high as 1% of the total population. Greater than 75% of patients present within the first month of life and 90% within the first year. Key factors to note during the history include a thorough prenatal and delivery history, discharge weight, feeding habits and duration, recent emesis (including amount and color), bowel movements, as well as other congenital anomalies. Bilious emesis remains the cardinal sign of malrotation with midgut volvulus. Of particular note, abdominal pain and distention are not prominent early features of malrotation; however, as volvulus develops with associated mesenteric compromise, pain, irritability, and abdominal tenderness become apparent. As malrotation is a primary developmental problem, it is not surprising that other congenital anomalies are observed in 30% to 60% of patients with malrotation as illustrated in **Table 2**.

While majority of patients with malrotation are diagnosed within the first month of life, a significant number of patients continue through childhood, adolescence, and even adulthood without diagnosis. Individuals >2 years old with undiagnosed malrotation often report intermittent abdominal cramps, poor weight gain, and, in advanced cases, malnutrition.

Initial assessment should begin with evaluation of age-specific vital signs, fluid status, and interaction with providers. Fever, tachycardia, lethargy, and dehydration all indicate severe illness requiring urgent intervention. A scaphoid abdomen is not uncommon although signs of distention, abdominal wall erythema, and focal/diffuse peritonitis are worrisome signs and often represent intestinal ischemia. Initial management should begin with stabilization/resuscitation, pain control, nasogastric tube insertion for proximal decompression, basic laboratory studies, and foley catheter placement.

An unstable child suspected of having malrotation with an acute abdomen requires no imaging modalities, but rather prompt transportation to the operating room. In a stable patient, initial imaging should begin with plain radiographs of the abdomen evaluating for signs of bowel obstruction, "double bubble," free intraperitoneal air, and gas/stool in the rectum.

The upper gastrointestinal series (UGIS) is the diagnostic test of choice to confirm the diagnosis of malrotation. Typically performed with barium or water-soluble contrast and placement of a nasogastric tube, contrast is slowly instilled into the stomach and

TABLE 1. Differential Diagnosis for Bilious Emesis in a Neonate

Malrotation with midgut volvulus
Duodenal atresia
Jejunal atresia
Incarcerated hernia
Necrotizing enterocolitis
Duodenal web
Meconium ileus/Meconium plug
Hirschsprung's Disease
Imperforate anus

its course through the foregut is monitored. Assistance of a pediatric radiologist and understanding of intestinal development will eliminate equivocal examinations and false interpretations, which occur in 15% of all upper GI studies performed for malrotation.

A normal UGIS illustrates a gentle C-shaped configuration of the duodenum, which crosses the midline and ascends to the level of the pylorus to form the duodenojejunal junction at the ligament of Treitz as illustrated in **Figure 1**. In patients with malrotation, the C-shape of the duodenum does not cross the midline and takes a caudal trajectory toward the right lower quadrant. In addition, the fourth portion of the duodenum does not rise to the level of the pylorus and the entire small bowel remains on the right side of the abdomen as illustrated in **Figure 2**. The key findings on the upper GI study include (1) abnormal position of the duodenojejunal junction, (2) corkscrew or spiral course of the distal duodenum and jejunum, and (3) location of the proximal jejunum in the right abdomen.

In addition to plain radiographs and upper GI studies, cross-sectional imaging and ultrasound examination can also be utilized. In patients with malrotation, the superior mesenteric vein lies to the left of the superior mesenteric artery and as midgut volvulus develops a "whirlpool" sign can be visualized. The use of ultrasound in children is noninvasive and easy to perform, but unfortunately neither specific nor sensitive to diagnose malrotation alone. Atypical vascular orientation or a "whirlpool" sign should alert the surgeon to

TABLE 2. Congenital Anomalies Associated with Malrotation

Intestinal atresia
Duodenal web
Congenital Diaphragmatic hernia
Gastroschisis
Omphalocele
Paraduodenal hernia
Heterotaxia syndrome
Meckel's diverticulum
Trisomy 21

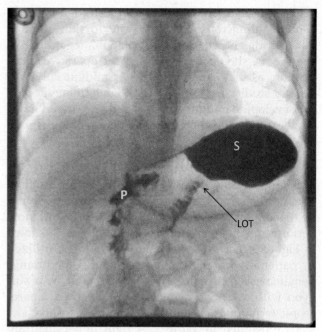

FIGURE 1 • Normal upper gastrointestinal series S, stomach; P, pylorus; LOT, Ligament of Treitz.

the possibility of malrotation, not used to confirm the diagnosis.

Diagnosis and Treatment

In a patient with tachycardia, hypotension, lethargy, peritonitis and acidosis emergent transportation to the operating room is needed. Preparation for operative intervention in patients without signs of systemic toxicity should include resuscitation, correction of

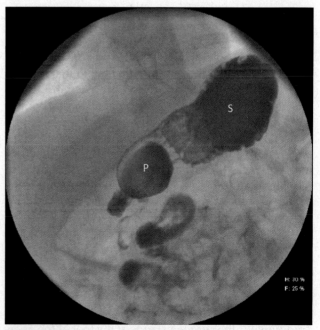

FIGURE 2 • Abnormal upper gastrointestinal series illustrating malrotation. S, stomach; P, pylorus.

electrolyte disturbances, and administration of intravenous antimicrobial therapy prior to skin incision. Patients diagnosed with malrotation, regardless of symptoms, should be scheduled for operative intervention, as they are susceptible to midgut volvulus. Several studies have attempted to determine the risk for developing midgut volvulus and have found it difficult to predict the risk based on radiographic imaging.

Surgical Approach

The surgical procedure for correction of malrotation, commonly known as Ladd's procedure, was first described by Dr. William Ladd in 1932 and now performed both open and laparoscopically as illustrated in **Figure 3**. The open technique should be utilized in patients with acute midgut volvulus, peritonitis, hematemesis, abdominal wall erythema or by a surgeon with a lack of comfort with advanced laparoscopic techniques. The procedure consists of five key steps illustrated in **Table 3**. A right upper-quadrant transverse incision is the preferred incision although a midline minilaparatomy may also be considered to gain entrance to the peritoneal cavity. The bowel should be eviscerated and carefully inspected for evidence of ischemia or perforation, and detorsed in a counterclockwise direction, often requiring one to three complete turns to fully reduce the volvulus. To assure complete detorsion and division of all coloduodenal bands, the proximal jejunum is grasped in the left hand and ileocecal junction in the right hand. The entire small bowel should then hang below the surgeon's hands in a "U" shape. The base of the mesentery should be widened by division of the anterior mesenteric leaflet. The small bowel is returned to the abdominal cavity and placed along the right lateral gutter and the colon along the left lateral gutter. Prophylactic appendectomy is also performed to prevent a future diagnostic dilemma. Potential pitfalls during the open Ladd's procedure are listed in **Table 3**. It is unnecessary to fix the bowel to the lateral abdominal wall with sutures after proper Ladd's procedure, as the bowel is rotated as far clockwise as possible and therefore not able to rotate any further. Several studies have clearly illustrated that fixation of the bowel to the lateral abdominal wall may actually increase the incidence of recurrent obstructions and offers no significant benefit to the patient.

In 1995, van der Zee and colleagues describe the first laparoscopic Ladd's procedure. A laparoscopic approach is not only safe and effective for the correction of malrotation but also leads to decreased hospital stay, decreased intravenous narcotic requirements, and earlier enteral feeding in both children and adults. Traditionally, the surgeon stands at the foot of the operating room table and three or four 5-mm laparoscopic

TABLE 3. Key Technical Steps and Potential Pitfalls for the Ladd's Procedure

Key Technical Steps
1. Entry into abdominal cavity and inspection of bowel.
2. Counterclockwise detorsion of midgut if volvulus present, potential bowel resection.
3. Division of coloduodenal bands (Ladd's bands).
4. Widening of midgut mesentery by division of the anterior mesenteric leaflet.
5. Prophylactic appendectomy.
6. Return of small bowel along right lateral gutter, colon along left lateral gutter.
7. Abdominal closure.

Potential Pitfalls
- Failure to completely reduce volvulus.
- Failure to divide all coloduodenal bands (Ladd's bands).
- Failure to place the small bowel along the right lateral gutter and colon along the left lateral gutter.
- Fixation of bowel to lateral abdominal wall.
- Failure to perform appendectomy.

ports are placed to aid in dissection. The steps to the laparoscopic technique are identical to those of the open technique as described above. An extracorporeal appendectomy can be performed through a port site to avoid placing a larger port, which would be needed for the laparoscopic stapler. The most difficult steps during the laparoscopic approach include the entry into the peritoneal cavity, confirmation of malrotation by identification of abnormally positioned anatomy, and detorsion of the small bowel. The surgeon should always have a low threshold for conversion should there be uncertainty regarding anatomy, acute midgut volvulus with fragile bowel, or failure to resolve the malrotation.

Special Intraoperative Considerations

If the bowel appears healthy upon entrance to the abdominal cavity, Ladd's procedure should be performed. However, if compromised bowel is encountered after the reduction of the volvulus, the surgeon has three main options including (1) resection of clearly necrotic bowel with primary anastomosis as illustrated in **Figure 4**, (2) return of compromised bowel to peritoneal cavity without resection, temporary abdominal closure with planned second-look laparatomy, and (3) resection of necrotic bowel with creation of stomas and planned additional resection if stomas become necrotic or elective stoma closure in several months. When the surgeon is faced with potential bowel resection, the ultimate goal should be preservation of the maximal length of intestine to prevent the serious complication of short gut syndrome. If repeat laparatomy is planned, it is recommended that a form of temporary abdominal closure be utilized to keep intra-abdominal pressure as low as possible.

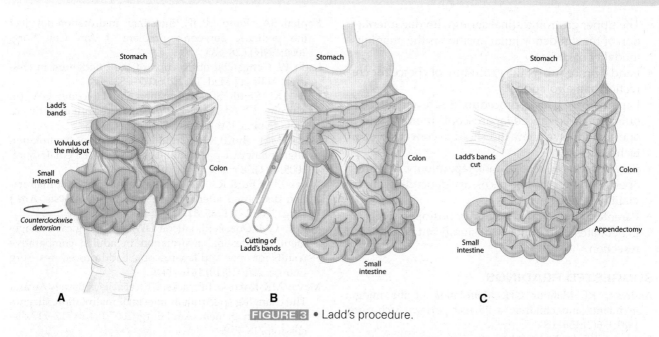

Stomach

Ladd's bands

Volvulus of the midgut

Small intestine

Colon

Counterclockwise detorsion

A

Stomach

Cutting of Ladd's bands

Colon

Small intestine

B

Stomach

Ladd's bands cut

Colon

Small intestine

Appendectomy

C

FIGURE 3 • Ladd's procedure.

Postoperative Management

With an uncomplicated patient, attention to providing appropriate analgesia, monitoring fluid status and resisting the urge for immediate enteral feeds is needed. Patients should have frequent vital sign measurements during the first 24 hours and in some cases may benefit from brief stay in an intensive care unit, especially if the patient had hemodynamic instability during the operative exploration or are <12 months old. Return of bowel function largely depends on degree and duration of preoperative obstruction and overall health of the patient, but generally enteral feeds can be started within 2 or 3 days. In general, patients who underwent laparoscopic Ladd's procedure can be fed 1 or 2 days earlier as compared to the open technique.

On the other hand, patients who have undergone Ladd's procedure for malrotation and were discovered to have had midgut volvulus requiring bowel resection are often critically ill and require admission to a critical care unit for support **(Figure 4)**. Parenteral nutrition is necessary if the neonate is to survive. Repeat laparotomy should be accomplished within the first 24 to 48 hours. If however the patient begins to decompensate as evident by hemodynamic instability, persistent acidosis, or necrotic-appearing stomas, return to the operating room should be much sooner than initially planned. The true incidence of recurrent midgut volvulus after Ladd's procedure is unknown but believed to be quite low, <1%. It must be kept in mind that these patients are susceptible to adhesive bowel obstruction as well.

TAKE HOME POINTS

• All children with bilious emesis should be suspected of having malrotation with midgut volvulus until proven otherwise.

• Older children and adults with malrotation often complain of chronic intermittent abdominal pain, cramps, nausea, and vomiting.

• A thorough history and physical examination are absolutely necessary with particular attention to vital signs, weight, fluid status, and evidence of peritonitis.

• A hypotensive neonate with bilious emesis and peritonitis should immediately be taken to the operating room for exploration.

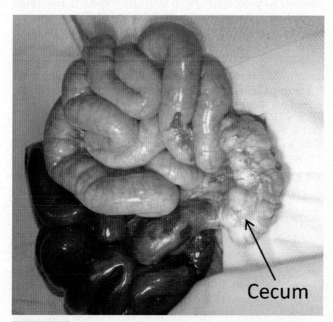

Cecum

FIGURE 4 • A 21-month-old male with malrotation and midgut volvulus.

- The upper gastrointestinal series with documentation of the duodenojejunal position is the imaging modality of choice.
- Ladd's procedure is the procedure of choice for correction of malrotation.
- Laparoscopic Ladd's procedure is safe and effective but requires advanced laparoscopic training, and one should have a low threshold to convert to open technique.
- Bowel resection, second-look laparotomy, and an open abdomen may be necessary depending on the viability of the bowel.
- Parenteral nutrition is necessary postoperatively in neonates who underwent significant bowel resection.

SUGGESTED READINGS

Andrassy RJ, Mahour GH. Malrotation of the midgut in infants and children: a 25-year review. Arch Surg. 1981;116(2):158–160.

Applegate KE, Anderson JM, Klatte EC. Intestinal malrotation in children: a problem-solving approach to the upper gastrointestinal series. Radiographics. 2006;26(5):1485–1500.

Bass KD, Rothenberg SS, Chang JH. Laparoscopic Ladd's procedure in infants with malrotation. J Pediatr Surg. 1998;33(2):279–281.

Bax NM, van der Zee DC. Laparoscopic treatment of intestinal malrotation in children. Surg Endosc. 1998;12(11):1314–1316.

Berdon WE, Baker DH, Bull S, et al. Midgut malrotation and volvulus: which films are most helpful. Radiology. 1970;96:375–383.

Draus JM Jr, Foley DS, Bond SJ. Laparoscopic Ladd procedure: a minimally invasive approach to malrotation without midgut volvulus. Am Surg. 2007;73(7):693–696.

Durkin ET, Lund DP, Shaaban AF, et al. Age-related differences in diagnosis and morbidity of intestinal malrotation. J Am Coll Surg. 2008;206(4):658–663.

Fraser JD, Aguayo P, Sharp SW, et al. The role of laparoscopy in the management of malrotation. J Surg Res. 2009;156(1):80–82.

James A, O'Neill J, Grosfeld JL, et al. Rotational anomalies and volvulus. In: Jaon Jr, ed. Principles of Pediatric Surgery. 2nd ed. St. Louis, MO: Mosby, 2004.

Kapfer SA, Rappold JF. Intestinal malrotation-not just the pediatric surgeon's problem. J Am Coll Surg. 2004;199(4):628–635.

Ladd W. Congenital obstruction of the duodenum in children. N Engl J Med. 1932;206:277–283.

Little DC, Smith SD. Malrotation. In: Holcomb GW III, Murphy JP, eds. Ashcraft's Pediatric Surgery. 5th ed. Philadelphia, PA: Elsevier, 2010:416–424.

Malek MM, Burd RS. Surgical treatment of malrotation after infancy: a population-based study. J Pediatr Surg. 2005;40(1):285–289.

Malek MM, Burd RS. The optimal management of malrotation diagnosed after infancy: a decision analysis. Am J Surg. 2006;191(1):45–51.

Matzke GM, Dozois EJ, Larson DW, et al. Surgical management of intestinal malrotation in adults: comparative results for open and laparoscopic Ladd procedures. Surg Endosc. 2005;19(10):1416–1419.

McVay MR, Kokoska ER, Jackson RJ, et al. Jack Barney Award. The changing spectrum of intestinal malrotation: diagnosis and management. Am J Surg. 2007;194(6):712–717;discussion 718–719.

Mehall JR, Chandler JC, Mehall RL, et al. Management of typical and atypical intestinal malrotation. J Pediatr Surg. 2002;37(8):1169–1172.

Millar AJ, Rode H, Cywes S. Malrotation and volvulus in infancy and childhood. Semin Pediatr Surg. 2003;12(4):229–236.

Pracros JP, Sann L, Genin G, et al. Ultrasound diagnosis of midgut volvulus: the "whirlpool" sign. Pediatr Radiol. 1992;22(1):18–20.

Prasil P, Flageole H, Shaw KS, et al. Should malrotation in children be treated differently according to age? J Pediatr Surg. 2000;35(5):756–758.

Smith SD. Disorders of intestinal rotation and fixation. In: Grosfeld JL, ed. Pediatric Surgery. Vol 2. 6th ed. Philadelphia, PA: Mosby Elsevier, 2006.

Strouse PJ. Disorders of intestinal rotation and fixation ("malrotation"). Pediatr Radiol. 2004;34(11):837–851.

van der Zee DC, Bax NM. Laparoscopic repair of acute volvulus in a neonate with malrotation. Surg Endosc. 1995;9(10):1123–1124.

Zerin J, DiPietro M. Superior mesenteric vascular anatomy at US in patients with surgically proved malrotation of the midgut. Radiology. 1992;183:693–694.

89 Neuroblastoma

ERIKA NEWMAN and IHAB HALAWEISH

Presentation

A 17-month-old male is brought by his parents to the emergency department with complaints of irritability, reduced appetite, and loose stools for the past 2 weeks. In addition, they note that his abdomen appears larger and more firm than usual. He is an otherwise healthy toddler who has been growing appropriately and meeting all milestones. He has had no unexplained fevers, weight loss, or abnormal skin lesions. The physical examination is significant for hypertension, abdominal distension, and a palpable abdominal mass in the left upper quadrant. A plain abdominal film shows displacement of the stomach medially and the left diaphragm superiorly. An abdominal ultrasound was obtained revealing a retroperitoneal mass.

Differential Diagnosis

The differential diagnosis of neuroblastoma (NB) is broad and varies according to the location of the mass. Suprarenal and retroperitoneal masses include NB, Wilms tumor, undifferentiated soft tissue sarcoma, and lymphoma. Metastatic disease in the bone marrow must be distinguished from lymphoma, osteosarcoma, Ewing's sarcoma, and primitive neuroectodermal tumors. NB is the most common tumor in infants and the most common extracranial malignancy in children, accounting for up to 8% to 10% of all childhood malignancies. Further imaging to characterize the nature of the mass is typically needed.

Workup

In addition to a complete abdominal and pelvic examination, including an evaluation for hypertension, the workup of NB involves a series of radiographic and chemical studies. A plain radiograph of the affected area may reveal stippled calcification within the tumor, common with NB. In children, ultrasound is typically the first imaging modality for solid masses and may reveal a lobulated mass of mixed echogenicity. Computed tomography (CT) with intravenous contrast can provide valuable information regarding the resectability of the mass as detailed by its relationship with surrounding structures and blood vessels. Large thoracic and abdominal tumors that encase any major blood vessels, encroach the spinal canal, or cross the midline are unresectable at diagnosis. CT may also help to define the extent of metastasis. Magnetic resonance imaging (MRI) will determine whether spinal extradural tumor extension has occurred. Bone scans and long bone plain radiographs will determine the presence of bone cortex metastasis. Iodine-123-labeled metaiodobenzylguanidine (MIBG) is metabolized by the medullary cells of the adrenal gland, and is useful in assessing primary tumors and metastatic disease. Bone marrow aspirates may show neuroblastic metastatic foci. A bone marrow biopsy of both iliac crests is often required in cases of negative bone marrow aspirates for adequate staging. Laboratory testing for the urine catecholamines homovanillic acid (HVA) and vanillylmandelic acid (VMA), which may be elevated in up to 95% of patients, is useful as tumor markers. In this case, a CT of the orbits, chest, abdomen, and pelvis reveals a large mass extending from the diaphragm to the pelvis **(Figure 1)**. There is also an infraorbital mass and lytic lesions in the right mandible, fifth rib, right humerus, iliac crest, and pubic ramus. MIBG shows enhancement in similar areas. Biopsy of the abdominal mass shows a small round blue-cell tumor consistent with NB. Cytogenetic analysis reveals MYC-N amplification and detection of loss of heterozygosity for chromosome 1p.

Discussion

NB is an embryonal cancer of the peripheral sympathetic nervous system with signs and symptoms reflecting the tumor site and extent of disease. Over 50% of cases occur in children <2 years and 90% of cases are diagnosed by 8 years of age. There are approximately 650 new cases in the United States each year. The majority of NB arises in the retroperitoneum (75%) with 50% in the adrenal gland and 25% in the abdominal and pelvic paravertebral ganglia. The remaining cases are at the paravertebral ganglia in either cervical or thoracic locations **(Figure 2)**. More than half of patients present with metastases to the long bones and skull, bone marrow, liver, lymph nodes, and skin.

NB arises from cells of the neural crest that form the adrenal medulla and sympathetic ganglia. The genetic event that triggers the pathogenesis of NB is most likely related to a series of prenatal and perinatal

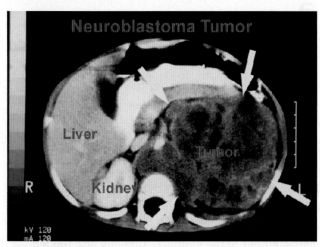

FIGURE 1 • Retroperitoneal NB that crosses the midline and encases the abdominal aorta and mesenteric vessels.

mutational events. NB exhibits extreme clinical heterogeneity from spontaneous regression in newborns to aggressive and metastatic disease in school-age children. There are several karyotypic abnormalities including chromosomal deletions, translocations, and gene amplifications that have been shown to affect prognosis. Aneuploidy of tumor DNA occurs and carries a favorable prognosis, whereas amplification of the N-myc oncogene (>10 copies) adversely correlates with prognosis independent of clinical stage in up to 30% of patients. Gain of 17q and deletion of the short arm of chromosome 1 (1p deletion) are also associated with poor prognosis.

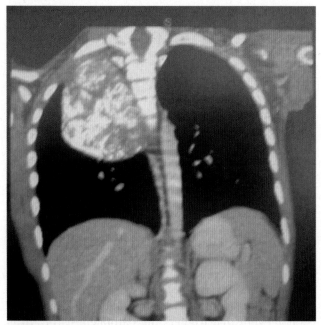

FIGURE 2 • Thoracic NB in the posterior upper mediastinum.

The clinical presentation of NB is insidious with vague symptomatology. Pain, due to primary or metastatic disease, is the most common symptom. Nonspecific symptoms include malaise, fever, sweating, weight loss, and growth retardation. Neurologic symptoms are less common and include Horner's syndrome due to invasion of superior cervical ganglion and paralysis due to spinal cord and nerve root compression. Opsomyoclonus syndrome is a paraneoplastic syndrome of autoimmune origin characterized by ataxia, opsoclonus ("dancing eyes"), myoclonus, and dementia. Orbital metastases with orbital proptosis, and periorbital ecchymoses ("raccoon eyes") are uncommon.

The diagnosis of NB is established from tumor tissue obtained by biopsy. Diagnosis can also be established by the presence of tumor cells in a bone marrow aspirate or biopsy. Histologically, immature neuroblasts appear as sheets of dark-blue nuclei with scanty cytoplasm in a delicate vascular stroma. Further differentiated masses contain ganglion cells with a more abundant stroma. Using the Shimada index, NB can be grouped into favorable or unfavorable histology on the basis of immunohistochemistry.

HVA and VMA in urine samples are elevated in 95% of cases and help establish the diagnosis. Evaluation of local disease is accomplished by ultrasound, CT, and MRI. During the workup for metastatic disease, bone scan has traditionally been used to detect cortical bone involvement and bone marrow aspirates or biopsies are used to establish marrow disease. MIBG can be used to evaluate the extent of bone or metastatic disease.

Diagnosis and Treatment

Patient stratification is important in guiding therapeutic options. The International Neuroblastoma Staging System (INSS) is the most widely accepted staging system and is the current standard for clinical trials **(Table 1)**. INSS takes into account the resectability of the tumor and the lymph nodal status.

The Children's Oncology Group (COG) has further developed a stratification system based on INSS stage, age, N-myc status, and Shimada histology that classifies patients into low risk, intermediate risk, and high risk **(Table 2)**. This provides the most accurate assessment and directs therapy for optimal outcomes.

Treatment modalities used in the management of NB are surgery, chemotherapy, and radiation therapy. In low-risk patients with stage 1 or 2 disease, surgery alone may be sufficient. Achieving complete macroscopic clearance is not essential as minor residual disease is usually stable with cure rates of >90% without further therapy. Chemotherapy is indicated in the event of relapse, or in the presence of N-myc amplification with unfavorable histology.

TABLE 1. International Neuroblastoma Staging System

Stage	Incidence (%)	Description
1	5	Tumor limited to site of origin
2A	10	Incompletely excised unilateral tumor. Negative nodes
2B	10	Unilateral tumor, complete or incomplete excision. Positive nodes
3	25	Unilateral tumor with contralateral nodes positive or tumor spread across the midline
4	60	Dissemination to distant lymph nodes, bone, bone marrow, liver, skin, or other organs
4S	5	Infants <1 y of age with stage 1, 2A/B primary tumor with spread to skin, liver, or bone

TABLE 2. Children's Oncology Group (COG) Risk Stratification for Neuroblastoma

Risk Stratification (COG)	Survival (%)
Low	90–100
Intermediate	75–98
High	20–69

In children with intermediate-risk disease and stage 3 or 4 disease, initial chemotherapy with chemotherapeutic agents such as cyclophosphamide, vincristine, dacarbazine, doxorubicin, cisplatin, and teniposide is mandatory, followed by surgical resection of the primary tumor. Radiation therapy is used for tumors with incomplete response to chemotherapy.

Treatment of children with high-risk disease includes induction with high-dose chemotherapy. In the event of response, resection of the primary tumor is attempted with administration of radiotherapy to the primary tumor bed. This is followed by myeloablative chemotherapy and stem cell rescue. Postchemotherapy treatment with 13-*cis*-retinoic to control minimal residual disease has been shown to improve outcomes in this group.

In some children with stage 4S disease without N-*myc* amplification, no treatment is necessary and the disease resolves spontaneously. Early treatment with chemotherapy or low-dose radiotherapy is required in the face of large tumors or hepatomegaly with mechanical obstruction, respiratory compromise, or liver dysfunction.

Surgical Approach

If the tumor appears resectable, without metastases, surgical resection is indicated with the goal of complete resection. Epidural anesthesia is often considered and provides excellent pain control in the postoperative period. For abdominal tumors, a full inspection of the liver with biopsy of any suspicious lesions and a sampling of lymph nodes are warranted for adequate staging and treatment planning. A minimum of 6 to 9 nodes should be obtained from the para-aortic region (hiatus to the bifurcation). The same principles apply to tumors in the cervical and thoracic regions, though sampling of contralateral nodes is not required. During thoracotomy for thoracic tumors or laparotomy for abdominal/pelvic

masses arising from the sympathetic ganglia, it may be impossible to avoid leaving small amounts of gross or microscopic residual disease along the nerve roots at the foramina. The areas are marked with titanium clips for postoperative monitoring. A small amount of residual disease with negative lymph nodes could still result in stage IIa disease with good prognosis.

For tumors with vascular encasement encountered intraoperatively, the tumor rarely invades into the tunica media of major blood vessels. The key principle is to identify major blood vessels early before they enter the tumor and then proceed with a careful and meticulous dissection is performed outside of the subadventitial plane with the scalpel.

Successful thoracic NB resection via a thorascopic approach has been utilized. The technique is useful for small (<6 cm), stage I lesions with favorable histology, and has been found to have similar local control and disease-free survival when compared to open thoracotomy.

Special Intraoperative Considerations

The most important factors of survival in NB are age at the time of diagnosis, N-MYC status, and stage. The current trend is to intensify therapy in the high-risk group and minimize therapy in low- and intermediate-risk patients. Current clinical trials are aimed at reducing toxic therapies in the intermediate-risk patients.

Case Conclusion

The patient's first chemotherapy course was complicated by the development of a right eye ptosis with sixth cranial nerve palsy and significant fluid retention that all resolved within the month. He tolerated subsequent cycles of chemotherapy without further events. He then underwent resection of the primary tumor, including dissection off of the right common iliac artery. His final stratification was stage IV, high risk. He went on to myeloablative chemotherapy and rescue bone marrow transplantation with complete response. He remains disease free at 6 months post therapy.

TAKE HOME POINTS

- NB is the most common tumor in infants and the most common extracranial solid neoplasm in all children.
- Low-risk disease may be cured with surgical resection alone.
- Current trials are focused on reducing chemotherapy and toxicity in intermediate-risk patients.
- N-myc amplification is associated with poor prognosis independent of patient age and tumor stage in up to 30% of patients.
- Complete surgical excision is the goal of operative therapy though effort should be made to preserve adjacent organs and the spinal canal.

SUGGESTED READINGS

Maris JM. Recent advances in neuroblastoma. N Engl J Med. 2010;362(23):2202–2211.

Maris JM, Hogarty DM, Bagatell R, et al. Neuroblastoma. Lancet. 2007;369:2106–2120.

O'neill JA. Principles of Pediatric Surgery. 2nd ed. St Louis, MO: Mosby, 2003.

Park JR. Neuroblastoma: biology, prognosis, and treatment. Pediatr Clin North Am. 2008;55(1):97–120.

Palpable Abdominal Mass in a Toddler

DOUGLAS C. BARNHART

Presentation

A 15-month-old boy who was born prematurely at 28 weeks' gestation is growing and developing normally. He has no other medical problems or long-term sequelae of prematurity. While giving him a bath, his mother notes a large mass that seems to be left sided. He is examined by his pediatrician who confirms the presence of large abdominal mass that is not tender. His vital signs including blood pressure are normal. Routine laboratories including a CBC and urinalysis are normal.

Differential Diagnosis

The sudden recognition of a large abdominal mass in an infant or a young child is not an uncommon occurrence and is the typical presentation for most intra-abdominal malignancies in this age group. These masses are often very large at presentation and are typically nontender and apparently asymptomatic. The most common malignancies of early childhood, which present with large abdominal masses, are Wilm's tumor (nephroblastoma), neuroblastoma, and hepatoblastoma. Less common primary pediatric renal tumors include congenital mesoblastic nephroma (infants < 6 months), clear cell sarcoma, rhabdoid tumor, and renal carcinoma. Rhabdomyosarcoma may also present with a large abdominal mass although this is more typically located in the pelvis as it often arises from the genitourinary tract. Less common abdominal malignancies in a young child are germ cell tumors and lymphoma.

It is important to recognize that not all palpable abdominal lesions in the young child are malignancies, however. Massive hydronephrosis can present with a large unilateral abdominal mass. It would be common though for these to be detected on prenatal ultrasound. Autosomal dominant polycystic kidney disease can present with bilaterally enlarged kidneys that may be palpable on physical examination. Large omental cysts, duplication cysts of the gastrointestinal tract, lymphatic malformations, and ovarian cysts may also present with abdominal fullness and possibly a palpable mass.

Workup

Given the lifelong risk of malignancy associated with radiation exposure in children, CT scans should be used judiciously. Abdominal ultrasound is the preferred initial study in a child presenting with a palpable abdominal mass. Most of the benign diagnoses can be made with the use of ultrasound alone. Patients with hydronephrosis, polycystic kidney disease, and ovarian cysts are likely not to require a CT scan for diagnosis and management. Children with solid or mixed (solid and cystic) lesions on ultrasound should undergo a CT scan with oral and intravenous contrast to characterize the organ of origin and anatomic extent of the mass. In some cases, it can be difficult to discern if a large tumor is arising from the liver (hepatoblastoma), adrenal gland (neuroblastoma), or kidney (Wilm's tumor).

Presentation Continued

The patient underwent a contrast CT scan that demonstrated a 7-cm mass arising from the left kidney. The CT scan demonstrated a "claw sign" in which the remaining renal parenchyma encircles the mass (Figure 1). This suggests a primary renal tumor even if the mass abuts and displaces the liver and the adrenal gland is not visualized. As Wilm's tumor can occur bilaterally (5% of all children with Wilm's tumors), it is important to assure that the contralateral kidney is normal. The CT scan often demonstrates compression of the inferior vena cava (IVC) by the mass. Wilm's tumor is prone to develop tumor thrombi, which can extend into the vena cava and even the right atrium. A Doppler ultrasound is typically obtained to evaluate the renal vein and the IVC. The lungs and liver are the most common sites of distant metastases. A chest CT is therefore obtained as part of the preoperative staging evaluation. The child's ultrasound demonstrated no signs of tumor thrombus in the IVC, and there were no distant metastases.

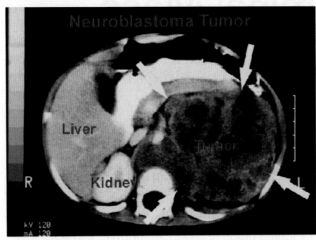

FIGURE 1 •The child's CT scan demonstrates a large solitary mass involving the left kidney. The renal parenchyma is displaced by the tumor. This "claw sign" is seen more clearly on the coronal images. The right kidney is normal. There was no evidence of hepatic or pulmonary metastases.

TABLE 1. Wilm's Tumor Staging	
Stage	**Description**
I	Tumor limited to the kidney and resected without disruption of the capsule or the biopsy
II	Tumor extends beyond kidney but is resected completely without spillage of tumor. Tumor may extend into renal sinus or beyond renal capsule but is contained within a pseudocapsule. All margins and lymph nodes are free of tumor.
III	Residual nonhematogenous tumor confined to the abdomen. Occurs in several ways: preoperative rupture, peritoneal implants, intraoperative spill, biopsy (preoperative or intraoperative), residual tumor left due to involvement of adjacent structures, resection margin positive on final pathology, lymph nodes involved.
IV	Hematogenous metastases (most commonly to lung or liver)
V	Bilateral renal tumors

Diagnosis and Treatment

Based on the age at presentation and appearance on CT scan, this toddler is presumed to have a Wilm's tumor and should be managed accordingly. The treatment of Wilm's tumor is multimodality and has been well defined initially through the National Wilm's Tumor Study and subsequently through Children's Oncology Group trials in North America. Similar organizations in Europe (SIOP–International Society of Paediatric Oncology) and the United Kingdom have conducted clinical trials as well. Essentially, all children are treated with surgical resection and chemotherapy. Radiation therapy is used to treat pulmonary metastases and selectively to enhance intra-abdominal local control. There are fundamental differences between North America and Europe in the approach to Wilm's tumor. The American approach favors upfront resection to provide immediate local control and accurate staging. This strategy may potentially diminish the required chemotherapy. The European strategy treats with chemotherapy presumptively without biopsy or initial resection in many cases. This strategy simplifies resection as there is often a dramatic response to chemotherapy. This may decrease the rate of intraoperative tumor rupture but confound accurate staging as lymph node status prior to treatment is unknown. The remainder of this discussion will focus on the American approach. All children with Wilm's tumor should be treated in a center with a multidisciplinary team.

Survival in children with Wilm's tumor is principally determined by the stage at presentation and the presence of diffuse anaplasia **(Table 1)**. More recent studies suggest that loss of genetic material at 1p and 16q may also be associated poorer outcomes. Children with favorable histology (lack of anaplasia) and lower stages (I–II) have excellent outcomes with standard two-drug chemotherapy (vincristine and dactinomycin). Typical therapy for children with higher stages of favorable histology Wilm's tumors adds a third drug such as doxorubicin. Children with favorable histology do well with even stage IV patients having overall survival near 90%. Anaplasia is associated with resistance to chemotherapy. These children do more poorly with overall survival in stage IV patients approximately 50%. Due to the markedly decreased survival associated with this histology, adjunctive chemotherapy regimens for these patients remain an active area of research.

Abdominal radiation therapy is used to improve local control in patients with local stage III disease. Whole-lung radiation is standard therapy for children with pulmonary metastases, but current research is directed to see whether this can be eliminated in those who have complete response to a more intensive chemotherapy regimen. Management of children with bilateral Wilm's tumors (stage V) requires preservation of renal function, while not jeopardizing oncologic cure. Decisions regarding biopsy and resection in these complicated children must be done as part of multidisciplinary approach and are beyond the scope of this discussion.

Decisions regarding local control are made independently of the presence of distant metastases. The three principal goals of laparotomy for Wilm's tumor are to (1) obtain accurate diagnosis and staging, (2) resect the primary tumor without causing local upstaging (i.e., tumor spillage), and (3) avoid resection of adjacent organs. Many Wilm's tumors present as very large masses, and size per se should not be considered a contraindication to upfront resection. Contraindications to initial resection include extensive venous tumor thrombus and invasion of adjacent organs. Tumor thrombus in Wilm's tumor can be extensive with involvement of the retrohepatic IVC and the right atrium. In such cases, operative biopsy and pre-resection chemotherapy are recommended as they typically reduce the thrombus facilitating resection. Tumor thrombus in the renal vein and infrahepatic vena cava can typically be extracted after obtaining vascular control of the IVC. The extent of tumor thrombus can be accurately characterized preoperatively using CT scan and ultrasound. In contrast, extension to adjacent organs can often not be determined preoperatively. With the exception of the adrenal gland, other involved organs should not be resected as a part of the initial operation. Rather in such cases, an operative biopsy should be performed and nephrectomy deferred until chemotherapy is given.

Surgical Approach

Given the large size and fragility of Wilm's tumors, generous exposure is required to avoid tumor rupture during resection. The importance of this cannot be overstated as tumor rupture will necessitate abdominal radiation even if the child was stage I or II preoperatively. Additionally, the large size of the mass frequently distorts relationships with adjacent visceral vessels making exposure essential for protection of the mesenteric and the contralateral renal vessels. The ureter must be resected with an adequate margin to assure that it is free of tumor. Finally, proper staging must include aortocaval lymph node sampling and inspection of the peritoneal surfaces.

In order to accomplish these goals, a generous transverse laparotomy is typically performed **(Table 2)**. For large right-sided tumors, a thoracoabdominal exposure may facilitate vascular control and mobilization of the tumor. A retroperitoneal, flank approach is not appropriate due to the large size of these tumors and the clinical significance of an intraoperative rupture. Laparoscopic resection is not appropriate for upfront resection but is being explored using the European approach of delayed resection after preoperative chemotherapy.

Upon entry into the peritoneal cavity, inspection and palpation is performed for staging, and all findings are documented. Any bloody fluid in the peritoneum is recorded and collected. The peritoneum is inspected for tumor implants. Either of these findings would suggest preoperative tumor rupture. The liver is inspected and palpated although most lesions would be identified on preoperative imaging. In the past, the contralateral kidney was exposed, inspected, and palpated on both the anterior and the posterior surfaces. This maneuver placed this typically normal and soon-to-be solitary kidney at risk of injury. Given the accuracy of current CT scans, this is not necessary and should be avoided. If there is no obvious invasion of adjacent organs on this initial examination, it is appropriate to begin mobilization for nephrectomy. In the case of obvious invasion of other organs, a wedge

---

TABLE 2. Key Technical Steps and Potential Pitfalls

Key Technical Steps

1. Generous transverse supraumbilical laparotomy or thoracoabdominal approach.
2. Inspection of peritoneum for evidence of rupture, peritoneal implants or other metastases.
3. Mobilize colon and duodenum to expose tumor and involved kidney.
4. Mobilize tumor and kidney without disruption of capsule.
5. Control renal artery and vein. Palpate vein to evaluate for tumor thrombus. Divide artery followed by vein.
6. Mobilize ureter into pelvis to allow resection en bloc.
7. Aortocaval lymph node sampling.

Potential Pitfalls

- Unnecessary biopsy of mass.
- Disruption of tumor capsule resulting in spillage of tumor.
- Resection of adjacent organs (except adrenal gland) (invasion should prompt biopsy and chemotherapy prior to resection).
- Misidentification and subsequent division of mesenteric or contralateral renal vessels.
- Failure to perform aortocaval lymph node sampling.

---

biopsy should be performed. A generous biopsy should be obtained as core needle biopsies may fail to detect anaplasia. Any type of biopsy is considered to cause rupture of the tumor and results in upstaging of the tumor (stage III). Therefore, a tumor that can be resected should not be biopsied simply to confirm the diagnosis prior to resection.

After resection is decided upon, the peritoneal reflection of the ipsilateral portion of the colon is divided to allow the colon to be mobilized medially. The duodenum is similarly mobilized to allow exposure of the renal hilum, IVC, and aorta. If the aorta can be exposed initially, the renal artery should be isolated and divided after mobilization and retraction of the renal vein. This is followed by ligation of the vein. In most cases, however, the tumor is sufficiently large that the IVC and the aorta will be obscured. In these cases, initial mobilization of the tumor will be required to allow access to the aorta and the IVC.

The tumor is mobilized typically in a gradual circumferential fashion. It is common for there to be neovascularity from the retroperitoneum. Vessel-sealing devices are helpful in this mobilization. Careful attention must be paid to avoid traction on the mass as the tumor capsule is easily disrupted resulting spillage of tumor. If the ipsilateral adrenal gland is adherent to the tumor, it should be resected along with the nephrectomy specimen. No attempt to separate the adrenal gland should be made if this may increase the risk of tumor rupture. As the nephrectomy specimen is circumferentially mobilized, the ureter will become apparent. The ureter should be dissected distally to allow resection en bloc with the nephrectomy specimen. The ureter is divided as distally as possible, but it is unnecessary to resect a cuff of bladder. Mobilization of the tumor allows it to be rolled medially to provide posterior exposure of the renal artery. Duplicated renal arteries are common and should be sought. Dissection of the renal vein allows it to be retracted to provide anterior exposure of the renal artery was well. With left-sided tumors, the gonadal vein may be divided to facilitate this exposure.

Ideally, the artery is ligated prior to division of the renal vein to avoid engorgement of the tumor. There can be marked distortion of the mesenteric and the contralateral renal vessels with large Wilm's tumors, so it is essential to achieve adequate exposure of the aorta to verify the anatomy prior to ligation of the purported renal artery. The renal vein should be palpated for tumor thrombus prior to ligation. If there is tumor thrombus present, proximal and distal control of the IVC must be obtained so that renal vein/IVC junction can be opened for a tumor thrombectomy. Typically, the tumor thrombus is not densely adherent and can be withdrawn through the venotomy with forceps. Division of the renal vessels and ureter provides access to any remaining retroperitoneal attachments that can be divided with electrocautery to complete the nephrectomy.

The nephrectomy specimen should be sent intact to pathology. As an important part of the pathologic staging of Wilm's tumor is a systematic microscopic examination of inked margins, bivalving the specimen in the operating room is contraindicated.

After removal of the nephrectomy specimen, the aorta and IVC are clearly visible allowing aortocaval lymph node sampling. As 41% of stage III tumors are due to lymph node involvement only, this node sampling is essential to correct staging. All visible aortocaval lymph nodes are removed, but it is not necessary to perform a formal lymph node dissection that may be associated with increased morbidity. Hemostasis is verified and lymphatic leaks sought prior to closure of the laparotomy.

Consideration should be given to placing a subcutaneous venous access port at the time of nephrectomy. This should be decided in discussion with the pediatric medical oncologist as some children with stage I tumors may be successfully managed with only a peripherally inserted central catheter. Additionally, a current study is investigating whether chemotherapy may be safely eliminated in infants with stage I smaller tumors. All others can typically be treated with a single lumen central venous access device.

Postoperative Care

Children may be admitted to the acute care floor or intensive care dependent upon local practice with particular attention to assuring adequate analgesia and fluid resuscitation. Many children will benefit from epidural analgesia if it is available. It is essential to assure adequate intravascular volume to provide perfusion to the now solitary kidney, and urine output should be carefully monitored typically with a Foley catheter. Most children's postoperative ileus is relatively brief (2 to 4 days) and nasogastric decompression is not routinely required. Small bowel: small bowel intussusception can occur in the immediate postoperative period in children who underwent resection of retroperitoneal tumors. This should be sought if the child seems to have a prolonged postoperative ileus or an immediate postoperative bowel obstruction.

Chemotherapy is typically initiated prior to discharge home from the operation (usually by postoperative day 5). After completion of chemotherapy and possible radiation therapy, surveillance is performed using chest and abdominal CT scans. Local recurrences in the renal bed are managed with resection and radiation in addition to chemotherapy.

Case Conclusion

The boy undergoes a laparotomy and is found to have an intact tumor capsule without evidence of metastatic disease. A tumor nephrectomy is performed without spillage. There was no involvement of the renal vein. Final pathology showed stage I favorable histology Wilm's tumor. He was treated with a standard course of vincristine and dactinomycin and is currently in remission.

TAKE HOME POINTS

- Wilm's tumor is the most common renal tumor in children. Renal masses in children are managed presumptively as Wilm's tumor.
- Outcomes are dependent on the stage and the presence or absence of diffuse anaplasia.
- Decisions about local control via nephrectomy are independent of hematogenous metastases.
- Preoperative or intraoperative biopsy should be avoided to not upstage tumor and mandate abdominal radiation.
- Primary resection of the tumor should be performed avoiding disruption of the tumor capsule or resection of adjacent organs.
- Aortocaval lymph node sampling is essential for accurate staging.
- Adjunctive chemotherapy is routine, while radiotherapy is used to supplement local control in stage III tumors and for pulmonary metastases.

SUGGESTED READING

Davidoff AM. Wilm's tumor. Curr Opin Pediatr. 2009;21(3): 357–364.

Ehrlich PF. Wilm's tumor: progress and considerations for the surgeon. Surg Oncol. 2007;16(3):157–171.

91 Hepatoblastoma

TERRY L. BUCHMILLER

Presentation

A 3-year-old previously healthy girl presents to her pediatrician with a right upper abdominal fullness discovered yesterday by her mother during bathing. She has seemed a bit more tired than usual after playing and has been eating less at mealtimes for 1 week. There have been no fevers, recent travel, and no other family members are ill.

On physical examination, she is listless, though well hydrated and afebrile. She has no scleral icterus and no adenopathy. Her lungs are clear to auscultation. A firm, nonmobile mass is palpated in the RUQ just under the costal margin. It is not tender but moves with respiration. Her abdomen is otherwise soft and nondistended, and she has no peritoneal signs.

Differential Diagnosis

The differential diagnosis of an right upper quadrant (RUQ) abdominal mass in a pediatric patient is broad and includes hydronephrosis, nephroblastoma (Wilms tumor), liver masses and tumors, choledochal cysts, intestinal duplication cysts, and retroperitoneal tumors. Liver masses include hemangiomas, focal nodular hyperplasia, and liver tumors, both benign and malignant. The most common malignant tumor in young children is the hepatoblastoma. Hepatocellular carcinoma more commonly seen in those over 5 years. Liver sarcomas, rhabdoid tumors, immature teratomas and choriocarcinomas are more uncommon.

Workup

Evaluation of a potential abdominal mass in children may include plain films to detect calcifications, displacement of the stomach or the intestine, and assessment of the bowel gas pattern. As these findings will likely be nonspecific, further imaging includes an abdominal ultrasound to narrow the differential diagnosis and ascertain organ involvement as well as characteristics of the mass. An abdominal CT with intravenous and oral contrast can further define vascular involvement and assess lymphadenopathy. MRI may ultimately be an important adjunct in hepatic lesions in determining tumor relationship to biliary anatomy and the hepatic vasculature. A chest x-ray or a CT should be obtained to rule out metastatic disease. Laboratory evaluation should include a CBC, electrolytes, serum transaminases, AFP, β-HCG, and a urinalysis. Serum AFP is produced in the fetal liver and yolk sac and declines to adult levels after age 6 months. Elevated AFP occurs in 90% of patients presenting with hepatoblastoma and can be used as an adjunct to assess response to treatment and disease recurrence.

Presentation Continued

CBC and electrolytes were normal. Her ultrasound showed normal kidneys without hydronephrosis and a solid mass measuring 4 × 4.5 cm confined to the right hepatic lobe with mildly increased vascular flow. An abdominal CT with contrast confirmed this solitary hepatic mass and showed no vascular impingement or invasion. There was no obvious adenopathy. The following day, the β-HCG returned at 1 (normal, < 6 mIU/mL) while the AFP was significantly elevated at >50,000 (normal, 1 to 15 ng/mL).

Diagnosis and Treatment

Based on the workup demonstrating a large solid hepatic mass in a toddler with a markedly elevated AFP, the single leading diagnosis is hepatoblastoma. Hepatoblastoma is the most common malignant hepatic tumor in children <3 years of age, and complete surgical resection offers the best chance for cure. However, approximately 20% of children with hepatoblastoma have metastatic disease at presentation. Hepatoblastomas are epithelial-based lesions that are either predominantly fetal (well differentiated), embryonal (immature/ poorly differentiated), mixed epithelial/mesenchymal, or anaplastic. A chest CT should be obtained to exclude pulmonary metastases. Evaluation by both a pediatric surgeon and a pediatric oncologist are warranted, and assessment for inclusion in clinical trials is encouraged.

Imaging is scrutinized to assess for primary tumor resection. If there is metastatic disease and/or obvious unresectability, then the tumor should be biopsied and neoadjuvant chemotherapy initiated. Restaging after chemotherapy will reassess for later resection. In select cases of bilobar disease in the absence of metastasis, primary liver transplantation may be considered.

Presentation Continued

The chest CT was negative and all abdominal imaging suggested the solitary tumor being contained in the right hepatic lobe. Therefore, the patient is a candidate for a formal right hepatic lobectomy.

Surgical Approach

Although preoperative imaging may suggest respectability, only surgical exploration is confirmatory. Nonanatomic liver resections are typically avoided because of a higher rate of incomplete resection and local relapse.

Operative steps include careful preparation with the placement of several large bore intravenous lines (preferably in the upper extremity), an arterial line, and a urinary catheter as blood loss should be anticipated. An epidural catheter for postoperative pain management should be considered. Blood products including packed RBCs, FFP, and platelets should be available. Positioning should allow the surgeon access to the neck, chest, abdomen, and groins.

A right subcostal incision is used to evaluate the tumor location and extent. The abdomen is explored for any regional or metastatic disease not detected on preoperative imaging studies. Suspicious extrahepatic lesions should be biopsied and sent for frozen section prior to resection. If the lesion is deemed resectable, an appropriate anatomic hepatic lobectomy or trisegmentectomy is undertaken.

The liver is completely mobilized by dividing the triangular ligament and attachments to the bare area, allowing anterior displacement of the liver and access to the retrohepatic vena cava. Attachments to the right adrenal and small branches to the IVC are divided. The IVC is mobilized and the resection plane assessed for vascular invasion. The hepatic veins are palpated to assure clearance from the tumor. Intraoperative ultrasound may be useful in completing the vascular assessment.

The porta hepatis is dissected and the appropriate branches of the hepatic artery, portal vein, and bile duct are isolated. Assuring resectability after complete vascular assessment, the respective portal structures are now ligated. After vascular ligation, a demarcation line is evident and the parenchyma is now divided. Anatomic liver resection is undertaken proceeding from the portal structures, up the retrohepatic cava, toward the hepatic veins. Many different techniques

TABLE 1. Key Technical Steps and Potential Pitfalls to Hepatic Lobectomy

Key Technical Steps
1. Right subcostal incision and full exploration.
2. Mobilize the liver anteriorly by dividing all attachments to the diaphragm and the abdominal wall.
3. The IVC is mobilized and, in addition to the hepatic veins, palpated to assure clearance from tumor. Intraoperative ultrasound may be a useful adjunct.
4. Perform portal dissection, and ligation of the appropriate branches of the hepatic artery, portal vein, and bile duct.
5. The parenchyma is divided following the line of vascular demarcation. Small vascular branches and bile ductules within the liver substance are ligated.
6. The hepatic veins are dissected within the liver substance. Once the appropriate branch is ligated, the final parenchymal attachments are divided completing specimen resection.
7. Small bile leaks and/or vessels on the remaining raw surface are ligated. Omental placement over the raw surface is optional.
8. Drain(s) are left and the abdomen closed.

Potential Pitfalls
- The major morbidity and mortality from pediatric liver resection is from intraoperative hemorrhage. Thorough preoperative evaluation and planning minimizes risk.
- Be aware of common anatomic variations of a replaced right or left hepatic artery.
- Inaccurate assessment of vascular invasion may lead to hemorrhage and tumor recurrence.
- Unexpected invasion of the remaining hepatic vein is the most common cause of positive resection margins, severe hemorrhage, and postoperative liver failure from the Budd-Chiari syndrome. Intraoperative US can improve assessment if uncertain.
- The course of the hepatic veins is extremely short as they originate close to the liver surface. Divide within the parenchyma if tumor margins allow. Supradiaphragmatic IVC control is encouraged should the ability to control the hepatic veins be challenging.

and instruments for parenchymal division exist subject to surgeon experience and preference. Small vascular branches and bile ductules within the liver substance are ligated as encountered. The hepatic veins should be approached by dissection within the liver substance. Once the hepatic vein(s) are ligated, the final parenchymal attachments are divided completing specimen resection.

The raw surface of the remaining liver is closely scrutinized and small bile leaks or vessels are ligated. The omentum may be placed over this raw surface in older children. Drain(s) are left.

The major morbidity and mortality with hepatic tumor resection is from intraoperative hemorrhage. Potential pitfalls include inaccurate assessment of vascular invasion leading to hemorrhage and tumor recurrence. Variations in vascular anatomy are common as the right hepatic artery arises from the superior mesenteric artery and the left hepatic artery from the left gastric artery in 15% each, respectively **(Table 1)**.

Special Intraoperative Considerations

Should tumor be suspected at the resection margin, intraoperative frozen section should be performed as complete resection is desired. Knowledge of hepatic segmental anatomy will assist in resection options.

Presentation Continued

The patient's right hepatic lobectomy was performed with a 150-mL blood loss and no transfusion requirement. Gross tumor resection was achieved and no suspicious extrahepatic lesions were encountered. She was extubated at the termination of the operation and taken to the ICU for management.

Postoperative Management

Most children readily adapt to major hepatic resection with compensatory hypertrophy. Postoperative hepatic insufficiency is manifest by hypoglycemia, hypoalbuminemia, and hypoprothrombinemia and requires meticulous surveillance. However, neonates remain a susceptible population. Intravenous fluids should contain 10% dextrose, and supplemental albumin and Vitamin K are provided as needed the first week. Close attention to vital signs, urine output, and hemoglobin levels assures no occult postoperative bleeding. Oral feeding may be resumed when the ileus resolves, typically within 2 to 3 days. When the patient is tolerating a regular diet, the abdominal drain can be removed when it is low volume and free from bile. Chemotherapy is usually initiated after several weeks to allow for hepatic regeneration and recovery.

Case Conclusion

Her recovery was uneventful and she maintained normal serum glucose levels. She was transferred to the floor where her ileus resolved on POD 3. Her nasogastric tube was removed, and her diet advanced. Her drain output was <30 mL of serous fluid and was removed on POD 6. She was discharged home on oral narcotics. Her final pathology returned as pure fetal-type hepatoblastoma with clear tumor margins. She is being closely observed without chemotherapy and monitored for tumor recurrence with serum AFP and imaging. A >85% cure rate is anticipated.

TAKE HOME POINTS

- More than 70% of all pediatric liver tumors are malignant, accounting for 1% of all pediatric malignancies. Hepatoblastoma is the third most common abdominal malignancy following neuroblastoma and Wilms tumor.
- Hepatoblastoma presents between ages 6 months to 3 years and can be associated with the Beckwith-Weidemann syndrome, familial adenomatous polyposis, hemihypertrophy, and a low birth weight. Serum AFP is elevated in 90%. Children with associated conditions should be considered for tumor screening with serum AFP and US to increase the likelihood of earlier detection.
- Multiple tumor staging systems exist that guide treatment. Approximately 20% have metastatic disease at presentation with lung, brain, and/ or bone marrow involvement. Only one-third to one-half of children diagnosed with hepatoblastoma have tumors amenable to primary resection.
- Diagnostic imaging with US, CT, and MRI is used and to assess resection. Chest CT is most commonly used to rule out pulmonary metastasis.
- Complete surgical resection remains the ultimate goal as the only effective cure.
- Several chemotherapeutic regimens exist that are based on cisplatin. Although most patients receive postoperative chemotherapy, it may be avoided in those with completely resected tumors with pure fetal histology. Radiation therapy has a very limited role.

- Preoperative chemotherapy may shrink bulky tumors making them more amenable to complete resection.
- The best survival rate approaches 95% in those with stage I disease (complete resection) with pure fetal histology. Overall survival rates are 75%.
- Children with unresectable tumors in the absence of metastasis may be strongly considered for liver transplantation. Transplantation is ultimately utilized in 6% of patients with hepatoblastoma and may be combined with neoadjuvant chemotherapy.

SUGGESTED READING

Essentials of pediatric surgery. In: Rowe M et al., eds. Liver Tumors. St Louis, MO: Mosby-Year Book, 1995:278–290.

92 Intussusception

SABINA SIDDIQUI and JAMES D. GEIGER

Presentation

A 9-month-old previously healthy male infant is brought to the emergency department with a 12-hour history of severe intermittent abdominal pain during which he would draw his knees up into his abdomen and become inconsolable. His mother tried various home remedies for colic, as he was playful and normal between episodes. She became concerned when he became more lethargic, had an episode of vomiting, and passed stool resembling currant jelly. On your evaluation of the child, he appears lethargic but is not in any acute distress. Initially, his abdomen is soft and mildly distended and not obviously tender. However, during the examination, his abdomen becomes distended and tender with a palpable, sausage-like mass in the right upper quadrant.

Differential Diagnosis

The differential diagnosis for this patient includes intussusception, incarcerated hernia, ruptured appendicitis, gastroenteritis, Meckel's diverticulitis, volvulus, and blunt abdominal trauma associated with abuse.

Workup

Presentation Continued

You order a CBC that shows a white blood cell count of 14.0 and a hematocrit of 45%. A chemistry panel shows a sodium of 150, potassium of 3.2, chloride of 120, bicarbonate of 20, a BUN of 18, and creatinine of 0.7. A plain abdominal film documents mild dilated loops of small bowel with a few air fluid levels with a paucity of gas in the right lower quadrant. You decide to order an abdominal ultrasound that shows concentric alternating echogenic and hypoechogenic bands (target sign) in the bowel in the right upper quadrant.

Routine laboratory tests are nonspecific in these patients, but the CBC and electrolytes can show evidence of dehydration or infection.

Plain abdominal radiograph may be normal, or show distal obstructive pattern with paucity of gas in the right lower quadrant related to a soft tissue mass in the right lower quadrant (Dance's sign), or, rarely, free air associated with perforation. Abdominal ultrasound will show coencentric echogenic and hypoechogenic bands (target or doughnut sign) on transverse view or a "pseudokidney" sign on oblique view of the intussuscepted bowel (Figure 1).

The diagnosis is confirmed with an abdominal ultrasound or an air-contrast enema. If the patient develops or presents with a surgical abdomen or is unstable, the contrast enema is contraindicated and the patient should be resuscitated and taken straight to the operating room.

Diagnosis and Treatment

Intussusception is the telescoping of one portion of the bowel (known as the intussusceptum) into an immediately adjacent segment (known as the intussuscipiens) (Figure 2). Edema and venous congestion lead to mucosal ischemia, which causes the "currant jelly" stools. While some cases may spontaneously reduce, without successful reduction, the ischemia may progress to full-thickness necrosis and rarely perforation.

Presentation Continued

While awaiting surgical consultation and an air-contrast enema, you order IV placement, a fluid bolus at 20 mL/kg, and a second-generation cephalosporin antibiotic.

The treatment algorithm for intussusception is dependent on the patient's clinical status. If the patient shows signs of advanced bowel obstruction, antibiotics and nasogastric tube decompression may be indicated. In the absence of hemodynamic instability, frank peritonitis or radiographic evidence of

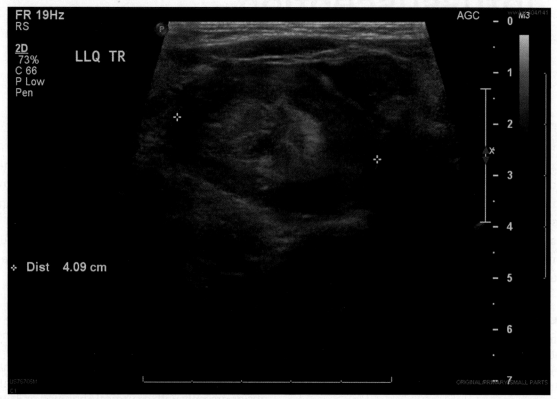

FIGURE 1 • Abdominal ultrasound illustrates a "target sign" with hypoechoic rim (edematous bowel wall) surrounding hyperechoic central area (intussusceptum and mesenteric fat).

perforation with free air, air-contrast enemas are both diagnostic and therapeutic. Enemas should be performed in consultation with a surgeon and a radiologist. A rectal tube is inserted and an adequate seal must be maintained to ensure success. Air is introduced with a manometer and pressure insufflation is carefully monitored not to exceed 120 mm Hg. Contrast enemas are sometimes utilized with barium or water-soluble contrast instilled up to a column of 100 cm above the patient. Enemas can be repeated up to three times before considered a failed maneuver **(Figure 3)**.

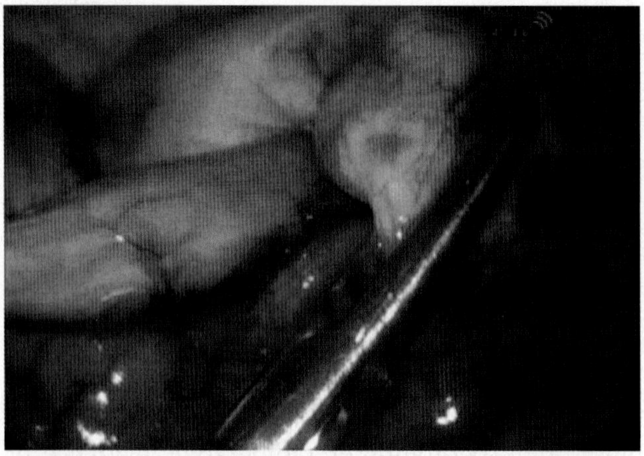

Presentation Continued

You achieve successful reduction on the first attempt and admit the child for observation and further resuscitation.

Successful reduction is determined both radiographically and clinically. On imaging, there is easy reflux of air into the small bowel and symptom improvement. Clinically, the child's abdominal pain resolves. Enemas are successful in up to 90% of cases. Upon successful reduction, the patient is admitted to the hospital for observation as 5% to 10% of cases will recur.

Presentation Continued

You are recalled to the patient's bedside 4 hours later for recurrent symptoms with intermittent pain. You attempt radiographic reduction, however without success this time. You reassure the mother and plan to take the child to the operating room.

FIGURE 2 • Intraoperative photograph shows intussuscepted ileum into the ascending colon. (Photo courtesy of Dr. Marcus Jarboe, with many thanks.)

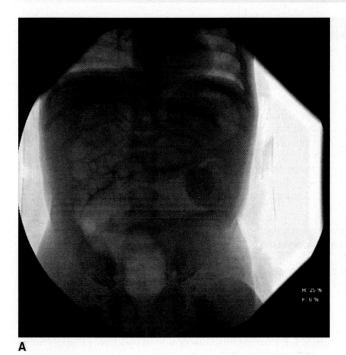
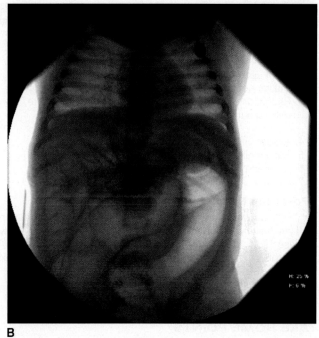

A

B

FIGURE 3 • Air-contrast enema demonstrates a long ileocolic intussusception with intussusceptum encountered in sigmoid colon (**left**) and reduced now to the splenic flexure (**right**).

Surgical Approach

Surgery is the initial therapy for the unstable patient or the patient who presents with frank peritonitis. Surgery is also indicated for patients who are unable to achieve reduction with enema therapy, have an identified lead point, or have had multiple recurrences.

Two surgical approaches are common: open and laparoscopic. In an open procedure, a transverse incision is made in the right upper quadrant and the intussuscepted mass is delivered into the wound. Reduction is performed with gentle finger pressure on the apex of the intussuscepted intestine in the descending or the transverse colon to "milk" out the intussusceptum. Care is taken not to pull the bowel out as the inflamed and edematous bowel is friable and may be damaged. Appendectomy is sometimes performed, but there is no clear data supporting this additional procedure. If the bowel shows evidence of frank necrosis or cannot be manually reduced, resection is performed with primary anastomosis. The bowel is run to ensure there is not a mechanical lead point.

In the laparoscopic approach, three ports are placed: one at the umbilicus, one in the right upper quadrant at the midclavicular line and one in the left lower quadrant at the midclavicular line. The bowel is inspected, reduction is performed by placing a grasper into the folded over intussusceptiens and 'unfolding' the tissue of the cecum while applying gentle counter-traction on the intussuscepted ileum. The bowel is run to identify a possible mechanical lead point or a perforation and necrosis. Appendectomy and resection are performed as indicated above (**Table 1**).

Special Intraoperative Considerations: (1) Necrotic bowel. After successful reduction, it is common for the bowel to appear nonviable at first. Warm saline and time may allow the appearance of the bowel to improve. It is important to be aware that lymphoid hypertrophy and mucosal edema may cause "thumbprinting" of the bowel, also making it appear nonviable. These lesions do not require resection. If the bowel continues to appear nonviable, a standard small bowel resection is performed including the cecum in some cases. (2) Irreducible lesion. Rarely, the intussusception is irreducible in the operating room. Rather than use excessive force and create a perforation with subsequent peritoneal contamination, an ileocolic resection can be performed. (3) The unidentified lead point— Most cases of intussusception are idiopathic, with no identifiable lesion in up to 85% of cases. Mechanical lead points can include Meckel diverticulum, intestinal polyp, enteric duplication cysts, intestinal tumor, or hemangioma. If a lead point is identified, resection is performed to prevent recurrence.

Case Conclusion

You successfully perform a laparoscopic reduction of the intussusception. The patient is returned to the floor in stable condition. The patient has a return of bowel and is started on clear liquids and advanced over the next day. He is discharged home postoperative day 3 tolerating a regular diet.

TABLE 1. Key Technical Steps and Potential Pitfalls in the Surgical Reduction of Intussusception

Key Technical Steps

Open Approach

1. Right upper-quadrant transverse incision.
2. Delivery of intussuscepted mass into wound.
3. Reduction of intussusception by gentle distal pressure, milking out intussusceptum.

4. Assess viability of small bowel.
5. Run small bowel and rule out presence of lead point.
6. ± Perform appendectomy.
7. Closure.

Laparoscopic Approach

1. Entry into abdomen at umbilicus and insufflation.
2. Trochars placed in right upper and left lower quadrants.
3. Reduction of intussusception by unfolding the intussusceptiens tissue while applying gentle counter-traction on the intussusceptum.
4. Assess viability of small bowel.
5. Run small bowel and rule out presence of lead point.
6. ± Perform appendectomy.
7. Closure.

Potential Pitfalls

- "Pulling" with forceful traction on proximal intussusceptum instead of milking it out leading to perforation of friable bowel.
- Lymphoid hyperplasia and edema causing "thumbprinting" may be misdiagnosed as nonviable bowel, it does NOT need to be resected.
- If unable to reduce intussusception manually, perform a ileocolic resection.

TAKE HOME POINTS

- Intussusception is the predominate cause of intestinal obstruction in children between 3 months and 2 years old.
- Patients with intussusception may present with the classic triad of colicky abdominal pain, vomiting, and red currant jelly stools.
- Air-contrast enema is diagnostic and therapeutic: 90% of cases are resolved nonoperatively.
- Operative indications include sepsis, peritonitis, recurrent intussusception, or failure of nonoperative reduction.
- During operative reduction, the technique is to apply pressure distally and "milk" the intussusceptum (distal bowel) from the intussusceptiens (proximal bowel).

SUGGESTED READINGS

Albanese CT, Sylvester KG. Pediatric surgery. In: Doherty Gerard M, ed. Current Diagnosis and Treatment: Surgery. 13th ed. McGraw-Hill Medical, 2009.

Daneman A, Alton DJ. Intussusception. Issues and controversies related to diagnosis and reduction. Radiol Clin North Am. 1996;34(4):743–756.

Daneman A, Navarro O. Intussusception. Part 2: an update on the evolution of management. Pediatr Radiol. 2004;34(2):97–108.

DiFiore JW. Intussusception. Semin Pediatr Surg. 1999;8:214.

Ein SH. Recurrent intussusception in children. J Pediatr Surg. 1975;10(5):751–755.

Hackam DJ, Grikscheit TC, Wang KS, et al. Pediatric surgery. In: Brunicardi FC, Andersen DK, Billiar TR, et al., eds. Schwartz's Principles of Surgery. 9th ed. McGraw-Hill Medical, 2009.

Kia K, Mona V, Drongowski R, et al. Laparoscopic versus open surgical approach for intussusception requiring operative intervention. J Pediatr Surg. 2004;40(1):281–284.

Llu KW, MacCarthy J, Guiney EJ, et al. Intussusception—current trends in management. Arch Dis Child. 1986; 61(1):75–77.

Ong NT, Beasley SW: The leadpoint in intussusception. J Pediatr Surg. 1990;25:640–643.

Ravitch M. Intussusception. In: Ravitch M, et al., ed. Pediatric Surgery. Chicago, IL: Yearbook Medical Publishers, 1979:992.

Saxton V, Katz M, Phelan E, et al. Intussusception: a repeat delayed gas enema increases the nonoperative reduction rate. J Pediatr Surg. 1994;29:588–589.

Skandalakis JE, Colborn GL, Weidman TA, et al. Small Intestine. In: Skandalakis JE, Colburn GL, Weidman TA, et al., eds. Skandalakis' Surgical Anatomy. Springer, 2002.

Stringer MD, Pablot SM, Brereton FJ. Pediatric Intussusception. Br J Surg. 1992;79:867–876.

Swischuk LE, Hayden CK, Boulden T. Intussusception: indications for ultrasonography and an explanation for the doughnut and pseudokidney signs. Pediatr Radiol. 1985;15:388–391.

93 Necrotizing Enterocolitis

RICHARD HERMAN and DANIEL H. TEITELBAUM

Presentation

Patient A: This infant is a former 32-week premature infant who is now 3 weeks old weighing 1,800 g. He presents with increased residuals after enteral feedings, emesis, and abdominal distension. He has had no fevers. Abdominal exam is soft, distended without signs of erythema.

Patient B: This infant is a former 24-week premature infant now 10 days old weighing 900 g who presents with fever and abdominal distension. Abdominal exam is distended, tender, and discolored.

Differential Diagnosis

Acute neonatal abdominal distension is concerning for necrotizing enterocolitis (NEC), especially in the premature infant. However, there are many other causes for neonatal abdominal distension. These can vary from other surgical emergencies to relative benign entities. Potential surgical diagnoses/emergencies begin by distinguishing between those infants presenting acutely with abdominal distension in the newborn period and those presenting a few days to weeks later. The former would include neonatal ascites, distal intestinal obstruction, or obstruction of the genitourinary system. The latter would include intestinal volvulus, isolated intestinal perforation, Hirschsprung's disease, or a partial obstruction of the gastrointestinal tract, such as an ileal stenosis. Nonsurgical pathologies include a functional ileus due to sepsis, bacterial or fungal, pseudomembranous colitis, or primary ascites or secondary ascites due to cardiac anomalies or other medical conditions.

Workup

After a full history and physical examination, both patients in Cases A and B will require a full set of laboratory values including a complete blood cell count, comprehensive metabolic panel, a blood gas, and routine abdominal radiographs (typically supine, and left and right decubiti films to assess for free air). Contrast enemas are contraindicated when considering a diagnosis of NEC; as such studies may result in colonic perforation. An upper gastrointestinal series is occasionally performed in a child where the diagnosis of a malrotation with volvulus is entertained.

Patient A has a slightly elevated white blood cell count of 27,000 cells/mm^3 and a mildly depressed platelet count of 90,000/mm^3. The abdominal radiograph shows pneumatosis intestinalis without evidence of pneumoperitoneum or portal venous gas **(Figure 1)**.

Patient B has a low white blood cell count of 3,000 cells/mm^3 and is also thrombocytopenic with a platelet count of 60,000/mm^3. The abdominal radiograph is significant for pneumoperitoneum **(Figure 2)**.

Discussion

NEC accounts for approximately 1% to 7% of all admissions to neonatal intensive care units, with infants weighing <1,500 g having an estimated incidence between 10% and 12%. Aside from prematurity and low birth weight, other risk factors include rapid initiation of feedings and certain medications, including indomethacin, theophylline, and aminophylline. About 90% of all cases of NEC occur after the initiation of enteral feedings; therefore, if a neonate has been NPO, development of NEC is less likely. The rate of advancing feeds has also been closely linked with the development of NEC. Certain nonspecific physical examination findings include lethargy, temperature instability, apnea, bradycardia, hypoglycemia, and shock. More specific abdominal findings include feeding intolerance (increased gastric residuals), abdominal distension, and blood per rectum (although not the most common cause for neonatal hematochezia). A fixed mass and palpable bowel loops are more concerning for necrotic intestine. Color change of the abdominal wall (darkened or erythematous) and scrotal color change to a reddish or a bluish hue are quite suggestive of advanced NEC. In the latter case, this may denote intestinal perforation with passage of meconium into a patent processus vaginalis. Vomiting and diarrhea can also been seen.

Though laboratory values are also nonspecific in the diagnosis of NEC, the following changes can be seen: an elevated or a depressed white blood cell count, thrombocytopenia, metabolic acidosis, and an elevated C-reactive protein. A depressed platelet count is quite common in neonates with septicemia of any cause, but a decline by more than 50% may suggest advanced

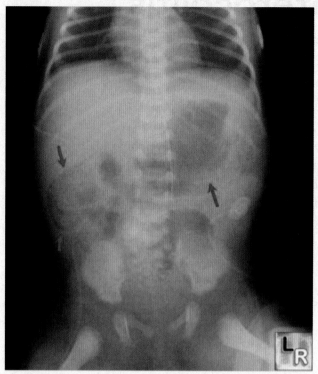

FIGURE 1 • Abdominal x-ray showing pneumatosis (*Red arrows*).

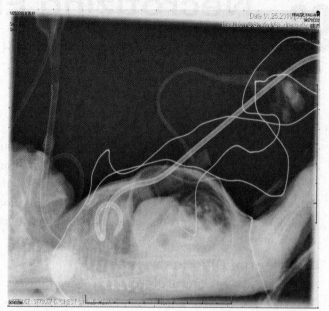

FIGURE 2 • Cross table lateral film showing pneumoperitoneum (*Green arrow*).

NEC. Radiologic signs include pneumoperitoneum, portal venous gas, pneumatosis, intraperitoneal fluid, and fixed bowel loops on serial radiographs. With good ultrasonographic imaging, NEC can be detected with sensitivity near 100% in some series. Ultrasonographic findings include stagnant, nonmobile bowel loops, target sign (signifying the abnormal loops), portal venous air, and abdominal fluid. Stagnant, nonmobile loops also suggest necrotic bowel.

Diagnosis and Treatment

The treatment of NEC can vary from nonoperative management to surgical intervention. Even among each of these pathways, variability exists. In the patients with a mild course, or low suspicion, a 1-week course of antibiotics is recommended. This can be prolonged up to 2 weeks in some of the more complicated cases. Patient A would fall into this category and would likely receive a 2-week course of antibiotics while being maintained NPO. Surgical intervention can also vary from peritoneal drain placement to laparotomy with bowel resection, which would be indicated for patient B. The indications for each of these approaches will be discussed later on in this chapter **(see Figure 3)**.

Surgical Approach

One of the foremost decisions to make in an infant with NEC is determining if a surgical intervention

is required. For all of the above-mentioned tests, the only absolute indication for surgery, whether it is a peritoneal drain placement or laparotomy, is pneumoperitoneum. Kosloske et al. described 12 criteria for operating in NEC and classified them into categories of best, good, fair and poor indicators for the need of surgical intervention **(Table 1)**.

Once the decision to operate is made, one must decide the surgical approach. Over the past decade, tremendous controversy has arisen regarding the most optimal intervention. While an exploratory laparotomy has typically been viewed as the gold standard of care, many surgeons have found that primary peritoneal drainage was an effective treatment of NEC. The earliest suggestion of the effective use of primary peritoneal drainage was first published by Ein et al. in 1977 as a means of stabilizing premature neonates with intestinal perforations. In 1994, Morgan et al. reported a 79% survival rate for infants <1,500 g treated with primary peritoneal drainage. These earlier studies led to a prospective, randomized, controlled trial by Moss et al. In this study, primary peritoneal drain placement in preterm infants <1,500 g demonstrated no difference in survival, or other clinically important early outcomes, compared to an open laparotomy. Another recent prospective randomized controlled trial by Rees et al., from 13 countries, demonstrated conflicting results from Moss's trial, where peritoneal drainage was found to be relatively ineffective. However, in the Rees trial, the study was limited to infants <1,000 g versus 1,500 g in the Moss study. However, differences are striking between the studies, as Rees et al. had a

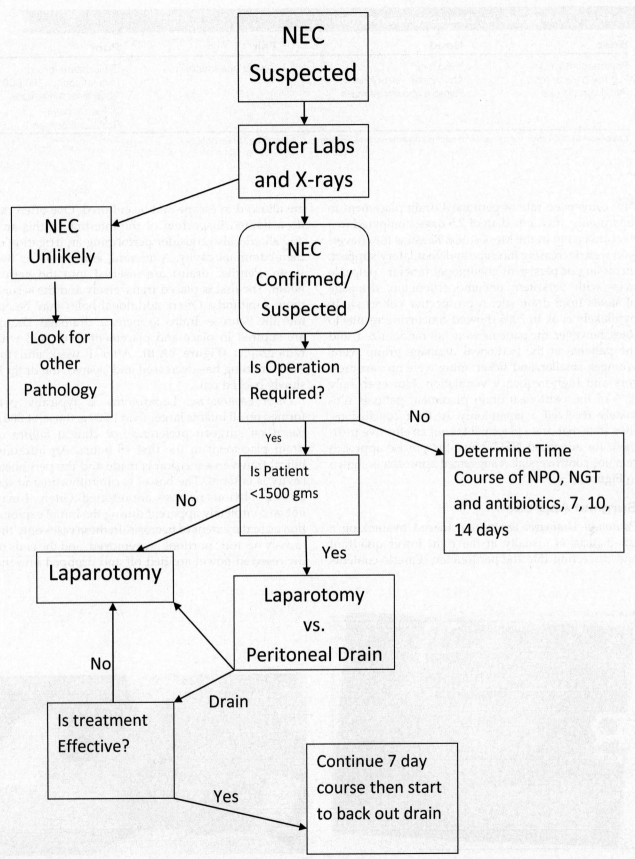

FIGURE 3 • Suggested management of NEC. Note, decision management may vary depending on the clinical presentation, and the weight threshold of 1,500 g is only a guideline. NEC, Necrotizing enterocolitis; NGT, nasogastric tube.

TABLE 1. Indications for Operative Intervention

Best	Good	Fair	Poor
Pneumoperitoneum	Fixed loop	Severe pneumatosis	Clinical deterioration
Positive paracentesis	Abdominal wall erythema		Platelet count <100,000
Portal venous gas	Palpable abdominal mass		Abdominal tenderness
			GI hemorrhage
			Gasless abdomen

Kosloske AM. Indication for operation in necrotizing enterocolitis revisited. J Pediatr Surg. 1994;29:663.

74% conversion rate of peritoneal drain placement to laparotomy after a median of 2.5 days, compared to a 9% conversion in the Moss study. Reasons for conversion were increasing inotrope and ventilatory support, increasing or persistent pneumoperitoneum, palpable mass with persistent pneumoperitoneum, drainage of stools from drain site. A prospective cohort study by Blakely et al. in 2006 showed concurring results to Rees; however, the patients were not randomized, and the patients in the peritoneal drainage group were, younger, smaller, and sicker; more were on vasopressors and high-frequency ventilation. However, only 23% of the peritoneal drain placement patients ultimately received a laparotomy. In their conclusions, they state that drain placement is not an effective treatment for advanced NEC. Thus, the precise approach remains controversial. A suggested approach is shown in **Figure 3**.

Surgical Approach

Peritoneal Drainage: Drains are placed by making a small incision, usually in the right lower quadrant and dissecting into the peritoneum. Enteric contents are allowed to escape and be cultured. One often can do a limited inspection of the intestine in this area and should also consider performing an irrigation of the abdominal cavity. Afterward, either one- or two ¼ -in. Penrose drains are inserted into the peritoneum. The first is placed transversely and the second more superiorly. Often, additional holes may be cut into the Penrose drains to increase drainage. Drains are sutured in place and placement confirmed with radiographs **(Figure 4A,B)**. After 1 week and the fluid draining has decreased and cleared, the drain is slowly backed out.

Open Laparotomy: Laparotomy is typically performed on all infants larger than 1,500 g, those <1,500 g based on surgeon preference, or clinical failure of drain placement in the first 48 hours. An infraumbilical transverse incision is made and the peritoneal cavity is entered. The bowel is carefully run and the areas of obvious necrosis are resected. Often, it may not be completely apparent during the initial exploration as to the extent of necrosis. In these cases only the grossly necrotic portions are removed, and the ends of the resected bowel are tied off and dropped into the

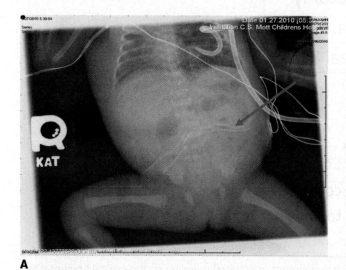
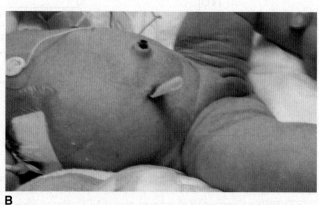

FIGURE 4 • **A:** Abdominal x-ray post peritoneal drain placement. (Drain marked with *arrow*.) **B:** View of peritoneal drain placement in right lower quadrant.

peritoneal cavity. A second-look laparotomy is then performed between 24 and 48 hours to examine questionable areas. The most proximal part of the bowel is brought up as an ostomy and the remaining viable portions of bowel re-anastomosed. Some authors have reported successful management by avoiding an ostomy and performing a primary anastomosis. While this may work with very limited disease, more diffuse NEC will almost always result in a diverting ostomy.

Each of the above procedures carries its own risk. For peritoneal drain placement, visibility is poor and hepatic injury, or small intestinal injury can occur during placement. Laparotomy complications include hepatic injury, intestinal leak, sepsis, bleeding due to a typical coagulopathic state, stoma necrosis, and recurrent NEC. Multiple complications can be seen with the creation of an ostomy in the neonate; infections, dehiscence, stenosis, hernias, prolapse, retraction, and bowel obstructions. In particular, most infants are coagulopathic and the liver lacks normal fibrose supportive structures. In these cases, even minor trauma to the liver may result in virtually noncontrollable hemorrhage. Correction of coagulopathy and even injection of fibrin glue directly into the liver fracture may be helpful; however, such injuries often may lead to significant morbidity or death.

Special Intraoperative Considerations

There are two main special intraoperative considerations in NEC. The first is that one must always consider bowel preservation and the prevention of short bowel syndrome if possible. Often, multiple blind loops or additional ostomies can be created, to facilitate saving as much bowel as possible. At times, a single proximal stoma may be performed, and the more distal bowel segments are joined together and allowed to heal. One may stent open these distal anastomoses over a silastic catheter.

The second consideration is to decide if one is dealing with NEC-totalis, the most severe case of NEC. This diagnosis is made when <10% of the bowel is viable. Most of these infants are <1,000 g and mortality has ranged from 42% to 100% depending on the series. If these infants survive, they will require long-term TPN, management of short bowel syndrome, and many ultimately need a small bowel transplant. When NEC totalis is encountered, immediate and very direct discussion with the parents is needed to decide whether ongoing treatment is desired. If there is minimal or no viable bowel the surgeon should seriously consider giving the parents an option not to continue care. This is important, particularly in a child who has other comorbidities that may make their quality of life substandard (e.g., severe intracranial hemorrhage).

Postoperative Management

For postoperative drain placement, the infant is kept NPO on total parenteral nutrition and antibiotics for approximately 14 days. The characteristics of the drain output are observed. After the output is minimal and no longer feculent in nature, the drain is slowing backed out starting 7 days after insertion. Removal is usually at a rate of 1 to 2 cm per day; the last part of the drain will usually fall out on its own. After 2 weeks have passed, feeds are slowly restarted. Feedings are generally started at a continuous infusion, and the hourly volume increases 1 mL daily. NEC strictures are common and occur in 9% to 36% of cases. In general, these strictures are found within the colon, most commonly at the splenic flexure, but as well on the left side of the colon. A contrast enema should be considered prior to the initiation of feeds and if the infant experiences feeding intolerance.

Any patient who has undergone drain placement needs to be closely monitored and evaluated for potential conversion to laparotomy. Conversion should be considered in any patient who fails to improve, or whose condition worsens. Deterioration of the clinical condition includes increasing vasopressor or ventilator requirements, organ failure including renal failure, persistent pneumoperitoneum, worsening coagulopathy, or a worsening lactic acidosis.

Postlaparotomy care is similar with respect to 2 weeks of NPO, TPN, and antibiotics. Feeds are then usually slowly restarted after gastrointestinal function has returned. If the proximal ostomy has a high output, then one should make an attempt to "refeed" the output from the ostomy into the mucous fistula. The reestablishment of gastrointestinal continuity is done approximately 8 weeks postoperatively. Prior to reestablishing continuity, a contrast enema study should be performed to check for strictures or other anatomic problems.

Case Conclusion

Patient A: Undergoes nonoperative management, is followed with routine x-rays, placed on antibiotics and NPO for 14 days. Feeds are slowly restarted and the patient is monitored for feeding tolerance.

Patient B: Undergoes placement of peritoneal drain, made NPO and given intravenous antibiotics. Starting postoperative day 7 the drain is slowly backed out. After a completed 2-week course of antibiotics, and return of bowel function, enteral feeds are slowly started after a contrast enema demonstrates no colonic stricture.

TAKE HOME POINTS

- Confirm diagnosis of NEC versus other pathology.
- Obtain appropriate imaging and laboratory values.
- Decide operative versus nonoperative management.
- For nonoperative management, decide duration.
- If operative management, decide on drain placement versus Laparotomy.
- Preserve as much bowel as possible.
- Be aware of post-NEC strictures.
- When reestablishing enteral feedings, begin a slow feeding course, advance of one ml of hourly feeds daily.

SUGGESTED READINGS

Blakely ML, Tyson JE, Lally KP, et al. Laparotomy versus peritoneal drainage for necrotizing enterocolitis or isolated intestinal perforation in extremely low birth weight infants: outcomes through 18 months adjusted age. Pediatrics. 2006;117(4):680–687.

Kim SS, Albanese CT. Necrotizing enterocolitis. In: Grosfeld J, et al., ed. Pediatric Surgery. 6th ed. Philadelphia, PA: Mosby Elsevier, 2006:1427–1453.

Kosloske AM. Indication for operation in necrotizing enterocolitis revisited. J Pediatr Surg. 1994;29:663–666.

Morgan LJ, Shochat SJ, Hartman, GE. Peritoneal drainage as primary management of perforated NEC in the very low birth weight infant. J Ped Surg. 1994;29:310–314.

Moss RL, Dimmitt RA, Barnhart DC, et al. Laparotomy versus peritoneal drainage for necrotizing enterocolitis and perforation. N Engl J Med. 2006;354(21):2225–2234.

Rees CM, Eaton S, Kiely EM, et al. Peritoneal drainage or laparotomy for neonatal bowel perforation? A randomized controlled trial. Ann Surg. 2008;248(1):44–51.

Rectal Bleeding in a Young Child

GAVIN A. FALK and OLIVER S. SOLDES

Presentation

An 18-month-old boy with an unremarkable past medical history presents to the emergency department (ED) with a 3-day history of episodic bright red bleeding per rectum. On examination, the child is quiet, tachycardiac, and normotensive. His abdomen is soft, nontender, and nondistended, without palpable masses. He does not seem to be in pain but appears pale and lethargic. He has not had any episodes of hematemesis. His distressed mother confirms that there is no family history of clotting disorders, inflammatory bowel disease, or polyposis syndromes. A nasogastric (NG) tube was placed and the aspirate is clear.

Differential Diagnosis

The causes of lower gastrointestinal (GI) bleeding in neonates (<30 days or age), infants (30 days to 1 year), children (1 to 12 years), and adolescents (>12–adults) are diverse and vary by age. Most causes in otherwise healthy children are self-limited. A child (1 to 12 years) who presents with bleeding per rectum has a differential diagnosis that includes anal fissures, Meckel's diverticulum (MD), inflammatory bowel disease, intestinal polyps, and intestinal duplications. Uncommon causes of rectal bleeding include arteriovenous malformation, varices due to liver disease, and upper GI bleeding from peptic disease. In a young child (< 4 to 5 years), MD is the most common cause of clinically significant lower GI bleeding. Occasionally, the degree of hemorrhage is impressive and may require transfusion.

Workup

After a full physical examination and comprehensive history taking, the patient undergoes further evaluation in the ED with basic laboratory tests including a complete blood count, coagulation studies, and type and screen. His serum hemoglobin is reported as 11 g/dL, with a normal platelet count and BMP. His PT/INR and APTT are within normal limits. The patient undergoes a Technetium (Tc) 99m pertechnetate scan ("Meckel's scan"), the diagnostic modality of choice to investigate for an MD with heterotopic gastric mucosa.

Discussion

Complications associated with MD are most readily understood in the context of the embryologic origin of these diverticula. MD is the most frequently encountered diverticulum of the small intestine **(Figure 1)**. It is a true diverticulum containing all of the layers of the normal small intestinal wall. During the embryologic development of the midgut, the omphalomesenteric (vitelline) duct connects the yolk sac to the intestinal tract and usually obliterates by the seventh week of life. Arrest of the obliteration of the duct may lead to a number of omphalomesenteric anomalies, the most common of which is MD. The blood supply of the MD is derived from the paired vitelline arteries. The left vitelline artery involutes and the right artery (which also gives rise to the superior mesenteric artery) may persist and travel to the tip of the diverticulum. Incomplete involution of the duct and vitelline artery remnants, with failure to separate from the abdominal wall, may produce connections to the base of the umbilicus. These may give rise to draining ileoumbilical vitelline duct fistulas, vitelline duct cysts, blind-ending umbilical sinuses, and fibrous umbilicodiverticular bands, depending on the extent of involution

The "rule of 2s" is often quoted as an aide-mémoire to the features of MD: The incidence is 2%; it is located within 2 ft of the ileocecal valve, is 2 in. in length, is usually symptomatic by 2 years of age, is two times as common in boys, and can contain two types of heterotopic mucosa. The heterotopic mucosa is most commonly gastric (80%) or pancreatic (5%) or both. The gastric mucosa is metabolically active and secretes hydrochloric acid. The pathogenesis of hemorrhage is thought to be ulceration of the ileum adjacent to the gastric mucosa **(Figure 2)**.

Although MD is the most common cause of significant rectal bleeding in young children, intestinal obstruction is actually the most frequent presenting symptom of MD (30% obstructive vs. 27% hemorrhagic presentation). Fibrous umbilicodiverticular bands to the abdominal wall produce a point of fixation around which the midgut volvulus may occur.

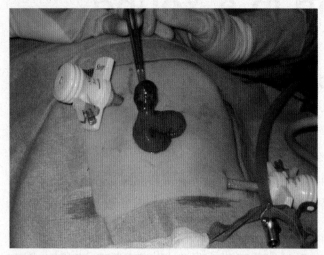

FIGURE 1 • The Meckel's Diverticulum is delivered via the umbilicus when laparoscopically assisted extracorporeal diverticulectomy is performed.

Mesodiverticular bands arising from vitelline artery remnants extending from the tip of the diverticulum to the mesentery may give rise to internal hernias. Heterotopic mucosa within the diverticula can act as a lead point for intussusception.

Inflammation related to the heterotopic mucosa may produce Meckel's diverticulitis, which may be confused with acute appendicitis and may rarely lead to perforation with peritonitis and abscess formation. Enteroliths within the diverticula and incarceration of an MD within an inguinal hernia (Littre's hernia) may also rarely occur.

Diagnosis and Treatment

Given the varied presentation of patients with MD, several different diagnostic modalities may be used in an attempt to arrive at the diagnosis. The correct diagnosis of MD is made more often in children presenting with bleeding versus other symptoms.

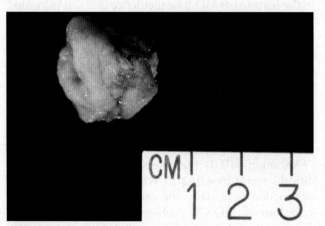

FIGURE 2 • Meckel's Diverticulum with heterotopic gastric mucosa. There is ulceration of the ileal mucosa adjacent to the heterotopic gastric mucosa.

Tc 99m nuclear scan is the most accurate way to detect the heterotopic gastric mucosa frequently found in MD. The usefulness of the Tc 99m Meckel's scan derives from the finding that approximately 95% of diverticula excised for bleeding contain gastric mucosa. The patient is injected intravenously with Tc 99m pertechnetate and a nuclear scan is performed. This isotope is selectively taken up by gastric mucosa and, if present, produces a positive scan **(Figure 3A,B)**. Scintigraphy has a sensitivity of 85%, specificity of 95%, and accuracy of 90% in children. Pentagastrin stimulation, H2 histamine blockers, and glucagon may enhance the accuracy of the scan. Angiography is infrequently used due to its invasive nature and because it is useful only if there is brisk active bleeding. Tagged red cells scans are less sensitive and specific than Meckel's scans and are seldom used.

Management of the Symptomatic MD

When the cause for presentation is hemorrhage, bleeding related to a MD is often episodic and surgery can usually be briefly delayed until the patient is stabilized and diagnostic evaluation can be performed. Intravenous hydration and volume resuscitation are a first step in management. Infrequently, a blood transfusion may be required. A NG tube should be inserted early in the evaluation to help rule out an upper GI source and confirm lower GI bleeding. A Meckel's scan should be obtained and, if positive, proceed to operation without delay. A child with an unexplained source of lower GI bleeding may require exploratory operative intervention (preferably laparoscopy) even if the nuclear scan is negative.

Management of an Incidentally Found MD

It is not definitely clear from the medical literature how a surgeon should proceed when they find an MD incidentally. The vast majority of incidentally discovered Meckel's diverticula will remain asymptomatic, especially if it has been asymptomatic into adulthood. The lifetime complications from Meckel's diverticula are estimated as 4% to 6%. An incidentally discovered Meckel's diverticula should be palpated. If there is an area of palpable thickening thought to be heterotopic mucosa, resection is usually indicated. In younger children, it can be argued that an incidentally found MD should be removed given the child's greater lifetime risk of developing complications. Asymptomatic incidentally discovered MD should generally only be resected under optimal conditions, in the absence of peritonitis and shock, because of the limited benefits and the small risk of suture line leak and peritonitis.

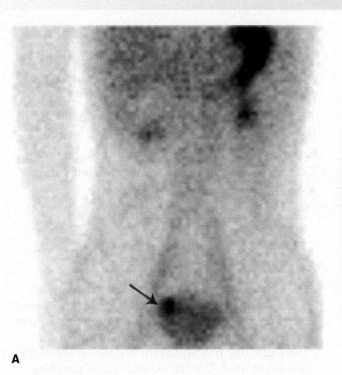

A

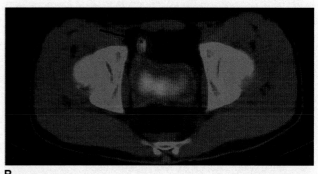

B

FIGURE 3 • **A, B** Meckel's scan demonstrating hetero-topic gastric mucosa. Heterotopic gastric mucosa within a MD with uptake of radiotracer. There is also uptake in the mucosa of the stomach and the bladder. Courtesy of Sankaran Shrikanthan, MD.

Surgical Approach

Surgical resection is the treatment of choice for symp-tomatic MD, and the approach is dependent on the patient's presentation and clinical condition **(Table 1)**. Preoperative intravenous antibiotics are administered. The operation for bleeding or intussuscepted MD can be performed either as an open, laparoscopic, or laparoscopic-assisted procedure with extracorporeal resection. In slender children, the diverticulum is read-ily externalized by minimally enlarging the umbilical trocar incision, allowing palpation, examination, and excision of the diverticulum by conventional technique while conferring the benefits of a small abdominal inci-sion. An initial minimally invasive approach is usually possible in children.

Regardless of approach, the first step is to inspect and assess the diverticulum. There is often a large mes-enteric vessel, which extends to the tip of the diver-ticulum that should be ligated. Resection of the MD can then be achieved either by diverticulectomy or segmental bowel resection and primary anastomosis by stapled or hand-sewn techniques. Open resection is generally performed via a transverse right lower-quad-rant incision. An incidental appendectomy is generally performed when this incision is used, to eliminate the diagnosis of appendicitis in the evaluation of abdomi-nal pain later in life.

When the patient presents with acute hemorrhage, it is safest to perform a wedge resection of the diverticu-lum and adjacent area of ileal ulceration is usually per-formed. The ileal mucosa should be visually inspected

to identify and control the sight(s) of bleeding. The closure is generally performed transversely by hand-sewn technique in young children but may be stapled if the base of the diverticulum is narrow and the bowel lumen is large enough to avoid narrowing. A segmental ileal resection is indicated if there is evi-dence of intestinal ischemia, extensive inflammation, irreducible intussusception, the base of the diverticu-lum is very wide, or there is palpable ectopic tissue near the diverticular opening. Ileal mucosa with sig-nificant ulceration and bleeding opposite the diver-ticulum (on the mesenteric side) usually requires segmental resection. In cases where diagnostic testing has failed to make a definitive diagnosis, an explor-atory laparoscopy is a safe way to proceed to localize the lesion.

Pitfalls associated with resection of a bleeding MD include failure to control hemorrhage from areas of adjacent ulceration if the diverticulum is excised with a stapler without opening the ileum and inspection of the mucosa. Longitudinal closure and simple wedge excision (diverticulectomy) of a wide-based diver-ticulum may create a stenosis. Leaks from suture or staple lines may occur and offset the limited benefits of excision of asymptomatic MD especially in acutely ill elderly patients, who are unlikely to develop com-plications of the MD late in life. Caution should be observed in placement of the primary laparoscopic tro-car in cases where attachment to the umbilical abdomi-nal wall is suspected (volvulus, draining ileoumbilical vitelline duct fistulas, vitelline duct cyst, or sinuses).

TABLE 1. Key Technical Steps and Potential Pitfalls in Resection of MD

Key Technical Steps

1. Laparoscopic, laparoscopically assisted extracorporeal or open technique.
2. With laparoscopically assisted extracorporeal technique, the diverticulum is easily delivered via a minimal umbilical incision in slender children.
3. Remove the appendix in open procedures with a right lower-quadrant incision.
4. If there is a mesenteric vessel to the tip of the diverticulum, it should be ligated prior to resection.
5. For a bleeding diverticulum, it is safest to begin with incision and wedge resection with direct inspection of the mucosa. Include adjacent ulcerated ileum in the resection.
6. For nonbleeding diverticula with a moderate or a narrow base width, stapler excision may be used.
7. Transverse resection and Heineke-Mikulicz type closure of the ileum is preferred to avoid narrowing the lumen.
8. Segmental resection and primary anastomosis is appropriate for wide diverticula, extensive ulceration and ulceration on the mesenteric ileal wall, or bulky heterotrophic mucosa that extends to the base of the diverticulum.
9. Standard anastomotic/closure technique for small bowel is utilized. In small-diameter bowel, a single layer hand-sewn technique may be advantageous to minimize luminal narrowing.

Potential Pitfalls

- Failure to control hemorrhage from areas of ulceration with stapler excision without direct examination of the ileal mucosa.
- Narrowing the lumen of the ileum.
- Leak at suture or staple lines.
- Perforation of the diverticulum or ileum with primary umbilical ports when a connection to the base of the umbilicus is suspected (volvulus, patent ducts).
- Unnecessarily large incisions.

A nonumbilical site for the primary trocar may be selected in these cases.

Postoperative Management

Postoperative care following Meckel's diverticulectomy or segmental resections consists of conventional care for small bowel surgery with supportive care consisting primarily of intravenous fluids, 1 or 2 doses of postoperative antibiotics, a brief period of nothing by mouth (NPO), and sometimes NG suction (segmental resections) until any ileus resolved. If a simple wedge resection or diverticulectomy is performed with laparoscopic or laparoscopically assisted extracorporeal technique, an NG tube is usually not needed and clear liquids may be initiated the following day.

Case Conclusion

The patient undergoes successful laparoscopic-assisted Meckel's diverticulectomy with wedge resection. At follow-up in the outpatient clinic 3 weeks later, the child was well, with no further bleeding, and a benign abdominal examination. Pathologic analysis of the surgical specimen confirms a gastric mucosa containing MD with ulceration. Further follow-up is unnecessary.

TAKE HOME POINTS

- MD is the most common cause of clinically significant rectal bleeding in young children (<4 to 5 years). Bleeding may be impressive and require transfusion.
- With the exception of tachycardia, hypotension, and pallor, the physical exam in patients with MD is often normal. The NG aspirate is usually clear.
- MD often presents with episodic painless rectal bleeding, but obstructive symptoms are more common (with volvulus, internal hernia, or intussusception). An acute abdomen (diverticulitis and perforation), or umbilical fistulas/cysts/sinuses may occur.
- A positive Meckel's nuclear scan is diagnostic in the child with significant lower GI bleeding and is the test of choice.
- Wedge resection of the diverticulum and adjacent ulceration with direct inspection of the ileal mucosa is safest in MD presenting with hemorrhage. A laparoscopically assisted extracorporeal approach is usually possible in the slender child.
- Segmental resection may be necessary to control hemorrhage from extensive ulceration, ulceration opposite the diverticulum, for ischemia, or when narrowing of the ileal lumen will result from diverticulectomy.

SUGGESTED READINGS

Brown RL, Azizkhan RG. Gastrointestinal bleeding in infants and children: Meckel's diverticulum and intestinal duplications. Sem Pediatr Surg. 1999;4:202–209.

Dassinger MS. Meckel's diverticulum. In: Mattei, P ed. Fundamentals of Pediatric Surgery. 1st ed. New York, NY: Springer, 2011.

Ruscher KA, Fisher JN, Hughes CD, et al. National trends in the surgical management of Meckel's diverticulum. J Pediatr Surg. 2011;46:893–896.

St. Vil D, Brandt ML, Panis S, et al. Meckel's diverticulum in children: a 20-year review. J Pediatr Surg. 1991;11:1289–1292.

Vane DM, West KW, Grosfeld JL. Vitelline duct anomalies: experience with 217 childhood cases. Arch Surg. 1987;122:542–547.

95 Omphalocele

EMILY M. FONTENOT and SEAN E. MCLEAN

Presentation

A 34-year-old primagravida female is referred to your office by her obstetrician after an abdominal wall defect with herniation of small bowel and liver was noted on her first-trimester ultrasound. She presents for counseling concerning the child's delivery and surgical options for repair. A fetal ultrasound is performed that revealed an omphalocele with no other anomalies. Karyotype was performed that revealed a normal male karyotype (46, XY). The mother continues along in her pregnancy with frequent ultrasounds, and the remainder of the pregnancy is unremarkable. She gives birth to a 38-week estimated gestational age male infant via normal spontaneous vaginal delivery with APGARS 8 and 9 at 1 and 5 minutes, respectively. His lower extremities and abdomen are placed into a sterile abdominal bag, and he is transferred to the neonatal intensive care unit.

Differential Diagnosis

Of the types of congenital abdominal wall defects, omphalocele and gastroschisis represent the most common. *Omphalocele* is a midline anterior abdominal wall fascial defect >4 cm. The rectus muscles are present and normal but insert widely on the costal margins and do not meet in the middle at the xiphoid. The resultant defect allows for herniation of the midgut and other abdominal viscera. The herniated organs are contained within a membranous sac that consists of peritoneum, Wharton's jelly, and amnion. The umbilical cord inserts on the apex of this membrane. *Small omphalocele* contains small bowel with or without stomach and has a fascial defect <5 cm. *Giant omphalocele* contains bowel, stomach, and liver and has a defect >5 cm. *Ruptured omphalocele* is the third presentation of omphalocele where the sac has ruptured *in utero* or during birth.

Gastroschisis is a full-thickness abdominal wall defect that occurs just to the right of a normally inserted umbilical cord. The herniated bowel and abdominal viscera are not covered by a membrane. The viscera are subjected to exposure to amniotic fluid during gestation.

There are other types of abdominal wall defects and syndromes that involve congenital abdominal wall abnormalities. An *umbilical hernia* is an abdominal wall defect caused by a persistent umbilical ring and is covered by skin. *Pentalogy of Cantrell* is a rare congenital abnormality characterized by omphalocele, anterior diaphragmatic hernia, malformation or absence of the pericardium, sternal cleft, and cardiac malformations. *Ectopia cordis thoracis* is due to partial or complete failure of midline fusion of the sternum resulting in the heart protruding from the chest through a split sternum. In contrast to the Pentalogy of Cantrell, the heart is not covered by a membrane in ectopia cordis thoracis. Lastly, *prune belly syndrome* is a constellation of anomalies including deficient or absent abdominal wall muscles, bilateral cryptorchidism, and a dilated dysmorphic urinary tract.

Workup

On physical examination, the newborn patient has a fascial defect of 6 cm with small bowel and liver herniated through his umbilicus and covered by a translucent sac with the umbilical cord inserted at its apex **(Figure 1)**. Chest x-ray, echocardiogram, renal ultrasound, and skeletal radiography are performed and note no abnormalities. Routine laboratory tests are run and are all within normal limits, including blood glucose of 115 mg/dL.

Discussion

Omphalocele occurs due to a failed midline fusion of the lateral embryonic folds and unsuccessful return of the midgut into the abdominal cavity. The incidence of omphalocele is 1 in 5,000 live births. Omphaloceles are more commonly seen in males, infants born to multiparous women, twin or multiple births, infants born to African American females, families with a history of omphalocele, and with advanced maternal age (>30 years). Omphalocele can present as a part of a syndrome (Beckwith-Wiedemann, OEIS [omphalocele, exstrophy, imperforate anus, and spinal anomalies], Gershoni-Baruch, Donnai-Barrow) or with an associated chromosomal abnormality (trisomy 13,14, 15, 18, or 21). Fifty percent to seventy percent of patients with an omphalocele will have at least one associated anomaly. Cardiac defects represent the most frequent anomaly occurring in 30% to 50% followed by

481

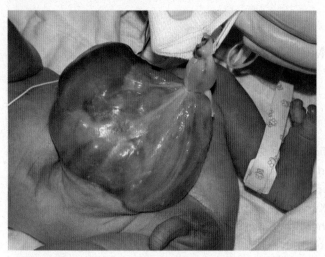

FIGURE 1 • Giant omphalocele with small bowel and large portion of the liver herniated through the defect.

musculoskeletal, gastrointestinal, and genitourinary abnormalities. Chromosomal abnormalities occur in 30%. Most frequently these are trisomies 13, 14, 15, 18, and 21. Omphalocele has also been seen with Turner's syndrome and triploidy. Beckwith-Wiedemann syndrome is associated with an umbilical defect, which is characterized by macroglossia, hyperinsulinemia, and organomegaly, as well as an increased risk of Wilms' tumor, hepatoblastoma, and neuroblastoma. The umbilical defect may result in omphalocele or umbilical hernia. Omphalocele is also part of the OEIS complex, which involves omphalocele, bladder exstrophy, imperforate anus, and spinal defects. Lower midline syndrome includes exstrophy of the bladder or cloaca, vesicointestinal fissure, colon atresia, imperforate anus, sacral vertebral defects, and lipomeningocele or meningomyelocele. Whether the size of the defect correlates with association of other anomalies remains to be determined and continues to be the subject of investigation.

Management

Management of omphalocele involves care of the fetus and mother upon discovery of the omphalocele during prenatal ultrasound. Omphalocele can first be detected by ultrasound at 10 to 14 weeks. The sensitivity of detecting an omphalocele on antenatal ultrasound is 75%. After the diagnosis is established, further prenatal testing is performed to assess for the presence of other congenital abnormalities and genetic alterations that may be life threatening or lead to fetal demise. Elevated maternal serum and amniotic fluid alpha fetoprotein can be found with omphalocele and other abdominal wall defects. Fetal karyotype is recommended due to the high incidence of chromosomal abnormalities associated with omphalocele. In a fetus

with omphalocele, there is a 50% chance of a congenital heart abnormality; thus, fetal echocardiography is recommended to evaluate for cardiac anomalies. Serial ultrasounds and close prenatal surveillance must be performed because the fetus with omphalocele is at increased risk for fetal growth retardation, polyhydramnios, and intrauterine death.

After the diagnosis of omphalocele is confirmed, prenatal counseling should be provided by a multidisciplinary team that includes a pediatric surgeon to provide the parents with an overview of the postnatal and surgical management of the future newborn patient. Delivery for omphalocele should occur in a tertiary care center with advanced neonatal and pediatric surgical support. Mode and timing of delivery is determined by the obstetrical team. There is no benefit to delivery prior to 37 weeks' gestation. During delivery there is a risk of dystocia, sac rupture, and injury to abdominal viscera; therefore, special care and preparation must be taken. Cesarean section should be performed for giant omphalocele. Vaginal delivery is appropriate for small omphalocele.

Initial postnatal care and management should focus upon stabilization of the newborn and prevention of injury to the sac and its contents. Rupture of the sac increases the risk of infection, intestinal injury, or hepatic trauma. With compromise of the sac or its contents, the option for delayed closure will be lost. After birth, the infant must immediately be evaluated for pulmonary or cardiac compromise by routine birth assessment. Some infants may require supplemental oxygen, or intubation and ventilator support. Patients with a giant omphalocele may be at risk for pulmonary insufficiency from pulmonary hypoplasia. Such patients may require prolonged ventilation, advanced modes of ventilator support, or extracorporeal life support.

Upon confirmation of cardiovascular and pulmonary stability, intravenous (IV) access is established. Peripheral IV catheters are sufficient for immediate postnatal resuscitation. Many infants with omphalocele will require parenteral nutrition; thus, early central venous access is preferable. Umbilical vessels should not be used for access because the course of the umbilical vessels is abnormal due to the omphalocele. Furthermore, the vessels are ligated at the time of repair.

With established access, patients are immediately placed on D10/0.25 normal saline IV fluid at a rate of 140 to 150 mL/kg/d. With the demonstration of adequate hydration, the fluid rate can be scaled back to a maintenance rate of 80 to 100 mL/kg/d. With an intact sac, fluid loss is not excessive. A ruptured sac can lead to high fluid loss. These patients should be maintained at the higher fluid rate (140 to 150 mL/kg/d); fluid boluses (20 mL/kg of 0.45 normal saline) should be administered when clinically indicated.

After fluid resuscitation has begun, two aspects of management are of particular importance in babies with omphalocele. First, the baby with omphalocele is at significant risk for hypothermia. Temperature must be closely monitored, temperature in the resuscitation room should be elevated, the newborn should be placed in an isolette with a warmer, and the omphalocele should be covered with plastic wrap to maintain body heat. Second, close glucose monitoring is essential. Due to the association between omphalocele and Beckwith-Wiedemann syndrome, tight glucose monitoring must be performed until the syndrome is ruled out.

Further management includes the placement of a replogle and urinary catheter for gastric and bladder decompression. Antibiotics and Vitamin K are administered. The baby is assessed by physical examination and appropriate imaging for other anomalies. After the initial resuscitation, all infants with omphalocele receive an echocardiogram to evaluate for heart abnormalities.

After the child is deemed stable, the membranous sac is evaluated to look for areas of disruption. The size of the fascial defect is also noted at this time. Next the omphalocele should be covered to protect the sac, to prevent insensible evaporative fluid loss, and to minimize heat loss. Wet gauze may accelerate hypothermia; thus, Xeroform or other nonadherent dressing should be placed around the sac. A second layer with dry mildly compressive gauze should be wrapped around the omphalocele. A third layer of plastic wrap may also be applied. If the child will require transfer to a tertiary care center, then the infant's lower extremities and abdomen should be placed into a sterile bowel bag in preparation for transfer. As long as the membrane is intact, closure is not paramount and should be delayed until the neonate has been stabilized and other anomalies have been ruled out. If the membrane has been violated, the viscera should be placed in a spring-loaded silo. The silo should be placed in the operating room or in a sterile setting at the isolette in the neonatal intensive care unit with the support of an operating room team.

Surgical Approach

Repair of omphalocele should be performed under planned and controlled circumstances. Prior to repair, a stable cardiopulmonary state must be achieved. The patient should be appropriately evaluated for cardiac defects by echocardiogram and other associated anomalies. Patients with Beckwith-Wiedemann syndrome require aggressive management of serum glucose. Children must have a karyotype performed. The presence of trisomy 13 or 18 may change the overall clinical plans for the patient (Table 1).

The goals of surgery for omphalocele are to reduce the viscera into the abdominal cavity and to close

---

TABLE 1. Key Technical Steps and Potential Pitfalls in Surgical Management of Omphalocele

Key Technical Steps

1. Sharp dissection of the membranous sac from the fascial and skin edges.
2. Reduction of the herniated viscera.
3. Primary closure of the fascia in a tension-free manner.
4. Primary closure of the skin.

Potential Pitfalls

- Increase in intra-abdominal pressure resulting in respiratory compromise or abdominal compartment syndrome.
- Injury to the liver capsule.
- Disruption of portal, mesenteric, or central venous blood.

---

the skin and fascia. Children with omphalocele will have a reduced abdominal domain. Forced placement of the viscera into the abdomen places the patient at risk for an abdominal compartment syndrome. The amount of viscera that requires reduction in relation to the size of the abdomen is a key factor in determining the timing and the type of surgical closure. Other equally important factors are the size of the fascial defect and the overall physiologic state of the patient.

For an omphalocele <5 cm, a primary closure is the best option. Closure involves removal of the sac at the level of the skin. If there is residual sac covering the liver, some sac can be left to avoid injury to the capsule of the liver. The umbilical vessels and urachus are suture ligated. Skin flaps are raised to expose the fascia. Some surgeons will manually stretch the muscles and fascia to increase abdominal domain. As the viscera are reduced, it is important to communicate with the anesthesiologist to avoid the creation of an abdominal compartment syndrome; furthermore, care must be taken with the liver during reduction to avoid torsion of the hepatic veins, disruption of portal vein inflow, or hemorrhage from injury to the liver capsule. With respiratory or hemodynamic compromise, temporizing measures must be taken for closure of the abdomen. The midgut should be reduced first followed by the liver. Once the viscera are reduced with no signs of compartment syndrome, the fascia is closed in the midline. If midline closure is not possible, transverse closure is acceptable. Simple or mattress stitches are placed through the abdominal wall (except skin) with absorbable suture. The skin is closed with a running absorbable suture. An umbilicoplasty is performed if there is sufficient skin.

Primary closure may not be an option due to an increase in abdominal pressure or a wide gap in the fascia. In such cases, there are multiple options for closure. Skin closure is a temporary closure strategy. Fascia is closed as permitted. Skin flaps are created and the edges closed. A small ventral hernia remains that is repaired at a later date. Another temporizing method is to bridge the fascia with nonabsorable (Gortex, Marlex), absorbable (Vicryl, Dexon), or biologic mesh (Alloderm, Surgisis). Skin flaps are mobilized to cover the mesh. Nonabsorbable graft is a temporary option. The mesh is removed and fascia closed after the child has grown. The potential complications with nonabsorbable mesh include infection, seroma, and fistula. Absorbable graft material (Vicryl, Dexon) provides favorable short-term results, but the repair will weaken over time leaving a ventral hernia. Such hernias should be repaired when the child has grown sufficiently to allow for a primary fascial closure. Biologic mesh will incorporate into the fascia and stimulate fibroblast in-growth. There are no large series for biologic mesh that have determined the efficacy and the complication rates.

Staged reduction and closure is employed for a small omphalocele that cannot be closed primarily, a large omphalocele with a high volume of herniated viscera, or a wide fascial defect. The key principle is to provide temporary coverage while the viscera are gradually reduced into the abdomen. Temporary coverage can be achieved with a silastic silo (sewn to the edges of the fascia) or a spring-loaded silo suspended from the isolette. Pressure is applied by placing ties or sutures on the silo to push the viscera into the abdomen. A third technique involves sewing sheets of gortex or silastic to opposite ends (or sides) of the fascia. The closure is gradually tightened by cutting out a portion of each sheet in the center and closing it with a new suture line. This is done every 2 to 3 days until the fascial edges are close enough to perform a primary closure.

For patients with a giant omphalocele or that are too unstable for surgery, the "paint and wait" technique with or without compression is the best option. The hernia sac is coated with an antimicrobial agent that allows the sac to toughen into an eschar. Currently, silver sulfadiazine (Silvadene) is the treatment of choice due to its broad-spectrum antimicrobial activity, little toxicity, and ease of daily application. Mercurochrome, Betadine, and silver nitrite are no longer used because they create metabolic and electrolyte derangements. The hernia sac is coated with an antimicrobial agent that causes the sac to toughen into an eschar. As the sac contracts, the infant continues to grow. A large ventral hernia develops that can later be repaired primarily, with muscle flaps or a biocompatible mesh. Compression can be added by wrapping an elastic bandage around the sac. The bandage should assume the conformation of a cone and is carried around the back of the patient to create compressive forces toward center of the abdominal cavity. The addition of elastic bandage compression may speed the process of reduction of the viscera and increase the likelihood of

a delayed primary fascial repair. "Paint and wait" usually takes 6 to 12 months before definitive closure is achieved.

Postoperative Management

Systemic antibiotics should be continued for 5 to 7 days following the procedure or until the prosthesis is removed. IV fluid at an initial rate of 140 mL/kg/h should be started and titrated for a urine output of at least 1 mL/kg/h. Parenteral nutrition by a central venous catheter should continue until bowel function returns. A prolonged ileus, as seen with gastroschisis, is not expected. If bowel function fails to return by 3 weeks, a contrast bowel study should be ordered to rule out other gastrointestinal pathology.

Case Conclusion

In the present patient, primary closure of the defect was not plausible. As our patient had no other pathology, we elected to perform a staged repair. Nonadherent gauze was placed over the Silvadene-coated membrane. An external compression bandage was then wrapped around the externalized viscera and around the infant **(Figure 2)**.

Over the next week, the viscera were slowly reduced. On the tenth day of life, the infant was taken to the operating room where the defect was closed primarily. Parenteral nutrition was continued until bowel function returned. The infant was discharged to home on day of life 21.

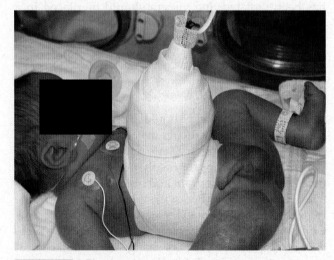

FIGURE 2 • Elastic compression bandages are placed around the omphalocele around the infant to gradually reduce the herniated viscera.

Complications

Many of the complications of omphalocele repair can be attributed to the increase in abdominal pressure that results from reduction of the herniated viscera into an abdomen with inadequate domain. Pulmonary compromise and abdominal compartment syndrome can result. It is not infrequent for these infants to develop indirect inguinal hernias following repair due to dilation of the internal ring from increased intra-abdominal pressure. There is no need for immediate repair as this may act as a "pop off" valve releasing excess pressure. Repair is delayed until comorbid conditions resolve. An increased incidence of gastroesophageal reflux may also occur due to the increase in pressure.

As with any abdominal operation, there remains a risk for adhesions to develop. Intra-abdominal wall infections may lead to wound separation, dehiscence, or sepsis. The presence of a prosthesis increases this risk. Complications related to catheter infection and decline in liver function from prolonged parenteral nutrition remain a threat. Due to abnormal fixation and rotation of the intestine, a child with an omphalocele has malrotation; however, corrective repair does not take place at the time of the abdominal wall defect repair. Therefore, complications related to malrotation and midgut volvulus are occasionally observed.

Outcomes

The overall mortality in live birth with omphalocele is 10% to 25%. There is no general consensus on whether there is a relation of the size of the defect to the outcome. However, an increase in the incidence of an unfavorable outcome has been shown with exteriorization of the liver. Outcomes related to omphalocele are dependent upon comorbid conditions. Infants with an isolated omphalocele, regardless of size, have a 75% to 95% survival. In those with a large omphalocele, prognosis and outcome are related to associated pulmonary complications (pulmonary hypoplasia).

TAKE HOME POINTS

- 50% to 70% of infants with omphalocele has an additional congenital anomaly with cardiac defects occurring in 30% to 50% of cases.
- Early strict glucose monitoring is paramount until Beckwith-Wiedemann syndrome can be ruled out.
- When the membrane is not ruptured, repair is delayed until other pathology is ruled out.
- The goal of repair is primary closure with no increase in intra-abdominal pressure.
- In the unstable infant, the "Paint and Wait" technique should be employed.
- Morbidity and mortality are largely due to concurrent anomalies.

SUGGESTED READINGS

Baird R, Gholoum S, Laberge J, et al. Management of a giant omphalocele with an external skin closure system. J Pediatr Surg. 2010;45(7):E17–E20.

Frolov P, Alali J, Klein M. Clinical risk factors for gastroschisis and omphalocele in humans: a review of the literature. Pediatr Surg Int. 2010;26(12):1135–1148.

Heider A, Strauss R, Kuller J. Omphalocele: clinical outcomes in cases with normal karyotypes. Am J Obstet Gynecol. 2004;190(1):135–141.

Isalm S. Clinical care outcomes in abdominal wall defects. Curr Opin Pediatr. 2008;20(3):305–310.

Kumar H, Jester A, Ladd A. Impact of omphalocele size of associated conditions. J Pediatr Surg. 2008;43(12):2216–2219.

Ledbetter D. Gastroschisis and omphalocele. Surg Clin North Am. 2006;86(2):249–260, vii.

Mac Bird T, Robbins J, Druschel C, et al.; National Birth Defects Prevention Study. Demographic and environmental risk factors for gastroschisis and omphalocele in the National Birth Defects Prevention Study. J Pediatr Surg. 2009;44(8):1546–1551.

Mann S, Blinman T, Douglas Wilson R. Prenatal and postnatal management of omphalocele. Prenat Diagn. 2008;28:626–632.

Marvin S, Owen A. Contemporary surgical management strategies for congenital abdominal wall defects. Semin Pediatr Surg. 2008;17(4):225–235.

Whitehouse J, Gourlay D, Masonbrink A, et al. Conservative management of giant omphalocele with topical povidone-iodine and its effects on thyroid function. J Pediatr Surg. 2010;45(6):1192–1197.

96 Gastroschisis

SAMIR K. GADEPALLI and JAMES D. GEIGER

Presentation

You are called to the delivery room of a newborn male with abdominal contents open to air. The term baby was born via vaginal delivery and had APGARs of 9 and 9 at 1 and 5 minutes, respectively. Prenatal events were significant for polyhydramnios and echogenic bowel seen on fetal ultrasound. Mother is an otherwise healthy 19-year-old G1P1 on prenatal vitamins. On examination, the child weighs 3.1 kg, has normal vital signs, and is in no acute distress. Abnormal physical examination findings include an open, mildly sunken fontanelle, intestinal contents seen protruding from a small 1- to 2-cm defect to the right of an intact umbilical cord without any covering, and bilateral undescended testicles.

Differential Diagnosis

Abdominal wall defects are found in 1 of 5,000 live births. Differences between an omphalocele and gastroschisis are highlighted by location of defect, structures seen outside, presence of a sac, and associated anomalies (see Table 1). Omphaloceles are found in the midline, have an amniotic sac as a cover, contain the intestine, often liver and other abdominal organs, and are within the umbilical stalk. Associated anomalies may include midline defects, such as cardiac or bladder/cloacal, and syndromes such as Beckwith-Weidemann (BW) or trisomy 13, 18, or 21. Prognosis and mortality vary with the presence of associated anomalies, especially the severity of any congenital heart disease and the size of the omphalocele. Gastroschisis is almost invariably found to the right of the umbilicus with only intestinal contents, without a sac, and associated anomalies, such as jejunal-ileal atresias, gastroesophageal reflux, or undescended testicles.

Workup

In patients with an omphalocele, the presence of associated anomalies must be excluded quickly. Bladder extrophy or Pentalogy of Cantrell can be readily seen on physical exam. Abnormal blood glucose and examination revealing an enlarged tongue can help identify BW syndrome, followed by an echocardiogram and renal ultrasound to find cardiac and renal anomalies, respectively. Chromosomal and prenatal amniocenteses are also helpful in certain situations. Spinal ultrasound and skeletal survey help to identify neural tube or musculoskeletal defects.

About 10% of gastroschisis patients are considered complicated with associated intestinal atresias. Atresia may be identified at the initial examination of the intestine, but if thickened, this can be difficult.

Abdominal x-rays and contrast studies aid in confirming intestinal atresias. In patients with gastroschisis, necrotizing enterocolitis is more common and can be identified using physical (abdominal distension, apnea, bradycardia, desaturations, abdominal wall erythema), laboratory (elevated white blood cell count, decreasing platelet counts), and radiographic (pneumatosis, portal venous gas, pneumoperitoneum) characteristics.

Diagnosis and Treatment

Priorities in the management of gastroschisis are to establish coverage for the intestinal contents, resuscitate and maintain intravascular volume, identify associated anomalies, and provide nutrition. At birth, intestinal coverage can be obtained with a bowel bag covering the entire baby until resuscitation has been completed. It is also important to make sure the mesentery is not twisted and the bowel is supported to avoid traction on the mesenteric vessels. Babies are usually born in a dehydrated state and are prone to further volume losses secondary to exposure of intestines; therefore, placing warm towels or a bowel bag can keep the intestines moist while maintaining body temperature.

Resuscitation involves placing an intravenous (IV) line and starting fluids usually at 150 mL/kg/d. Establishing an IV can be a challenge, and occasionally, an intraosseous, saphenous vein cutdown, or central-line venipuncture may be required. Once fluids are started, electrolytes must be closely followed to ensure abnormalities can be quickly corrected. Finally, a nasogastric tube and a Foley catheter serve as usual adjuncts, especially when complete reduction of intestinal contents is attempted.

Establishing nutrition and achieving goal enteral nutrition in patients with gastroschisis remains a

TABLE 1. Differences Between Omphalocele and Gastroschisis

	Omphalocele	Gastroschisis
Location of defect	Midline	Right of umbilicus
Presence of sac	Present	Absent
Contents	Usually liver, intestine	Intestines only; Liver rare
Associated anomalies	Midline (cardiac, bladder) Syndromes (trisomy, BW)	Intestinal atresias

BW-Beckwith-Weidemann.

challenge. Associated anomalies, such as intestinal atresia, can complicate the management of gastroschisis and are not always diagnosed at birth. The presence of matted, thickened bowel is not uncommon and the presence of an atresia can go unrecognized prior to final closure. Intestinal function is usually delayed in these patients, complicating the picture. A contrast study can help identify if an atresia exists, while parenteral nutrition is provided until intestinal continuity can be reestablished. When enteral nutrition is initiated, periods of intolerance are common and slow steady advancement is preferred. Bilious aspirates do not always reflect an obstruction as bile reflux and gastroparesis are common. Emesis is a better indicator of feeding intolerance but also may represent a sign of developing necrotizing enterocolitis, which can occur more frequently in this population **(Figure 1)**.

Surgical Approach

After an IV is established, options for reduction of contents and abdominal wall closure can be considered. Options for closure are placement or construction of a silo with gradual reduction of contents until abdominal domain is reestablished versus primary closure

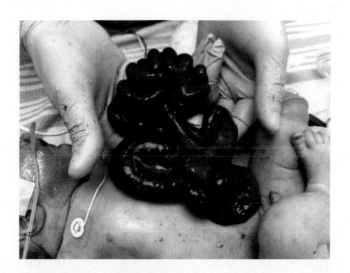
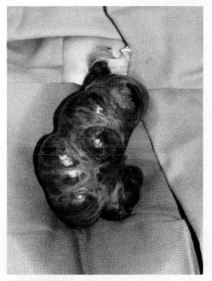
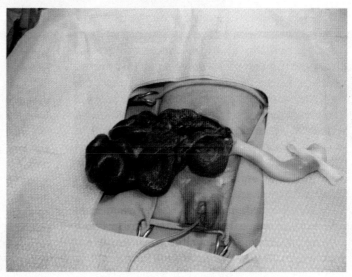

FIGURE 1 • Different types of gastroschisis defects represent the variation in bowel morphology.

with or without the use of a patch (biologic or mesh). A nasogastric tube and rectal tube with irrigation can be used to decompress the bowel to increase room in the peritoneal cavity. A key component for the decision is the creation of an abdominal compartment syndrome. If upon reduction of abdominal contents, the peak pressures increase dramatically or increased tension is required to close the wound, the prudent approach would be placement of a silo and gradual reduction **(Figure 2)**.

The key steps in abdominal closure are decompressing the bowel, running the bowel to identify any atresias or perforations, undermining the fascia, closure of the fascia and skin, and creation of an umbilicus **(Table 2)**. Potential pitfalls include perforation of the bowel, which is fragile in its matted, exposed state; therefore, maneuvers to decompress the bowel should be limited to irrigation and gentle manipulation. Another pitfall is the closure of the defect under tension, which can create an abdominal compartment syndrome with respiratory compromise, decreased urine output, and potential intestinal ischemia and dehiscence.

Special Intraoperative Considerations

As suggested above, the presence of an atresia can dramatically change the course of the operation. Options for management when an atresia is encountered include resection and primary anastomosis, creation of an ostomy, and reduction with delayed management of the atresia in a second operation. The strategy chosen is determined by the overall status of the patient, condition of the bowel, and presence of other anomalies.

In a patient with matted, edematous, thickened bowel, creation of an ostomy may not be a feasible option, and with a large-size discrepancy between proximal and distal segments, reduction of contents and returning for a second surgery may be the ideal option. Babies can be easily decompressed for several weeks with an atresia allowing for improvement in the quality of the bowel and allow the child to grow

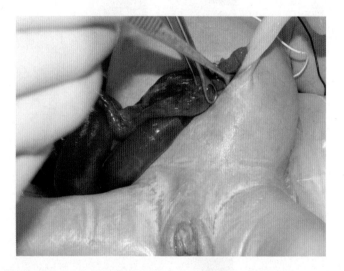

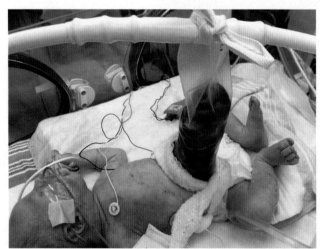
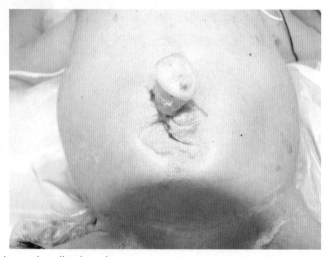

FIGURE 2 • The bowel can be placed in a silo, partially reduced, or primarily closed.

TABLE 2. Key Technical Steps and Potential Pitfalls to Abdominal Wall Closure

Key Technical Steps
1. Decompressing bowel.
2. Running bowel to identify any atresias.
3. Undermining fascia.
4. Closure of fascia and skin.
5. Creation of umbilicus.

Potential Pitfalls
- Inadvertent bowel injury.
- Abdominal compartment syndrome.

- The presence of liver in a midline abdominal wall defect is likely to be an omphalocele.
- Intestinal atresias can occur in 10% of patients and pose a significant challenge to the management of patients with gastroschisis.
- Abdominal compartment syndrome can occur with aggressive attempts at reduction of intestinal contents and abdominal wall closure and can be prevented with gradual reduction.
- Wound breakdown and feeding intolerance are common postoperative problems that require carefully throughout management strategies.
- Mortality is <10% and in general occurs as a result of intestinal failure and complications of total parenteral nutrition.

on parenteral nutrition. If the liver is severely affected by parenteral nutrition, the child has poor weight gain and growth, or the bowel cannot be adequately decompressed for the time period, an operation is warranted sooner; otherwise, 6 to 8 weeks is a commonly chosen endpoint to avoid inflammatory adhesions and bowel injury at re-operation.

Postoperative Management

Feeding intolerance is a common problem in gastroschisis secondary to any combination of gastroesophageal reflux, gastroparesis, intestinal dysmotility, shortened intestinal length, and bacterial overgrowth increasing the potential for necrotizing enterocolitis. The presence of an atresia must be excluded using a contrast study. If bacterial overgrowth is suspected from recurrent episodes of enterocolitis or malabsorption, cycling enteral antibiotics can be useful. Gastroesophageal reflux and dysmotility can usually be addressed with nonoperative measures including elevation of the head, small and frequent meals, histamine blockers, proton pump inhibitors, and promotility agents, such as metoclopramide or erythromycin. Occasionally, a combination of partial parenteral and enteral nutrition is required.

Wound infection and dehiscence are common complications to anticipate after gastroschisis closure. Close observation of the wound and perioperative antibiotic use are essential steps in the closure. Frequently, undermining the wound creates an area of erythema and ecchymosis around the wound and increases concern of infection especially after a period of initial silo placement. Delayed closure of the skin is useful when mesh is not exposed on the underlying fascia and there is tension present on the skin during initial closure.

TAKE HOME POINTS

- Fundamentals in the management of gastroschisis at birth include coverage of intestinal contents, maintenance of body temperature, and early, aggressive resuscitation.

SUGGESTED READINGS

Barlow B, Cooper A, Gandhi R, et al. External silo reduction of the unruptured giant omphalocele. J Pediatr Surg. 1987;22:75.

Bethel CA, Seashore JH, Touloukian RJ, et al. Cesarean section does not improve outcome in gastroschisis. J Pediatr Surg. 1989;24:1–3; discussion 3–4.

Boyd PA, Bhattacharjee A, Gould S, et al. Outcome of prenatally diagnosed anterior abdominal wall defects. Arch Dis Child Fetal Neonatal Ed. 1998;78:F209–F213.

Brown MF, Wright L. Delayed External Compression Reduction of an Omphalocele (DECRO): an alternative method of treatment for moderate and large omphaloceles. J Pediatr Surg. 1998;33:1113–1115; discussion 1115–1116.

de Lorimier AA, Adzick NS, Harrison MR, et al. Amnion inversion in the treatment of giant omphalocele. J Pediatr Surg. 1991;26:804–807.

Driver CP, Bruce J, Bianchi A, et al. The contemporary outcome of gastroschisis. J Pediatr Surg. 2000;35:1719–1723.

Dunn JC, Fonkalsrud EW. Improved survival of infants with omphalocele. Am J Surg. 1997;173:284–287.

Dunn JC, Fonkalsrud EW, Atkinson JB, et al. The influence of gestational age and mode of delivery on infants with gastroschisis. J Pediatr Surg. 1999;34:1393–1395.

Greenwood RD, Rosenthal A, Nadas AS, et al. Cardiovascular malformations associated with omphalocele. J Pediatr. 1974;85:818–821.

Hatch EI, Baxter R. Surgical options in the management of large omphaloceles. Am J Surg. 1987;153:449–452.

Heider AL, Strauss RA, Kuller JA, et al. Omphalocele: clinical outcomes in cases with normal karyotypes. Am J Obstet Gynecol. 2004;190:135–141.

Hong AR, Sigalet DL, Guttman FM, et al. Sequential sac ligation for giant omphalocele. J Pediatr Surg. 1994;29:413–415.

Huang J, Kurkchubasche AG, Carr SR, et al. Benefits of term delivery in infants with antenatally diagnosed gastroschisis. [see comment]. Obstet Gynecol. 2002;100:695–699.

Koivusalo A, Lindahl H, Rintala RJ, et al. Morbidity and quality of life in adult patients with a congenital abdominal wall defect: a questionnaire survey. J Pediatr Surg. 2002;37:1594–1601.

Koivusalo A, Rintala R, Lindahl H, et al. Gastroesophageal reflux in children with a congenital abdominal wall defect. J Pediatr Surg. 1999;34:1127–1129.

Koivusalo A, Taskinen S, Rintala RJ, et al. Cryptorchidism in boys with congenital abdominal wall defects. Pediatr Surg Int. 1998;13:143–145.

Krasna IH. Is early fascial closure necessary for omphalocele and gastroschisis? J Pediatr Surg. 1995;30:23–28.

Lenke RR, Hatch EI Jr. Fetal gastroschisis: a preliminary report advocating the use of cesarean section. Obstet Gynecol. 1986;67:395–398.

Mahour GH, Weitzman JJ, Rosenkrantz JG, et al. Omphalocele and gastroschisis. Ann Surg. 1973;177:478–482.

Minkes RK, Langer JC, Mazziotti MV, et al. Routine insertion of a silastic spring-loaded silo for infants with gastroschisis [see comment]. J Pediatr Surg. 2000;35:843–846.

Molik KA, Gingalewski CA, West KW, et al. Gastroschisis: a plea for risk categorization. J Pediatr Surg. 2001;36:51–55.

Mollitt DL, Ballantine TV, Grosfeld JL, et al. A critical assessment of fluid requirements in gastroschisis. J Pediatr Surg. 1978;13:217–219.

Saxena AK, Hulskamp G, Schleef J, et al. Gastroschisis: a 15-year, single-center experience. Pediatr Surg Int. 2002;18:420–424.

Schlatter M, Norris K, Uitvlugt N, et al. Improved outcomes in the treatment of gastroschisis using a preformed silo and delayed repair approach. J Pediatr Surg. 2003;38:459–464; discussion 459–464.

Schwartz MZ, Tyson KR, Milliorn K, et al. Staged reduction using a Silastic sac is the treatment of choice for large congenital abdominal wall defects. J Pediatr Surg. 1983;18:713–719.

Singh SJ, Fraser A, Leditschke JF, et al. Gastroschisis: determinants of neonatal outcome. Pediatr Surg Int. 2003;19:260–265.

Snyder CL, Miller KA, Sharp RJ, et al. Management of intestinal atresia in patients with gastroschisis. J Pediatr Surg. 2001;36:1542–1545.

97 Tracheoesophageal Fistula

STEVEN W. BRUCH

Presentation

A newborn baby boy, born to a healthy 28-year-old female at 37 weeks' estimated gestational age with APGAR scores of 8 and 9, had difficulties with his first feed. He coughed and sputtered after the feeding appearing to choke and then almost immediately spit up all of the feeding. There was no bile in the emesis. A nasogastric tube was passed but met resistance. A chest x-ray revealed the tube curled up at the thoracic inlet, a slightly distended stomach, but otherwise a normal abdominal gas pattern.

Differential Diagnosis

Failure to tolerate feeds and an x-ray showing a nasogastric tube coiled in a proximal esophageal pouch with air in the bowel is typical in a baby born with esophageal atresia (EA) and a distal tracheoesophageal fistula (TEF). There are five variations of EA with or without TEF as seen in **Figure 1**, with the most common being EA with a distal TEF. An iatrogenic esophageal perforation can mimic an EA with difficult passage of a nasogastric tube. These perforations are almost always in the proximal esophagus and heal on their own with intravenous antibiotics, nothing per mouth, and placement of a tube past the perforation into the stomach to help drain the saliva.

Workup

Preoperative workup attempts to answer three questions: Are there associated anomalies? What side of the chest is the arch of the aorta located? And what is the exact anatomy of the trachea, esophagus, and their connections?

Anomalies associated with EA and TEF include chromosomal anomalies and a sequence of anomalies referred to as the VACTERL sequence that includes **v**ertebral, **a**norectal, **c**ardiac, **t**racheal, **e**sophageal, **r**enal, and **l**imb anomalies. A karyotype will look for chromosomal anomalies the most frequent being trisomies 13 and 18, which are lethal, and trisomy 21, Down's syndrome. The VACTERL anomalies are evaluated with physical exam looking for the anorectal anomalies, usually imperforate anus, plain x-rays for the vertebral and limb anomalies, an abdominal ultrasound for renal anomalies and to look for tethering of the spinal cord, and an echocardiogram for cardiac abnormalities.

The echocardiogram is also used to locate the aortic arch. If the arch is located on the right side, it makes it difficult to complete the esophageal anastomosis over the arch when approached through a right-sided thoracotomy. In that event, a left thoracotomy allows a more tension-free esophageal anastomosis.

The anatomy of the trachea and esophagus can be defined in a number of ways. The initial plain x-ray determines if a distal TEF is present. If there is a gasless abdomen as seen in **Figure 2**, there is no distal TEF, whereas if there is gas in the bowel, a connection between the trachea and the distal esophagus is present. A proximal fistula can be evaluated with a "pouchogram," rigid bronchoscopy, or both. A pouchogram depicted in **Figure 3** involves placing a small amount of barium in the proximal esophageal pouch to evaluate the size of the pouch and to look for a connection between the proximal esophageal pouch and the membranous portion of the trachea. A small pouch implies that fluid swallowed by the fetus exited the pouch via a proximal fistula, therefore not providing the pressure required to distend the proximal esophageal pouch. Rigid bronchoscopy will allow visualization of the distal fistula, which is usually seen at the carina as shown in **Figure 4**. A close look should be undertaken for a proximal fistula, which is rare and quite a bit more subtle than the distal fistulas. An H-type fistula often is suspected later than the neonatal period and is diagnosed with an esophagram as seen in **Figure 5**, and/or rigid bronchoscopy.

Diagnosis and Treatment

With the diagnosis made and the workup completed, the newborn is taken to the operating room for repair of the EA and TEF. In children with EA without a distal TEF, a gastrostomy tube placement with evaluation of the gap length between the two ends of esophagus is the first step in treatment. If the gap length is ≥3 vertebral bodies, repair is delayed. With growth, the gap length may shorten allowing primary repair, or remain "long" leading to the creation of an esophageal spit fistula in the left side of the neck and an eventual esophageal replacement with either a gastric or colon conduit.

Surgical Approach

A right posterolateral thoracotomy is used unless a right-sided aortic arch is identified on echocardiography,

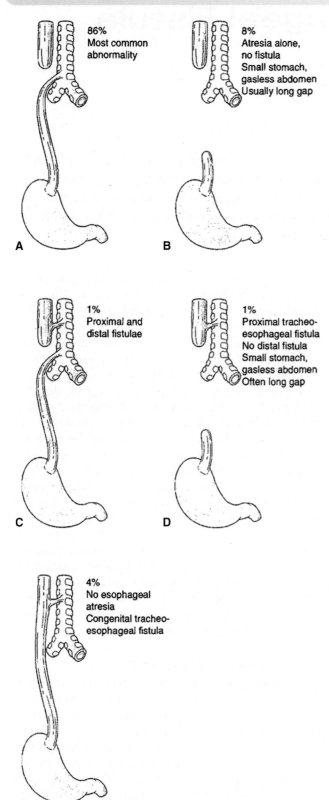

86%
Most common
abnormality

8%
Atresia alone,
no fistula
Small stomach,
gasless abdomen
Usually long gap

1%
Proximal and
distal fistulae

1%
Proximal tracheo-
esophageal fistula
No distal fistula
Small stomach,
gasless abdomen
Often long gap

4%
No esophageal
atresia
Congenital tracheo-
esophageal fistula

FIGURE 1 •The five varieties of EA with and without tracheoesophageal fistulas with their rates of occurrence. (**A**) EA with a distal TEF. (**B**) Pure EA. (**C**) EA with a proximal and a distal tracheoesophageal fistula. (**D**) EA with a proximal TEF. (**E**) H-type TEF.

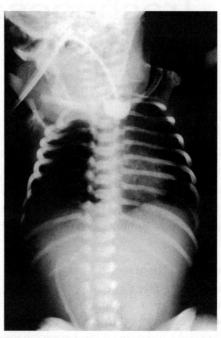

FIGURE 2 •The gasless abdomen of pure EA. The proximal pouch is outlined with contrast.

when a left posterolateral thoracotomy provides optimal exposure. A muscle-sparing technique minimizes rib cage and spinal abnormalities later in life. The chest is entered through the fourth interspace using a retropleural approach. This allows for more easy retraction of the lung during the case and prevents intrapleural soilage in case of an anastomotic leak post operatively. The azygos vein is identified and divided exposing the connection between the trachea and the distal esophagus. The esophagus will distend with each breath helping identify its location. The fistula is divided as close to the tracheal wall as feasible with Prolene sutures. The proximal pouch is then searched for asking the anesthesiologist to push on the nasogastric tube in the pouch. The proximal esophagus will be located at the thoracic inlet. A suture, used to provide traction, is placed through the esophageal pouch and the nasogastric tube. The proximal pouch is dissected fully as proximal as possible keeping in mind the possibility of coming across a proximal fistula between the pouch and the membranous portion of the trachea. The dissection should avoid opening the membranous tracheal wall by staying on the thick muscular wall of the esophageal pouch. At this point, an assessment of the length of the gap between the two ends of the esophagus should be made. If the two ends can be brought together, an anastomosis is performed. If extra length is required, the distal esophagus may be mobilized. Although the blood supply to the distal esophagus, which is segmental from the descending aorta, is more tenuous than that

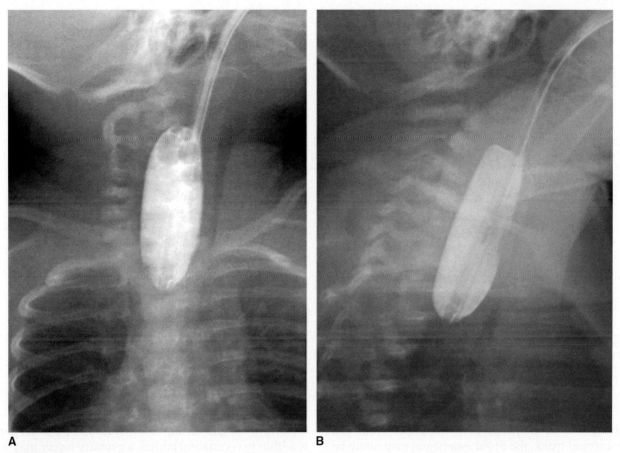

A   B

FIGURE 3 • AP (**A**) and lateral (**B**) views of a pouchogram revealing no connection between the upper esophageal pouch and the trachea.

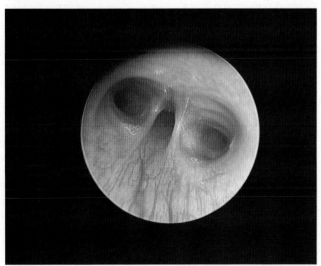

FIGURE 4 • Bronchoscopic view of the distal TEF emanating from the carina between the right and the left mainstem bronchi.

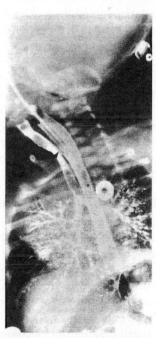

FIGURE 5 • Esophogram demonstrating an H-type TEF denoted by the *arrow*. Contrast placed in the esophagus entered the tracheobronchial tree via the H-type fistula.

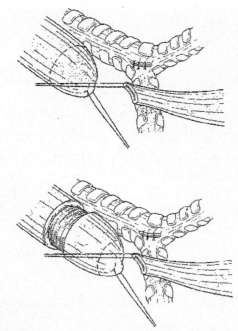

FIGURE 6 • Use of a circular esophageal myotomy on the upper pouch to gain length and close the esophagus primarily.

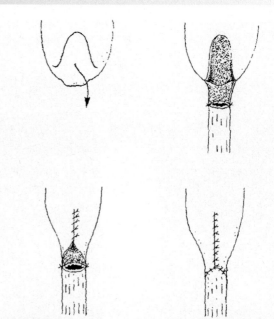

FIGURE 7 • Use of an anterior muscle flap of the upper pouch to gain length and close the esophagus primarily. (Reprinted from Gough MH. Esophageal atresia—Use of an anterior flap in the difficult anastomosis. J Pediatr Surg. 1980;15(3):310–311, with permission from Elsevier.)

of the proximal esophagus, which arises from the thyrocervical trunk, the distal esophagus may safely be mobilized if length is required after complete mobilization of the proximal esophagus. Other techniques to gain length include circular myotomies of the proximal pouch and tubularization of the proximal pouch as seen in **Figures 6 and 7**. When adequate length is obtained, an eight-stitch anastomosis is performed with absorbable suture material. The five back row sutures are placed, and a nasogastric tube is placed through the anastomosis and into the stomach. Then, the remaining three anterior sutures are placed to complete the anastomosis as shown in **Figure 8**. A chest tube is placed and the thoracotomy incision is closed. Recently, thoracoscopic techniques have been developed to complete the repair in a minimally invasive fashion.

Special Intraoperative Considerations

Babies born with pure EA without a connection between the trachea and the distal esophagus present unique problems. The gap between the two ends of the atretic esophagus is often too long to bridge in the neonatal period. The first operative step in a pure EA is the placement of a gastrostomy tube to gain access to the stomach for enteral feeds. The stomach in these babies is very small making the placement technically challenging. When the gastrostomy tube is placed, an estimate of the gap length can be obtained by placing a tube in the upper pouch and a neonatal endoscope in the distal esophagus via the gastrostomy site and

looking at the gap distance with fluoroscopy. If the gap is within two vertebral bodies, a primary repair may be attempted. Most of the time, this gap will be too long to close, and the baby will be nursed with a Replogle tube in the proximal pouch, the head of the bed elevated 45°, and using the G-tube for feedings. Evaluation of the gap length should then be carried out every 4 to 6 weeks. Most agree that if the gap is not close enough to attempt repair by 3 months of age, then it is time to think about an esophageal replacement. This would include creating a spit fistula in the left neck in preparation for a gastric transposition or a colon conduit. The spit fistula allows sham feeds in these babies while they await their replacement operation. An option to consider prior to going to replacement of the esophagus is the "Foker" technique. This technique uses tension on the esophageal ends over time to lengthen the proximal and distal esophageal remnants. Multiple sutures with pledgets are placed on the proximal and distal esophageal ends. These sutures are then brought out the back of the baby (the lower pouch sutures out the upper back, and the upper pouch sutures out the lower back) where they are placed on traction and shortened a small incremental amount each day until the ends are close enough to allow primary anastomosis as shown in **Figure 9**.

On occasion, babies with EA are born with premature lungs and ventilation becomes difficult. The premature lungs require increased peak inspiratory pressures to adequately ventilate. This may result in a large portion

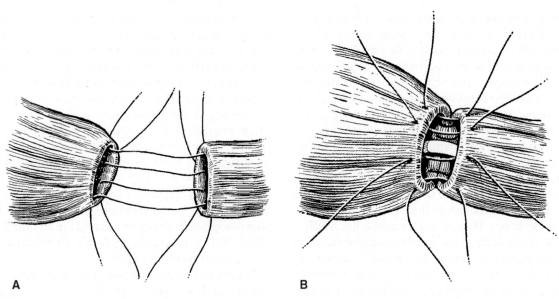

A   **B**

FIGURE 8 • Esophageal anastomosis. **A:** Posterior sutures placed. **B:** Nasogastric tube is passed and anterior sutures complete the anastomosis.

of each mechanical breath going down the fistula rather than to the lungs because the air will travel the path of least resistance. This can be a difficult problem to manage. Attempts can be made to place the tip of the endotracheal tube past the fistula opening. This can

rarely be sustained as a solution because of the mobility of the endotracheal tube, and the close relationship of the TEF and the carina. There are several other options to control this problem. Placement of a Fogarty catheter that is inflated into the fistula opening with rigid

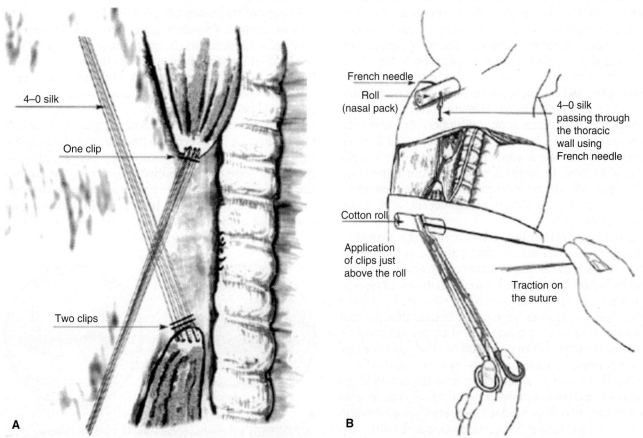

A   **B**

FIGURE 9 • The "Foker" technique. **A:** Sutures placed in upper pouch and distal esophagus. Metal clips are placed to track the position of the esophageal ends using plain x-ray. **B:** Sutures are brought out the back and traction is used over time to lengthen the two segments of the esophagus.

bronchoscopy followed by reintubation often temporizes the situation. However, the Fogarty often inadvertently slips out of position causing this method to fail. Another option is to place a gastrostomy tube and put the end of the tube to underwater seal, thus increasing the resistance of the fistula tract and allowing more air into the lungs. At the time of gastrostomy tube placement, a Rumel tourniquet may be placed around the gastroesophageal junction and brought out the upper abdomen. This can be used to intermittently occlude the esophagus again forcing air into the mainstem bronchi rather than down the fistula. A more long-term solution is to divide the fistula through a right posterolateral thoracotomy. This should improve the respiratory status of the baby. If the anesthesiologist can then easily ventilate and oxygenate, the definitive repair can be done. If the baby does not improve after the fistula is divided, the distal esophagus should be stretched cranially and tacked to the prevertebral fascia with permanent sutures and the chest closed. This allows a definitive repair later when the baby has grown and the respiratory issues have resolved.

Postoperative Management

In the postoperative period, the baby is nursed with the head of the bed elevated and meticulous care is taken to keep the oropharynx suctioned of saliva to prevent aspiration and pneumonia. Some surgeons will feed enterally through the tube across the anastomosis into the stomach. A contrast study of the esophagus is performed about 1 week after the operation to look for a leak. If no leak is present, the tube is removed, feeds are begun, and the chest tube is removed if no formula or saliva is seen draining. If there is a leak, large or small, the baby remains on antibiotics, the chest tube remains in place, and the study is repeated 1 week later until no leak is seen. These postoperative leaks seal with time. In addition to a leak, four more complications should be anticipated: stricture formation, gastroesophageal reflux, tracheomalacia, and recurrence of the TEF.

Stricture formation is common occurring in up to 40% of repairs. The stricture is almost always at the anastomosis although rarely a primary cartilaginous esophageal stricture may be present in the distal esophagus in association with a TEF. Strictures are initially dilated with balloon dilators, or tapered bougie dilators that can be used over a guide wire (Savory dilators) or passed blindly (Maloney dilators). If a gastrostomy tube is present, Tucker dilators may be attached to a string that traverses the stricture from the mouth to the stomach and pulled through the stricture. A child with a stricture that fails to stay open after serial dilation should be evaluated for gastroesophageal reflux disease, as the stricture will not resolve until the reflux is adequately managed.

Gastroesophageal reflux occurs very commonly in this patient population, up to 70% of the time. Reflux is initially managed medically with a proton pump inhibitor with or without the addition of an H2 blocker. If medical management fails, a fundoplication may be necessary. Care must be taken when fashioning a fundoplication in these children. The distal portion of the esophagus in TEF patients does not peristalse well and a fundoplication can lead to difficulties with dysphasia. Most pediatric surgeons will use a "floppy" Nissen fundoplication in these patients, although some prefer a partial wrap. Occasionally, these children will have a relatively short esophagus due to the initial repair and require a Collis-Nissen fundoplication to gain adequate length for a proper fundoplication.

Tracheomalacia can mimic gastroesophageal reflux disease in this patient population and occurs in up to 20% of babies born with TEF. Tracheomalacia occurs due to weakening of the tracheal cartilage resulting in "fishmouthing" of the trachea with expiration as seen on bronchoscopic view in **Figure 10**. Rigid bronchoscopy with the baby spontaneously breathing will diagnose tracheomalacia. Most babies will grow out of the malacia, but those with severe tracheomalacia require an aortopexy to stent open the trachea as seen in **Figure 11**.

Recurrent tracheoesophageal fistulas occur in up to 10% of repairs. If suspected in children with respiratory issues around feeds or frequent pneumonias, it can be diagnosed with an esophagram or using a combination of rigid bronchoscopy and esophagoscopy. The best contrast study to identify a recurrence is a prone pullback esophagram where the study is done with the child lying prone allowing gravity to reveal the connection between the trachea and the esophagus. The use of rigid bronchoscopy and esophagoscopy will sometimes identify a recurrent fistula, but they are often difficult to pick up. In those difficult cases, placing methylene blue into the trachea and ventilating allow the dye to pass through the fistula

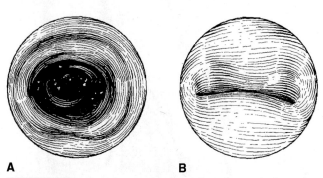

A   **B**

FIGURE 10 • Bronchoscopic view of tracheomalacia. **A:** Open trachea during inspiration. **B:** The "fish mouth" collapse of the trachea during expiration.

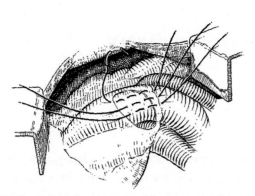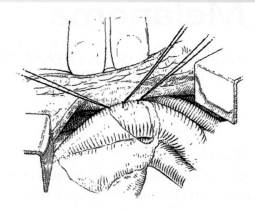

FIGURE 11 • Aortopexy involves suturing the adventitia of the aorta to the sternum. This stents open the trachea in the babies with severe tracheomalacia.

if present into the esophagus where the blue dye can be seen with esophagoscopy. A recurrent fistula can be approached initially endoscopically. The fistula is identified; the mucosa is removed as best as possible mechanically or with argon beam coagulation, and then an adhesive is placed bronchoscopically to occlude the fistula. If this fails an open procedure is required to separate the trachea and esophagus, repair the fistula, and place viable tissue between the suture lines. Usually, a flap of pericardium works well to prevent future recurrences.

Survival is excellent with a near-term infant without cardiac anomalies. However, prematurity and the presence of a significant cardiac defect reduce the expected survival. Infants weighing >1,500 g at birth without major congenital cardiac anomalies have a 97% survival rate. If the infant is either born <1,500 g or has a major cardiac anomaly, the survival rate decreases to 59%. Infants who weigh <1,500 g at birth and have a major cardiac abnormality have only a 22% chance of survival.

Case Conclusion

On the second day of life, the baby underwent successful repair of the EA and TEF. The contrast study at 1 week showed no leak. Feeds were initiated and tolerated well, and he was discharged home. During the transition from formula to baby food, he developed some vomiting and dysphasia. A stricture was identified at the area of the anastomosis that underwent serial dilation and remained open. Other than having a "hot dog" that was underchewed get caught at the anastomotic site at age 3 requiring upper endoscopy and retrieval, he has done well and is taking all of his nutrition by mouth and thriving.

TAKE HOME POINTS

- EA and/or TEF is identified at birth with emesis and failure to pass a nasogastric tube.
- Plain film confirms EA with the tube in the proximal pouch and presence of a distal TEF when there is air seen in the abdomen.
- Evaluation involves excluding associated anomalies including chromosomal and VACTERL anomalies, identifying the location of the aortic arch, and delineating the anatomy of the trachea, the esophagus, and their connections.
- Repair involves a right muscle-sparing posterolateral thoracotomy using a retropleural approach.
- Identification of the fistula and creation of an esophageal anastomosis with minimal tension provide the technical challenge.
- The anastomosis is studied at 1 week and allowed to heal on its own if a leak is identified. The leak should be retropleural and drained adequately with the chest tube.
- Postoperative complications include anastomotic leaks, strictures, gastroesophageal reflux, tracheomalacia, and recurrent TEFs.

SUGGESTED READINGS

Bruch SW, Hirschl RB, Coran AG. The diagnosis and management of recurrent tracheoesophageal fistulas. J Pediatr Surg. 2010;45:337–340.

Harmon CM, Coran AG. Congenital anomalies of the esophagus. In: Grosfeld JL, O'Neil JA Jr, Coran AG, et al., eds. Pediatric Surgery. 6th ed. Philadelphia, PA: Mosby Elsevier, 2006:1051–1081.

MacKinlay GA. Esophageal atresia surgery in the 21st century. Semin Pediatr Surg. 2009;18:20–22.

Spitz L, Bax NM. Esophageal atresia with and without tracheoesophageal fistula. In: Spitz L, Coran AG, eds. Operative Pediatric Surgery. 6th ed. London, UK: Hodder Arnold, 2006:109–120.

98 Melanoma

SEBASTIAN G. DE LA FUENTE, TIMOTHY W. MCCARDLE,
and VERNON K. SONDAK

Presentation

A 37-year-old woman noted a pigmented lesion on her left arm approximately 3 months ago. She sought the attention of a dermatologist who performed an excisional biopsy of the lesion. Pathology was consistent with malignant melanoma, Clark level II, with a Breslow depth of 0.8 mm without ulceration. The tumor mitotic rate was measured at 2 mitoses/mm². Margins from the biopsy were negative but close (<1 mm). Her physical examination only reveals a well-healed scar at the biopsy site with no palpable lymphadenopathy.

Epidemiology

Approximately 131,810 new cases of melanoma are predicted to be diagnosed in 2012 in the United States, with 55,560 expected to be noninvasive cases (melanoma *in situ*) and 76,250 invasive melanomas. The incidence of melanoma has been increasing steadily over the last few decades. Melanoma is 10 times more common in whites than in African Americans, with a mean age at diagnosis of 55 years, but it can affect any age group. The most common primary sites are on the extremities of women and on the trunk in men. Currently, malignant melanoma accounts for 5% of all skin cancer but is responsible for most skin cancer–related deaths, with 9,180 deaths predicted for 2012.

Even though the causes of melanoma are not fully understood, it is well established that exposure to sunlight, specifically ultraviolet (UV) radiation, is a significant factor for developing melanoma. While sunburns are primarily due to UVB (280 to 320 nm) radiation, UVA has been shown to induce mutations in various cell lines and is also considered a carcinogen. The highest-risk population is fair-skinned individuals who burn easily with sun exposure. Other risk factors for developing melanoma are shown in **Table 1**.

Workup

The initial evaluation of patients presenting with suspicious skin lesions should include a complete history and physical examination focusing on the characteristics of the lesion as well as the status of the regional lymph nodes. Suspicious lesions are those presenting with geometric asymmetry, irregular borders, a variety of colors within the same lesion, diameter larger than 6 mm, or lesions that have changed over time (evolution) **(Table 2) (Figure 1)**. The presence of itching, bleeding, or ulceration should also raise concern. Melanoma typically arises *de novo* from normal skin, but it can also arise in a preexisting nevus. It is important to emphasize that not all melanomas are visibly pigmented. Amelanotic melanomas lack the classic dark or multicolored appearance of most melanomas, which can lead to delays in recognition.

Suspicious skin lesions should be biopsied to establish the definitive diagnosis. Whenever possible, excisional biopsy with 1 to 2 mm margins of normal skin extending down to subcutaneous fat is recommended. If excisional biopsy is undesirable due to the size of the lesion or its anatomic location (e.g., face, ears, digits, palm, etc.), incisional or punch biopsy may be performed **(Figure 2)**. Shave biopsies should ideally include enough of the underlying dermis to allow determination of the depth of the lesion. Blood tests or imaging studies are generally not necessary in patients who are diagnosed with clinically localized melanomas and no symptoms of metastatic disease, except as needed to evaluate the patient's overall medical status or suitability for general anesthesia.

Staging

Staging of melanoma is based on clinical and pathologic features and is determined according to the TNM classification **(Table 3)**. Clinical staging is based on the initial primary tumor biopsy, a complete physical examination, and, where indicated, imaging studies and laboratory tests. Pathologic staging includes the histologic results of definitive surgical procedures such as sentinel node biopsy and radical lymphadenectomy. Patients with clinical stage I and II (localized) melanoma are those with no clinical or radiologic evidence of regional or distant metastases. Clinical stage III patients are those with regional metastases, manifesting as enlarged lymph nodes or satellite or in-transit disease or both. Clinical stage IV is reserved for patients with distant metastases. Pathologic stages I

TABLE 1. Risk Factors for Malignant Melanoma

Skin type and color:
- Whites with red or blond hair or fair skin are at increased risk.

UV light exposure:
- Blistering sunburns
- Use of sunlamps
- Tanning beds

Personal history of melanoma:
- 1%–2% of people with melanoma will develop a second one at some point.

Familial:
- 10% of all people with melanoma have a family history of melanoma.

Multiple atypical nevi

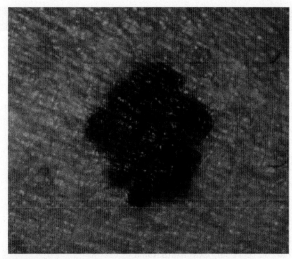

FIGURE 1 • Malignant melanoma presenting with asymmetry, irregular borders, and a variety of colors.

and II comprise patients with no histologic evidence of nodal involvement after undergoing sentinel lymph node biopsy. Pathologic stage III patients have histologic evidence of metastatic disease in regional lymph nodes or intralymphatic sites.

The T component of the TNM system, addressing the primary tumor, incorporates the Breslow thickness of the melanoma, the presence or absence of ulceration **(Figure 3)**, and, in melanomas ≤1 mm thick, the mitotic rate. In the case presented above, the patient has a nonulcerated 0.8-mm melanoma with a mitotic rate >1 mitosis/mm²; therefore, her tumor is classified as a T1b melanoma.

Other histopathologic features have prognostic implications and should be routinely described on the pathology report. These include the presence or absence of regression, microsatellitosis, vertical growth phase, angiolymphatic invasion, and tumor-infiltrating lymphocytes **(Table 4) (Figure 4)**.

Surgical Management

The fundamental principle in the treatment of primary cutaneous melanoma consists of wide excision of skin and subcutaneous tissues down to or including fascia with a radial margin measured from the edges of the biopsy scar or of any residual pigmented lesion. This

excision margin is determined by the depth and anatomical location of the primary tumor **(Table 5)**. Wide excision done by itself (i.e., without an accompanying lymph node biopsy or dissection) can often be performed under local anesthesia, with intravenous sedation if necessary. The resected specimen is oriented and sent for permanent pathologic examination. In most cases, the resulting defect can be closed primarily, but skin grafts or local skin flaps may be needed when primary closure is not feasible.

The most common first site for metastatic disease is in the lymph node basin draining the primary tumor site. Before the development of sentinel lymph node biopsy, most patients presenting with melanomas of 1.5 mm or greater in Breslow thickness were subjected to elective regional lymphadenectomy. This was done for both

TABLE 2. The ABCDEs of Melanoma Recognition

A. Asymmetry
B. Border irregularity
C. Color variation
D. Diameter of >6 mm
E. Evolution (change in lesion)

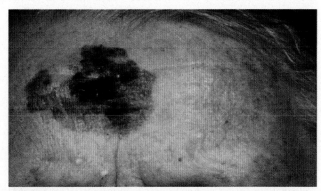

FIGURE 2 • Forehead melanoma diagnosed with punch biopsy.

TABLE 3. Seventh Edition AJCC Staging Classification

Primary Tumor (T)

TX: primary tumor cannot be assessed
T0: no evidence of primary tumor
Tis: melanoma *in situ*
T1a: melanomas 1.0 mm or less in thickness without ulceration and mitosis $0/mm^2$
T1b: melanomas 1.0 mm or less with either ulceration or mitosis ≥ 1 $mitosis/mm^2$
T2a: melanomas 1.01–2.0 mm without ulceration
T2b: melanomas 1.01–2.0 mm with ulceration
T3a: melanomas 2.01–4.0 mm without ulceration
T3b: melanomas 2.01–4.0 mm with ulceration
T4a: melanomas >4.0 mm without ulceration
T4b: melanomas > 4.0 mm with ulceration

Regional Lymph Nodes (N)

NX: nodes cannot be assessed
N0: no regional node metastasis detected
N1a: one node with micrometastasis
N1b: one node with macrometastasis
N2a: 2–3 nodes with micrometastases
N2b: 2–3 nodes with macrometastases
N2c: in-transit/satellite metastases without nodal metastases
N3: four or more nodes with metastasis, or matted nodes, or in-transit/satellite metastases with nodal metastases

Distant Metastasis (M)

M1a: metastases to skin, subcutaneous tissue, or distant lymph nodes with normal LDH
M1b: metastases to lungs with normal LDH
M1c: all other visceral metastases with normal LDH or any metastases with elevated LDH

	Clinical Staging				Pathologic Staging		
Stage 0	Tis	N0	M0	0	Tis	N0	M0
Stage IA	T1a	N0	M0	IA	T1a	N0	M0
Stage IB	T1b	N0	M0	IB	T1b	N0	M0
	T2a	N0	M0		T2a	N0	M0
Stage IIA	T2b	N0	M0	IIA	T2b	N0	M0
	T3a	N0	M0		T3a	N0	M0
Stage IIB	T3b	N0	M0	IIB	T3b	N0	M0
	T4a	N0	M0		T4a	N0	M0
Stage IIC	T4b	N0	M0	IIC	T4b	N0	M0
Stage III	Any T	≥N1	M0	IIIA	T1-4a	N1a	M0
					T1-4a	N2a	M0
				IIIB	T1-4b	N1a	M0
					T1-4b	N2a	M0
					T1-4a	N1b	M0
					T1-4a	N2b	M0
					T1-4a	N2c	M0
				IIIC	T1-4b	N1b	M0
					T1-4b	N2b	M0
					T1-4b	N2c	M0
					Any T	N3	M0
Stage IV	Any T	Any N	M1	IV	Any T	Any N	M1

Adapted from the American Joint Committee on Cancer (AJCC). AJCC Cancer Staging Manual. 7th ed. New York, NY: Springer Science and Business Media LLC, 2010, www.springer.com

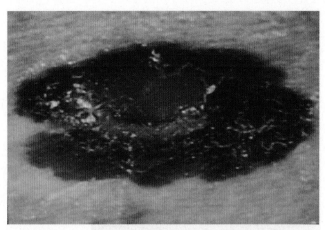

FIGURE 3 • Malignant melanoma, Clark level 4 with a Breslow depth of 6 mm presenting with an area of ulceration in the center of the lesion.

therapeutic and staging purposes, because the status of regional lymph nodes is the most important prognostic factor for survival. The observation in clinical trials that elective lymphadenectomy did not provide survival benefit and was associated with significant morbidity, such as lymphedema, wound infection, and nerve injuries, led to the development of lymphatic mapping and the sentinel lymph node biopsy procedure in the early 1990s. Current guidelines recommend sentinel lymph node biopsy for patients with clinically node-negative melanomas that are at least 1 mm in thickness. If the primary melanoma is <1 mm deep, sentinel lymph node biopsy is considered in patients of young age, in the presence of ulceration, or with tumors with mitotic rate of at least 1/mm². If only a partial biopsy has been done, especially if substantial residual pigmented lesion is present, this may also be an indicator for sentinel lymph node biopsy in thin tumors.

Sentinel lymph node biopsy involves preoperative radionuclide lymphoscintigraphy and intraoperative injection of isosulfan blue dye. Preoperative lymphoscintigraphy, utilizing intradermally injected tracers such as ^{99m}Tc-sulfur colloid, permits determination of the lymphatic drainage patterns and allows

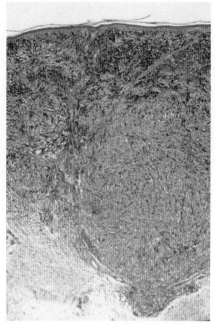

FIGURE 4 • Malignant melanoma in vertical growth phase (i.e., nests within the dermis are larger than the largest intraepidermal nests and mitotically active). A non-brisk lymphocytic host response is present.

identification of those basins at risk for melanoma metastasis **(Figure 5A)**. A new technique that combines single photon emission computed tomography with computer tomography (SPECT/CT) for localization of sentinel nodes provides considerably more anatomic detail than conventional lymphoscintigraphy **(Figure 5B,C)**.

Patients are typically injected 1 to 2 hours prior to the operation, allowing enough time for the tracer to travel to the basin of interest. The sentinel lymph node is identified intraoperatively with the aid of a handheld gamma counter. Additionally, intradermal administration of 0.5 to 1 mL of isosulfan blue dye (Lymphazurin 1%) around the intact tumor or biopsy site immediately preceding the procedure facilitates localization of the sentinel lymph node during surgery. The combination of dye and radiolabeled colloid solution allows the

TABLE 4. Histopathologic Factors Associated with Melanoma Prognosis

- Tumor thickness
- Ulceration
- Phase of tumor growth (radial versus vertical growth phase)
- Mitotic rate
- Angiolymphatic invasion
- Regression
- Tumor-infiltrating lymphocytes
- Solar elastosis
- Satellitosis

TABLE 5. Recommended Surgical Margins for Invasive Melanoma Based on Prospective Randomized Trials*

Tumor Thickness	Margin Recommendation
<1.0 mm	1.0 cm
1.0–2.0 mm	1.0–2.0 cm depending on ability to achieve primary closure
>2.0 mm	2.0 cm

*Randomized trials included only patients with primary melanomas located on the trunk and proximal extremities. In other locations, (e.g., hands, face, etc.), 1.0 cm margins may be acceptable even for thicker tumors.

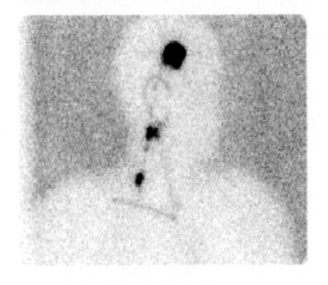

RT LAT Pix:2.4mm 99m Technetium

A

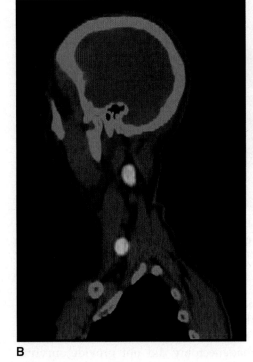

B

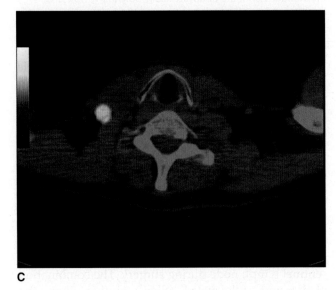

C

FIGURE 5 • **A:** Conventional planar lymphoscintigraphy in a patient with a 2.1-mm nonulcerated melanoma of the temporal scalp. Images are taken after injecting ^{99m}Tc-sulfur colloid intradermally into the primary melanoma site. Note the anatomical landmarks defined on the scan by the technologist (ear, sternocleidomastoid muscle, and clavicle) for orientation purposes.
B: Sagittal image from 3D SPECT-CT lymphoscintigraphy of the same patient as in (**A**), demonstrating uptake in upper and lower cervical lymph nodes and more clearly demonstrating the relationship of the nodes to the ear, sternocleidomastoid muscle, and clavicle.
C: Axial image from 3D SPECT-CT lymphoscintigraphy of the same patient as in (**A**) and (**B**), showing the relationship of the upper sentinel lymph node to the undersurface of the sternocleidomastoid muscle.

surgeon to identify the sentinel lymph node in more than 98% of cases. Removed nodes are then carefully evaluated using hematoxylin and eosin staining and immunohistochemistry techniques with antibodies to one or more melanoma marker epitopes such as S100, HMB45, and MART-1/Melan-A. Complications of sentinel lymph node biopsy include hematoma, wound infection, and seroma, although serious adverse effects are very uncommon.

Follow-up

Controversy exists among clinicians regarding the frequency and duration of postoperative surveillance in

patients with history of melanoma. Most experts would recommend following these patients every 3 to 6 months for the first 3 years and annually thereafter. This schedule is influenced by a variety of factors such as the stage of the primary melanoma, number of lymph nodes involved, any prior history of melanoma, the presence of multiple atypical moles, or a family history of the disease. For asymptomatic patients, some authors recommend a chest x-ray and lactate dehydrogenase (LDH) levels every 6 to 12 months, but their value has never been shown, and we do not routinely obtain these tests.

The main goal of any surveillance program includes identification of new primary or recurrent disease at an early stage that would allow potential curative resection. Skin cancer education including potential deleterious effects of sun exposure and the need for appropriate protection, such as sun avoidance, protective clothing, and broad-spectrum sunscreens, should be promoted among melanoma patients and their families. Routine self–skin examination and assessment of lymph node basins is of great value, since many patients presenting with recurrence find the disease themselves.

Presentation Continued

A 75-year-old man with a history of a thin melanoma in the thigh 2 years ago presents with enlarged ipsilateral inguinal nodes. At the time of the original diagnosis, he was treated with excision with adequate resection margins, but a sentinel lymph node biopsy was not performed. The patient did not have complaints other than occasional headaches and a few episodes of visual changes.

Workup

The use of routine blood work and imaging studies for patients with clinical stage I or II disease is of low yield. Patients presenting with more advanced stages or with symptomatology of metastatic disease should be evaluated more extensively. Currently available blood tests such as LDH serum levels have low sensitivity and specificity. In patients with stage IV disease at presentation, elevated serum values of LDH are associated with reduced survival rates. Regardless of the stage of the original melanoma, patients with suspected recurrence should undergo a complete physical examination including a full dermatologic evaluation and assessment of all lymph node groups. In patients with prior surgery, the status of the scars at the primary and lymph node resection sites as well as the presence of lymphedema should be documented. When a melanoma patient presents with an enlarged lymph node, the preferred diagnostic modality is a fine needle aspiration (FNA) of the node. If this cannot be performed or if the FNA is nondiagnostic, an open biopsy is the next step, orienting the incision so as to facilitate a subsequent lymph node dissection.

The use of imaging studies in the initial staging of the patient with advanced or recurrent disease includes computed tomography and positron emission tomography (PET) scans. PET scanning is sensitive for detecting metastatic melanoma deposits as small as 5 to 10 mm in size but is nonspecific. The use of PET/CT fusion scans provides improved anatomic definition but does not eliminate false-positive results. Pelvic CT scans are often recommended in the setting of inguinofemoral lymphadenopathy to evaluate for the presence of intrapelvic disease. Brain magnetic resonance imaging (MRI) is recommended when patients have neurologic symptoms and for patients with palpable nodes or distant disease.

Surgical Management of Node-Positive Disease

The current recommendation for melanoma patients with regional lymph node metastases and no evidence of distance disease is complete lymphadenectomy, which includes removal of all nodes of the involved nodal basin. In patients with inguinal metastasis, such as the case above, superficial inguinal node dissection (inguinofemoral lymphadenectomy) is indicated at a minimum. This technique involves en bloc resection of all inguinal lymphatic tissue contained within the femoral triangle, as well as the node-bearing tissue superior to the inguinal ligament but superficial to the external abdominal oblique aponeurosis. The decision making about adding a pelvic node dissection, that is, performing a superficial and deep inguinal node dissection (ilioinguinal lymphadenectomy), remains controversial. Some authors recommend routine biopsy of Cloquet's node to predict involvement of pelvic lymph nodes. In our experience, we have found this approach to be of very limited value. Radiographic evidence of pelvic nodal metastasis is an absolute indication for ilioinguinal lymphadenectomy, but we tend to perform this in most patients with palpable inguinal nodes.

The most common complications following inguinofemoral and ilioinguinal lymphadenectomy include wound infections and seroma, lymphedema, and deep vein thrombosis. Preoperative antibiotics are routinely used, but postoperatively antibiotics are only given if signs or symptoms of infection develop. To prevent the femoral vessels from being exposed in the event of a wound disruption, the sartorius muscle is often detached from its origin on the anterior superior iliac spine and transposed, suturing it to the inguinal ligament to cover the femoral vessels. The severity of lymphedema can be minimized by the use of fitted gradient compression stockings, using limb measurements obtained preoperatively, in the first few months postoperatively and as needed thereafter. Typically, inguinal lymphadenectomy patients are kept on bed rest overnight but are asked to ambulate starting on postoperative day 1. Frequent leg elevation when the patient is not ambulating helps as well. Low molecular weight heparin administration and early ambulation may decrease the rate of postoperative DVT.

Adjuvant Therapy and Treatment of Metastatic Disease

The majority of patients with early-stage melanoma will be cured by excision alone. Current recommendations for adjuvant therapy for patients with stage IIB or III melanoma include interferon alpha therapy or enrollment in clinical trials. Interferon alpha treatment has been consistently shown to improve relapse-free survival by approximately 20% to 30%, and in some analyses overall survival by a smaller amount. Recently, a large European randomized trial involving more than 1,250 patients with stage III melanoma showed a statistically significant improvement in relapse-free survival, but not overall survival, in patients treated with pegylated interferon. Due to its much longer half-life, pegylated interferon allows weekly injections as opposed to daily or three times per week injections for standard interferon, but in the European study it was given for 5 years rather than one. Whenever possible, patients with melanoma should be referred for clinical trials that may allow developing better therapies for the future.

Adjuvant radiation therapy can be considered in certain situations. For desmoplastic melanoma with neurotropic spread, radiation to the primary site is often used. Radiation to the regional node basin is also often recommended in the face of risk factors for postlymphadenectomy regional recurrence, which include extracapsular extension, four or more involved lymph nodes, maximum nodal metastasis size ≥3 cm, or recurrent disease in the nodal basin after complete lymphadenectomy. Radiation therapy is also used in the treatment of brain metastases and may be useful in palliating other symptomatic metastases.

Dramatic changes in the management of patients with metastatic melanoma have occurred over the last few years with the introduction of two new targeted agents. Ipilimumab, an antibody directed against cytotoxic T-lymphocyte antigen 4 (CTLA4), has been shown to improve overall survival for patients with unresectable metastatic melanoma when given alone or combined with dacarbazine. More recently, selective inhibition of the mutant BRAF V600E protein with vemurafenib was shown in a phase III study to dramatically prolong progression-free and overall survival compared to dacarbazine. About 50% of patients with metastatic melanoma have tumors that harbor the BRAF V600E gene mutation, so patients with metastatic disease should routinely have their tumors undergo mutational analysis to determine if targeted therapy is an appropriate consideration. Patients treated with vemurafenib or other selective BRAF inhibitors such as dabrafenib develop cutaneous squamous cell carcinomas, particularly keratoacanthoma-type lesions, at a greatly increased frequency.

TAKE HOME POINTS

- Early recognition and treatment are associated with more favorable outcomes.
- The presence of ulceration and the mitotic count determines T1a versus T1b in melanomas ≤1 mm, and these factors influence surgical decision making in these patients.
- The most important prognostic factor for clinically localized melanoma is the status of the lymph nodes draining the primary site.
- Postoperative surveillance relies mostly on physical examination, with imaging studies performed when metastatic disease is suspected.
- New therapies have shown improved overall survival in patients with metastatic disease.
- Whenever possible, patients with advanced melanoma should be referred for clinical trials that would allow developing even better therapies for the future.

SUGGESTED READINGS

Gershenwald JE, Ross MI. Sentinel-lymph-node biopsy for cutaneous melanoma. N Engl J Med. 2011; 364;1738–1745.

Morton DL, Cochran AJ, Thompson JF, et al. Multicenter Selective Lymphadenectomy Trial Group. Sentinel node biopsy for early-stage melanoma: accuracy and morbidity in MSLT-I, an international multicenter trial. Ann Surg. 2005;242:302–311.

Paek SC, Griffith KA, Johnson TM, et al. The impact of factors beyond Breslow depth on predicting sentinel lymph node positivity in melanoma. Cancer. 2007;109:100–108.

Rao NG, Yu HH, Trotti A III, et al. The role of radiation therapy in the management of cutaneous melanoma. Surg Oncol Clin N Am. 2011;20:115–131.

Sondak VK, Flaherty LE. Targeted therapies: improved outcomes for patients with metastatic melanoma. Nat Rev Clin Oncol. 2011;8:513–515.

Zager JS, Hochwald SN, Marzban SS, et al. Shave biopsy is a safe and accurate method for the initial evaluation of melanoma. J Am Coll Surg. 2011;212:454–460.

99 Melanoma Presenting with Regional Lymph Node Involvement

MICHAEL S. SABEL

Presentation

A 45-year-old woman presented to her dermatologist after noticing a suspicious lesion on her left thigh. An excisional biopsy performed in the office demonstrated a 1.8-mm superficial spreading melanoma with ulceration. The patient now presents to your office for surgical management. On physical examination, there is a well-healed longitudinal scar on the left thigh and a palpable 1.5-cm, mobile, firm lymph node in the left groin.

Differential Diagnosis

All patients diagnosed with invasive melanoma should undergo a thorough physical examination, paying particular attention to the regional draining lymph node basins. Approximately 5% of patients will present with clinically apparent regional lymph node involvement at the time of diagnosis. Still others develop palpable lymphadenopathy months or years after excision of a primary melanoma, while occasional patients present with nodal metastasis in the absence of a detectable primary tumor. Regional lymph nodes may become enlarged due to infection, inflammation, or reactive hyperplasia, particularly after an excisional biopsy of the primary tumor has been performed. However, any palpable nodes that are larger than 1 to 1.5 cm in size, hard, or fixed to adjacent structures must be considered suspicious for metastatic involvement. Metastatic nodal involvement can be reliably verified in most cases with a fine needle aspiration (FNA) biopsy. Excisional biopsy should be reserved for situations in which the node is clinically suspicious, but the aspiration biopsy is negative or indeterminate because the complications of an open biopsy (including seroma, infection, and scarring) can interfere with the performance of a subsequent lymph node dissection. If an excisional biopsy is performed, it is important to orient the incision so that it can be readily re-excised during the complete node dissection if the node proves to be involved with tumor.

(FNA of the palpable node confirms the presence of metastatic melanoma)

Workup

Unfortunately, once melanoma has spread to the lymph nodes, there is a steep drop-off in survival. However, node-positive melanoma is a potentially curable disease, and an aggressive surgical approach is warranted. Patients, such as this one, with biopsy-proven palpable nodal involvement, should undergo wide local excision of the primary tumor and complete lymph node dissection if there is no radiologic evidence of distant metastases.

A metastatic workup should be performed to evaluate any patients presenting with clinical stage III disease. The most important part of this workup is a detailed history and physical examination. The history should include a thorough review of symptoms, focusing on symptoms consistent with metastatic disease, including any neurologic symptoms from possible brain metastases. In addition to the history and physical examination, all patients with clinically evident stage III disease should have a serum lactate dehydrogenase (LDH) level measurement and at minimum a chest x-ray. Many surgeons, however, would recommend staging of these patients with a CT scan of the chest/abdomen/pelvis, PET scan, or PET/CT. Several retrospective studies have suggested that these studies can lead to a change in surgical management in 15% to 35% of cases, with PET/CT outperforming either PET or CT alone. For patients, such as the present one, with palpable inguinal adenopathy, a CT scan of the abdomen and the pelvis not only may evaluate for intra-abdominal metastasis but can also identify enlarged pelvic lymph nodes that might convert an inguinal node dissection to an inguinal-iliac dissection. CT scan or MRI of the brain is not routinely necessary in asymptomatic patients.

It is important to note that with both CT scans and PET scans, false-positive findings are common; histologic confirmation of an abnormal lesion should be obtained whenever feasible before concluding a patient has stage IV disease and abandoning a potentially curable surgical approach.

The patient is asymptomatic and physical examination shows no evidence of metastatic disease. A serum

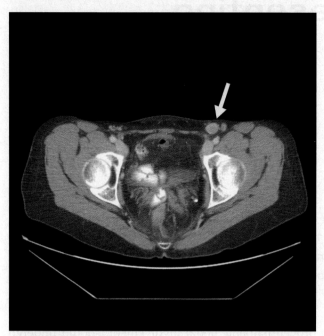

FIGURE 1 • CT scan demonstrating lymphadenopathy (*arrow*) in a patient with melanoma.

LDH level and CT scan of the chest, abdomen, and pelvis show no areas suspicious for metastatic disease and no enlarged pelvic lymph nodes. The enlarged inguinal lymph node was visualized **(Figure 1)**.

Surgical Approach

For patients with palpable disease in the axilla, a complete axillary lymph node dissection should include levels I, II, and III to provide the best regional control. In a very thin person, anterior retraction of the pectoralis major and minor muscle may allow for adequate dissection of the level III nodes. However, in most individuals, it may be necessary to divide the pectoralis minor. To do so, the pectoralis major is retracted anteriorly and the fascia on either side of the tendon of the pectoralis minor is incised. With a finger behind the muscle to protect the axillary artery and vein, the insertion of the pectoralis minor is divided with electrocautery.

For patients with palpable disease in the groin, the extent of lymphadenectomy ("superficial" vs. "superficial and deep") is controversial. Some surgeons advocate complete superficial and deep inguinal lymph node dissections in all patients with palpable adenopathy. Others reserve deep dissection to those patients with a positive Cloquet's node, or three or more involved nodes. Still others only perform deep groin dissections when there is radiographic evidence of pelvic adenopathy. If a deep groin dissection is to be performed together with a superficial dissection, this can be accomplished through one skin incision by obliquely dividing the external and internal oblique muscles to expose the pelvic retroperitoneum, or alternatively by dividing the inguinal ligament. Dividing the ligament is particularly useful in cases of extensive disease low in the pelvis along the distal external iliac vessels. Although it is simpler to divide the ligament over the femoral vessels, wound healing may be improved if the inguinal ligament is detached from the anterior superior iliac spine **(Table 1)**.

The patient undergoes a wide excision of the melanoma with 2-cm margins and a superficial and deep inguinal lymph node dissection. Three of eleven inguinal nodes and zero of five deep nodes are positive for lymph node metastases. There is no evidence of extracapsular extension.

Postoperative Management

After a complete node dissection, there is a risk of recurrence in and around the dissected bed. The risk of regional recurrence increases with the size and number of involved nodes, and the presence of extracapsular extension. Some have advocated the use of adjuvant

---

TABLE 1. Key Technical Steps and Potential Pitfalls in Superficial and Deep Inguinal Lymph Node Dissection

Key Technical Steps

1. The patient is positioned supine with the leg flexed and externally rotated in the frog-leg position.
2. An oblique, slightly S-shaped incision is created starting medial to the anterior superior iliac spine and coursing to a point 1–2 cm below the apex of the femoral triangle. An ellipse of skin over the palpable mass is included in the resection.
3. Progressively thicker flaps are raised laterally to the sartorius muscle, medially to the adductor longus and superiorly to a line from the pubic tubercle to the anterior superior iliac spine.
4. The lymph node–bearing tissue is then excised from over the femoral nerve, artery, and vein and off of the external oblique aponeurosis.
5. A deep dissection can be performed by creating a separate incision in the external oblique aponeurosis or by dividing the inguinal ligament.
6. The peritoneum is retracted medially to expose the iliac fossa. The iliac nodes are dissected off the common and external iliac vessels. The obturator nodes are dissected off the posterior surface of the external iliac vein.
7. After closure over a deep drain, the sartorius is mobilized and transposed to sit over the exposed femoral vessels.
8. A superficial drain is placed and the incision is closed.

Potential Pitfalls

- Injury to the spermatic cord structures or the contents of an unexpected hernia.
- Injury to the femoral or iliac neurovascular structures.
- Injury to the ureter.
- Bleeding from the obturator and iliac veins.

radiation to the dissected nodal basin. A recently completed prospective randomized trial demonstrated that radiation to the basin after radical lymph node dissection does decrease regional recurrence rates, although this does not appear to impact overall survival. Therefore, it is reasonable to consider postoperative radiation in patients with extracapsular extension, multiple involved lymph nodes (≥2 cervical or axillary nodes or ≥3 inguinal nodes), or large nodes (≥3 cm in the neck or axilla or ≥4 cm in the groin), but the risks and benefits of adjuvant radiation must be carefully weighed. Given the higher risk of recurrence and lower morbidity of radiation after a neck dissection, the threshold for adjuvant radiation for cervical metastases is lower. On the other hand, adjuvant radiation after an inguinal node dissection is associated with significant morbidity and should be reserved for patients with a very high risk of relapse.

Patients with clinically evident regional metastases are also at a high risk of distant metastases, and most patients in this situation will ultimately die of their disease. Therefore, adjuvant therapy should be considered. Although multiple systemic therapies have been studied, none had demonstrated a benefit in reducing the risk of relapse or death for high-risk melanoma patients until the introduction of high-dose interferon alpha-2b (IFNα-2b). Three randomized studies have demonstrated an improvement in disease-free survival with high-dose interferon (HDI), while two of the three demonstrated an improvement in overall survival. However, significant toxicities of HDI and the equivocal results of some of the trials have made the use of IFNα-2b controversial. Serious side effects include flu-like symptoms (malaise, fevers, chills, arthralgias), fatigue, depression, liver function abnormalities, nausea and vomiting, and neutropenia and infectious complications. Based on the available data, all patients with high-risk melanoma should have a balanced discussion concerning the potential risks and benefits of adjuvant HDI. Participation in clinical trials is strongly encouraged for patients who opt not to be treated with IFNα-2b.

TAKE HOME POINTS

- Approximately 5% of melanoma patients will present with clinically involved regional nodes.
- FNA of suspicious nodes is recommended to document regional involvement. Excisional biopsy can interfere with the subsequent node dissection.
- Workup should include a thorough history and physical examination, serum LDH level and staging, which can be accomplished by CT, PET scan, or CT/PET.
- Patients without definitive evidence of distant disease should undergo complete lymph node dissection. In the axilla, this typically involves levels I, II, and III. In the groin, some surgeons routinely perform a superficial and deep dissection, while other surgeons limit the deep dissection to patients with evidence of iliac or pelvic disease.
- Adjuvant radiation to the regional basin may be considered for patients at high risk of regional recurrence (multiple nodes, extracapsular extension); however, the risks (lymphedema, wound complications) must be carefully weighed against the benefits (decreased regional recurrence, no improvement in overall survival).
- All stage III melanoma patients should be referred to a medical oncologist for consideration of adjuvant therapy with HDI. Patients who opt not to be treated with interferon should be encouraged to participate in clinical trials.

100 Merkel Cell Carcinoma

MICHAEL S. SABEL

Presentation

A 69-year-old woman presents to her primary care physician when she notices a firm, nontender, red mass on her left forearm (**Figure 1**). She first noticed it a few weeks ago, and in the interval, it has grown rapidly. An excisional biopsy performed under local anesthesia demonstrates a Merkel cell carcinoma (MCC). She is referred to your office for further evaluation and treatment.

Differential Diagnosis

MCC is a rare but aggressive skin cancer, which is also called *neuroendocrine carcinoma of the skin* or *small cell carcinoma of the skin*. MCC is rare, with only approximately 500 new cases each year and an annual incidence of 0.6 per 100,000 (based on Surveillance, Epidemiology and End-Results [SEER] data). They are most common among older individuals, with an average age at diagnosis of 69 years and only 5% of patients below the age of 50. They typically present as an intracutaneous nodule or plaque that has grown rapidly over a few weeks to months. It can be flesh-colored, red, or purple. While it sometime ulcerates, the overlying skin is frequently intact. They are most common on sun-exposed areas, with approximately 50% on the face and neck, 40% on the extremities, and 10% on the trunk. The differential includes lipoma, keratoacanthoma, epidermal cysts, pyogenic granuloma, basal cell carcinoma, squamous cell carcinoma, amelanotic melanoma, lymphoma cutis, and metastatic carcinoma of the skin.

Workup

Approximately 70% of MCC patients present with localized disease, while 25% will have palpable regional lymphadenopathy at presentation and 5% present with distant metastases. As with any patient with a new cutaneous or subcutaneous lesion, a thorough history and physical examination including a complete skin and lymph node examination is warranted. However, MCC is rarely suspected clinically at the time of presentation. The diagnosis is made on excisional biopsy. Microscopically, MCC tumors arise in the dermis and frequently extend into the subcutaneous fat. The tumor is composed of small blue cells with round-to-oval, hyperchromatic nuclei and minimal cytoplasm. There are three variants: intermediate (the most common), small cell, and trabecular. The small cell variant is identical to other small cell carcinomas and must be distinguished from metastatic small cell carcinoma. This can be accomplished through immunohistochemistry. Merkel cell tumors express CAM 5.2

and cytokeratin (CK) 20. CK7 and thyroid transcription factor-1 (TTF-1), which is typically found on bronchial small cell carcinomas, are absent on MCC. The intermediate type can often be confused for melanoma or lymphoma. MCC is invariably negative for S-100 and leukocyte-common antigen, which distinguishes it from these.

MCC typically metastasizes to the regional lymph nodes, skin, lung, brain, bone, and liver. Patients with clinically involved lymph nodes or symptoms suggestive of distant metastases should have a computed tomography (CT) scan of the chest, abdomen, and pelvis. CT scan of the chest should also be considered in patients with the small cell variant to exclude the presence of a lung mass suspicious for small cell lung cancer. Otherwise, for patients who have clinically localized disease, a chest x-ray alone is reasonable. The use of routine imaging studies in asymptomatic patients with clinically localized MCC is associated with a low rate of detecting true disease and a high false-positive rate, generating additional tests or biopsies and increasing patient anxiety without impacting overall survival.

On history, the patient is otherwise asymptomatic and physical examination reveals no evidence of in-transit, regional, or distant metastases. There are no other suspicious skin lesions. Review of the biopsy results confirms MCC, measuring 3.5 cm. Chest x-ray shows no pulmonary lesions.

Diagnosis and Treatment

MCC is considered to be both radiosensitive and chemosensitive. Therefore, treatment of MCC should proceed in a multidisciplinary fashion. The initial treatment is usually surgical. Because of the high rate of local recurrence, margins of 2 to 3 cm have historically been recommended. However, low local recurrence rates have been reported after margin-negative excision with more narrow margins. For lesions <2 cm in greatest dimension, margins of 1 cm are typically adequate. For lesions >2 cm, a 2-cm margin is recommended when

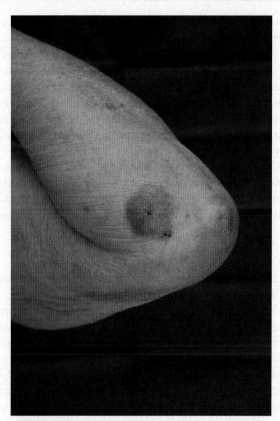

FIGURE 1 • Merkel cell carcinoma.

feasible. For patients with MCC in cosmetically sensitive areas, where even 1-cm margins would be difficult, Mohs micrographic surgery has been reported to have comparable local control rates.

All patients with clinically localized MCC should undergo sentinel lymph node biopsy (SLNB) in conjunction with wide excision. Approximately 20% to 30% of clinically node-negative MCC patients are SLNB positive, and the pathologic lymph node status is the most consistent predictor of survival. Because MCCs have a histologic appearance of a small cell, approximately the size of a lymphocyte, they can be extremely difficult to detect within the lymph nodes using standard hematoxylin and eosin (H&E) staining alone. Therefore, immunohistochemical analysis of the sentinel nodes, in particular with anti-CK-20, is essential. For patients having Mohs surgery, it may be preferable to perform the Mohs surgery after the patient has undergone SLNB.

Surgical Approach

Preoperative planning is critical to determine whether the patient will be able to be closed primarily. If not, then reconstruction with either a split-thickness skin graft or a rotational flap should be considered. The likelihood of postoperative radiation to the primary site should be taken into account when deciding the optimal method for reconstruction.

Prior to being taken to the operating room, the patient should undergo a perilesional injection of technetium sulfur colloid and lymphoscintigram. In the operating room, blue dye (either Lymphazurin or Methylene Blue) is injected intradermally around the lesion. In cases where shine-through may impact the ability to find the sentinel lymph node, the wide excision should be performed first. One- to two-centimeter margins, depending on the size of the primary tumor, are measured around the tumor (or scar from the prior biopsy). If primary closure is feasible, an ellipse is drawn around the lesion with a 3.5 to 1 ratio of length to width. After excision, the skin flaps are elevated to allow primary wound closure. If primary closure is not likely, then either a rotational flap is marked out preoperatively or a donor site for a split-thickness skin graft is prepped out. After changing gowns, gloves, and instruments, the SLNB is performed.

If there is any concern regarding the margin status, it may be preferable to place a temporary graft, such as Integra, until the final pathology results are known. The patient can then return to the operating room for a skin graft or rotational flap once it is known that negative margins have been attained **(Table 1)**.

The patient undergoes wide resection without the need for a skin graft. Two axillary sentinel lymph nodes are identified. The final pathology report reveals no residual MCC in the primary specimen and two of two lymph nodes are positive for metastatic disease, evident on both H&E and immunohistochemical staining.

For patients who have clinically involved lymph nodes and no evidence of distant metastasis, complete lymph node dissection (CLND) should be performed at the time of wide resection. For clinically node-negative patients who undergo SLN biopsy and are found to harbor metastases, CT scan may be considered to rule out distant disease. If negative, CLND is typically considered. As MCC is a radiosensitive tumor, radiation therapy to the regional basin alone can be considered in cases where CLND may be excessively morbid or for patients with minimal tumor burden in the SLN. Failure to treat the lymph node basin after a positive SLN has been associated with high recurrence rates, although the impact on overall survival is unknown. Presentation to a multidisciplinary tumor board on a case-by-case basis is recommended.

Case Conclusion

The patient returns to the operating room for a completion node dissection. None of the 24 lymph nodes contain metastatic MCC.

TABLE 1. Key Technical Steps and Potential Pitfalls in Wide Excision and SLNB for MCC

Key Technical Steps

1. Preoperative planning for primary closure versus skin graft or rotational flap.
2. Preoperative injection of Tc^{99} colloid sulfur and lymphoscintigram and intraoperative injection of blue dye.
3. Wide excision first, if necessary, to minimize impact of shine-through on the SLNB.
4. Measure adequate margins around the lesion (or scar) and excise down to and including the fascia.
5. Undermine flaps for primary closure or perform skin graft or rotational flap. Consider temporary graft if margin status is a concern.
6. Change position (if necessary), gowns, gloves, and instruments for performance of the SLNB.

Potential Pitfalls

- Unable to close the primary site.
- Inability to detect the sentinel lymph node.
- Positive tumor margins.

Postoperative Management

MCC is radiosensitive and radiation therapy is often part of the treatment algorithm. Adjuvant radiation is critical if surgical margins are positive or relatively narrow. Adjuvant radiation may be omitted for small primary tumors (<2 cm) if clear margins are obtained. For primary tumors ≥ 2 cm, even with negative margins, adjuvant radiation should be strongly considered.

Radiation can also be used for the regional basin. As stated above, radiation may be considered as an alternative to completion node dissection for patients with minimal tumor burden within a positive SLN; however, CLND is typically considered first-line treatment. Adjuvant radiation after CLND is not necessary for patients with microscopic disease within the SLN. This combination may be considered for patients with extensive lymph node disease or extracapsular extension. However, the benefits of reducing regional recurrence must be weighed against the increased morbidity of surgery and radiation, the most significant of which is lymphedema.

Although MCC is generally considered a chemosensitive tumor, adjuvant chemotherapy is the least studied treatment modality for MCC and currently has no established role in the treatment of local or regional disease.

TAKE HOME POINTS

- MCC is a relatively rare, but highly aggressive, cutaneous malignancy that is more common among the elderly.
- Workup, including immunohistochemical staining of the biopsy, is needed to differentiate from amelanotic melanoma, lymphoma cutis, metastatic carcinoid, and metastatic small cell lung cancer.
- MCC can be treated with surgery, radiation, and in some cases chemotherapy, so a multidisciplinary approach is strongly recommended.
- Local disease is treated by wide excision with clear margins and often followed by adjuvant radiation.
- Clinically node-negative patients should undergo SLNB in addition to wide excision. Patients with a positive SLN typically undergo CLND, although radiation to the involved basin may also be considered.
- CLND followed by radiation should be considered for patients with extensive lymph node involvement or extracapsular extension.

101 Nonmelanoma Skin Cancer

ANASTASIA DIMICK

Presentation

A 65-year-old white male presents with a slowly enlarging, tender 1.5-cm hyperkeratotic erythematous nodule on his left forearm. The patient first noticed the lesion about 3 months ago. He has severe photodamage (atrophic skin with numerous lentigines and senile purpura). Because of his occupation as a farmer, he has a chronic history of significant sun exposure. Previous medical history is significant for actinic keratoses (precancerous skin lesions for squamous cell carcinoma) on the face and hands, which have been treated with liquid nitrogen or cryotherapy **(Figure 1)**. Family history is significant for melanoma in his father.

Differential Diagnosis

In this clinical context, the most likely diagnosis is squamous cell carcinoma of the skin **(Figure 2)**. Other diagnostic possibilities include basal cell carcinoma **(Figure 3)**, basosquamous cell carcinoma, and melanoma. Clinical features of this lesion that point to squamous cell carcinoma are the erythematous color, the presence of hyperkeratosis or rough crusty skin, and tenderness. Melanomas can be hyperkeratotic in rare instances and sore or pruritic but are typically dark brown or black and asymptomatic. There is an uncommon variant of melanoma called amelanotic, which lacks pigment on clinical exam. These lesions may have a clinical appearance similar to basal cell carcinomas, which are usually pearly pink with telangiectatic vessels. The diagnosis of amelanotic melanoma is virtually always made on histopathologic grounds. Basosquamous cell carcinomas have clinical features of both basal cell carcinomas and squamous cell carcinomas.

Workup

The patient underwent a cutaneous biopsy in the outpatient clinic. Pathology was consistent with well-differentiated squamous cell carcinoma.

Discussion

Squamous cell carcinoma is the second most common type of skin cancer in the United States. Basal cell carcinoma is the most common type of skin cancer in the United States. Together, these nonmelanoma skin cancers account for over 3 million cases per year. The vast majority of these cancers are caused by ultraviolet light exposure. As the population ages, the incidence is expected to increase. Risk factors for developing skin cancer include previous history of skin cancer, family history of skin cancer, fair skin (Fitzpatrick I [always burns, never tans] and Fitzpatrick II [usually burns, tans with difficulty]), severe sunburn history, excessive occupational or avocational sun exposure, and immunosuppressed state. Patients that have undergone organ transplantation have a significantly higher risk of developing skin cancer, particularly squamous cell carcinoma. Candidates for organ transplantation should receive pretransplant counseling on skin cancer prevention and a complete skin examination to identify and treat any precancerous growths, such as actinic keratoses, and cancerous lesions. Squamous cell carcinomas may also arise in burn scars, chronic ulcers, previously irradiated sites, and certain inflammatory conditions of the skin such as discoid lupus erythematosus or genital lichen sclerosus et atrophicus. Although less common than squamous cell carcinomas induced by ultraviolet radiation, these squamous cell carcinomas tend to have a more malignant course.

Diagnosis and Treatment

The diagnosis of skin cancer is confirmed with a skin biopsy. There are two main histopathologic subtypes of squamous cell carcinoma: well-differentiated and poorly differentiated. In general, the prognostic outcome for well-differentiated squamous cell carcinomas is good, while poorly differentiated squamous cell carcinomas tend to behave aggressively and are more likely to metastasize. In addition, other features associated with increased metastatic potential are tumor diameter greater than 2 cm and tumor depth greater than 2 mm. The overall metastatic rate of solar induced squamous cell carcinoma is <5%. Squamous cell carcinomas of the scalp, ears, and lips have a higher metastatic rate of approximately 10% to 15%. Other squamous cell carcinomas, which behave more aggressively, are those with histologic evidence of perineural invasion. Adjuvant radiation therapy should be considered to lower the risk of metastases of squamous cell carcinomas with perineural invasion.

511

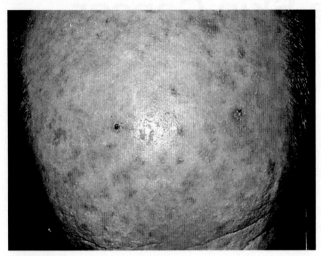

FIGURE 1 • Actinic keratoses.

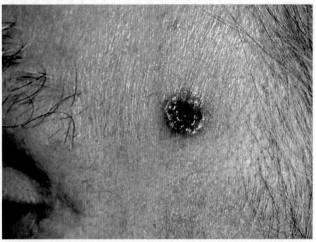

FIGURE 3 • Basal cell carcinoma. (From Goodheart HP, MD. Goodheart's Photoguide of Common Skin Disorders. 2nd ed. Philadelphia, PA: Lippincott Williams & Wilkins, 2003, FIGURE 22.17.)

The mainstay of treatment for squamous cell carcinoma is excision with histopathologic confirmation of clear or negative margins. Unlike melanoma, there are no standardized excisional margins for squamous

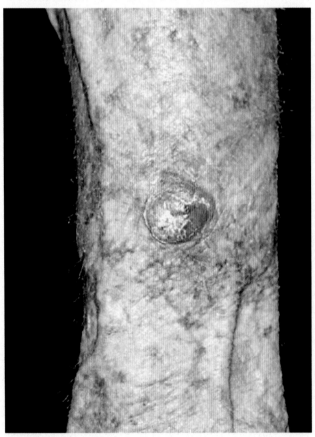

FIGURE 2 • Squamous cell carcinoma. (From Goodheart HP, MD. Goodheart's Photoguide of Common Skin Disorders. 2nd ed. Philadelphia, PA: Lippincott Williams & Wilkins, 2003, FIGURE 22.10.)

cell carcinoma. Adequate excisional margins typically range from 4 to 10 mm. Another treatment modality is Mohs micrographic surgery. Mohs micrographic surgery should be considered for squamous cell carcinomas on the face, especially those involving the H-zone (temple, midface, perioral, periorbital and periauricular regions) and neoplasms on the trunk and the extremities, which are larger than 2 cm. Mohs micrographic surgery usually results in the lowest risk of recurrence. Recurrent squamous cell carcinomas should be referred for Mohs micrographic surgery.

Treatment of basal cell carcinoma is similar to squamous cell carcinoma. In addition, electrodesiccation and curettage is an acceptable therapeutic option for small (<2 cm) basal cell carcinomas with nonaggressive histopathologic subtypes on the trunk and extremities. There are different histopathologic subtypes of basal cell carcinomas including superficial, nodular, micronodular, infiltrative, and morpheaform. Micronodular, infiltrative, and morpheaform are considered to be the aggressive growth patterns because they are more likely to recur after treatment because of ill-defined borders. Mohs micrographic surgery is the preferred therapeutic option for these basal cell carcinomas.

After successfully treating the squamous cell carcinoma, further follow-up is warranted. The patient should undergo a complete skin and lymph node examination to ensure that there are no other concerning lesions or lymphadenopathy. In addition, the patient should receive counseling on the importance of performing monthly self–skin examinations and practicing sun safety techniques such as avoiding the sun between the hours of 11 AM and 4 PM, wearing sun protective clothing, and applying a broad-spectrum sunscreen with an SPF of 15 or higher.

TAKE HOME POINTS

- Squamous cell carcinoma is the second most common type of skin cancer in the United States.
- The vast majority of these cancers are caused by ultraviolet light exposure.
- The mainstay of treatment for squamous cell carcinoma is excision with histopathologic confirmation of clear or negative margins.
- After successfully treating the squamous cell carcinoma, further follow-up is warranted. The patient should undergo a complete skin and lymph node examination to ensure that there are no other concerning lesions or lymphadenopathy.

102 Necrotizing Soft Tissue Infections

MICHELLE K. MCNUTT and LILLIAN S. KAO

Presentation

A 45-year-old-man with a history of diabetes and hypertension presents to the emergency room with right leg pain and fever. His vital signs are as follows: systolic blood pressure of 90 mm Hg, heart rate of 120 beats per minute, and temperature of 101.9°F. On physical exam, his right leg has erythema extending from his ankle to midcalf. Furthermore, he has edema extending to his knee with significant pain on palpation despite cutaneous anesthesia. His laboratory values include a white blood cell (WBC) count of 18,000 with 23% bands, serum sodium concentration of 130 mmol/L, creatinine of 2.1, glucose of 300 mg/dL, and base deficit of 6 mEq/L.

Differential Diagnosis

The differential diagnosis of necrotizing soft tissue infections (NSTIs) is broad and includes nonnecrotizing cellulitis, impetigo, furuncles, carbuncles, folliculitis, skin changes of chronic venous insufficiency, insect and spider bites, or malignancy. In contrast to the other diagnoses in the differential, failure to promptly identify and treat an NSTI may result in significant short- and long-term disability, limb loss, and/or death.

Discussion

NSTIs represent a wide spectrum of diseases that can involve the skin, subcutaneous fat, superficial or deep fascia, muscle, or any combination of these structures that result in tissue death. Other descriptive terms for NSTIs include clostridial myonecrosis, gas gangrene, Meleney's ulcer, and flesh-eating infections. Fournier's gangrene refers to an NSTI involving the perineum. These terms all refer to an aggressive soft tissue infection that requires prompt diagnosis and surgical debridement to prevent complications such as sepsis, multiple organ failure (MOF), and death. Despite advances in medical and surgical care, the average mortality rate remains high, ranging from 10% to 23.5% in recent studies.

There are three clinical subtypes of NSTIs. Type I infections are the most common form of disease and are polymicrobial in nature. The causative microbes are a combination of gram-positive aerobes (*Staphylococcus*, *Streptococcus*, *Enterococcus*), gram-negative aerobes (*Pseudomonas*, *Escherichia coli*, *Enterobacter*, *Klebsiella*, etc.), anaerobes (*Bacteroides*, *Clostridium*), and fungi (Candida, mucormycoses). These organisms not only act synergistically but can also produce virulence toxins that increase tissue destruction. Type II, or monobacterial, NSTIs are frequently caused by β–hemolytic streptococci, *Clostridium perfringens*, and *Staphylococcus aureus*. Salt-water acquired NSTIs occur when a skin wound is infected with *Vibrio vulnificus* and are referred to as type III NSTIs. While type III infections are uncommon, these may progress rapidly to MOF and cardiovascular collapse within 24 hours and must be recognized and treated quickly.

Workup

The most important components in the diagnostic evaluation of NSTIs are a high index of suspicion and a thorough physical exam. Findings suspicious for NSTI include erythema, tense edema, vesicles or bullae, necrosis, grayish wound drainage, crepitus, ulcers, cutaneous anesthesia, and pain disproportionate to physical exam findings. Early NSTIs may present with subtle superficial findings on exam. By the time cutaneous manifestations such as blisters, bullae, crepitus, or skin necrosis are present, there may have been a significant delay in diagnosis and operative debridement. Since delay in diagnosis is associated with increased mortality, the physician must maintain a high index of suspicion during the initial evaluation. Systemic toxicity (fever, tachycardia, tachypnea, and diaphoresis) and progression of infection despite antibiotic therapy should also alert the physician to a possible NSTI.

An evaluation of past medical history is also important. While patient comorbidities such as chronic renal insufficiency, diabetes, coronary artery disease, peripheral vascular disease, and immunosuppressive conditions may serve as risk factors, NSTIs may develop in the absence of any past medical history. Other risk factors may include a history of traumatic injury, intravenous drug use, or prior surgery.

Laboratory evaluation should include an electrolyte panel, complete blood cell count with differential, and blood gas analysis. Superficial wound cultures are not helpful in directing antibiotic therapy and should not be obtained. Laboratory findings associated with NSTIs include azotemia, hypocalcemia, hyponatremia, leukocytosis, thrombocytopenia, and metabolic acidosis. A serum lactate level above 54.1 mg/dL and a serum sodium level <135 mEq/L have been associated with a higher mortality rate. C-reactive protein may be elevated as well.

Radiographic evaluation is rarely necessary to diagnose an NSTI. Soft tissue gas may be seen on plain radiographs, but the absence does not exclude the diagnosis. MRI findings of thickened fascia, fluid collection, and deep fascial rim enhancement can help differentiate NSTI from cellulitis, but should be combined with clinical findings for diagnostic accuracy. Radiographic evaluation should never delay prompt surgical debridement.

Diagnosis and Treatment

Adjunctive tests to history and physical exam findings are not necessary for the presumptive diagnosis of NSTI. The triad of crepitus, skin blistering, and radiographic evidence of soft tissue gas has a sensitivity of over 80% for the diagnosis of NSTI; thus, these three signs serve as a helpful screening tool. Rapid surgical exploration remains the gold standard for diagnosis and should be performed if NSTI is suspected. Intraoperative findings suggestive of an NSTI include thrombosis of small blood vessels (obliterative endarteritis), swollen gray fascia (liquefactive necrosis), and the ability to easily dissect fascia away from normally adherent tissue (loss of tissue planes). If the diagnosis is still uncertain, deep tissue fascial biopsy with frozen section analysis may be confirmatory. Histologic changes consistent with NSTIs include tissue necrosis, fibrinous vascular thrombosis, polymorphonuclear infiltration, and microorganisms within destroyed tissue.

The laboratory risk indicator for necrotizing fasciitis (LRINEC) score measures nonspecific biochemical and inflammatory markers and can aid in the early recognition of necrotizing infections **(Table 1)**. A numerical score is assigned based on six laboratory parameters: C-reactive protein, total WBC count, hemoglobin concentration, sodium level, creatinine, and glucose. A score of ≥6 should raise the suspicion of necrotizing fasciitis (positive predictive value, 92% and negative predictive value, 96%), and a score of ≥8 is strongly predictive of the disease. The LRINEC score was derived from a single-center retrospective study and requires

TABLE 1. Laboratory Risk Indicator for Necrotizing Fasciitis Score

Variables, Units	Score
C-reactive protein, mg/L	
<150	0
≥150	4
Total white cell count, per mm³	
<15	0
15–25	1
>25	2
Hemoglobin, g/dL	
>13.5	0
11–13.5	1
<11	2
Sodium, mmol/L	
≥135	0
<135	2
Creatinine, µmol/L	
≤141	0
>141	2
Glucose, mmol/L	
≤10	0
>10	2

further validation with prospective studies. Despite this limitation, the LRINEC score remains a useful tool for the early detection of NSTI, and an elevated score should alert the physician to a patient at increased risk of having an NSTI.

Patients with NSTI often present with systemic toxicity and vital sign abnormalities that require optimization in concert with surgical debridement. Electrolyte abnormalities should be corrected, hyperglycemia treated with insulin, intravascular volume status optimized with fluid resuscitation, and broad-spectrum antibiotics initiated. Operative exploration should not be delayed in the unstable patient. A diagnostic incision and even therapeutic exploration can be performed at the bedside in the unstable patient.

NSTI patients should be treated initially with broad-spectrum antibiotics that can then be narrowed, based on cultures. There are no data to support the use of one initial antibiotic regimen over another; however, most combinations include penicillins or cephalosporins with either an aminoglycoside or a fluoroquinolone, plus an antianaerobic agent, such as clindamycin or metronidazole. As the incidence of methicillin-resistant *S. aureus* NSTIs is increasing, vancomycin or linezolid may be used empirically until culture results are available. Aminoglycosides and vancomycin should be appropriately dosed and monitored in patients with renal insufficiency. Patients with cirrhosis or saltwater and seafood exposure are at increased risk for developing *Vibrio* infections. *Vibrio* is a gram-negative bacillus and is susceptible to doxycycline, as well as other antibiotics, with gram-negative activity.

Surgical Approach

Definitive therapy for NSTIs requires prompt surgical debridement and excision of all infected tissue to a margin of normal healthy tissue. This initial surgical debridement is of paramount importance and should be performed in an urgent fashion.

Since the underlying soft tissue destruction is frequently more severe than the superficial physical exam findings, the initial incision should be extensile, thus allowing the surgeon to extend the incision as necessary based upon intraoperative findings. Excision of all infected and necrotic tissue is necessary. Margins of excision should be carried out to grossly normal tissue, characterized by the lack of inflammation and purulence and the presence of normal bleeding. A tissue biopsy should be sent to pathology to confirm the diagnosis and help tailor the antibiotic regimen postoperatively. After irrigation and surgical hemostasis, the wound should be packed open with Kerlix or gauze, or, alternatively, a negative pressure wound therapy system may be used for temporary soft tissue coverage.

NSTIs may progress rapidly despite surgical debridement; therefore, most patients benefit from reexploration in 24 hours, or sooner as clinically indicated, to confirm adequacy of debridement and absence of progression. The wound is explored in the operating room on a scheduled basis, and soft tissue coverage is delayed until no further debridement is necessary. Once the wound is healthy with no progression of infection and the patient's systemic toxicity has resolved, the wound may be closed. Wound closure may require a combination of rotational flaps and skin grafting depending on the size of the soft tissue defect **(Table 2)**.

TABLE 2. Key Technical Steps and Potential Pitfalls in Surgical Debridement for NSTI

Key Technical Steps
1. Extensive incision.
2. Aggressive excision of all necrotic tissue.
3. Excision margin to grossly normal tissue.
4. Consideration of guillotine amputation or disarticulation in presence of systemic toxicity and hemodynamic instability.
5. Repeat surgical debridement until infection controlled.
6. Soft tissue coverage with primary closure, skin graft, or rotational flap.

Potential Pitfalls
- Inadequate initial debridement.
- Failure to excise necrotic fascia.

Special Intraoperative Considerations

In Fournier's gangrene, a colostomy may be considered if fecal soilage is contaminating the open wound. This can be accomplished with either open or laparoscopic techniques with diverting transverse or sigmoid colostomy. With aggressive infections involving the extremities, a damage-control guillotine amputation or disarticulation may be indicated in the setting of systemic toxicity and hemodynamic instability to control the infection. Heart disease, shock (systolic blood pressure <90), and clostridial infections have been identified as three independent predictors of limb loss with NSTIs. The possibility of amputation should always be discussed with the patient or the family preoperatively.

Postoperative Management

Patients with an NSTI are best monitored in an intensive care unit setting. Aggressive fluid resuscitation and broad-spectrum antibiotic therapy should continue in the postoperative period. Continuous hemodynamic monitoring with the use of arterial and central lines may be necessary. Renal function, glucose control, and acid–base status should also be carefully monitored. Rapid clinical resolution frequently occurs following appropriate surgical debridement of the necrotic tissue, particularly if the infection is diagnosed at an early stage. Failure of resolution or clinical deterioration should raise the suspicion of progressive spread of infection and prompt a repeat exploration in the operating room.

Broad-spectrum antibiotics should be tailored to culture-specific therapy once tissue biopsy results are available and the patient has clinically improved. Antibiotics may be discontinued after clinical resolution and operative confirmation of control of infection.

The use of hyperbaric oxygen therapy (HBO) for NSTIs remains controversial. Randomized trials are lacking, and observational studies have demonstrated conflicting results. HBO cannot be recommended as routine therapy without further prospective trials. HBO may be considered with isolated clostridial infections in combination with surgical debridement, but it should never delay appropriate surgical debridement or interfere with resuscitation.

Another controversial therapy is the use of intravenous immunoglobulin for the treatment of streptococcal NSTIs. Proposed mechanisms of action involve the production of antibodies to neutralize circulating streptococcal antibodies and the interaction with proinflammatory cytokines to minimize the systemic inflammatory response. Additional studies are required before this therapy can be recommended.

Case Conclusion

The above patient was immediately treated with broad-spectrum antibiotics, insulin, and intravenous fluid resuscitation and was taken to the operating room within 6 hours of initial evaluation. All four muscle compartments were involved with infection and necrosis, and he had persistent hypotension and tachycardia in the operating room despite aggressive fluid resuscitation. A guillotine below-knee amputation was performed and he was transferred to the intensive care unit. He had four subsequent debridements and wet to dry dressings were used for temporary coverage of his wound. He required vasopressors and ventilator support initially postoperatively. He required dialysis for acute kidney failure that resolved during the course of his hospital stay. After his infection had resolved and his nutritional status was optimized, he underwent formal above-knee amputation. He was discharged home on postoperative day 16.

TAKE HOME POINTS

- The physician must maintain a high index of suspicion for prompt diagnosis.
- Delay in diagnosis and treatment increases morbidity and mortality.
- The most important therapy is immediate surgical debridement.
- Supportive therapy includes aggressive fluid resuscitation and broad spectrum antibiotics to cover gram-negative, gram-positive, and anaerobic bacteria.
- Repeat surgical debridements every 24 to 48 hours until infection is controlled.
- Mortality remains relatively high, ranging from 10% to 23.5% despite aggressive therapy.

Acknowledgments

Lillian S. Kao is supported by an NIH K23 Career Development Award (K23RR020020-05).

SUGGESTED READINGS

Anaya DA, McMahon K, Nathens AB, et al. Predictors of mortality and limb loss in necrotizing soft tissue infections. Arch Surg. 2005;140(2):151–157.

Elliott DC, Kufera JA, Myers RA. Necrotizing soft tissue infections. Risk factors for mortality and strategies for management. Ann Surg. 1996;224(5):672–683.

Elliott DC, Kufera JA, Myers RA. The microbiology of necrotizing soft tissue infections. Am J Surg. 2000;179:361–366.

May AK, Stafford RE, Bulger EM, et al. Treatment of complicated skin and soft tissue infections. Surg Infect. 2009;10(5):467–499.

Sarani B, Strong M, Pascual J, et al. Necrotizing fasciitis: current concepts and review of the literature. J Am Coll Surg. 2009;208(2):279–288.

Wong CH, Khin LW, Heng KS, et al. The LRINEC (laboratory risk indicator for necrotizing fasciitis) score: a tool for distinguishing necrotizing fasciitis from other soft tissue infections. Crit Care Med. 2004;32(7):1535–1541.

103 Extremity Mass (Sarcoma)

TIMOTHY L. FRANKEL and ALFRED E. CHANG

Presentation

A 35-year-old previously healthy man presents to his primary care physician noting a lump on his anterior leg, present for the past 2 months. It is not tender and he denies any recent trauma to the area. The mass has slowly increased in size over 2 months and is now approximately 5 cm in diameter **(Figure 1)**. Examination reveals a firm lesion fixed to the surrounding tissue with no obvious overlying skin changes. He has full range of motion of his knee and ankle with no obvious neurovascular deficits. There is no inguinal adenopathy or lesions elsewhere.

Differential Diagnosis

Masses located on either the arm or the leg can arise from a variety of malignant and benign pathologies. Benign lesions include lipomas, sebaceous cysts, neurofibromas, etc. Their treatment involves marginal excision when lesions are symptomatic, growing, or for diagnosis. Occasionally, trauma may result in mass formation from either inflammation or hematoma. A careful history can help identify this diagnosis, but a thorough exam is needed as trauma can often expose a previously unidentified malignancy and can in rare circumstances contribute to their growth as in the case of desmoid tumors.

Malignant lesions are classified according to their tissue of origin and may be initially grouped as either sarcomas of the bone or soft tissue sarcomas (STS). Bony sarcomas include osteosarcomas, Ewing sarcomas, malignant fibrous histiosarcoma (MFH) of the bone, and giant cell tumors. They are distinguished from STS by their firmness and fixation to underlying bone. The principal treatment of bony sarcomas is wide resection or rarely amputation with adjuvant chemotherapy. While primary osteosarcomas are often resistant to radiotherapy, it can be useful in the treatment of Ewing sarcoma when resection is not possible as in the case of axial skeletal involvement.

STS comprise the majority of malignant extremity masses. They often grow silently and only come to attention when they become visible or cause pain and loss of function due to distortion of surrounding structures. It is this reason that retroperitoneal sarcomas can go unnoticed until they are very large in size. The most important characteristics in the prognosis of STS are size, location, and grade. Open or large bore core needle biopsy is needed to make an appropriate diagnosis and guide further therapy. STS can be classified as originating from any mesenchymal structures of the extremity including fat, smooth or skeletal muscle, vessels, or nerves. MFH is the most common

STS, accounting for roughly 30% of the annual incidence **(Table 1)**. Typically occurring in the fifth and the sixth decades of life, these tumors are defined by their storiform growth pattern and infiltration of histiocytes. Over the past decade, the incidence of MFH has declined as advances in histology have led to reclassification of tumors to different subtypes.

Liposarcomas are derived from adipocytes and make up 15% of STS diagnosed in the United States annually. There are a variety of subtypes ranging from the slow-growing well-differentiated and myxoid liposarcomas to the more aggressive dedifferentiated and pleomorphic variants. Because therapy differs depending on which form is encountered, a well-trained pathologist is crucial in ensuring appropriate care is given. Low-grade liposarcomas are treated with surgical resection alone as metastases are rare and chemotherapy and radiotherapy are often ineffective. Higher-grade lesions may benefit from adjuvant or neoadjuvant radiation therapy, which will be discussed later. Leiomyosarcoma is the third most common STS and represents malignant growth of smooth muscle cells. They may occur throughout the body, but are commonly found where smooth muscle cell density is highest, such as the uterus. As with other STS, surgical resection represents the cornerstone of treatment with chemotherapy reserved for advanced disease. Rhabdosarcomas are rarely seen in adults, but represent the most common pediatric solid tumor. They arise from skeletal muscle progenitor cells and grow and metastasize rapidly. Unlike other STS, surgery alone rarely leads to cure, but multimodality therapy with the addition of chemotherapy and radiation has led to a 70% cure rate even in advanced disease. Rhabdosarcomas can be divided into embryonal or alveolar subtypes based on their histology with the former having a more favorable prognosis. Angiosarcomas occur most often on the scalp or the face in the eighth and the ninth decades of life. Risk factors include old age, prior exposure to

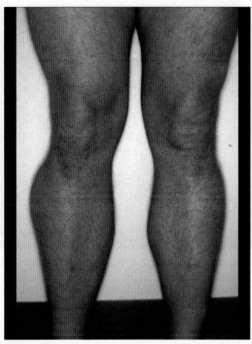

FIGURE 1 • A 35-year-old man presents with a right leg mass.

TABLE 2. Results of Randomized Trials of Adjuvant Radiation Following Sarcoma Resection		
Author (n)	Local Recurrence w/ or w/o Radiation	Survival w/ or w/o Radiation
Pisters et al. (1996) (n = 164)	18% vs. 31% at 5 y	84% vs. 81% at 5 y
Yang et al. (1998) (n = 141)	1% vs. 24% at 10 y	74% vs. 75% at 10 y

cell morphologies are present. These lesions have an aggressive behavior and therefore require wide resection and radiation therapy for control **(Table 2)**.

Workup

A thorough history and physical examination is important in differentiating benign versus malignant soft tissue lesions of the extremity. The character and rate of growth of the mass is elicited as well as any overlying skin changes or functional abnormalities of the limb. Lesions that have shown no growth over many years can often be treated with careful observation unless symptomatic. The decision on whether to next proceed directly to biopsy versus radiologic studies depends largely on the suspicion of malignancy. If a benign lesion such as lipoma is suspected, excisional biopsy is both diagnostic and therapeutic avoiding the need for costly imaging. When radiographic studies are needed, magnetic resonance imaging (MRI) is the primary modality for imaging extremity sarcomas. It allows delineation of muscle compartments, measurement of tumor size, and proximity to surrounding structures. Malignant lesions tend to be heterogeneous and enhanced on T2-weighted images, whereas benign masses appear similar to surrounding tissues **(Figure 2)**. When MRI is unavailable or in patients with metallic implants, computed tomography (CT) can be used.

All extremity masses in which malignancy is suspected should be biopsied and the tissue sent for pathologic analysis. There are four accepted methods of biopsy: fine needle aspiration (FNA), core needle biopsy, and incisional or excisional biopsy. FNA is performed by cleaning the skin immediately over the mass and infiltrating the subcutaneous tissue with local anesthetic. Next, a 22-gauge needle attached to a 3-mL syringe is inserted into the mass and negative pressure applied. The needle is retracted and advanced multiple times until debris is seen within the syringe. This is then extruded onto a slide for immediate review by a trained cytopathologist. Benefits of this procedure are its low morbidity and ability to be performed in an outpatient clinic provided a cytopathologist is immediately

ionizing radiation, and chronic lymphedema. The latter is an important cause of morbidity following axillary or inguinal lymphadenectomy and is thought to be one factor contributing to a rise in the incidence of this STS. Wide excision followed by adjuvant radiation is the treatment of choice for angiosarcoma, but local recurrence is common and the morbidity from reresection high. Synovial sarcoma is an STS that can occur throughout the body and whose histologic features resemble those of synovial cells. There are two subtypes: monophasic, which are dominated by spindle cells, and biphasic, where spindle and epithelial

TABLE 1. Soft Tissue Sarcoma Subtypes with Annual Incidence	
STS Subtype	Annual Incidence (%)
MFH	28
Liposarcoma	15
Leiomyosarcoma	12
Unclassified	11
Synovial Sarcoma	10
Malignant peripheral nerve sheath	6
Rhabdomyosarcoma	5
Fibrosarcoma	3
Ewing's Sarcoma	2
Angiosarcoma	2
Epithelioid, clear cell sarcoma, alveolar soft part, hemangiopericytoma	1

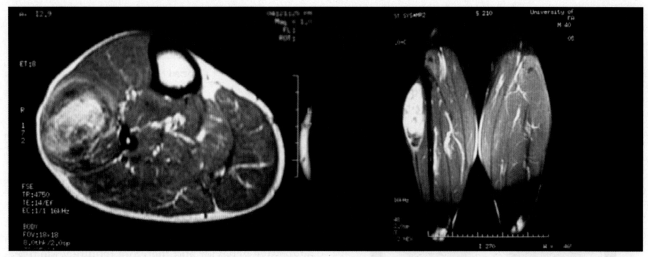

FIGURE 2 • MRI of lower-extremity mass can show features of the tumor, such as necrosis and proximity to surrounding structures such as vessels and bones.

available. Unfortunately, due to the small amount of tissue obtained, diagnostic uncertainty may still exist and information regarding grade and subtype of tumor may be lacking. Hence, FNA biopsies are reserved to document local recurrence or metastatic lesions. Core needle biopsy is performed in a similar fashion and can also take place in the outpatient setting. A larger bore needle is inserted into the lesion percutaneously and tissue cores removed for histologic analysis. Complication rate is low and the larger volume of tissue and retention of architecture allows for greater diagnostic certainty. When lesions are difficult to palpate or are in close proximity to vital structures, image-guided biopsies may be performed. With both FNA and core biopsy, the insertion point should be immediately above the lesion of interest and the needle tract removed with the specimen during operative extirpation.

Incisional or excisional biopsy is reserved for cases in which FNA and core biopsy fail to establish a diagnosis. Depending on the size of the lesion and proximity to vessels, nerves, and joints, the lesion is either completely removed (lesions <3 cm) or a small wedge taken (lesions >3 cm) for histologic analysis. It is important when performing either incisional or excisional biopsies to orient the incision along the longitudinal axis of the limb to facilitate future re-resection. In addition, meticulous hemostasis should be achieved to avoid a hematoma that may dissect through tissue planes and potentially seed the area with tumor cells. Ideally, the biopsy should be done by the surgeon who will ultimately execute the definitive operation and is trained in the management of STS.

Once tissue is obtained and a diagnosis made, imaging and histology are used to stage the patient for treatment planning. Important characteristics used in STS staging include size (<5 cm or >5 cm), tumor grade (low vs. high), and distant metastatic spread. Patients should undergo imaging of the extremity for operative planning as well as a high-resolution chest CT scan to evaluate for pulmonary metastases. The incidence of regional nodal involvement is very low (<5%). Histologic subtypes that are associated with higher risks for nodal involvement include epithelioid and clear cell sarcomas, which if documented is equated with systemic spread of disease. Ideally, all information should be discussed at a tumor board, where pathology and radiographs can be reviewed and input from surgeons and medical and radiation oncologists can be used to formulate a treatment plan.

Diagnosis and Treatment

Presentation Continued

Core needle biopsy of the mass is performed revealing a high-grade synovial sarcoma. MRI and CT scan confirm the mass to be 6 cm in size and confined to the anterior tibialis with no evidence of metastatic disease found **(Table 3)**.

The treatment of STS depends on the pathologic classification and stage of the tumor. Classically, small, low-grade tumors can be treated with wide excision including 2-cm margins, with no adjuvant therapy needed. For high-grade tumors, or those >5 cm, treatment should be multimodal and include surgical resection with the addition of radiation therapy. Multiple trials over the past three decades have shown improved local control in patients with resected sarcomas when radiation therapy is added. Survival, however, has been unaffected as most patients die of metastatic disease present at the time of primary tumor resection. The decision on preoperative versus

TABLE 3. Key Technical Steps and Potential Pitfalls to Treatment of Soft Tissue Sarcomas

Key Technical Steps

1. Biopsy is obtained via core needle or open approach.
2. MRI is used to evaluate size and proximity to vital structures.
3. Incision for both biopsy and operation should be made along the longitudinal axis of the limb to aid in future operations.
4. Lesions should be resected with 2–3 cm of normal tissue and include surrounding fascia.
5. If abutting the bone, periosteum should be taken.
6. If closure will create undo tension, a myocutaneous flap may be used.
7. High-grade or large tumors should receive adjuvant radiation +/– chemotherapy.
8. Biannual surveillance imaging including local site and chest should be performed for rapid identification and treatment of local and distant recurrences.

Potential Pitfalls

- Biopsies should be read by pathologists trained in soft tissue sarcomas to ensure appropriate diagnosis and grade of tumor is identified.
- Incisions made circumferentially on extremities lead to wider reresections and undo morbidity as these scars need to be included with the specimen.
- Ideally, the biopsy should be performed by the surgeon who is planning the definitive operation.

postoperative radiation remains controversial and is the subject of ongoing clinical trials. Chemotherapy is used in patients with stage IV disease, large high-grade tumors and occasionally in the neoadjuvant setting to reduce tumor size allowing for a less morbid operation.

The goal of operative intervention should be removal of the tumor to microscopically negative margins while preserving physiologic function. Prior to 1980, the standard therapy for extremity STS was amputation. Marginal resection of the tumor (removing the tumor along the capsule) was associated with a high local recurrence rate of >80%. Wide excision with a rim of normal tissue was associated with a local recurrence rate of close to 50%. Hence, radical excision involving amputation including the joint above the sarcoma or a radical muscle compartment resection was the standard of care, which was associated with a local recurrence rate of 7% to 18%. In the past, single institution studies reported that radiation may be a useful adjuvant treatment to reduce local recurrence rates associated with wide excisions. In 1982, Rosenberg et al. reported a randomized trial of patients undergoing either limb-sparing surgery involving wide excision with radiation therapy versus amputation. Although local recurrence was seen only in the limb-salvage group, there was no difference in overall survival.

This study changed the standard of care for sarcoma resection reserving amputation only for those patients in whom potentially curative resection would render the extremity unusable.

As with open biopsies, the initial incision should be made along the longitudinal axis of the extremity allowing for less tension on the skin following closure (**Figure 3**). If a large defect is anticipated, consultation with plastic surgery should be considered preoperatively and incisions made that facilitate free or rotational myocutaneous flap coverage. This often allows for a superior functional and cosmetic outcome and can be useful when neoadjuvant radiation has been given. The mass is identified and resected along with a 2 cm of surrounding uninvolved tissue. If fascial planes are encountered, these should be removed with the specimen. Nerves and arteries should be preserved if removal will significantly impact limb function. Arterial reconstruction can be considered if gross

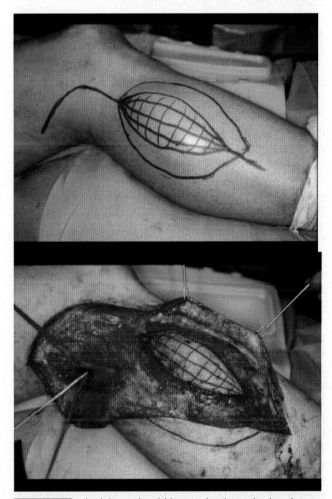

FIGURE 3 • Incisions should be made along the longitudinal axis of the extremity to aid in closing. Exposure of nearby nerves and vessels (vessel loop marks the peroneal nerve and the anterior tibial artery) is crucial to prevent loss of function to the limb.

tumor encasement is found. If bone is encountered, the involved periosteum should be removed and the cortical bone left intact. The skin and soft tissue are reapproximated if possible or reconstruction is performed. Once the specimen is removed, it should be taken to the pathologist with careful inking of all margins to assess if the tumor is close to the margins. If certain margins are felt to be close by gross inspection or frozen section analysis, additional margins can be taken at that time. If margin status is unclear, wounds can be temporarily left open and managed with vacuum-assisted closure devices or cellular collagen matrices until pathologic review is complete and closure can be safely performed. Metallic clips are placed along the borders of the tumor for subsequent radiation therapy if the patient has not received preoperative radiation. Usually, the skin flaps are closed over suction drains with their exit sites placed so that subsequent radiation fields will include them. Depending on the extent of operation, patients typically spend 1 to 2 days in the hospital and are discharged home with physical therapy.

Following surgery, patients are given time to recover and external-beam radiation therapy initiated 4 to 6 weeks after surgery. The standard dose is 60 to 70 Gy in 1.8 to 2.0 Gy/d fractions to an area 5 to 7 cm surrounding the original tumor. Preoperative radiation has shown some benefit as tissue oxygenation is improved and margin assessment easier. There is an association, however, with greater surgical morbidity and no proven increase in efficacy.

The role of adjuvant chemotherapy for STS remains controversial. Although strong data exist in pediatric rhabdosarcomas, reports in adult tumors have been conflicting. In a randomized trial comparing anthramycin- and ifosfamide-based chemotherapy to surgery alone, there was an improvement in disease-free and overall survival. However, a large meta-analysis of 14 trials evaluating the use of adjuvant chemotherapy for STS found an improvement in disease free survival but no change in overall survival. The standard approach for most centers is doxorubicin and ifosfamide-based chemotherapy for four to six cycles in high-risk patients without significant medical comorbidities.

Isolated limb perfusion (ILP) is a way to deliver high-dose chemotherapy to an affected limb with minimal systemic exposure. The technique involves isolation of the inflow and outflow vessels to the limb and cannulation with large infusion catheters. The inflow and outflow cannulas are connected to a heart lung bypass machine equipped with a membrane oxygenator, heater, and roller pump. High-dose chemotherapy can then be administered to the leg and cleared from blood prior to returning to the systemic vasculature. During ILP, doses in excess of 10 times the maximal tolerated systemic dose can be achieved with a fraction of the systemic short- and long-term toxicities. When adverse

events are encountered, they typically involve burns or blistering to the extremity occasionally requiring amputation.

In 1988, Di Filippo et al. published a series of 64 patients with extremity sarcomas treated with hyperthermia and melphalan, actinomycin, or cisplatinin. Of the 55 patients available for evaluation, 29 were deemed initially unresectable operative candidates (locally advanced disease with no extralimb metastases). Following ILP, 17 (59%) of these patients had sufficient tumor reduction to allow limb-sparing surgery, while 12 went on to amputation. A similar study by Eroglu et al. reported on 37 patients with STS of extremity, 14 of which were considered unresectable at the time of presentation. Patients were treated with ILP using a combination of cisplatin and doxorubicin and followed for response and toxicity. The objective response in this group was 78.6% with a complete response (CR) of 14.3% and a partial response (PR) of 64.3%. Very little systemic toxicity was noted and wide excision was possible in 11 of the 14 patients (78.6%).

Postoperative Management

After resection and adjuvant therapy, patients with STS should be routinely surveyed for evidence of local and distant recurrence. Evidence shows that early recognition and prompt treatment of recurrent disease can improve long-term survival. Patients should be seen every 3 months for the first 2 years with thorough history and physical exams. Any abnormalities should be followed up with imaging and biopsy when necessary. Because lungs represent the most common site of disease spread, patients should receive a high-resolution chest CT scan and extremity MRI semiannually for 2 years.

When patients recur locally, they should be aggressively treated with re-resection or amputation. If adjuvant radiation therapy was not given, it can be used following re-resection to improve local control. Despite aggressive local control, overall mortality is dictated by the development of metastatic disease. Between 20% to 40% of patients with resected STS will develop distant metastases, typically in the first 2 to 3 years. The standard treatment for disseminated disease is chemotherapy, typically with doxorubicin and ifosfamide. When patients present with limited number of metastases to a single body compartment, surgical metastasectomy represents the only option for cure. For this to be considered, the patient must be sufficiently fit for surgery and have a reasonable disease-free interval. In a retrospective review of data from a multi-institutional European sarcoma study, 255 selected patients underwent metastasectomy for STS. The 3- and 5-year overall survival rates were 54% and 38%, respectively, and early stage primaries with long disease-free periods were independent predictors of survival.

Case Conclusion

Following resection with adjuvant radiation therapy, imaging surveillance was performed semiannually. During his 18-month visit, he was found to have two suspicious lesions on chest CT located in the right lower lobe. He underwent successful thoracoscopic wedge resection of the two lesions and has remained free of disease.

SUGGESTED READINGS

Cormier JN, Pollock RE. Soft tissue sarcomas. In: Brunicardi FC, Andersen DK, Billiar TR, et al., eds. Schwartz's Principles of Surgery. 9th ed. New York, NY: McGraw-Hill, 2009, Chapter 36.

Frustaci S, Gherlinzoni F, De Paoli A, et al. Adjuvant chemotherapy for adult soft tissue sarcomas of the extremities and girdles: results of the Italian randomized cooperative trial. J Clin Oncol. 2001;19:1238–1247.

Kubitz SM, D'adamo DR. Sarcoma. Mayo Clinic Proc. 2007;82(11):1409–1432.

Pisters PW, Harrison LB, Leung DH et al. Long-term results of a prospective randomized trial of adjuvant brachytherapy in soft tissue sarcoma. J Clin Oncol. 1996;14(3):859–868.

Rosenberg SA, Tepper J, Glatstein E, et al. The treatment of soft-tissue sarcomas of the extremities. Ann Surg. 1982;196:305–315.

Sarcoma Consensus Conference. Limb-sparing treatment of adult soft-tissue sarcomas and osteosarcomas. JAMA. 1985;254(13):1791–1794.

Sarcoma Meta-analysis Collaboration. Adjuvant chemotherapy for localised resectable soft-tissue sarcoma of adults: meta-analysis of individual data. Lancet. 1997; 350:1647–1654.

van Geel AN, Pastorino U, Jauch KW, et al. Surgical treatment of lung metastases: The European Organization for Research and Treatment of Cancer-Soft Tissue and Bone Sarcoma Group study of 255 patients. Cancer. 1996;77:675–682.

Yang JC, Chang AE, Baker AR et al. Randomized prospective study of the benefit of adjuvant radiation therapy in the treatment of soft tissue sarcomas of the extremity. J Clin Oncol. 1998;16(1):197–203.

104 Retroperitoneal Sarcoma

CHANDU VEMURI and SANDRA L. WONG

Presentation

A 50-year-old man with a history of hypertension presents for evaluation of an enlarging scrotal mass, thought to be an inguinal hernia. On examination, he has a large left scrotal mass that is firm, nontender, and not reducible. He is also noted to have firmness throughout the entire abdomen but has no abdominal pain. He reports some fatigue, early satiety, and a 15-lb unintentional weight loss over the past year, though he has increasing abdominal girth. Otherwise, he is active and continues to work full time.

Differential Diagnosis

Patients with retroperitoneal sarcoma typically present with nonspecific symptoms and will often have an abdominal mass on physical examination. Some symptoms are specific to mass effect on nearby structures. Because of the location, diagnosis is often delayed, and the majority of patients have tumors that are larger than 10 cm in size at time of initial evaluation. Retroperitoneal masses are usually malignant and about one-third of these masses are sarcomas. The differential diagnosis includes germ cell tumors, lymphoma, and other tumors of retroperitoneal solid organs, including endocrine cancers and renal cell carcinoma.

Workup

Occasionally, the mass is appreciated on cross-sectional imaging performed for other reasons, but otherwise a CT scan of the abdomen and the pelvis with oral and IV contrast is the preferred initial radiographic evaluation. Complete workup involves a detailed history and physical examination, including assessment of diffuse lymphadenopathy, scrotal exam, and serum laboratory studies to selectively evaluate excessive endocrine hormone production, elevated germ cell tumor markers (e.g., alpha-fetoprotein (AFP), beta-human chorionic gonadotrophin (β-hCG), and lactate dehydrogenase.

In this patient, physical examination was only remarkable as noted above. CT scan of the abdomen and pelvis was significant for a massive retroperitoneal mass extending through the left inguinal canal into the scrotum (Figure 1). The radiologic appearance was consistent with liposarcoma given the predominantly fatty appearance with linear septa. A CT-guided core needle biopsy confirmed a low-grade well-differentiated liposarcoma. CT scan of the chest did not demonstrate any evidence of pulmonary metastasis. Laboratory values were normal, including a creatinine of 0.8 mg/dL. He was referred for surgical resection.

Discussion

Presenting symptoms can include vague abdominal or back pain and weight loss, as well as symptoms specific to location of the tumor such as early satiety if there is mass effect on the stomach or venous obstruction of the lower extremity from a pelvic tumor. Biopsy of suspicious masses can be performed preoperatively to establish a diagnosis. Biopsy, with a core needle biopsy approach if possible, is mandatory if there is a question about the diagnosis, if there is consideration for neoadjuvant treatment, or if the tumor is felt to be unresectable.

Imaging should be directed to preparation for surgical resection. Magnetic resonance imaging (MRI) is an alternate modality that is sufficient, but not necessary, for these patients. Workup should also include evaluation of metastatic disease, most commonly to lungs or liver. Plain chest radiographs can be used to evaluate for pulmonary metastasis, but CT should be performed if any abnormalities are seen or if the sarcoma is considered a high risk for metastasis. Positron emission tomography scans do not have a defined role in assessment of retroperitoneal sarcoma.

Diagnosis and Treatment

The cornerstone of treatment for localized disease is complete surgical resection. This patient was felt to have a resectable retroperitoneal sarcoma and this was recommended. Resection should include involved intra-abdominal/retroperitoneal structures with anastomoses and reconstruction as appropriate. Sarcomas with critical vascular involvement, peritoneal implants, involvement at the root of the mesentery, or spinal cord involvement are usually considered unresectable. Incomplete resections with microscopically positive margins lead to an increased risk of local recurrence, which represents a common form of treatment failure. Great care must be taken to ensure complete resection without capsular intrusion during the index operation. Repeat resection for recurrent disease is

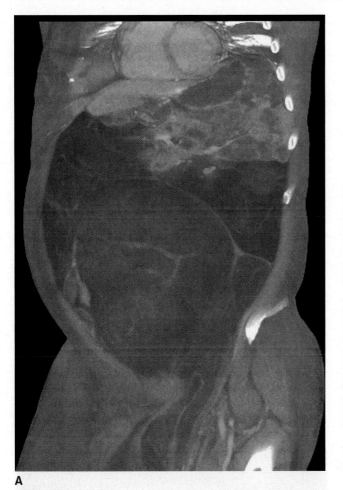

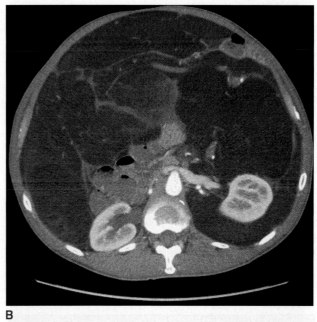

A   **B**

FIGURE 1 • Case presentation. **A:** Retroperitoneal/intra-abdominal sarcoma occupying the majority of the abdominal cavity is demonstrated on angled sagittal views from a CT scan. Note displacement of the intra-abdominal contents superiorly and extension of the tumor into the scrotum via the inguinal canal. **B:** Selected axial view of the liposarcoma demonstrating a homogeneous fatty appearance with linear septa. Note anterior displacement of the descending colon (*arrow*).

recommended, especially if interval surveillance is able to detect early recurrences. Unfortunately, recurrent disease often predicts further recurrences, which often become increasingly more aggressive in terms of tumor biology and more technically difficult to resect with successive operations.

Retroperitoneal sarcomas are relatively uncommon neoplasms derived from mesenchymal cells, with only an estimated 10,000 new cases of soft tissue sarcoma in the United States each year. Only 10% to 15% of these cases will be of retroperitoneal origin. More than 50 different histologic subtypes have been described, but the most commonly seen retroperitoneal sarcomas are liposarcomas or leiomyosarcomas. Prognosis is largely dictated by the ability to achieve complete surgical resection, and median survival for patients who undergo complete resection is 60 months compared to 24 months for those undergoing incomplete resection. Other factors associated with decreased survival include high histologic grade, large tumor size, and older patient age.

Multimodality treatment approaches, including systemic chemotherapy and radiation therapy, merit consideration since resection alone has unsatisfactory outcomes in high-risk tumors. There are good data to support the use of radiation in conjunction with limb-sparing procedures for extremity sarcomas. However, radiation to the retroperitoneum is complicated by dose-limiting toxicity to abdominal viscera, which are uniquely radiosensitive, and by very large treatment fields. For this reason, preoperative radiation approaches have been considered to improve rates of local control and reduce recurrences. When the sarcoma is *in situ*, bowel and other structures are displaced and out of the intended radiation field, allowing for more effective use of radiation. It is unlikely that radiation would change the size of the tumor or change the scope and/or extent of the planned operation. Many small series have demonstrated the safety and feasibility of radiation for selected patients with high-risk retroperitoneal sarcomas, and studies using standard external-beam radiation therapy,

TABLE 1. Resection of Retroperitoneal Sarcoma

1. Midline laparotomy.
2. Thorough exploration to verify resectability.
3. Complete exposure of sarcoma and surrounding structures.
4. Resection of mass with en bloc resection of contiguous organs and vessels.
5. Placement of metal clips in resection bed.
6. Reconstruction (bowel, major vessels) as needed.
7. Abdominal closure.

Potential Pitfalls

1. Inadequate preoperative imaging to determine involvement of major intra-abdominal structures
2. Inadequate exposure of vessels for vascular control in a field with limited exposure due to the size of tumor
3. Rupture of tumor

brachytherapy approaches, or intraoperative electron-beam radiotherapy approaches are ongoing to evaluate their efficacy in disease outcomes. The use of systemic chemotherapy for most histologic subtypes of retroperitoneal sarcoma remains controversial. Response rates are relatively low, and there is no demonstrated improvement in overall or disease-specific survival with either neoadjuvant or adjuvant chemotherapy regimens. Some commonly used cytotoxic agents include doxorubicin and ifosfamide. There is limited experience with combined chemoradiation treatments.

Surgical Approach and Special Intraoperative Considerations

Retroperitoneal sarcomas, by definition, can originate from mesenchymal tissues throughout the retroperitoneum. Hepatic sarcomas, intra-abdominal desmoid tumors (desmoids fibromatosis), and gastrointestinal stromal tumors should be considered separately since these tumors have a different presentation and management strategies. Because the location and extent of retroperitoneal sarcomas vary greatly, the surgical approach must be tailored to each patient.

A midline incision is most commonly used for access since standard laparotomy provides excellent exposure of viscera, vascular structures, and the retroperitoneum (Table 1). Upon entering the abdomen, thorough evaluation is made to ensure that the mass is resectable. Often, mobilization of intra-abdominal structures is necessary for this assessment. Once this decision has been made to proceed, further dissection should be

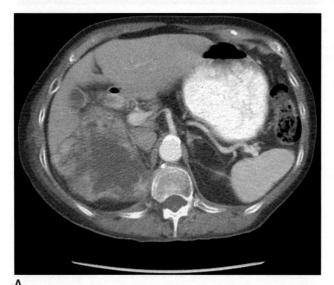

A

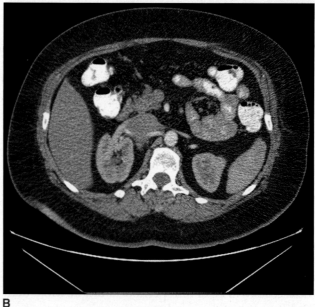

B

FIGURE 2 • Select cases of retroperitoneal sarcoma requiring resection of contiguous structures. **A:** This is a 78-year-old woman with a right-sided 10.1 × 8.7 cm retroperitoneal leiomyosarcoma involving the superior pole of the right kidney and extending to the posterior aspect of the liver. Preoperative treatment with radiation therapy led to internal necrosis of the tumor, as seen on the posttreatment/preoperative CT scan. Resection included en bloc right nephrectomy. There was no involvement of the hepatic parenchyma. **B:** This is a 55-year-old woman who presenting with worsening right-sided back pain. After many sessions with physical therapy and a chiropractor, she underwent evaluation with a thoracic/lumbar spine MRI. After finding a retroperitoneal mass, she underwent a CT of the abdomen and the pelvis, which demonstrated a mass involving the right renal vessels and the IVC. She underwent segmental resection of the IVC with en bloc right nephrectomy. The IVC was reconstructed using an interposition tube graft and the kidney was autotransplanted after the uninvolved kidney was dissected free from the involved portions of the renal vein and artery. (*Continued*)

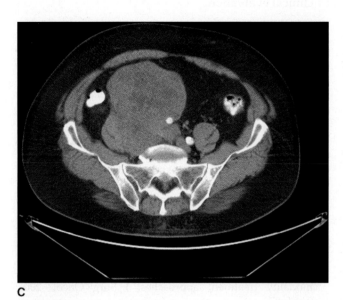
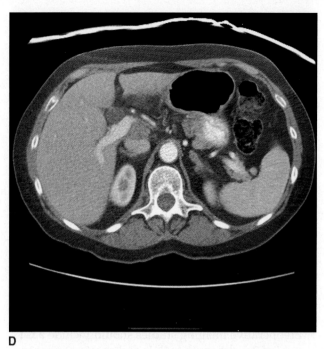

C

D

FIGURE 2 • **C:** This is a 66-year-old man with a high-grade leiomyosarcoma of the right retroperitoneum/pelvis discovered after an episode of abdominal pain. He was also noted to have right lower-extremity edema, likely due to venous compression. On CT scan, encasement of the right iliac vessels and suspected involvement of the right ureter are noted. He underwent resection of the sarcoma with en bloc resection of the right ureter, right common and external iliac artery and vein with end-to-end ureteral reconstruction (Boari flap), and vascular reconstruction of the vessels with prosthetic grafts. **D:** This is a 66-year-old woman with biopsy-proven leiomyosarcoma incidentally found during a laparoscopic cholecystectomy. The 3-cm mass is noted to straddle the portal vein and the IVC. Because of the extent of vascular involvement, this sarcoma was deemed unresectable. The patient was relatively asymptomatic and declined palliative treatment. She developed liver metastases 2 years after initial diagnosis.

carried out in a manner to best visualize the entirety of the mass and ensure ability to obtain vascular control if necessary during the course of dissection. Structures such as bowel, mesentery, ureters, and major vessels should not be divided until resection is known to be possible. Tumors with critical vascular involvement, peritoneal implants, involvement at the root of the mesentery, or spinal cord involvement are usually unresectable; debulking procedures are usually not considered.

Exposure in the retroperitoneum is often limited by large tumors. With the insidious growth pattern of sarcomas, contiguous structures may have to be resected en bloc to assure complete removal of tumor. Resection of colon, small bowel, kidney, adrenal gland, and inferior vena cava (IVC) must often be considered as part of the procedure depending on the location and growth pattern of the sarcoma. En bloc nephrectomy is necessary in many cases even though the renal parenchyma is rarely invaded. Bowel resection is often necessary because of the extent of involvement of the mesentery/mesocolon.

Once the tumor is resected, metal clips should be placed in the resection bed to allow for later identification of the anatomic limits of the tumor. Necessary reconstructive procedures are performed at this time **(Figure 2)**. Bowel

anastomoses are usually performed without incident. Major vascular reconstruction techniques have been described, including primary repair or use of prosthetic graft replacements, though ligation of many vessels is generally well tolerated. Because the risk of nodal metastasis is virtually nonexistent, lymphadenectomy is unnecessary. The abdomen is closed in the standard fashion. Drains are rarely needed.

Postoperative Management

Immediate postoperative management of these patients is dictated by the extent of resection, noting that postoperative ileus is common with long procedures or if there was extensive displacement of bowel by the sarcoma.

The long-term care of these patients requires surveillance with physical exam and imaging every 3 to 6 months for the first 2 to 3 years and then annually thereafter. Interval of surveillance may vary based on the expected risk of recurrence (dependent on completeness of surgical resection and histopathologic features) and underlying performance status of the patient. Recurrences are difficult to detect without cross-sectional imaging. Follow-up should also include chest imaging for detection of metastatic disease.

Case Conclusion

This patient underwent resection of a 13 kg, 52 × 47 × 14 cm well-differentiated liposarcoma with en bloc colon resection due to extensive involvement of the descending and sigmoid mesocolon. Because of the extent of inguinal involvement, the defect in the groin was repaired to obviate problems with an inguinal hernia. His postoperative course was uncomplicated and he noted an improvement in his prior symptoms.

TAKE HOME POINTS

- Differential diagnosis must include germ cell tumors, lymphoma, other malignancies of retroperitoneal solid organs including endocrine cancers and renal cell carcinoma.
- Preoperative imaging studies should include a CT scan of the abdomen/pelvis and chest imaging to evaluate for the presence of pulmonary metastases.
- The cornerstone of treatment is complete surgical resection. En bloc resection of contiguous structures may be necessary.
- Recurrence rates are high. Patients should be followed closely with cross-sectional imaging and clinical evaluation.

SUGGESTED READINGS

Hollenbeck ST, Grobmyer SR, Kent KC, et al. Surgical treatment and outcome of patients with primary inferior vena cava leiomyosarcoma. J Am Coll Surg. 2003;197:575–579.

Jaques DP, Coit DG, Hajdu SI, et al. Management of primary and recurrent soft tissue sarcoma of the retroperitoneum. Ann Surg. 1990;212:51–59.

Jemal A, Siegel R, Xu J, et al. Cancer statistics, 2010. CA Cancer J Clin. 2010;60:277–300.

Karakousis CP. Refinements of surgical technique in soft tissue sarcomas. J Surg Oncol. 2010;101:730–738.

Liles JS, Tzeng CW, Short JJ, et al. Retroperitoneal and intra-abdominal sarcoma. Curr Probl Surg. 2009;46:445–503.

Pisters PWT, O'Sullivan B. Retroperitoneal sarcomas: combined modality treatment approaches. Curr Opin Oncol. 2002;14:400–405.

Raut CP, Pisters PW. Retroperitoneal sarcomas: combined-modality treatment approaches. J Surg Oncol. 2006; 94:81–87.

105 Penetrating Chest Injury

ALBERT CHI and ADIL H. HAIDER

Presentation

A 22-year-old male presents to the emergency room with multiple stab wounds to the head, back, and left upper arm. Emergency medical services (EMS) vitals are BP 100/P, HR 104, RR 26, O$_2$, and Sats 97% on room air. Physical examination on arrival reveals that the patient is speaking, but has diminished breath sounds on right, abdomen is soft, has 2+ symmetric pulses distally, and is moving all four extremities. He complains of chest pain and increasing shortness of breath. Initial emergency department (ED) vitals are BP 77/56, HR 126, and Sats 96% on 100% nonrebreather mask.

Differential Diagnosis

When managing unstable patients with penetrating chest injuries, trauma teams must rapidly and accurately intervene with potential life-saving procedures. The airway, breathing, and circulation of trauma run hand in hand in the case of the hypotensive patient with an undetermined underlying cause. Three diagnoses must be considered that need immediate intervention: (1) pericardial tamponade, (2) tension pneumothorax, and (3) ongoing blood loss (e.g., hemorrhage from great vessels, pulmonary hilum, lung parenchyma, or intercostal artery). As interventions and surgical approach are very specific for each of these processes, quick assessment and judgment are necessary.

Workup

In the unstable patient, clinical suspicion and physical exam findings (i.e., breath sounds absent or present, muffled or distant heart sounds) are relied on. Do not delay chest tube thoracostomy tube placement or needle decompression for suspected tension pneumothorax. In the case of suspected cardiac tamponade, a quick Focused Assessment Sonography for Trauma (FAST) pericardial view can determine the presence of fluid surrounding the heart. *A clinical caution*: even with a negative pericardial window, a cardiac injury can still be present if the pericardial wound communicates with the thorax, decompressing into the chest. In the stable patient, portable upright anterior posterior chest x-ray should be performed with FAST as an adjunct. Computed tomography can be considered for stable patients after primary survey is performed.

Discussion

In this patient, with a penetrating wound to the chest, decreased breath sounds on the side of injury and hypotension, a tension pneumothorax should be assumed. Immediate steps to decompress this must be undertaken.

Chest-Needle Decompression

A simple pneumothorax is the most common thoracic injury after penetrating chest trauma and frequently results from an injury to the lung parenchyma. Without an adequate vent for decompression, increased intrathoracic pressure may result in kinking of the vena cava, decreased venous return to the heart, and cardiovascular collapse. In the prehospital setting, needle decompression is frequently performed on injured patients with a suspected tension pneumothorax. It can be inserted rapidly, with little additional risk to the patient, and is an adequate temporizing measure until a formal tube thoracostomy can be performed.

Key Steps

1. Locate the second intercostal space and the midclavicular line.
2. Prepare site with Chlorhexidine solution or an alcohol swab.
3. Make a puncture with 14-G catheter or angiocatheter from central line kit if additional length is needed secondary to body habitus.
4. Advance until rush of air is encountered and remove needle while stabilizing catheter.
5. Placement of one-way valve if available
6. Confirm resolution of pneumothorax.

Pitfalls

1. Fourteen-gauge catheter length is 1¼ inches, and many patients' chest walls may require greater length to enter the chest cavity.
2. May cause additional injury to lung parenchyma or even reports of hilar vessel injury from chest-needle decompression

Thoracostomy Tube

Drainage of the pleural space by means of a chest tube is the commonest intervention in thoracic trauma, and it provides definitive treatment in the majority of cases. While a relatively simple procedure, it carries a significant complication rate, reported as between 2% and 10%. While many of these complications are relatively minor, some require operative intervention and deaths still occur (e.g., from laceration of neurovascular bundle in inferior surface of ribs).

A chest tube is indicated to drain the contents of the pleural space. Usually this will be air or blood, but may include other fluids such as chyle or gastric/esophageal contents. Chest tube insertion is also appropriate to prevent the development of a pleural collection, such as after a thoracotomy or to prevent a tension pneumothorax in the ventilated patient with rib fractures.

Absolute Indications

- Pneumothorax (*tension, open, or simple*)
- *Hemothorax*
- Traumatic arrest (bilateral)

Relative Indications

- Rib fractures and positive pressure ventilation
- Profound hypoxia/hypotension and penetrating chest injury
- Profound hypoxia/hypotension and unilateral signs to a hemithorax

Key Steps

1. Place the patient's ipsilateral arm over head to maximize exposure.
2. Don mask, gown and gloves; prep and drape area of insertion, if time allows.
3. Select site for insertion: midaxillary line, between fourth and fifth ribs and the same level of the nipple in males and inframammary line in females.
4. Infiltrate insertion site with local anesthetic, make a 3- to 4-cm incision through skin and subcutaneous tissues between the fourth and fifth ribs, parallel to the rib margins.
5. Use a Kelly clamp to push through the pleura and open the jaws widely, again parallel to the direction of the ribs.
6. Insert finger through your incision and into the thoracic cavity. Make sure you are feeling lung (or empty space) and not liver or spleen.
7. Grasp end of 36 french chest tube with the Kelly forceps (convex angle toward ribs), and insert chest tube through the hole made in the pleura.
8. After tube has entered thoracic cavity, remove Kelly, and manually advance the tube posteriorly and toward the apex of the thoracic cavity.
9. Connect chest tube to pleurovac and place to wall suction.
10. Suture in place with a nonabsorbable suture and place an occlusive dressing.

Pitfalls

- Must confirm with manual palpation of lung parenchyma. An incision placed too low can inadvertently place thoracostomy tubes intra-abdominal and not intrathoracic.
- Blood loss on initial insertion of chest tube. Placement of an additional clamp at the distal end of the chest tube during insertion decreases the amount of spillage and aids in the measurement of estimated blood loss.
- Be careful of potential injury to the chest tube inserter from rib fractures—double gloving is recommended.

Diagnosis and Recommendations

The indications for thoracotomy after traumatic injury typically include persistent shock, arrest at presentation, and ongoing thoracic hemorrhage. Operative intervention due to ongoing hemorrhage is most commonly performed after 1,500 mL of blood output on initial chest tube insertion or continued hourly blood loss of 250 mL or more for 3 consecutive hours after tube thoracostomy. Evidence of gastric contents could also represent an esophageal injury, and massive air leak from chest tube could suggest a bronchial tracheal injury.

Emergent thoracotomy is performed by an anterolateral approach as this provides the most rapid access to the heart and mediastinum. However, if there is time for operative planning, then the incision that provides the best exposure for the suspected injuries should be used.

Anterolateral Thoracotomy

Key Steps to Thoracotomy

1. Place patient in supine position with arms extended.
2. Place double-lumen endotracheal tube by anesthesia if time and stability allow; for injuries to the left chest, the endotracheal tube can be advanced in the right mainstem bronchus keeping the left lung collapsed.
3. Make the incision in the fourth intercostal space starting at the sternal border to the midaxillary line.
4. Anatomic landmarks of the fourth intercostal space is just below the nipple and the inframammary fold in males.
5. Enter the chest with three bold strokes of the knife: the first divides the skin and the subcutaneous tissue, the second through the pectoralis anteriorly and serratus laterally, and the third is through the intercostal muscles entering the pleural space (**Figure 1**).

Pitfalls

- Exposure of certain structure is not always optimal with this standard thoracotomy incision.
- If the Finecetto/rib retractor is placed with the bar/spin mechanism toward the sternum, then it may obstruct extension of the incision across the sternum (clamshell thoracotomy) if required.

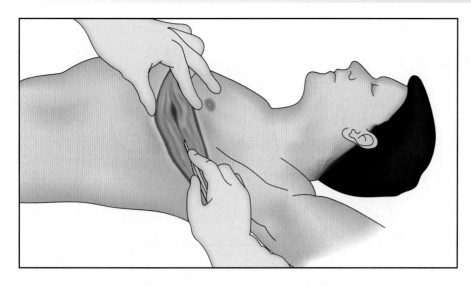

FIGURE 1 • The emergent left anterolateral thoracotomy incision should follow the intercostal space.

Resuscitative Thoracotomy

The best survival results with this procedure are seen in patients who undergo ED thoracotomy for thoracic stab injuries with isolated cardiac stab wounds and arrive with signs of life in the ED. Factors such as mechanism of injury, location of major injury, and signs of life should be taken into account when deciding whether to perform resuscitative thoracotomy in the ED.

Accepted Indications

- Penetrating thoracic injury
  - Traumatic arrest with previously witnessed cardiac activity (prehospital or in-hospital)
  - Unresponsive hypotension (BP < 70 mm Hg)
- Blunt thoracic injury
  - Unresponsive hypotension (BP < 70 mm Hg)
  - Rapid exsanguination from chest tube (>1,500 mL)

Relative Indications

- Penetrating thoracic injury
  - Traumatic arrest without previously witnessed cardiac activity
- Penetrating nonthoracic injury
  - Traumatic arrest with previously witnessed cardiac activity (prehospital or in-hospital)
- Blunt thoracic injuries
  - Traumatic arrest with previously witnessed cardiac activity (prehospital or in-hospital)

Additional Steps to ED Thoracotomy

1. Create a window and using the Mayo scissors cut along the intercostals avoiding the neurovascular bundle on the inferior portion of the rib cage.
2. Place rib spreader into the incision with the handle toward the axilla and open to expose the workspace.
3. Mobilize the lung by cutting the inferior pulmonary ligament.
4. Manually palpate posterior ribs and palpate the spine; the thoracic aorta should be the first tubular structure encountered.
5. To crossclamp the aorta, open the parietal pleural and place a vascular clamp across. If a nasogastric tube (NGT) is present, the NGT can be used to identify the esophagus.
6. If cardiac tamponade or a cardiac injury is suspected, open the pericardium.
7. To open the pericardium, pinch the left lateral aspect with your finger or clamp anterior to the phrenic nerve and open widely parallel to the nerve sliding scissors along the pericardium.

Pitfalls

- Injury to the aorta, the intercostal arteries, or the esophagus during aortic clamping
- Injury to the phrenic nerve when opening the pericardium

Other Thoracotomy Approaches

The choice of thoracic incision **(Figure 2)** for trauma repair is based on the anatomic location of injury and physiologic status. There are many incisions available for thoracic trauma. These include anterolateral thoracotomy, transsternal anterolateral "clamshell" thoracotomy, posterolateral thoracotomy, "book incision" (anterolateral thoracotomy, partial upper sternotomy to a supraclavicular extension), and median sternotomy.

The left anterolateral thoracotomy is the utility incision for resuscitation under circumstances of acute deterioration or cardiac arrest. This incision allows exposure for opening the pericardium, open cardiac massage, clamping of the descending thoracic aorta, and treatment of a large percentage of cardiac and left lung injuries.

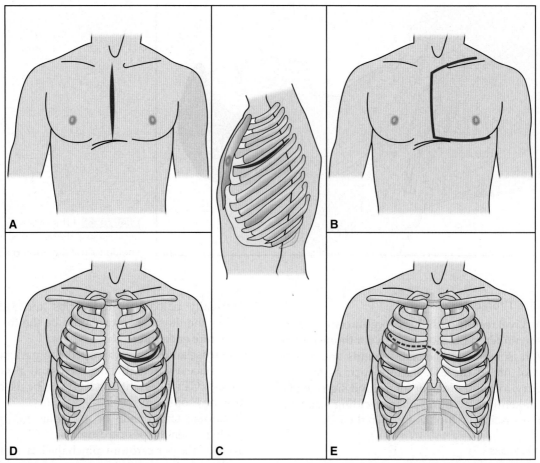

FIGURE 2 • Thoracic incisions for trauma include (**A**) median sternotomy, (**B**) book thoracotomy, (**C**) posterolateral thoracotomy, (**D**) anterolateral thoracotomy, and (**E**) extension of an anterolateral thoracotomy across the sternum.

A left posterolateral thoracotomy allows much greater exposure to the left hilum, including the hilar pulmonary artery, vein, and bronchus. It is also ideal exposure for the descending aorta.

A right posterolateral thoracotomy is indicated for right hilar injuries and also gives excellent exposure of the thoracic portion of the esophagus.

Posterolateral thoracotomy requires the patient to be repositioned in the lateral position and may exacerbate hemodynamic instability in hypovolemic patients. It is particularly well suited for approaching posterior lung parenchymal lacerations and intercostal vessel injuries.

The "book" or "trap door" incision is seldom used but can be considered for exposure of left-sided thoracic outlet injuries. It has the advantage of providing exposure of a long segment of the left common carotid and left subclavian artery. The anterolateral thoracotomy component of this incision can be made above or below the breast, and attention must be paid to the internal mammary artery. The current approach for the management of left subclavian artery injuries is to gain proximal control via anterolateral thoracotomy in the left third interspace combined with a separate clavicular incision for definitive repair.

The standard median sternotomy incision provides excellent exposure to the heart and proximal great vessels, including the ascending aorta innominate artery, and left common carotid artery. It is recommended primarily for anticipated isolated anterior cardiac injuries where there is no need to repair injuries to other organ systems. Further exposure can be obtained with extension into either the supraclavicular area or the neck.

A clamshell thoracotomy provides almost complete exposure to both thoracic cavities. In general, the indication for performing a clamshell thoracotomy is when access is needed to both sides of the chest. For example:

• To improve exposure and access to the heart (especially right-sided structures) following a left anterolateral thoracotomy performed for profound hypotension or traumatic arrest
• To provide access to the right chest in transmediastinal injuries or multiple penetrating injury to both the left and the right chest
• To allow cardiac massage following a right-sided thoracotomy

The only part of the thoracic cavity that is not easily reached through a clamshell incision is the very superior mediastinal vessels. If there is an injury here, the sternum can be split to provide wide exposure to this area.

Intraoperative Management of Specific Injuries

Pulmonary Tractotomy for Penetrating Lung Injury

1. Once the hemithorax is entered, control of the pulmonary hilum can be accomplished with finger occlusion or a clamp. The purpose is prevent passage of air into the systemic circulation as well as hemostatic control.
2. Place a lung clamp on either side of the tract created by the knife or the bullet.
3. Insert a gastrointestinal anastomosis stapler through the entrance and exit wound of the lung.
4. Fire the stapling device to fully expose the injury tract.
5. Directly ligate bleeding vessels or exposed bronchi with 3-0 Vicryl figure eight sutures.

Pitfalls

- Large unsealed areas of the lung may cause persistent blowing air leaks leading to an unplanned reoperation.

Intercostal Bleeding

1. Identify the area of injury.
2. Place a circumferential suture around the rib with an absorbable suture and large needle from within the chest cavity.
3. If necessary, a straight needle may be used to place a suture around the rib and skin and then back into the pleural cavity to get control of the vessels. These sutures can typically be removed after 48 hours.
4. Both ends of the intercostals artery must be ligated.

Pitfalls

- Including the neurovascular bundle may cause rib pain.

Massive Pulmonary Hilar Bleed

1. Attempt to control bleeding with manual pressure, hemostatic suture, or rapid resection of the bleeding segment.
2. If hilar clamping is the only option, hold ventilation to allow manual grasping of the hilum with your nondominant hand.
3. Place Satinsky clamp around the entire hilum.
4. If unable to place clamp, twist the lung to rapidly control the hilum without a clamp.

Pitfalls

- Phrenic nerve injury during clamping
- Hilar clamping is not well tolerated by patient in shock.

Pneumonectomy: Due to the substantial alterations in cardiopulmonary physiology, outcomes after traumatic pneumonectomy are very poor. Thus, this procedure should be reserved only for patients where lung salvage is not possible. That being said the decision to proceed with this highly morbid procedure should be taken quickly and decisively as delaying this usually results in mortality.

Case Conclusion

Based on EMS reports, a chest x-ray plate was present on the ED stretcher upon arrival of the patient, and an x-ray was shot even before the automated blood pressure was measured. As hypotension was noted along with decreased breath sounds on the side of injury, the ED staff immediately performed needle decompression resulting in a rush of air and immediate improvement of blood pressure and ability to breath. The digital x-ray in **Figure 3** appeared on the screen after needle thoracostomy and demonstrates the large tension pneumothorax prior to decompression. Note how the mediastinal structures have been shifted into the left chest. A right chest tube was then placed, which drained approximately 2 L of frank blood on insertion. This prompted emergent transfer of the patient to the operating room for a right-sided posterolateral thoracotomy. Upon exploration, a posterior intercostal artery laceration due to the stab wound was found, but no pulmonary injury was noted. The intercostal artery was ligated with large sutures placed around the rib. Two chest tubes were placed intraoperatively and managed expectantly. The importance of rapid operative intervention can be gauged from the fact that the patient's initial pH on arterial blood gas was 7.09. Intraoperatively, the patient was resuscitated with 1:1:1 ratio of packed red blood cells, fresh frozen plasma, and platelets. By the end of the case and with reversal of hemorrhagic shock, the patient's arterial pH had normalized to 7.32. The patient was discharged home on postoperative day 4 without complications.

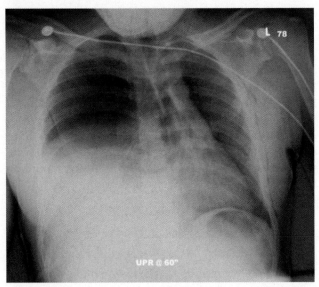

FIGURE 3 • Chest X-ray prior to needle thoracostomy, which demonstrates a large tension pneumothorax.

TAKE HOME POINTS

- In patients with altered hemodynamics after penetrating chest injury, immediate action directed at reversing the most likely cause of instability must be taken.

- Negative FAST exam does not rule out a pericardial violation or a cardiac injury.
- Most patients with penetrating injury (up to 75%) are simply managed with a tube thoracostomy.
- If 1,500 mL of blood drains out of chest tube immediately, then the patient most likely needs an operative intervention.
- In the operating room, choice of incision is dictated by suspicion of injured structures.

SUGGESTED READINGS

Mattox KL, Wall MJ Jr, LeMaire SA. Injury to the thoracic great vessels. In: More EE, Feliciano DV, Mattox KL, eds. Trauma. 5th ed. New York: McGraw-Hill, 2004:571–581.

Rhee PM, Acosta J, Bridgeman A, et al. Survival after emergency department thoracotomy: review of published data from the past 25 years. J Am Coll Surg. 2000;190:288–298.

Wall MJ, Hirshberg A, Mattox KL. Pulmonary tractotomy with selective vascular ligation for penetrating injuries to the lung. Am J Surg. 1994;168:665–669.

Wall MJ Jr, Soltero E, Mattox KL. Penetrating trauma. In: Pearson FG, Cooper JD, Deslauruers J, et al., eds. Thoracic Surgery. 2nd ed. New York, NY: Churchill Livingstone, 2002:1858–1863.

106 Stab Wound to the Neck

GINA M.S. HOWELL and JASON L. SPERRY

Presentation

A 25-year-old female involved in a domestic dispute presents to the emergency department with a stab wound to the left neck. On admission, she is normotensive, protecting her airway, has no signs or symptoms of respiratory difficulty, and is neurologically intact. Focused neck examination reveals a single 2-cm wound anterior to the sternocleidomastoid (SCM) muscle at the level of the thyroid cartilage. There is a small, pulsatile hematoma with an associated bruit, and a moderate amount of crepitus on palpation. Plain films demonstrate subcutaneous emphysema, no tracheal deviation, and no pneumothorax.

Differential Diagnosis

Penetrating trauma in the cervical region can result in significant morbidity and mortality, as it is a relatively unprotected area with a high density of vital structures. Specific injury patterns depend upon the anatomic level of injury (Table 1). This patient has a Zone II injury placing her at risk for damage to the carotid and vertebral arteries, jugular veins, vagus nerve, larynx, trachea, esophagus, and spinal cord.

Workup

The initial evaluation of every trauma patient should adhere to the principles of the Advanced Trauma Life Support–directed primary survey with rapid assessment of the airway as the ultimate priority. Translaryngeal endotracheal intubation by a skilled practitioner is the preferred method of airway control, but one must be prepared to provide an emergency surgical airway if necessary. The focused physical examination that follows should assess for signs and symptoms of significant vascular and aerodigestive tract injury (Table 2). "Hard" signs mandating immediate operative exploration without the need for additional diagnostic workup include shock/hypotension, active hemorrhage, expanding or pulsatile hematoma, bruit, loss of pulse, neurologic deficit, significant subcutaneous emphysema, respiratory distress, or air leaking through the neck wound. Plain chest and cervical radiographs are typically taken for all patients during this initial assessment primarily to evaluate for serious injuries (e.g., pneumothorax, hemothorax, tracheal deviation) requiring expeditious treatment.

In stable patients with wounds that penetrate the platysma but who do not need immediate exploration, further radiographic and endoscopic evaluation is usually recommended to evaluate for surgically significant injuries. Though practice patterns vary among institutions, computed tomography (CT) has become the backbone of modern trauma evaluation and is often used as the initial diagnostic study. The addition of intravenous contrast (computed tomographic angiography [CTA]) makes this modality even more useful for determination of injury track, proximity to vital structures, and is the preferred method over conventional arteriography and duplex ultrasonography for the detection of vascular injuries (Figure 1). As an adjunct to CT, it is also prudent to formally evaluate the esophagus with barium contrast esophagography (Figure 2) or esophagoscopy, with many centers utilizing both techniques on a routine basis. Suspicion of laryngotracheal injury warrants laryngoscopy and bronchoscopy.

Diagnosis and Treatment

This patient has a penetrating wound in Zone II. She likely has a significant vascular injury based on the finding of a pulsatile hematoma and associated bruit. In addition, she may also have an injury to her aerodigestive tract as evidenced by subcutaneous emphysema on clinical and radiographic examination. She is not unstable and does not require emergent intubation, but does have "hard" signs of injury, and therefore, should go immediately to the operating room for exploration. Cervical immobilization is unnecessary due to the extremely low likelihood of unstable spine fracture in this setting, and can actually be harmful by interfering with serial neck examination and potential life-saving maneuvers.

Discussion

It is universally accepted that all patients with hemodynamic instability or hard signs of injury require emergent operation without the need for additional diagnostic workup. There is variability, however, in

TABLE 1. Anatomic Zones of the Neck and Associated Injuries

Zone	Landmarks	Important Structures
I	Clavicle—cricoid cartilage	Great vessels, proximal carotid artery, vertebral artery, lung, trachea, esophagus, thoracic duct, spinal cord, cervical nerve trunks
II	Cricoid cartilage—angle of mandible	Carotid artery and branches, jugular veins, vertebral artery, larynx, trachea, esophagus, vagus nerve, spinal cord
III	Angle of mandible—skull base	Distal internal carotid artery, vertebral artery, jugular veins, pharynx, salivary glands, cranial nerves

the management of patients who do not fall into this category. The era of mandatory exploration for every penetrating neck wound and its high associated nontherapeutic exploration rate has certainly passed, but may still serve as the most appropriate strategy in situations where immediate radiologic and endoscopic capabilities are not readily available. Selective operative management, on the other hand, relies upon serial observation and ancillary studies to effectively diagnose or rule out injuries requiring surgical intervention. There is a negligible rate of missed injury with this approach and is the strategy advocated by most, particularly for injuries that may involve Zones I and III because of the difficulty in examining and exposing these areas. Simple observation alone should be exercised with caution even in asymptomatic patients with no signs of significant injury, as some injuries

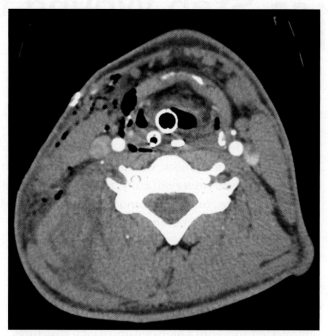

FIGURE 1 • CTA of the neck. CTA is the initial diagnostic study of choice in the evaluation of penetrating neck wounds that do not require immediate exploration. This image demonstrates subcutaneous emphysema concerning for injury to the aerodigestive tract.

(e.g., esophageal) are often clinically occult at the time of presentation. A suggested management algorithm for penetrating neck injuries is depicted in **Figure 3**.

Surgical Approach

A standard Zone II neck exploration is performed under general anesthesia with the patient positioned supine on the operating room table with arms tucked, neck extended, and head rotated to the contralateral side **(Table 3)**. A vertical neck incision along the anterior border of the SCM muscle is routinely utilized **(Figure 4)**. Once the dissection is carried through skin, subcutaneous tissue, and platysma, posterolateral retraction of the SCM provides exposure to all vital structures. Unless there is another obvious injury requiring immediate attention, the vascular structures are typically explored first by opening the carotid sheath. Division of the middle thyroid and facial veins will facilitate complete visualization the carotid artery, which lies deep and medial to the internal jugular vein. Attention is then turned to the aerodigestive tract with care taken not to injure the recurrent laryngeal nerve, which lies in the tracheoesophageal groove. Mobilization of the esophagus is accomplished by dissecting in the posterior areolar plane and then encircling the esophagus with a Penrose drain to facilitate rotation and circumferential inspection. The larynx and trachea should be visualized and palpated for signs of injury. This may require mobilization of the thyroid and/or division of strap muscles.

TABLE 2. Clinical Signs and Symptoms of Significant Injury

Vascular	Respiratory	Digestive
Hemodynamic instability[a]	Airway compromise[a]	Hematemesis
Pulsatile hematoma[a]	Air bubbling from neck wound[a]	Odynophagia
Expanding hematoma[a]	Significant subcutaneous emphysema[a]	Dysphagia
Active hemorrhage[a]	Hemoptysis	Subcutaneous emphysema
Bruit	Dysphonia	
Neurologic deficit	Tracheal tenderness	
Pulse deficit	Dyspnea	

[a]Indicates hard sign of injury mandating operative exploration.

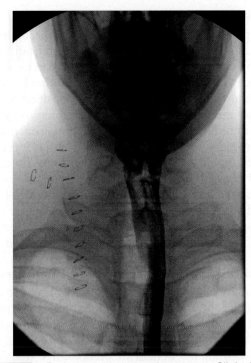

FIGURE 2 • Barium contrast esophagogram. Clinical exam alone is unreliable in excluding esophageal injury. Formal evaluation with barium esophagogram and/or esophagoscopy is recommended to minimize the consequences of missed injury or delay in diagnosis. This image demonstrates a normal study without evidence of contrast extravasation.

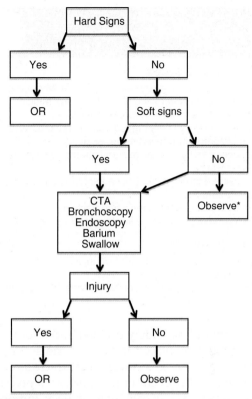

FIGURE 3 • Suggested management algorithm for Zone II penetrating injuries. *Observation alone should be exercised with caution, as some injuries may be clinically occult at the time of presentation.

Intraoperative esophagoscopy and bronchoscopy are often utilized to supplement direct open examination and minimize the incidence of missed injuries.

Management of Common Zone II Injuries

Vascular Injury

It is currently recommended that all common and internal carotid artery injuries should be repaired, even in patients presenting with significant neurologic deficits, as early revascularization has consistently been associated with improvement or stabilization of neurologic symptoms. Proximal and distal control of the common, external, and internal carotid arteries must be obtained before definitive repair. If exposure is less than ideal, vascular control can be accomplished with a Fogarty balloon catheter. Prior to clamping, consideration should be given to heparinization provided there are no contraindications. Shunting is usually unnecessary in the typical young trauma patient, but should be employed if there is suspicion for cerebral malperfusion or evidence of poor back bleeding.

Sharp penetrating weapons typically result in relatively clean injuries that are amenable to primary repair with minimal debridement. Arteriorrhaphy can be accomplished with interrupted 6-0 polypropylene sutures. If the laceration is circumferential, an end–end repair may be performed. If the injury is near the bifurcation of the common carotid into its internal and external branches, a patch angioplasty will help minimize the development of stenosis. Large perforations or defects are unlikely from this mechanism, but if present are treated with segmental resection and interposition graft. Saphenous vein conduit is preferred for this purpose due to superior long-term patency compared with polytetrafluoroethylene.

Whenever possible, internal jugular vein injuries should be repaired. However, if the patient is unstable or simple repair is not feasible this vessel can be ligated unilaterally with minimal morbidity. Similarly, the external carotid artery may be safely ligated secondary to extensive collateral circulation. Due to difficult access, bleeding from the vertebral vessels is best managed by temporary control of hemorrhage in the operating room, followed by immediate transfer to the arteriography suite for embolization.

Esophageal Injury

Expeditious diagnosis is critical in limiting the morbidity and mortality associated with esophageal injuries. If detected within the first 12 to 24 hours, the vast majority of full-thickness stab wound injuries can be repaired primarily in a two-layer fashion.

TABLE 3. Key Technical Steps and Potential Pitfalls in Zone II Neck Exploration

Key Technical Steps
1. Neck incision along anterior border of SCM muscle.
2. Open carotid sheath and divide facial and middle thyroid veins to expose carotid artery.
3. If carotid artery injury present, obtain proximal and distal control before definitive repair.
4. Inspect internal jugular vein and attempt primary repair if necessary.
5. Mobilize esophagus and place Penrose drain to rotate circumferentially.
6. Palpate and visualize larynx and trachea.
7. Perform esophagoscopy and/or bronchoscopy.

Potential Pitfalls
- Vagus or recurrent laryngeal nerve injury.
- Missed esophageal injury.
- Difficulty obtaining proximal or distal control of carotid artery.

The area should be widely drained and a local muscle flap should be placed to buttress the suture line, particularly if there is a concomitant tracheal or vascular injury. In the event of the latter, it is preferable to place drains via a contralateral neck incision to avoid the catastrophic consequences associated with blowout of a fresh carotid repair. Severely destructive injuries requiring esophageal exclusion with gastrostomy and jejunostomy are extremely rare. After any repair, a barium swallow should be performed between postoperative days 5 and 7 before initiating oral intake.

Tracheal Injury

Most penetrating tracheal injuries that occur as the result of stab wounds occur without significant tissue loss and can be repaired primarily. This can be accomplished in a single layer utilizing 3-0 absorbable sutures in an interrupted fashion. Again, interposition of well-vascularized tissue (omohyoid or SCM muscle) is essential to minimize risk of fistula formation. Concomitant tracheostomy is not routinely indicated to protect a tracheal repair. If performed, tracheostomy should be placed one ring distal to the injury and should be limited to severe crush injuries, major laryngeal injuries, tears that traverse >1/3 of the circumference, or when prolonged postoperative ventilatory support is anticipated. Early extubation is safe and recommended.

Special Intraoperative Considerations

It is not uncommon to find injuries that traverse more than one zone, requiring additional access incisions. Unfortunately, this is not always known beforehand in the patient who proceeds directly to the operating room without the benefit of preoperative diagnostic imaging. Zone I injuries may necessitate a median sternotomy, a supraclavicular incision with resection of the head of the clavicle, or a combined "trapdoor" approach involving the addition of an anterolateral thoracotomy. Zone III injuries are notoriously difficult to expose, requiring cephalad extension of a standard vertical Zone II incision with possible disarticulation or partial resection of the mandible and in some instances limited craniotomy. Commonly utilized surgical incisions are illustrated in **Figure 4**.

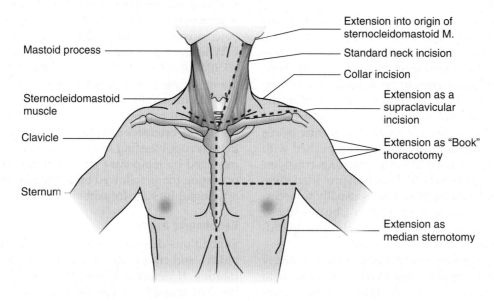

Mastoid process

Sternocleidomastoid muscle

Clavicle

Sternum

Extension into origin of sternocleidomastoid M.

Standard neck incision

Collar incision

Extension as a supraclavicular incision

Extension as "Book" thoracotomy

Extension as median sternotomy

FIGURE 4 • Incisions for exposure of penetrating neck injuries.

Postoperative Management

Patients will typically be monitored in the intensive care unit during the immediate postoperative period where frequent neurologic assessment and hemodynamic monitoring can be performed. Early postoperative complications related specifically to neck exploration can include hemorrhage, recurrent laryngeal nerve injury, and esophageal leak. Unilateral recurrent laryngeal nerve injury will produce hoarseness and require formal evaluation by an otolaryngologist with laryngoscopy. Postoperative hemorrhage can be rapidly fatal if not recognized promptly. The confined space of the neck can result in airway compromise if bleeding is not controlled. Fortunately, leak in the cervical esophagus typically results in localized abscess amenable to drainage, whereas leak involving the thoracoabdominal esophagus can result in fulminant mediastinitis, which is often fatal.

Case Conclusion

The patient undergoes standard central neck exploration. After evacuation of a moderate-sized hematoma, you find a clean-based laceration of her internal carotid artery and internal jugular vein, both of which are amenable to primary repair. You also find a small anterior tracheal tear, which is also repaired primarily. The esophagus is visualized externally and internally with flexible endoscopy and there is no evidence of injury. The patient is extubated immediately after the operation and taken to the intensive care unit for monitoring. A barium swallow performed on postoperative day 1 confirmed no evidence of esophageal injury, and an oral diet is begun. The patient is discharged home on postoperative day 5.

TAKE HOME POINTS

- Assessment and management of the airway is the top priority.
- Hemodynamic instability or "hard" signs of injury require immediate surgical exploration.
- Both mandatory exploration and selective operative management can be equally justified in the appropriate clinical setting for Zone II injuries.
- Esophageal injuries are often clinically occult at presentation, and early diagnosis is important to minimize associated morbidity and mortality.
- All common and internal carotid injuries should be repaired.
- In the setting of multiple repairs, well-vascularized flaps should be utilized to protect suture lines.

SUGGESTED READINGS

Demetriades D, Theodorou D, Cornwall E, et al. Evaluation of penetrating injuries of the neck: prospective study of 223 patients. World J Surg. 1997;21:41–47.

Tisherman SA, Bokhari F, Collier B, et al. Clinical practice guideline: penetrating zone II neck trauma. J Trauma. 2008;64:1392–1405.

107 Burns

JEFFREY S. GUY

Presentation

You are informed of a patient who is being transported to your facility. By report, the patient is a 22-year-old male who was involved in an explosion of a small building suspected to be a methamphetamine lab. Prehospital providers report that the patient is awake and breathing spontaneously. He has burns on the front of his chest, abdomen, and bilateral legs from his groin to his toes.

Differential Diagnosis

Making a differential diagnosis for a burn injury may seem odd to some. After all the diagnosis of a burn injury should be obvious to most, including those with minimal medical training. The hazard in caring for those with burn injury is essentially becoming entranced in the grotesque nature of the burn injury and not identifying occult potential life threats in a timely fashion.

In structure fires, victims may be hit by falling debris, fall through collapsing floors, or escape upper floors by jumping through windows. Patients may get burned after a motor vehicle crash (MVC), and focusing on the burn may delay rapid and appropriate treatment of commonly encountered traumatic injuries. Patients presenting with major burn injuries should undergo a methodical evaluation for traumatic injuries employing the concepts taught in advanced trauma life support (ATLS). Any injury that can occur following a fall, assault, or MVC should be sought in a burned patient.

The most dreaded complication in the early management of the burned patient is loss of the patency of the airway from airway edema. Failure to detect airway edema in a timely fashion can be catastrophic.

In this case, the patient may likely to have been exposed to hazardous materials and be at risk for a chemical burn. A patient contaminated with hazardous materials presents unique challenges to the medical providers as well as the receiving institution. If the patient inadequately decontaminated, bringing the patient into the hospital emergency department (ED) risks the safety of the medical providers as well as other patients within the ED. A contaminated patient must be decontaminated prior to entry into the ED, and providers providing decontamination and medical care during this phase of care must don appropriate level of personal protective equipment.

Chemical burns that are not adequately decontaminated will continue to cause injury to the patient during transport to the hospital and evaluation within the ED. Therefore, appropriate contamination needs to be immediate and of an adequate magnitude to reduce the risk of ongoing tissue injury or systemic toxicity to the patient. If a contaminated patient is brought into the ED, the safety of other patients, visitors, is jeopardized. Furthermore, contamination of the health care facility can cause closure of the ED until it can be made safe by decontamination.

Workup

The initial evaluation and treatment of the burned victim should follow the principles taught in ATLS. A systemic evaluation to identify and treat immediate life threats is then followed by a head-to-toe examination. Often, providers not experienced in caring for severe burns may focus on the horrific nature of the sights and smells associated with the burn. This mistake is similar to that which is commonly made in the evaluation of the pregnant trauma patient; providers will commonly and erroneously center their evaluation on the fetus instead of the more immediate life-threatening injury to the mother.

All clothing and jewelry must be removed as these may retain residual heat and continue to injure the patient. In the early hours after a burn injury, accurate determination of burn depth is deceptively difficult. Some burns are easily determined as full thickness, while others are more indeterminate.

The patient needs to be fully exposed to quantify the magnitude of the burn injury. To fully determine the size of the burns, the burns will require local debridement. Prior to debridement, the burn often appears more superficial than it actually is. Another problem occurs when a provider erroneously determines that a normal or a superficially injured area is blackened by soot.

Local wound debridement prior to arrival at the burn center may not be appropriate, but providers should take measures to accurately estimate burn size. Underestimations of burn size will likely lead to inadequate fluid resuscitation and complications of prolonged hypovolemic shock. Overestimation of burn size will produce the complication of excessive fluid administration.

Diagnosis and Treatment

Perhaps to many, making the diagnosis of a burn would seem rather straightforward. However, with an injury of this magnitude, there are several limb- and life-threatening complications that can develop rapidly. In addition to the diagnosis of "burn," the patient might also develop (1) toxic asphyxiation, (2) airway obstruction, (3) smoke inhalation, (4) circumferential burns of the torso preventing respiration, or (5) limb-threatening limb ischemia from circumferential limb burns. Furthermore, appropriate triage and fluid treatment depend on accurately estimating burn size.

Airway

The highest priority is for the provider to determine the patency of the airway. Following an inhalation injury, the mucosa of the trachea can become edematous increasing the patient's work of breathing, as well as the patency of the airway lumen. Inhalation injury should be suspected in patients with burns to the face or chest, singeing of facial hair, soot in the mouth or sputum, or change in the character of their voice. A patient with swelling of the upper airway or epiglottis will have drooling, and seek a sitting, forward-leaning position. If airway edema is a concern, the patient should be intubated.

Smoke Inhalation

The leading cause of death from structure fires is complications from smoke inhalation. However, smoke injury, when it is the only injury, has a mortality rate of <10%. When combined with burn injuries, the mortality of smoke inhalation increases to 20%. The presence or absence smoke inhalation is a greater predictor of survival than the size of the burn or the age of the patient. The diagnosis of smoke inhalation should be considered in patients who were in structure fires or were rescued from an enclosed space fire. The presence of soot in the sputum is known as carbonaceous sputum. Bronchoscopy is commonly used to identify soot below the level of the vocal cords and confirm smoke inhalation.

Burned patients who present with a decreased mental status are likely to have experienced some magnitude of asphyxiation or intoxication. Fire requires heat, oxygen, and fuel. In a structure fire, the flames consume the oxygen in the environment and produce several toxic gases. In a structure fire, the percentage of oxygen in the ambient environment is frequently less than the ambient 21%. Also, two asphyxiates associated with structure fires are carbon monoxide and hydrogen cyanide (HCN).

Carbon monoxide (CO) is a colorless, odorless gas that binds with hemoglobin more than 210 times stronger than oxygen. Patients who have been involved in structure fires may suffer from carbon monoxide toxicity. CO toxicity is the leading cause of poisoning deaths in the United States. The symptoms of CO toxicity are nonspecific and include headaches, nausea, and dizziness. In the most severe cases of CO poisoning, patients will experience weakness, seizures, coma, arrhythmias, hypotension, and eventually death.

The complex of carbon monoxide and hemoglobin is known as carboxyhemoglobin. On room air, the half-life of carboxyhemoglobin is 250 minutes. On 100% oxygen by an endotracheal tube, the half-life is reduced to 60 minutes. With hyperbaric oxygen at two atmospheres, the half-life is reduced to 27 minutes.

A patient with thermal injuries, smoke inhalation, and carbon monoxide toxicity requires complex and aggressive care by experienced providers. Use of hyperbaric oxygen remains controversial and of questionable benefit in such critically injured patients. At present time, there is universal agreement that application of 100% oxygen is beneficial to these patients.

Cyanide Toxicity

HCN is produced from the burning of many materials in the environment. HCN poisons cellular respiration at the level of the electron transport chain or oxidative phosphorylation. The net result is anaerobic metabolism and the development of lactic acidosis. A simple chemical laboratory test is presently lacking; however, most medical centers send a sample to a reference lab to obtain plasma cyanide levels. The treatment of suspected cyanide poisoning must occur rapidly. Given the absence of confirmatory laboratory tests, medical providers must make a decision to treat for cyanide poisoning based on the historical information and nonspecific metabolic findings. In the event of cyanide toxicity, the patient may demonstrate lactic acidosis and an increase in oxygen saturation on the venous blood gas.

Rapid treatment of suspected cyanide poisoning is required to avoid neurologic complications or death. The modern treatment includes the use of hydroxocobalamin (Cyanokit), which is an analogue of vitamin B_{12}. This modern antidote chelates the cyanide. This antidote is well tolerated, but has the peculiar side effect of causing a red discoloration of the skin and urine. Hydroxocobalamin interferes with the accuracy of many common laboratory tests, such as electrolyte and hepatic panels.

Burn Depth

Burn depth determination is deceptively difficult. The appearance of the burns can change dramatically in the first 48 hours. Burn depth is categorized based on the anatomical regions of the skin injured. Superficial burns (first degree) involve only the epidermis, typically appears as reddened skin, and will heal typically within a week with minimal treatment. Partial-thickness burns (second-degree burns) involve the epidermis and varying depth of the underlying dermis. Partial-thickness burns will blister and will have a red glistening appearance of the wound beds.

These wounds may take 2 to 3 weeks to close and may produce some degree of scarring. Partial-thickness burns may require surgery. Full-thickness burns are characterized by destruction of both the epidermis and the dermis and will commonly appear as white, gray, or black and are leathery in texture.

Burn Size Estimation

In adults, perhaps the easiest and best-known method of determining burn size is the rule of nines. Each major body region comprises approximately 9% of the total body surface area (TBSA). This rule does not apply to children because children have differing body proportions that change as the child ages. For instance, infants have proportionally larger heads and smaller lower extremities compared to an adult. To estimate burn size in children, a diagram such as the Lund-Browder chart is required.

Perhaps the most commonly deployed method of determining burn size in adults is the rule of nines. The premise of the rule of nines is that in adults each major body region is approximately 9% TBSA. These major regions include entire head, entire arm, anterior chest, posterior chest, anterior abdomen, posterior abdomen, thigh, and lower leg. The entire palm *of the patient* (not the palm of the provider) approximates 1% of the TBSA. The area of the genitalia also approximates 1% TBSA.

Fluid Resuscitation

Most providers are aware that a burn injury is capable of producing severe and even life-threatening hypovolemia. After a major burn injury, the walls of the capillaries lose integrity and predispose the victim to hypovolemia. This loss of intravascular fluid from the microcirculation is often called leaky capillary syndrome. This is initiated by the release of proinflammatory mediators and reactive oxygen species from the nonviable burned tissue. The overall biologic effect of these mediators includes microvascular changes consistent with capillary leak syndrome, vascular stasis, and decreased cardiac output. Baxter et al. demonstrated that burned animals had a decrease in measured cardiac output that is refractory to treatment with intravenous fluid, vasopressors, and inotropic support. Myocardial depression typically improves in 4 to 8 hours from the time of injury.

The resuscitation of burn shock is a reactionary therapy to the pathophysiologic response to a severe injury. Burn resuscitation does nothing to abrogate or reverse the pathophysiologic events that created the burn shock. There are several formulae that can be used to estimate the amount of fluids and rates required to treat burn shock. What all of the formulae have in common is the changing fluid requirements of the patient in the first several hours after burn injury.

To calculate a patient's resuscitative fluid needs, one needs the weight of the patient in kilograms and the percent body surface area burned (% TBSA). Perhaps the most well-known and applied resuscitation formula is the Parkland. Applying this formula, the amount of fluid administered to the victim is 4 mL/kg/% TBSA burn. One-half of the total calculated fluid needs are administered in the first 8 hours after the injury. Therefore, if the patient does receive therapy for the first 2 hours after the injury, the first half of the fluids should be administered over 6 hours. The second half of the calculated fluid need is given in remaining 16 hours.

Our patient is an 80-kg male who has a 54% TBSA burn at midnight. Calculating a Parkland formula would look like the following:

Total 24 hour fluid needed:
4 mL/kg/% burn or 80 kg × 54% burn = 17,280 mL over 24 hours
Fluid needed from midnight to 8:00 AM—first 8 hours from injury/first 8 hours of resuscitation
17,280 mL/2 = 8,640 mL first 8 hours
8,640 mL/8 h = 1,080 mL/h
Fluid needed from 8:00 AM to midnight—hours 8 to 24
17,280 mL/2 = 8,640 mL for remaining 16 hours
8,640 mL/16 h = 540 mL/h
If the same patient who was burned at midnight but required 2 hours of transport only received 500 mL prior to arrival at the burn center.
17,280 mL/2 = 8,640 mL first 8 hours
8,640 mL – 500 mL = 8,140 mL
8,140/6 h = 1357 mL/h

Formal fluid resuscitation is typically reserved for those patients with burns >20% TBSA; only burns of this severity are associated with the capillary leak syndrome. For burns <20%, patients can commonly be managed by providing them with 150% of their calculated maintenance rate.

Presentation Continued

This patient was described as being burned on the anterior trunk (both chest and abdomen) and both legs from groin to toes. Applying the rule of nines to determine estimated burn size, this patient has 54% TBSA burn.

Adequacy of resuscitation is usually determined by urine output and systemic blood pressure. Placement of a Foley catheter is appropriate to evaluate the urine output on an hourly basis. A urine output of 0.5 mL/kg/hr is usually adequate. To avoid complications of excessive fluid administration, consider decreasing the fluid rate when the urine output exceeds 1 mL/kg/hr. In children and the elderly, one should strive for the urine output to be at least 1 mL/kg/hr since the kidneys of these patients have a decreased ability to concentrate solutes. The most commonly used fluid for burn resuscitation is Lactate Ringers. Many burn providers avoid normal saline because large volumes of saline are associated with the development of a hyperchloremic metabolic acidosis.

Circumferential Burns

Skin that has sustained full-thickness burns contracts and is less elastic than normal skin. Circumferential burns of the limbs are limb threatening, and circumferential burns of the thorax are life threatening. In the case of thoracic burns, the skin contracts around the torso and produces a profound decrease is chest wall compliance. When an intubated patient is on volume mode ventilation, a marked increase in the peak inspiratory pressure may occur. When ventilating the patient with an Ambu bag, the bag will be rigid and near impossible to compress. With time and ongoing fluid resuscitation, this will progress increasing the patient's work of breathing to the point of respiratory embarrassment. Escharotomy of chest wall burns produces an immediate and profound improvement in compliance and improves ability to ventilate. When performing escharotomies on a ventilated patient, pressure control modes should be avoided because once the escharotomy incision have been made, the immediate improvement in chest wall compliance may produce a marked increase in tidal volume and risk of pneumothorax.

With circumferential burns of the limb, the burn eschar contracts while the underlying tissues are becoming edematous. This causes obstruction of venous outflow of the burned limb while the arterial flow remains open. This amplifies the rate of edema formation up to the point where the arterial inflow is obstructed. Escharotomy of the limb is required to reestablish distal blood flow and maintain limb viability.

Surgical Approach

Escharotomies

Limb escharotomies should be done in a timely fashion, typically within 4 hours of injury, to reduce the likelihood of limb-threatening ischemia. With circumferential burns of the chest, decompressive escharotomies may need to be performed rapidly to avoid respiratory embarrassment where patients are unable to be ventilated.

On limbs, escharotomies can be performed readily with an electrocautery. The incisions should be positioned on the true medial and lateral aspects of the limb. In a severely burned arm, the true anatomic position the arm occurs when the arm is held with the palm up. Escharotomies of the hands should be done after consultation with the receiving burn center.

Escharotomies of circumferential chest wall burns will produce an almost immediate increased in chest wall compliance. When patients are being mechanically ventilated with a pressure-control mode, failure to anticipate improvement in chest wall compliance will result in pulmonary barotrauma.

Burn Excision

Full-thickness burns are necrotic tissue, and this dead tissue is the source of significant systemic effects causing the patient to be profoundly ill. Early surgical excision of the burn wound will reduce both morbidity and mortality.

The details of the burn excision will vary with the anatomical region of the body burned, the age of the patient, as well as the overall physiologic status of the patient. Operative care of the large burns should only occur in specialized centers with a large volume of experience providing both the operative and the perioperative care to these types of patients. A general rule for burn excision has been to limit the operative time to <2 hours to limit both blood loss and hypothermia. Patients are then returned to the operating room every 24 to 48 hours until all the burn has been excised.

The timing of surgery with patients with smoke inhalation is complicated by the "honeymoon" period experienced by these patients. With smoke inhalation, the patients will have a period of 48 to 72 hours prior to developing significant pulmonary problems that may complicate transport to the operating room, as well as increasing the hazards of performing such an operation. Therefore, in patients with smoke inhalation, one should attempt to surgically excise as much as burn as safely possible prior to the respiratory status deteriorating.

In patients with critical burns, early trips to the operating rooms should remove the greatest mass of burned tissue. Early trips to the operating room should focus on those anatomical areas that allow for both rapid and large debridement. Excision of burns from areas such as the hands, feet, or face should be delayed because these areas take considerably greater time to perform a careful excision. Areas that require more time for excision are usually delayed until the patient is in a more favorable physiologic state.

Burn excision can be associated with considerable blood loss; therefore, attempts to limit hemorrhage should be made. Tourniquets and topical hemostatic agents should be deployed whenever feasible. Burn patients easily become hypothermic and typically large areas of the body are exposed during operative procedures. All maneuvers to maintain the patient's body temperature should be deployed.

Once the burn wounds have been excised, the surgeon has numerous options for closure of the wounds. Preservation of patient function is more important than cosmetic outcome. A functional outcome that the patient can use for performance of activities of daily living is more important than producing an outstanding-looking hand that is essentially useless to the patient.

Donor skin is taken with various depths based on the area to be covered as well as the need to possible reharvest the site in the case of larger burns. Skin grafts that are taken very thin are perhaps more likely to take on the wound bed, but due to the small amount of dermal tissue in the skin graft, the amount of contracture of the graft will be greater. Donor sites taken thicker will have more dermis and will contract less; therefore, these types of thicker grafts are more desirable in areas of high mobility, such as the hands, antecubital fossa, neck, and face. Donor sites are typically taken at 0.010 to 0.012 inch thick, and for areas needing thicker grafts the thickness is commonly 0.018 inch. As a general rule, donor sites taken at 0.010 inch take about 10 to 14 days to heal.

A skin graft that is applied in a sheet fashion will commonly contract about 30%, and a graft that is meshed 1.5:1 will commonly retain the original size of the donor site. Faces and necks are universally grafted with thick sheet grafts or full-thickness grafts. Hands are commonly grafted with either sheet or nonexpanded 1:1 split-thickness grafts. Expanded mesh grafts are used to a variable degree based on the amount of donor sites available for harvest and the areas to be grafted.

Over the past 15 years, the use of dermal implants has increased in the acute operative care of the burn wound. A split-thickness skin graft has the entire epidermal layer and varying thickness of the dermis. The thicker the dermis the greater time required for the donor site to heal, but greater dermis means less contracture of the grafts and a greater functional outcome. Dermal implants are commonly considered for use in areas of high function or cosmetic considerations. There are two dermal implants used for autografting, one biologic and one synthetic. When a dermal substitute is used, a staged operative approach is used. During the first operation, the wound is excised and the dermal substitute applied to the wound bed. Following an interval to allow the implant to vascularize, autografts are applied over the dermal substitute **(Table 1)**.

Postoperative Management

The success of a technical procedure in the operating room is highly dependent on the care provided after surgery. Meticulous nursing care and therapy by experienced providers is required to optimize the functional

---

TABLE 1. Key Technical Steps and Potential Pitfalls in Burn Excision

Key Technical Steps

1. Timing of operation is important. Operating too early on a patient may lead to a poorly resuscitated patient. In contrast, operating on a patient too late may be associated with a massive systemic inflammatory response syndrome or complications from smoke inhalation.
2. Large and broad areas should be excised early to maximize the mass of debrided tissue early.
3. Limit excisions to 20% TBSA or 2 hours of operating room time.
4. Tangential excision will result in large blood losses.
5. Application of allografts to excised wounds will limit heat loss and abrogate hypermetabolism.
6. Best donor site is the back. Mesh 1.5:1 will make graft size approximately that of the donor site. 3:1 will expand to about twice the original size.
7. When grafting the face or neck, use donors from scalp or upper back, and nonmeshed skin.
8. Graft sites used for central lines early in the reconstructive process.

Potential Pitfalls

- An excision of 20% TBSA can be associated with a total blood volume loss.
- Hypothermia should be avoided by warming all intravenous fluids, OR fluids, and the use of warmers.
- In critical patients who cannot tolerate graft loss, wound excision should be carried down to fascia.

---

outcome for the patient. Performing operative care on a burn patient at an institution not equipped to provide this high level of specialized postoperative care will result in poorer results. In the early postoperative period, unit protocols focusing on wound care and therapeutic positioning are designed to increase grafting success and maximize range of motion of injured areas.

Following autografting, the wounds are dressed with topical antibiotics and complex dressings. When dressing a fresh skin graft, the layer immediately adjacent to the graft is a nonadherent layer such as Adaptic, Xeroform, Vaseline gauze, or fine mesh gauze. The next layer typically consists of an antibiotic layer followed by several rolls of Kerlix to serve as an antishear layer and finally a layer for compression with an elastic dressing, such as an ACE or Coban wrap.

The process of wound healing and scar remodeling is a protracted process. Patients are taught a series of range of motion of exercises in an effort to maximize functional recovery. In serious burns that cross joints, the patient will need to perform therapy on a daily basis to maintain range of motion and preserve function. These patients require evaluation in the postoperative period by a therapist experienced in care of the burned victim. In an effort to reduce hypertrophic scarring, most burn centers use custom-fitted pressure garments.

TAKE HOME POINTS

- The presence of smoke inhalation is a greater predictor of mortality than the age of the patient and the size of the burns.
- Circumferential burns of the chest wall can decrease pulmonary compliance producing respiratory embarrassment.
- Burn excision of 20% can result in the loss of a total blood volume.
- The maximal area of excision that should be performed in one operation is 20% TBSA or a maximal operating time of 2 hours.
- Burn resuscitation with normal saline can produce a hyperchloremic metabolic acidosis.
- Carbon Monoxide is the leading cause of poisoning deaths in the United States.

SUGGESTED READINGS

Ballard-Croft C, Horton JW. Sympathoadrenal modulation of stress-activated signaling in burn trauma. J Burn Care Rehabil. 2002;23(3):172–182.

Baxter C, Cook WA, Shires GT. Serum myocardial depressant factor of burn shock. Surg Forum. 1966;17:1–2.

Baxter C, Shires GT. Physiological response to crystalloid resuscitation of severe burns. Ann N Y Acad Sci. 1968;150:874–894.

de La Cal MA, et al. Pneumonia in patients with severe burns: a classification according to the concept of the carrier state. Chest. 2001;119(4):1160–1165.

Demling RH. Burns. Fluid and electrolyte management. Crit Care Clin. 1985;1(1):27–45.

Demling RH. Fluid resuscitation after major burns. JAMA. 1983;250(11):1438–1440.

DesLauriers CA, Burda AM, Wahl M. Hydroxocobalamin as a cyanide antidote. Am J Ther. 2006;13(2):161–165.

Dyess DL, et al. Modulation of microvascular permeability by 21-aminosteroids after burn injuries. J Burn Care Rehabil. 2000;21(5):406–413.

Holm C. Resuscitation in shock associated with burns. Tradition or evidence-based medicine? Resuscitation. 2000;44(3):157–164.

Horton JW, et al. Hypertonic saline-dextran suppresses burn-related cytokine secretion by cardiomyocytes. Am J Physiol Heart Circ Physiol. 2001;280(4):H1591–H1601.

Leape LL. Initial changes in burns: tissue changes in burned and unburned skin of rhesus monkeys. J Trauma. 1970;10(6):488–492.

Lee J, et al. Potential interference by hydroxocobalamin on cooximetry hemoglobin measurements during cyanide and smoke inhalation treatments. Ann Emerg Med. 2007;49(6):802–805.

Shimizu S, et al. Burn depth affects dermal interstitial fluid pressure, free radical production, and serum histamine levels in rats. J Trauma. 2002;52(4):683–687.

Shirani KZ, et al. Update on current therapeutic approaches in burns. Shock. 1996;5(1):4–16.

Williams WG. Pathophysiology of the burn wound. In: Herndon D, ed. Total Burn Care. New York, NY: W.B. Saunders, 2002:514–522.

108 Blunt Abdominal Trauma from Motor Vehicle Crash

CARLA KOHOYDA-INGLIS and STEWART C. WANG

Presentation

A 32-year-old man with no significant past medical history presents as the unrestrained driver of an older, mid-sized, four-door sedan involved in a severe head-on motor vehicle crash with a large tree **(Figure 1)**. Bystanders found the man unresponsive and pulled him from the vehicle. On arrival of Emergency Medical Services (EMS), the man was responsive only to painful stimuli, had labored respirations, and was bleeding from the mouth. On EMS examination, the patient's abdomen was firm, but not distended, with positive bowel sounds.

Differential Diagnosis

Care of injured patients begins with assessment at the scene by emergency responders to get the right patient to the right place in the right amount of time. This patient met Field Triage Decision Scheme step 1 (Physiologic) criteria with decreased level of consciousness (Glasgow Coma Scale (GCS) ≤ 13) and was appropriately transported to a high-level trauma center.

Unlike penetrating trauma, blunt trauma such as motor vehicle crashes may cause internal injuries in multiple body compartments with little external evidence. Initial evaluation (primary survey) of the patient in the emergency room focuses on quickly identifying and treating life-threatening injuries that affect *A*irway, *B*reathing, *C*irculation, *D*isability (neurologic) **(Table 1)**.

On arrival to the trauma center, EMS reported a large amount of damage to the steering wheel and that the patient had been restrained by an automatic shoulder belt but had not used the available lap belt. There was 13 inches of intrusion in the toepan area **(Figure 2)**. Passenger compartment intrusion >12 inches at the occupant site or 18 inches anywhere in the vehicle is associated with a high risk of severe injury (Injury Severity Score (ISS) > 15) to that occupant and is part of step 3 of the Guidelines for the Field Triage of Injured Patients.

On primary survey, he was awake and alert, but complaining of right lower chest and right upper abdominal pain. His vital signs were BP 110/80, RR 12, HR 95, T36.7. Physical examination revealed decreased breath sounds in the right chest and tenderness on palpation on the right lower chest wall and the right upper abdomen without peritoneal signs. Focused abdominal sonography for trauma (FAST) ultrasound exam showed fluid at the right hepatorenal fossa with right-kidney irregularity. Portable chest x-ray (CXR) showed fluid in the right chest; pelvis x-ray was normal. A chest tube was placed for the right hemothorax with 900-mL initial output and slow subsequent output.

Workup

In the absence of indication for immediate surgical exploration (e.g., hemodynamic instability with positive FAST or high chest tube output), 3-D imaging to detect occult internal injuries from blunt trauma is the next priority. CT scans in this patient showed the following:

(1) A large complex liver laceration extending completely through the medial segment of the left lobe and into the lateral segment of the left lobe and the right lobe **(Figure 3A)**.

(2) Poorly perfused right kidney, narrowing of the right renal artery with extravasation of intravenously administered contrast material from the right renal artery, and a large right perinephric hematoma **(Figure 3B)**.

Initial Management

Surgical management of the multiply injured patient involves the principles of quick stabilization and resuscitation followed by prioritized treatment of individual injuries. With control of the airway and ability to ventilate the patient, the highest priority is to control hemorrhage, especially arterial bleeding. The presence of active contrast extravasation (arterial bleeding) from the right kidney on abdominal CT mandates immediate intervention. Experience over the past few decades has shown that many solid abdominal organ injuries can be managed without open abdominal exploration and also that hemorrhage control with interventional radiologic techniques provides better organ salvage rates than open operations, which frequently result in organ removal (e.g., nephrectomy, splenectomy) rather than repair to control bleeding. Since there were no immediate hard indications for open exploration (hemodynamic instability, hollow organ injury, penetrating

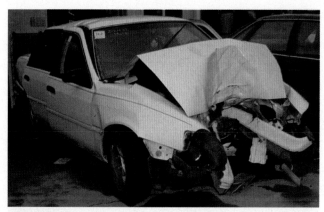

FIGURE 1 • Vehicle damage from frontal crash into large tree.

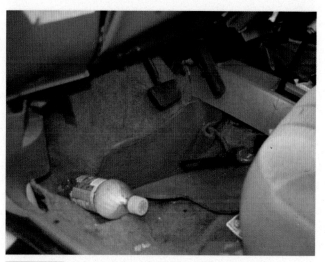

FIGURE 2 • Interior damage with >12 in of toepan intrusion into the driver's space. This meets step 3 (Mechanism of Injury) criteria for field triage and is associated with significant risk of severe injury.

mechanism), this patient underwent radiologically guided embolization of the right kidney and liver with successful control of the bleeding **(Figures 4 and 5)**. The patient was then admitted to the ICU for supportive care.

While hemorrhage control is paramount as indication for surgical intervention in the initial postinjury period, the sequelae of organ injury in the days following may also require intervention. It is also important to reassess the patient for injuries missed during the initial assessment. Bile leak is common following large liver injuries and must be controlled (washout and drain placement, often laparoscopic) to avoid bile peritonitis. A HIDA scan is a sensitive test for bile leakage. In this patient, screening HIDA scan on post injury day 3 showed bile extravasation from the liver with drainage into the right chest tube via the pleural cavity. A clinical diagnosis of right diaphragmatic injury was made. Right-sided diaphragm injuries from blunt trauma are much less common than injuries to the left side. Small isolated right diaphragm injuries may not require operative repair since they are much less likely to develop complications such as organ herniation due to the large liver buttressing it underneath. However, due to the interval development of increased liver elevation on CXR as well as the complication of bile leak into the pleural cavity, operative repair was indicated in this case.

Operative Management

The patient was explored through a midline abdominal incision. The liver was found to be partially herniated into the right chest **(Figure 6)**. In order to safely reduce the fractured liver back into the abdominal cavity, the midline abdominal incision was extended into the right chest (thoracoabdominal incision) to allow the liver to be pushed down from above. The large diaphragm tear was easily repaired with pledgeted sutures **(Figure 7)**. The thin, pliable nature of the diaphragm can result in significant disorientation of torn edges, and optimal repair is facilitated by alignment of the edges with tags, stay sutures, or clamps during the repair. The right pleural cavity was irrigated and drainage maintained with a chest tube. Source control and drainage is an important surgical principle when tissues have been damaged and contents contaminate body cavities. The gallbladder was found to be partially avulsed in the line of the liver laceration and was resected. Multiple drains were placed to drain the leak from bile ducts too small to control individually. The abdominal cavity volume was insufficient to allow primary fascial closure following the reduction of the liver due to the intestinal swelling induced by injury and operation. Closure of the fascia with resultant increased abdominal compartment pressures would have compromised renal as well as pulmonary function in this patient with significant injuries to both of those organ systems and also increased the chances for incisional dehiscence. The fascia was bridged with a temporary dressing and closed at a subsequent operation. Temporary closure techniques (e.g., V.A.C., ABThera) have simplified the management of complex trauma patients requiring abdominal operations for damage control.

TABLE 1. Primary Survey of the Injured Patient

Primary Survey of the Injured Patient

A	Airway with cervical spine protection
B	Breathing and ventilation
C	Circulation with hemorrhage control
D	Disability (neurologic evaluation)
E	Exposure/environmental control

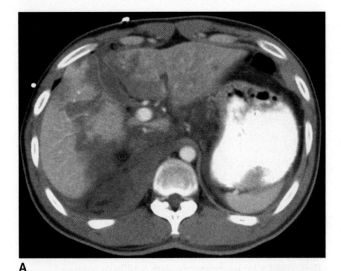

A

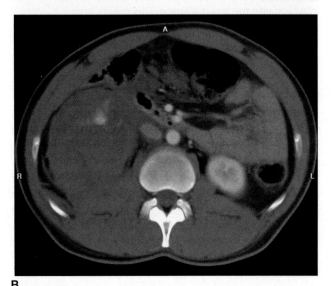

B

FIGURE 3 • CT scan images from the patient in the scenario demonstrating (**A**) large complex liver laceration and (**B**) large perinephric hematoma with contrast extravasation.

TAKE HOME POINTS

- The ABCDs take top priority: Airway, Breathing, Circulation, Disability.
- Indications for urgent laparotomy following blunt trauma include
  - Hemoperitoneum in the setting of hemodynamic instability
  - Perforation of hollow viscus or peritonitis
- At urgent laparotomy, the primary objective is damage control of bleeding and peritoneal soilage. It is better to do a partial operation for damage control than to complete a large complex operation on a sick, unstable, multiply injured patients.
- Most solid organ injuries can be managed without open operation; advances in 3-D medical imaging and

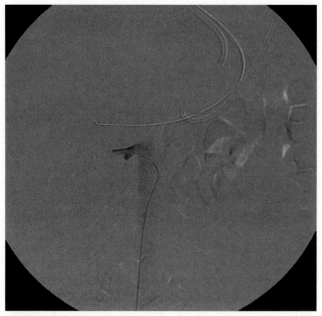

FIGURE 4 • Bleeding from the right renal artery was controlled after placement of 5- and 8-mm coils.

interventional radiologic techniques have markedly decreased the need for open abdominal exploration.
- Not all clinically important injuries will be immediately diagnosable, even with extensive 3-D scanning. Follow-up evaluations and a high index of suspicion are essential.

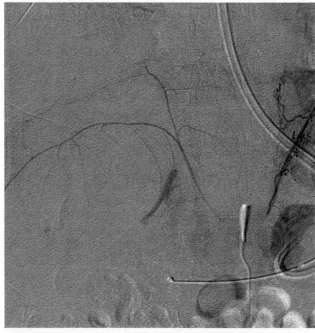

FIGURE 5 • Extravasation from a descending branch of the right hepatic artery. This was subsequently controlled with injection of Gelfoam.

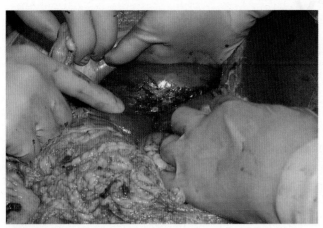

FIGURE 6 • Large liver laceration found on abdominal exploration.

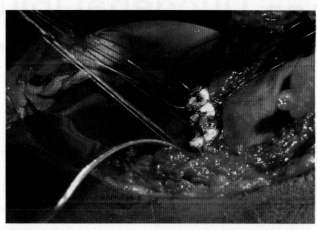

FIGURE 7 • Repair of diaphragm with pledgeted sutures.

SUGGESTED READINGS

Demetriades D, Velmahos GC. Indications for and techniques of laparotomy. In: David Feliciano, Kenneth Mattox, Ernest Moore, eds. Trauma. 6th ed. New York, NY: McGraw-Hill Professional, 2007:607–622.

Franklin GA, Casós SR. Current advances in the surgical approach to abdominal trauma. Injury. 2006;37(12): 1143–1156.

Lee JC, Peitzman AB. Damage-control laparotomy. Curr Opin Crit Care. 2006;12(4):346–350.

Sasser SM, Hunt RC, Sullivent EE, et al. National Expert Panel on Field Triage, Centers for Disease Control and Prevention (CDC). Guidelines for field triage of injured patients. Recommendations of the National Expert Panel on Field Triage. MMWR Recomm Rep. 2009;58(RR-1):1–35.

109 Duodenal Injury

FILIP BEDNAR and MARK R. HEMMILA

Presentation

A 22-year-old man is brought to the hospital by ambulance after being stabbed during a domestic dispute. He arrives in the emergency room with a kitchen knife sticking out of his abdomen in the right upper quadrant. By report, the knife has a blade at least 10 in long. The knife blade is now buried in his abdominal wall up to the handle. His initial SBP is 80 mm Hg.

Differential Diagnosis

This patient has a penetrating mechanism of injury with possible traumatic injuries to the abdomen, retroperitoneum, and chest region. Vital structures and injuries that could prove rapidly lethal include pericardial tamponade, tension pneumothorax, and arterial or venous laceration. It is imperative to consider and evaluate for these injuries during the initial assessment in the trauma bay.

Workup

The primary survey focuses on airway, breathing, circulation, neurologic deficit, and exposure using the Advanced Trauma Life Support protocol. This patient may or may not require endotracheal intubation in the emergency room. He should have large bore IV access established but not receive significant crystalloid fluid administration until operative intervention is underway. A focused abdominal sonography for trauma (FAST) exam quickly evaluates the patient's pericardial space for evidence of pericardial fluid and/or tamponade. A flat-plate chest radiograph will reveal the presence of a hemothorax or pneumothorax requiring chest tube placement. It is important to logroll this patient, examining for additional evidence of injury. If time permits, a blood sample should be obtained for blood type and crossmatch. Type-specific or O negative blood products should be available for immediate administration, if necessary.

Presentation Continued

In the present case, FAST exam is negative for pericardial blood but positive for a fluid stripe between the liver and the kidney in the right upper quadrant of the abdomen. Chest x-ray shows no hemothorax or pneumothorax. Given the mechanism of injury and fascial penetration, this patient has a clear indication for immediate operative exploration.

His ER workup should be expeditious and ideally last <10 minutes. The knife should be left in place and prepped into the operative field. The surgeon should be prepared to explore for injuries to the liver, biliary system, duodenum, inferior vena cava (IVC), right kidney, stomach, small bowel, colon, and vascular system in retroperitoneal zones 1 (central abdomen) and 2 (flank).

Treatment

A generous midline laparotomy is the standard approach for trauma in this circumstance (Table 1). The patient should be surgically prepped and draped from the sternal notch to the groin. One leg should be prepped and draped into the field from the groin to the knee. Endotracheal intubation, if not already performed, should occur just prior to skin incision. Blood products must be available. Entry into the abdomen should be accomplished quickly and safely, typically using a scalpel with limited passes to divide the skin, subcutaneous tissue, and fascia. Next, the peritoneum is sharply divided over the length of the incision both cephalad and caudad with heavy scissors. An examination of the position of the knife blade, trajectory, and injuries is quickly made prior to removing the knife. All four quadrants should be rapidly packed off with laparotomy sponges and the small bowel eviscerated toward the midline. Once all four quadrants are packed, a careful exploration and systematic control of significant acute hemorrhage is performed one quadrant at a time. If time permits, allowing the anesthesia team to catch up with blood product administration prior to starting the exploration can be helpful to the patient. The most likely vascular structures to be injured under these circumstances include the intrahepatic vasculature, the portal triad, IVC, right renal pedicle, celiac axis, superior mesenteric vessels, aorta, and the pancreaticoduodenal complex of blood vessels.

TABLE 1. Key Technical Steps and Potential Pitfalls to a Duodenal Injury Repair

Key Technical Steps

1. Midline laparotomy from xiphoid to the pubic symphysis.
2. Rapid packing of all four quadrants.
3. Careful exploration and hemostasis by quadrants.
4. Mobilization of the hepatic flexure medially.
5. Kocher and/or Cattell-Braasch maneuvers to fully expose the entire duodenum.
6. Damage control vs. definitive repair.
7. External drainage of suture lines and provision of feeding access.
8. Consider delayed closure and second look laparotomy once stable to reassess bowel viability and exploration for other occult injuries.

Potential Pitfalls

- Failure to control acute hemorrhage from vascular structures surrounding the duodenum prior to duodenal assessment.
- Deciding between damage control approach and definitive repair based on patient's status and other injuries.
- Protection of the right ureter and kidney during medial visceral rotation.
- Avoidance of iatrogenic vascular and pancreatic injuries during the duodenal mobilization and assessment.
- Failure to plan for pancreatic or duodenal leak.

Duodenal Exposure

Once initial hemostasis has been obtained and the patient has been adequately resuscitated, a systematic exploration of the abdominal viscera is performed. In this case, the surgeon has to have a high suspicion for duodenal and pancreatic injuries along with the other abdominal viscera in the area of the penetration. Exposure of the duodenal loop and pancreatic head is achieved using a combination of the Kocher and the Cattell-Braasch maneuvers **(Figure 1)**. The surgeon may also elect to divide the ligament of Treitz to further expose the fourth portion of the duodenum and the duodenojejunal junction. To begin the exposure, the retroperitoneal attachments of the hepatic flexure of the colon and the gastrocolic ligament are initially divided to gain access to the lateral aspect of the second portion of the duodenum. A Kocher maneuver is performed by incising the peritoneum laterally to the duodenal C-loop and then mobilizing the duodenum and the pancreatic head medially. This will allow visualization of the majority of the first, second, and a portion of the third section of the duodenum.

The Cattell-Braasch maneuver is a full right to medial visceral rotation including the right colon and small bowel. To perform this maneuver, the white line of Toldt is incised lateral to the right colon and the right colon and cecum are mobilized medially. Attention must be given to identify and protect the right ureter in

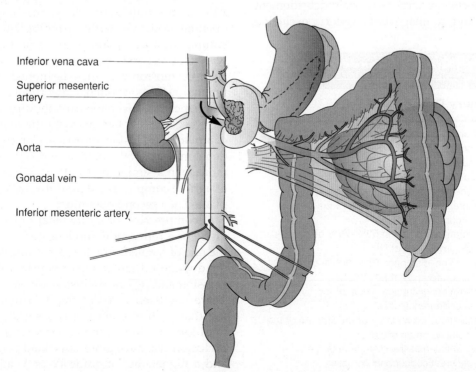

Inferior vena cava

Superior mesenteric artery

Aorta

Gonadal vein

Inferior mesenteric artery

FIGURE 1 • The Cattell-Braasch and Kocher maneuvers allow rotation of the right colon and the small intestine completely away from the right retroperitoneum, allowing exposure of the duodenum and the pancreatic head, as well as the vascular structures and kidney. (From Mulholland. Greenfield's Surgery. Philadelphia, PA: Lippincott, Williams and Wilkins, 2006.)

Clinical Scenarios in Surgery

the process. This maneuver allows the surgeon access to the base of the bowel mesentery, which is also mobilized from the right lower quadrant to the ligament of Treitz. This exercise will further expose the third and the fourth portions of the duodenum with additional mobilization provided by division of the ligament of Treitz itself. Once the full medial visceral rotation is performed, the surgeon also has access to all of the right-sided retroperitoneal organs and vascular structures including the IVC, right renal complex, and the superior mesenteric blood vessels.

Injury Assessment and Repair

With full exposure and the patient stabilized, the surgeon has to assess the degree of duodenal injury before selecting the proper repair or damage control approach. Duodenal injuries are graded **(Table 2)** and it is important to ascertain the location of the laceration in relation to the other nearby anatomic structures. A crucial maneuver is to assess whether the duodenal papilla is involved as this will determine whether a simple or a complex repair is required. If uncertainty exists, a cholecystectomy and an on-table cholangiogram can be performed to assess the common bile duct. Passing a balloon catheter ("biliary Fogarty") or a similar small catheter through the cystic duct stump following cholecystectomy and feeding it distally can prove to be a simple maneuver to identify the relationship of the ampulla to the area of injury.

Options for repair of a duodenal laceration include simple primary closure with or without debridement, simple repair and drainage with pyloric exclusion,

TABLE 2. AAST Grading of Duodenal Injuries

Grade	Injury Description
I	Intramural hematoma–involving single portion of the duodenum
	Laceration–partial thickness, no perforation
II	Intramural hematoma–involving more than one portion of the duodenum
	Laceration–disruption <50% of the circumference
III	Laceration–disruption 50%–75% of the circumference of D2
	Laceration–disruption 50%–100% of the circumference of D1, D3, D4
IV	Laceration–disruption >75% of the circumference of D2
	Laceration–involvement of the ampulla or the distal common bile duct
V	Laceration–massive disruption of the pancreaticoduodenal complex
	Vascular–devascularization of the duodenum

Advance one grade for multiple injuries up to grade III. D1, first portion of duodenum; D2, second portion of duodenum; D3, third portion of duodenum; D4, fourth portion of duodenum.

Roux-en-Y duodenojejunostomy, duodenal diverticularization (antrectomy, oversewing of duodenum, and loop gastrojejunostomy), and a full pancreaticoduodenectomy for massive injuries of the pancreaticoduodenal complex. In general, the simplest repair that gets the job done and an operation that will "fail well" is preferred. Performance of a Whipple for trauma should be the option of last resort and is best conducted in stages. All of these repairs should have consideration given to supplementation of the repair with buttressing of vulnerable suture lines and strategic placement of external drainage devices. Drainage of the pancreas and attention to provision of feeding access for the patient in the form of a nasojejunal tube, gastrojejunostomy tube, or a distal feeding jejunostomy are imperative.

Most simple duodenal injuries are closed primarily without tension using a single- or double-layer closure technique in a transverse fashion to avoid narrowing the bowel lumen. Suture lines may be buttressed with an omental flap or a serosal flap by oversewing with a loop/limb of jejunum. Another option for more extensive lacerations or perforations of the duodenum, which cannot be closed primarily, is to create a Roux limb of jejunum and use it to repair the luminal defect by constructing a duodenojejunostomy in a side-to-side fashion. Pyloric exclusion can offer protection of a fresh suture line and temporarily redirect gastric outflow **(Figure 2)**. To create pyloric exclusion, a distal longitudinal gastrostomy is made on the anterior surface of the stomach. The pyloric ring is grasped with an Allis clamp, pulled into the stomach, and the pyloric opening oversewn with a running 2-0 or 3-0 Prolene suture. Another option is to staple the pylorus shut with a thoracoabdominal (TA) stapler. A draining loop gastrojejunostomy is then fashioned. More complex repairs such as duodenal diverticularization (biliary and pancreatic diversion from the affected duodenum) have become less favored with the more frequent use of a pyloric exclusion approach. Complex type III duodenal injuries (>50% of the duodenal circumference or more than a simple perforation) will require selection of a more complex repair and this may be best accomplished at a second operation.

Decompression of a duodenal repair with an antegrade or a retrograde duodenostomy tube can reduce the rate of fistula formation. Most simple lacerations of the duodenum can be repaired primarily, and decompression and pyloric exclusion are often not necessary. There has been a recent trend in literature suggesting that pyloric exclusion is associated with greater morbidity. However, the patients who receive pyloric exclusion also have more associated pancreatic injuries and a higher rate of grade IV or V injuries. No prospective randomized trials are available to answer this question definitively.

The most important goal in selecting any repair or drainage procedure of the duodenum lies not only in

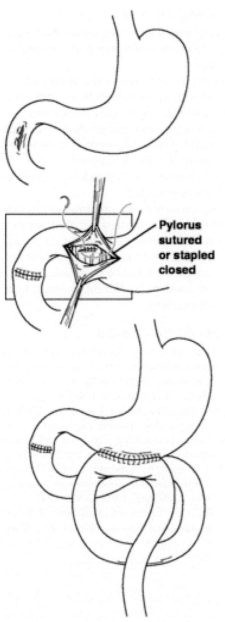

Pylorus
sutured
or stapled
closed

FIGURE 2 • The pyloric exclusion procedure: primary repair of the duodenal injury, protective closure of the pylorus, and gastrojejunostomy to reestablish enteric continuity.

understanding how it will work but often in how it will affect the patient if it fails. The second key aim is to be constantly aware of the overall state of the patient. If the patient is moving toward the lethal triad of hypothermia, acidosis, and coagulopathy, damage control will become the primary goal with reconstructions reserved for a later operation.

Special Intraoperative Considerations

Isolated injury to the duodenum is rare and injury to the duodenum is typically associated with injuries to other vital structures in the area. The surgeon may encounter severe hemorrhage from portal structures, the aorta, the IVC, the superior mesenteric or celiac vessels, or the renal vessels. Exsanguination from any of these is

the most rapid mode of death from this type of injury. During the Kocher and Cattell-Braasch maneuvers, the surgeon must be ready to obtain control of vascular structures in the area. Frank bleeding or a large hematoma should warrant the surgeon taking appropriate steps to gain proximal and distal vascular control prior to further exploration. The Pringle maneuver will provide control of portal and hepatic hemorrhage. The superior mesenteric and pancreaticoduodenal vessels may be controlled by manual occlusion of the supraceliac aorta and compression of the pancreaticoduodenal complex with tightly rolled laparotomy sponges after the Kocher and Cattell-Braasch maneuvers. Right renal hilum injuries may be exposed by mobilizing the kidney out of Gerota's fascia. Full aortic clamping may be necessary depending on the extent and location of the vascular injury. Walking the clamps to isolate just the area of injury once vascular control has been achieved will lessen the ischemic burden. IVC injuries may be repaired primarily, if properly visualized. In these scenarios, more definitive duodenal or pancreatic repair will often have to be delayed to a later time, and simple drainage with temporizing measures will suffice for initial control of the area. Resuscitation, stabilization, and avoidance of the lethal triad of hypothermia, acidosis, and coagulopathy are important.

Postoperative Management

Patients are typically admitted to the ICU after an initial trauma laparotomy and stabilization. Critical care goals include proper resuscitation and warming of the patient with reversal of any significant coagulopathy. Monitoring for ongoing hemorrhage is essential. Many patients will be admitted with an open abdomen secondary to perioperative resuscitation and massive visceral swelling. Management of the open abdomen requires care, diligence, and constant attention to avoid an enterocutaneous fistula. If the abdomen is open, the surgeon should plan for reexploration within the next 12 to 48 hours based on the patient's response to resuscitation. Tube feeding may begin within 24 to 48 hours of injury, provided the patient has stabilized and a repair of the injury has been performed.

Postoperative complications after a duodenal injury include duodenal narrowing, duodenal leak with attendant abscess formation, and occult injury to other surrounding viscera, most notably the pancreas or biliary tree. Useful diagnostic studies to evaluate for these complications may include upper GI contrast studies, CT scan, ERCP, MRCP, and HIDA scans. Long-term duodenal narrowing with functional obstruction will most likely require a definitive operative repair with duodenorrhaphy, Roux-en-Y duodenojejunal reconstruction, or gastrojejunostomy. Duodenal leaks are a common occurrence despite adequate vascularity and buttressing of the repair. Drainage of suture lines will allow for the formation of a stable fistula tract. Duodenal fistulas will often close spontaneously and a definitive repair or fistula closure operation should be delayed until patient has fully recovered from his acute injuries. Presence of distal feeding access in the form of a feeding jejunostomy or a nasojejunal tube is absolutely necessary and should be considered as part of the initial operation, if allowed by the patient status. Pancreatitis can lead to dehiscence of suture lines. Vascular repairs near the pancreas should utilize native tissue rather than prosthetic graft material whenever possible. Protecting the repair with tissue coverage from omentum is extremely wise. Pancreatic duct or biliary tract injuries may require stents, or drainage tube placement involving endoscopic or radiologic techniques in addition to operative interventions as necessary.

Case Conclusion

On operative exploration, the injured man was found to have a lateral laceration of the second portion of his duodenum without associated vascular injuries. The duodenal defect was repaired primarily in two layers. In performing the repair, the duodenum was closed in a transverse direction and the suture line covered by omentum. The site was also drained externally using a closed-suction drain. Despite these precautions, the patient did develop a duodenal leak, which was well controlled with the closed suction drain. Enteral nutrition was provided via a nasojejunal tube placed at the time of operation. By 6 weeks after his initial operation, his duodenal leak had resolved and he was tolerating oral intake.

TAKE HOME POINTS

- Duodenal injuries are frequently associated with injuries to other surrounding viscera and vascular structures.
- Proper exposure to assess the duodenal injury is essential and is achieved with a combination of the Kocher and Cattell-Braasch maneuvers.
- Definitive repair or damage control measures are performed based on the overall patient status and the extent of the duodenal injury.
- External drainage of all duodenal repairs suture lines is recommended.
- Feeding access must be obtained to provide the patient with the necessary nutrition for proper recovery. This feeding access should be capable of functioning even if the duodenal repair fails.
- A high suspicion must be maintained postoperatively for duodenal repair breakdown, leak, and abscess formation.

SUGGESTED READINGS

Carrillo EH, Richardson JD, Miller FB. Evolution in the management of duodenal injuries. J Trauma. 1996;40:1037–1045.

Ivatury RR, Nassoura ZE, Simon RJ, et al. Complex duodenal injuries. Surg Clin North Am. 1996;76:797–812.

Seamon MJ, Pieri PG, Fisher CA, et al. A ten-year retrospective review: does pyloric exclusion improve clinical outcome after penetrating duodenal and combined pancreaticoduodenal injuries? J Trauma. 2007;62:829–833.

Snyder WH, Weigelt JA, Watkins WL, et al. The surgical management of duodenal trauma: precepts based on a review of 247 cases. Arch Surg. 1980;115:422–429.

Velmahos GC, Constantinou C, Kasotakis G. Safety of repair for severe duodenal injuries. World J Surg. 2008;32:7–12.

Weigelt JA. Duodenal injuries. Surg Clin North Am. 1990;70:529–539.

110 Pelvic Fracture

AVI BHAVARAJU and OLIVER L. GUNTER

Presentation

A 45-year-old male was involved in a high-speed motor vehicle collision. He was a restrained driver and required prolonged extrication. During transport, he exhibited altered mental status and was unable to provide any history. On arrival to the emergency department, initial vital signs were pulse 150, blood pressure 60/palp, respiratory rate of 30, and unobtainable oxygen saturations.

He was intubated in the emergency department and resuscitated with crystalloid and blood products. Chest x-ray (CXR) was negative; pelvis x-ray (PXR) showed diastases of the pubic symphysis and the right sacroiliac joint, a left sacral fracture, and pubic rami fractures. Additional injuries included bilateral humerus fractures and a femur fracture (Figure 1).

Differential Diagnosis

This patient presents with shock from blunt trauma. The differential diagnosis in this setting includes the following:

1. Hemorrhage
   a. Thorax
   b. Abdomen
   c. Pelvis
   d. Retroperitoneum
   e. Extremity/long bone
   f. External
2. Tension pneumothorax
3. Cardiac tamponade
4. Spinal cord injury
5. Myocardial ischemia or arrhythmia

Workup

Immediate priorities include securing the **A**irway and assessing **B**reathing and **C**irculation (ABCs) in accordance with Advanced Trauma Life Support (ATLS) guidelines. History and physical examination, when available, may alert to the possibility of a pelvic fracture. If the patient is awake and alert, he may complain of pelvic, hip, or lower back pain exacerbated by position or lower-extremity movement. Abnormal rotation or shortening of a lower extremity and instability over the pelvic ring are physical findings indicative of a potential pelvis fracture. Blood at the urethral meatus may indicate bladder or urethral disruption, which occur with high frequency in association with pelvis fractures.

Important laboratory tests include type and screen, complete blood count, electrolytes, coagulation studies, and resuscitation markers (blood gas, lactate, and base deficit).

Screening radiographs in the emergency department are helpful to identify the source of shock. Lateral cervical spine, chest, and pelvis films can help direct resuscitation and treatment plans. Abdominal ultrasound can identify hemoperitoneum, particularly in the setting of blunt trauma. Computerized tomography (CT) is an invaluable diagnostic tool for evaluating multisystem trauma patients. The addition of intravenous contrast makes CT a rapid and sensitive imaging modality to evaluate sources of hemorrhage. Extravasation of contrast in proximity to pelvis fractures may indicate active bleeding that requires further management.

In the patient presented above, CT scan revealed an "open-book" pelvis fracture with 1.5 cm of pubic diastasis, bilateral sacral fractures, a right superior pubic ramus fracture, right sacroiliac diastasis, a left acetabular fracture, and bilateral inferior pubic rami fractures. Active contrast extravasation was seen in the anterior pelvis and around the bladder with a large associated pelvic hematoma (Figures 2 and 3).

Based on the CT findings and clinical picture suggesting class IV shock, he was resuscitated and taken to interventional radiology for emergent pelvic angiography. Findings included pseudoaneurysms with contrast extravasation from both internal pudendal arteries and the left sacral artery. There were no concurrent intra-abdominal injuries requiring operative intervention. Bilateral internal pudendal artery and left sacral artery coil embolization was completed; the patient was then sent to the ICU for continued resuscitation and stabilization (Figures 4 and 5).

Discussion

Once a pelvis fracture has been diagnosed on an anteroposterior pelvis radiograph, additional imaging may further characterize the fracture pattern and identify

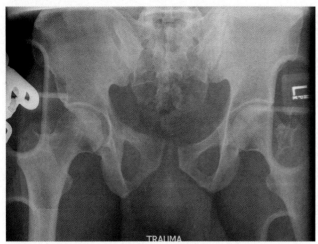

FIGURE 1 • AP pelvis film obtained in emergency department.

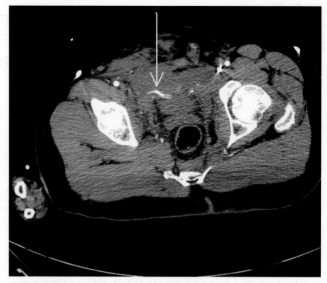

FIGURE 3 • Axial CT image showing contrast extravasation.

other associated injuries. Pelvic inlet and outlet views show fractures of the pelvic ring, while oblique projections better demonstrate acetabular injuries. CT imaging of the pelvis with reconstructed views is useful for operative planning and identifies more subtle fractures with high sensitivity.

Pelvis fractures may be classified into five categories based on mechanism and predominant force vectors:

1. Anterior–posterior compression (APC) injuries
2. Lateral compression (LC) injuries
3. Vertical shear injuries

4. Combined mechanical injuries
5. Acetabular fractures

Grading is from one to three in order of increasing severity of ligamentous and bony injuries. Those with significant ligamentous disruption and diastasis are often referred to as "open-book" fractures.

While lower-grade injuries may be managed nonoperatively with weight-bearing (WB) restriction, more severe injuries require surgical stabilization.

The patient in our scenario underwent bilateral percutaneous iliosacral screw fixation to repair his pelvic

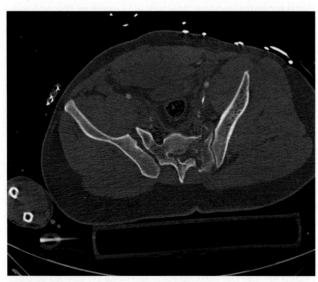

FIGURE 2 • Axial CT image showing the left sacral fracture and right SI diastasis.

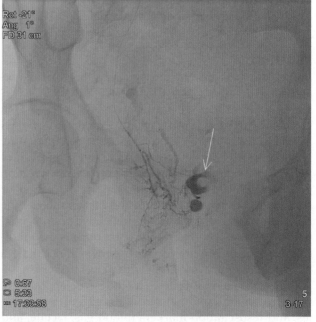

FIGURE 4 • IR image showing right internal iliac pseudoaneurysm.

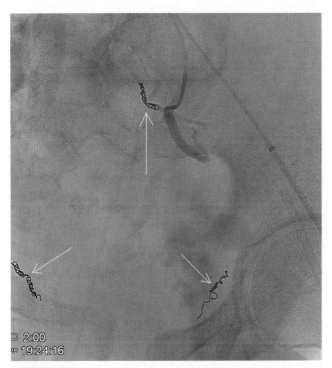

FIGURE 5 • Postembolization IR image.

ring injuries and open reduction and internal fixation of his extremity fractures **(Figure 6)**.

CT scan with IV contrast is a useful imaging modality for patients with multiple injuries. Contrast extravasation indicates active hemorrhage and demonstrates pelvic or retroperitoneal hematomas. Most pelvis fracture–related bleeding will tamponade and cease spontaneously; however, severe injuries may require arteriography and embolization to control hemorrhage.

Disruption of the pelvic ring increases the pelvic volume. In the setting of pelvis fracture–related bleeding, patients may benefit from closed reduction to reduce

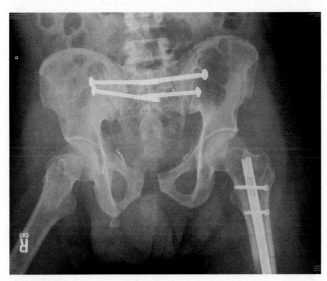

FIGURE 6 • Post-op AP pelvis.

the pelvic volume and tamponade ongoing hemorrhage. This is achieved with external fixation devices, commercially available pelvic binders, or with a sheet tightly wrapped around the pelvis.

Surgical Approach

The initial management of a patient with pelvic injuries should begin with a thorough assessment according to ATLS guidelines. The mechanism of injury and the physiologic state of the patient determine the subsequent course. For hemodynamically stable patients, the initial management is WB restriction and formal orthopedic evaluation.

Hemodynamically unstable patients must be evaluated and managed systematically. Patients in shock must have the source of hemorrhage identified and controlled in the midst of ongoing resuscitation. Adequacy of resuscitation should be monitored simultaneously. Life-threatening injuries should be addressed in order of severity as they are identified.

Although pelvic injuries can be associated with significant hemorrhage, associated injuries are common and must be evaluated. Screening radiographs can rule out intrathoracic or pelvic injuries. If a pelvis fracture is found, external reduction of the pelvic ring is a useful temporizing maneuver to minimize ongoing bleeding. Abdominal ultrasound can expeditiously identify patients that require immediate laparotomy. Evaluation and splinting of long bone injuries minimizes fracture-related bleeding. Lacerations with significant external hemorrhage can be controlled with external pressure or a tourniqet. If the patient can be stabilized, further imaging may be indicated. CT imaging of the brain, spine, and torso is an invaluable tool (particularly in the setting of polytrauma) with the addition of IV contrast to rule out solid organ injury and bleeding.

Signficant pelvic hemorrhage can be difficult or impossible to control, primarily because of anatomic inaccessibility of the injured vessels. Although external reduction combined with either intra- or extraperitoneal packing may be utilized, arteriography with embolization can selectively embolize individual vessels. This method is obviously preferable to nonselective operative ligation of one or both internal iliac arteries. An aortogram with bilateral iliac runoff, followed by selective angiography of both internal and external iliac systems is the initial approach taken. If contrast extravasation is seen, selective embolization with coils or foam should be performed. Strong consideration should be given to embolizing vessels that have evidence of vessel spasm or an abrupt cutoff since these usually represent signs of injury. This approach is successful in upward of 80% to 90% of patients. It is essential to continue the resuscitation throughout the hemorrhage control process until appropriate endpoints are met to prevent the lethal combination of hypothermia, coagulopathy, and acidosis. Recurrent instability may require reassessment and repeat angiography to assess for rebleeding. Inability to control pelvic hemorrhage by means of external reduction, pelvic packing, angioembolization, or operative ligation is associated with high mortality **(Tables 1 and 2)**.

Special Intraoperative Considerations

Patients with pelvis fractures undergoing laparotomy require special consideration, as the technique utilized may differ from the standard laparotomy for trauma. If an external compression device is present, exposure can be severely limited, and great care must be taken when deciding to remove this device as the patient may hemorrhage from re-expansion of the pelvic volume. If possible, the standard laparotomy incision should be limited to a supraumbilical incision, as extending below the semilunar line may disrupt anterior extension of a pelvic hemtoma, leading to further hemorrhage. Damage control techniques of rapid control of hemorrhage followed by temporizing measures with delayed reconstruction should be considered for patients who are severely physiologically compromised.

Intraoperative control of pelvic bleeding is technically challenging and often ineffective. Ligation of the hypogastric arteries is one technique to control pelvic arterial bleeding, but may be complicated by difficult exposure and distorted anatomy in the face of an extensive retroperitoneal hematoma. Venous pelvic

bleeding usually arises from cancellous bone or the sacral venous plexus, is diffuse in nature, and difficult or impossible to control with ligation. This type of pelvic bleeding is best controlled by tamponade. Management of pelvic bleeding during laparotomy is done by tightly packing the pelvis via an intraperitoneal approach in combination with temporary abdominal closure. Postoperatively, the patient may need to be managed with angiography and embolization if there is continued hemorrhage. Once stabilized, the patient can be returned to the operating room for reexploration. At this time, the pelvic packing can be removed, bowel continuity can be restored, and any additional injuries can be addressed. Definitive closure follows traditional principles of damage control laparotomy. At this point, stabilization of the pelvis fracture, either internal or external, may be considered in conjunction with orthopedics.

Open pelvic fractures deserve special consideration. An open pelvis fracture involves direct communication between a fracture fragment and the rectum, vagina, or skin of the perineum or groin. While open pelvis fractures only account for 5% of all pelvis fractures, the mortality of this injury has been estimated at 50% and can acutely result from uncontrolled bleeding from the fracture site because the wound is open to the enviornment and receives no internal tamponade. Initial management should focus on control of acute hemorrhage and wound management. Associated regional injuries are common and may include injuries to the bladder, urethra, vagina, and anorectum, which may increase the risk of infection and the complexity of subsequent reconstruction. Consideration should be given to fecal and urinary diversion to reduce the risk of pelvic sepsis and to facilitate operative repair of the fractures.

Postoperative Management

Postoperative management of pelvic fractures involves a multifaceted approach to patient care. They key elements to consider are WB status, prophylaxis of deep venous thrombosis (DVT), postoperative complications, and long-term follow-up. Postoperative WB status is highly variable, but most unstable pelvis fractures require several weeks of lower-extremity non–weight bearing.

The incidence of DVT in patients with pelvic trauma is reported as high as 60%. Routine DVT prophylaxis is recommended. DVT prophylaxis may be mechanical (ambulation, sequential compression devices) or chemical (e.g., low molecular weight heparin, coumadin).

The most frequent complication after severe pelvis fracture is sciatic or lumbosacral nerve injury (10% to 15% incidence). Nonunions and malunions also occur. Pain and pelvic or limb deformity are the most common complaints from patients. Females may have higher rates of urinary symptoms, cephalopelvic disproportion, and gynecologic pain.

TAKE HOME POINTS

- Classification of pelvis fractures
  - LC—grade I, II, III
  - APC—grade I, II, III
  - Vertical shear
  - Combined mechanism
- Imaging modalities
  - X-rays—AP, inlet, outlet, oblique/judet
  - CT abdomen/pelvis
    - IV contrast enhanced to evaluate for intra-abdominal injuries
    - Noncontrast with thin cuts and reconstructed views
- Initial workup should follow ATLS guidelines.
- High rate of concurrent truncal injuries requires full trauma workup and evaluation.
- Indications for angioembolization
  - Contrast extravasation on CT
  - Uncontrolled pelvic hemorrhage identified intraoperatively
  - Recurrent pelvic hemorrhage
- Orthopedic management pearls
  - Temporary pelvic stabilization for hemodynamically unstable patients
    - Bed sheet
    - Pelvic binder
    - External fixator
  - Definitive repair by an orthopedic surgeon
  - Early initiation of DVT prophylaxis
  - Limitation of weight bearing as necessary

SUGGESTED READINGS

Burgess AR, Eastridge BJ, Young JW. Pelvic ring disruptions: effective classification system and treatment protocols. J Trauma. 1990;30(7):848–856.

Dalal SA, Burgess AR, Siegel JH, et al. Pelvic fracture in multiple trauma: classification by mechanism is key to pattern of organ injury, resuscitative requirements, and outcome. J Trauma. 1989;29(7):981–1000.

Davis JW, et al. Western trauma association critical decisions in trauma: management of pelvic fracture with hemodynamic instability. J Trauma. 2008;65:1012–1015.

Geerts WH, Code KJ, Jay RM, et al. A prospective study of venous thromboembolism after major trauma. N Engl J Med. 1994;331:1601–1606.

Guillamondegui OD, et al. Pelvis fractures. In: Cameron J, ed. Current Surgical Therapy. 8th ed. Philadelphia, PA: Mosby Elsevier Science, 2004.

111 Airway Emergency

DEREK T. WOODRUM and DAVID W. HEALY

Presentation

A 65-year-old woman is brought to the emergency department as a level I trauma after being thrown from a horse. At the scene, emergency responders placed the patient in a cervical collar and administered high-flow oxygen via face mask. In the emergency department, her pulse-oximetry saturation is 92% and she has partially obstructed (snoring, noisy) breathing. Due to hypotension and a focused abdominal sonogram positive for free fluid, she is taken directly to the operating room for an exploratory laparotomy. Intravenous and arterial access are already in place.

After rapid sequence induction of anesthesia in the operating room, direct laryngoscopy is performed with in-line cervical stabilization and cricoid pressure after removing the anterior portion of the cervical spine collar. The laryngoscopist is unable to visualize the vocal cords or pass an endotracheal tube into the trachea. The saturations begin to fall into the 80s.

Discussion

An airway emergency is one of the most critical, time-sensitive situations encountered by surgeons and anesthesiologists. This case occurred in the operating room in a "controlled" setting, but a surgeon will very likely be involved in many cases involving airway management during their careers. Smaller hospitals may not have in-hospital 24-hour anesthesia services, and emergency airway management may fall to the surgical team. Even when a full complement of help is available, the surgical team may be the first responder to an airway emergency on rounds, in the trauma bay, or in offsite locations like radiology or in burn debridement rooms. Finally, the surgical team will occasionally be called upon for a surgical airway in the operating room, in settings of trauma or impossible ventilation/impossible intubation.

The purpose of this chapter is to highlight salient points when approaching an airway emergency. It is crucial that the physician has a previously thought-out and well-understood approach to airway management. We discuss preinduction airway evaluation, rapid sequence induction for standard intubation, and what to do when intubation is unsuccessful. Surgical airway management is also reviewed.

Differential Diagnosis

This patient's hypoxia is likely caused by several factors including hypoventilation from partial airway obstruction, depressed mental status, and opioid administration. Other factors need consideration, including pulmonary contusion, aspiration, pneumothorax or hemothorax associated with rib fractures, depressed cardiac output from cardiac contusion, tamponade, or aortic dissection.

Workup

In an airway emergency, there is very little time for additional workup. A preexisting chest radiograph can diagnose pneumothorax, hemothorax, or widened mediastinum—but the main focus should be on the airway exam. The goal in an urgent situation is to maintain oxygenation while simultaneously identifying predictors of difficult ventilation and intubation. This risk stratification will help guide immediate and subsequent airway management. If a patient is hypoxemic with little or no ventilatory effort, the airway should be supported by chin lift with or without an oral pharyngeal airway while oxygen is applied.

The airway exam is performed to specifically aid in the prediction of three situations: difficult mask ventilation, difficult intubation, and difficult surgical airway. **Table 1** lists risk factors for difficulty with each of these three procedures. The ability to mask ventilate is supremely important in maintaining gas exchange and in saving a patient's life. It may be continued for some time if intubation is unsuccessful. **Figure 1** illustrates the Mallampati scoring system, which is a description of how much of the oropharynx can be visualized. A Class III (no visualization of the uvula but the soft palate can be seen) or Class IV (even the soft palate cannot be visualized) Mallampati score alerts to the likelihood of *both* difficult mask ventilation and intubation with direct laryngoscopy. Alternative airway devices and airway expert consultation should be obtained immediately.

TABLE 1. Risk Factors for Difficult Mask Ventilation, Difficult Intubation, and Difficult Cricothyroidotomy

Difficult Mask Ventilation	Difficult Intubation	Difficult Cricothyrotomy
Mallampati 3 or 4	Mallampati 3 or 4	Surgery to neck
Obesity	Limited extension	Hematoma or infection
Sleep apnea	Cervical collar	Obese and access (e.g. flexion scoliosis)
Presence of beard	Hospital bed	Radiation
Prior neck radiation	Limited mandibular protrusion	Tumors (including thyroid goiter)

The recommended brief airway exam in the emergency setting includes assessment of mouth opening, Mallampati class, and mandibular protrusion (ability to extend the lower teeth anterior to the upper teeth). Presence or absence of teeth is noted, and neck mobility—particularly extension—is assessed if the patient has a cleared cervical spine.

Rapid Sequence Induction

After the airway exam is completed and urgent calls for assistance are made, preoxygenation is performed prior to induction of anesthesia. This is best carried out utilizing a nonrebreathing mask with collapsible air reservoir. In a patient breathing spontaneously, an Ambu bag is not ideal for preoxygenation as it is difficult to draw oxygen from the self-expanding bag. If the airway is partially obstructed but respiratory effort is present, a jaw thrust/chin lift maneuver should be performed. After preoxygenation and application of cricoid pressure, general anesthesia should be induced to optimize intubating conditions. **Table 2** lists the common emergency induction agents and muscle relaxants. The comparative advantages and disadvantages are outside the scope of this chapter, but etomidate is used frequently for its property of hemodynamic stability on

induction. The use of succinylcholine or rocuronium in the doses listed will provide optimal intubating conditions within 60 seconds. Contraindications to succinylcholine are listed below. Due to these contraindications, rocuronium is frequently used in rapid sequence induction of anesthesia. It will provide approximately 30 to 45 minutes of muscle relaxation. However, the patient will not return to spontaneous ventilation in that time; waking the patient up if intubation is not successful will not be an option.

Succinylcholine is a widely used and relatively safe muscle relaxant, but the potential complications should be known. Any provider administering it *must* be familiar with the absolute contraindications and avoid its use in patients with burns, hyperkalemia, upper motor neuron lesions, neuromuscular disorders, and those with a personal or family history of malignant hyperthermia.

Unable to Ventilate

In the case scenario of this chapter, intubation was not successful after rapid sequence induction and direct laryngoscopy. In this situation, a well thought-out backup plan must be readily instituted. **Figure 2** illustrates a flow diagram of how to manage an unsuccessful

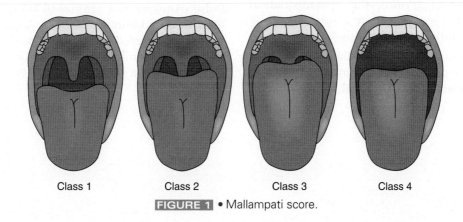

Class 1   Class 2   Class 3   Class 4

FIGURE 1 • Mallampati score.

TABLE 2. Common Emergency Induction Agents and Muscle Relaxants

Induction Agent	Dose
Etomidate	0.2-0.3mg/kg IV
Sodium thiopental	3-5mg/kg IV
Propofol	2-3mg/kg IV
Ketamine	1-2mg/kg IV
Muscle Relaxant	**Dose**
Succinylcholine	1-1.5mg/kg IV
Rocuronium	0.6-1.2mg/kg IV

intubation. It is a modification of the American Society of Anesthesiologist's Difficult Airway Algorithm, focusing on the goals of maintaining gas exchange and oxygen saturation as the airway is managed. Key points are noted in the text following the flow chart.

1. If the initial intubation attempt is unsuccessful, the pulse-ox reading should be noted while optimizing intubation conditions for subsequent attempts. If the saturation is already dropping below 90%, *further intubation attempts should not be attempted.*

2. Oxygenation and ventilation with bag mask should be attempted immediately, while calling for a surgical airway kit and preparing for surgical airway. A surgical airway is not the next step, but parallel preparations should be made.

3. If the bag-mask ventilation is successful, the patient is "re"preoxygenated before subsequent attempts at intubation utilizing alternate airway techniques by an airway expert familiar with alternate devices.

4. If bag-mask ventilation is unsuccessful, a laryngeal mask airway (LMA) should be placed. If LMA placement is successful and ventilation through the LMA is adequate, an airway expert may then consider trans-LMA intubating techniques.

5. If LMA placement is unsuccessful, or inadequate at providing effective oxygenation, a surgical airway should be promptly established (see below).

Of critical importance is the immediate call for help from experienced providers if the initial attempt at intubation is unsuccessful. The goal is oxygenation and gas exchange, and this should be accomplished with bag-mask ventilation if intubation is not successful. We recommend against the use of advanced alternative airway devices (video laryngoscope, intubating supraglottic airways, fiberoptic intubations, etc.) by inexperienced providers. Just as an anesthesiologist is unlikely to safely perform an appendectomy (even after observing the procedure hundreds of times), it is unlikely that a surgical team member will be successful in using advanced, alternative airway devices in a critical situation. The strong focus should remain on oxygen delivery and airway patency—this is the reason for LMA placement if intubation and bag-mask ventilation are unsuccessful.

Surgical Approach

If intubation is unsuccessful and mask ventilation is inadequate to permit additional attempts by alternate airway methods, a surgical airway should be performed without delay. Two methods are commonly employed: kit-based wire-guided cricothyroidotomy **(Figure 3 and Table 3)** and open cricothyroidotomy **(Table 4)**. Wire-guided technique utilizing a Melker cricothyrotomy kit is very common and is widely available. Benefits to the kit-based technique include wide availability, provider familiarity, and rapid placement. The open approach may take longer to perform and involves more dissection time .

Postoperative Management

After establishing a definitive airway—that is, a cuffed tube in the trachea—placement is confirmed by listening for bilateral breath sounds and checking for return of end-tidal CO_2. The latter is accomplished either by observing color change on an in-line device, or by return of CO_2 to a gas analyzer on an anesthesia machine. However, blood must be flowing to the lungs in order for CO_2 delivery. In the setting of very low cardiac output (exsanguination, massive MI, or PE) or in cardiac arrest without CPR, CO_2 will not be detected even if the airway is correctly positioned. Pulse oximetry and arterial blood gas sampling are used in an adjunctive manner. A chest x-ray (CXR) should be ordered to confirm position and to check for adequate inflation of all lung lobes (an emergency operation should not be delayed for a CXR, of course).

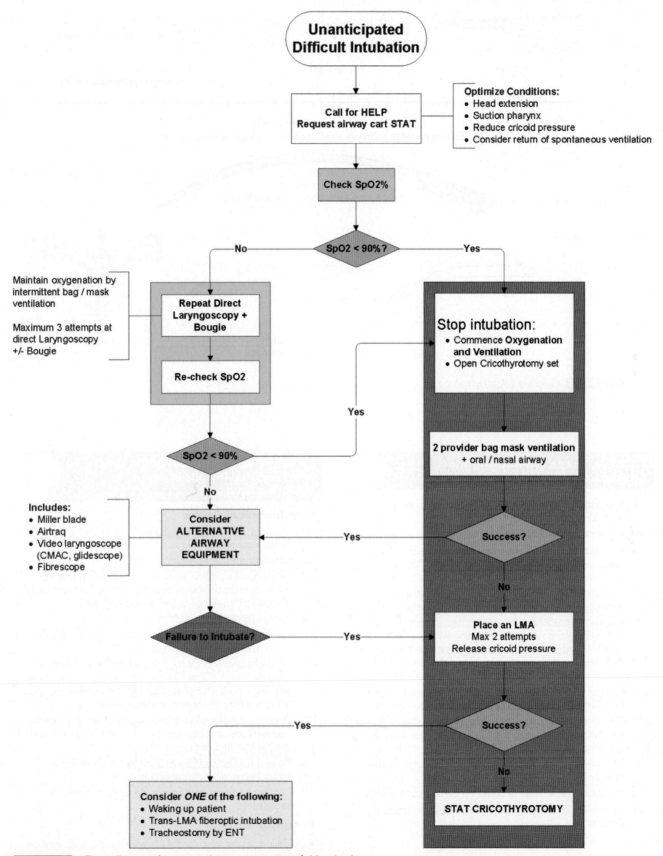

FIGURE 2 • Flow diagram for managing an unsuccessful intubation.

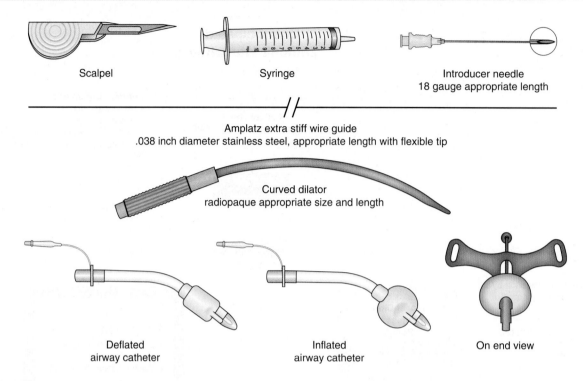

FIGURE 3 • Melker cricothyrotomy kit.

TABLE 3. Steps When Using the Melker Cricothyrotomy Kit

1. Shoulder roll to optimize position (do not extend neck in cervical spine injury)
2. Rapid disinfectant skin prep
3. Palpation of cricothyroid membrane (start in sternal notch, palpate upward along the trachea. The first cartilaginous prominence is the cricoid cartilage).
4. Vertical midline incision. This is not a percutaneous technique—it is a wire-assisted *open* procedure.
5. Needle is introduced through pretracheal tissues through the cricothyroid membrane where air will readily withdraw into the syringe. A syringe half-filled with saline will return bubbles when the needle tip is intratracheal.
6. The guidewire is advanced into the trachea (as in modified Seldinger technique for central venous access).
7. The curved dilator is loaded through the deflated airway catheter, and this combined unit is advanced over the wire into the trachea.
8. The wire and the dilator are removed from the airway catheter.
9. The balloon is inflated and bag ventilation commences.
10. Placement and position are verified as in orotracheal intubation.

TABLE 4. Key Technical Steps and Potential Pitfalls in Open Cricothyroidotomy

Key Technical Steps

1. Shoulder roll to optimize position (do not extend neck in cervical spine injury).
2. Rapid disinfectant prep.
3. Palpation of cricothyroid membrane (start in sternal notch, palpate upward along the trachea. The first cartilaginous prominence is the cricoid cartilage).
4. Vertical midline incision.
5. Spread tissues rapidly, down to the cricothyroid membrane. Exposure may be difficult.
6. Horizontal incision through the cricothyroid membrane and placement of tracheal dilator if available. If not available, use the back handle of a *separate* scalpel handle without a blade to hold open the membrane.
7. Place a cuffed tracheostomy tube (or a standard endotracheal tube) through the cricothyroid membrane and remove the obturator.
8. Place the inner cannula to allow connection to the Ambu bag or anesthesia circuit.
9. Confirm end-tidal carbon dioxide (cardiac output is necessary).

Potential Pitfalls

- Trauma to lateral vascular structures or wrong level incision if a transverse incision is used. These are two reasons for vertical midline incision in the emergency setting.
- False passage of tracheostomy tube.

TAKE HOME POINTS

- Immediate consultation with an airway management expert gives the greatest chance for successful outcome in emergency airway management.
- Rapid sequence induction followed by direct laryngoscopy (accompanied by in-line cervical stabilization if cervical spine stability is uncertain) is the current standard of care.
- An understanding of the failed airway algorithm (memorized!) is crucial for logical, safe, and sequential handling of the emergency airway.
- Alternative airway devices beyond a standard LMA require previous experience for successful placement. Their use is not recommended in an emergency without prior familiarity.

SUGGESTED READINGS

Hung O, Murphy M. Context sensitive airway management. Anesth Analg. 2010;110(4):982–983.

Kheterpal S, et al. Incidence and predictors of difficult and impossible mask ventilation. Anesthesiology. 2006;105(5):885–891.

Melker JS, Gabrielli A. Melker cricothyrotomy kit: an alternative to the surgical technique. Ann Otol Rhinol Laryngol. 2005;114(7):525–528.

Melker kit video. http://www.cookmedical.com/cc/resources.do?id=4813. Accessed 10/1/2010.

112 Acute Renal Failure

APRIL E. MENDOZA and ANTHONY G. CHARLES

Presentation

A 63-year-old man presents to the emergency room complaining of an acute-onset abdominal pain. He described the pain as initially located in the left lower quadrant but now generalized. He has now developed some nausea and vomiting. His last bowel movement was a day prior to presentation. He admits to fever and chills and has been diaphoretic. He denies prior episodes of similar abdominal pain.

His past medical history is significant for non–insulin-dependent diabetes mellitus for over 10 years controlled with an oral hypoglycemic and essential hypertension managed with an angiotensin-converting-enzyme (ACE) inhibitor. His past surgical history is significant for an appendectomy 45 years ago. He has never undergone a screening colonoscopy. He has no known allergies.

His vitals revealed a temperature of 100°F, pulse rate of 120 per minute, respiratory rate of 32, and a blood pressure of 90/53. Physical exam showed an obese man, in acute painful distress. He has no jugular venous distension and his chest exam was unremarkable. Abdominal examination revealed generalized abdominal tenderness with rebound and guarding. The remainder of the exam revealed warm extremities with brisk capillary refill and no evidence of edema. Abdominal radiographic series revealed free air under the diaphragm.

He is diagnosed with a perforated viscous. Exploratory laparotomy confirms perforated sigmoid diverticulitis with extensive abdominal soilage. He undergoes a sigmoid colectomy and Hartman's procedure. The following morning, he remains mechanically ventilated. His vitals have remained stable; however, he has become oliguric with a urine output of only 20 mL per hour.

Differential Diagnosis

Acute kidney injury (AKI) describes the full spectrum of renal dysfunction that is characterized by the RIFLE criteria. It is based on the extent of injury utilizing the serum creatinine, glomerular filtration rate (GFR), and urine output. The RIFLE criteria consist of five categories of renal dysfunction: Risk, Injury, Failure, Loss, and End-stage renal disease.

The RIFLE Criteria

- Risk—1.5-fold increase in the serum creatinine or GFR decrease by 25% or urine output <0.5 mL/kg/h for 6 hours
- Injury—twofold increase in the serum creatinine or GFR decrease by 50% or urine output <0.5 mL/kg/h for 12 hours
- Failure—threefold increase in the serum creatinine or GFR decrease by 75% or urine output of <0.5 mL/kg/h for 24 hours, or anuria for 12 hours
- Loss—complete loss of kidney function (need for renal replacement therapy [RRT]) for more than 4 weeks
- ESRD—complete loss of kidney function (e.g., need for RRT) for more than 3 months

Postoperative oliguria indicates AKI. Oliguria is defined as urine output <0.5 mL/kg/h in adults or <1.0 mL/kg/h in children weighing <10 kg. Early identification of the etiology can prevent further progression of renal injury. Always consider the possibility of preexisting renal disease in surgical patients, as this carries a higher risk of developing postoperative acute renal failure.

Etiology of AKI is organized into three groups: prerenal, renal, and postrenal. With respect to the patient presented above, we discuss the range of possible causes of his new oliguria.

Prerenal

Hypoperfusion of the kidneys from shock states is the hallmark of prerenal kidney dysfunction. All causes of renal hypoperfusion should be entertained. Hypovolemia and volume depletion should be high on the differential as a cause of this patient's oliguria owing to third spacing from peritonitis and his emergent abdominal surgery.

Redistributive shock, such as cardiogenic or septic shock, particularly in patients with a longstanding history of diabetes and hypertension may result in poor

TABLE 1. Renal Etiologies of Acute Kidney Injury

Acute interstitial nephritis	Drugs (antibiotics), NSAIDS
Papillary necrosis	Analgesics, infection, diabetes mellitus
Acute cortical necrosis	Profound shock
Glomerulonephritis	Immunologic
Vasculitides	Hypersensitivity reactions, diffuse intravascular coagulation, malignant hypertension
Intrarenal shunting	Hepatorenal syndrome

renal perfusion. Abdominal compartment syndrome with evidence of increased bladder pressures, hypotension, and increased peak inspiratory pressures on the ventilator must also be considered. Persistent hypoperfusion of the kidney may lead to acute tubular necrosis (ATN).

Renal

Renal causes of acute renal dysfunction describe diseases of the renal parenchyma usually ATN. The etiology of ATN is numerous, but potential causes in the surgical patient include ischemia and nephrotoxins such as myoglobin, hemoglobin, contrast media, antibiotics (aminoglycosides, cephalosporins, sulfonamides, vancomycin), and anesthetic agents (methoxyflurane, enflurane). Other causes are listed in **Table 1** and should be considered if the etiopathogenesis of the renal failure remains obscure.

Postrenal

Postrenal causes of renal dysfunction can usually be quickly identified by physical examination. Removing or replacing the urinary catheter can usually diagnose an enlarged prostate or a clogged catheter. Physical

Presentation Continued

The patient is extubated the following morning and is awake, but confused. Physical examination reveals normal heart and chest sounds. His abdomen is mildly distended and generalized edema is present. He denies pain except for tenderness at the incision site on palpation. His central venous pressure (CVP) ranges from 4 to 6 cm H2O. His current blood pressure recordings have been between 100 to 110 mm Hg systolic and 50 to 80 mm Hg diastolic. Review of the chart shows a preoperative creatinine of 1.5 mg/dL with a postoperative creatinine now at 3.2 mg/dL.

examination can identify a full bladder, or a bladder scan can be used in the case of obese patients. Direct ureteral injury has an incidence of 1% to 2% during abdominal surgery. Injury ranges from ligation, transection, devascularization, and partial laceration of the ureter. Though rare, usually bilateral ureteral injury will present with significant acute renal dysfunction.

Workup

The initial diagnostic evaluation for acute renal dysfunction should start with a review of the patient's history and a physical examination. Adjunctive invasive monitoring, urinary catheterization, trends in urine and serum chemistry (sodium, potassium, urea, and creatinine), urine microscopy, and ancillary tests such as bladder and renal ultrasonography have an additional role in identifying and categorizing the cause of renal dysfunction and subsequent renal failure.

Examination

Assessing the neurologic function, perfusion status, and signs of volume overload gives the clinician a better idea of the cause, severity, and progression of renal dysfunction. This patient has some signs of volume overload as evidenced by peripheral edema, which could be caused from cardiac or renal failure. Indeed, cardiac failure could be the cause of the renal failure. His abdomen is mildly distended, but not tense to suggest abdominal compartment syndrome. Neither rectal nor stomal exam reveals melena, frank blood, or evidence of prostate enlargement.

The bladder is not palpable. His catheter was flushed to ensure no obvious obstruction in the tubing **(Table 2)**.

Laboratory and Ancillary Testing

In all surgical patients, it is imperative to initially consider prerenal causes of renal failure. If the patient's CVP is low, with associated hypotension and tachycardia, a fluid challenge test may be a useful to determine the cause, particularly if the patient responds by increasing urine output. With new-onset oliguria, the clinician should also be prompted to obtain urine electrolytes, as well as a urinary analysis (UA) **(Table 3)**.

The addition of urine electrolytes especially urinary sodium and creatinine is imperative. If renal failure exists, this test can demonstrate whether the origin is prerenal or renal; the two most common causes in the acute setting. These values allow the clinician to calculate fractional excretion of sodium (FeNA).

In many situations, calculating the fractional excretion of urea or FeUrea may be more appropriate and accurate. It is well described that the use of diuretics,

TABLE 2. Physical Exam and Possible Indications of AKI

Physical Exam	Possible Indications
Vitals signs	
Temperature	Possible infection
Blood pressure	Hypertension: nephrotic syndrome, malignant hypertension
	Hypotension: hypovolemia, redistributive shock
Heart rate	Tachycardia: shock, arrythmias
	Bradycardia: inadequate renal perfusion
Weight loss/gain	Fluid overload or hypovolemia
Mouth	dehydration
Neck	Distended jugular veins: fluid overload possible cardiac origin Collapsed jugular veins: hypovolemia
Chest	Pulmonary crackes/rales: fluid overload New murmurs/rubs: heart failure, endocarditis, pericarditis
Abdomen	Bladder fullness, masses: genitourinary obstruction
Rectum	Enlarged prostate
Skin	Rash: interstitial nephritis; Findings of atheroembolic events

such as furosemide and bumetanide, can falsely elevate the excretion of sodium. Liver cirrhosis and other medical problems also affect the excretion of sodium. Urea and nitrogen byproducts remain relatively constant and should be considered in these circumstances **(Table 4)**.

Cardiac dysfunction remains a potential cause of oliguria. In this patient, an EKG, cardiac enzymes, echocardiography, chest radiograph, and serum chemistry panel should also be considered. Invasive monitoring can complement exam findings and give a better idea of volume status. These tests may correlate physical exam findings.

Renal ultrasonography can be useful if the initial workup cannot help guide the diagnosis. This is a quick, noninvasive method to evaluate obstructive causes of renal failure and can also identify signs chronic disease.

TABLE 3. Common Urinary Analysis Findings and Possible Indications

Muddy brown/granular casts	ATN
Epithelial cell casts	ATN
Red cell casts	Vasculitis, glomerulonephritis
Proteinuria	Glomerular disease
Uniform, round RBC[a]	Extrarenal bleeding
Dysmorphic RBC	Glomerular disease

[a]RBC: red blood cell

TABLE 4. Key lab findings of Pre-renal and Renal causes of AKI

Laboratory Test	Pre-renal Findings	Renal Findings
BUN to creatinine ratio	>20:l	10–20:1
Urine specific gravity	>1.020	1.010–1.020
Urine sediment	Hyaline casts	Granular/epithelial casts
Urine sodium	>20 mEq/L	
FeNa percent	<1%	>2%
FeUrea percent	<35%	>35%

FeNa = Una × Pcr/Pna × Ucr multiply by 100
FeUrea = Uurea × Pcr/Purea × Ucr multiply 100

Invasive Tests

Invasive tests that contribute to management of renal failure include central venous and arterial monitoring, and/or pulse contour continuous cardiac output (PiCCO). Renal biopsy should rarely be warranted in the acute setting. It is reserved for when all tests and workup have remained unrevealing and the condition continues without improvement. It is also useful for the evaluation of acute glomerulonephritis/vasculitis or isolated hematuria with proteinuria.

Presentation Continued

His urine output has continually decreased now with a total of 50 cc of urine in 24 hours, although he has received several liters of fluid. He is 15 L positive and now has crackles bilaterally on chest exam with increasing extremity edema. His CVP is elevated at 15. Cardiac enzymes and BNP (brain natriuretic peptide) are within normal limits, and he has had no EKG changes consistent with evolving heart disease. His creatinine has climbed to 6 mg/dL from his baseline of 1.5 mg/dL. His BUN (blood urea nitrogen) is approaching 70 mg/dL, and his ABG (arterial blood gas) reveals a pH of 7.25. A UA shows epithelial cell casts. RRT is now considered the next best step in his management.

Diagnosis and Treatment

The patient is diagnosed with acute renal failure secondary to ATN. Underresuscitation in the face of sepsis, emergent surgery and third spacing likely resulted in renal dysfunction and ischemic injury that

TABLE 5. Indications for Renal Replacement Therapy

Acidosis refractory to medical therapy
Acute, severe electrolyte changes (commonly hyperkalemia)
Intoxications (methanol, ethanol)
Volume overload
Uremia-any of the below symptoms or findings
    Encephalopathy
    Severe azotemia (BUN: >100 mg/dL)
    Significant bleeding
    Uremic pericarditis

further evolved into ATN. Underlying renal insufficiency made him especially susceptible to this injury.

Early identification and supportive measures are the only treatment options. It is important to reduce further injury and stop any potentially nephrotoxins. Once supportive measures prove futile and renal dysfunction continues, RRT should be initiated.

Indications for RRT are seen in **Table 5**.

Clinical Approach to Acute Renal Dysfunction

Adequate perioperative resuscitation is crucial for preventing renal dysfunction. Invasive monitoring may prove a helpful adjunct in surgical patients with AKI. It is well known that the mortality is increased in this subset of critically ill patients.

Key clinical components.

1. Ensure proper perioperative resuscitation, minimize exposure to nephrotoxins, monitor fluid balance.
2. Examine the patient.
3. Employ the trends in serum and urine chemistry to help confirm the diagnosis and guide therapeutic endpoints.
4. Consider adjunctive monitoring such as echocardiogram prior to invasive monitoring.
5. Consider the need for RRT if patient meets criteria.

Figure 1 describes the initial workup and management of patients with clinical findings consistent with AKI.

Pitfalls in management include

1. Failure to examine the patient and review preexisting comorbidities
2. Indiscriminate use of diuretics in the face of hypotension and underresuscitation
3. Prolonged use of diuretics when patient meets criteria for dialysis
4. Ignoring respiratory status in acute renal failure
5. Misinterpreting information gathered from invasive monitoring

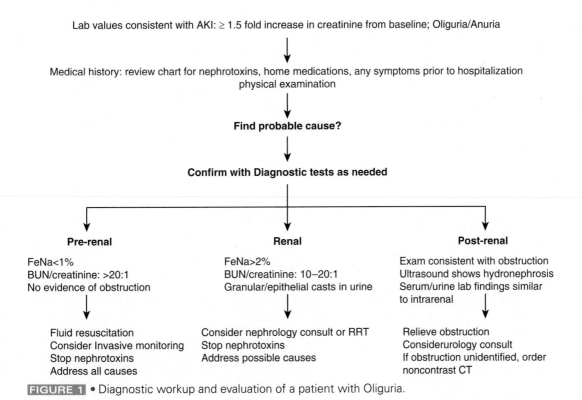

Lab values consistent with AKI: ≥ 1.5 fold increase in creatinine from baseline; Oliguria/Anuria

↓

Medical history: review chart for nephrotoxins, home medications, any symptoms prior to hospitalization physical examination

↓

Find probable cause?

↓

Confirm with Diagnostic tests as needed

Pre-renal

FeNa<1%
BUN/creatinine: >20:1
No evidence of obstruction

↓

Fluid resuscitation
Consider Invasive monitoring
Stop nephrotoxins
Address all causes

Renal

FeNa>2%
BUN/creatinine: 10–20:1
Granular/epithelial casts in urine

↓

Consider nephrology consult or RRT
Stop nephrotoxins
Address possible causes

Post-renal

Exam consistent with obstruction
Ultrasound shows hydronephrosis
Serum/urine lab findings similar to intrarenal

↓

Relieve obstruction
Considerurology consult
If obstruction unidentified, order noncontrast CT

FIGURE 1 • Diagnostic workup and evaluation of a patient with Oliguria.

Case Conclusion

The patient was started on RRT. His preexisting comorbidities made him susceptible to acute renal dysfunction and ultimately renal loss when his clinical course was complicated by hypotension and sepsis. The patient required dialysis for 6 weeks and eventually regained renal function. His favorable outcome is likely a result of proper resuscitation and the appropriate use of RRT.

TAKE HOME POINTS

- Use baseline chemistries to assess renal function.
- Ensure adequate perioperative resuscitation.
- Surgical patients must be assumed to have a prerenal cause until proven otherwise.
- All types of redistributive shock are also prerenal causes of AKI and failure.
- Be cognizant of comorbidities.
- Avoid nephrotoxic medications-aminoglycosides, IV contrast, etc.

- Diuretics may be utilized only after correction of shock.
- Use of diuretics does not alter the course of renal failure.
- Consider RRT when patient meets criteria.
- Renal failure is associated with increased mortality in surgical patients.

SUGGESTED READINGS

Bellomo R, Ronco C, Kellum JA, et al. Acute renal failure-definition, outcome measures, animal models, fluid therapy and information technology needs: the Second International Consensus Conference of the Acute Dialysis Quality Initiative (ADQI) Group. Crit Care. 2004;8:204–212.

Diskin CJ, Stokes TJ, Dansby LM, et al. The comparative benefits of the fractional excretion of urea and sodium in various azotemic oliguric states. Nephron Clin Pract. 2010;114:145–150.

Madaio MP. Renal biopsy. Kidney Int. 1990;38:529.

Mullin RJ. Acute renal failure. In: Cameron JL, ed. Current Surgical Therapy. Philadelphia, PA: Mosby, 2008;1200–1206.

Stafford RE, Cairns BA, Meyer AA. Renal failure. In: Souba WW, Fink MP, Jurkouch GS, et al., eds. ACS Surgery: Principles and Practice. New York, NY: WebMD professional publishing, 2006;1408–1412.

113 Adrenal Insufficiency

STEVEN R. ALLEN and HEIDI L. FRANKEL

Presentation

A 67-year-old female was involved in a motor vehicle crash 7 days ago. Her injuries included a closed head injury consisting of a subarachnoid hemorrhage and bilateral tibia/fibula fractures. She was able to be extubated at postinjury day 3; however, she required reintubation 24 hours previously (using rapid sequence methodology employing etomidate and succinylcholine) for increasing respiratory difficulty. Over the past 24 hours, she has become hemodynamically unstable with progressive tachycardia and hypotension despite adequate fluid.

Differential Diagnosis

A broad differential diagnosis is pertinent to identify and treat all potential etiologies leading to her hemodynamic instability. Due to the patient's intubation and underlying pulmonary disease, ventilator-associated pneumonia leading to sepsis and septic shock must be highly considered. Other pulmonary causes, such as a pulmonary embolism (PE), may also contribute to this clinical picture. Additionally, with her age and multiple comorbidities, one must consider an acute cardiac event, such as a myocardial infarction (MI). Her orthopedic injuries also predispose her to fat emboli. Adrenal insufficiency (AI) must be considered as she was intubated with etomidate, which has been found to cause AI, although less likely after a bolus dose.

age. Neurologically, she is arousable but does not consistently follow commands. Her cardiac exam demonstrates a regular rhythm but tachycardic.

On further workup, blood cultures were consistently negative. Her white blood count was within normal limits of 11,000 and hemoglobin was stable at 9.7. The electrolyte panel demonstrated a sodium of 131 and potassium of 5.3. The CT scan of the chest was negative for a PE and her echocardiogram demonstrated an ejection fraction of 65% with no obvious wall motion abnormalities and cardiac enzymes were not elevated.

Presentation Continued

Her past medical history is significant for chronic obstructive pulmonary disease, rheumatoid arthritis for which she takes 15 mg of prednisone daily, hypertension, and diabetes. Her vital signs demonstrate a temperature of 38.6°C, a heart rate of 130, and blood pressure of 85/40. Her blood pressure was responsive but dependent on continuous Levophed administration. Her respiratory rate is 25 on the ventilator with a FiO$_2$ of 0.6, PEEP of 7.5, and pressure support of 10 to 12. Her current oxygen saturation is 92%. She has received three 1-L boluses of crystalloid to affect her hemodynamic status with no improvement. Her current central venous pressure is 10 and her urine output is only 10 mL per hour. On physical exam, she is an obese woman who appears her stated

Diagnosis and Treatment

In the face of hemodynamic instability unresponsive to fluid resuscitation and dependent on vasopressors and having ruled out other etiologies including sepsis, PE, and acute MI, AI is the one likely diagnosis that remains. AI seems relevant in light of her chronic steroid use and severe stress from injury. Other signs that suggest the diagnosis of AI include persistent, unexplained fever, weakness, and the inability to wean the ventilator support as well as hyponatremia and hyperkalemia. Other tests that may point toward the diagnosis of AI include mild eosinophilia with mean eosinophil counts of 3.5% versus 0.9% in those with normal adrenal function. These laboratory abnormalities are, however, more likely in the face of chronic AI.

Adrenal function may be assessed by several tests although none are considered to be extremely reliable. The random cortisol level may be helpful. Cortisol is normally secreted in a diurnal cycle. However, this diurnal variation is often lost in the critically ill patient. Cortisol may be checked at any time in the critically ill patient for this reason. Within the literature, many values have been proposed as the appropriate minimum value (range, 10 to 34 µg/dL); however, many would agree that a random cortisol over 18 is a normal response to stress.

The adrenocorticotropic hormone (ACTH) stimulation test may also be diagnostic and has been used over the past four decades. This test is conducted by administering 250 µg of ACTH (cosyntropin) either intravenously or intramuscularly. Cortisol levels are measured before and then 30 and 60 minutes after administration of the cosyntropin. This test may be performed at any time of the day. Some have proposed a low-dose version of the ACTH stimulation test where only 1 µg of cosyntropin is administered intravenously. Due to the low dose, it is thought that it is more sensitive for partial AI. This has not been proven and the preferred test is the standard dose of 250 µg.

The "delta 9" may be helpful in making the diagnosis of AI. In a multicenter, randomized trial, Annane demonstrated that those patients who showed a change in baseline cortisol levels by 9 µg/dL at 30 or 60 minutes during the ACTH stimulation test had lower mortality rates if they received corticosteroids. This test is thought to demonstrate adrenal reserve in the face of critical illness or sepsis but does not assess the integrity of the hypothalamic–pituitary–adrenal axis. It is also argued that those patients that are maximally stressed may be effectively secreting the maximum amount of cortisol. Therefore, while it may be sufficient, the delta value may not be very high and may be <9 µg/dL. The utility of the delta 9 may be limited for this reason. The recent multicenter CORTICUS trial did not report outcome differences between responders and nonresponders to a stimulation test, hence does not advocate for performance of this test.

Free cortisol may also be helpful in identifying AI. More than 90% of cortisol is bound to proteins including cortisol-binding globulin and albumin. Experts would agree that the active portion of cortisol is that which is free, or not bound to proteins. Delayed test results make this test impractical in critically ill patients. More work must be done to assess the true utility of this test and to develop a more clinically relevant test.

Other tests exist but should not be utilized in the critically ill population and include the insulin tolerance test and metyrapone test. The insulin tolerance test may lead to profound hypoglycemia, while the metyrapone test may exacerbate an adrenal crisis.

Presentation Continued

Since the differential diagnosis had been narrowed to include AI without any other obvious cause of the hemodynamic instability, random cortisol level was 10 µg/dL. Additionally, a standard ACTH stimulation test was performed. At 60 minutes after injection, the cortisol level was 17 mg/dL. The change in cortisol levels was less than the proposed 9 mg/dL. It was determined that our patient was indeed suffering from AI.

Treatment of AI

AI may be separated into AI in those who regularly take exogenous corticosteroids for other medical problems such as rheumatoid arthritis or asthma, also known as secondary AI and acute AI. Faced with the effects of AI, one must appropriately supplement the patient with corticosteroids. For those on chronic steroids in the face of stress from critical illness, one should consider increasing the dose of corticosteroids. How long one should supply the elevated dose or whether an elevated dose is even required is not well described in the literature.

Hydrocortisone is the corticosteroid of choice as both prednisone and cortisone require hydroxylation to obtain the active compound of prednisolone and cortisol, respectively. One must consider the replacement of mineralocorticoids as well in AI. This is not necessary if hydrocortisone is used due to the combined activity of both glucocorticoids and mineralocorticoids. However, the major protocol difference between two large trials that had discordant results in patients with septic shock was that the "positive" trial also included use of a mineralocorticoid in addition to administration of hydrocortisone.

The administration of hydrocortisone (150 to 200 mg daily for 5 to 7 days) has been shown to lead to a decreased vasopressor requirement as well as improved organ dysfunction, fewer ventilator days, fewer ICU days, and most importantly lower 28-day mortality. The exact dose is controversial as many studies have demonstrated positive effects with varying dosages ranging from 50 mg every 6 hours to 100 mg every 8 hours with a treatment length of 1 to 5 days.

A 2002 study by Annane et al. demonstrated a 28-day survival benefit in patients with septic shock and AI who received hydrocortisone and fludrocortisone with no difference in adverse events between the study group and the placebo control group. However, one must use caution as a more recent study known as the CORTICUS trial demonstrated no significant difference in mortality between patients who received hydrocortisone versus placebo. Additionally, there was no difference in patients who did not have a response to the ACTH stimulation test compared to those who did respond. While shock was reversed more quickly in those who received hydrocortisone, there was no survival benefit. A recent meta-analysis by Annane confirmed these results.

Case Conclusion

The patient was treated with 50 mg of hydrocortisone every 6 hours for 5 days. Within several hours of her first dose of steroids, her hemodynamic status stabilized and the pressor support was weaned without incident and she was subsequently extubated. She was transitioned from hydrocortisone to oral prednisone as her condition improved and she was able to take medications by mouth. She was later discharged from the intensive care unit in stable condition on her home dose of prednisone.

TAKE HOME POINTS

- AI may present with subtle signs that mimic other clinical etiologies including sepsis, pulmonary embolus, and acute MI.
- One must establish a broad differential diagnosis in order appropriately rule out each of the life-threatening entities.
- Clinical signs may include hypotension, tachycardia, and fever as well as weakness and an inability to wean the patient from the ventilator.
- Laboratory studies that may point toward AI include hyponatremia and hyperkalemia as well as a mild eosinophilia, although these are more common in those with chronic AI.
- The diagnosis of AI may be made by a random cortisol level as well as the results of the standard ACTH stimulation test.

- While the absolute cortisol level may point to the diagnosis, the "delta 9" rule may also help discriminate the actual diagnosis.
- Treatment with hydrocortisone at a dose of 50 to 100 mg every 6 to 8 hours is considered the preferred standard. The length of the treatment course is dependent on the patient's clinical response.

SUGGESTED READINGS

Annane D, et al. Corticosteroids in the treatment of severe sepsis and septic shock in adults: a systematic review. JAMA. 2009;301:2362–2375.

Annane D, et al. Effect of treatment with low doses of hydrocortisone and fludrocortisone on mortality in patients with septic shock. JAMA. 2002;288:862–871.

Annetta M, et al. Use of corticosteroids in critically ill septic patients: a review of mechanisms of adrenal insufficiency in sepsis and treatment. Curr Drug Targets. 2009;10:887–894.

Cooper MS, Stewart PM. Adrenal insufficiency in critical illness. J Intensive Care Med. 2007;22:348–362.

Cooper MS, Stewart PM. Corticosteroid insufficiency in acutely ill patients. N Engl J Med. 2003;348:727–734.

Edwin SB, Walker PL. Controversies surrounding the use of etomidate for rapid sequence intubation in patients with suspected sepsis. Ann Pharmacother. 2010;44: 1307–1313.

Grossman AB. Clinical review#: the diagnosis and management of central hypoadrenalism. J Clin Endocrinol Metab. 2010;95:4855–4863.

Hamrahian A. Adrenal function in critically ill patients: how to test? When to treat? Cleve Clin J Med. 2005;72: 427–432.

Johnson KL, Rn CR. The hypothalamic-pituitary-adrenal axis in critical illness. AACN Clin Issues. 2006;17:39–49.

Marik PE, et al. Recommendations for the diagnosis and management of corticosteroid insufficiency in critically ill adult patients: consensus statements from an international task force by the American College of Critical Care Medicine. Crit Care Med. 2008;36:1937–1949.

Nylen ES, Muller B. Endocrine changes in critical illness. J Intensive Care Med. 2004;19:67–82.

Rivers EP, et al. Adrenal insufficiency in high-risk surgical ICU patients. Chest. 2001;119:889–896.

Sprung CL, et al. Hydrocortisone therapy for patients with septic shock. N Engl J Med. 2008;358:111–124.

114 Acute Respiratory Distress Syndrome (ARDS)

PAULINE K. PARK, KRISHNAN RAGHAVENDRAN, and
LENA M. NAPOLITANO

Presentation

A 65-year-old female, with a history of chronic renal failure requiring hemodialysis, underwent an urgent left hemicolectomy for a partially obstructing colon cancer. On postoperative day 5, she develops fever, abdominal pain, and leukocytosis. Abdominal radiographs confirm extensive pneumoperitoneum. Emergent laparotomy confirms anastomotic disruption. Resection of the anastomosis with end-colostomy and Hartman's procedure is performed. The patient develops worsening severe hypoxemia in the operating room, with a PaO_2 of 85 mm Hg on FiO_2 1.0. She is maintained intubated and mechanically ventilated and is admitted to the surgical intensive care unit (ICU) postoperatively.

Differential Diagnosis

This patient has severe hypoxemia and acute respiratory failure. It is important to establish a definitive diagnosis in patients with severe hypoxemia, as definitive treatment strategies must be aligned with the diagnosis. The differential diagnosis of severe hypoxemia in this patient includes the following:

- Bacterial pneumonia
- Aspiration pneumonia or pneumonitis
- Pulmonary embolus
- Heart failure
- Pulmonary edema
- Transfusion-associated acute lung injury (TRALI)
- Acute respiratory distress syndrome (ARDS)

Any patient with the acute onset of bilateral pulmonary infiltrates and severe hypoxemia in the absence of evidence of cardiogenic pulmonary edema should be evaluated for ARDS. ARDS is a syndrome defined by (1) the presence of bilateral pulmonary infiltrates of acute onset, (2) $PaO_2{:}FiO_2$ (P/F) ratio of ≤200, and (3) no evidence of left atrial hypertension.

Workup

The workup for ARDS includes diagnostic imaging and laboratory tests to exclude the other potential diagnoses of the acute hypoxemic respiratory failure. ARDS is ultimately a clinical diagnosis, excluding other etiologies of the severe hypoxemia. ARDS-associated mortality rates remain high, at approximately 40%, and therefore an early diagnosis is critical to initiation of optimal management.

Chest Radiograph

This patient had a normal chest radiograph preoperatively and developed bilateral infiltrates with the development of abdominal sepsis **(Figure 1)**. Pneumonia generally demonstrates a lobar infiltrate rather than bilateral infiltrates.

Transthoracic Echocardiography

This diagnostic test is used to evaluate for cardiogenic pulmonary edema. This patient's echocardiogram demonstrated a hyperdynamic state with an estimated ejection fraction of 70% and no evidence of left ventricular dysfunction, left atrial hypertension, or valvular disease. This is consistent with her diagnosis of abdominal sepsis and does not confirm a diagnosis of heart failure. There is no evidence of right heart strain or right ventricular dysfunction that may be present in patients with pulmonary embolus.

Laboratory Tests

Arterial blood gas confirms hypoxemia, PaO_2 of 85 mm Hg on FiO_2 1.0, which confirms a PaO_2/FiO_2 ratio ≤200 mm Hg. No other specific laboratory tests confirm a diagnosis of ARDS. Brain (B-type) natriuretic peptide (BNP) levels are elevated in acutely decompensated heart failure, so low levels may be indicative of a diagnosis of ARDS.

Sputum

Respiratory cultures should be obtained to evaluate for possible bacterial or aspiration pneumonia as the etiology of the patient's acute respiratory failure.

Electrocardiogram

Electrocardiogram (EKG) reveals sinus tachycardia with no conduction abnormalities. In patients with pulmonary embolus or acute cor pulmonale, a right heart strain pattern may be present. EKG is also helpful to evaluate for possible acute myocardial infarction.

Chest Computed Tomography Scan

Computed tomographic (CT) pulmonary angiography is used to diagnose pulmonary embolism and may also be useful in identification of effusion, pneumothorax, or posterior dependent atelectasis that can help to guide treatment strategies. Some patients with severe hypoxemia will not be stable for transport for CT imaging. Four (4)-extremity venous duplex scan may be considered to evaluate for extremity venous thrombosis, which would warrant initiation of systemic anticoagulation, but this does not provide a definitive diagnosis of pulmonary embolism as the etiology of the severe hypoxemia.

Diagnosis

This patient has ARDS, meeting all of the criteria for the ARDS definition including bilateral infiltrates on chest radiograph, hypoxemia ($PaO_2/FiO_2 \leq 200$ mm Hg), and no evidence of cardiogenic pulmonary edema (Table 1). The ARDS is likely secondary to the abdominal sepsis from anastomotic leak.

Pathophysiology

ARDS is characterized by diffuse alveolar damage and hyaline membranes representing epithelial injury and increased permeability of the endothelium and epithelium. This results in the accumulation of protein- and neutrophil-rich pulmonary edema in the lung interstitium and in the distal airways. Additional mechanisms impair the removal of pulmonary edema fluid and inflammatory cells from the lung (Figure 2).

Treatment

Treatment of the Cause

The first priority in management of ARDS is treatment of the underlying cause or precipitating event. In this patient, treatment of the abdominal sepsis is required, including broad-spectrum empiric antibiotics, surgical source control, resuscitation, and cardiorespiratory support.

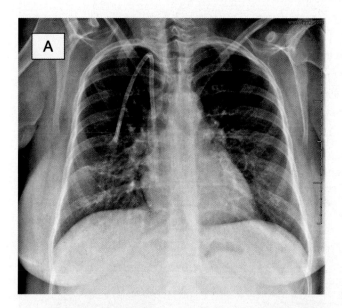

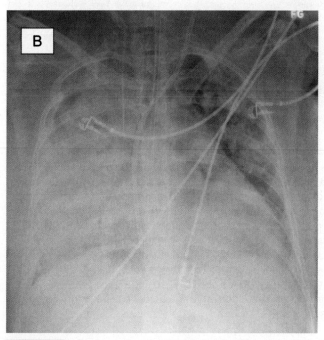

FIGURE 1 • Preoperative chest radiograph (A) and on ICU admission (B).

TABLE 1. The American-European Consensus Conference (AECC) Definition of Acute Lung Injury (ALI) and ARDS Developed in 1994	
ALI Criteria	**Timing**: Acute onset **Oxygenation**: $PaO_2/FiO_2 \leq 300$ mm Hg (regardless of positive end-expiratory pressure [PEEP] level) **Chest radiograph**: Bilateral infiltrates seen on frontal chest radiograph Pulmonary artery wedge: ≤18 mm Hg when measured or no clinical evidence of left atrial hypertension
ARDS Criteria	Same as ALI except: **Oxygenation**: $PaO_2/FiO_2 \leq 200$ mm Hg (regardless of PEEP level)

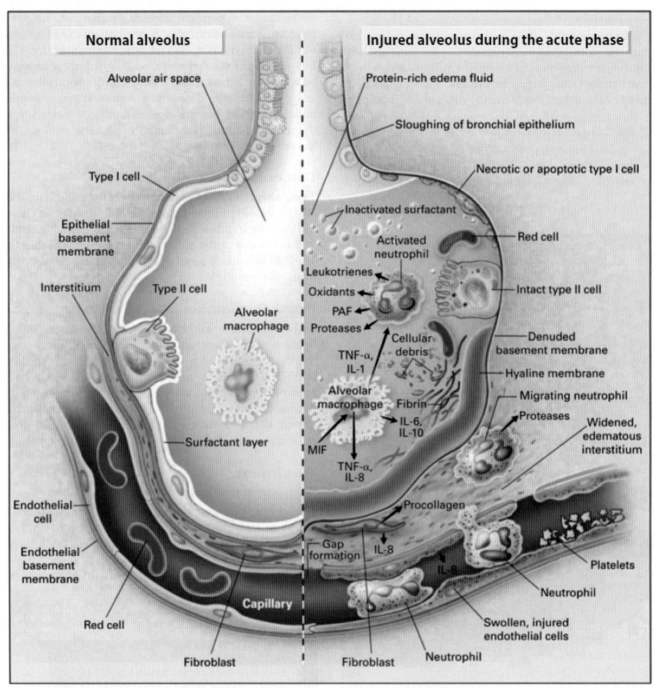

FIGURE 2 • **(A)** The normal alveolus and **(B)** the injured alveolus in the acute phase of acute lung injury and the acute respiratory distress syndrome. In the acute phase of the syndrome **(B)**, there is sloughing of both the bronchial and alveolar epithelial cells; protein-rich hyaline membranes form on the denuded basement membrane. Neutrophils adhere to the injured capillary endothelium and marginate through the interstitium into the air space, which is filled with protein-rich edema fluid. In the air space, alveolar macrophages secrete cytokines; interleukin (IL)-1, -6, -8, and -10; and tumor necrosis factor α (TNF-α), which act locally to stimulate chemotaxis and activate neutrophils. IL-1 can also stimulate the production of extracellular matrix by fibroblasts. Neutrophils can release oxidants, proteases, leukotrienes, and other proinflammatory molecules such as platelet-activating factor (PAF). A number of anti-inflammatory mediators are also present in the alveolar milieu including IL-1 receptor antagonist, soluble TNF receptor, autoantibodies against IL-8, and cytokines such as IL-10 and -11 (not shown). The influx of protein-rich edema fluid into the alveolus leads to the inactivation of surfactant. MIF, macrophage-inhibitory factor. (Adapted from the Massachusetts Medical Society, with permission.)

Respiratory Support with Mechanical Ventilation

The goal of mechanical ventilation is to increase oxygenation while minimizing the risk of further lung injury, known as ventilator-induced lung injury. Low tidal volume (6 mL/kg) ventilation is associated with a significant reduction in mortality **(Table 2)** and is the standard ventilator management of ARDS. This strategy allows for permissive hypercapnia. With the development of the National Institutes of Health (NIH)-sponsored ARDS Clinical Trials Network, large well-controlled trials of ARDS therapies have been completed. Thus far, the only treatment found to improve survival rates in such a study is a mechanical ventilation strategy using low tidal volumes. If the

ARDS patient has persistent hypoxemia, additional strategies including recruitment maneuvers (RM), "open lung" ventilation with higher end-expiratory pressure (PEEP), and mechanical ventilation with higher mean airway pressures (airway pressure release ventilation or high-frequency oscillatory ventilation) are considered.

Therapies Targeted at the Lung Injury

The use of a fluid-conservative strategy after patients with ARDS are no longer in shock was associated with improved oxygenation and a significant reduction in the duration of mechanical ventilation, and no difference in 60-day mortality or nonpulmonary organ failures. Therefore, conservative volume management

---

TABLE 2. Low Tidal Volume Ventilation Strategy from ARDS Network (www.ardsnet.org)

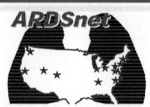

NIH NHLBI ARDS Clinical Network
Mechanical Ventilation Protocol Summary

INCLUSION CRITERIA: Acute onset of
1. $PaO_2/FiO_2 \leq 300$ (corrected for altitude)
2. Bilateral (patchy, diffuse, or homogeneous) infiltrates consistent with pulmonary edema
3. No clinical evidence of left atrial hypertension

PART I: VENTILATOR SETUP AND ADJUSTMENT
1. Calculate predicted body weight (PBW)
   Males = 50 + 2.3 [height (inches) - 60]
   Females = 45.5 + 2.3 [height (inches) -60]
2. Select any ventilator mode
3. Set ventilator settings to achieve initial V_T = 8 ml/kg PBW
4. Reduce V_T by 1 ml/kg at intervals $\leq$ 2 hours until V_T = 6ml/kg PBW.
5. Set initial rate to approximate baseline minute ventilation (not > 35 bpm).
6. Adjust V_T and RR to achieve pH and plateau pressure goals below.

OXYGENATION GOAL: PaO$_2$ 55-80 mmHg or SpO$_2$ 88-95%
Use a minimum PEEP of 5 cm H_2O. Consider use of incremental FiO_2/PEEP combinations such as shown below (not required) to achieve goal.

Lower PEEP/higher FiO2

FiO$_2$	0.3	0.4	0.4	0.5	0.5	0.6	0.7	0.7
PEEP	5	5	8	8	10	10	10	12

FiO$_2$	0.7	0.8	0.9	0.9	0.9	1.0
PEEP	14	14	14	16	18	18-24

Higher PEEP/lower FiO2

FiO$_2$	0.3	0.3	0.3	0.3	0.3	0.4	0.4	0.5
PEEP	5	8	10	12	14	14	16	16

FiO$_2$	0.5	0.5-0.8	0.8	0.9	1.0	1.0
PEEP	18	20	22	22	22	24

PLATEAU PRESSURE GOAL: $\leq$ 30 cm H_2O
Check Pplat (0.5 second inspiratory pause), at least q 4h and after each change in PEEP or V_T.
If Pplat > 30 cm H_2O: decrease V_T by 1ml/kg steps (minimum = 4 ml/kg).
If Pplat < 25 cm H_2O and V_T< 6 ml/kg, increase V_T by 1 ml/kg until Pplat > 25 cm H_2O or V_T = 6 ml/kg.
If Pplat < 30 and breath stacking or dys-synchrony occurs: may increase V_T in 1ml/kg increments to 7 or 8 ml/kg if Pplat remains $\leq$ 30 cm H_2O.

pH GOAL: 7.30-7.45
Acidosis Management: (pH < 7.30)
  If pH 7.15-7.30: Increase RR until pH > 7.30 or $PaCO_2$ < 25 (Maximum set RR = 35).

If pH < 7.15: Increase RR to 35.
  If pH remains < 7.15, V_T may be increased in 1 ml/kg steps until pH > 7.15 (Pplat target of 30 may be exceeded).
  May give $NaHCO_3$
Alkalosis Management: (pH > 7.45) Decrease vent rate if possible.

I: E RATIO GOAL: Recommend that duration of inspiration be $\leq$ duration of expiration.

and titrated diuretic administration (furosemide [Lasix], bumetamide [Bumex]) with either intermittent administration or continuous infusion can be considered. In patients with nonuniform infiltrates, positioning the patient with the good lung down can improve oxygenation by improving perfusion to the more aerated portion of the lung.

Supportive Therapies

Patients with ARDS require adequate sedation and analgesia, usually administered by IV continuous infusion titrated to effect. In critically ill patients with severe ARDS (defined as P/F ratio <150), early administration of a neuromuscular blocking agent (cisatracurium) for 48 hours improved the adjusted 90-day survival and increased the time off the ventilator without increasing muscle weakness. Neuromuscular blockade may be required in these severe cases, but prolonged neuromuscular blockade has been associated with myopathy and neuropathy in critically ill patients. Measures to reduce ventilator-associated pneumonia (VAP) are instituted, as ARDS patients can require prolonged mechanical ventilation and are at high risk for VAP. Early mobilization and physical therapy to reduce ICU-acquired weakness is an important component of care. All ARDS patients require nutritional support, and enteral nutrition is preferred as it is associated with decreased infectious complications in ICU patients. In some, but not all studies, administration of a specialized enteral nutrition formula (with omega-3 fatty acids [eicosapentaenoic acid, gamma-linolenic acid] and antioxidants) was associated with improved outcomes (reduced mortality, increased ventilator-free and ICU-free days, reduced organ failure and improved oxygenation).

Critical Care Approach to ARDS Rescue Strategies

The ARDS rescue strategies **(Table 3)** described below are implemented in ARDS patients with severe life-threatening hypoxemia (PaO$_2$/FiO$_2$ ≤100 mm Hg) that are not responsive to the standard ARDS management strategies reviewed above.

TABLE 3. Rescue Strategies for Severe Hypoxemia and ARDS

Recruitment maneuvers
Prone positioning
Inhaled nitric oxide
Inhaled prostacyclin and other vasodilatory prostaglandins
Extracorporeal membrane oxygenation (ECMO)

Recruitment Maneuvers

Recruitment maneuvers (RM) attempt to increase the amount of aerated lung to improve gas exchange. RM are performed by sustained inflation with continuous positive airway pressure (i.e., 30 cm H$_2$O PEEP for 30 seconds) or controlled ventilation at increased airway pressure. RM can improve oxygenation, but may also result in transient adverse events (hypotension, hypoxemia) or pneumothorax, and have not been shown to improve survival.

Prone Positioning

The prone position improves oxygenation in 70% to 80% of patients with ARDS, and maximal improvements are seen in the most hypoxemic patients. Both alveolar recruitment and end-expiratory lung volume increase with prone position, with improved ventilation/perfusion matching. A review of all published meta-analyses on the efficacy of prone position in ARDS concluded that prone ventilation was associated with reduced mortality only in the cohort of patients with severe hypoxemia, defined as PaO$_2$/FiO$_2$ ≤100 mm Hg.

Inhaled Nitric Oxide

Inhaled nitric oxide (INO) is a selective pulmonary vasodilator that improves oxygenation by increasing blood flow in ventilated areas to improve ventilation/perfusion matching. A meta-analysis of 12 trials and 1,237 patients confirmed that INO significantly increased oxygenation that persisted through day 4 of treatment, but no significant effect of INO on hospital mortality was identified.

Inhaled Prostacyclin and Other Vasodilatory Prostaglandins

Prostacyclin is a selective pulmonary vasodilator and inhibitor of platelet aggregation. When aerosolized, its vasodilatory action improves ventilation/perfusion matching in the lung, resulting in improved oxygenation and no effect on systemic arterial blood pressure. Inhaled iloprost is a more stable analog of prostacyclin and is approved by the FDA for pulmonary hypertension, and can be used instead of INO in ARDS patients with severe hypoxemia to improve oxygenation.

Extracorporeal Membrane Oxygenation

Extracorporeal membrane oxygenation (ECMO) is considered in patients with severe refractory hypoxemia unresponsive to all ARDS management strategies. Veno-venous ECMO is the most common strategy employed, with a 50% survival rate reported in 1,473 adults with ARDS treated with ECMO from the Extracorporeal Life Support Organization (ELSO).

The CESAR trial was a multicenter trial performed in the United Kingdom that randomized 180 patients to conventional mechanical ventilation versus ECMO and demonstrated that ARDS management with a standardized algorithm including ECMO in an expert center resulted in improved 6-month outcome (death or severe disability at 6 months, 63% vs. 47%; RR, 0.69; 95% CI, 0.05–0.97; p = 0.03). But compliance with a low tidal volume ventilation strategy was not mandated in the control cohort. The precise role of ECMO in ARDS as a salvage therapy remains unclear.

Special Considerations

Complications in ARDS patients are common. Clinicians must pay careful attention to early recognition of potential complications, particularly pneumothorax and VAP. VAP is a common risk factor for development of ARDS and almost 60% of patients with ARDS from other risk factors can develop VAP. Evaluation for other common infectious complications (central line–associated bloodstream infection, catheter-associated urinary tract infection) in ICU patients should be considered if fever and/or leukocytosis develop during the ICU stay.

Follow-up

It has been documented that ARDS patients who survive have significant functional impairments during initial recovery, but most achieve near-normal lung function at 1 year, which persists without deterioration at 5 years. The major disability in these patients is a combination of exercise limitation, physical and psychological sequelae, and decreased physical quality of life. ARDS patients should have follow-up to assess the recovery of their pulmonary function. Chest radiograph, pulmonary function tests, and chest CT imaging are all considered dependent on the patient's clinical condition at follow-up.

Case Conclusion

This patient with sepsis-associated ARDS was treated with low tidal volume ventilation, conservative fluid administration, prone positioning, and sepsis management. She required 12 days of mechanical ventilation and was successfully weaned and extubated. Quantitative lower respiratory tract cultures obtained by bronchoalveolar lavage were negative for bacterial pathogens. She completed a course of systemic antibiotics for treatment of abdominal sepsis due to secondary peritonitis. She did not require supplemental oxygen on discharge home. Arterial blood gas confirmed adequate oxygenation on room air.

TAKE HOME POINTS

- ARDS definition includes the acute onset of bilateral infiltrates, PaO_2/FiO_2 ≤200 mm Hg (regardless of PEEP level) and no clinical evidence of left atrial hypertension.
- ARDS can be caused by both direct (pulmonary) and indirect (nonpulmonary) etiologies.
- Any patient with the acute onset of bilateral pulmonary infiltrates and severe hypoxemia in the absence of cardiogenic pulmonary edema should be evaluated for ARDS.
- ARDS-associated mortality rates remain high, at approximately 40%, and therefore an early diagnosis is critical to initiation of optimal management.
- Low tidal volume (6 mL/kg) ventilation is associated with decreased mortality in ARDS.
- A fluid-conservative management strategy, supplemented with targeted diuretic administration, is associated with improved ICU outcomes in ARDS.
- ARDS rescue strategies should be considered in patients with severe life-threatening hypoxemia (PaO_2/FiO_2 ≤100 mm Hg) that are not responsive to the standard ARDS management strategies.

SUGGESTED READINGS

Brower RG, Matthay MA, Morris A, et al. Ventilation with lower tidal volumes as compared with traditional tidal volumes for acute lung injury and the acute respiratory distress syndrome. N Engl J Med. 2000;342(18): 1301–1308.

Herridge MS, Tansey CM, Matte A, et al. Canadian critical care trials group. Functional disability 5 years after acute respiratory distress syndrome. N Engl J Med. 2011;364: 1293–1304.

Napolitano LM, Park PK, Raghavendran K, et al. Nonventilatory strategies for patients with life-threatening 2009 H1N1 influenza and severe respiratory failure. Crit Care Med. 2010; 38(4 suppl):e74–e90.

Papazian L, Forel JM, Gacouin A, et al. ACURASYS study investigators. Neuromuscular blockers in early acute respiratory distress syndrome. N Engl J Med. 2010;363(12): 1107–1116.

Peek GJ, Mugford M, Tiruvoipati R, et al.; for the CESAR trial collaboration. Efficacy and economic assessment of conventional ventilator support versus extracorporeal membrane oxygenation for severe adult respiratory failure (CESAR): a multicenter randomized controlled trial. Lancet. 2009;374:1351–1363.

Pipeling MR, Fan E. Therapies for refractory hypoxemia in acute respiratory distress syndrome. JAMA. 2010;304(22): 2521–2527.

Raghavendran K, Napolitano LM. ALI and ARDS: advances and challenges. Crit Care Clin. 2011;27:xiii–xiv.

Stewart RM, Park PK, Hunt JP, et al.; NHLBI ARDS Clinical Trials Network. Less is more: improved outcomes in surgical patients with conservative fluid administration and central venous catheter monitoring. J Am Coll Surg. 2009;208(5):725–735.

Wiedemann HP, Wheeler AP, Bernard GR, et al. Comparison of two fluid-management strategies in acute lung injury. N Engl J Med. 2006;354:2564–2575.

115 Ventilator-associated Pneumonia

KRISHNAN RAGHAVENDRAN

Presentation

A 28-year-old male was involved in a motor vehicular accident traveling at 60 miles per hour. He sustained a significant traumatic brain injury (Glasgow coma scale of eight), was intubated at site, and transported to the ED. Subsequent workup revealed multiple cerebral contusions with no midline shift, infiltrates in the base of the right lung zones, mild hypoxia, and a femur fracture. He was then admitted to the intensive care unit (ICU) and was managed with supportive care including monitoring of intracranial pressure, mechanical ventilation, early nutrition and appropriate prophylaxis for prevention of venous thromboembolism, and stress-related mucosal disease. On the fourth day following trauma, he had a fever of 101°F, a leukocytosis of 21,000, and a new-onset infiltrate in the right upper lobe.

Differential Diagnosis

Presence of fever, leukocytosis, and a new infiltrate in a patient who has been endotracheally intubated and mechanically ventilated should raise a strong suspicion for ventilator-associated pneumonia (VAP). The patient at the time of initial presentation had evidence of hypoxia with an infiltrate in the lung, and this should raise the possibility of aspiration-induced lung injury. Aspiration-induced pneumonitis may manifest signs similar to infection, but a major aspiration event is unlikely at a point where patient has been intubated with a cuffed tube. However, aspiration pneumonitis is a risk factor for development of aspiration pneumonia. Isolated pulmonary contusion without any other evidence of thoracic trauma is unlikely and is not likely to manifest fever and leukocytosis. Pulmonary infarctions secondary to pulmonary embolism should also be considered in the differential diagnosis. Finally, acute development of a dense infiltrate in the right upper lobe should also raise the possibility of migration of the endotracheal tube down the right main stem bronchus with resultant occlusion of the right upper lobe bronchus and subsequent collapse. However, a collapse is not associated with fever or leukocytosis.

VAP, defined as a pulmonary infection occurring after at least 48 hours of mechanical ventilation, is the leading cause of death in the ICU, with estimated prevalence rates of 10% to 65% and mortality rates of 25% to 60%. The incidence of VAP varies from series to series, and in general, the incidence varies from 5 to 25/1,000 ventilator days. VAP remains a major cause of mortality and morbidity in the critically ill patient and comprises the second commonest nosocomial infection in the ICU. In spite of significant advances that have been made in recent years to reduce the incidence of VAP in most ICUs, it still is considered the major cause of mortality and increased economic burden associated with the mechanically ventilated patient. The crucial aspect in the management of VAP relies on prompt and accurate diagnosis.

Workup

This patient underwent a bronchoscopy and quantitative bacteriology from the bronchoalveolar lavage (BAL). A Gram stain from the lavage was additionally obtained. A chest x-ray showed the tip of the endotracheal tube was visualized at 4 cm above the carina.

The timing or the clinical criteria used to diagnose VAP are variable. Most ICUs either follow the CDC criteria (fever, leukocytosis, and new-onset infiltrate) or a variation of clinical pulmonary infection score. The latter scoring system takes into consideration fever, leukocytosis, nature of tracheal secretions, lung infiltrate, and oxygenation with/without BAL Gram stain finding of neutrophils or bacteria. Once the clinical suspicion of VAP is entertained, a bacteriologic workup is then initiated.

Determination of specific bacteriology and early initiation of appropriate broad-spectrum antibiotics remain the cornerstone of diagnosis and treatment of VAP. Sputum Gram stain and culture are considered inappropriate, as they are neither sensitive nor specific. The specimen used for quantitative bacteriology should be obtained either through a bronchoscope or by the use of a coaxial catheter that is inserted blindly through the endotracheal tube. The latter approach,

TABLE 1. Bacteriology of Isolated Organisms from a Single Center Study

Organism	Number of Episodes of VAP (Percentage)
Pseudomonas aeruginosa	38 (20.3)
Staphylococcus aureus (MSSA and MRSA)	33 (17.6)
Group A, B, C Streptococci	32 (17.1)
Haemophilus influenza	16 (8.5)
Klebsiella sp	7 (3.4)
Escherichia coli	7 (3.4)
Streptococcus pneumoniae	7 (3.4)
Other gram negatives (including Acinetobacter sp, Serratia, Stenotrophomonas)	32 (17.1)

TABLE 2. Measures to Prevent VAP and Components of VAP Bundle

A. *Nonpharmacologic*
Avoidance of endotracheal intubation (using noninvasive ventilation methods when possible)
Early weaning of mechanical ventilation
Appropriate staffing levels in the ICU
Subglottic suctioning
Avoid unnecessary manipulation/changes of the ventilatory circuit
Drain ventilatory circuit/use heat and moisture exchangers
Semierect positioning
Prevent gastric distension/check gastric volumes and residual feeds
Biofilm prevention on the endotracheal tubes
Hand washing/disinfection

B. *Pharmacologic*
Use of chlorhexidine
Antibiotic cycling
Limit use of antibiotic prophylaxis
Shorter course of empirical antibiotic therapy
Stringent protocols for blood transfusions

C. *Components of VAP bundle*
Head of Bed (HOB) elevated > 30°
Scheduled readiness to wean assessment
Sedation vacation/appropriate sedation
Deep Venous Thrombosis (DVT) prophylaxis
Stress ulcer prophylaxis

called the mini-BAL, does not involve a bronchoscope, and the diagnostic yield is considered similar to conventional bronchoscopy. Additionally, some ICUs use a protective brush inserted via a bronchoscope to obtain direct cultures from the affected area of the lung. The brush is then retrieved and directly plated onto the culture media. Significance is attributed to observed bacterial burden of more than 10^4 CFU/mL.

Diagnosis and Treatment

Regardless of the diagnostic modality used to ascertain the specific bacteriology, early initiation of appropriate broad-spectrum antibiotic therapy should be initiated as soon as the cultures are obtained. VAP is broadly classified into early (<4 ventilator days) and late (>4 ventilator days). The bacteriology of early VAP involves Enterobacteriaceae or gram-positive organisms such as methicillin-sensitive *Staphylococcus aureus* (MSSA). The appropriate antibiotic of choice includes second-generation cephalosporins, fluoroquinolones, or extended-spectrum penicillins as a single agent. Late VAP is invariably due to resistant organisms including but not limited to methicillin-resistant *Staphylococcus aureus* (MRSA), *Pseudomonas* species, or *Acinetobacter* species **(Table 1)**. A combination therapy of vancomycin plus beta lactams (third-generation cephalosporins, carbapenems) or fluoroquinolones +/– aminoglycosides is recommended.

With improved understanding of the pathogenesis of VAP, major strides have been taken in recent years in the institution of prevention strategies for VAP. A detailed list of methodologies used to prevent VAP and items included in the VAP bundle is provided in **Table 2**.

Case Conclusion

The patient was diagnosed with VAP on the fourth day following trauma. Patient was started on ceftriaxone at the time of diagnosis. The quantitative cultures were consistent with 10^5 CFU/mL of *Klebsiella pneumoniae*. The antibiotics were discontinued after 8 days at which time the white count and fever had subsided. The ventriculostomy catheters were removed on the sixth day following trauma and patient continued to improve clinically. He was extubated on the ninth posttrauma day and was subsequently transferred to an adult rehabilitation facility.

TAKE HOME POINTS

- The bacteriology of early and late VAP is very different and should inform antibiotic selection.
- It is important to obtain quantitative bacteriology from the lower respiratory tract prior to initiation of antibiotics.

- The initiation of antibiotics should be prompt and broad spectrum and also depend on typical microbiograms of the individual ICU.
- The duration of treatment should be 5–14 d.
- De-escalation or discontinuation of antibiotics should be considered once the quantitative cultures are finalized.

SUGGESTED READINGS

American Thoracic Society, Infectious Diseases Society of America. Guidelines for the management of adults with hospital-acquired, ventilator-associated, and healthcare-associated pneumonia. Am J Respir Crit Care Med. 2005;171(4):388–416.

Chastre J, Fagon JY. Ventilator-associated pneumonia. Am J Respir Crit Care Med. 2002;165(7):867–903.

Iregui M, Ward S, Sherman G, et al. Clinical importance of delays in the initiation of appropriate antibiotic treatment for ventilator-associated pneumonia. Chest. 2002;122(1):262–268.

Kollef MH. Prevention of hospital-associated pneumonia and ventilator-associated pneumonia. Crit Care Med. 2004;32(6):1396–1405.

Raghavendran K, Wang J, Bellber C, et al. Predictive value of sputum gram stain for the determination of appropriate antibiotic therapy for VAP. J Trauma. 2007;62(6):1377–1383.

116 Septic Shock

PAMELA A. LIPSETT

Presentation

A 68-year-old man presents to the emergency department with severe acute abdominal pain located in his left lower quadrant for the last 2 days. He has had a fever to 101°C, diarrhea 4 days ago, and now constipation for the last day. He has not vomited, but he has been nauseated and has been unable to take solid food or liquids. He has made little urine in the last day. He reports a history of acute diverticulitis requiring two previous hospitalizations in the last year and hypertension controlled with medication. He is unable to give a more complete history because of increasing confusion. His vital signs reveal an elevated temperature to 101.5°C, a pulse of 128, a respiratory rate of 32, and a blood pressure of 74/38 mm Hg. His examination demonstrates an acutely ill appearing man in pain and respiratory distress. He is mildly confused but without focal neurologic findings. He is tachypneic with rapid shallow respiratory efforts but clear lungs. His oxygen saturation is 90% on 60% face mask. His cardiac examination is normal save for his depressed blood pressure and elevated heart rate. His abdominal examination reveals a distended abdomen that is rigid and painful to palpation both generally and especially in the left lower quadrant where there is a suggestion of fullness. His stool is guaiac negative. His extremities are cool with pulses not palpable.

Differential Diagnosis

As is often the case, two issues must be immediately addressed; the patient is in shock and the shock is most likely related to the abdominal pain. The magnitude of the systemic illness suggests that this patient has an abdominal catastrophe. With a rigid abdomen and signs of shock, the possibility of a perforated viscous with intra-abdominal contamination is considered as well as all of the more general causes of peritonitis. In this age group, the most common etiologies of a rigid abdomen and pneumoperitoneum are related to diverticulitis, a perforated ulcer, or even appendicitis. A history of diverticulitis makes this diagnosis most likely, but the broad differential related to an acute abdomen must be considered. Identification of the specific etiology and source control is an essential element of ultimate treatment for this patient, but he has signs and symptoms of shock, which must be addressed expeditiously.

Shock is defined as inadequate tissue perfusion. While shock maybe classified in many ways, it is commonly classified as shown in **Table 1**. With the history of poor intake and diarrhea, this patient may have had an element of dehydration, but it is unlikely that his very depressed blood pressure is entirely due to hypovolemia. Of note, his diastolic pressure is quite low suggesting vasodilatation rather than vasoconstriction. Moreover, the combination of fever and abdominal pain suggests infection due to abdominal contamination and resulting distributive (i.e., septic)

shock. Due diligence in considering cardiac and noncardiogenic causes is appropriate; however, investigation should not delay action in ensuring resuscitation. Further studies are required to address the etiology of shock and to define the most likely contributing cause.

Workup

Laboratory evaluation demonstrates an elevated white blood cell (WBC) count of 24,000/mm³, hemoglobin of 15.0 g/dL, and a depressed platelet count of 100,000. Electrolytes reveal a sodium of 142, potassium 3.4, chloride 100, bicarbonate 20, glucose 180 mg/dL, blood urea nitrogen 48, and serum creatinine of 1.8 mg/dL. Lactate is elevated to 4.9, arterial blood gas is 7.30/30/60. A plain radiograph is fairly unremarkable. A computerized tomographic (CT) scan without contrast demonstrates an inflammatory mass in the sigmoid colon with pericolonic fluid extending into the pelvis and a small amount of localized free air adjacent to the colon. A cardiogram shows sinus tachycardia without acute changes. A chest radiograph shows a modest respiratory effort, but clear lungs.

Discussion

The Surviving Sepsis Campaign (SSC) has defined two endpoints for consideration in the treatment of septic shock: one to be completed by 6 hours (the resuscitation bundle) and one by 24 hours (the management bundle). The composition of these bundles

TABLE 1. Differential Diagnosis of Shock

Hypovolemic	Extracardiac Obstructive	Cardiogenic	Distributive
Hemorrhagic Trauma Gastrointestinal	Extrinsic vascular compression Mediastinal tumors	Myocardial Infarction Myocarditis Cardiomyopathy Pharmacologic/toxic Drugs (beta blockers, calcium channel blockers, etc.) Intrinsic depression	Infection/inflammation/ tissue injury

Nonhemorrhagic
 Dehydration
 Vomiting
 Diarrhea
 Burns
 Polyuria
 Diuretic use, diabetes
  insipidus, etc.
	Elevated intrathoracic
	 pressure
	 Tension
	  pneumothorax
	 Positive-pressure
	  ventilation
		Mechanical
		 Valvular stenosis
		 Valvular regurgitation
		 Ventricular septal defects
		 Ventricular aneurysm
			Sepsis

Third-space losses Peritonitis, ascites	Vascular flow obstruction Pulmonary embolism Air embolism Tumors Aortic dissection Acute pulmonary hypertension Pericardial tamponade Pericarditis	Arrhythmias	Pancreatitis
			Trauma Burns Anaphylaxis Snake bite, medication Neurogenic Spinal cord trauma Endocrine Myxedema coma Adrenal insufficiency

recommended in the SSC guidelines is shown in **Table 2**. Notably, the SSC guidelines last published in 2004 are currently being revised and are expected for publication within the next year. Based on studies that have been published since 2004, it is very likely that the degree of support for some of the prior recommendations will change and new recommendations will follow.

Use of the elements of the SSC or "bundle" has decreased mortality from more than 50% to as low as 37.5%. Further details of management of septic shock will be discussed in the next section. Source control for intra-abdominal sepsis while essential and important is secondary to the initial resuscitation and stabilization of a patient in septic shock. The description of the CT scan suggests that this patient has Hinchey stage III disease **(Table 3)**, and an intervention will be required once he has been resuscitated. While open surgery has classically been applied to the treatment of complicated diverticulitis, staged percutaneous treatment with

one-staged repair has been reported with increasing success, as high as 91% of patients in a recent report.

Diagnosis and Treatment

Severe sepsis is defined as the presence of infection and end-organ dysfunction, hypoperfusion, or hypotension. Septic shock is one step further into critical illness with refractory hypotension or hypoperfusion in spite of adequate fluid administration. Signs of systemic hypoperfusion in this case include an elevated serum lactate (>4 mm/L), oliguria, mental confusion, and a decreased PaO_2/FIO_2 ratio (60/60 = 100). The patient should be approached with therapies consistent with the SSC guidelines. Given the poor condition of the patient at presentation, immediate attention should be focused on support of his respiratory effort with additional oxygen (100% face mask). He is likely to require intubation and mechanical ventilation to decrease the work of breathing and to administer additional positive pressure given his very poor and concerning

TABLE 2. Surviving Sepsis Bundle Components

Resuscitation Bundle to be Completed by 6 h

1. Measure serum lactate
2. Obtain blood cultures before the administration of antibiotics.
3. Broad-spectrum antibiotics should be administered within 3 h for an emergency department admission and within 1 h for nonemergency department intensive care unit admissions.
4. If the patient is hypotensive, deliver a minimum of 500–1000 mL of crystalloid (or colloid equivalent) over a 30-min period.
   If the patient remains hypotensive in spite of fluid resuscitation:
5. Achieve and maintain a mean arterial pressure of >65 mm Hg.
6. Achieve central venous pressure of >8 mm Hg.
7. Achieve central venous oxygen saturation of >70%.

Management Bundle to be Completed by 24 h

1. Administer IV hydrocortisone 300 mg/d for 7 d in three divided doses to patients with refractory hypotension despite adequate fluid replacement and vasopressors.
2. Administer protein C activated (drotrecogin alfa) to patients with septic shock, ≥2 sepsis-induced organ failures, and no contraindications.
3. Maintain glucose control greater than lower limit of normal with a target value of 150 mg/dL (8.3 mm/L).
4. Maintain the median value of inspiratory plateau pressures <30 cm H_2O for mechanically ventilated patients.

PaO_2/FIO_2 ratio. Adequate intravenous (IV) access must be obtained and fluids should be rapidly administered to restore blood volume, which is decreased from antecedent volume loss from diarrhea, poor oral intake, and capillary leak with loss into the peritoneal cavity and into the microcirculation. His metabolic acidosis must be reversed. Isotonic fluids (or colloids) should be administered to restore blood volume and

perfusion pressure. The SSC guidelines suggest that the central venous pressure should be >8 mm Hg. A meta-analysis of 29 studies published in 2008 found among early resuscitation studies quantitative or goal-directed resuscitation when compared with standard resuscitation resulted in a significant decrease in mortality (odds ratio [OR] 0.50, 95% confidence interval [CI] 0.37 to 0.69). However, while the use of SVO_2 is suggested by the SSC guidelines, this is not universally accepted. A large trial of patients with adult respiratory distress syndrome (ARDS) did not demonstrate any benefit of a pulmonary artery catheter over a central venous catheter.

If the patient remains hypotensive after fluid resuscitation, vasopressors are typically added. The SSC guidelines suggest that either dopamine or norepinephrine is an appropriate agent. More recently, a randomized controlled trial compared dopamine versus norepinephrine in 1,629 patients with shock, the majority with sepsis. While there was no difference in mortality between the two groups, the incidence of adverse events (arrhythmias) was significantly greater in the dopamine group. The role of vasopressin in the treatment of septic shock is less certain as a large randomized trial did not show any benefit in mortality but did show that vasopressin may reduce progression to renal failure and mortality in patients at risk of kidney injury who have septic shock.

Following the acquisition of blood cultures, patients who are in septic shock should have broad-spectrum antibiotics administered in short order (<1 hour). For the patient in this scenario, expected pathogens include enteric gram-negative bacteria, facultative aerobic gram-positive organisms, and anaerobes. Resistant pathogens are unlikely to be present in the patient described. However, patients who develop septic shock in the hospital, after recent hospitalization or following a stay in a long-term care facility, are

TABLE 3. Hinchey Stage for Diverticulitis

Stage	Definition	Treatment
Stage I	Small (<4 cm) confined pericolic or mesenteric abscess	Antibiotics, nothing by mouth/clear liquids
Stage II	Large pericolonic abscess (>4 cm) often extending to the pelvis	Antibiotics, nothing by mouth, percutaneous drainage followed by elective one-stage procedure with controlled infection
Stage III	Rupture of a pericolonic abscess causing purulent peritonitis	As above if sepsis is controlled, otherwise laparotomy if sepsis continues. Resection of involved colon and reanastomosis, with or without diversion. A laparoscopic approach maybe possible.
Stage IV	Free rupture of an inflamed diverticulum causing feculent peritonitis	As above with exploratory laparotomy in most cases, possible one- or two-staged procedure. Classic three-staged procedure largely abandoned.

all at increased risk of resistant pathogens. Empiric selection of antibiotics should consider epidemiologic risk factors noted. Depending on the etiology of septic shock, appropriate initial antibiotic selection has been linked to improved survival; thus, broad-spectrum agents are initially selected. The Surgical Infection Society guidelines for intra-abdominal infections of moderate to severe severity would indicate that several choices of antibiotics would be appropriate for the case patient. For single agents, these would include imipenem-cilastatin, meropenem, doripenem, and piperacillin–tazobactam. Experts should be familiar with the pharmacodynamic and kinetic issues of antibiotic administration in critically ill patients. Hospital systems should be organized so that a patient who has just been identified as having septic shock can rapidly receive appropriate antibiotics. Administration of antibiotics within 1 hour has been demonstrated to have a significant survival benefit.

One of the controversial issues in the management of patients in septic shock is whether a critically ill patient should receive low-dose steroids (<300 mg of hydrocortisone). While there are conflicting trials on the subject, the SCC guidelines recommend the use of steroids for a short period (7 days) in patients with septic shock who are unresponsive to fluids and vasoactive agents. Current data would suggest that patient survival is not changed when using steroids, but that time requiring vasopressors is reduced when hydrocortisone is used. An adrenal stimulation test is not required and administration of steroids may be beneficial when used for more than 100 hours but <7 days. Fludrocortisone does not appear to be necessary.

Currently, the use of activated protein C (APC) is recommended by the SSC guidelines for patients who qualify by severity of illness and who do not have a contraindication. However, more recent data from clinical trials and a Cochrane Collaborative concluded that APC did not reduce the risk of death in adult patients with severe sepsis (pooled RR: 0.97, 95% CI: 0.78, 1.22). Further APC use was associated with an increased risk of bleeding (RR: 1.47, 95% CI: 1.09, 2.00). It seems unlikely that APC will be included in the next SSC update.

The control of blood glucose has undergone much study and debate over the last decade. While tight glucose control (80 to 110 mg/dL) appeared to be of significant benefit to patients when considering both survival and morbidity, more recent studies have not demonstrated overall survival benefit and have suggested significant harm secondary to hypoglycemia episodes when glucose is controlled too tightly. Thus, a target glucose of <150 seems appropriate.

Patients with severe sepsis and septic shock are likely to develop respiratory failure ARDS. Should a patient develop ARDS, low tidal volume (<6 mL/kg of predicted body weight) with management of the ventilator to achieve an inspiratory plateau pressure of <30 cm H_2O has been shown to improve survival. This is an element of treatment that has not been well translated into clinical practice but has strong data supporting improved survival.

Once this patient has had adequate resuscitation, source control of the intra-abdominal process must be achieved. The specific surgical management of a patient with complicated diverticulitis is presented in an earlier chapter. Given the severity of this patient's presentation, a staging temporizing procedure with percutaneous drainage would be an appropriate initial treatment in many patients.

Special Considerations

Some patients with complicated diverticulitis will present with Hinchey stage IV disease with gross fecal contamination. Patients in this category will need rapid resuscitation, operative intervention, and source control. One study suggested that survival is improved when source control occurs within 6 hours.

Patients who develop sepsis and septic shock following a surgical procedure often show warning signs that can be identified by careful observation of their postoperative course. Typically in a patient who is developing a complication, the normal postoperative ebb and flow metabolism is disrupted, and patients may be identified by an extraordinary initial stress response and fluid requirement, failure to diurese in a timely fashion, and signs of infection developing such as worsening glucose control, mental confusion or delirium, rising WBC, and fever. These high-risk patients should undergo a careful examination and directed laboratory and radiograph studies as appropriate.

Patients with end-organ dysfunction or failure at baseline are at increased risk of death following an episode of sepsis or septic shock. Management of patients in this group should carefully consider known organ failure and selection of strategies for support streamlined appropriately. For example, patients with cardiac disease at baseline and poor ejection fraction may need early beta agonist support, though attempts at establishing supranormal oxygen delivery do not appear warranted. Another important consideration is a patient with worsening renal function who develops septic shock. While searching for a source of infection a CT scan may seem appropriate, the use of IV contrast should be very carefully considered as to the risk benefit relationship in what additional information the IV contrast may infer versus the harm of IV contrast when a patient already has compromised renal blood flow due to shock. This is especially important when the presentation of an acute pulmonary embolus may be confused with septic shock. Often the discriminating feature is that sepsis is not "suddenly occurring," and often the antecedent signs mentioned above have been present but are unrecognized.

Postoperative Management

Once a patient is stabilized, source control should be obtained. This can be accomplished by percutaneous drainage in many patients, while open surgery will be required in some. For patients with a closed space infection such a cholangitis or pyelonephritis, early drainage and decompression is necessary if the patient remains unstable. In patients in whom a device is associated with the septic source, the device (e.g., central line) may need to be removed as part of the treatment algorithm.

Ongoing support in an ICU is needed following intervention until organ dysfunction has resolved. While the exact duration of antibiotics will depend on source and degree of source control, with the exception of endovascular infections, the need for antibiotics beyond 14 days suggests inadequate source control or a secondary infection or complication. Most patients will require 5 to 10 days of antibiotics with an ongoing study to identify whether a time-based treatment philosophy or symptom-based (resolution of fever, WBC, local signs) should dictate duration of therapy for complicated intra-abdominal infections.

Case Conclusion

This patient was intubated initially and placed on ARDS protocol settings. He received 14 L of crystalloids in addition to norepinephrine to support intravascular volume and blood pressure. Following blood cultures, piperacillin–tazobactam was administered within 1 hour of his presentation. His urine output improved from 5 to 10 mL/h to 35 mL/h before he went to interventional radiology for percutaneous drainage of his pelvic abscess. Within 4 hours of his drainage procedure while receiving ongoing fluid, his norepinephrine requirement abated, so steroids were not administered. His ventilatory requirement continued for the next 3 days, but following a spontaneous breathing trial on day 4, he was successfully liberated from the ventilator. He began to spontaneously diurese on day 2.5 and was assisted with diuretics to remove the fluid (total 20 L) he had gained while in shock. He was transferred to the ward for rehabilitation on day 5 after presentation in septic shock.

TAKE HOME POINTS

- A patient with shock should be recognized immediately and treatment begun based on first principles.
- Support of failing or dysfunctional organ systems should be a treatment priority based on typical priorities of airway, breathing, and circulation. This often means that the patient should receive the administration of oxygen, mechanical ventilation, and aggressive administration of fluids, vasoactive agents, and antibiotics.
- Surviving sepsis guidelines provide evidence-based treatment strategies that are based on 6-and 24-hour time points. These guidelines will be updated in 2012.
- Initial resuscitation should precede any attempt at source control beyond antibiotic administration.

SUGGESTED READINGS

Acute Respiratory Distress Syndrome Network. Ventilation with lower tidal volumes as compared with traditional tidal volumes for acute lung injury and the acute respiratory distress syndrome. N Engl J Med. 2000;342(18):1301–1308.

De Backer D, Biston P, Devriendt J, et al. Comparison of dopamine and norepinephrine in the treatment of shock. N Engl J Med. 2010;362:779–789.

Dellinger RP, Carlet JM, Masur H, et al. Surviving Sepsis Campaign guidelines for management of severe sepsis and septic shock. Intensive Care Med. 2004;30(4):536–555.

Dharmarajan S, Hunt SR, Birnbaum EH, et al. The efficacy of nonoperative management of acute complicated diverticulitis. Dis Colon Rectum. 2011;54:663–671.

Ferrer R, Artigas A, Levy M, et al. Improvement in process of care and outcome after a multicenter severe sepsis educational program in Spain. JAMA. 2008;299(19):2294–2303.

Jones AR, Brown MD, Trzeciak S, et al. The effect of quantitative resuscitation strategy on mortality patients with sepsis: a meta-analysis. Crit Care Med. 2008;36(10):2734–2739.

Marti-Carvajal AJ, Sola I, Lathyris D, et al. Human recombinant activated protein C for severe sepsis. Cochrane Database Syst Rev. 2011;(4):CD004388.

117 Abdominal Compartment Syndrome

REBECCA PLEVIN and HEATHER L. EVANS

Presentation

A 28-year-old man is in a high-speed motorcycle collision with a large truck. He is intubated in the field for loss of consciousness and suspected closed head injury and has one episode of hypotension en route to the hospital. In the emergency room, he is noted to have a right arm laceration, an unstable pelvis, and a large scalp laceration. He immediately undergoes angiographic embolization of his bilateral internal iliac arteries and is transferred to the ICU, where he receives 15 L of crystalloid, 6 units of packed red blood cells, 8 units of FFP, and two 6-packs of platelets. After his blood pressure normalizes, he undergoes CT scan of the head, chest, abdomen, and pelvis, revealing a small subarachnoid hemorrhage and an open book pelvic fracture. There are no intra-abdominal injuries, but the intestines are noted to be edematous. An external fixation device is placed on the pelvis for stability. In the next 24 hours, the patient develops progressive hypoxemic respiratory failure and increasing peak airway pressures, persistent hypotension unresponsive to further fluid resuscitation, oliguria, and rising creatinine. On physical exam, his abdomen is distended and tense to palpation.

Differential Diagnosis

While creating the differential diagnosis of abdominal distention and organ failure following trauma, the clinician must first rule out life-threatening causes of these symptoms. In this patient who is persistently hypotensive despite massive volume resuscitation, the immediate concern is a missed intra-abdominal injury. Blood vessel injury leading to hemoperitoneum or bowel ischemia could cause this patient's symptoms. Hollow viscus injury and intraperitoneal contamination with bowel contents must also be considered given the patient's mechanism of injury and current presentation, which could be due to septic causes.

Ileus is common following severe trauma, particularly in the setting of massive fluid resuscitation. It is typically self-limited and improves with time. However, ongoing shock and fluid resuscitation could prolong the duration of an ileus. Other less benign causes of abdominal distention, such as *Clostridium difficile* colitis, must also be ruled out. This bacterial infection can lead to massive bowel wall edema and ileus, which would explain the patient's progressive abdominal distention and septic symptoms. *C. difficile* is less likely in a newly hospitalized patient, but as there is no background information about his prior health and antibiotic history, colitis must remain on the differential to avoid missing a catastrophic complication such as bowel perforation. This infection should be placed higher on the differential if the patient receives antibiotics for sepsis or has a significant leukocytosis, even in the absence of diarrhea.

Bowel obstruction is possible given the patient's abdominal distention. Physical exam would help elucidate inciting factors such as an abdominal wall hernia or scars suggestive of prior abdominal surgery. In the absence of these factors or other chronic medical conditions, bowel obstruction in a young man is less likely. Abdominal distention is a frequent first sign of Ogilvie's syndrome (acute colonic pseudo-obstruction), but it does not typically present this early in the hospital course.

In addition to abdominal distention, the patient developed rapid multisystem organ failure (MSOF). The clinician must consider a systemic inflammatory response such as transfusion-related acute lung injury (TRALI) or adult respiratory distress syndrome in the differential. In addition to MSOF, each of these conditions can cause ileus due to release of inflammatory mediators and result in abdominal distention.

Workup

The first step in working up this patient is to obtain laboratory studies, specifically a complete blood count to evaluate for a drop in hemoglobin and hematocrit. Significant hematocrit decrease would necessitate surgical exploration of the abdomen to locate a bleeding source. Exploratory laparotomy would also be warranted if the patient showed peritoneal signs, as an unrecognized hollow viscus injury and intraperitoneal contamination would quickly lead to sepsis and death if unrecognized. In the absence of immediate indications for operative intervention, imaging studies would be useful. Plain radiographs of the abdomen to look for free air or ultrasound to look for free fluid are faster than CT scan and do not require the patient to be moved from the ICU. Of course, if he were stable enough, a CT scan would provide important additional information about the patient's injuries.

In the absence of immediate indicators for surgical intervention, the adequacy of the patient's resuscitation should be evaluated. Given his MSOF and hypotension, sepsis is within the differential, so the patient must be optimized from a medical standpoint while the clinician searches for an infectious source. Central monitoring must be placed and resuscitation started with resuscitation endpoints according to the Surviving Sepsis Campaign guidelines.

There are a number of possible explanations for the sudden increase in peak airway pressures. Pneumothorax must be ruled out by chest x-ray (CXR), and respiratory therapy should be involved to evaluate for airway obstruction with airway secretions or foreign body. Bronchoscopy should be conducted if foreign body (e.g., a missing tooth) is high on the differential. The patient's decreased urine output should be investigated by checking the position of the Foley catheter and ruling out catheter obstruction. Obtaining urine electrolytes and calculating the fractional excretion of sodium (FeNa) would be useful to evaluate for acute tubular necrosis.

Presentation Continued

As part of his workup, a central venous catheter was placed and the central venous pressure measured at 15 mm Hg. Peak airway pressures on the ventilator >50 mm Hg, and CXR did not show a pneumothorax or evidence of airway plugging. The patient's urine output remained <5 mL/h. When he was stable enough for transport, a follow-up CT scan was done and was negative for free air or missed solid organ injuries. However, the CT did show distended, edematous bowel, moderate ascites, and narrowing of the inferior vena cava (IVC). The patient had a Foley catheter placed during his initial trauma workup and bladder pressures were measured. The initial bladder pressure was six, and as the patient's abdominal distention increased his bladder pressure rose to 18. The bladder pressure was 23 when the patient

began exhibiting signs of renal, cardiovascular, and respiratory compromise.

Based on this workup, the patient was surmised to have abdominal compartment syndrome (ACS), but unrecognized injury could not be completely ruled out, as a hollow viscus injury might not show up on CT scan and might cause the patient's ascites. Diagnostic paracentesis (and possible therapeutic) is one option at this point, but due to the patient's significant bowel edema, exploratory laparotomy and decompression of the abdomen was deemed the more appropriate next step.

Discussion

ACS is defined as "sustained intra-abdominal pressure (IAP) >20 mm Hg (with or without an abdominal perfusion pressure [APP] <60 mm Hg) that is associated with new organ dysfunction/failure." Intra-abdominal hypertension (IAH) also involves elevated IAP but does not result in organ dysfunction. IAH is defined as a pathologic sustained IAP ≥12 mm Hg. IAH is graded based on the degree of hypertension (Table 1). Risk factors for ACS include massive fluid resuscitation and tissue edema, abdominal surgery, ileus, sepsis, and hemorrhage. ACS is therefore most often found in the most critically ill of ICU patients. The prevalence of IAH and ACS has varied from study to study based on the criteria used to define each condition, but in a multicenter point prevalence study the prevalence of IAH and ACS was found to be 50.5% and 8.2%, respectively.

The different types of ACS are differentiated by their respective causes. Primary ACS occurs after injury or disease of the abdominopelvic organs leads to increased IAP, such as with hemorrhage from a large liver laceration or a ruptured abdominal aortic aneurysm. Secondary ACS results from factors external to the abdominal compartment. ACS following massive fluid resuscitation and resulting bowel edema is a classic example of secondary ACS. IAH can be broken down into hyperacute, acute, subacute, and chronic based on the length of time over which the condition

TABLE 1. Grading System for Intra-Abdominal Hypertension

Grade I: IAP 12–15 mmHg
Grade II: IAP 16–20 mmHg
Grade III: IAP 21–25 mmHg
Grade IV: IAP ≥25 mmHg

develops (seconds, hours, days, and months to years, respectively). Hyperacute IAH is usually the result of physiologic processes such as sneezing or Valsalva. Chronic IAH occurs in pregnancy, liver failure, ascites, and intra-abdominal tumor. These subtypes, of course, do not always require intervention.

While measurement of IAP is the gold standard for diagnosing ACS, CT scan can provide useful clues to the diagnosis. Intrahepatic IVC narrowing may occur as a result of abdominal pressure preventing adequate filling. Bowel walls may appear thickened secondary to edema and the diaphragms may appear elevated. The patient may have a "round belly sign," defined as an anteroposterior:transverse ratio >0.8 when measured at the level where the left renal vein crosses the aorta.

ACS is clinically significant because it increases a patient's risk of developing respiratory, cardiovascular, renal, gastrointestinal, and neurologic dysfunction. These conditions are associated with increased ICU time and morbidity, and IAH/ACS are independent predictors of mortality in ICU patients. IAH and ACS are most frequently diagnosed using modifications of the Kron technique, whereby bladder pressure is measured using a urinary catheter (**Table 2**). There are several commercially available products for measuring bladder pressures. "Home-made" devices to measure bladder pressure can also be assembled, but it is important to remember that these devices have downsides, including potentially less reliable results, increased risk of urinary tract infection, and increased time required to obtain data.

It is important to note that there are several factors that may affect IAP. Pregnancy and morbid obesity can cause chronically elevated IAP. In hospitalized patients, sepsis, abdominal surgery, and mechanical ventilation may lead to elevated IAP. In order to be considered diagnostic for ACS, the elevated IAP pressure must be sustained and associated with a new pathologic process in one or more organ systems.

Nonoperative Management

Nonoperative management in the early stages of IAP may prevent further progression to ACS and save the patient from undergoing a decompressive laparotomy (**Table 3**). There are two main techniques by which IAP can be managed. The first is by decreasing the "mass effect" of intra-abdominal contents on tissue perfusion. By removing unnecessary contents from the abdomen, there is more space for edematous bowel. This allows the bowel to take up more space in the abdominal cavity without increasing abdominal pressure and decreasing tissue perfusion. The second mechanism involves improving abdominal wall compliance to increase abdominal cavity volume. The type of intervention chosen depends on many factors, including the reason for ACS developing, other diagnoses in the differential, and patient comorbidities. For example, if missed injury remains a concern, surgery is appropriate, whereas surgical intervention should be avoided if possible in a patient with severe cirrhosis or other severe medical comorbidities.

Surgical Treatment

When medical management of IAH fails and a patient develops ACS, surgical decompression of the abdomen is warranted. The goal is to decrease IAP with the aim of improving perfusion to the affected organs. There is no consensus among experts regarding an IAP value that requires surgical intervention. Rather, surgery is necessary when there is evidence of organ dysfunction despite optimal medical therapy using the methods described above. Delaying decompression leads to further tissue ischemia, organ failure, and increased mortality.

TABLE 2. The Modified Kron Technique for Measuring Bladder Pressure

Measuring Bladder Pressure

1. Insert 18-gauge IV catheter into the culture port of the Foley catheter, remove needle.
2. Attach IV catheter to pressure tubing.
3. Attach tubing to 1-L NS, 60-mL Luer lock syringe, and disposable pressure transducer.
4. Position patient supine and zero transducer at the midaxillary line.
5. Inject 25 mL saline into the urinary bladder and clamp Foley catheter distal to the culture port.
6. Measure bladder pressure at end-expiration.

TABLE 3. Nonoperative Management of Increased IAH

Techniques for Nonoperative Management of ACS

Decrease mass effect	Evacuate intraluminal contents: NGT, colonic decompression, minimize enteral nutrition, prokinetic agents
	Remove space-occupying lesions: surgical debridement/excision, percutaneous drainage of fluid collections
	Optimize fluid status: avoid excessive IVF, target daily fluid balance net even to negative 3 L, diuresis, hemofiltration
	Optimize tissue perfusion: keep APP ≥60 mm Hg with judicious IVF, vasoactive medications
Increase abdominal wall compliance	Adequate sedation/analgesia, reverse Trendelenburg/elevate head of bed, remove constrictive abdominal dressings, pharmacologic paralysis

TABLE 4. Key Technical Steps to Creating an Abdominal Vacuum Pack

Key Technical Steps

1. Incise ~1-in slits in a variety of locations on a large plastic drape.
2. If possible, drape the exposed bowel with omentum.
3. Lay the drape flat in a subfascial position, taking care to cover all abdominal contents and to pack the drape into the paracolic gutters.
4. Cover drape with sterile gauze.
5. Place two flat Jackson-Pratt drains on top of the gauze.
6. Cover the wound with sterile towels and an iodine impregnated polyurethane drape (3 M Ioban; 3 M Healthcare, St. Paul, Minnesota) and place drains to low continuous suction.

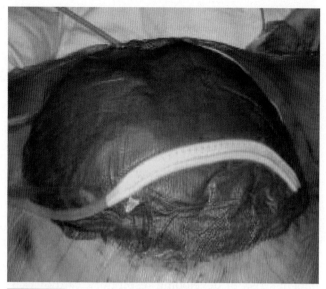

FIGURE 1 • Vacuum-packed abdomen.

Surgical treatment consists of decompressive laparotomy. If space-occupying lesions are present, they should be evacuated at this time. In the past, the abdomen was often closed primarily, but there has been a shift toward staged closure in order to avoid closing the fascia immediately. Using a temporary abdominal closure (TAC) decreases the risk of ACS recurrence, facilitates a second look into the abdomen if necessary, and is often easier than attempting to close the abdomen when significant bowel edema is present.

Methods of addressing the abdomen following decompressive laparotomy include prosthetic mesh, the Bogota bag, vacuum packing (often used in damage control laparotomy following trauma, see **Table 4**), and negative pressure systems such as vacuum-assisted closure devices. In addition to decreasing the risk of further ACS and allowing access to the abdomen if needed, vacuum packs and negative pressure devices have the additional benefit of removing abdominal exudate **(Figure 1)**. However, care must be taken with wound vacuums to apply the devices correctly in order to minimize the risk of enterocutaneous fistula formation.

Postoperative Management

Patients are still at risk for ACS after surgical decompression. If the fascia is closed, either by primary approximation or with prosthetic mesh, IAP may again become elevated. Even with vacuum packs or negative pressure system, recurrent ACS is possible, particularly if massive fluid resuscitation continues. It is thought that these systems do not always allow for necessary expansion of intra-abdominal volume during postoperative resuscitation and reactive tissue edema.

Because patients remain at risk for ACS following decompressive laparotomy, postoperative care focuses on decreasing IAP by the same methods described above (see "Nonoperative Management"). Bladder

pressures should be monitored postoperatively, and the clinician must remain vigilant for further signs of organ dysfunction that could indicate a repeat episode of ACS. Repeat ACS episodes are an indication for second look and release of the TAC.

Patients who undergo laparotomy for ACS need eventual abdominal closure. However, prolonged hospitalization with an open abdomen/vacuum pack often leads to tissue contraction and loss of domain, which makes it difficult or impossible to close the abdomen in a one-stage procedure. These patients may require mesh to augment fascial closure, skin grafting to achieve complete soft tissue coverage, and finally component separation to maintain long-term abdominal wall integrity. Each step may require months of preparation and recovery. Patients with ACS can undergo treatment from months to years before the abdomen is completely "closed."

Case Conclusion

The patient is taken to the operating room and undergoes exploratory laparotomy. No intra-abdominal sources of bleeding or other injuries are identified, but the patient's intestines are boggy and edematous. A vacuum pack is placed intraoperatively and the patient returns to the ICU for hemodynamic monitoring including bladder pressure measurements every 4 hours. He is taken back to the operating room for reapplication of the vacuum pack the following day after his peak pressures and acute renal failure, which had improved slightly the prior day, worsen overnight in conjunction with bladder pressure increase from 21 to 40. His bowel is increasingly edematous, but there is no frank intestinal necrosis. Over the following weeks, the patient's fascia is partially closed, and he is left with a midline abdominal incisional hernia that is repaired with Vicryl mesh once his bowel edema decreases. He stabilizes hemodynamically, his renal function improves, and he is successfully extubated. He is discharged to a skilled nursing facility with wound vacuum in place over his midline soft tissue defect, which decreases in size over several months. Split-thickness skin grafting is used to cover the remaining exposed subcutaneous tissue, and 1 year later, the patient returns to the operating room for component separation and restoration of abdominal wall integrity.

TAKE HOME POINTS

- ACS affects multiple organ systems; therefore, during evaluation of a patient with increased IAP, it is important to rule out other causes of injury to each affected organ system.
- IAH: sustained pathologic IAP ≥12 mm Hg. ACS: sustained pathologic IAP >20 mm Hg accompanied by new organ dysfunction/failure.
- The modified Kron technique is the gold standard for measuring IAP, whereby the intracystic pressure is measured after injecting 25 mL of saline into the urinary bladder.
- IAH may be treated nonoperatively by evacuating intraluminal contents, increasing abdominal compliance, optimizing fluid status, and optimizing tissue perfusion.

- Surgical decompression is necessary when signs of organ dysfunction emerge despite best nonoperative management. TAC is advocated by many in order to decrease the risk of subsequent ACS episodes and facilitate second looks.
- Bladder pressures should be measured even after decompressive laparotomy because compartment syndrome can occur even with TAC.
- Enterocutaneous fistulae are a known complication of temporary negative pressure dressings.

SUGGESTED READINGS

Al-Bahrani AZ, et al. A prospective evaluation of CT features predictive of intra-abdominal hypertension and abdominal compartment syndrome in critically ill surgical patients. Clin Radiol. 2006;62:676–682.

Cheatham ML. Nonoperative management of intraabdominal hypertension and abdominal compartment syndrome. World J Surg. 2009;33(6):1116–1122.

Dellinger R, et al. Surviving Sepsis Campaign: international guidelines for management of severe sepsis and septic shock: 2008. Intensive Care Med. 2007;34(1):17–60.

Gracias V, et al. Abdominal compartment syndrome in the open abdomen. Arch Surg. 2002;137:1298–1300.

Kron IL, Harman PK, Nolan SP. The measurement of intra-abdominal pressure as a criterion for abdominal re-exploration. Ann Surg. 1984;199(1):28–30.

Malbrain ML. Different techniques to measure intra-abdominal pressure (IAP): time for a critical re-appraisal. Intensive Care Med. 2004;30(3):357–371.

Malbrain ML, et al. Prevalence of intra-abdominal hypertension in critically ill patients: a multicentre epidemiological study. Intensive Care Med. 2004;30(5):822–829.

Malbrain ML, et al. Results from the international conference of experts on intra-abdominal hypertension and abdominal compartment syndrome. I. Definitions. Intensive Care Med. 2006;32(11):1722–1732.

Reintam A, et al. Primary and secondary intra-abdominal hypertension–different impact on ICU outcome. Intensive Care Med. 2008;34(9):1624–1631.

Sugrue M. Abdominal compartment syndrome. Curr Opin Crit Care. 2005;11(4):333–338. (Review.)

Sugrue M, Buhkari Y. Intra-abdominal pressure and abdominal compartment syndrome in acute general surgery. World J Surg. 2009;33(6):1123–1127.

118 Nutritional Support in the Critically Ill Surgery Patient

KYLE J. VAN ARENDONK and ELLIOTT R. HAUT

Presentation

A 35-year-old multisystem trauma victim presents after a high-speed motorcycle crash. After undergoing embolization for bleeding secondary to his open book pelvic fracture, he developed abdominal compartment syndrome requiring decompressive laparotomy. The operation revealed multiple liver lacerations and a small bowel perforation that was primarily repaired. Over the next several days, he experienced a significant systemic inflammatory response and multiple organ dysfunction syndrome requiring the use of vasopressors and mechanical ventilation.

Discussion

The above patient suffering from major multisystem trauma is a common scenario managed by the surgical critical care team. One of the many challenges facing the team is finding a way to provide nutrition through the long ICU course that invariably ensues. The first two issues that must be addressed are when to begin nutrition and via what route that nutrition should be provided.

Timing. The benefits of early enteral nutrition in the critically ill and injured patients have been well established. Ideally, enteral nutrition should be initiated within the first 24 to 48 hours following ICU admission. Early provision of enteral nutrition dampens the inflammatory response and is associated with lower mortality, decreased morbidity, and improved outcomes.

Enteral versus Parenteral. The enteral route is preferred over the parenteral route whenever possible because of both the benefits of enteral nutrition and the risks associated with parenteral nutrition. Enteral nutrition has been shown to stimulate the production of secretory IgA, preserve upper respiratory tract immunity, maintain the intestinal brush border, preserve gut-associated lymphoid tissue, and prevent the translocation of bacteria across the intestinal wall, all leading to a decrease in infectious complications in surgical ICU patients.

Enteral nutrition also avoids the many risks inherent to parenteral nutrition, including mechanical complications of central venous access placement (i.e., pneumothorax, hemothorax, arterial puncture, etc.), line sepsis, electrolyte disturbances, and liver dysfunction. With the use of parenteral nutrition, gut disuse leads to mucosal atrophy, bacterial overgrowth, diminished blood flow, and decreased gut immunity, all of which may lead to increased translocation of bacteria across the intestinal wall.

Enteral Nutrition

Routes for Enteral Nutrition: Enteral feeds can be provided through several routes. Gastric feeds can be provided via an orogastric or a nasogastric tube or via a gastrostomy tube, placed either surgically, endoscopically (percutaneous endoscopic gastrostomy [PEG] tube) or percutaneously via interventional radiology. Postpyloric feeds can be given via a nasoduodenal or a nasojejunal tube, a surgical jejunostomy tube, or a PEG tube with a jejunal extension (PEG-J).

Bedside placement of nasoduodenal tubes can be time-consuming and at times difficult. The critical care and surgical teams should plan ahead whenever possible and have a nasoduodenal tube placed intraoperatively under direct manipulation in patients undergoing laparotomy who are expected to need enteral nutrition access. When a nasoduodenal feeding tube is placed in the ICU, a two-step procedure should be utilized to avoid inadvertent bronchial placement and the potential complications that can result **(Table 1 and Figure 1)**. In addition, taking the small amount of extra time to secure the tube to the nose (i.e., via a commercial device such as the AMT bridle™) after placement is confirmed can increase the likelihood that the enteral tube stays in position through periods of patient agitation and patient repositioning.

No evidence exists for a mortality benefit with postpyloric feeds rather than gastric feeds. Most studies have also failed to show a significant difference in the rate of ventilator-associated pneumonia with postpyloric feeds, although lower rates of regurgitation and aspiration have been seen. Given these concerns over the risk of aspiration with gastric feeds, some providers suggest that critically ill patients at high risk of aspiration should preferentially be fed via a postpyloric route, especially if showing signs of intolerance to

TABLE 1. Two-step Procedure for Nasoduodenal Feeding Tube Placement

1. Prior to placement, estimate the length of tube needed to extend just below the patient's carina (typically about 30 cm).
2. With the stylet in, insert the tube to the measured length and obtain a chest x-ray to confirm that the tube is midline (in the esophagus) rather than extending laterally (toward the lung) into either bronchi **(Figure 1A)**.
3. After midline position is confirmed by x-ray, advance the tube with the stylet to the desired position.
4. Obtain an abdominal x-ray to confirm successful positioning **(Figure 1B)**.
5. Reposition as needed.
6. When correct placement is confirmed, fasten the tube securely and remove the stylet.
7. Begin tube feeds.

gastric feeds. However, gastric feeds can still be used safely in the majority of patients.

Monitoring of Enteral Feeding: One way to monitor the tolerance of gastric feeds and possible risk of aspiration is to measure gastric residual volumes, which can be checked approximately every 6 hours and are considered acceptable when less than approximately 200 to 300 mL (exact values vary by institution). Repeated high gastric residuals should encourage the transition to postpyloric feeding, although repeatedly holding tube feeds when gastric residuals are high in the absence of any clinical signs of feeding intolerance is discouraged.

A common problem in the ICU patient receiving enteral feeds is the frequent stopping of enteral feeds for frequent, often daily, trips to the operating room or to diagnostic testing. Tube feeds at an hourly goal rate cannot provide full nutrition when they are routinely infusing for only a small portion of each 24-hour period. If these patients are already intubated or have a tracheostomy in place, the need for anesthesia induction for intubation is precluded and tube feeds can therefore safely be left running during these periods in order to maximize nutritional support. In the case of postpyloric feeding, the risk of aspiration even when induction of anesthesia is required is exceedingly low. Nutrition should therefore be continued during procedures or diagnostic testing whenever possible.

Enteral Nutrition in Specific Patient Population: Clinical scenarios do exist in which enteral nutrition must be avoided. For example, bowel perforation, bowel obstruction, and discontinuity of the gastrointestinal tract (i.e., damage control surgery) preclude enteral feeding. However, research is showing the number of these conditions is fewer than previously thought. In cases of acute pancreatitis, enterocutaneous fistulae, and the open abdomen, enteral nutrition now has been shown to be safe and even beneficial, in contrast to the historical teaching to avoid enteral feeds in these situations.

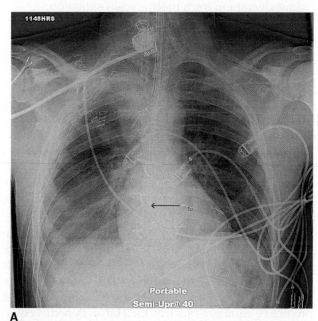

A

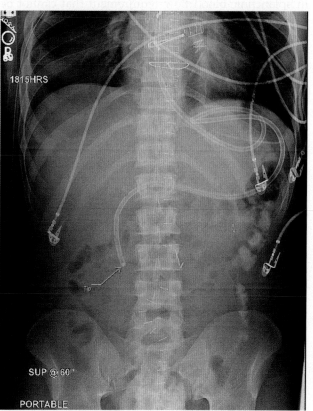

B

FIGURE 1 • Radiographs showing (**A**) initial insertion of the feeding tube into the distal esophagus to confirm midline positioning beyond the carina and (**B**) advancement of the feeding tube into a postpyloric position.

For acute pancreatitis, increasing evidence shows that early enteral nutrition improves outcomes. Gastric and jejunal feeds may even provide similar benefit, contrary to intuition that would suggest that gastric feeds would stimulate the pancreas and worsen the inflammatory response. For proximal enterocutaneous fistulae, enteral feeds can be provided distal to the fistula. For more distal fistulae, proximal enteral feeds can be given, and the length of small bowel present prior to the fistula will determine if enteral nutrition will be adequate. In these cases, as well as in cases of short gut syndrome, the addition of "supplemental" parenteral nutrition may be necessary.

Historically, enteral nutrition has also been delayed for several days until bowel function has returned (as marked by presence of bowel sounds, passage of flatus, etc.) after any gastrointestinal surgery. In the general ICU population, however, these signs are not necessarily reliable, and enteral nutrition should not be delayed based upon the lack of bowel sounds or passage of flatus and stool.

Finally, enteral nutrition should be avoided in patients with significant hemodynamic instability. In patients requiring vasopressor support or large-volume fluid or blood product resuscitation, enteral nutrition is typically withheld until the patient is more hemodynamically stable and fully resuscitated. Although ischemic bowel is a rare complication of enteral nutrition, theoretically enteral nutrition may require an increase in splanchnic blood flow requirement that cannot be supported in low cardiac output states. For this reason, hemodynamic instability has been considered a contraindication to early enteral feeding. However, enteral support is often provided to patients on stable low doses of vasopressors while watching carefully for any signs of intolerance.

Parenteral Nutrition

When early enteral nutrition is *not* possible, decision making depends on the patient's nutritional status prior to admission to the ICU. No nutritional support is necessary for the first 7 days in previously healthy patients without evidence of malnutrition, after which parenteral nutrition should then be initiated. However, if patients have evidence of malnutrition prior to the episode of critical illness, parenteral nutrition should be initiated as soon as possible. Parenteral nutrition can be stopped once enteral nutrition has begun and is able to provide a majority of the patient's energy requirements.

Parenteral nutrition can also be used to supplement enteral support in cases in which enteral support cannot meet a patient's full caloric requirements after approximately 7 days. Maintaining at least a portion of patients' nutritional support via the enteral route is important, as even "trickle" or "trophic" feeds (usually considered

10 to 30 mL/h) may be beneficial in maintaining the intestinal brush border and preventing mucosal atrophy.

Parenteral nutrition requires adequate venous access. Peripheral parenteral nutrition (PPN) is a lower osmolality solution that can safely be given through a peripheral vein, although it is rarely able to provide full nutritional support. PPN is often used as a bridge until full enteral support can be achieved or adequate venous access is obtained for central parenteral nutrition (CPN). CPN consists of a high osmolality solution that can provide full nutrition but must be given through a central venous line.

Several approaches can help decrease line sepsis when using parenteral nutrition. Lines should be placed in a standardized fashion using a checklist to ensure adherence to best practices for sterility. A peripherally inserted central catheter or a single lumen central line is preferred over the use of any multiple lumen catheters because of the lower risk of line sepsis. The subclavian vein is preferred (vs. internal jugular or femoral) given its lower rate of infection. The central line should be a new line inserted with a fresh stick rather than changed over a guide wire at a preexisting central line site. Ideally, the central line should be limited to provision of parenteral nutrition ("dedicated") without any other use (i.e., blood draws or medication administration).

Presentation Continued

After a long course in the SICU, this patient was slowly weaning from mechanical ventilation. His prealbumin was measured to be 25 (normal range, 18 to 38). His nitrogen balance was calculated to be positive. A metabolic cart was completed, and his respiratory quotient (RQ) was 1.1. His tube feeds were adjusted appropriately. His glycemic control, initially maintained with an insulin drip, was converted to a subcutaneous regimen.

Calculating Nutritional Requirements

Energy requirements vary based on the clinical situation, but a general estimate is 25 to 30 kcal/kg/d. Higher energy requirements can be seen in patients with burns, sepsis, and multisystem trauma. Energy requirements can also be calculated using published predictive equations such as the Harris-Benedict equation **(Table 2)**, which gives a measure of resting energy expenditure (REE) that can then be adjusted by an activity or a stress factor to calculate total daily energy expenditure **(Table 3)**. Finally, indirect calorimetry can

TABLE 2. Useful Formulas

Harris-Benedict equation (kcal/24 h) for estimating resting energy expenditure (REE)	REE (men) = 66.5 + (13.8 × weight in kg) + (5 × height in cm) − (6.8 × age)
	REE (women) = 655 + (9.6 × weight in kg) + (1.8 × height in cm) − (4.7 × age)
Caloric content of nutrients/ infusions	Carbohydrate: 4 kcal/g
	Dextrose: 3.4 kcal/g
	Protein: 4 kcal/g
	Fat: 9 kcal/g
	Ethanol: 7 kcal/g
	Propofol: 1.1 kcal/mL
	10% lipid solution: 1.1 kcal/mL
	20% lipid solution: 2 kcal/mL
Nitrogen balance	Nitrogen balance = (protein intake ÷ 6.25) − (UUN + 4)
Respiratory quotient (RQ)	Carbohydrate: 1.0
	Protein: 0.8
	Fat: 0.7
	Underfeeding: <0.7
	Overfeeding: >1.0

UUN = urine urea nitrogen

TABLE 4. Sample Calculations

	Goal: provide 70-kg patient with 25 kcal/kg/d and 1.0 g protein/kg/d
	70 kg × 25 kcal/kg/d = 1,750 kcal/d
	70 kg × 1.0 g protein/kg/d = 70 g protein/d
Tube feeds	Chosen tube feed contains 1.5 kcal/mL and 0.06 g protein/mL
	1,750 kcal/d ÷ 1.5 kcal/mL = 1,167 mL/d
	1,167 mL ÷ 24 h = 49 mL/h
	1,167 mL × 0.06 g protein/mL = 70 g protein
	The tube feeds can be run continuously at 49 mL/h, which will provide 25 kcal/kg/d and 1.0 g protein/kg/d.
CPN	Chosen CPN solution contains 70 g amino acids and 285 g dextrose in 1,000 mL and will be added to 250 mL of 20% lipid emulsion.
	Total volume = 1,250 mL
	1,250 mL ÷ 24 h = 52 mL/h
	70 g amino acid × 4 kcal/g = 280 kcal
	285 g dextrose × 3.4 kcal/g = 969 kcal
	250 mL × 2 kcal/mL = 500 kcal
	Total kcal/d = 1,749
	1,749 kcal/d ÷ 70 kg = 25 kcal/kg/d
	The CPN can be run continuously at 52 mL/h, which will provide 25 kcal/kg and 1.0 g protein/kg/d.

CPN = central parenteral nutrition

also be used. Indirect calorimetry uses a "metabolic cart" to measure the amount of oxygen consumed and carbon dioxide eliminated in order to calculate a patient's actual (as opposed to predicted) REE. In order to maintain accuracy, indirect calorimetry is typically limited to patients who are on mechanical ventilation and who are at a relatively steady state.

Carbohydrates, protein, and fat provide 4, 4, and 9 kcal/g, respectively. Ethanol provides 7 kcal/g. In clinical settings, dextrose, with 3.4 kcal/kg, should typically be used rather than carbohydrate in calculations. For parenteral nutrition, 10% and 20% lipid solutions contain 1.1 and 2 kcal/mL, respectively. In the ICU setting, infusions of propofol also provide significant calories that must be considered (1.1 kcal/mL) (Table 2). In general, approximately 60% of calories should come from carbohydrate, 25% to 30% from fat, and 10% to 15% from protein. Protein seems to be the nutrient most important for wound healing, immune function, and preventing the loss of lean body mass. Critically ill patients are therefore often given

TABLE 3. Approximate Stress Factor Multipliers for REE

Elective surgery	1.2
Multisystem trauma	1.3–1.5
Sepsis	1.5–1.8
Burns	1.5–2.0

additional protein based upon either simple equations (estimating 1 to 2 g/kg/d of protein need) or by calculating their actual nitrogen balance (see example in **Table 4**).

Monitoring Adequacy of Nutritional Support

The concept of nitrogen balance is based on the balance between anabolism and catabolism. Providing nutritional support to the critically ill patient is meant to shift this balance to the anabolic state so that the patient's protein does not need to be utilized for gluconeogenesis (catabolism). The ideal state of positive nitrogen balance is then a greater intake of nitrogen than excretion of nitrogen, while a negative nitrogen balance is to be avoided. Nitrogen balance is calculated by subtracting total nitrogen losses (urine, stool, insensible losses) from nitrogen intake **(Table 2)**. Nitrogen intake is calculated based on 6.25 g of protein containing 1 g of nitrogen, while nitrogen losses are estimated by measuring a 24-hour urine urea nitrogen (UUN) and adding an estimate of stool and insensible losses.

Adequacy of nutrition can also be estimated using the respiratory quotient (RQ), which is calculated via indirect calorimetry. The RQ is the ratio of carbon dioxide produced to oxygen consumed. Each of the major nutrients has a unique RQ: protein (RQ = 0.8), fat (RQ = 0.7), and carbohydrates (RQ = 1.0). Pure carbohydrate metabolism therefore has an RQ of 1.0, while pure fat oxidation has an RQ of 0.7. The ideal RQ on an individual patient is approximately 0.8. An RQ under 0.7 represents underfeeding with resulting lipolysis and ketosis. An RQ over 1.0 represents overfeeding **(Table 2)**.

Reassessment of the adequacy of nutritional support in meeting requirements should be done at regular intervals. In addition to indirect calorimetry and the other methods mentioned, a number of laboratory values also serve as markers of adequate nutrition. Albumin and transferrin levels have half-lives of approximately 20 and 10 days and so do not serve as ideal markers of changes made in the short term. Prealbumin is a more useful marker with its shorter half-life of about 2 days. Retinol-binding protein is a relatively new marker with an even shorter half-life of about 12 hours. Unfortunately, however, each of these markers also reflects the acute phase response to critical illness and therefore may not accurately reflect nutritional status in the ICU setting.

Critically ill patients should have their glucose levels monitored closely. Strict glucose control, keeping glucose levels 80 to 110 mg/dL, was accepted as the standard of care after one large trial showed reduced sepsis, reduced ICU length of stay, and lower hospital mortality with strict control compared to "conventional" therapy (keeping glucose levels <200 mg/dL). However, more recently, another large trial has brought this practice into question after showing increased mortality in patients receiving strict glucose control compared to a more lenient approach (keeping glucose levels <180 mg/dL), thought to be due to a difference in episodes of hypoglycemia. Many institutions have now relaxed their goal for glucose control to approximately 100 to 150 mg/dL, although these targets may be different for specific patient populations (i.e., cardiac surgery) and change frequently with newly emerging research.

Overfeeding and Refeeding Syndrome

Overfeeding patients in the critical care setting should be avoided with the same vigilance that underfeeding is avoided. Overfeeding can cause harmful metabolic consequences, including hyperglycemia and hypertriglyceridemia. In addition, overfeeding can have deleterious effects on weaning from mechanical ventilation by burdening the patient with an extra load of carbon dioxide that must be expired. This diagnosis must be considered and ruled out in any patient who does not have another more obvious cause for failure to wean.

When initiating nutritional support in the critically ill, the critical care team must avoid the risk of refeeding syndrome. This condition typically occurs when the sudden introduction of nutrition in a relatively malnourished patient stimulates the release of insulin, causing phosphate, potassium and magnesium to shift intracellularly. The diagnosis is made when hypophosphatemia, hypokalemia, and hypomagnesemia are discovered after initiation of nutritional support in at-risk patients, such as those with prolonged malnutrition, excessive gastrointestinal losses, chronic alcohol abuse, metastatic cancer, and recent abdominal surgery, all of which lead to depletion of the above electrolytes. Refeeding syndrome can result in generalized muscle weakness and difficulty in weaning the patient from mechanical ventilation due to the depletion of ATP stores resulting from hypophosphatemia. The condition can be avoided by slowly reintroducing nutrition in patients at high risk of developing the syndrome.

Immunonutrition

More recently, the focus has shifted from nutritional *support* to nutritional *therapy* as a way to augment the immune system and dampen the systemic inflammatory response. In high-risk patients, immune-modulating enteral feeds containing supplements such as arginine, glutamine, omega-3 fatty acids and antioxidants such as selenium, vitamin C, and vitamin E have been studied. Additional research is needed regarding each of these individual additives, but immune-modulating formulas appear to have a variety of clinical benefits in the critically ill.

Case Conclusion

After weaning from mechanical ventilation, this patient was transferred from the ICU to the regular care floor. His tube feeds were continued while he regained swallowing function with the help of speech and language pathologists. He was able to support his nutrition with an oral diet before transfer to a rehabilitation facility.

Conclusion

The importance of appropriate nutritional support in the critically ill cannot be overemphasized. Failure to provide adequate nutrition has been shown to increase morbidity and mortality in the ICU. Appropriate nutritional support in the critically ill limits the inflammatory response and decreases the rate of ICU complications.

TAKE HOME POINTS

- Early nutrition is beneficial in critically ill patients.
- Enteral nutrition is preferable to parenteral nutrition whenever possible.
- Consider risks of gastric versus postpyloric feeding.
- Overfeeding should be avoided as much as underfeeding.
- Use objective data (i.e., laboratory values, nitrogen balance, and indirect calorimetry) to guide changes in nutritional support.

SUGGESTED READINGS

Al-Omran M, Albalawi ZH, Tashkandi MF, et al. Enteral versus parenteral nutrition for acute pancreatitis. Cochrane Database Syst Rev. 2010;(1):CD002837.

Finfer S, Chittock DR, Su SY, et al. Intensive versus conventional glucose control in critically ill patients. N Engl J Med. 2009;360(13):1283–1297.

Gramlich L, Kichian K, Pinilla J, et al. Does enteral nutrition compared to parenteral nutrition result in better outcomes in critically ill adult patients? A systematic review of the literature. Nutrition. 2004;20(10):843–848.

Marderstein EL, Simmons RL, Ochoa JB. Patient safety: effect of institutional protocols on adverse events related to feeding tube placement in the critically ill. J Am Coll Surg. 2004;199(1):39–47; discussion 47–50.

McClave SA, Martindale RG, Vanek VW, et al. Guidelines for the provision and assessment of nutrition support therapy in the adult critically ill patient: Society of Critical Care Medicine (SCCM) and American Society for Parenteral and Enteral Nutrition (A.S.P.E.N.). JPEN J Parenter Enteral Nutr. 2009;33(3):277–316.

Mehanna HM, Moledina J, Travis J. Refeeding syndrome: what it is, and how to prevent and treat it. BMJ. 2008;336(7659):1495–1498.

Ziegler TR. Parenteral nutrition in the critically ill patient. N Engl J Med. 2009;361(11):1088–1097.

119 Acute Liver Failure

BERNARD J. DUBRAY and CHRISTOPHER D. ANDERSON

Presentation

You are the on-call surgeon covering a rural community when you receive a page from the local emergency room (ER). The ER physician states there is a young girl he would like you to evaluate. "Eight years old. Her mother brought her in complaining that her skin has turned yellow and she's been itching incessantly over the last 12 hours." The emergency department (ED) physician goes on to explain his examination and notes that she has a "quite a tremor" along with "gingival bleeding."

You arrive on the scene and conduct a thorough history and physical examination. This was a previously healthy girl who this morning awoke complaining of itching along with nausea and some malaise. Throughout the course of the day, her mother noted the change in skin color. When prompted, the girl admits her urine has also been "coke-colored." On exam, you note scleral icterus as well as the gingival bleeding the ED physician had told you about. A nonlateralizing pill-rolling tremor is also present. This does not extinguish with movement, and when you ask the girl to walk across the room, she stumbles slightly. Her chest is clear and heartbeat regular. Your abdominal exam is notable for hepatomegaly.

In light of your findings, you probe the mother further prior to initiating a workup. She reveals that her sister "had a liver problem" when she was young, but "she got a transplant and is doing fine now."

Differential Diagnosis

Interference with the metabolism and excretion of bilirubin results in clinical jaundice, which can be categorized as prehepatic, hepatic, or posthepatic. Development of a differential diagnosis requires a thorough understanding of the physiologic mechanisms involved and should include the most likely, as well as the most morbid, diagnoses. The combination of acute jaundice and coagulopathy in an adolescent should raise the suspicion for hepatic dysfunction. Further workup and management, however, is dependent upon the precise etiology, which differs quite dramatically between adults and adolescents (Table 1). In adults, almost 50% of the cases of acute liver failure (ALF) can be attributed to acetaminophen overdose versus <20% in children. Other common causes in adults include nonacetaminophen drug toxicity and acute hepatitis B virus. Etiologies common in children include infectious hepatitis, metabolic disease, and autoimmune disease.

Evidence of palmar erythema, clubbing, gynecomastia, testicular atrophy, ascites, or spider nevi suggests a chronic component to hepatic dysfunction. Slit lamp examination can detect Kayser-Fleischer rings in patients presenting with Wilson's disease. Their presence, however, is only seen in 50% to 60% of patients with isolated hepatic involvement compared to 90% of patients with neurologic involvement.

Detection and monitoring of hepatic encephalopathy are another important exam tool that can guide further workup and management. Patients should undergo an initial assessment but then have serial examinations to detect subtle changes. Categorization of hepatic encephalopathy is based on changes in behavior, cognition, and neurologic exam and ranges from stages 0 (minimal to no evidence of encephalopathy) to 4 (coma) (Table 2).

Workup

The preliminary diagnostic workup in a patient suspected of having ALF begins with a battery of biochemical tests aimed at differentiating the possible etiologies. General tests to assess blood counts, electrolytes, and renal function are important. More specific tests include the liver function panel as well as a coagulation profile. Further laboratory tests that help differentiate etiologies of liver failure include a hepatitis panel, acetaminophen level, serum ceruloplasmin level, and serum copper level.

The development of encephalopathy within 8 weeks of liver injury in a person with a previously normal liver defines fulminant disease. The treatment of patients in this category is largely supportive but is dictated by the severity of the liver failure. Admission to a highly skilled, intensive care unit is necessary in all patients with fulminant liver failure in order to monitor the effects on multiple organ systems. Principles of care are aimed at ameliorating reversible causes of hepatocellular injury while supporting the multiorgan complications of liver failure.

TABLE 1. Differential Etiologies of ALF

Differential Etiologies of ALF	Common Examples in Children	Common Examples in Adults
Toxic	Acetaminophen, wild mushrooms, valproic acid, pyrrolizidine alkaloids	Acetaminophen, wild mushrooms, valproic acid
Infectious/viral	Herpes simplex, adenovirus, enterovirus, and paramyxovirus, and Epstein-Barr virus	Hepatitis A, hepatitis B, other viral hepatitis
Autoimmune	Autoimmune hepatitis, hemophagocytic lymphohistiocytosis, celiac disease, primary sclerosing cholangitis	Autoimmune hepatitis
Metabolic	Galactosemia, tyrosinemia, mitochondrial disorders, fatty acid oxidation disorders, Wilson's disease	Acute fatty liver of pregnancy, Reye's syndrome, Wilson's disease
Vascular/other		Budd-Chiari syndrome, ischemic hepatitis

ALF secondary to acetaminophen toxicity is an example of a potentially reversible injury. Hepatic glutathione stores are reduced following acetaminophen overdose, which are restored by administering N-acetylcysteine. If given within 8 hours of ingestion, N-acetylcysteine is likely to prevent serious hepatotoxicity and death from acetaminophen overdose.

The young girl's initial laboratory investigations are notable for a moderate transaminitis, elevated total bilirubin, and an INR of 3.5. Additionally, the patient's serum ceruloplasmin level is <5 mg/dL. Given the constellation of laboratory findings, your suspicion for a case of fulminant Wilson's disease is elevated.

Wilson's disease is a rare autosomal recessive genetic disorder of copper accumulation that typically presents in a 4:1 female:male ratio in patients between 5 and 50 years of age. Reduced biliary excretion of copper leads to its accumulation in the liver as well as other tissues, principally the brain. Hepatic dysfunction is the usual presenting feature; however, neuropsychiatric and hematologic complaints may also be involved.

The time course of presentation is variable, but can be acute, especially in children.

Diagnosis is dependent upon a high degree of clinical suspicion and can be made through a combination of physical and laboratory findings. The classic presentation of a young patient with decreased ceruloplasmin level and Kayser-Fleischer rings is only seen in about 50% of those diagnosed with Wilson's disease. Guidelines for diagnosing Wilson's disease have been proposed by the American Association for the Study of Liver Diseases and are useful in nonfulminant cases.

Whereas patients diagnosed with Wilson's disease following workup for elevated liver enzymes can undergo medical treatment to increase copper excretion, management of fulminant cases is similar to all causes of fulminant hepatic failure.

Diagnosis and Treatment

The onset of hepatic encephalopathy distinguishes fulminant liver failure from acute liver dysfunction. Any patient admitted with liver dysfunction who develops encephalopathy should be moved to an intensive care unit in a hospital with a liver transplant program. Nitrogenous substances that produce ammonia within the gastrointestinal tract are thought to contribute to the development of hepatic encephalopathy. Ammonia, which is a known neurotoxin, is efficiently cleared from the portal circulation in the healthy liver. Buildup, however, can occur in cases of ALF and contribute to encephalopathy. Medical treatments aim to either remove nitrogenous substances or prevent ammonia production, and are most effective in patients with a component of chronic liver failure.

Cerebral edema develops in 75% to 80% of patients with grade IV encephalopathy, which can have devastating consequences in ALF. Cerebral edema results in increased intracranial pressure (ICP) and brainstem herniation, which are among the leading causes of mortality from ALF. Initial management

TABLE 2. Stages of Hepatic Encephalopathy

Stage	Clinical	Reflexes	Neurologic
0	None	Normal	Normal
1	Confusion, mood disturbances, forgetfulness	Normal	Tremor, apraxia
2	Drowsy, inappropriate, decreased inhibitions	Hyperreflexive	Dysarthria, ataxia
3	Stuporous	Hyperreflexive, (+) Babinski	Rigidity
4	Comatose	Absent	Decorticate or decerebrate

focuses on reducing excess stimulation, protein intake, and avoiding sedating medications. Head elevation, hyperventilation, and hyperosmolarity are additional adjuncts in treatment. ICP monitoring in ALF remains controversial due to its invasive nature and failure to improve survival. Epidural catheters can significantly reduce bleeding complications and offers the safest approach. Currently, over 50% of U.S. transplant programs routinely use ICP monitoring to guide therapy in ALF.

Metabolic disturbances are common in ALF and include acid–base disorders as well as electrolyte abnormalities. An inability of the failing liver to clear lactate results in a lactic acidosis; however, this is often coupled with a respiratory alkalosis, producing a mixed acid/base disorder. Additionally, hypoglycemia can manifest as the liver begins to lose its ability to perform hepatic gluconeogenesis. Especially in the pediatric patient, maintenance of serum glucose is a paramount component of clinical management. Common electrolyte disturbances include hyponatremia, hypophosphatemia, and hypokalemia.

Hematologic complications arise from ALF as the ability of damaged hepatocytes to synthesize the proteins is diminished. Both pro- and anticoagulant proteins are reduced, which may explain the low risk of bleeding despite the elevations in PT/INR. Although there remains clinical management debate, many authors advocate avoidance of aggressive correction of coagulopathy except in cases of active bleeding. The correction of coagulopathy has not been shown to improve mortality and the volume load from plasma transfusion may worsen cerebral edema.

With advanced critical care monitoring and support, spontaneous recovery from ALF has increased from 15% to 40%. The introduction of liver transplantation improves survival to 60%, though deciding who will benefit from transplant remains problematic. Selection of patients for orthotopic liver transplantation (OLT) for ALF attempts to identify those least likely to have spontaneous recovery. Allografts remain a precious resource

Presentation Continued

Despite supportive care in a highly skilled intensive care unit, the young girl shows signs of decompensation. Whereas in the ER she was conversant, she now appears lethargic and listless. A repeat coagulation profile reveals that her INR has jumped from 2.5 to almost 9. With her mother at the bedside, you explain that the girl's liver is failing and without a transplant, she will almost certainly die.

TABLE 3. King's College Criteria

Acetaminophen	Nonacetaminophen
List for OLT if • pH < 7.3 • Arterial lactate > 3.0 mm/L following fluid resuscitation OR all three occur within 24 hours 1. Grade 3 or 4 encephalopathy 2. INR > 6.5 3. Creatinine > 3.4 mg/dL	List for OLT if • INR > 6.5 OR any three: • Age <10 or >40 • Jaundice >7 days before encephalopathy • INR > 3.5 • Bilirubin > 17 mg/dL • Unfavorable cause: Wilson's disease, idiosyncratic drug reaction, halothane toxicity, seronegative hepatitis

and the 1-year survival for those transplanted for ALF is less (60% to 80%) than those transplanted for chronic disease (80% to 90%). Multiple systems have been developed to help determine who is likely to have spontaneous recovery from ALF and while no system is flawless, the King's College criteria are the most widely accepted in predicting death/need for transplantation (Table 3).

Surgical Approach

Liver transplantation is a highly coordinated, multidisciplinary endeavor. Explanation regarding U.S. policy on organ allocation, donor hepatectomy, and organ preservation is beyond the scope of this chapter. The remainder will briefly describe the techniques of recipient hepatectomy and engrafting (Table 4).

TABLE 4. Key Technical Steps and Potential Pitfalls to Orthotopic Liver Transplantation

Key Technical Steps
Recipient Hepatectomy
1. Bilateral subcostal incision with midline extension.
2. Division of ligamentous attachments of the liver.
3. Skeletonization and division of the porta hepatis.
4. Isolation and division of retrohepatic cava.

Engraftment
1. Anastomosis of suprahepatic and infrahepatic vena cava.
2. Anastomosis of portal vein.
   • Portal reperfusion.
3. Anastomosis of hepatic artery.
   • Arterial reperfusion.
4. Biliary anastomosis.

Potential Pitfalls
• Difficult dissection in setting of cirrhosis or previous abdominal surgery.
• Excessive bleeding from coagulopathy, varices, and portal hypertension.
• Donor–recipient size mismatch.

Bicaval Liver Transplantation

OLT classically utilizes a bicaval technique, using vena cava interposition, and consists of the recipient hepatectomy followed by engraftment of the donor liver. Exposure is gained through a bilateral, subcostal incision with an upper midline extension—aptly referred to as the "Mercedes incision." Following inspection for any contraindication to transplant (i.e., extrahepatic malignancy), the ligamentous attachments of the liver can be divided for an unobstructed view of the porta hepatis. Essential dissection of the porta includes isolation and division of the common hepatic artery, common bile duct and portal vein.

With the liver free from ligamentous attachments, the retrohepatic cava can be encircled and clamped to gain vascular control. Division of the suprahepatic and infrahepatic vena cava frees the specimen, which can be removed from the operative field. The donor allograft, which has been prepared on the back table during the recipient hepatectomy, is then introduced into its orthotopic position in the right, upper quadrant. Anastomosis of the supra- and infrahepatic vena cava is performed using nonabsorbable, monofilament suture in a running fashion. As the infrahepatic caval anastomosis is nearing completion, the portal vein is flushed with either normal saline or lactated ringers solution to clear the graft of air and intravascular perfusate. Following completion of the portal anastomosis, if there is no evidence of bleeding, the bicaval clamps can be removed and the graft reperfused with portal circulation.

Depending on the arterial anatomy of the donor, the recipient hepatic artery is typically anastomosed at the junction of the gastroduodenal artery. Principles utilized during the venous anastomoses are adhered to for arterialization. Finally, the bile duct is reconstructed either primarily or via a Roux-en-Y biliary enterostomy.

Caval Preservation Techniques

The "piggyback" technique of OLT is an alternative method of venous reconstruction that obviates the need for venovenous bypass. Improvements in hemodynamic stability are achieved by keeping the retrohepatic cava in place, thus allowing increased venous return during the case. Instead of encircling the supra and infrahepatic cava during the recipient hepatectomy, the hepatic veins are isolated and ligated. A cloaca is then fashioned from the divided hepatic veins to receive the donor suprahepatic cava. After oversewing the infrahepatic donor vena cava, the remainder of the case proceeds as in the classic technique. The addition of a temporary portocaval anastomosis to the piggyback techniques is often employed. This improves hemodynamic stability and decreases mesenteric congestion during the anhepatic phase of the operation.

Split Liver Transplantation

Given the shortage of quality allografts for transplant, the utilization of split livers has become an important method to meet recipient demand. The liver is typically divided at the falciform ligament with the left lateral section going to a child and the remaining portion going to an adult. Utilization of this method requires an optimal graft and is not recommended in the setting of steatosis or extended criteria donors.

Special Intraoperative Considerations

Venovenous Bypass

Some centers that utilize the classic bicaval technique will bypass routinely, while others selectively. Centers that use venovenous bypass selectively have specific indications for bypass including hypotension following test clamp of the vena cava despite appropriate volume resuscitation, significant intraoperative mesenteric or intestinal edema, or fulminant hepatic failure. Venovenous bypass decompresses the splanchnic circulation while preserving cardiac preload from the lower extremities during the anhepatic phase. Cannulation of the femoral vein by Seldinger's technique bypasses systemic venous return from the lower extremities, which is received by the intrajugular vein. Likewise, the portal vein may be cannulated to bypass the portal venous system.

Portal Vein Thrombosis

Cases of thrombosed portal veins may be encountered frequently during the recipient engrafting and require special consideration. In the majority of cases, a portal endovenectomy can be performed to restore adequate inflow via the portal vein. When a thrombectomy or an endovenectomy cannot be performed, donor iliac veins vessels provide a suitable conduit, which can be anastomosed to the recipient superior mesenteric vein to bypass the thrombosis.

Aberrant Arterial Anatomy

Replaced hepatic arteries occur in 15% to 20% of the general population and require construction of a common inflow channel to receive the recipient hepatic artery. During the donor hepatectomy, iliac vessels are harvested should aberrant anatomy require vascular reconstruction in the recipient. Should the inflow be insufficient from the recipient, donor iliac vessels can also be used to fashion a conduit from the native aorta to the donor liver.

Biliary Considerations

Often the recipient bile duct is not suitable for end-to-end anastomosis, which can present an intraoperative challenge. In such circumstances, a Roux-en Y choledochojejunostomy should be fashioned to complete the biliary reconstruction. Patients with primary biliary disorders (e.g., primary sclerosing cholangitis) will also require a biliary–enteric anastomosis to avoid using a diseased recipient bile duct.

Postoperative Management

Attention in the early postoperative period is focused on graft function. Signs that the new liver is working include production of bile in the operating room, ability to wean vasopressor support, awakening from anesthesia, clearance of lactic acidosis, and normalization of liver function tests. Within the first 24 hours, the serum transaminases will be elevated but then should trend toward normal. Additionally, one should appreciate normalization of INR and resolution of hypoglycemia as the graft begins to assume its synthetic and endocrine functions. Deviations from the typical postoperative course should be taken seriously and evaluated fully.

Allograft Dysfunction

Functional delays from donor steatosis or prolonged preservation times can be anticipated in some cases following OLT. This, however, must be distinguished from structural problems. Whereas functional delays typically respond to supportive measures, structural problems are often related to vascular complications, which only worsen and have the potential to jeopardize the allograft. Failure to clear neurologically, hemodynamic instability, increasing liver function tests, and hypoglycemia are signs of graft dysfunction that deserve full evaluation.

Vascular Complications

Vascular complications following OLT can be devastating and are related to either inflow or outflow problems. Complications with hepatic inflow typically stem from either hepatic artery or portal vein thrombosis. Many centers routinely examine the liver with Doppler ultrasound 24 hours postoperatively to assess vessel patency, although rising serum transaminases should alert the clinician to the possibility of thrombosis. Early portal vein thrombosis or hepatic artery thrombosis (HAT) should prompt surgical exploration when detected. However, successful thrombectomy and restoration of allograft function is difficult and these patients usually require early retransplantation.

Allografts that are salvaged are at increased risk of biliary complications and cholangiopathy following HAT as the blood supply to the bile duct is potentially compromised. Hepatic outflow problems produce a Budd-Chiari–like syndrome. Acute presentations elevate transaminases and cause hepatic congestion, whereas chronic obstruction presents with ascites and portal hypertension.

Case Conclusion

The patient was listed for liver transplantation emergently (Status 1 listing). A donor organ became available within 48 hours, and the patient underwent OLT using a bicaval technique. Her mental status normalized within 3 days, and she remains clinically well now 3 years following transplant.

TAKE HOME POINTS

- Coagulopathy in the setting of recent onset of jaundice should raise the clinical suspicion for hepatic dysfunction and/or impending failure.
- Development of encephalopathy in a patient with acute hepatic dysfunction should prompt transfer to an intensive care unit in a hospital with a liver transplant program.
- OLT is a technically demanding operation that requires adaptability and ingenuity to reconcile disparities in donor–recipient anatomy.

SUGGESTED READINGS

Koffron A, Stein JA. Liver transplantation: indications, pretransplant evaluation, surgery, and posttransplant complications. Med Clin North Am. 2008;92(4):861–888, ix.

Lee WM. Acute liver failure. N Engl J Med. 1993;329(25):1862–1872.

Stravitz RT. Critical management decisions in patients with acute liver failure. Chest. 2008;134(5):1092–1102.

Trey C, Davidson CS. The management of fulminant hepatic failure. Prog Liver Dis. 1970;3:282–298.

Vaquero J, et al. Complications and use of intracranial pressure monitoring in patients with acute liver failure and severe encephalopathy. Liver Transpl. 2005;11(12):1581–1589.

120 Variceal Bleeding and Portal Hypertension

BRENDAN J. BOLAND and ANDREW S. KLEIN

Presentation

A 55-year-old man with a history of chronic hepatitis C infection is brought into the emergency department after several bouts of hematemesis at home. His family says that he repeatedly vomited a large amount of dark red blood and had not been feeling ill before the hematemesis. His blood pressure is 80/40 mm Hg, and his heart rate is 108 beats per minute. He is awake and responsive but appears confused. Physical examination reveals slight scleral icterus, a mildly distended but soft abdomen, and splenomegaly.

Differential Diagnosis

Gastroesophageal varices should be the first consideration in the patient with an upper gastrointestinal bleed and a documented history of liver disease. About half of patients with cirrhosis have varices, and the risk of developing varices increases with evidence of hepatic decompensation. Varices are a direct consequence of portal hypertension. They can develop throughout the length of the gastrointestinal tract but most commonly are detected at or just proximal or distal to the gastroesophageal junction. Variceal bleeding is a particularly lethal complication of portal hypertension. The 6-week mortality after an episode of bleeding exceeds 20%.

Bleeding from gastroesophageal varices typically is brisk and classically presents with effortless, recurrent hematemesis, melena, or both. Varices should be strongly suspected as a source in any patient with history or stigmata of liver disease. Clinical exam signs may include jaundice, spider angiomata, palmar erythema, caput medusae, splenomegaly, and/or ascites. A Mallory Weiss tear or severe esophagitis can present similarly, and both are common in patients with heavy alcohol use; however, the bleeding is usually less severe and self-limited. Peptic ulcer of the duodenum or stomach is the single most common cause of severe upper gastrointestinal bleeding and needs to be a consideration even in the patient with liver disease. A history of dyspepsia, infection with *Helicobacter pylori*, or nonsteroidal anti-inflammatory drug use are risk factors for ulcers. Regardless of the cause of bleeding, the initial goals are the same— resuscitation and endoscopy for diagnosis and treatment.

Soon after arrival in the emergency room, the patient becomes increasingly confused. His disorientation progresses rapidly to somnolence and he is difficult to arouse with verbal stimulation.

Workup

Securing the patient's airway is particularly important in the setting of the moderate-to-severe encephalopathy that should be suspected clinically. Endotracheal intubation prevents aspiration of blood and gastric contents and ensures a stable airway for endoscopy. Resuscitation should begin concurrently with placement of multiple large caliber venous catheters either peripherally or centrally. Blood tests should include a complete blood count, serum electrolytes, a liver profile, and a prothrombin time to rule out the presence of thrombocytopenia, coagulopathy, electrolyte abnormalities, or renal dysfunction that frequently occur in cirrhotic patients in the setting of acute hemorrhage. Blood and blood products (fresh frozen plasma and platelets) are transfused as indicated, but over transfusion should be avoided as elevated systemic venous pressure increases the risk of variceal bleeding. A hemoglobin level of approximately 8 to 10 g/dL is ideal.

Endoscopy

The cornerstone of the initial workup is endoscopy and should be done within 12 hours of admission. When varices are identified, endoscopic ligation (banding) is the preferred treatment. The varix is suctioned into a channel in the endoscope and a band is deployed, strangulating the varix and causing thrombosis. If banding cannot be performed for technical reasons, endoscopic sclerotherapy with a chemical sclerosant such as sodium tetradecyl sulfate, sodium morrhuate, ethanolamine oleate, or absolute alcohol can be attempted.

Presentation Continued

The patient is stabilized hemodynamically and undergoes esophagogastric endoscopy. He is found to have actively bleeding grade III esophageal varices that are successfully banded. There is evidence of moderate portal hypertensive gastropathy. His hemoglobin is 8 g/dL and his INR is 1.8.

Diagnosis and Treatment

Pharmacologic Treatment

Pharmacologic therapy with a splanchnic vasoconstrictor is initiated during the initial resuscitation. Vasopressin is a potent vasoconstrictor and effectively lowers portal pressure but is associated with multiple side effects including peripheral, cardiac, and mesenteric ischemia. Terlipressin is a synthetic analogue of vasopressin that has been shown to reduce mortality in acute variceal bleeding with significantly fewer side effects, but is not currently available in the United States. Octreotide, a somatostatin analogue, is safe and widely available and is currently considered the pharmacologic treatment of choice for most cases of acute variceal bleeding **(Table 1)**.

Prophylactic antibiotics have been shown to lower mortality and should be administered. Norfloxacin given orally is the first-line recommendation, but oral intake is usually impractical in the acute setting, and ciprofloxacin or levofloxacin can be given intravenously. Ceftriaxone has been shown to be superior to norfloxacin at preventing bacterial infection in patients with more advanced cirrhosis.

Transjugular Intrahepatic Portosystemic Shunts

Combination endoscopic and pharmacologic therapy controls bleeding in 80% to 90% of patients.

TABLE 1. Pharmacologic Treatment of Bleeding Gastroesophageal Varices

Drug	Dose	Comments
Octreotide	50 µg IV bolus, 50 µg/h IV	Somatostatin analogue widely available, favorable safety profile
Vasopressin	0.2–0.8 U/ml	Potent vasoconstrictor, ischemic complications limits usefulness, needs to be given with IV nitroglycerin
Terlipressin	2 mg IV q4h	Vasopressin analogue, less side effects, shown in randomized trials to lower mortality, not available in the United States

Nonresponders may be treated with portosystemic shunts. These procedures create a connection between the portal and the systemic venous circulations, thereby decompressing the hypertensive portal circulation. Transjugular intrahepatic portosystemic shunt (TIPSS) is an interventional radiologic procedure that creates an intrahepatic fistula between a branch of the portal vein and a hepatic vein. A stent graft is then deployed, maintaining the connection. It successfully controls bleeding in over 90% of patients that fail first-line therapy but has a high rate of stenosis that requires frequent monitoring and reintervention (up to 80%). The use of covered stent grafts shows promise in significantly reducing the rate of stenosis. As TIPSS lowers the portal–systemic venous pressure gradient, it also can control refractory ascites and is often used in the elective setting for this purpose.

Balloon Tamponade

Balloon tamponade is an important temporizing tool in the refractory case or as a bridge to definitive therapy, but its use is associated with potentially fatal complications including esophageal/gastric necrosis or perforation, particularly when inserted by inexperienced personnel.

Surgical Approach

With the advent of TIPSS, the use of surgical shunts in the setting of acute bleeding has diminished. However, surgical shunts continue to have a role when lack of local expertise or technical issues make TIPSS impossible. Since long-term surgical shunt patency surpasses that of TIPSS, the former may be preferable when continuing follow-up is problematic. Liver transplantation is the preferred therapy for patients suffering from the complications of portal hypertension who also have decompensated hepatic function. In this instance TIPSS, not surgical shunt, is generally preferred to control the portal hypertension as a bridge to ultimate liver transplantation.

Portocaval Shunts

There are two types of surgical shunts: selective, which preserve prograde flow through the portal vein to the liver, and nonselective, which divert all portal flow to the systemic circulation. The prototypical nonselective shunt is the side-to-side portocaval shunt. Because they completely bypass the liver, nonselective shunts have the drawback of possibly worsening or causing encephalopathy. They are, however, a good treatment for ascites as they decompress the portal vein and the hepatic sinusoids. Portocaval shunts may create significant technical challenges for patients who ultimately require liver transplantation. The porta hepatis becomes a reoperative field at the time of transplantation, and dismantling the portocaval shunt can be problematic for even the most experienced surgeon. In patients who may eventually undergo liver transplantation, who fail TIPPS, the mesocaval shunt using an interposition graft is preferred (see below). The only truly selective shunt is the distal splenorenal shunt. It maintains antegrade flow through the portal vein and decompresses gastroesophageal varices through the short gastric, left gastroepiploic and splenic veins into the systemic venous drainage of the left renal vein. As no portal blood is diverted to the systemic circulation, encephalopathy is not a consequence. It has no effect on ascites and therefore is a poor choice in patients where this is an issue.

Preoperatively, detailed anatomic information regarding the anatomy of the portal circulation needs to be obtained through a CT scan with a portal venous phase, an MRI with contrast, or the venous phase of a superior mesenteric angiogram. If a selective shunt is being considered, ultrasound or mesenteric angiography should be done to confirm that there still is prograde flow to the liver. Surgery in any patient with portal hypertension is challenging. The surgeon and the anesthesiologist must be prepared for potential massive blood loss.

Mesocaval Interposition Shunt

The mesocaval shunt is considered the easiest and safest of the mesenteric decompressive operations, and therefore a good choice in the emergency setting (see **Table 2**). It avoids dissection in the porta hepatis, and therefore does not complicate later liver transplantation. It can be performed through a midline or subcostal incision. The superior mesenteric vein (SMV) is found by opening the root of the transverse mesocolon to the right of the superior mesenteric artery. The SMV is cleared and mobilized from the neck of the pancreas inferiorly, small braches ligated, while larger branches can be controlled with vessel loops. The infrarenal inferior vena cava (IVC) is identified by mobilizing the second and third portions of the duodenum. The IVC is cleared anteriorly and laterally to allow for placement of a side-biting clamp without tension. An anterior venotomy is made and a narrow ellipse of IVC is excised. An interposition graft of 12- to 18-mm ringed polytetrafluoroethylene (PTFE) is anastomosed first to the IVC and then to the anterior aspect of the SMV, using fine monofilament nonabsorable suture. In order to place the anastomosis anteriorly on the SMV, above its main branch points, the graft should assume a "C"-shaped configuration. From the IVC, the graft travels inferiorly in relation to the duodenum, then anteriorly across its third portion and the uncinate process of the pancreas. It is important to recognize that the IVC and the SMV are *not* parallel structures, and the end

TABLE 2. Key Technical Steps and Potential Pitfalls

Mesocaval Interposition Shunt
Key Technical Steps
1. Right subcostal or midline laparotomy.
2. Open root of mesocolon and clear superior mesenteric vein (SMV) from neck of pancreas inferiorly.
3. Mobilize third portion of duodenum and clear anterior surface of inferior vena cava (IVC).
4. Interposition graft to anterior surface of IVC, travels inferior then anterior to duodenum, oblique anastomosis to anterior SMV. The IVC and the SMV are not parallel.
5. Surgeon and assistant work carefully to minimize tension during SMV anastomosis.

Potential Pitfalls
- Bleeding from branches of SMV or IVC during dissection.
- Graft too long or short.
- Anastomosis to branch of SMV, not main trunk.

Distal Splenorenal shunt
Key Technical Steps
1. Left subcostal incision.
2. Lesser sac entered, splenic vein is identified inferior to pancreas.
3. Splenic vein mobilized from SMV distally for 7 cm.
4. Splenic vein divided near SMV, coronary, and right gastroepiploic vein divided.
5. Left renal vein identified and cleared.
6. Splenic to renal vein anastomosis.

Potential Pitfalls
- Bleeding during dissection of splenic vein.
- Injury to pancreas.
- Collaterals from portal to systemic circulation left behind (coronary, right gastroepiploic).

of the PTFE graft must be cut on a bias to accommodate this discrepancy. The SMV is often thin walled, and tearing this vein can be minimized by placing stay sutures at the toe and heal of the anastomosis; performing the right side of the anastomosis from inside the vessel, rostral to caudal, while the assistant coapts the SMV and the PTFE graft assuring that there is no tension; and then finally running the left or outside portion of the anastomosis. The surgeon should avoid the tendency to take large bites of the SMV wall as this will "flatten" the back wall of the SMV and diminish the patency of the anastomosis or even occlude the SMV. The length of the graft is particularly important—too long and it may bend on itself; too short and it may distort or kink the SMV. At the conclusion of the procedure, the effectiveness of the shunt in decompressing the portal circulation should be confirmed by obliquely inserting a 25-gauge needle attached to IV extension tubing into the PTFE graft and measuring the pressure gradient with and without a vascular clamp occluding the graft on the IVC side. If effective, the pressure in the shunt with the clamp off should be within several mm Hg of the patient's central venous pressure.

Distal Splenorenal Shunt

Technically, the distal splenorenal shunt is a challenging operation and is most appropriate for elective surgery and not for a patient who is actively hemorrhaging (see **Table 2**). It disconnects the portal system from the esophageal venous plexus and drains the varices onto the renal vein. The operation is performed through a left subcostal incision. The lesser sac is entered through the gastrocolic ligament, and mobilizing the inferior border of the pancreas cephalad identifies the splenic vein. The splenic vein is fully mobilized from the confluence with the SMV for a distance of 6 to 7 cm. This requires the ligation and division of numerous small splenic vein branches to the pancreas as well as the inferior mesenteric vein (IMV). To minimize bleeding or inadvertent tearing of these fragile branches, which can then retract into the pancreas, ligating the pancreatic side with very fine sutures should be performed before tying the splenic vein side. Care should also be taken to divide the coronary vein and the right gastroepiploic vein, as these are important communications with the perioesophageal venous plexus. The left renal vein is then identified, inferiorly and somewhat deeper to the splenic vein. The left adrenal and gonadal veins are ligated and divided. The splenic vein is divided close to the portal confluence, and the portal side is oversewn. The splenic vein is then swung down to the left renal vein and a side-to-side running anastomosis is performed.

Special Intraoperative Considerations

Patients who have been fluid-resuscitated after sustaining a major hemorrhage may develop significant retroperitoneal edema that in the setting of thickened mesentery that often accompanies portal hypertension may make the identification of the SMV difficult. Use of an oblique incision in the retroperitoneum (as opposed to a longitudinal one) just lateral to the palpated SMA often solves this dilemma. If not, the surgeon should remember that when the duodenum is Kocherized and the connective tissue inferior to the third portion of the duodenum is dissected from the patient's right to left, the first major vascular structure encountered is the SMV.

Preoperative imaging of the splanchnic venous system is occasionally misleading. An SMV that appeared to be an appropriate target for placement of a mesocaval shunt may, upon actual inspection, prove to be sclerosed or recanalized from previous thrombosis. Keeping in mind the primary goal of the operation, which is to decompress the varices that are the source of life-threatening bleeding, when such unsuspected anatomic variations are encountered, the surgeon must be prepared to choose an alternate procedure such as a central or distal splenorenal shunt or portocaval shunt.

Postoperative Management

Patients must be monitored for signs of hepatic decompensation, coagulopathy, and encephalopathy postoperatively if a mesocaval shunt has been performed. Rarely, the shunt may need to be revised or ligated if these complications occur. Doppler ultrasound is useful to demonstrate patency. A comprehensive guide to the care of patients with cirrhosis and hepatic dysfunction is complex and beyond the scope of this chapter.

Case Conclusion

The patient is subsequently readmitted three times with recurrent variceal hemorrhage. Mesenteric angiography demonstrates hepatopetal flow in the portal vein. A distal splenorenal shunt is performed. At 12 months postoperatively the patient has not had recurrent hemorrhage.

TAKE HOME POINTS

- Gastroesophageal varices are the likely source of acute upper GI bleeding in patients who have a known history of cirrhosis or who have clinical stigmata of chronic liver disease.
- Early endoscopy is the key to accurate diagnosis.
- Endoscopic banding is first-line treatment for bleeding esophageal varices.
- Octreotide is the preferred pharmacologic treatment for bleeding gastroesophageal varices.
- TIPSS is effective in decompressing the portal venous system but has limited durability and is often best used as a bridge to transplantation.
- For patients who require a surgical shunt and who may be candidates for a liver transplant in the future, the mesocaval "C" shunt is the preferred surgical procedure.

SUGGESTED READINGS

Cameron JL, Sandone C. Shunts in Atlas of Gastrointestinal Surgery second edition. Hamilton 2007 BC Decker.

Elwood DR, Pomposelli JJ, Pomfret EA, et al. Distal splenorenal shunt: preferred treatment for recurrent variceal hemorrhage in the patient with well compensated cirrhosis. Arch Surg 2006;141:385–388.

Garcia - Tsao G, Bosch J. Management of Varices and Variceal Hemorrhage in Cirrhosis. N Eng J Med 2010 362;9:823–832.

Knechtle SJ. Portal Hypertension: From Eck's fistula to TIPS. Ann Surgery 2003;238:S49–55.

121 End-Stage Renal Disease (Renal Transplantation)

LEIGH ANNE REDHAGE and DEREK MOORE

Presentation

A 56-year-old male with polycystic kidney disease and hypertension arrives at your transplant center for evaluation. His nephrologist predicts he will require dialysis in the next 4 months and recommends him for evaluation for renal transplantation.

Differential Diagnosis

Causes for end-stage renal disease (ESRD) and therefore potential kidney transplant are numerous and can be grouped into several major categories including glomerulonephritis, hereditary, metabolic, toxic, multisystem disease, congenital, tumors, and chronic obstruction. Most patients have undergone a workup for their chronic kidney disease with a nephrologist and arrive to see a transplant surgeon with a diagnosis regarding the etiology of the renal failure. The first successful kidney transplant was performed between identical twins in Boston in 1954. Since then, with the advent of immunosuppression, transplants for ESRD from both living and deceased donors have increased in number to around 13,000 annually in the United States.

Workup

The workup for a potential transplant candidate involves a detailed history and physical as well as appropriate laboratory studies and imaging as indicated. Key components of the history include information regarding the etiology of renal failure, the length of time on dialysis, and the amount of urine the patient makes, if any. Other pertinent past medical history includes cardiac and pulmonary disease, cancer, and infections. In addition, information about prior transplants and transfusion of blood products must be obtained due to the affect on the degree of sensitization to human leukocyte antigens (HLA) and the ease of obtaining a negative crossmatch to potential donors. The physical exam should focus on elements of the patient's anatomy that might preclude them from safe transplantation, especially severe peripheral vascular disease or prior deep vein thrombosis (DVT) that might manifest as diminished femoral and pedal pulses or lower extremity swelling.

Testing for all potential transplant candidates involves both evaluation for safety of the operative procedure and assessment for risk factors, such as active infection or malignancy, associated with adverse outcomes in the setting of immunosuppression. Laboratory studies include complete blood count, comprehensive metabolic panel, coagulation panel, HLA typing, and viral serologies (HBV, HCV, HIV, CMV). Additionally, all patients should have a chest radiograph, EKG, and tuberculosis skin test. All transplant candidates undergo psychosocial evaluation to screen for characteristics that may be associated with medication or post-operative care noncompliance. Other testing is primarily related to recommended screening exams based on patient age and gender: colonoscopy for all patients greater than 50 years old, Pap smear if female without prior hysterectomy, mammogram if female over 40 years old, and PSA if male over 50 years old. If the patient has not made urine for over 5 years, a voiding cystourethrogram may be considered to assure adequate bladder volume for anastomosis of the donor ureter. Some centers perform a CT scan on all patients on dialysis more than 5 years to evaluate for renal cell carcinoma. For a history of systemic lupus erythematous or DVT, patients should undergo a hypercoagulable workup; for those with a history of DVT, a venous phase CT is recommended to evaluate for patency of the iliac veins. Patients with viral serology positive for hepatitis C virus are referred to a hepatologist and undergo a liver biopsy and screening for hepatocellular carcinoma.

Diagnosis and Treatment

Once a patient is cleared for transplantation, investigation for potential donors ensues. The two options for donors include living (either related or unrelated) and deceased. Donors must be healthy themselves and undergo a detailed history and physical as well as any age-appropriate testing. Compatibility of donors and recipients is based on HLA/major histocompatibility complex haplotypes both type I and type II. For patients with willing living donors who are not a satisfactory match, some transplant centers are willing to arrange paired matches. Transplant candidates without living donors are placed on the list for deceased donor renal transplant.

Preoperative history and physical should include updates since the last clinic visit as well as repeat labs, chest x-ray, and EKG as some patients may be close to a year from their last clinic visit when a kidney becomes available. Patients on dialysis should have their fluid status and electrolytes evaluated for possible preoperative dialysis, although most on their routine dialysis schedule will not. Preoperative consent should include not only transplantation but also induction of immunosuppression, which will begin during the transplantation operation.

Immunosuppression includes two phases for transplant recipients: induction and maintenance. Induction regimens differ depending on transplant centers but most include antithymocyte immunoglobulin with steroids. The maintenance phase usually includes a calcineurin inhibitor (cyclosporine or tacrolimus), mycophenolate mofetil, and prednisone, although some centers have had success with steroid avoidance protocols.

Surgical Approach

In the operating room, a three-way Foley catheter is placed so that sterile saline can be infused to fill the bladder prior to anastomosis of the ureter. Transplanted kidneys are generally placed into the right iliac fossa with anastomosis of the renal artery and vein to the right iliac vessels unless contraindicated due to recipient anatomy, prior operation or transplantation, or known vascular disease. The right side is chosen preferentially because the right external iliac artery and vein are often more superficial than the left. In type I diabetics who may be candidates for pancreas transplantation, the kidney is placed on the left side to preserve the right for an eventual pancreas allograft. The Gibson transplant incision is a gently curving incision from the symphysis pubis to just superior and medial to the anterior superior iliac spine (ASIS). The layers of the abdominal wall are incised until the retroperitoneal space is reached. The inferior epigastric vessels are often divided. The spermatic cord is retracted medially in males; the round ligament is divided in females. The external iliac vessels are isolated with care taken to ligate all crossing lymphatics to prevent lymphocele. Proximal and distal control of the artery and vein are achieved with atraumatic vascular clamps. The donor kidney is then taken off ice, but attempts are made to keep it cold while the anastomosis is being completed. The renal artery and vein are then sewn to the external iliac artery and vein in an end-to-side fashion with fine monofilament nonabsorbable suture **(Table 1)**.

After the vascular anastomoses are complete and the kidney is reperfused, attention is turned to the ureter. The three-way Foley is clamped and the bladder distended with irrigation, so it can be identified.

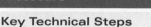

TABLE 1. Key Steps and Potential Pitfalls to the Kidney Transplant Procedure

Key Technical Steps

1. Three-way Foley with flush inserted prior to prep.
2. Right (or left if anatomic limitation to right) gently curving or "hockey stick"–shaped incision from two fingerbreadths superior to the syphilis pubis and two fingerbreadths medial to the anterior superior iliac spine.
3. Divide inferior epigastric vessels.
4. Reach retroperitoneal space and stay extraperitoneal by sweeping down the peritoneum medially.
5. Dissect external iliac vessels carefully dividing surrounding lymphatics to gain proximal and distal control.
6. Donor renal artery and vein are sewn to the external iliac artery and vein in an end-to-side fashion with fine monofilament suture, followed by reperfusion of the kidney.
7. Bladder distended with fluid and detrusor muscle and bladder mucosa opened.
8. Mucosa-to-mucosa neoureterocystostomy is performed over a ureteral stent with absorbable suture.
9. Detrusor muscle of the bladder is then closed loosely with absorbable suture.
10. Anastomoses checked and hemostasis obtained.
11. Incision closed in several anatomic layers.

Potential Pitfalls

- Twisting of the donor vessels during anastomosis.
- Anastomosing the ureter to the colon or the rectum instead of the bladder.
- Multiple or short donor vessels requiring careful anastomosis.
- Living donor vessels do not have Carrel patch.
- Inadequate reperfusion of the kidney.

A large-gauge needle is inserted into the presumed bladder to ensure proper identification. The detrusor muscle and the bladder mucosa are opened, and a mucosa-to-mucosa neoureterocystostomy is performed over a ureteral stent with absorbable suture. The detrusor muscle of the bladder is then closed loosely over the neoureterocystostomy with absorbable suture. Hemostasis is achieved and the incision is closed. After closing the muscular layer over the kidney, a Doppler is used to confirm good flow to the kidney. A closed suction drain may be left to evaluate for collection of lymph, urine or blood, but is not required.

Postoperative Management

Postoperative management of renal transplant patients requires adequate fluid resuscitation. Patients who receive a living donor transplant will often have a large diuresis the night of the operation and may require hourly mL per mL replacement intravenous fluid based on the amount of urine output. Relative hypotension should be treated aggressively to avoid compromising renal perfusion. Other postoperative orders include strict ins and outs, daily weights, morning labs including immunosuppressant levels, pain medications (avoid morphine due to active metabolite that is cleared renally), immunosuppression medications, antiviral prophylaxis, DVT prophylaxis, and Foley catheter instructions (usually left in place until postoperative day 3).

Postoperative graft function can be described as immediate, slow, or delayed. Immediate graft function is common in living donor transplants. Patients have immediate urine output and decreasing serum creatinine. Slow graft function is subjective and defined as oliguria (although not seen in those patients producing urine from their native kidneys) and a serum creatinine that does not fall initially. Delayed function describes a patient that requires dialysis in the first week posttransplant.

As with any operative intervention, complications can occur following renal transplantation **(Table 2)**. Several complications can occur in the more immediate postoperative period including wound infection, seroma, and lymphocele. Wound infection occurs uncommonly in renal transplant recipients, but the risk of wound infection may be significantly increased in obese patients. Treatment consists of drainage of the infection and antibiotics. Seromas are sterile collections of fluid usually in the subcutaneous space. Symptomatic collections can be treated with aspiration, although this runs the risk of infecting the sterile collection and the fluid often reaccumulates. Serial aspirations or percutaneous drainage may be required for treatment of seromas.

Lymphoceles usually occur in the subfascial plane, and are due to accumulation of lymph leakage created by the disruption of the lymphatics surrounding the iliac vessels during intra-operative dissection. Often lymphoceles are small and asymptomatic but can be large and cause pain, swelling, ureteral obstruction, venous obstruction leading to DVTs or renal vein thrombosis, or urinary incontinence from compression of the bladder. Diagnosis is made by ultrasound and often reveals a round, septated cystic mass. Treatment is not required for small, asymptomatic lymphoceles. For collections concerning for a urine leak, infection, or compression of the kidney, percutaneous drainage

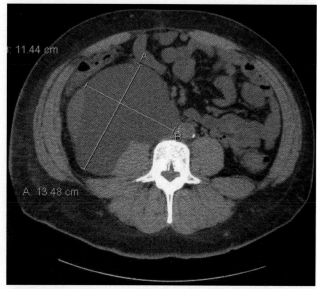

FIGURE 1 • Right groin lymphocele following kidney transplantation.

is necessary. The aspirate should be tested for creatinine to rule out urine leak. Obstructive or infected lymphoceles are managed with infusion of a sclerosing agent or surgical intervention with marsupialization externally or internally into the peritoneal cavity (see **Figure 1** for CT image of lymphocele).

Vascular complications include bleeding, renal vein or artery thrombosis, and renal artery stenosis. Graft thrombosis occurs within the first 2 to 3 days postoperatively and may be related to surgical technique, although patients with a history of a hypercoagulable state are at higher risk. Compression of the renal hilum by a large fluid collection or hematoma can contribute to vascular thrombosis. Symptoms include oliguria (although unreliable if the patient's native kidneys were still producing urine), graft swelling, tenderness, and hematuria, Laboratory tests reveal rising serum creatinine. Evaluation is best achieved with a transplant ultrasound with Doppler, although a radioisotope nuclear medicine scan may also be used. Arterial or venous thromboses often require transplant nephrectomy. Renal artery stenosis is usually a late complication occurring 3 months to several years postoperatively. Diagnosis is made via transplant ultrasound with Doppler. Treatment is first with percutaneous angioplasty followed by surgical intervention as needed.

Urologic complications include urinary extravasation and ureteral obstruction. Urine leaks can occur at the level of the bladder, ureter, or renal calyx and presents as copious drainage through a JP drain or fluid drainage from the incision. Both drainage fluid and serum creatinine should be checked, and a Foley catheter should be placed. The fluid from a urine leak will have a creatinine that is significantly higher than the serum creatinine. If the urine leak is small, Foley

TABLE 2. Potential Complications Following Renal Transplantation

Potential Complications
- Seroma
- Lymphocele
- Urinary extravasation
- Ureteral obstruction
- Ureteral stenosis
- Bleeding
- Renal artery or vein thrombosis
- Renal artery stenosis

catheter placement and bladder decompression may allow the leak to seal. Large leaks require percutaneous nephrostomy tube placement and stenting if the intraoperative stent was removed or no stent was used. Some urine leaks require definitive surgical repair. Repair of the ureter should be performed over a double-J stent.

Ureteral obstruction presents with impaired graft function and oliguria. The obstruction can be secondary to compression by clots, lymphoceles, fibrosis, or ureteral stenosis. Diagnosis can be made by ultrasound that demonstrates hydroureter. A retrograde pyelogram may show the area of obstruction. Obstruction is managed surgically by evacuating the hematoma, lymphocele, or collection causing the obstruction. Similar to the treatment of urine leaks, percutaneous stent placement followed by surgical intervention may be required for ureteral stenosis.

Postoperatively in the outpatient setting, patients require labs every few days to check immunosuppressant levels as well as graft function. Transplant recipients follow up initially with the surgeon, but once all surgical issues are resolved, care often returns to the nephrologist. Nephrologists often manage long-term management of immunosuppressants and concerns for rejection.

TAKE HOME POINTS

- Transplant candidates must tolerate a large operation, have adequate anatomy for transplantation, and be healthy enough to start immunosuppression.
- Intraoperatively, tension-free, wide anastomoses are necessary.
- Careful attention to postoperative urine output and blood pressure; aggressive fluid resuscitation may be needed to replace urinary losses.
- Complications require prompt attention and management.

SUGGESTED READINGS

Greco F, Hoda MR, Alcaraz A, et al. Laparoscopic living-donor nephrectomy: analysis of the existing literature. Eur Urol. 2010;58(4):498–509.

Kayler L, Kang D, Molmenti E, et al. Kidney transplant ureteroneocystostomy techniques and complications: review of the literature. Transplant Proc. 2010;42(5):1413–1420.

Pascual J, Zamora J, Galeano C, et al. Steroid avoidance or withdrawal for kidney transplant recipients. Cochrane Database Syst Rev. 2009;(1):CD005632.

Ponticelli C, Moia M, Montagnino G. Renal allograft thrombosis. Nephrol Dial Transplant. 2009;24(5):1388–1393.

Rajiah P, Lim YY, Taylor P. Renal transplant imaging and complications. Abdom Imaging. 2006;31(6):735–746.

Case Conclusion

Your patient receives a living unrelated donor kidney, tolerates the procedure well and had immediate urine output in the OR after the ureter was anastomosed. He recovers without complication and was discharged home on postoperative day 3. He calls the clinic 1 week later due to swelling of his right leg and a new palpable mass in his right lower abdomen. He returns to clinic and a CT scan is performed that shows a round cystic septated mass concerning for a lymphocele. Because it is causing compressive symptoms, he is taken to the OR for a laparoscopic marsupialization of the lymphocele. He responds favorably to the marsupialization and has resolution of his symptoms.

122 Melanoma of the Head and Neck

ANDREW KROEKER, ANDREW SHUMAN and ERIN MCKEAN

Presentation

A 57-year-old caucasian man presents with an irregular pigmented lesion on the left frontotemporal scalp. The patient noticed that the lesion grew over the previous 6 months. Initially, the area of concern was round and uniform in color. As the lesion increased in size, the border became more irregular and began to display different shades of brown. The area has been nontender and without bleeding or ulceration, but the patient describes the lesion as mildly pruritic.

Workup

The diagnostic workup of a suspicious pigmented cutaneous lesion includes a detailed medical history and physical examination. An early symptom frequently associated with malignant lesions is pruritis. Symptoms associated with more advanced lesions include ulceration, pain, and bleeding. A focused history includes questioning the patient about prior sun exposure, the use of tanning beds, work history, a history of significant blistering sunburns, or a personal and family history of skin cancer.

On examination, the mnemonic **ABCD(E)** has been used in the evaluation of a pigmented lesion suspicious for melanoma. This includes *A*symmetric shape, *B*order irregularity, *C*olor variation, and *D*iameter >6 mm. *E*volution has been added to the screening metric and refers to the change in character over time. A melanoma displaying some of these pathologic characteristics is shown in **Figure 1**. Although a useful guide, it is important to recognize that some uncommon subtypes of melanoma are not captured by this screening tool. These include desmoplastic, amelanotic, and nodular variants.

A biopsy should be performed on all lesions that are worrisome to either the patient and/or caregiver. Initially, excisional biopsy with 1 to 2 mm margins that fully encapsulates the suspicious tissue should be undertaken when possible. If complete excisional biopsy is not possible due to size or anatomic constraints, a full-thickness incisional or punch biopsy should be completed in the thickest portion of the lesion. Shave biopsy should be avoided since this limits evaluation of tumor depth and therefore makes appropriate staging more difficult. The specimen should be evaluated by a pathologist experienced in cutaneous disease in order to make an appropriate histologic diagnosis. Once a diagnosis of melanoma is confirmed, a histopathologic template should be reported as recommended by the AJCC. This includes information such as tumor depth, mitotic rate, angiolymphatic invasion, ulceration, and perineural spread. To complete the initial diagnostic workup, any patient diagnosed with melanoma of the head and neck should undergo a comprehensive exam by a dermatologist.

Melanoma arising from the mucosal surfaces of the body is felt to be a distinct pathologic entity from the cutaneous version. This is a rare subtype that accounts for roughly 1% of all cases of melanoma. Unlike the cutaneous version, the incidence of mucosal melanomas is not changing significantly. Common sites include the nasal cavity and the oral cavity; therefore, presenting symptoms include complaints specific to those areas, including epistaxis and nasal obstruction. Many lesions remain asymptomatic during the initial course of disease. The differential diagnosis of a pigmented mucosal lesion includes amalgam tattoos, oral mucosal nevi, melanotic macule, oral mucosal nevi, melanoacanthoma, and mucosal melanoma.

The diagnostic evaluation of mucosal melanoma is similar to cutaneous melanoma. A complete head and neck exam including fiberoptic nasopharyngoscopic examination of all mucosal surfaces should be undertaken. Computed tomography scan of the head and neck and a chest radiograph to evaluate for lung metastases are typically utilized. Much like the cutaneous counterpart, any suspicious pigmented mucosal lesion should be biopsied. Also, similar immunohistochemical stains are also employed, including S-100, vimentin, and HMB-45. There is a distinct AJCC staging profile for mucosal melanoma.

The patient undergoes excisional biopsy of the suspicious lesion. Histopathologic review demonstrates malignant melanoma invading to a depth of 2.7 mm with no microscopic evidence of ulceration. There is no clinical evidence for regional or distant metastatic disease. No second primary lesions were noted on

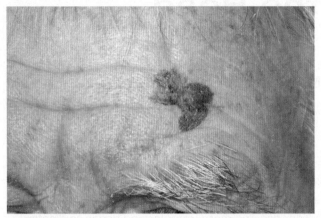

FIGURE 1 • Typical melanoma of the head and neck. (Courtesy of Timothy Johnson, MD; University of Michigan Department of Dermatology.)

formal cutaneous evaluation. The patient's melanoma is staged as T2N0M0.

Diagnosis and Treatment

Classification of melanoma based on traditional TNM stage was recently updated in the seventh edition of the *AJCC Cancer Staging Manual*. Breslow depth (depth of tumor invasion below the basement membrane) is the primary determinant of T stage and is described in detail in **Table 1**. Tumor depths of 1.0, 2.0, and 4.0 mm remain as thresholds for the four stages; the updated staging system has removed Clark level. Each stage is further subclassified into either "a" for tumor without ulceration or "b" for tumor with ulceration. For prognostic purposes, further distinction is made within T1 lesions with regards to mitotic figures per mm^2 of tissue. Nodal disease staging includes one node for N1 disease, two to three nodes for N2 disease, and greater than three nodes for N3 disease. Selective lymphadenectomy has played an important role in the accurate staging of certain subpopulations with melanoma. Lymphoscintigraphy followed by lymphatic mapping and sentinel lymph node biopsy (SLNB) (sentinel lymphadenectomy) remain important components of melanoma staging and should be used or discussed with the patient in defining occult stage III disease among patients who present with clinical stage IB or II melanoma. Clinical staging is reviewed further in **Table 2**.

Melanoma is a disease with a high metastatic potential. However, the propensity for distant metastatic spread is directly related to disease stage. The diagnostic workup of TI disease requires a complete history and physical examination. For more advanced disease, chest x-ray, lactate dehydrogenase, and liver function tests are often employed to exclude distant disease in patients with clinically negative nodal disease and are more strongly recommended in clinically positive nodal disease. Further imaging studies should

be ordered as clinical scenarios warrant. Stage IV disease often necessitates a complete metastatic workup including cross-sectional imaging of the brain, neck, chest, abdomen, and pelvis, and/or FDG-PET scans.

Primary Site

Once the diagnosis of melanoma has been confirmed, a wide local excision (WLE) of the lesion should be performed. This is executed with 1-cm margins for lesions <1 mm in depth (T1) and 2-cm margins for lesions >1 mm (T2 to T4). No survival benefit has been shown for wider margins. The depth of excision should include the entire epidermis and dermis, as well as the underlying subcutaneous tissues to the level of the underlying fascia. Extension of the excision into deeper tissue planes should be performed only if tumor invasion is evident. Branches of the facial nerve should be identified and preserved unless they are clinically involved. Tumor margins may be appropriately adjusted when the lesion abuts critical structures such as the eyelids. Meticulous pathologic attention to the tumor margin is crucial, and frozen sections are notoriously unreliable for melanoma. In certain cases, a "square" procedure may be recommended, in which a complete circumferential evaluation of the surgical margin is undertaken in order to ensure clear margins prior to final excision and reconstruction.

Many WLE sites can be closed primarily, although the defect size and location may necessitate reconstruction with skin grafts, local advancement flaps, or larger regional flaps. In general, reconstruction that involves tissue rearrangement should be delayed until pathologic margins are definitively cleared. While some centers report success with Mohs surgery for melanoma, the majority of institutions prefer to await final standard pathologic analysis.

Surgical management is also the mainstay of treatment for mucosal melanoma. However, unlike primary cutaneous disease, complete surgical resection of mucosal lesions is often difficult secondary to tumor site and associated morbidity. Neck dissection is typically performed in N+ cases. Adjuvant radiation therapy may improve locoregional control for mucosal melanoma, although there is no proven improvement in overall survival; chemotherapy is typically only utilized in the palliative setting.

Nodal Disease

Evaluation of cervical metastatic disease has been extensively studied and recommendations continue to evolve. Therapeutic lymphadenectomy is indicated in clinically positive nodal disease. As a general rule, a primary scalp/facial lesion anterior to an imaginary line drawn from one tragus to the other will drain anteriorly through the parotid basin and anterior neck, and lesions posterior to this imaginary line will drain to the

TABLE 1. AJCC TNM Cutaneous Melanoma Guide—2010

Classification

T	Thickness (mm)	Ulceration Status/Mitosis
Tis	N/A	N/A
T1	≤1.00	a: without ulceration and mitosis <1/mm^2
		b: with ulceration or mitosis ≥1/mm^2
T2	1.01–2.00	a: without ulceration
		b: with ulceration
T3	2.01–4.00	a: without ulceration
		b: with ulceration
T4	≥4.01	a: without ulceration
		b: with ulceration

N	No. of Metastatic Nodes	Nodal Metastatic Burden
N0	0	N/A
N1	1	a: micrometastasis[a]
		b: macrometastasis[b]
N2	2–3	a: micrometastasis[a]
		b: macrometastasis[b]
N3	≥4 metastatic nodes, or matted nodes, or intransit metastases/satellites with metastatic nodes	a: micrometastasis[a]
		b: macrometastasis[b]

M	Site	Serum LDH
M0	No distant metastases	N/A
M1a	Distant skin, subcutaneous, or nodal metastases	Normal
M1b	Lung metastases	Normal
M1c	All other visceral metastases	Normal
	Any distant metastases	Elevated

[a]Micrometastasis: diagnosed after SLNB.
[b]Macrometastasis: clinically detectable nodal metastases confirmed pathologically.
Adapted from the American Joint Committee on Cancer (AJCC). AJCC Cancer Staging Manual. 7th ed. New York, NY: Springer Science and Business Media LLC, 2010. www.springer.com

posterolateral neck. Therefore, superficial parotidectomy and selective neck dissection are recommended for anterior lesions, and posterolateral neck dissection is recommended for posterior lesions.

Currently, there is no conclusive evidence that prophylactic complete regional lymphadenectomy is beneficial in patients with clinically negative nodal disease. However, approximately 15% to 20% of patients at initial presentation harbor occult metastatic disease. It is accepted that in early lesions (depth <1.2 mm) without clinical evidence of nodal disease, there is generally no indication for lymphadenectomy. With lesions between 1.0 and 3.5 mm depth of invasion, SLNB may be warranted.

Sentinel node biopsy involves preoperative intradermal injection of a radiolabeled colloid tracer. This is followed by lymphoscintigraphy to map the nodal drainage basins of interest. At the onset of surgery, the surgeon injects the lesion intradermally with blue dye to assist in the visual confirmation of the sentinel nodes. Intraoperatively, once the primary lesion has been completely excised, the surgeon uses the nuclear medicine imaging, the presence of blue dye within the nodes of interest, as well as the scintigraphy probe to assist in localization of the sentinel lymph nodes. Typically, specimens are processed for pathologic review by permanent section, which usually involves both traditional H&E staining and melanoma-specific immunohistochemical stains. Patients with known metastatic disease or those who have previously undergone WLE or had surgical manipulation in the area of concern are not candidates for SLNB. In the hands of a surgeon experienced in head and neck oncology, sentinel nodes within the parotid bed and neck can be

TABLE 2. AJCC Cutaneous Melanoma Staging Guidelines—2010

	T1a	T2a	T1b	T2b	T3a	T4a	T3b	T4b
N0	1A	1B		IIA		IIB		IIC
N1a	IIIA		IIIB		IIIA		IIIB	
N2a								
N1b	IIIB		IIIC		IIIB		IIIC	
N2b								
N2c				IIIB				
N3				IIIC				
M1a				IV				
M1b								
M1c								

safely and successfully excised with appropriate facial nerve dissection and monitoring.

Adjuvant and Palliative Treatment

The role of immune modulators in melanoma has been studied extensively. Adjuvant interferon α2b has been shown in some studies to increase disease-free and overall survival in stage III disease. This therapy is not without significant side effects, and close monitoring, appropriate patient selection, and counseling by a medical oncologist are crucial.

Distant metastatic disease confers a very poor prognosis. There is a limited role for surgery in management of these difficult cases, although there may be a role for surgical palliation in specific clinical scenarios. Specific prognostic indicators are used in stage IV disease and include the number and location of anatomic sites involved with distant disease, as well as the length of time elapsed from primary excision to recurrence; mean 5-year survival in stage IV disease is approximately 6% to 7% **(Figure 2)**.

Melanoma is generally resistant to external beam radiation and cytotoxic chemotherapy. Adjuvant radiation therapy may play a role in the prevention of local disease recurrence in selected cases; however, there is no evidence for an overall survival benefit. The use of chemotherapy remains controversial, as no regimen has been shown to alter long-term survival. The primary role for both chemotherapy and radiation is in the palliative setting. Recent advances in targeted therapies, including both monoclonal antibodies that promote an antitumor T-cell response and inhibitors of gene products associated with oncogene function, have shown promise toward improving survival in stage IV disease.

The patient undergoes WLE with 2-cm margins followed by local tissue rearrangement. Sentinel lymph nodes located in this superficial parotid lymphatic

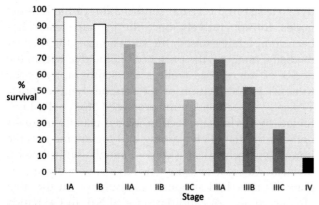

FIGURE 2 • Cutaneous melanoma—5-year survival based on AJCC TNM stage

basin and in level 2 of his right neck were biopsied and sent for permanent pathology.

Discussion

The lifetime risk of developing melanoma is almost 40 times greater than it was just 75 years ago. The incidence of melanoma continues to rise faster than any other malignancy. It affects people of all ages, with approximately one-quarter of new cases diagnosed in patients <40 years of age. The head and neck is a frequent primary site, with close to one-quarter of all cases occurring in this region. Risk factors implicated in the development of melanoma involve both environmental exposures and genetic predisposition. Both fair skin and a history of significant sun exposure are correlated with increased incidence of melanoma. Furthermore, the presence of numerous and/or large congenital nevi and a prior personal or family history of melanoma correspond to an increased relative risk. Although present in a minority of cases of melanoma, genetics also play an important role. The most common mutation involves the p16 tumor suppressor gene. The autosomal recessive disorder, *Xeroderma pigmentosa*, also confers a significantly increased risk of melanoma.

Histologic subtypes exist within cutaneous melanoma. Common variants include superficial spreading and nodular subtypes. The term lentigo maligna correlates to melanoma *in situ* and is thought to be the precursor to invasive lesions known as lentigo malignant melanoma. Less common subtypes include amelanotic, desmoplastic, and desmoplastic-neurotropic melanoma. The utility of these subclassifications is limited, however, as prognosis is more highly correlated with the depth of tumor invasion than histologic subtype. It is also important to recognize the distinction between cutaneous melanoma and melanoma originating in mucosal surfaces of the body. Mucosal melanoma is thought to behave more aggressively and carries a poorer overall prognosis than cutaneous primary disease. Furthermore, a small percentage of melanomas will present with regional or distant metastatic disease in the absence of a known primary site. After an attempt to find the primary lesion is made, these cases should be approached similarly to patients with known primary lesions and metastatic disease.

Surveillance

Early identification of local and regional recurrence as well as new primary lesions is the primary goal of oncologic surveillance. It is important to instruct patients about the warning signs of melanoma and the need to perform monthly self-examinations. Although late recurrence (>10 years from the time of initial diagnosis) is relatively uncommon, it still occurs with moderate regularity and therefore necessitates indefinite surveillance. Follow-up guidelines from the National

Comprehensive Cancer Network vary based upon stage. Melanoma *in situ* lesions require, at minimum, annual skin examinations by a health care provider indefinitely. More advanced-stage cancers require a focused history and physical exam every 3 to 6 months for 2 years, then every 3 to 12 months for 2 years, followed by annual exams indefinitely. Imaging and laboratory studies may be used to evaluate any concerning symptoms, or at the discretion of the individual provider.

Case Conclusion

The patient is seen in postoperative follow-up to discuss the final pathology and staging. Both sentinel lymph nodes were negative for melanoma. No adjuvant therapy is recommended. He is scheduled for routine follow-up in 3 months' time.

TAKE HOME POINTS

- Surgery is the primary treatment modality for melanoma.
- Timely identification and excision of malignant lesions is crucial.
- Surgery requires in-depth anatomical knowledge and experience in order to dissect and preserve critical neurovascular structures, and to appropriately respect aesthetic issues while remaining oncologically sound.
- Appropriate histopathologic and clinical staging is necessary for both risk stratification and selection of appropriate treatment modalities.

SUGGESTED READINGS

Balch CM, Gershenwald JE, et al. Final version of 2009 AJCC melanoma staging and classification. J Clin Oncol. 2009;27:6199–6206.

Balch CM, Soong SJ, Smith T, et al. Long-term results of a prospective surgical trial comparing 2 cm vs. 4 cm excision margins for 740 patients with 1–4 mm melanomas. Ann Surg Oncol. 2001;8:101–108.

Barth A, Wanek LA, Morton DL. Prognostic factors in 1,521 melanoma patients with distant metastases. J Am Coll Surg. 1995;181:193–201.

Brand CU, Ellwanger U, Stroebel W, et al. Prolonged survival of 2 years or longer for patients with disseminated melanoma, an analysis of related prognostic factors. Cancer. 1997;79:2345–2353.

Byers RM. Treatment of the neck in melanoma. Otolaryngol Clin North Am. 1998;31:833–839.

Chang AE, Karnell LH, Menck HR. The national cancer database report on cutaneous and noncutaneous melanoma: a summary of 84,836 cases from the past decade. Cancer. 1998;83:1664–1678.

Flaherty KT, Puzanov I, et al. Inhibition of mutated, activated BRAF in metastatic melanoma. N Engl J Med. 2010;363:809–819.

Hodi FS, O'Day SJ, et al. Improved survival with ipilimumab in patients with metastatic melanoma. N Engl J Med. 2010;363:711–723.

Kirkwood JM, Ibrahim JG, Sosman JA, et al. High-dose interferon alfa-2b significantly prolongs relapse-free and overall survival compared with the GM2-KLH/QS-21 vaccine in patients with resected stage IIB-III melanoma: results of Intergroup Trial E1694/S9512/C509801. J Clin Oncol. 2001;19:2370–2380.

Morton DL, Thompson JF, et al. Sentinel-node biopsy or nodal observation in melanoma. N Engl J Med. 2006;355:1307–1317.

Rigel DS, Friedman RJ, Kopf AW, et al. ABCDE—an evolving concept in the early detection of melanoma. Arch Dermatol. 2005;141:1032–1034.

Schmalbach CE, Johnson TM, Bradford CR. The management of head and neck melanoma. Curr Probl Surg. 2006;43:781–835.

Schmalbach CE, Nussenbaum B, et al. Reliability of sentinel lymph node mapping with biopsy for head and neck cutaneous melanoma. Arch Otolaryngol Head Neck Surg. 2003;129:61–65.

Stern SJ, Guillamondegui OM. Mucosal melanoma of the head and neck. Head Neck. 1991;13:22–27.

Surveillance, Epidemiology and End Results. (2003). http://seer.cancer.gov.

Wagner Marcus MD, Morris Christopher G. MS002E Mucosal melanoma of the head and neck. Am J Clin Oncol. 2008;31:43–48.

Wornom IL, Smith JW, Soong SJ, et al. Surgery as palliative treatment for distant metastases of melanoma. Ann Surg. 1986;204:181–185.

123 Head and Neck Cancer

MATTHEW SPECTOR and ERIN MCKEAN

Presentation

A 55-year-old man with a 50 pack-year smoking history presents with hoarseness for 3 months. This has been progressive in nature and is associated with mild dysphagia, odynophagia, and weight loss. He denies shortness of breath but does report two-pillow orthopnea. On physical exam, he has inspiratory stridor without stertor or retractions. Otologic, nasal, oral cavity, and oropharyngeal examination is unremarkable. He has a 3-cm left level 2 neck mass that is firm, nontender, and mobile. Flexible fiberoptic laryngoscopy reveals an exophytic lesion of the left aryepiglottic fold extending inferiorly onto the false and true vocal cord. There is fixation of the left vocal cord.

Differential Diagnosis

New-onset hoarseness in a smoker with other concerning symptoms should be considered a cancer until proven otherwise. Breathing or swallowing problems are not uncommon as tumors become more advanced. Tumors of the glottic portion of the larynx often present early, as small tumors significantly affect the voice in this region, while other laryngeal subsites (supraglottic or subglottic) may be quite large before detected clinically.

There are other destructive processes of the upper aerodigestive tract that can mimic cancer, and biopsy is important to confirm diagnosis. Infectious processes (laryngitis or thrush), congenital anomalies (laryngocele), and autoimmune diseases (Wegener's granulomatosis, sarcoidosis, amyloidosis) can have presentations similar to cancer.

Workup

The patient undergoes further evaluation with a CT scan of his neck and chest to evaluate the extent of local, regional, and distant disease. There is no cartilage invasion of the larynx, and there is a single lymph node in the left neck that is 2 cm **(Figure 1)**. There is no metastatic disease in the chest. The patient is staged as a T3N1M0 (stage 3).

Approximately 30% to 50% of patients with supraglottic tumors, 6% to 18% of patients with glottic tumors, and 4% to 27% of patients with subglottic tumors will have regional metastasis at their initial presentation. Many centers are also using positron emission tomography (PET) scans, although this is not currently the standard of care to evaluate the primary tumor. All patients should undergo operative direct laryngoscopy, esophagoscopy with biopsies under general anesthesia for treatment planning and to confirm absence of a second primary tumor (up to 10%

of patients). These tests and procedures are routinely performed to allow appropriate staging for treatment planning (see below) **(Figure 2)**.

The workup of an unknown primary tumor (a patient presents with regional metastasis without evidence of primary tumor location) deserves specific mention. First, a thorough head and neck exam, including fiberoptic nasopharyngoscopy and laryngoscopy, is warranted. A fine needle aspiration biopsy of the neck mass should be performed, either directly or with ultrasound guidance, to confirm the diagnosis. A contrast-enhanced CT of the neck and chest including the skull base should be performed to attempt and identify the primary tumor. If no primary tumor is identified with anatomic (CT) imaging, PET scanning may aid in diagnosis. Some may choose to perform a PET/CT alone if clinical evaluation fails to identify a primary tumor site. The patient should then be taken to the operating room for direct laryngoscopy, esophagoscopy, tonsillectomy (if tonsils are present), and biopsies directed by the previous workup. The most common sites for an unknown primary tumor are the tonsils and the tongue base, followed by the nasopharynx and hypopharynx. The advantages of identification of the primary tumor include directed treatment, thereby sparing the patient treatment-related effects in uninvolved areas, as well as adequate treatment of a small primary tumor before it advances.

Discussion

Head and neck cancer is the fifth most common cancer with over 600,000 cases diagnosed each year. Men are affected five times as often as women. Head and neck cancer can be divided into subsites including the larynx, pharynx (nasopharynx, oropharynx, and hypopharynx), and oral cavity. Risk factors for all head and neck cancers include tobacco and alcohol, which work

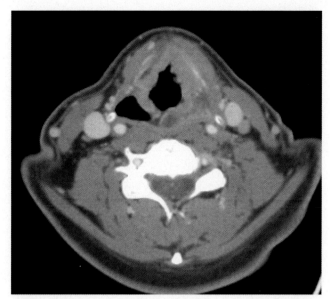

FIGURE 1 • CT scan of a primary squamous cell carcinoma of the supraglottic larynx. The contrast-enhancing lesion involves the left arytenoids, aryepiglottic fold, and false vocal cord.

synergistically to increase risk. Human papilloma virus has also been shown as causative to the oropharynx subsite, and these patients generally have a better prognosis.

Overall survival rates are dependent upon tumor subsite and stage at diagnosis. Patients are staged based on the American Joint Committee on Cancer (AJCC) guidelines using the TNM classification system. Stages I and II represent early local disease without regional or distant metastasis. Stages III and IV represent advanced disease with either a locally aggressive tumor or a metastatic disease (regional or distant) **(Table 1)**.

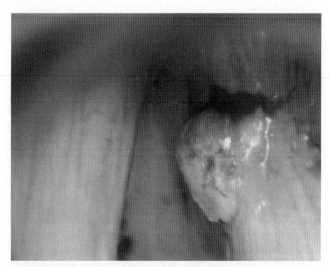

FIGURE 2 • Intraoperative direct laryngoscopic view of cancer: T1 squamous cell carcinoma of the right true vocal cord. (Photo courtesy of Norman Hogikyan, MD.)

Diagnosis and Treatment

Timely diagnosis and appropriate workup is important in the proper management of head and neck cancer patients. Referral to a head and neck cancer surgeon

TABLE 1. AJCC TNM Staging for Larynx Cancer

AJCC TNM Staging for Larynx Cancer

Supraglottis

T1	Tumor limited to one subsite of supraglottis with normal vocal cord movement
T2	Tumor invades >1 adjacent subsite of supraglottis or glottis or oropharynx, without fixation of larynx
T3	Tumor limited to larynx with vocal cord fixation and/or invasion of postcricoid area, preepiglottic tissue, paraglottic space, and/or minor thyroid cartilage invasion (inner cortex)
T4a	Tumor invades through the thyroid cartilage and/or beyond the larynx
T4b	Tumor invades prevertebral space, encases carotid artery, or invades mediastinal structures

Glottis

T1	Tumor limited to vocal cords (+/– anterior or posterior commissure) with normal vocal cord movement
T1a	Tumor limited to one vocal cord
T1b	Tumor on both vocal cords
T2	Tumor extends to supraglottis or subglottis, without fixation of larynx
T3	Tumor limited to larynx with vocal cord fixation and/or invasion of postcricoid area, preepiglottic tissue, paraglottic space, and/or minor thyroid cartilage invasion (inner cortex)
T4a	Tumor invades through the thyroid cartilage and/or beyond the larynx
T4b	Tumor invades prevertebral space, encases carotid artery, or invades mediastinal structures

Subglottis

T1	Tumor limited to subglottis
T2	Tumor extends to vocal cord(s) with normal or impaired mobility
T3	Tumor limited to larynx with vocal cord fixation
T4a	Tumor invades through the thyroid cartilage and/or beyond the larynx
T4b	Tumor invades prevertebral space, encases carotid artery, or invades mediastinal structures

Regional Lymph Nodes

N0	No regional lymph node metastasis
N1	Metastasis in a single ipsilateral node, 3 cm or less in greatest diameter
N2	
N2a	Metastasis in a single ipsilateral node, >3 cm but <6 cm in greatest diameter
N2b	Metastasis in multiple ipsilateral nodes, none >6 cm
N2c	Metastasis in bilateral or contralateral nodes, none >6 cm
N3	Metastasis in a lymph node, >6 cm in greatest dimension

Adapted from the American Joint Committee on Cancer (AJCC). AJCC Cancer Staging Manual. 7th ed. New York, NY: Springer Science and Business Media LLC, 2010, www.springer.com

is most appropriate, and discussion at a head and neck oncology tumor board allows for decisive treatment. There should be a high suspicion for cancer in patients with a neck mass over 50 years of age and patients with previous smoking and/or alcohol history who have new speech or swallowing complaints.

Treatment

According to the AJCC guidelines, surgery or radiation therapy are acceptable options for early stage (I, II) disease. These tumors are limited in their extent, and there is no evidence of regional or distant metastasis. Multimodality treatment is necessary for advanced stage (III, IV) disease, as these tumors are either locally aggressive or have metastasized. Options may include surgery followed by radiation or chemoradiation. It is important to note that each subsite of head and neck cancer (e.g., oral cavity, oropharynx, nasopharynx, hypopharynx, larynx, salivary glands, nose and paranasal sinuses) has a different staging system, prognosis, and varying treatment recommendations. Surgical approaches are specifically tailored to the tumor, and reconstruction must be considered in preoperative planning. Speech and swallowing outcomes, as well as cosmesis, should be a factor in choosing local, regional, or free tissue reconstruction options. Pretreatment dental and speech pathology consultations should be obtained.

Surveillance

Consistent with National Comprehensive Cancer Network (NCCN) guidelines, patients are followed every 1 to 3 months for the first year, every 2 to 4 months for the second year, and every 4 to 6 months until the fifth year. At this point, the patient is considered to be cured of disease and can follow up yearly or on an as-needed basis. A key factor in oncologic surveillance is to encourage patients to be seen early if they develop new pain (or worsening pain) at the primary site, new otalgia, dysphagia, odynophagia, hoarseness, significant weight loss, hemoptysis, or hematemesis.

Case Conclusion

The patient was staged as a T3N1M0 (stage 3) squamous cell cancer of the supraglottic larynx. Options for chemoradiation versus primary surgery with postoperative radiation were discussed. The patient successfully underwent surgical excision of his tumor with total laryngectomy, bilateral selective neck dissections of levels II to IV, cricopharyngeal myotomy, tracheoesophageal puncture for later speech rehabilitation, and placement of a temporary Dobhoff feeding tube. He was discharged on postoperative day 5 uneventfully and was allowed to swallow soft foods at 3 weeks after surgery. His pathology showed one involved lymph node without extracapsular spread or perineural invasion, and he received adjuvant radiation therapy **(Figure 3)**.

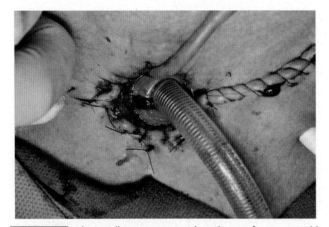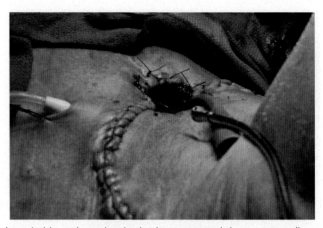

FIGURE 3 • Immediate postoperative views of stoma and incisions (with endotracheal tube in stoma and then removed). This is now the patient's only airway, with complete removal of the larynx and thus disconnection with the upper airway. A red rubber Robinson catheter is seen in the tracheoesophageal puncture site, maintaining an opening for later voice prosthesis placement. (Photos courtesy of Norman Hogikyan, MD.)

TAKE HOME POINTS

- Early stage (I, II) tumors can be treated with single modality therapy, while advanced stage (III, IV) are treated with multimodality therapy. Adequate diagnosis and staging are key to determining the appropriate therapy.
- Timely referral to a head and neck surgeon is important to begin treatment.

SUGGESTED READINGS

Bailey BJ, Calhoun KH, Derkay CS, et al. Head and Neck Surgery – Otolaryngology. Vol. 2, Section 4. ISBN 978-0781729086.

Cummings CW, Haughey BW, Thomas JR, et al. Cummings Otolaryngology: Head and Neck Surgery. ISBN 978-0323019859.

Edge SB, Byrd DR, Compton CC, et al. AJCC Cancer Staging Manual. 7th ed. 2010. ISBN 978-0-387-88440-0.

Galer CE, Kies MS. Evaluation and management of the unknown primary carcinoma of the head and neck. J Natl Compr Canc Netw. 2008;6(10):1068–1075.

NCCN Guidelines for head and neck cancer care. National Comprehensive Cancer Network Web site. http://www.nccn.org/professionals/physician_gls/PDF/head-and-neck.pdf.

Index

Page numbers in *italics* denote figures; those followed by a t denote tables.